NOV 1999

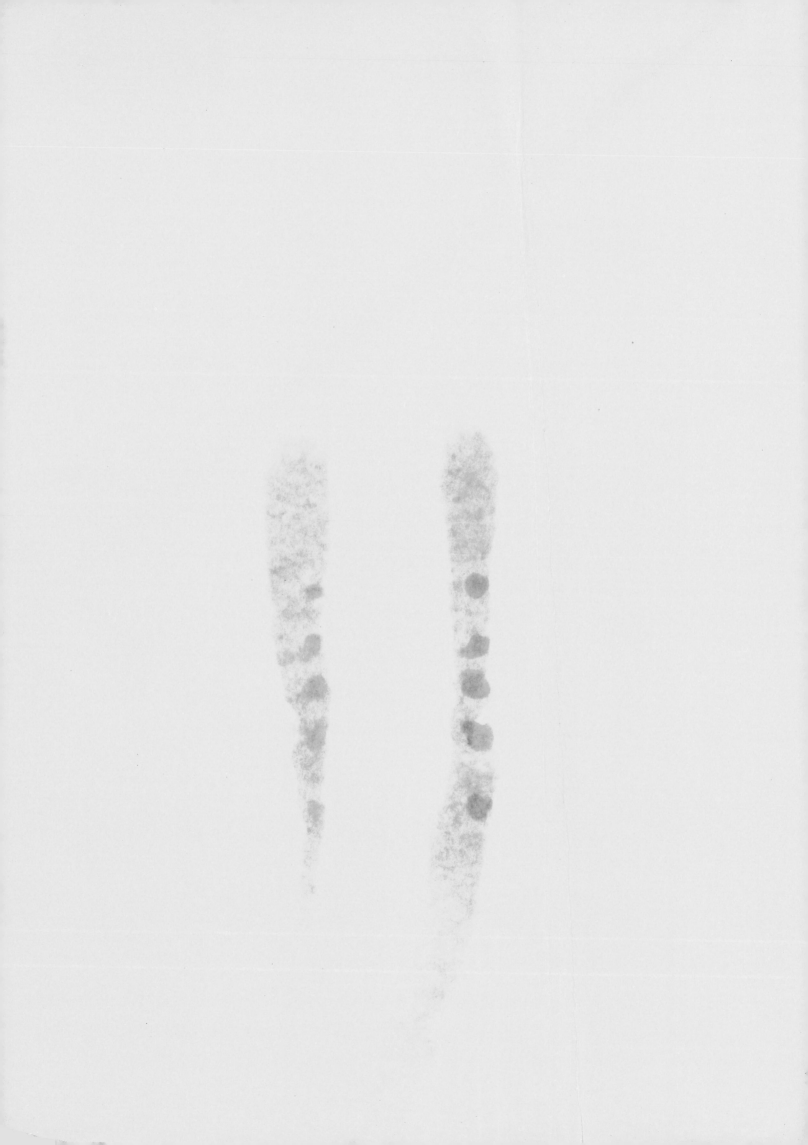

AMERICAN SURGERY
An Illustrated History

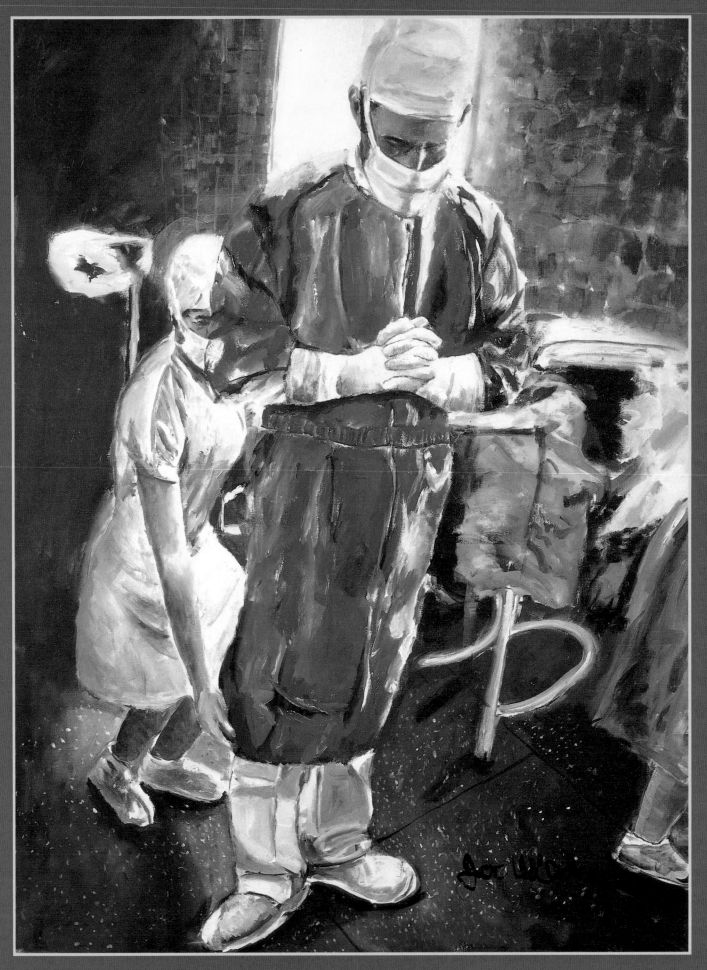

"Contemplation Before Surgery" by Joseph R. Wilder (1987). Surgery is a mystical craft, which often defies explanation. To be allowed with consent to cut into another human being's body, to gaze at the depth of that person's suffering, and to excise the demon of disease—such doing assumes an awesome responsibility. *(Collection of the artist)*

AMERICAN SURGERY
An Illustrated History

by

IRA M. RUTKOW, M.D., M.P.H., DR.P.H.

with 451 illustrations, including 171 in full color

Stanley B. Burns, M.D., Photohistorian

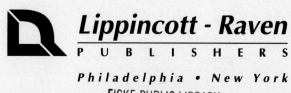

Lippincott - Raven
PUBLISHERS

Philadelphia • New York

Acquisitions Editor: Lisa McAllister
Developmental Editor: Emilie Linkins
Manufacturing Manager: Dennis Teston
Production Manager: Bernadine Richey
Interior Designer and
    Production Editor: Shelley Himmelstein
Production Assistant: Graceanne Malloy
Cover Designer: Jeane Norton
Indexer: Ann Cassar
Compositor: Shelley Himmelstein, Inc.
Printer: Toppan Printing Co.

Printed in Singapore

9 8 7 6 5 4 3 2 1

Library of Congress Cataloging-in-Publication Data

Rutkow, Ira M.
    American surgery: an illustrated history/by Ira M. Rutkow
        p. cm.
    Includes bibliographical references and index.
    ISBN 0-31676-352-7
    1. Surgery—United States—History. I. Title.
RD27.3.u6r87 1998   97-17654
617'.0973—dc21   CIP

To my wonderful family:
my wife *Beth*,
our children *Lainie* and *Eric*,
my parents *Bea* and *Al Rutkow*.

They are my beacons to the world of the past.

CONTENTS

SURGICAL SPECIALTIES AND BIOGRAPHIES

PREFACE

To surgeon, sufferer, and society, the flowering of surgery has proved to be a central theme in our shared human experience. Long associated with religious overtones, it is the very mystification of surgery and the veil of the operating room that fascinate the lay person with his or her own inevitable date with a surgical knife. Such an evolutionary partnership is what induced Henry J. Bigelow, a nineteenth-century Harvard professor of surgery, to exclaim, "Why is the amphitheatre crowded to the roof on the occasion of some great operation, while the silent working of some drug excites little comment? Mark the hushed breath, the fearful intensity of silence, when the blade pierces the tissues, and the blood wells up to the surface. Animal sense is always fascinated by the presence of animal suffering."

Continuing through today, the public's insatiable interest with virtually all things surgical portends a greater understanding of the history of surgery. Affirming this mandate is the simple fact that major events in the development of the American profession of surgery closely mirror significant occurrences in the history of our country. Assuredly, a case can be made for stating the now obvious: certain aspects of modern surgery, such as body sculpting, organ transplantation, and open heart surgery, can be regarded as cultural icons. That surgery closely reflects the value structures of our society, validates the importance of understanding our surgical heritage.

As surgery comes ever nearer to paralleling the pathways of modern society, so must the writing of medical history go beyond the simple narration of a great doctor's life or the straightforward understanding of the development of clinical or surgical techniques. With the hagiographic haze slowly being lifted, it is no longer acceptable for surgical history to be expounded upon as little more than an unrelated series of contributions by individual physicians. There can be little dispute with the modern assumption that medical history involves not only clinical content but ethical, political, and socioeconomic elements as well. Yet, to place this modern view of surgical history within the broad sweep of social change requires an understanding of the recondite technical problems that littered the surgical landscape. Unquestionably, owing to their clinical expertise, surgeons have knowledge and experience that place them in a unique position to help assess historical fact and direct surgical historical inquiry.

During my training as a general surgeon (1975–1982), I was always fascinated by the many stories the attending surgeons told about their past colleagues. In turn, the ability to trace the evolution of what I did as a surgeon and to understand its historic rationale provided an unforgettable intellectual satisfaction. However, the paucity of oral vignettes about eighteenth- or nineteenth-century American surgeons always seemed odd. Clearly, the older a person is the more history he or she has been personally exposed to. The simple passage of time makes the older surgeon a store-house of half a century of surgical history as well as a link to yet even earlier times and surgeons. So, the dearth of historic lore remained curious until I gradually began to understand that an in-depth appreciation of what truly shaped American surgery and its professional mores and organizations was lacking. This seems emphasized by an established practice that minimalizes historical intellectualism within the current body of surgery and surgical education. Undoubtedly, specific individuals remain committed to teaching and revealing to their students the importance of understanding the past. Nonetheless, passing comments that studying surgical history is, at best, a waste of time are too often heard!

As my own historical interests increased, I began doing research into American surgical history and collecting the written works of my surgical forebears. I became acquainted with a body of literature that was surprising in its originality and crudely eloquent in style. Unfortunately, my historical forays were thwarted by the simple fact that an all-encompassing history of American surgery had never been written. In fact, the history of surgery in this country had been minimally chronicled by both general and medical historians. Understandably, those who have never toiled in this vineyard of surgical history would be surprised at its zigzagging trail. Distressingly, it seemed as if the ingenuity and boldness with which early American surgeons approached seemingly insolvable surgical problems would remain almost unrecognized in American history.

I regard the opportunity to write this book, *American Surgery: An Illustrated History* as a unique honor. To understand and set forth the past of one's profession is to better comprehend that discipline's present and anticipate its future. As I would learn, there is no way to separate present-day surgery and one's own practice routines from the experiences of all the surgeons and all the years that have gone before. Accordingly, the opportunity to organize such a vast project was an undertaking that I approached with utmost respect for, and homage to, a multitude of surgical ancestors.

I have planned *American Surgery: An Illustrated History* to be a compendium of surgical tales as well as an iconographic journey. The written chronicle contains three major levels of historical content within two overall sections. The first section consists of an in-depth chronological detailing of the history of American surgery. Because I found it difficult to weave the evolution of specific specialties within such a narrative, I used the last third of the book to relate each specialty's individual story. This organization of the work provides a better balance for understanding the whole of surgery and, at the same time, the organizational details and clinical highlights of specialization.

With regard to the three levels of historical content, the first and most rudimentary stratum provides an understanding of significant developments within the whole of American history that occurred during a particular surgical era. In this regard, time lines about daily life and history and politics serve as prologues to various chapters. In addition, famous Americans from all walks of life who were born during the surgical era under discussion are listed. With a quick glance, the reader is able to determine what well-known events were taking place and which personalities were alive. More important, many chapters begin with a written background section describing that era's socioeconomic and political milieu. When such nonmedical historical information is made available, the placement of surgical history within the context of evolving American history becomes an easier task.

The second level concerns the important process of surgical professionalization and specialization of American surgery. In fact, it serves as the book's leitmotif. Up through the last decades of the nineteenth century, surgical intervention was disdainfully looked upon as little more than a frightening technical exercise within the broad expanse of medicine. At what point was surgery no longer considered a mere physical craft but instead a true science based on legitimate research corroborated by independent clinical observations? What of the complex interaction between economic, institutional, political, and social factors relative to the professionalization of the surgeon and his technical skills? To what extent did events external to the world of surgery, most notably wars and technological advances, foster this evolving surgical independence? When did the American public perceive a professional division between physician and surgeon? Most important, when did the concept of surgical specialization become an integral part of the surgical health care delivery system? Was specialization a function of the modern era, or did vestiges of more focused clinical acumen exist in earlier times?

The final historical level consists of a detailed understanding of the lives of the great surgeons. Although biographies alone do not constitute an adequate medical history, surgeons have long been inspired by the courageous exploits of past scalpel wielders. Admittedly, there is a grand tradition of reading about the lives of the famous, and an understandable thrill still exists in studying the likes of Valentine Mott, J. Marion Sims, Samuel D. Gross, William Halsted, and Evarts Graham. Accordingly, more than a thousand biographical entries invest the daily lives and professional activities of past surgeons with renewed meaning. Because the historian is both raconteur and gossip, biographies serve as a fitting centerpiece for my surgical tale.

Although surgery as a subject matter in American art is quite rare, it possesses a rich, albeit unacknowledged, iconography that can illuminate this book's three levels of historic focus. Surgical themes, outside of official and often banal portraiture, tend to illustrate surgery as a manual craft. Such representations, often produced without specific medical intent, can also reflect clinical customs of the time. They reveal how surgeons dressed, what their offices looked like, and what constituted early operating theaters. From these images, information can be obtained on subjects rarely discussed in medical literature. I have, therefore, collected a potpourri of illustrations and photographs, many of which have never before been published, to help visualize the development of American surgery. The captions are intentionally quite detailed and narrate this "picture book" within the whole of the project. Even though aesthetics, rather than clinical surgical accuracy or importance, has served as a major criterion in selecting various works, this collection presents a thematic hierarchy of our evolving surgical sciences. Most important, however, this gathering represents the first extensive assemblage of artwork showing the relationship between science, society, and surgeon.

The publication of *American Surgery: An Illustrated History* marks the personal culmination of almost two decades of book collecting and historical surgical research, both in the United States and in Europe. In many respects it is a natural sequel to my *Surgery: An Illustrated History* (1993), but it more fully updates the surgeons' saga through the 1990s. After all, the history of world surgery in the twentieth century is more a tale of American triumphs than it ever was in the eighteenth or nineteenth centuries. The actual writing of the text and selection of illustrations took place from April 1995 through October 1996.

In researching this book, I consulted innumerable primary sources. Important information was also obtained from secondary references and from the writing and thoughts of others. I owe a special debt of gratitude to the many physicians and non-physicians who authored works on medical history. In particular, I have especially relied upon the following: Davis' *Fellowship of Surgeons* (1960), Derbyshire's *Medical Licensure and Discipline in the United States* (1969), Gerdts' *The Art of Healing: Medicine and Science in American Art* (1981), Howell's *Technology in the Hospital* (1995), Kaufman et al.'s *Dictionary of American Medical Biography* (1984), Kelly and Burrage's *Dictionary of American Medical Biography* (1928), Ludmerer's *Learning to Heal* (1985), Pernick's *A Calculus of Suffering* (1985), Rosen's *The Specialization of Medicine* (1944),

Rosenberg's *The Care of Strangers* (1987), Shafer's *The American Medical Profession* (1936), Shryock's *Medicine and Society in America* (1960) and *Medicine in America* (1966), Starr's *The Social Transformation of American Medicine* (1982), Stevens' *American Medicine and the Public Interest* (1971), and Warner's *The Therapeutic Perspective* (1986).

Many individuals are owed a great debt of gratitude for their assistance. Among them are Kevin Crawford and Charles Greifenstein of the College of Physicians of Philadelphia, Lois Black of the New York Academy of Medicine, Richard J. Wolfe of The Francis A. Countway Library of Medicine, and Robin Siegel of CentraState Medical Center in Freehold, New Jersey. The photographic expertise of Nancy Smith was greatly appreciated. Of course, I must extend special acknowledgments to my office manager, Susan Disbrow, for aiding me in the completion of this project. To Jeremy Norman, rare medical book dealer and historical scholar extraordinaire, go my sincerest thanks for sharing his thoughts about the philosophy of writing surgical history. Stanley B. Burns, M.D., receives my heartfelt appreciation for serving as photohistorian and assuring that my captions were accurate relative to the history of medical photography. His assistance in procuring such a wide range of medical illustrations was truly invaluable and contributed to the sweeping scope of the book. Through Stanley B. Burns' efforts, The Burns Collection and Archive houses the nation's largest private collection of early medical photography. Finally, the staff at Lippincott-Raven Publishers must also be recognized for their more than outstanding efforts in publishing a book of this scale. Among many, the labors of Lisa McAllister, Emilie Linkins, Shelley Himmelstein, and Graceanne Malloy should be applauded.

Ira M. Rutkow
Marlboro, New Jersey

Surgeons must be very careful

When they take the knife!

Underneath their fine incisions

*Stirs the Culprit - **Life!***

—Emily Dickinson (circa 1859)

pre-1500	1500	1550	1600	1650	1700	1750	1800	1850

Leif Ericson (fl. 11th cent.) reaches North America *(1000)*

Christopher Columbus (1446–1506) discovers the West Indies and possibly North America *(1492)*

John Cabot (1450–1498) sails to the North American coast *(1497)*

Juan Ponce de Leon (1460?–1521) discovers Florida *(1513)*

Giovanni da Verrazano (1485?–1527?) enters New York harbor *(1524)*

Alvar Núñez Cabeza de Vaca (1490?–1557?) explores Gulf Plains from Florida to Mexico *(1530)*

Jacques Cartier (1491?–1557?) navigates the St. Lawrence River *(1535)*

Francisco Vásquez de Coronado (1510–1554) explores Arkansas plains and Grand Canyon region *(1541)*

Hernando De Soto (1500?–1542) discovers Mississippi River *(1541)*

Martin Frobisher (1535?–1594) searches North American coast for a Northwest passage *(1576)*

Francis Drake (1545?–1596) voyages around the world, including a landing on the North American Pacific coast *(1579)*

Walter Raleigh (1552?–1618) explores Virginia coast *(1584)*

An estimated 1,000,000 Native Americans live north of the Rio Grande *(1600)*

Bartholomew Gosnold (?–1607) explores New England coast and discovers Cape Cod *(1602)*

Samuel de Champlain (1567?–1635) sails up the St. Lawrence River *(1603)*

Henry Hudson (?–1611) explores Chesapeake Bay, Delaware Bay, and the Hudson River *(1609)*

Opechancanough, chief of Virginia's Powhatan tribe, leads a furious rampage, which ends in the killing of 347 English colonists *(1622)*

An account of the Huron Indians is published containing a dictionary of their language *(1632)*

Colonists attack a Pequot village in Connecticut and burn alive almost 700 Native Americans *(1637)*

Roger Williams authors a dictionary of the language of New England Indians *(1643)*

First Protestant service for Native Americans held in Massachusetts *(1646)*

First Native American church established in Massachusetts *(1660)*

First Native American, Caleb Cheeshateaumuck, graduates from Harvard College *(1665)*

Jacques Marquette (1637–1675) and Louis Joliet (1645–1700) explore the Mississippi River *(1673)*

Native American tribes under Philip, son of Massasoit, are subdued after a year of vicious attacks in New England *(1676)*

Robert Cavelier de LaSalle (1643–1687) travels to the mouth of the Mississippi River *(1681)*

French and Native Americans attack and burn English settlement at Schenectady, New York *(1690)*

French and Native Americans massacre 50 settlers at Deerfield, Massachusetts, and carry off 100 more *(1704)*

Tuscarora Indians massacre more than 150 settlers in North Carolina *(1711)*

Carolina militiamen, aided by friendly Native Americans, attack and kill more than 300 Tuscarora Indians *(1712)*

Yamasee Indians massacre more than 200 settlers in South Carolina *(1715)*

Iroquois Confederation of Six Nations (Mohawk, Oneida, Onondaga, Cayuga, Seneca, and Tuscarora tribes) makes treaty with Virginia settlers *(1722)*

Settlers build Fort Dummer in Vermont to provide protection against Native Americans *(1724)*

Iroquois Confederation cedes Ohio Valley territory to Britain *(1744)*

French and Native Americans ambush and defeat colonial militiamen and British regulars near Fort Duquesne *(1755)*

First reservation for Native Americans established in New Jersey *(1758)*

Cherokee Indians massacre the garrison at Fort Loudoun on the Tennessee River *(1760)*

Cherokee and Iroquois tribes negotiate treaties *(1768)*

1700	1750	1800	1850	1900	1950	2000	2050	2100

DAILY LIFE AND EVENTS

Native Americans armed by the British attack settlements in the Northwest Territory *(1791)*

U.S. Army defeats Native Americans at Fallen Timbers, and armed resistance in the Northwest Territory is broken *(1794)*

Publication of *Edgar Huntly,* the first mystery novel to have a Native American as a character *(1799)*

Native Americans defeated at the Battle of Tippecanoe *(1811)*

Shawnee chief Tecumseh defeated and killed at the Battle of the Thames *(1813)*

Creek Indian War ends with Native American defeat at the Battle of Horseshoe Bend *(1814)*

Seminole Indians attack settlers in Florida and Georgia *(1817)*

Sequoya, also known as George Guess, develops an Indian alphabet used to teach thousands of Cherokees to read and write *(1821)*

Creek Indians reject treaty ceding to the United States government all their lands in Georgia *(1824)*

Creek Indians sign Treaty of Washington, which voids previous treaty and cedes less land *(1826)*

Congress passes the Indian Removal Act *(1830)*

State militia and U.S. troops massacre Black Hawk's Sauk tribe at Bad Axe River *(1832)*

George Catlin exhibits his "Gallery of Indians," a series of 500 paintings and sketches *(1837)*

U.S. cavalry troops forcibly relocate Cherokees from Georgia via the "Trail of Tears" to eastern Oklahoma *(1838)*

Seminoles are unwillingly displaced to Indian Territory in eastern Oklahoma after their crops and villages are destroyed by United States troops *(1842)*

Commencment of the Navaho Conflicts, with final victory won by United States troops under Kit Carson in 1863 *(1846)*

Massacre of Marcus Whitman and 12 other missionaries in the Pacific Northwest *(1847)*

The Spanish introduce silversmithing to the Navajo tribe *(1850)*

Sioux Indians give all their land in Iowa and most of their holdings in Minnesota to the United States government *(1851)*

Commencement of the Sioux Wars, which lasted until 1890, involving such Native American tribal chiefs as Little Crow, Sitting Bull, Crazy Horse, Red Cloud, and Big Foot *(1854)*

Native Americans and allied Mormons massacre 140 non-Mormon emigrants at Mountain Meadows, Utah *(1857)*

The Southern Plains Wars, involving the Arapaho, Comanche, and Cheyenne under Chief Black Kettle, the Kiowa under Chief Satanta, and the Ute under Chief Ouray, lasts until 1879 *(1860)*

Apache warfare breaks out, led by Chiefs Cochise, Victorio, Mangas Coloradas, and Geronimo, and persists until 1900 *(1861)*

The sculpture *Indian Hunter* is placed in New York City's Central Park *(1864)*

Congress establishes reservation in Indian Territory (now Oklahoma) for the five "civilized" tribes: the Cherokees, Chickasaws, Choctaws, Creeks, and Seminoles *(1867)*

Congress passes the Indian Appropriation Act, nullifying all prior treaties and making all Native Americans wards of the nation *(1871)*

The Modoc War and execution of Chief Captain Jack (Kintpuash) *(1872)*

George Custer's defeat and death at the Battle of the Little Big Horn *(1876)*

The Nez Percé War and flight of Chief Joseph *(1877)*

Helen Hunt Jackson's *A Century of Injustice* is published concerning the mistreatment of Native Americans *(1881)*

The Apache under Geronimo leave their Arizona reservation and resume warfare against settlers, ending with the tribe's surrender in 1886 *(1885)*

The Dawes Act provides lands to individual Native Americans in an effort to discourage them from living in tribes *(1887)*

Portion of Indian Territory is opened to settlers *(1889)*

Murder of Sitting Bull and massacre of 200 Sioux at Wounded Knee *(1890)*

Indian Territory land forcibly ceded to the United States government by the Sauk, Fox, and Potawatomi tribes is opened to settlers by presidential proclamation *(1891)*

The orchestral piece *Indian Suite* is first performed *(1892)*

Cherokee land between Kansas and Oklahoma, purchased by the United States government in 1891, is opened to settlement *(1893)*

Warfare and disease reduce Native American population to 400,000 *(1900)*

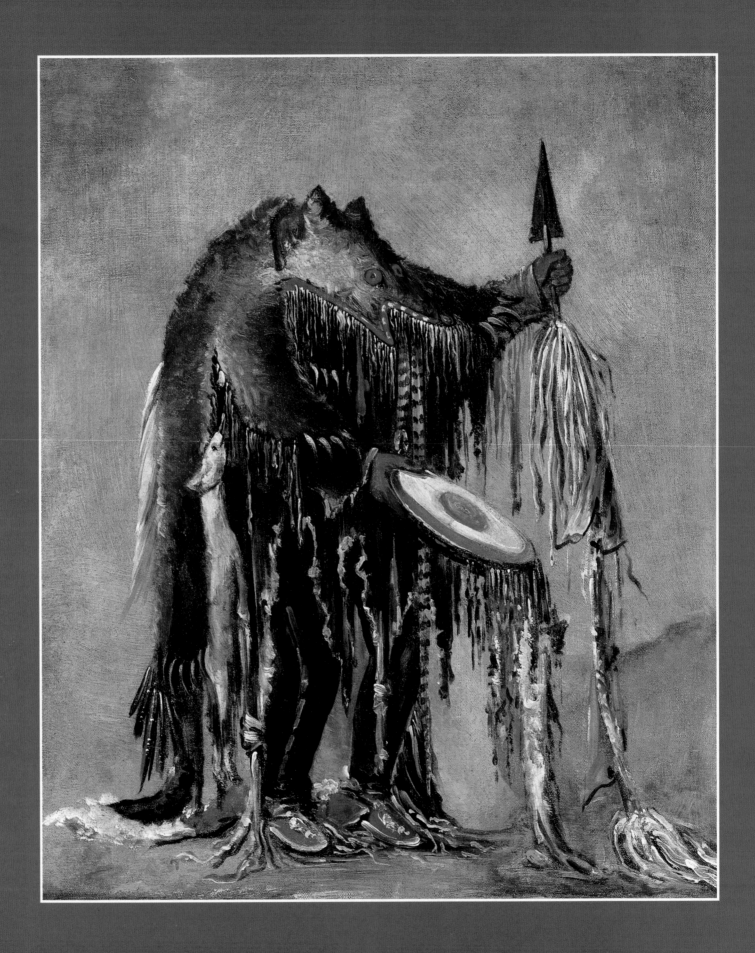

CHAPTER 1

NATIVE AMERICAN SURGERY

*S*urgery as a method of healing initially developed apart from treatments based on medication. As in all early civilizations, this once simple division of "medicine and surgery" was evident in prehistoric and aboriginal Native American societies. Hackneyed stereotypes of "gourd-rattling, drug-induced, wildly dancing incantators" have been shown to be false by contemporary observations and anthropologic research. It has been revealed that American Indians had an understanding of simple surgical problems that occasionally rivaled that of their colonial conquerors. For instance, their treatment of common wounds and the resultant healing process was every bit as skillful and successful as that of any European physician/surgeon.

In eighteenth- and nineteenth-century America, it was a commonly accepted observation that Native Americans appeared to recover more rapidly from gunshot, arrow, knife and other sharp injuries than their European counterparts. Numerous anecdotal reports concern wounded Native Americans, discharged from military hospitals so that they might die among their own people, who soon made rapid and supposedly "miraculous" recoveries once Indian medicine men began their particular form of treatment. No scientific rationale has ever been provided for this mystery of healing, but a folk belief has persisted that Native Americans possessed some sort of natural immunity to the usual infections that made wounds fatal to the early settlers. It was even speculated that "red" men, because of their outdoor life, were a more fit species than "white" men.

For the Native American, superstition, at least relative to bodily injury, was often superseded by practical therapeutic renderings. Early nineteenth-century written descriptions of the treatment of projectile wounds reveal both a pragmatism and an ingenuity approaching that of any European wound surgeon:

> When a [Choctaw] is wounded with a bullet or an arrow, the medicine man first sucks the wound then spits out the blood.... In their dressings, they do not use lint or compresses. Instead, to make the wound suppurate, they blow into it powder made of a root. Another root powder is used to dry and heal the wound, and still other roots are used in a solution with which the wound is bathed to help prevent gangrene.

> A [Flathead] squaw first sucked the wound perfectly dry, so that it appeared white as chalk; and then she bound it up with a piece of dry buck-skin as soft as woolen cloth, and by this treatment the wound began to heal, and soon closed up, and the part became sound again. The sucking of it so effectually may have been from an apprehension of a poisoned arrow.

The surgical acumen of the aboriginal Native Americans was probably derived partly from attempts at performing the most primitive of all known major surgical

1. *(facing page)* "Medicine Man, Performing His Mysteries Over a Dying Man" by George Catlin (1796–1872), painted in 1832. A Blackfoot shaman wears a bearskin garment while invoking an incantation over a wounded tribesman. Catlin originally worked as a portrait painter in Philadelphia but began to travel widely through North America studying various native peoples. The Blackfoot were members of three tribes of Algonquian Indians who lived in Montana and Saskatchewan, east of the Rocky Mountains. Stereotypes aside, Native American treatments for traumatic injuries were just as advanced as certain European methods. *(National Museum of American Art, Washington, DC/Art Resource, New York)*

operations, trephination of the human skull. A common belief is that trephining by prehistoric man was little used north of present-day Mexico. However, trephined skulls have been located as far away as Alaska, and other specimens have been reported from Michigan, Illinois, New Mexico, and Georgia. The importance of trephining in pre-Columbian North American aboriginal culture remains unclear, since few of these specimens demonstrate postoperative healing. More importantly, there is little archeological evidence to suggest that native North Americans utilized trephination subsequent to the sixteenth century.

What mattered was that *pari passu* with trephining was the necessity for additional technical decisions having to be made relative to overall wound care. How should bleeding be controlled? In what manner should a wound be covered? Was a primitive form of anesthesia available? Although much remains a mystery, it is known that Native Americans had at their disposal various herbs and plant extracts to stem bleeding, soothe wounds, alleviate pain, and hasten the recovery process. Among the most widely acknowledged botanical preparations and other natural medicinals were hellebore, applied locally; poultices made from tobacco, jimsonweed, white pine, or common elder; fir balsam employed as a salve; and pleurisy root, which was chewed and applied to a wound or powdered and blown into it. Slippery elm was particularly effective for its mucilaginous but nonirritative properties:

> When it is desirable to extract a ball, they introduce a piece of the slippery elm bark as far into the wound as is practicable, which is suffered to remain, till the sought for object is obtained, or no danger is likely to result by suffering it to remain.... The slippery elm bark beaten to a pulp and applied to the wounded part, is the usual remedy among the Osages for the extraction of a ball, thorn, &c.

Various types of dressings were employed in the protection of wounds. Larger injuries were sutured. For instance, the Dakota, Tuscarora, and Winnebago tribes closed lacerations and deeper injuries with threads of sinew on needles made from animal bone. To facilitate healing from the "bottom up," certain tribes inserted a thin membrane of bark between the cut skin surfaces before placing the sutures. In this way, granulation would start at the deepest part of the wound and assure a more rapid and complete recovery. Delaware Indians used a decoction of both hickory and sarsaparilla barks as wet dressings.

Although Native Americans had no scientific knowledge of antisepsis and asepsis, they appreciated the value of cleanliness in the treatment of open wounds. Numerous contemporary observers noted the use of both boiled and cold water to cleanse injuries. The Dakota and Apache tribes were particularly vigilant in using cold water as an almost constant wash in the treatment of compound fractures. The Choctaws of present-day Alabama, Louisiana, and Mississippi used a solution of boiled pennywort and sweet gum tree roots to help prevent wound gangrene. Native

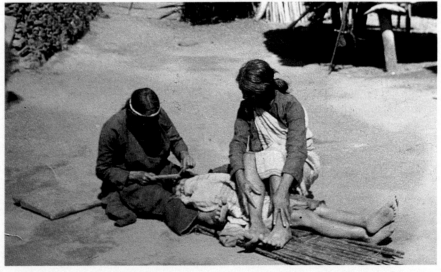

2. It was unusual for Native Americans to be photographed while undergoing a surgical operation. In this illustration, taken by an unknown photographer (circa 1900), the exact nature of this particular procedure is difficult to discern, but it apparently involves the region of the head and neck. Although the patient might have been given an anesthetic concoction to render her less sensible, the assistance of another individual was needed nonetheless to keep her from moving. *(Courtesy of Stanley B. Burns, M.D., and The Burns Collection and Archive)*

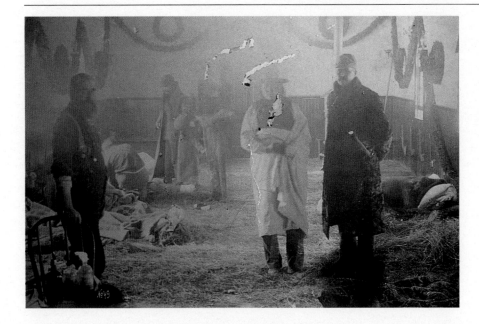

3. On December 29, 1890, hundreds of Sioux men, women, and children were slaughtered by the United States Army's 7th Cavalry at Wounded Knee Creek in South Dakota. This silver print was taken in a nearby church, where some of the wounded had been evacuated. Because the scene was lighted only by candles, the photograph was taken at a slow shutter speed and appears somewhat grainy and not sharp. Yet, it is a haunting image, showing cavalrymen apparently tending to their victims, while the sadness of that fateful day in Native American history permeates the picture. *(Courtesy of Stanley B. Burns, M.D., and The Burns Collection and Archive)*

Americans of the western Great Lakes were reported to have bathed gunshot and arrow injuries with copious amounts of warm water in which various drugs were diluted. The practice of taking water into their own mouths and spitting it over wounds was employed by Blackfoot medicine men.

Hemostasis was obtained with several ingenious methods. Although herbal, animal, and mineral substances were employed by virtually all Native American tribes as hemostatic agents, a most intriguing scheme was the use of spiderwebs to arrest bleeding. For the Haidahs, Kwakiutls, Apaches, Mohegans, and other widely scattered tribes, the packing of a wound with a spiderweb worked because the silk filaments provide a gossamer-like lattice network upon which a stable blood clot could be formed. Not surprisingly, this method was also practiced by European surgeons. However, the historical evidence seems to indicate that the Native American and European cultures developed the technique independently of one another. A variant on the theme of spiderwebs was to pack a wound with the spores or pulverized heads of different species of puffballs.

Various Missouri River and Plains tribes utilized the styptic properties of smooth sumac leaves and berries, mixed with herbal roots, to form an unsophisticated astringent to arrest mouth bleeding. More novel was the ability of the Cherokees to control certain types of bleeding with a plaster of buzzard's or eagle's down. The Mescaleros, an Apache people formerly ranging through modern-day Texas and eastern New Mexico, utilized scrapings from the insides of freshly tanned hides as a form of topical coagulant. American Indian expertise in hemostasis is best summed up by one nineteenth-century observer who stated, "I have known them to stop hemorrhages which I am persuaded would otherwise have proved fatal."

Knowledge of anatomy is one of four basic prerequisites to the development of surgery as a useful medical procedure. Like anesthesia, antisepsis, and the control of arterial and venous bleeding, a detailed understanding of anatomy is essential to the successful performance of any type of surgical operation. Living in the outdoors, the average Native American probably knew more about animal anatomy than the average European of his day. However, there is nothing to suggest that Indian medicine men or shamans possessed any detailed understanding of the human form to permit more than the performance of the most minor of surgical procedures.

One nineteenth-century percipient wrote, "neither did I ever see them...make the skeletons of their kings and great men's bones," while another frontiersman stated explicitly, "Indians are wholly ignorant in anatomy and their knowledge of surgery is very superficial." Similarly, there is no evidence to suggest that Native Americans performed postmortem examinations to determine cause of death or as an attempt to understand human structure and function. Yet, aboriginal Native

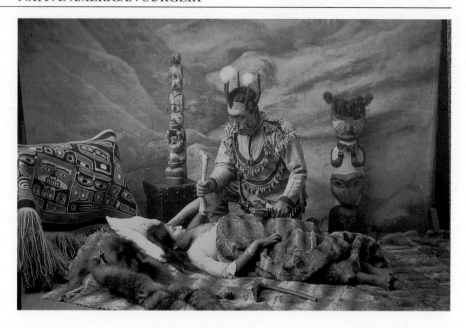

4. The Tlingit are a group of Indian peoples of the islands and coast of southeastern Alaska, including chiefly the Auk, Chilkat, Sitka, Stikine, Tongass, and Yakutat. One of the tribe's shamans examines a woman's exposed breast prior to providing an incantation (circa 1908). *(Courtesy of Stanley B. Burns, M.D., and The Burns Collection and Archive)*

Americans were believed to have understood through analogy with the animals they killed that blood circulated throughout the body owing to the action of the heart, that the lungs were organs of respiration, and that if the kidneys were destroyed life would cease. Some physical anthropologists even believe that prehistoric Native Americans understood the brain to be the organ of thought and essential for human existence.

Minor surgery, in its most rudimentary form, was observed among numerous tribes. In particular, lancing, scarification, and bloodletting were widely practiced. Employing porcupine quills and maguey thorns, medicine men and shamans would open the veins of the right arm for maladies of the trunk and those of the left arm for affected extremities. Rattlesnake fangs were commonly employed to introduce "medicine" under the skin. The Chippewas used an instrument consisting of several such "needles" fitted into a wood handle:

> This was used in treating "dizzy headache," neuralgia, or rheumatism in any part of the body. In giving the treatment the medicine was "worked in" with the needles. If only a small part were to be "gone over" it was customary to hold a knife in the left hand and to use the blade as a guide for the needles. These were "worked up and down" close to the blade, "which kept the medicine from spreading." The remedy used most often…was…hazel stalks or cedar wood burned to a charcoal and a small quantity of the charcoal or ash mixed with an equal quantity of dried gall of a bear…. The dark spots seen on the temples of many Indians are left by the charcoal in this medicine.

With flints or obsidian flakes serving as scalpels, the treatment of furuncles and small abscesses was remarkably similar across widely separated tribes. Fomenting poultices of warmed cornmeal or cooling plasters of "bruised" herbs were applied to boils, which would then be lanced once suppuration had reached a painful stage. The Indians of the Great Lakes region were known to have incised and drained small empyemas. Naiuchi, a renowned Zuni medicine man of the late nineteenth century, was observed opening a large breast abscess. He gave the woman a decoction of jimsonweed, which provided a "twilight" type of anesthesia. With a flint knife, Naiuchi incised the abscess, explored the loculated cavity with his finger, and evacuated a "large quantity" of purulent material. In 1896, an incision and drainage of a left groin abscess was described in which the wound was cleansed with water and packed with "pinon gum, kernels of squash seeds and mutton grease."

Because of superstition and for religious reasons, therapeutic amputation of an extremity was usually avoided. However, a case among the nineteenth-century Chippewa is mentioned in which a young man, whose lower extremities had been frostbitten when he was a child, eventually underwent bilateral amputation. It was said that the procedure was completed with a common knife and that the only dressing was tree bark. A more sinister and unique form of "amputation as punishment" was practiced by the Iroquois of western New York and by various North Carolina tribes. To readily identify and retain prisoners, members of those tribal nations mutilated their captives by cutting away "half of the foot." To accomplish this, an incision was made along the dorsum of the appendage at the metatarsal-phalangeal junction and carried proximal to the head of the metatarsal bones. Amputation was performed at this point, and a skin flap was rolled downward over the exposed joints and either wrapped or sutured closed. The disfigured detainees were said to have been able to walk, albeit with difficulty, and to have left such characteristic footprints that they were easy to track following any escape attempts. Another form of "punishment" amputation has been described as "cutting off half of their feet lengthwise so that they would not be able to run away." As an interesting aside, these Native American "punishment" amputations were also known to have included the use of sinew ligatures to control hemorrhage.

American Indians were quite successful in treating sprains, dislocations, and fractures. Understanding the principles of traction–counter traction, they were ingenious and skillful in providing unique types of immobilization. As one Western settler wrote, "fractures and dislocations are not rare among them, but they are pretty dexterous in reducing them." Most medicine men would immediately set broken bones and apply some type of form-fitting splint. Paddings of wet clay or rawhide were used, as well as slats of wood. The Ojibwas, a people of the region around Lake Superior and westward, would wash a fractured arm with warm water and grease it with various types of animal fat. After a warm poultice of wild ginger and spikenard had been applied, the extremity was covered with cloth and bound with thin cedar splints.

The Pima of what is now southern Arizona created splints from the flat, elastic ribs of the giant cactus. In a method that presaged the Europeans' use of plaster-of-

5. Basing his work on real-life observations of sixteenth-century Native Americans in Florida, Theodore DeBry (circa 16th century), a Flemish engraver, portrays various ways in which the members of this tribe cured their sick. On the left, a man is being prepared for some type of minor surgical procedure, possibly a bloodletting. The tribesman in the center is smoking tobacco, probably intended to help combat an infection, while on the right, an individual lies on his stomach inhaling the smoke of burning seeds with presumed medicinal properties. *(The Beinecke Rare Book and Manuscript Library, Yale University)*

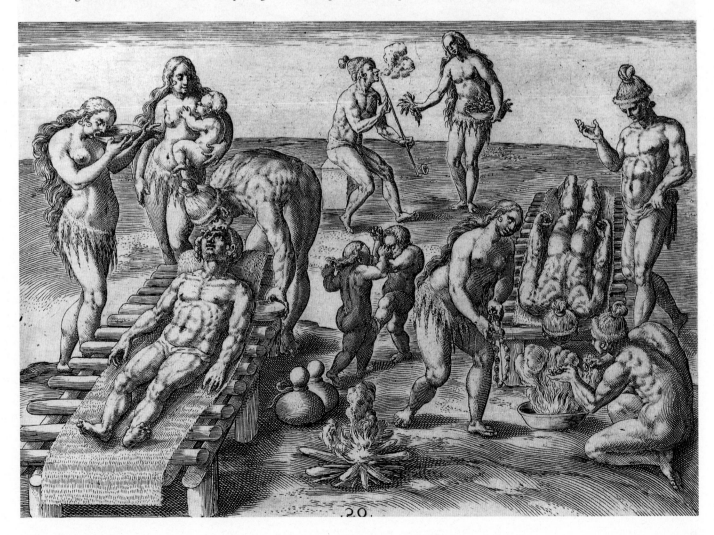

Paris dressings, the Shoshoni of present-day southern Utah and neighboring states created splints of fresh rawhide. The leather was soaked in warm water until soft. After the fracture was reduced, the rawhide was molded to the extremity, surplus hide was trimmed away, and the assemblage was held in place by leather thongs. Subsequent to its drying, the rawhide splint became an immovable cast no different from the best of modern appliances. Not infrequently, slats or windows were cut in these devices to allow treatment with soothing washes and poultices for compound fractures.

Understanding the importance of muscular relaxation in reducing a dislocated extremity, members of the Ottawa and Chippewa tribes administered decoctions that nauseated the patient. As described by one observer, "They are acquainted with the advantage of relaxing the skeletal muscles in dislocations; for in cases where they do not readily succeed, they nauseate the patient to a most distressing degree, and then find very little difficulty in replacing the luxated bone." Even the art of reducing a dislocation of one's own hip was understood: "If an Indian has a dislocation when hunting alone, he creeps to the next tree and tying one end of his strap to it, fastens the other to the dislocated limb and, lying on his back, continues to pull until it is reduced."

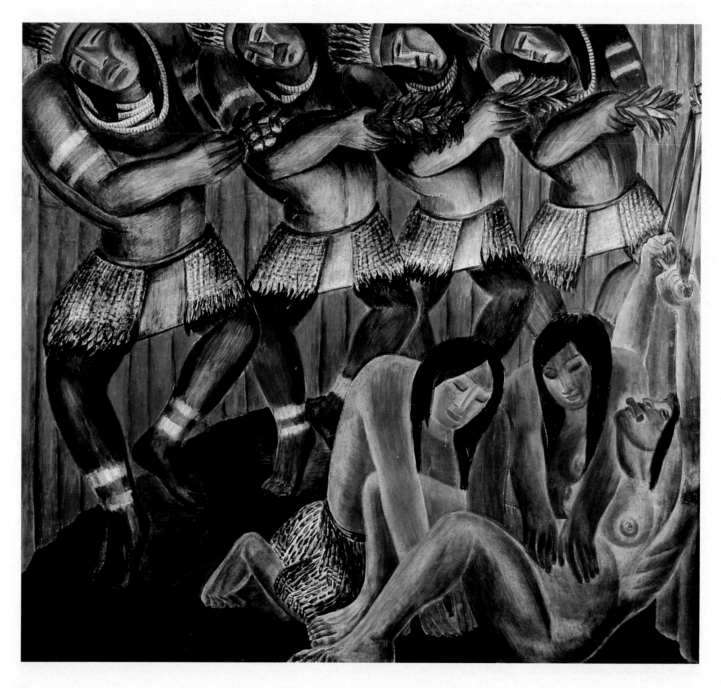

6. "California Native American Birth Scene." Bernard B. Zakheim (1896–1985) completed this fresco (circa 1935–1938) using partial funding from the New Deal's Works Progress Administration. Located in Toland Hall at the University of California Medical Center, San Francisco, this particular vignette from a much larger twelve-panel work shows two squaw-midwives assisting at childbirth by applying fundal pressure on the abdomen of the mother-to-be. The patient bites a stick while pulling on overhead ropes to augment her expulsive efforts. Four herb-holding shamans aid her exertions by providing prayer and a ceremonial dance. *(Courtesy of Masha Zakheim and the University of California Medical Center, San Francisco)*

Of the many surgical problems that Native Americans were forced to treat, their expertise with gunshot and arrow wounds was particularly evident. As far back as 1639, a newly settled New Englander noted that "some of them have been shot in the mouth, and out of the ear, some shot in the breast; some run through the flank with darts, and other desperate wounds, which either by their rare skill in the use of vegetative, or diabolical charms, they cure in a short time." In the mid-nineteenth century, Native Americans indigenous to Michigan were said to cleanse gunshot wounds with vegetable decoctions introduced via a bladder-and-quill syringe. More importantly, great care was taken to assure that premature closing of the wound's external orifice did not occur. By the introduction of a "tent" made from the bark of slippery elm, suppuration could continue unabated. Native Americans also attempted the extraction of foreign bodies:

> When a ball simply lodges beneath the integuments, they extract it with the point of the scalping knife or the handle of their bullet moulds, which from its shape, is the better qualified of the two. When however the ball is lodged more deeply, or has penetrated in a circuitous direction, it is permitted to come out by the slower process of suppuration; or to remain within a sac naturally formed by the surrounding muscular integuments…. They also make incisions with the knife of the surface, whenever it heals too fast for the more deep seated parts in the wound…. Osages…sometimes apply the pounded roots of the gall of the earth plant to wounds, inflammation generally follows, and the foreign body is easily extracted.

An intriguing interface of Native American medical failure and European surgical acumen occurred in 1535, when Alvar Núñez Cabeza de Vaca (1490?–1557?), a shipwrecked Spanish explorer, removed an arrowhead from an aboriginal's thoracic cavity. In this first recorded surgical operation in the American Southwest, Cabeza de Vaca achieved a complete cure, making him famous among his captors and leading to his eventual safe return to Western civilization. The operative report was included in his 1542 accounting of the ill-fated expedition:

> They brought a man to me and said that a long time ago he had been wounded with an arrow through the right shoulder, and the arrowhead was lodged over the heart. He said that it gave him much pain…. I touched him, felt the arrowhead, and saw that it traversed the cartilage. With a knife I opened his chest to that spot and saw that the point was crosswise and was very difficult to remove. I continued to cut, inserted the point of the knife, and with great difficulty I finally extracted it…. With a deer bone, using my knowledge of surgery, I took two stitches, following which he bled profusely all over me. With hair from an animal skin I staunched the flow of blood…. Because of this operation they had many dances and festivities…. On another day I cut the Indian's two stitches and he was well. The wound I had made was no more apparent than a crease in the palm of the hand. He said he felt neither pain nor any discomfort.

The surgical site was probably in the area of the anterior mediastinum, and the bleeding that Cabeza de Vaca so vividly describes undoubtedly resulted from puncture of the internal mammary vessels with his deer-bone needle. With this "miraculous" cure, the Spaniard gained psychological control over the Indians and all "that they considered valuable or cherished."

In most respects, prehistoric Native Americans were as inventive and efficient in the art and craft of surgery as other prescientific peoples throughout the world. Their surgical techniques appear to have included essentially all the rudimentary surgical devices and methodologies known in Europe prior to the first explorations of the North American continent. It would not be incorrect to state that among some Native American tribes, surgical knowledge and skill clearly equaled or surpassed the state of the healing arts in the Old World. By the late nineteenth century, one apodictic fact was well recognized: Western settlers had copied from their vanquished Native American foes much of their knowledge regarding the surgical treatment of all types of injuries.

COLONIAL AMERICA, 1607–1783

1600	1650	1700	1750	1800	1850

DAILY LIFE

Tobacco planted *(1612)*

First slaves *(1619)*

First criminal is executed by hanging *(1634)*

Harvard College *(1636)*

Bay Psalm Book printed *(1640)*

Jewish immigrants arrive in New Amsterdam *(1654)*

Wigs become fashionable *(1660)*

First sports trophy is presented to the winner of a horse race on Long Island *(1668)*

Mail service begins between New York and Boston *(1673)*

Paper money issued in Massachusetts *(1690)*

Salem witchcraft trials *(1692)*

Yale College *(1701)*

Boston News Letter, first continuous weekly newspaper *(1704)*

New York City slave revolt with execution of 100 individuals *(1712)*

First company of English actors appears at Williamsburg *(1716)*

Blackbeard, the pirate, is captured in North Carolina and his head brought back on a pole *(1718)*

Quakers demand abolition of slavery *(1727)*

Poor Richard's Almanac (1732)

Fire destroys half of Charleston *(1740)*

Princeton University *(1746)*

First legal society, the New York Bar Association *1747)*

Stagecoach line established between Philadelphia and New York City *(1756)*

First Chambers of Commerce in New York and New Jersey *(1763)*

Mason-Dixon line *(1766)*

Large-scale street lighting begins in Boston *(1773)*

Postal system established with Benjamin Franklin as Postmaster General *(1775)*

Common Sense published *(1776)*

Stars and Stripes adopted as Continental Congress flag *(1777)*

Bank of North America established in Philadelphia *(1782)*

The Pennsylvania Evening Post, the first daily newspaper *(1783)*

COLONIAL POPULATION

1630	=	5,700
1670	=	114,500
1690	=	213,000
1720	=	474,000
		(Boston 12,000, Philadelphia 10,000, New York 7,000)
1750	=	655,000
1780	=	2.7 million

HISTORY AND POLITICS

Jamestown *(1607)*

Plymouth colony and Mayflower Compact *(1620)*

Island of Manhattan purchased for $24 *(1626)*

Puritans arrive at Massachusetts Bay and settle in Salem *(1628)*

Rhode Island General Assembly agrees on code of civil law that separates church and state *(1647)*

Maryland Assembly passes Act of Toleration for Christians *(1649)*

Colony of New Jersey *(1665)*

King William's War, with England and France seeking control of eastern North America *(1689)*

North Carolina separates from South Carolina *(1712)*

British governor quells riot by poor in Philadelphia *(1726)*

Molasses Act places prohibitive duties on sugar, rum, and molasses *(1733)*

Governor of Virginia sends George Washington to demand French withdrawal from Ohio Territory *(1753)*

French and Indian War *(1756)*

Treaty of Paris ends the French and Indian War *(1763)*

The Sugar Act *(1764)*

COLONIAL AMERICA, 1607–1783

1600	1650	1700	1750	1800	1850

HISTORY AND POLITICS

The Stamp Act *(1765)*
British troops occupy Boston *(1768)*
Boston Massacre *(1770)*
Boston Tea Party *(1773)*
First Continental Congress *(1774)*
Battle of Lexington and Concord,
Battle of Bunker Hill *(1775)*
Declaration of Independence *(1776)*
Articles of Confederation *(1777)*
Battle of Monmouth *(1778)*
Bonhomme Richard, under John Paul
Jones, wins naval victory against the
British frigate *Serapis (1779)*
Battle of Yorktown *(1781)*
Benjamin Franklin, John Adams,
and John Jay negotiate peace
treaty with British in Paris *(1782)*
Treaty of Paris, with Great Britain
recognizing the United States
(1783)

FAMOUS AMERICANS
HEROES, POLITICIANS AND STATESMEN

Peter Minuit *(1580–1638)*
Miles Standish *(1584–1656)*
John Rolfe *(1585–1622)*
Virginia Dare *(1587–?)*
John Winthrop *(1588–1649)*
John Endecott *(1589–1665)*
Peter Stuyvesant *(1610–1672)*
William Penn *(1644–1718)*
James Oglethorpe *(1696–1785)*
Samuel Adams *(1722–1803)*
Crispus Attucks *(1723–1770)*
George Washington *(1732–1799)*
Martha Washington *(1732–1802)*
Daniel Boone *(1734–1820)*
Robert Morris *(1734–1806)*
John Adams *(1735–1826)*
Paul Revere *(1735–1818)*
Patrick Henry *(1736–1799)*
John Hancock *(1737–1793)*
Ethan Allen *(1738–1789)*
Haym Salomon *(1740–1785)*
Benedict Arnold *(1741–1801)*
Thomas Jefferson *(1743–1826)*
Abigail Adams *(1744–1818)*
John Jay *(1745–1829)*
John Paul Jones *(1747–1792)*
James Madison *(1751–1836)*
George Rogers Clark *(1752–1818)*
Betsy Ross *(1752–1836)*
Nathan Hale *(1755–1776)*
Alexander Hamilton *(1755–1804)*
John Marshall *(1755–1835)*
James Monroe *(1758–1831)*
John Jacob Astor *(1763–1848)*
John Quincy Adams *(1767–1848)*
Andrew Jackson *(1767–1845)*
Dolley Madison *(1768–1849)*
DeWitt Clinton *(1769–1828)*
William Henry Harrison *(1773–1841)*
Meriwether Lewis *(1774–1809)*
Henry Clay *(1777–1852)*
Stephen Decatur *(1779–1820)*
Zebulon Pike *(1779–1813)*
John C. Calhoun *(1782–1850)*
Martin Van Buren *(1782–1862)*
Daniel Webster *(1782–1852)*

COLONIAL AMERICA, 1607–1783

	1600	1650	1700	1750	1800	1850

FAMOUS AMERICANS

SCIENTISTS AND INVENTORS

Jared Eliot *(1685–1763)*

Benjamin Franklin *(1706–1790)*
John Winthrop *(1714–1779)*
Benjamin Banneker *(1731–1806)*
David Rittenhouse *(1732–1796)*
William Bartram *(1739–1823)*
David Bushnell *(1750–1824)*
Benjamin Thompson *(1753–1814)*
Oliver Evans *(1755–1819)*
John Barrow *(1764–1848)*
Robert Fulton *(1765–1815)*
Eli Whitney *(1765–1825)*

THEOLOGIANS AND PHILOSOPHERS

Nathaniel Ward *(1578?–1652)*
John Cotton *(1585–1652)*
Anne Hutchinson *(1591–1671)*
Roger Williams *(1603–1683)*
John Eliot *(1604–1690)*
Increase Mather *(1639–1723)*
Cotton Mather *(1663–1728)*
Jonathan Edwards *(1703–1758)*
Sarah Osborn *(1714–1796)*
John Woolman *(1720–1772)*
Ezra Stiles *(1727–1795)*
Elizabeth Ann Bayley Seton
(1774–1821)

EDUCATORS, SCHOLARS, AND REFORMERS

James Logan *(1674–1751)*
Paul Dudley *(1675–1751)*
Thomas Prince *(1687–1758)*
John Mitchell *(1690–1768)*
John Peter Zenger *(1697–1746)*
Issac Greenwood *(fl. 1st half 18th cent.)*
Thomas Clap *(1703–1767)*
William Smith *(1727–1803)*

AUTHORS

John Smith *(1580–1631)*
William Bradford *(1590–1657)*
Anne Dudley Bradstreet *(1612–1672)*
Michael Wigglesworth *(1631–1705)*
Edward Taylor *(1644?–1729)*
Sarah Kemble Knight *(1666–1727)*
William Byrd II *(1674–1744)*
Mercy Warren *(1728–1814)*
Hector St. John Crèvecoeur *(1735–1813)*
Thomas Paine *(1737–1809)*
John Trumbull *(1750–1831)*
Judith Murray *(1751–1820)*
Timothy Dwight *(1752–1817)*
Philip Freneau *(1752–1832)*
Phyllis Wheatley *(1753–1784)*
Joel Barlow *(1754–1812)*
Noah Webster *(1758–1843)*
Susanna Rowson *(1762–1824)*
Charles Brockden Brown *(1771–1810)*
Washington Irving *(1783–1859)*

COLONIAL AMERICA, 1607–1783

	1600	1650	1700	1750	1800	1850

VISUAL ARTISTS AND ARTISANS

John Smibert *(1688–1751)*
Joseph Blackburn *(1700–1763)*
John Greenwood *(1727–1792)*
Benjamin West *(1738–1820)*
John Singleton Copley *(1738–1815)*
Charles Willson Peale *(1741–1827)*
Winthrop Chandler *(1747–1790)*
Ralph Earl *(1751–1801)*
Gilbert Stuart *(1755–1828)*
John Trumbull *(1756-1843)*
Charles Bulfinch *(1763–1844)*
Reuben Moulthrop *(1763–1814)*
Benjamin Latrobe *(1764–1820)*
Duncan Phyfe *(1768–1854)*
Raphaelle Peale *(1774–1825)*
Rembrandt Peale *(1778–1860)*
Edward Hicks *(1780–1849)*
Thomas Sully *(1783–1872)*

PERFORMING ARTISTS

Charles Pachelbel *(1690–1750)*
Edward Enstone *(fl. 1st half 18th cent.)*
Francis Hopkinson *(1737–1791)*
William Selby *(1738–1798)*
William Billings *(1746–1800)*
John Harris *(fl. 2nd half 18th cent.)*
Alexander Reinagle *(1756–1809)*
Gottlieb Graupner *(1767–1836)*
Benjamin Carr *(1769–1831)*
John Wyeth *(1770–1858)*
Francis Scott Key *(1780–1843)*
Ananias Davisson *(1780–1857)*

BUSINESSMEN AND INDUSTRIALISTS

James Franklin *(1697–1735)*
William Stiegel *(1729–1785)*
Antonio Mèndez *(fl. 2nd half 18th cent.)*
John Cruger *(fl. 2nd half 18th cent.)*
Mathew Carey *(1760–1839)*
Francis C. Lowell *(1775–1818)*
Abel Porter
(fl. 1st half 19th cent.)

FAMOUS AMERICANS

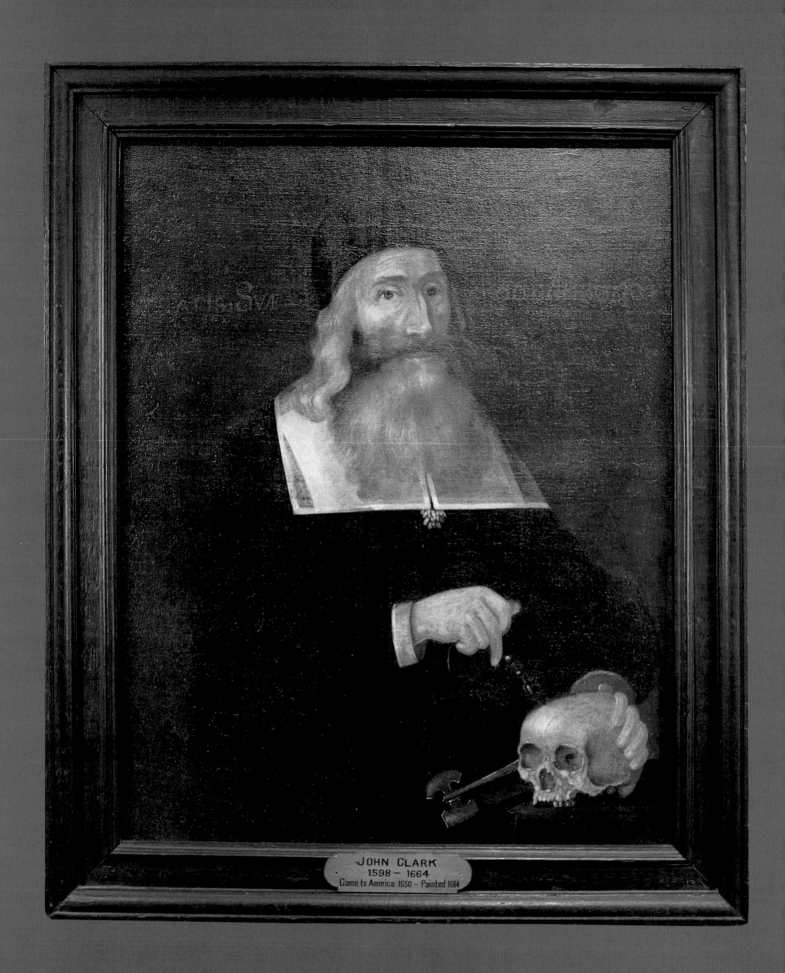

JOHN CLARK
1598 — 1664
Came to America 1650 – Painted 1664

CHAPTER 2

SURGICAL PRACTICE IN COLONIAL AMERICA 1607–1783

*D*aily life in colonial America was extremely harsh. Bitterly cold winters and oppressively hot summers meant an uncertain future for many settlers. Over half of the passengers on the 1620 voyage of the Mayflower died within three months of their landing. Of the nearly 1,700 colonists who settled in Jamestown prior to 1618, only 600 survived five years. By the beginning of the eighteenth century, 100,000 individuals had emigrated to the colony of Virginia. Yet, its population in 1701 was only 75,000 inhabitants! Disease was rampant: epidemics such as bubonic plague, diphtheria, dysentery, influenza, malaria, scarlet fever, smallpox, and yellow fever swept the land. There was no mistaking the fact that the continent of North America proved a hostile environment.

These difficulties were compounded by the fact that for the new colonists, one of the most evident societal problems was a dearth of physicians. The elite European medical doctor with a university educational background was generally unwilling to permanently settle in the New World. Such men were often landed gentry and had no economic, political, or religious need to emigrate. In colonial America there were few opportunities worthy of their prestige. Similarly, the European medical underclass of less well educated apothecaries, barber-surgeons, and surgeons were generally unwilling to leave their geographically and financially stable professional strongholds.

Accordingly, from 1607 to at least the time of the American Revolution, the colonists were left with a void of formally educated physicians and surgeons to attend to their medical needs. This situation was first described by John Smith (1580–1631), founder of the Jamestown colony when, in 1609, he received a burn from a gunpowder explosion. Although the severity of Smith's burn remains a matter of historical conjecture, he returned to England supposedly "because there was neither chirurgeon or chirurgerye in the fort."

For the first century and a half, following successful settlements, the art, craft, and profession of medicine were relegated to a position of little recognition or encouragement. Medical science, in any creative or pragmatic sense, was nonexistent in the colonies. Instead, the health-related problems of the growing populace were served by three classes of minimally prepared caregivers: colonial governors, clerics, and a wide range of self-educated "physicians," secular preachers, and schoolmasters. For the latter two groups, most of their work was poorly performed; as a consequence, little is known of their day-to-day medical and surgical activities. By the nineteenth century, health care providers and the generally unregulated aspects of colonial society had set undefined patterns of general medical practice. Firmly entrenched in the social and economic structure of America's emerging communities, these patterns of clinical practice would thwart the process of medical and surgical specialization for the next century.

1. *(facing page)* John Clark (1598?–1664), as painted (circa 1664) by Augustine Clement. Clark's portrait bears an inscription stating that his age is 66, but since his date of birth is uncertain, it cannot be ascertained whether the painting is a memorial rendering or not. Clark was the first in a dynasty of Boston physicians and surgeons that spanned seven generations through the turn of the nineteenth century. Born in England, he emigrated to New England about 1650. Clark is said to have received a "diploma" in England for his success in cutting for bladder stone. The inclusion in the Clement painting of a skull and trephination instruments as well as a Hey's saw (lying on the table) seems to imply that Clark was capable of performing most surgical operations of that era. While portraits of doctors abound in the nineteenth century, they are rare in pre-Revolutionary America. Accordingly, this painting is considered the earliest known portrayal of an American physician-surgeon and is among the first portraits painted in North America. *(The Francis A. Countway Library of Medicine)*

THE ROLE OF THE COLONIAL GOVERNORS

That colonial governors were able to provide reasonably well for the medical needs of their constituency speaks well for the quality of their leadership. The governors were among the best educated of the settlers and, from a layman's perspective, were as familiar with the European scientific and medical literature as any individual of their time. Among the most notable, John Winthrop (1588–1649), first governor of the Massachusetts Bay Colony, and his son, John Winthrop, Jr. (1606–1676), governor of the Connecticut Colony, were particularly well informed. The elder Winthrop, who is described as having a "piety of the self-accusing puritanic type" was extremely concerned about the obvious medical difficulties in settling North America. In 1643, he wrote Edward Stafford (?–1651) of London, who was known for his scientific interest although not a physician, for medical instructions regarding treatment of the more common diseases and injuries. Stafford's reply was lengthy and contained advice on the use of various cathartics and sudorifics. It also provided some of the earliest instructions on surgical treatment found in the New World:

> For a broken bone, or a joynt dislocated, to knit them; take ye barke of elme, or witch-hazle; cutt away the outward part, and cutt ye inward redd barke small, and boyle it in water, till it be thick that it will rope; pound well, and lay of it hott, barke and all upon ye bone or joynt, and tye it on; or with ye mussilage of it, and boyle armoniak make a playster and lay it on....

> For burning with gunn powder or otherwise - take ye inner green rine of elder, in latine sambucus, sempervive, and mosse that groweth on an old thacht howse top, of each alike; boyle them in stale lotium and sallet oyle, so much as may cover them four fingers; let all the lotium boyle cleane away, and straine very well; put new herbes and lotium as before, boyle that likewise away, and straine it as before. Then to that oyle adde barrowes grease until it come to be an oyntment, with which annoynt a paper, and lay it to ye burning annoynting the place also with a feather....

> For soare brests, take yolkes of eggs and honie alike, beat them till they be very thinn; then with wheat flower beat them, till it be as thick as hony: spread it upon flax, and lay it upon the breast, defending the nipple with a plate of lead as bigg as an halfe crowne, and a hole in it so begg that ye nipple may come out - renewe it every twelve hours: and this will breake and coole the brest. When it breakes, tent it with a salve of rosin, wax & turpentine alike quantitie....

Stafford's letter, taken mostly from John Gerard's (1545–1612) early seventeenth-century *The Herball, or, Generall Historie of Plantes*, consisted of generally ineffective treatments indicative of the lingering effects of Galen, Paracelsus, and medieval medical thought. However, the knowledge received from Stafford's reply was as competent as could be expected at that time. From such information it can be reasonably presumed that Winthrop's ability to treat patients and dispense medical advice approached that of the average European physician. In reality, there was little that a seventeenth-century physician could do to thwart most disease processes. Clinical medicine had not advanced to the stage where mankind's most dreaded medical problems—communicable conditions—were either understood or treatable. Although no information is available about Winthrop's surgical skills, at the time of his death an estate inventory included "3 sirenges - 2 treepans." It can be inferred that the governor thought it wise to have at least a few surgical instruments available as part of his technical armamentarium.

John Winthrop, Jr., was better known throughout the New England colonies for his medical skills than his father. Educated at Trinity College, Dublin, the younger Winthrop was a fellow of the Royal Society of London and counted among his many European correspondents the renowned alchemist Kenelm Digby (1603–1665). As governor of the Connecticut colony, he noted the scarcity of physicians and surgeons. So far as his scientific studies enabled him, he expressed a willingness to provide medical advice, and he was consulted by numerous individuals who wrote

Articles of Agreement Indented and made the eighteenth day of May anno Domini one thousand seven hundred and thirty six Between Zabdiel Boylstone of Boston in the County of Suffolk Practitioner in Physick & Surgery of the one part, and Joseph Lemmon of Charlestown in the County of Middlesex Esqr on the other part:—

Whereas Joseph Lemmon Junr Son of the said Joseph Lemmon Esqr hath lived with the said Zabdiel Boylstone in order to be Instructed by him in the arts Businesses or Mysterys of Physick and Surgery ever since the first of March last, and purposes to continue to live with the said Boylstone until the first day of March one thousand seven hundred and thirty seven if the said Boylstone shall so long live: whereupon It is agreed by and between the said Zabdiel Boylstone and Joseph Lemmon Esqr as follows viz

Imprimis The said Zabdiel Boylstone Doth Covenant and agree for himself to teach and Instruct the said Joseph Lemmon Junr in the arts, Mysterys and Businesses of Physick & Surgery during the term of two years from the first day of March last, provided the said Boylstone should live so long, and if the said Joseph Lemmon Junr shall incline so long to live with and continue in the said Boylstones Employ; and also to find and provide for him good sufficient and suitable Dyot and lodging during the said two years, or so long as the said Lemmon shall see cause to live with the said Boylstone

In

In Consideration whereof the said Joseph Lemmon for himself his Executors and admrs doth hereby Covenant and agree to and with the said Zabdiel Boylstone to pay him two hundred pounds in full Satisfaction for his Board Dyot and Lodging and for the Instruction which the said Boylstone shall give him in the said Mysterys of Physick and Surgery during the term of two years ending in March 1737 vizt one hundred pounds thereof upon demand; and the remaining sum of one hundred pounds on or before the first day of March next, if the said Boylstone and Joseph Lemmon Junr shall be then living. And further the said Joseph Lemmon Esqr doth hereby Covenant and agree to find and provide for his said Son suitable and sufficient apparel and washing during the time he shall be and remain in the Service or Employ of the said Boylstone. In witness whereof the said parties to these presents have hereunto interchangeably set their hands and Seals the day and year first herein before written

Signed Sealed & Delivered in presence of us.

Gillam Tailer

Recd of Joseph Lemmon One Hundred pounds of the within Consideration

Boston May 18 1736

---

lengthy letters explaining their medical conditions. Winthrop, Jr., prescribed among other things an electuary of centipedes, anise, calomel, elder, elecampane, guaiacum, horseradish, iron, jalap, niter, powdered coral, rhubarb, rubila, sulphur, the anodyne mithradate, unicorn horn, and wormwood. Whether he performed much in the way of actual "hands-on" medicine is difficult to ascertain. Certainly, the extant letters between him and his constituents seem to indicate that Winthrop, Jr., did not perform even the simplest of surgical procedures.

THE ROLE OF THE CLERGY

Next to the governors, the clerics were a leading force in early colonial medicine. Like their civilian counterparts who dispensed clinical advice, the clerics practiced little in the way of actual surgical operations, although some are believed to have been excellent phlebotomists. Among the most notable of the clerical group were Thomas Thacher (1620–1678), Increase Mather (1639–1723), and the latter's son, Cotton Mather (1663–1728).

Thomas Thacher, minister of the Old South Church in Boston and regarded as the outstanding Puritan preacher of his time, became the first colonist to author a work solely on a medical topic. In 1677, Thacher produced a broadside that described the essential characteristics of smallpox, together with its treatment and a recommended diet. He was quite deliberate in informing the reader that he was not a physician and that most of the information was obtained from the writings of the English physician Thomas Sydenham (1624–1689). Since newspapers were not yet printed in the colonies, it is believed that Thacher's papersheet was intended primarily for posting or for use as a circular for public instruction during an epidemic of smallpox in the winter of 1677–1678.

2. In early eighteenth-century America there were no medical schools. The only options for medical education and training were attendance at a European institution or apprenticeship with an American practitioner. These are the first and last pages of the rare original articles of indenture of Joseph Lemmon, Jr., to Zabdiel Boylston. The document provides that Lemmon's father, a lawyer, will pay Boylston two hundred pounds "during the term of two years" for his son's instruction "in the Arts Businesses or Mysterys of Physick and Surgery." Boylston is to be responsible for young Lemmon's room and board. Lemmon's father further agrees to provide his son "suitable and sufficient apparel and washing." (*The Francis A. Countway Library of Medicine*)

Whether the Mathers performed surgical operations is a matter of historical conjecture. However, they were closely identified with the earliest attempts to introduce inoculation, which was then considered the equivalent of a surgical operation, as preventive treatment against smallpox in the colonies. Increase Mather was born in Dorchester, Massachusetts, and studied at Harvard College and Trinity College in Dublin. Politically and religiously conservative, Mather was a vigorous proponent of scientific research, and from 1685 to 1701 he served as rector of Harvard University. He was pastor of the Second (or North) Church of Boston and vigorously opposed those clergymen who attempted to liberalize Puritan doctrine and church organization. In 1684, Mather authored his *Remarkable Providences Illustrative of the Earlier Days of American Colonisation*. In this work, he provides what is probably the first written account of an emergency surgical operation performed in the colonies:

> Remarkable was...Abigail Eliot...of Boston....when she was a child under a cart, an iron hinge...happened to strike her head...and pierced into the skull and brain.... Able chyrurgeons were sent for—in special Mr. Oliver and Mr. Pratt. The head being uncovered, there appeared just upon the place where the iron pierced the skull, a bunch as big as a small egg. A question arose, whether the skin should not be cut....This, Mr. Pratt inclined unto, but Mr. Oliver pleading that then the air would get to the brain, and the child would presently die. Mr. Oliver was desired to undertake the cure; and thus was his operation: He gently drove the soft matter of the bunch into the wound, and pressed so much out as well he could....The skull wasted where it was pierced....The skin was exceeding tendr, so that a silver plate...was always kept in the place to defend it from any touch or injury....This child lived to be the mother of two children, and she was not by this wound made defective in her memory or understanding.

THE EUROPEAN BACKGROUND OF AMERICAN MEDICAL PRACTICE

The two surgeons written about by Mather, Mr. Oliver and Mr. Pratt, represented a final group of important early colonial health care providers: regularly appointed physicians and surgeons who accompanied expeditions to colonize the New World. For instance, in 1628, the Court of Assistants of the Guild of Barber-Surgeons in London made the following appointment relative to Pratt:

> A Proposicon beeinge made to Intertayne a surgeon for [the] plantacon Mr. Pratt was ppounded as an abell man vp [on] theis Condicons Namely That 40lb should be allowed him viz for his Chest 25s Rest [for] his owne sallery for

3. A pristine circular amputation set (circa 1770) by Savigny of London. The house of Savigny was arguably the best surgical instrument maker in England at this time, and its shop on Pall Mall was frequently visited by many American students and physicians. Since there were virtually no instrument fabricators in the colonies, North American surgeons were dependent on using implements made in Europe. The configuration of this set, with its Santo Domingo mahogany carrying case and smooth ebony handles, was typical of those employed by American surgeons during the time of the Revolution. *(Collection of Alex Peck, Antique Scientifica)*

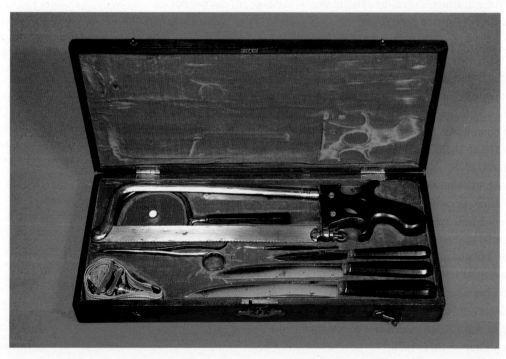

the first yeere prouided yt he [continue] 3 yeeres the Comp. to bee at Charge of transporting his wiffe & a ch [ild] have 20' a yeere for the other 2 yeers & to build him a Ho [use at] the Comp Chardge & to allott him 100 acrs of ground but if he stay but one yeere then the comp to bee at chardge of his bringing back for England & he to Leaue his seru [ant] and the Chist for the Comp service.

John Pratt fulfilled his three-year obligation with the Massachusetts Bay Company and then settled in Cambridge. Little is known of his professional activities, but on his return voyage to England, in 1645, his ship went down off the coast of Spain and he drowned. Of Oliver there is little further information other than that he resided in Boston from 1632 to 1644.

Although the clinical aspects of colonial medicine were largely dependent on English and Continental traditions, the socialization and professionalization processes were to be distinctly American. Unlike European society, which had long accepted the presence of individuals who dedicated their lives to the art and craft of surgery (e.g., medieval surgeons in the Confraternity of Sts. Cosmas and Damian; itinerant incisors for cataract, hernia, and bladder stones; Henry VIII's establishment in 1540 of the Royal Commonality of Barber-Surgeons; Louis XV's 1731 proclamation endowing the Académie Royale de Chirurgie, including yearly publication of its Mémoires; and the passage of a bill by England's Parliament, to which the royal signature was affixed in 1745, forming a Company or Corporation of Surgeons), the United States did not see the formation of such organizations until well after the Civil War.

In reality, there was never a demonstrable repudiation of European medical distinctions (i.e., separation of physician from surgeon), nor was there a truly new American type of medical practice. Instead, since so few European medical men ventured to colonial North America, a cadre of mostly self-educated settlers were forced to deliver rudimentary health care, using as a role model the English surgeon-apothecary or "general practitioner."

In mid- to late eighteenth-century England, the Royal College of Physicians, the Company of Surgeons, and the Society of Apothecaries controlled most aspects of health care delivery. Because there were relatively small numbers of English doctors who had actually received a university-granted M.D. and were members of the Royal College of Physicians, the country's growing requirement for more health care personnel fell to the larger population of non–university–educated surgeons and apothecaries. To be able to give better care to all types of patients, and to become more knowledgeable about surgical diseases and their treatment, the apothecaries joined with the surgeons. Conversely, the typical English country surgeon, distinct from the then emerging class of elite London hospital surgeons of high professional rank, knew little concerning pharmaceutical medicine and was compelled by circumstances to obtain an apothecary's license. Thus, by the time of the American Revolution, there existed in England a new and rapidly growing class of general practitioners, or surgeon-apothecaries.

Inevitably, the practice of medicine and surgery in colonial North America assumed characteristics different from those of European medical and surgical practice. In the colonies there was a low level of sophistication, and persons behaving like the English surgeon-apothecaries, but even less formally educated, soon found themselves, by default, in possession of the "profession" of medicine. These general practitioners eagerly assumed the status of "physicians." The citizenry began to address them as "doctor," even though very few colonial health care providers held a university degree. Most medical practitioners had simply received their medical training through nothing more than poorly structured proprietary apprenticeships or courses of self-learning. Undoubtedly, these minimally trained American "surgeon-apothecaries" or general practitioners were not averse to the sobriquet of "doctor" or "physician," since it masked the fact that North Americans were taken care of by individuals viewed in England as second-class personnel.

Men and women of all rank served as doctors. Any attempts at preserving the boundary between profession and trade fell by the wayside. In the colonies, it was plainly more convenient as well as more profitable to be a jack of all trades. This duality of purpose was never more evident than in the advertisements of eighteenth-century American "physicians." Robert Hutchings of Petersburg, Virginia, advertised a new supply of materials for carrying on the trade of a tailor, hairs and material for peruke-makers, and also "a large assortment of elixirs, such as Bostock's daffeys, Squires…with printed directions how to use them." In the same state, John Payras was regarded as the community's "doctor" but also sold "drugs, tea, sugar, olives, grapes, anchovies, raisins and prunes." Jean Pasteur began the practice of surgery, barbering, and wigmaking in Williamsburg in 1700. A Mrs. Hughes, "late from the West Indies," advertised that having settled in Norfolk, she would practice midwifery but also cured "ringworm, scald head, piles, and worms" while making "ladies' sacks, dresses, cloaks, bonnets, etc." Finally, a visitor to Fredericksburg in 1732 observed that a Mrs. Levistone was most memorable for her double billing as "doctoress and coffee woman."

Unlike the European countries, the colonies had essentially no dividing lines between physician and surgeon. Since there were few apothecaries, it was necessary for the dispensers of American health care to also act as both pharmacists and surgeons. Not until the mid-eighteenth century would institutions of higher learning be founded and provide for the formal education of individuals interested in studying medicine. Certainly, an organized profession of surgeons did not exist in colonial America, so an examining body such as London's Company of Surgeons appeared unnecessary.

Although barber-surgeons were not unheard of in the early colonies, their number was quite small. They were known to complete the difficult and burdensome work of minor surgery, particularly tooth extraction, incision of abscesses, and phlebotomy. Of the barber-surgeons who sailed to North America, the first known was Giles Heale (?–1653), hired as ship's surgeon when the *Mayflower* was chartered for its 1620 voyage. Heale remained at Plymouth colony through that first terrible winter of 1620–1621, but his exact medical and surgical duties, once he was on shore, remain a mystery.

The *Mayflower* sailed the year after Heale had completed an apprenticeship in the Guild of Barber-Surgeons of London, under the barber-surgeon Edward Blaney. Whether Heale was seeking adventure, desired experience in clinical practice, or merely needed the financial support such a job would provide remains unknown. According to the regulations of the barber-surgeons, it was strictly promulgated that a surgeon be part of the ship's company on any passenger vessel completing voyages "beyond seas." It was evidently Heale's duty to look after the general health of the crew and passengers. What he did once on land is uncertain. The mystery of Heale's shore duties is compounded by the presence of Samuel Fuller (1580–1633) on the *Mayflower*. Fuller was officially considered the *Mayflower's* physician, but in fact he held no medical diploma, and he was also considered the group's deacon. Yet, the men, women, and children in the Massachusetts Bay Colony continually referred to him as "Dr."

Heale returned to England on the *Mayflower* in April, 1621, and practiced in London for the remainder of his professional life. The saga of Heale and Fuller is most notable in that the "physician," who held no formal medical degree and had no known medical training, was viewed with greater respect than the "surgeon" with seven years' clinical apprenticeship. This subserviency of surgeon to physician was a European tradition that would not last long in the wilderness of North America. One indisputable fact remains: the first formally licensed medical practitioner in the Massachusetts Bay Colony was a barber-surgeon, who probably performed minor surgical procedures when called for.

Barber-surgeons were also among the early Dutch and Swedes along the Delaware River and could be found in virtually every colony. However, before long an evident rift developed between barber-surgeons and physician-surgeons similar to the professional animosities found in Europe. As is noted in Dutch records from New Amsterdam in 1652, initiatives were begun to strictly limit the work of barber-surgeons. Once these measures were accomplished, the barber-surgeon rapidly vanished from the colonial scene:

> On the petition of the chirurgeons of New Amsterdam that none but they alone be allowed to shave; the director and council understand that shaving alone doth not appertain exclusively to chirurgery, but is an appendix thereunto; that no man can be prevented operating on himself, nor to do another the friendly act provided it be through courtesy, and not for gain which is hereby forbidden....ship-barbers shall not be allowd to dress any wounds nor administer any potions on shore without the previous knowledge and special consent of the petitioners.

THE BEGINNINGS OF PROFESSIONALIZATION

By its very nature, early American medicine was forced to have a practical tendency. Unlike in Europe, there were few bone-setters, cataract couchers, herniotomists, or lithotomists roaming the frontier. Colonial governments made few attempts to regulate or legislate the practice of seventeenth-century American medicine. Yet, by 1700, the tenor of colonial medicine was beginning to change. An apprentice system of medical learning was in place, and the general practitioners trained in that fashion were overtly pragmatic in their therapeutic decision making. Medicine divorced itself from the influence of the governors and clerics. Apothecary shops came into existence, though they were few, and legitimate attempts to legislate the fledgling health care system were initiated. By the end of the eighteenth century, medical schools and hospitals were being formed, and sporadic medical literature indigenous to the American colonies was being published.

Advertisement.

For the benefit of any that has or may have Occasion. HEnry Hill Distiller in the Town of Boston New-England, having had a Child grievously afflicted with the Stone, apply'd himself to Mr. Zabdiel Boylston of the said Boston. Practitioner in Physick and Chirurgery; who on the 24th of June last, in presence of sundry Gentlemen, Physicians and Chyrurgeons, Cut the said Child, & took out of his Bladder a stone of considerable bigness, and with the blessing of God in less than a months time has perfectly Cured him, and holds his Water: This is his third Operation performed in the Town on Males and Females, and all with good success: He likewise pretends to all other Operations in Surgery. Which Operation the said Hill could not omit to make Publick.

ng-Lane Sold at the Post-Office in Cornhill. 1710.

For the Publick Good of any that have or may have Cancers——These may Certify, That my Wife had been labouring under the dreadful Distemper of a Cancer in her Left Breast for several Years, and altho' the Cure was attempted by sundry Doctors from time to time, to no effect; And when Life was almost despair'd of by reason of its repeated bleedings, growth & stench, and there seemed immediate hazard of Life, we send for Doctor Zabdial Boylston of Boston, who on the 28th of July 1718. (in the presence of several Ministers & others assembled on that Occasion) Cut her whole Breast off; and by the Blessing of GOD on his Endeavours, she has obtained a perfect Cure.

I deferred the Publication of this, left it should have broke out again. Edward Winslow.

Rochester, Octob. 14th. 1720.

4. Advertisements from the *Boston News-Letter* (July 17–July 24, 1710) *(top)* and the *Boston Gazette* (November 21–November 28, 1720) *(bottom)* that are the first published accounts of elective surgical operations performed in North America. Both operations were performed by Zabdiel Boylston; the earlier advertisement describes a procedure for bladder stone and the second is for a mastectomy. *(Massachusetts Historical Society)*

With the establishment of licensing standards and medical schools, American physicians hoped to create a profession that approached European standards. The need for such measures was evident in this plaintive description of medical practice in New York City in 1758:

> Few physicians among us are eminent for their skills. Quacks abound like locusts in Egypt...this is less to be wondered at, as the profession is under no kind of regulation. Loud as the call is, to our shame be it remembered, we have no law to protect the lives of the King's subjects from the malpractice of pretenders. Any man, at his pleasure, sets up for physician, apothecary, and chirurgeon. No candidates are either examined, licensed, or sworn to fair practice.

The first legislation calculated to control the practice of physicians and surgeons was enacted in Virginia. Like most early legislative remedies, this Act of 1639 was little more than a pro forma attempt at regulation:

> That it should be lawfull and free for any person or persons...where they should conceive the acco't of the phisitian or chirurgeon to be unreasonable either for his pains or for his druggs or medicines, to arrest the said phisitian or chirurgeon...the said phisitian should declare upon oath the true value worth and quantity of his druggs and medicines administred for the use of the patient...should it be sufficiently proved...that a phisitian or chirurgeon had neglected his patient, or that he had refused...his helpe and assistance to any person or persons in sickness or extremity...the said phisitian or chirurgeon should be censured...for his neglect or refuse all.

Two decades later, the Virginia Assembly enacted a statute specific to the regulation of "chirurgions accounts." Although lacking in true punitive measures, the law did state that "if it shall appear by evidence that the said...chirurgeon hath neglected his patient while he was under cure, the court shall censure him to pay so much as they in their discretion shall think reasonable." The first actual bill concerning professional fees was authorized by the Virginia House of Burgesses in September 1736. This law was an important step in the evolution of American surgery because the bill attempted to remedy the abuses of excessive fees and unreasonable prices for surgical operations and pharmaceuticals. In addition, within its regulatory language, surgeons and apothecaries who had obtained their education solely through an apprenticeship or other form of self-learning were clearly distinguished from "those persons who have studied physic in any university and taken any degree therein:"

> Whereas the practice of phisic in this colony, is most commonly taken up and followed, by surgeons, apothecaries, or such as have only served apprenticeships to those trades, who often prove very unskilful in the art of a phisician; and yet do demand excessive fees...and do too often, for the sake of making up long and expensive bills, load their patients with greater quantities thereof, than are necessary or useful...Be it therefore enacted...no practicer in phisic...shall recover, for visiting any sick person, more than the rates hereafter mentioned:

Surgeons and apothecaries, who have served an apprenticeship to those trades...	£	s	d
For every visit, and prescription, in town, or within five miles,	00	5	00
For every mile, above five, and under ten,	00	1	00
For a visit, of ten miles,	00	10	00
And for every mile, above ten,	00	00	06
With an allowance for all ferriages on their journeys.			
To surgeons, for a simple fracture, and the cure thereof,	02	00	00
For a compound fracture, and the cure thereof,	04	00	00

But those persons who have studied phisic in any university, and taken any degree therein...	£	s	d
For every visit, and prescription, in any town, or within five miles,	00	10	00
If above five miles, for every mile more, under ten,	00	1	00
For a visit, if not above ten miles,	1	00	00
And, for every mile, above ten,	00	1	00
With an allowance of ferriages, as before.			

Up through the time of the Revolution, the apprenticeship method remained the primary manner for young men to prepare themselves for clinical practice. The duration of apprenticeships varied considerably, as did the degree of formality in the arrangements between preceptor and student. In most instances, the apprentice read books recommended by his teacher, who was himself an autodidact in the ways of medicine. No formal study of anatomy was made, and cadaver dissection was limited. There was no instruction in physiology or the emerging science of pathology. Obstetric cases were usually handled by midwives. This was an era of American individualism, with each physician literally practicing his own brand of clinical medicine.

In reality, apprenticeship was a form of indentured servitude on the part of a young man. Since an apprenticeship was commonly begun at the early age of fourteen to seventeen years, frequently the student also received concurrent instruction in the humanities, either at an academy or from a neighboring clergyman. With propriety, the preceptee was expected to pulverize bark and roots, make and spread plasters, and prepare tinctures, ointments, and various extracts. From a surgical standpoint, the apprentice was sometimes entrusted with bleeding, pulling teeth, and dressing minor wounds, and usually he assisted his preceptor with whatever surgical operations he might perform. All this had to be dutifully performed in order for him to receive a certificate of proficiency and a written statement attesting to his good character.

There was little doubt that the apprentice's education was only as good as his preceptor's personal medical library and overall committment. In contrast with European medical education, which was more theory than practice, the American apprenticeship at least provided daily practical contact with patients. Despite its crudeness, preceptor-based learning remained central in the United States, even after the establishment of medical schools, which initially were strictly supplemental in nature.

In Europe, the physician was a university-educated man, whereas the surgeon was little more than a skilled craftsman. Physicians and surgeons were usually from different social classes, and this brought about professional jealousies, which festered during inevitable collaborations. Not until the mid-nineteenth century would an equalization of the two professions occur in Europe. In America, the apprentice-trained doctor was both physician and surgeon. Therefore, sharp distinctions of class, education, and service were obviated by the pressure of circumstance and rarely existed in the national medical psyche. From a negative standpoint, the apprenticeship had definite professional limitations. It provided only a "certificate of character and proficiency." A university education would be necessary if medicine were ever to become a learned profession, with its devotées receiving a "certificate of authority." Samuel Gross (1805–1884), doyen of mid-nineteenth century American surgery, incisively described his own preceptorial misadventures:

> My preceptor...had...considerable pretension to scientific knowledge...The understanding was that I was to remain under his tuition for three years, inclusive of two lecture terms, and that he was to receive, as an office fee, two hundred dollars, for which he was to furnish me with the use of certain books, and to examine me once a week on such branches as I might be studying. His library was small, and its contents of little value. He had no apparatus of any kind, plates or diagrams, no specimens in materia medica, or anatomical preparations; nothing, in short, but a skeleton...it soon became apparent to me that such instruction...had little value, and fell far short of what a student had a right to expect from his preceptor. Perhaps, however, this was not his fault, but the fault of the vicious system of office pupilage, still prevalent in nearly all sections of this country, a system which cannot be too pointedly condemned...

With a growing populace and an obvious need for some type of stronger governmental regulation, the first well-considered act to delineate the educational requirements for a physician was passed in New York in 1760. It stated that, "no one... shall practice as a physician or surgeon... before he shall have first been examined... and approved of... by one of His Majesty's council, the judges of the supreme court, the King's attorney-general, and the mayor of the city." Of course, the law had minimal impact because of the lack of medical knowledge on the part of the examiners. Not until 1792 did the New York State legislature pass the earliest act calling for true educational requirements:

> ...no one should practise physic or surgery...before he should have both attended the practice of some reputable physician for two years, if a graduate of a college, or for three years if not a graduate, and been examined, admitted, and approved by the Governor, Chancellor, Judges of the Supreme Court, Attorney-General, Mayor, and Recorder, or any two of them, taking to their aid three respectable physicians with whome the candidate had not lived to acquire medical information

Medical schools were first established in the mid-eighteenth century and included the University of Pennsylvania (1765), King's College, now Columbia University (1767), and Harvard University (1782). Still, concerted activity to organize physicians and surgeons and to meet their educational and clinical needs was minimal. Medical societies, initially envisioned as licensing authorities, were in their infancy; the state medical society of New Jersey (1766) was the first of these, but the Massachusetts Medical Society (1781) was more active in organizing physicians and promoting education.

EARLY MEDICAL PUBLISHING

The first printing press in America was established in Cambridge in 1639, under the auspices of Harvard College. However, few health care practitioners had anything original to present. Therefore, it is not surprising that few textbooks of medicine or surgery were authored by American physicians before the Revolutionary War. For those who could afford textbooks, many imported European works were available. Among the favored texts were those by the anatomists Albinus, Cheselden, Cowper, Monro *primus* and *secundus*, and Winslow. Medicine was learned from the works of Boerhaave, van Swieten, and Sydenham; the surgical favorites were treatises by Heister and Pott.

By the beginning of the eighteenth century, medical information and important professional announcements were being disseminated through newspaper and magazines. From 1704, when the *Boston News-Letter* was first published, through 1783, almost two hundred different newspapers appeared in the colonies. The sheer volume of these daily and weekly periodicals is staggering, considering the size of the colonial population. It has been estimated that scattered through these quarter million pages of newsprint are some 10,000 items of medical interest to the practitioner and the patient. For instance, in the *Boston News-Letter* for the week of July 17–24, 1710, a small announcement appeared on the back page detailing the events of the first publicly recorded elective surgical operation in colonial North America:

> For the benefit of any that has or may have Occasion, Henry Hill Distiller in the Town of Boston New-England, having had a child grievously afflicted with the Stone, apply'd himself to Mr. Zabdiel Boylstoun of the said Boston, Practitioner in Physick and Chirurgery; who on the 24th of June last, in presence of sundry Gentlemen, Physicians and Chyrurgeons, Cut the said Child & took out of his Bladder a stone of considerable bigness and with the blessing of God in less than a months time has perfectly Cured him, and holds his Water: This is his third Operation performed in the Stone on Males and Females, and all with good success: He likewise pretends to all other Operations in Surgery. Which Operation the said Hill could not omit to make Publick.

Whether Hill placed the advertisement because he was pleased with the results or at the request of Boylston remains unknown. However, in 1720, a similar piece regarding a mastectomy on the wife of an Edward Winslow appeared in the *Boston Gazette*, once again mentioning Boylston as surgeon ("he cut her whole breast off"). Examination of these colonial newspapers reveals that major surgical operations

5. *(facing page)* Sylvester Gardiner as portrayed by John Singleton Copley (1738–1815), one of the most popular American portrait painters of his day. Merchants and other businessmen constituted the bulk of Copley's patrons, while ministers and public officials also figured in fair numbers, in addition to a smattering of military personnel. Only three of Copley's subjects were physicians: Joseph Warren, painted about 1765, and Nathaniel Perkins and Sylvester Gardiner, both painted in the early 1770s. Gardiner was born in 1717 in Rhode Island and received his medical education and training in Great Britain. Having been a student of London's William Cheselden, he very likely had many opportunities to observe and assist his mentor with lithotomies, for which he later became renowned in the colonies. Gardiner returned to America in 1744 and was considered one of the best-trained physicians in the Boston area. A shrewd businessman, he became a wealthy entrepreneur but, unfortunately for him, was an outspoken loyalist. By 1776, he had lost most of his wealth, and he fled to Canada and eventually England, where he received a crown pension. Finally, in 1785, Gardiner returned to the United States and attempted to regain many of his former holdings, but he died a year later in Newport, Rhode Island. *(Private Collection)*

were being undertaken, albeit on a modest scale. For instance, *The Boston Evening-Post* for December 1767 reported the repair of a strangulated hernia with "opening of the intestinal cavity, performed successfully" by John Bartlett, and *The New-York Mercury* for May 1756 told of "extracting the stone from the human bladder" by Doctor Bard. Colonial physicians and surgeons used newspapers and magazines as important marketing tools to further their clinical reputations (e.g., *The Pennsylvania Journal, or Weekly Advertiser*, March 1780: "Doctor Yeldall…Wens, hair lip. Operation performed in one minute and the cure completed in four days") and as referral sources. In some instances, the misdeeds of the medical profession were also brought to the attention of an unwary public (e.g., *The Georgia Gazette*, August 1774: "Letter from Dr. Felix Pitt in defence of his actions, regarding some accusations of his 'having underhanded dealings' with a young man apprentice").

By studying colonial medical literature, one can make a clearer determination of the degree of early American cultural dependence on European medical ideas. For example, some European textbooks were highly regarded and were reprinted in

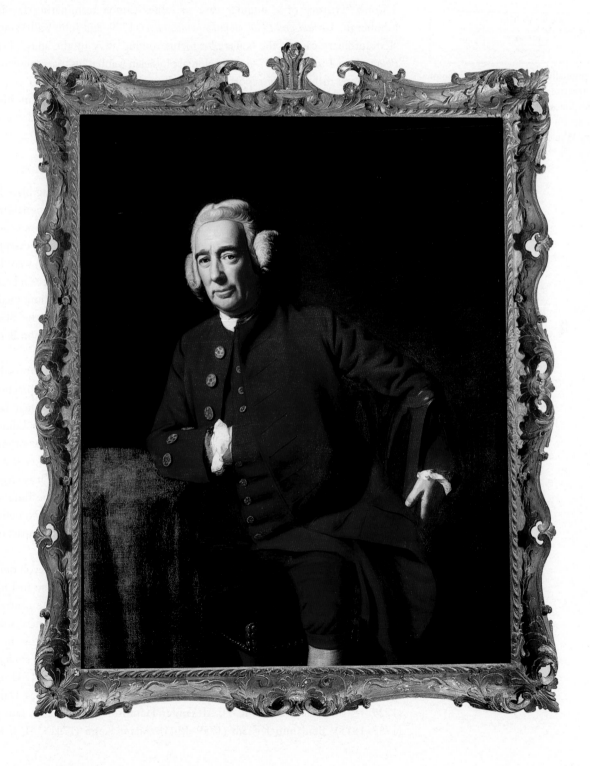

```
PLAIN  CONCISE

PRACTICAL  REMARKS

ON THE TREATMENT OF

WOUNDS  AND  FRACTURES;

TO WHICH IS ADDED, A SHORT

A  P  P  E  N  D  I  X

ON

CAMP AND MILITARY HOSPITALS;

PRINCIPALLY

Defigned for the Ufe of young MILITARY SURGEONS,
in NORTH-AMERICA.

By  JOHN  JONES,  M. D.
Profeffor of Surgery in King's College, New York.

NEW-YORK:
Printed by JOHN HOLT, in Water-Street, near the
Coffee-Houfe.
M,DCC,LXXV.
```

6. The exceptionally rare 1775 first edition of the earliest treatise on surgery published in America. John Jones' *Practical Remarks* was the standard guide for surgical care during the Revolutionary War. (*Author's Collection*)

colonial America, including editions that were translations from foreign languages and abridgements, such as William Cullen's *Lectures on the Materia Medica* (London 1773, Philadelphia 1775), William Northcote's *Extracts from the Marine Practice of Physic and Surgery* (London 1771, Philadelphia 1776, Boston 1777), John Ranby's *Nature and Treatment of Gun-Shot Wounds* (London 1744, Philadelphia 1776, Boston 1777), and Gerard van Swieten's *Diseases Incident to Armies* (Vienna, 1758, Philadelphia 1776, Boston, 1777).

Although American medical literature was in its infancy, a scattering of publications by colonial authors were printed abroad. In most instances, these works represented the graduation theses of American-born students who received European medical educations and medical diplomas. The remainder were usually case reports communicated to well-known English physicians. Among them were Isaac Hall's "Uncommon tumour of the thigh, successfully extirpated," Edinburgh, *Medical and Philosophical Commentaries*, 1775; George Martin's "Reflections and observations on the seminal blood vessels," Edinburgh, *Medical Observations and Essays*, 1742; James Tilton's "History of a singular case of rabies canina terminating favourably, Edinburgh, *Medical and Philosophical Commentaries*, 1779; and John Still Winthrop's "Extraordinary case of the bones of a foetus coming away by the anus," London, *Philosophical Transactions*, 1745. If a colonial physician wanted his cases, observations, or opinions to be widely reported within the colonies themselves, no exclusively medical periodicals were available. Consequently, he was forced to submit his work to a nonmedical weekly or monthly "magazine" such as the *American Museum* or the *Philadelphia Monthly Magazine*.

EARLY MEDICAL EDUCATION

A most important change in the tenor of colonial medicine was taking place by the mid- to late eighteenth century. There was a growing sense of professionalism with an ever-growing struggle to achieve clinical respectability. Knowledge was becoming increasingly exact and its applications more appropriate. Hospitals, exemplified by the Pennsylvania Hospital in Philadelphia, the first in the colonies, were beginning to open. One evidence of this attempt to increase the prominence and stability of medicine as a profession was that sons were following their fathers into medicine. By 1770, there were several renowned medical families, including the Blachlys, Budds, and Elmers in New Jersey, the Shippens in Philadelphia, and John Bard and his son Samuel in New York.

About this time an increasing number of Americans began to study abroad, with the ultimate goal of returning to the colonies and establishing medical practices. In general these young men came from wealthy backgrounds and with their family's support were able to absorb the financial burden of living in London or Edinburgh for an extended period. Compared with the force of Americans who continued to obtain their medical knowledge through apprenticeship or self-education, the number of individuals who studied abroad was quite small. For instance, it is estimated that there were about 3,500 medical practitioners in America at the time of the Revolution. However, fewer than 10 percent were doctors of medicine. Nonetheless, this cadre of foreign-educated physicians would have an extraordinary impact on the future direction of medicine and surgery in the United States.

From the time of the earliest settlement of the colonies to the Revolution, the greatest percentage of medical students who studied in Europe did so in England and Scotland. Most of the foreign-educated students came from the central and southern colonies; the numbers from New England were smaller. These students represented their homeland quite well and made favorable impressions on the leading teachers of the European countries. The young American medical students of this era included such future prominent personalities as Samuel Bard (1742–1821), Thomas Bulfinch (1728–1802), Thomas Dale (1700–1750), Thomas Dale, Jr. (1729–1816), Isaac Hall (1746–?), Alexander Hamilton (1712–1756), James Jay (1732–1815), Benjamin Kissam (1759–1803), Adam Kuhn (1741–1817), James

M'Clurg (1746–1823), John Morgan (1735–1789), John Moultrie (1729–1798), John Redman (1722–1808), Nicholas Shippen (1736–1808), James Smith (1731–1812), Benjamin Waterhouse (1754–1846), and William Charles Wells (1757–1817). The European experience became a decisive one to these future leaders. They compared medicine in America with medicine in Europe, noted the plusses and minuses, and returned to the colonies with a resolve to reform the fledgling profession.

THE SEPARATION OF SURGERY FROM INTERNAL MEDICINE

The most influential of this new breed of American physician was John Morgan, the first colonial health care provider to formally attempt to separate the practice of internal medicine from that of surgery. Morgan served a six-year medical apprenticeship with John Redman of Philadelphia. Upon its completion, Morgan volunteered to act as surgeon to the provincial troops of Pennsylvania in their campaign during the war between the French and the English. In 1760, as the scion of one of those rare colonial families that had the financial wherewithal to allow a son to formally study medicine in England, Morgan traveled abroad, studying first in London with William Hunter (1718–1783) and later in Edinburgh. Letters of introduction from Benjamin Franklin (1706–1790) provided Morgan with an entrée to many elite English physicians. In Edinburgh, Morgan fulfilled the requirements at the university's famed medical school and received his doctor of medicine degree (M.D.) in 1763. From Edinburgh, he went to Paris, where he lectured to members of the Parisian College of Surgery on suppuration and also presented methods employed by the Hunter brothers to inject and preserve anatomical specimens. To complete his journey, Morgan traveled to Italy, where he made the acquaintance of the eighty-two-year-old anatomist and pathologist Giovanni Morgagni (1682–1771).

Like many of his fellow colonists who were studying medicine in Europe, Morgan realized the utter necessity of establishing a school of medicine in his native country. Armed with a letter of endorsement from Thomas Penn (1702–1775), son of William Penn (1644–1718), and through the assistance of John Penn (1729–1795), a grandson, who was lieutenant governor of the Pennsylvania colony, Morgan introduced the concept to the trustees of the College of Philadelphia. His project met with immediate approval, and in May 1765, Morgan was elected professor of the theory and practice of physick in the new institution–the initial step in what would soon become the medical department of the University of Pennsylvania. Later that month, Morgan delivered his celebrated *A Discourse Upon the Institution of Medical Schools in America*, the first North American publication on medical education.

When Morgan resettled in Philadelphia, it had long been customary for physicians to practice all branches of medicine, including surgery, and to prepare and furnish their own medicines. Having worked with the new breed of elite hospital-based London surgeons, such as John Hunter (1728–1793), Percivall Pott (1714–1788), and Samuel Sharp (1700–1780), Morgan began to question that tradition and recommended a separation of pharmacy and surgery from the practice of medicine. He wanted to establish a proper professional hierachy in medicine, but the socio-political foundation on which the European professional system was built did not exist in medically unsophisticated America.

Morgan was adamant in his demands for change. He justly noted, "The general of any army should be acquainted with every part of military science....[Still] there is no need that he should...dig in a trench...No more then is a physician obliged, from his office, to handle a knife with a surgeon...The levelling of all kinds of practitioners so much with illiterate pretenders...tends...to make a vile trade of physic, instead of a noble profession, which, as it certainly is, so it ought to be esteemed." In his attempts to improve the level of American surgical skills, Morgan brought David Leighton, an English apothecary and surgeon, to America. Morgan publicly announced that henceforth he would refuse all surgical cases and the furnishing of medicines. He insisted that any of his future patients in need of surgical care or pharmaceuticals would have to avail themselves of the services of Leighton or another apothecary or surgeon. Much to his own financial disadvantage, Morgan remained true to his word and never again performed any type of surgical procedure. However, his plan to separate general medical practice from surgery and apothecary was met with skepticism and outright opposition from most of his fellow practitioners. No further information is available concerning the professional career of Leighton and his ultimate impact on the practice of surgery in Philadelphia. Morgan would go on to become a medical director of the Continental Army, and he was eventually involved in a professional imbroglio surrounding the misappropriation of funds. In the final analysis, Morgan's revolutionary ideas caused no discernible alteration in the manner of health care delivery in the colonies.

SMALLPOX INOCULATION

In 1721, the population of Boston was slightly more than 12,000. It had been almost twenty years since the city had undergone a major outbreak of smallpox. During those two decades the population had doubled, and many children were immunologically unprotected. In April 1721, a maritime fleet that had arrived from Barbados brought with it the beginnings of a new epidemic. Smallpox soon appeared in the city and by autumn had spread into the neighboring towns, especially Roxbury, Charlestown, and Cambridge. The terrors of smallpox in eighteenth-century colonial America were recurrent and devastating. The epidemics were especially hard on the young and the elderly; death rates ranged from 15 to 50 percent. Destructive abscesses required surgical drainage, and disfigurement was a common sequela. Although the biochemical concept of immunity was not yet understood, the scars from a prior attack of smallpox were known to ensure virtual safety from reinfection in those who nursed the sick.

Early in the epidemic, Cotton Mather had read, in the *Philosophical Transactions* of the Royal Society of London, of a method employed in Turkey and neighboring countries to prevent smallpox by inoculating healthy individuals with material taken from a pock of a patient with active smallpox. Mather attempted to interest several medical practitioners in Boston in this new "surgical process." The physicians, led by William Douglass (1691–1752), a Scottish immigrant who held the degree of doctor of medicine, ridiculed the idea, treating the concept with outright scorn and equating it with murder.

Despite the setback, Mather decided to visit Zabdiel Boylston, a successful practitioner in Boston and long-time friend of the Mather family. Boylston had been educated in medicine by his father, Thomas (1644–?), and was among the busiest physicians in New England. Considered particularly erudite, Boylston was interested in zoology and botany and carried on an extensive correspondence with the English physician and bibliophile Hans Sloane (1660–1753). Mather proposed to Boylston the deliberate inoculation of healthy young people. The intent was to produce a mild form of smallpox from which the patient would recover and, as a result, be protected against a more severe attack.

Why Mather singled out Boylston over other physicians remains a mystery. It is possible that Mather looked upon inoculation as a form of surgical operation and therefore one needing the services of a "surgeon." Boylston, although not a surgeon per se, was known to have successfully performed such difficult surgical operations as the removal of bladder stones and simple mastectomy as part of his general medical practice. Against vocal and violent opposition, Boylston decided to implement Mather's proposal. On June 26, 1721, Mather had his own six-year-old son, Thomas, and two of the family's African-American servants inoculated. Shortly thereafter, all three came down with mild cases of smallpox, from which they completely recovered. They soon began to demonstrate resistance to further infection. Nevertheless, the public outcry was horrendous. Boylston was even forced to go into hiding for two weeks after a threat of public hanging.

The results of Boylston's efforts were slowly recognized. By early in 1722, he had inoculated 247 persons, and two other physicians in Roxbury and Cambridge had

AN
Historical ACCOUNT
OF THE
SMALL-POX
INOCULATED
IN
NEW ENGLAND,

Upon all Sorts of Persons, *Whites*, *Blacks*, and of all Ages and Constitutions.

With some Account of the Nature of the Infection in the NATURAL and INOCULATED Way, and their different Effects on HUMAN BODIES.

With some short DIRECTIONS to the UN-EXPERIENCED in this Method of Practice.

Humbly dedicated to her Royal Highness the Princess of WALES,
By *Zabdiel Boylston*, F. R. S.

The Second Edition, Corrected.

L O N D O N:

Printed for S. CHANDLER, at the Cross-Keys in the *Poultry*.
M. DCC. XXVI.

Re-Printed at *B O S T O N* in *N. E.* for S. GERRISH in *Cornhil*, and T. HANCOCK at the Bible and Three Crowns in *Annstreet*. M. DCC. XXX.

7. Title page of Zabdiel Boylston's 1730 treatise on smallpox inoculation. *(The Francis A. Countway Library of Medicine)*

inoculated an additional 39. Of these 286 inoculated persons, only six died (2 percent), and several of them were supposed to have been infected prior to the treatment. In contrast, there were 5,759 cases of smallpox in Boston and 844 deaths—a mortality rate of almost 15 percent. The epidemic of 1721–1722 came to an inglorious end, but with an important measure of vindication for Boylston and Mather.

Boylston was a true scientific investigator, who spent much time analyzing his results. He maintained meticulous records of his patients and their clinical courses. After the 1721–1722 epidemic, Boylston and Mather jointly authored, and Boylston published, a twenty-two-page pamphlet entitled *Some Account of What is Said of Inoculating or Transplanting the Small Pox…with some Remarks Thereon*. Although practically the whole of the tract is from Mather's previous writings on the subject, Boylston contributed the important five-page "Remarks" section describing in detail the practice of inoculation among African Americans in Boston. Boylston provided careful descriptions of the symptoms, fever, prognosis, and the best times to obtain good results from inoculations. He clearly demonstrated from carefully gathered statistics that the mortality from inoculation was much lower than that from the epidemic. Two years later, Boylston was invited to London by Sloane. As the physician with the largest experience with inoculation in the world, Boylston was accorded many honors. He even lectured before the Royal College of Physicians and was elected a member of the Royal Society of London.

Whether Boylston performed any inoculations in Europe remains unknown. There has always been speculation that Boylston was involved in an attempt to inoculate certain members of the royal family, but no written records exist to verify such a rumor. At the request of the Royal Society, Boylston recounted his experience with inoculation in a small treatise, *An Historical Account of the Small Pox Inoculated in New England, Upon All Sorts of Persons, Whites, Blacks, and of All Ages and Constitutions* (1726). First published in London, this extremely rare work was dedicated to Caroline, Princess of Wales and daughter of King George I (1660–1727). Boylston was particularly adamant about using statistical tables to analyze patient outcomes, and his treatise was a masterpiece of early American scientific investigation.

Boylston soon returned to Boston but was not accorded the celebrity status he had enjoyed in London. In 1730, a second, corrected edition of his treatise was published in Boston. The revised text provides a thorough accounting of his experiences with inoculation, beginning in June 1721, and specifically answers the criticisms of Douglass. Through unstated means, presumably payment from the British royal family for his professional services, Boylston had acquired great wealth, which eventually permitted him to retire from active clinical practice in 1752.

Although the concept of inoculation would not be accepted for some time throughout the North American colonies, Boylston eventually saw his method adopted by many colonial physicians. In fact, inoculation played a key role in saving the Continental Army from a medical disaster. In 1776, the specter of smallpox infecting the colonial forces was a major concern of George Washington (1732–1799). That same year, colonial authorities believed that British troops had purposely helped spread the infection of smallpox in Boston so as to cause panic among American fighting men and prevent their invading the city. The threat of disease was beginning to undermine the effectiveness of the entire military effort. Washington knew he could utilize immune troops (i.e., those who had contracted smallpox in the natural way), but their number was too small. In a tactical judgement, worthy of the greatest medical decisions conceived by any military man, Washington had mass inoculations carried out during the first three months of 1777 on virtually all of his troops scattered from New York to Virginia. With private homes serving as treatment centers, this grand surgical experiment proved an unqualified success and helped lead to the American victory at Yorktown.

In 1801, Benjamin Waterhouse (1754–1846) brought cowpox inoculation, termed "vaccination," to the United States via its innovator, Edward Jenner (1749–1823) of England. The medical establishment and American society as a whole soon embraced this safer method, partly because of the lengthy history of success with direct inoculation. Vaccination was no longer considered a form of surgery, and by the end of the first decade of the nineteenth century it had rapidly become incorporated into the standard practice of medicine.

SURGICAL INSTRUMENTS

It is sometimes difficult to appreciate how different the practice of surgery in the seventeenth, eighteenth, and nineteenth centuries was from that performed today. For instance, the technical armamentarium of the colonial physician-surgeon was quite simple. There are records of surgical chests containing nothing more than "instruments, clysters, syringes, basins, galli-pots and salvatories." Not much was needed, because the routine performance of surgical operations can hardly be said to have existed until well after the Revolutionary War. The early records of colonial surgery are chiefly concerned with nothing more than the treatment of burns, dislocations, fractures, frostbites, ulcers, and wounds. Few men of standing possessed the necessary qualifications to be considered more "surgeon" than "physician."

Even when the physician was widely known for his surgical skills, records indicate that little in the way of actual operative surgery was completed. For instance, Isaac Senter (1753–799) of Newport, Rhode Island, was well known for his surgical skills. Senter kept accurate records of his clinical practice, but his entries for 1787 reveal only thirty-nine notations for what could be considered surgical procedures. They included numerous simple drainages of abscesses, sixteen tooth extractions, the reduction of six limb fractures, the draining of one hydrocele, and the reduction of two incarcerated hernias. Postoperative care of the surgical patient was minimal at best. Francis Haddon's (?–1680) treatment of a patient undergoing a leg amputation was to prescribe two cordials on the day of the operation and an intestinal purge four days later, with frequent ointments and external applications. Some two months later, with the patient still slow to heal, Haddon found it necessary to bleed the individual. Purging and bleeding became the trademark treatments of the colonial physician-surgeon.

To appreciate why Senter performed so few surgical operations is to realize the pain and suffering that each patient had to endure in this preanesthetic era. Why call on a surgeon to drain an abscess or extract a tooth? There was no more or less pain if a member of the family completed the task. Most importantly, no surgical fee would be asked for! Despite the meager volume of operative cases, Senter must have lived fairly well, because he was known to have customarily received $20 for a thigh amputation, $14 for inoculating a husband and wife against smallpox, and $4.50 for setting a fractured femur.

For the most part, surgery remained little more than a crude, unpromising branch of medicine. Yet, despite the lowly status of surgery as a healing art, it would be wrong to convey the impression that important events were not shaping the future evolution of American surgery. Highly heralded surgical procedures were being completed, including Silvester Gardiner's (1707–1786) removal of a bladder stone via the "lateral approach" (1741), John Bard's successful treatment of an abdominal pregnancy (1759), James Robertson's (1742–1814) management of scalped-head injuries via bone drilling to promote the formation of "proud flesh," or granulation tissue (1770s), and John Warren's (1753–1815) performance of an amputation at the shoulder joint (1781).

THE REVOLUTIONARY WAR

Of the many illustrious physicians in the colonial era, John Jones (1729–1791) can be regarded as the most renowned of the "chirurgeons." Author of the first true surgical work written by an American and printed in North America, Jones was born in Jamaica, Long Island, New York. The son of a physician, he was initially educated at home. At the age of eighteen he was sent to Philadelphia to begin medical studies as an apprentice to his uncle, Thomas Cadwalader (1708–1779), a distinguished physician and the first teacher of practical anatomy in the colonies. After a four-year preceptorship, Jones completed his medical education by traveling to Europe for the years 1751–1752.

In London, Jones studied at St. Thomas' Hospital under William Cheselden (1688–1752) and Samuel Sharp, at St. Bartholomew's with Percival Pott and Edward Nourse (1701–1761), and at St. George's Hospital with William Bromfield (1712–1792) and William Hunter. Continuing his grand tour of the Continent, Jones decided to obtain a formal doctor of medicine degree by enrolling in the University of Rheims. Graduating in May 1751, Jones supposedly authored a graduation thesis in French concerning surgical wounds. No copies of this thesis exist, and there has always been uncertainty about whether it was truly ever written. Jones traveled on to Paris, where he remained until April 1752, attended the anatomical lectures of Antoine Petit (1718–1794), and walked the wards of the Hotel Dieu, where Henri-Francois LeDran (1685–1770) and Claude LeCat (1700–1768) practiced. Continuing his educational tour, Jones went to Leyden, where he worked with Bernhard Albinus (1697–1770), and completed his journey in Edinburgh, watching Alexander Monro *primus* (1697–1767) perform anatomical dissections.

Jones resettled in New York City, where his unusually good education soon helped establish his excellent reputation. He was the first to perform the surgical operation of lithotomy in that city, and his fame was soon noted in several colonies. Jones began his career in public service in 1755, when he volunteered for the New York State Militia at the outbreak of the French and Indian War and served until the end of hostilities.

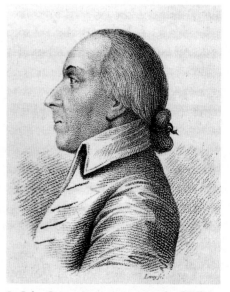

8. John Jones, in an engraving by William Leney (1769–1831), from the *American Medical and Philosophical Register* (1814). *(Historical Collections, College of Physicians of Philadelphia)*

9. John Warren conducted a series of anatomical lectures at the "dissecting theatre in the University at Cambridge." Paul Revere (1735–1828) engraved the certificate issued for attendance to the talks. Decorated with two skeletons, it contains the earliest depiction in the colonies of an anatomical dissection: a very straightforward if somewhat crude drawing of a corpse laid out on a table while the surgeon/anatomist completes his studies. *(Courtesy of the American Antiquarian Society)*

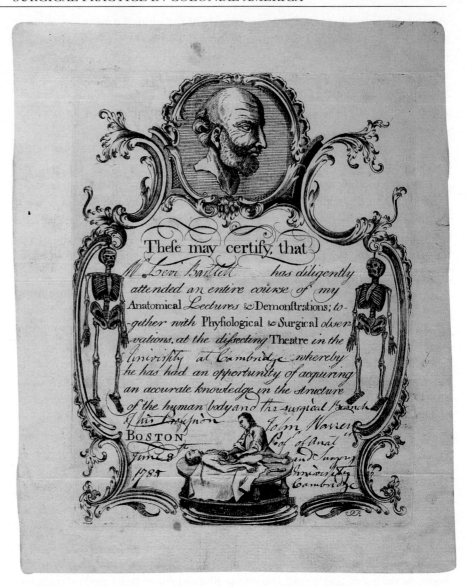

In 1767, Jones was named Professor of Surgery in the newly organized medical department of King's College in New York City. With a faculty consisting of, among others, Peter Middleton (?–1781), Professor of the Theory of Physic; John Van Brugh Tennent (1737–1770), Professor of Midwifery; and Samuel Bard, Professor of the Practice of Physic, the institution was among the most celebrated in the colonies. The majority of the faculty were Tories, which soon led to political difficulties. Putting politics aside, the school had the distinction of being the first in the colonies to provide a "complete" faculty of six professors offering courses in all subjects, and in May 1770 it awarded the first degree of doctor of medicine granted in the colonies.

Jones became the second professor of surgery in the colonies, the first having been William Shippen (1736–1808) at the University of Pennsylvania. No examples of Shippen's earliest lectures survive, but Jones' introductory remarks (November 1769) to his course in surgery provide information on medical teaching in the colonies and what was expected of surgeons. The didactic lecture, read from manuscript, was the customary method of teaching, and Jones' remarks were eagerly copied by his students:

> Surgery…may with great propriety be divided, into medical, & manual….The first, comprehends, an infinite variety of diseases, which require the assistance, of both internal, & external applications…the last, is confin'd to those cases, which admit of relief, from the hand alone, or assisted with instruments. Hence it will appear very evident, how necessary it is for the student in surgery to make himself thoroughly acquainted with all those branches of medicine,

which are requisite to form, the most accomplished physician; to which must be superadded some peculiar qualifications, to constitute the surgeon, of real merit, & abilities...there must be a happiness as well as art, to compleat the character of the great surgeon.... He ought to have firm steady hands, & be able to use both alike...a strong clear sight...& above all, a mind, calm & intrepid, yet humane, & compassionate, avoiding every appearance of terror & cruelty to his patients, amidst the most severe operations...what must we think of the insolence, & malevolence of those who represent [surgery] as a low mechanic art, which may be taught a butchers boy in a fortnight...under the protection of the liberal patrons of this medical institution, Ignorance, & imposture will no longer be able, to combat truth & error...

After taking a short respite in London in 1770, Jones, joined by Bard and others, petitioned the New York City Council for a charter to found a public hospital. Permission was granted in 1771, and the cornerstone of the New York Hospital was laid two years later. The events of the Revolutionary War disrupted the medical school, and in 1775 the partially finished hospital building was burned by British troops. With New York City captured by the British, Jones left the city in September 1776, never to return. He traveled to Albany, where he accepted a commission as a "surgeon" in the Continental Army. Two years later, Jones was sent to Philadelphia, where he was discharged from the army in 1781.

Difficulty with asthma prevented Jones from being active in the field, but he was instrumental in organizing the medical department of the army. However, Jones' major contribution to the Revolutionary War effort was his writing in 1775, *Plain Concise Practical Remarks on the Treatment of Wounds and Fractures*. As the first "surgical" work written by an American, the Remarks became the physician's *vade mecum* and accepted guide to surgical practice during the hostilities.

Finding the climate in Philadelphia more suitable for his asthma, Jones settled there permanently. In 1780, following the resignation of John Redman, one of the physicians of the Pennsylvania Hospital, Jones was unamiously elected by the managers to fill the vacancy. He was also appointed consulting physician to the Philadelphia Dispensary and was even elected first president of the city's Humane Society. When the College of Physicians of Philadelphia was formed in 1787, Jones was nominated first vice-president and contributed (posthumously) a paper on anthrax to the first volume of the College's *Transactions* (1793).

Jones was attending physician to George Washington and served as Benjamin Franklin's (1706–1790) doctor during the latter's final days. He even published a short account of Franklin's terminal illness in the *Pennsylvania Gazette* of April 21, 1790. Jones was afflicted with a painful bladder stone during the last years of his life, but he was always said to have continued indulging "in those *jeux d'esprit*, and entertaining anecdotes, which were the delight of all who heard them." He succumbed to pneumonia and was buried in the Arch Street burial ground of the Religious Society of Friends. All traces of his grave were lost during the mass burials of victims of the 1795 yellow fever epidemic in Philadelphia.

Jones' *Remarks* is among the rarest of American surgical texts: fewer than a dozen copies of the ninety-two-page first edition are known to exist. It was initially published in New York City, and a slightly expanded second edition bound with van Swieten's *Diseases Incident to Armies* was issued in 1776 in Philadelphia. Although historians have long criticized Jones' effort as being little more than a condensation of the teachings of LeDran, Pott, and other European surgeons, the fact remains that within this octavo-sized work was summarized the best surgical opinion of that era in simple and practical prose. It would be hard to imagine that this easily transported book could not have been of tremendous value for the numerous young, inexperienced Continental Army surgeons, who were without access to any other contemporary surgical literature. As Jones so eloquently noted in the preface:

The present calamitous situation of this once happy country, in a peculiar manner, demands the aid and assistance of every virtuous citizen; and though few men are possessed of those superior talents, which are requisite, to heal

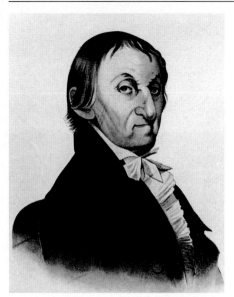

10. James Thacher *(Author's Collection)*

such might evils as now threaten the whole body politic with ruin and desolation; yet, every man has it in his power to contribute something towards so desireable an end; and if he cannot cure the fatal disease of this unfortunate country, it will, at least, afford him some consolation, to have poured a little balm into her bleeding wounds. Influenced by these motives, I have endeavoured to select the sentiments of the best modern surgeons upon the treatment of those accidents, which are most likely to attend our present unnatural contest.

The ten chapters include discussions of "wounds in general," "inflammation," "division of wounds," "penetrating wounds of the thorax and abdomen," "simple fractures," "compound fractures," "amputation," "blows on the head," "injuries arising from concussion or commotion," and "injuries arising from a fracture of the skull." Despite his reliance on European surgical writings, Jones does provide several original notes, including a successful case of trephining for delirium eighty days following a head injury.

Although the Revolutionary War cannot be regarded as a crucial event in the evolution of American surgery, certain advances were made in the treatment of battlefield injuries. The care of the patient after surgery was more carefully supervised than in the past. Increased attention was given to possible complications, although the appearance of "laudable pus" continued to be inappropriately regarded as a sign of adequate healing. Jones preferred to dilate wounds to facilitate drainage, and he advocated immediate amputation when the heads of bones were broken or capsular ligaments were torn.

Perhaps no other descriptions of surgery during the Revolutionary War are more graphic than those in James Thacher's (1754–1844) *Military Journal During the American Revolutionary War* (1823). Thacher was one of the most influential, but least flamboyant, physician-surgeons of his time. Born in Barnstable, Massachusetts, he served a four-year apprenticeship under Abner Hersey (1721–1787). Immediately following completion of his apprenticeship and soon after the battle of Bunker Hill, Thacher was appointed surgeon's mate under John Warren (1753–1815). He served with distinction in the Continental Army and was eventually promoted to the position of surgeon. Although his *Journal* does not have a specific section on surgery, it provides numerous interesting anecdotes from the standpoint of a Revolutionary War surgeon. Included are the scalping and subsequent treatment of a wounded soldier and observations on a gunshot injury to the sole of the foot obtained while the wounded soldier was fleeing from the enemy—an act Thacher describes as "cowardice treason." Thacher describes a scene (October 24, 1777) following the battle of Saratoga after 5,000 British troops led by General John Burgoyne (1722–1792) surrendered to Major Generals Philip Schuyler (1733–1794) and Horatio Gates (1728–1806):

> This hospital is now crowded with officers and soldiers from the field of battle; those belonging to the British and Hessian troops, are accommodated in the same hospital with our own men, and receive equal care and attention. The foreigners are under the care and management of their own surgeons...We have about thirty surgeons, and mates; and all are constantly employed. I am obliged to devote the whole of my time from eight o'clock in the morning to a late hour in the evening, to the care of our patients. Here is a fine field for professional improvement. Amputating limbs, trepanning fractured skulls, and dressing the most formidable wounds, have familiarized my mind to scenes of woe. A military hospital is peculiarly calculated to afford examples for profitable contemplation, and to interest our sympathy and commiseration. If I turn from beholding mutilated bodies, mangled limbs and bleeding, incurable wounds, a spectacle no less revolting, is presented, of miserable objects, languishing under afflicting diseases of every description-here...awful harbingers of approaching dissolution...emaciated bodies and ghastly visage...

From 1784 until his death, Thacher remained in private practice in Plymouth, Massachusetts. He is best remembered for his prolific writings, including *The American New Dispensatory* (1810) and *American Modern Practice* (1817). His books were widely regarded for reflecting the best available medical information of the early nineteenth century. Renowned for his clarity of organization and writing style, Thacher authored the first biographical dictionary of American physicians, *American Medical Biography* (1828). As an introduction to this work, Thacher wrote a little appreciated but well documented history of medicine in the United States.

BIOGRAPHIES OF COLONIAL AND REVOLUTIONARY SURGEONS

Names that recur most commonly in the accounts of surgery in Colonial and Revolutionary times include Thomas Bond, John Bard, James Lloyd, William Shippen, James Tilton, Samuel Bard, William Baynham, and John Warren. **Thomas Bond** (1713–1784) was instrumental in founding the first medical school and first hospital in the colonies. He was apprenticed to Alexander Hamilton (1712–1756) of Annapolis, and in 1738–1739 he completed his medical education by studying in London and Paris. Bond settled in Philadelphia, where he became particularly interested in municipal health affairs, primarily as a port physician. Although his practice would be classified as that of a general practitioner, Bond was well known for his surgical skills: "he reduced and splinted fractures, incised breasts, and imposthumated livers, scarified 'mortifying' feet, amputated legs, tapped not only legs but both chest and abdomen, [and] operated for stone in the bladder..." In 1751, Bond and Benjamin Franklin founded the Pennsylvania Hospital, which was the first such institution in the colonies to be devoted exclusively to the care of the sick. Bond was also a founding member of the American Philosophical Society (1743). Not known for his clinical writings, Bond left little in the way of memorable literary efforts.

John Bard (1716–1799) was the first physician in colonial America to perform a human dissection for the purpose of instructing young medical students. He received his own medical education as an apprentice to John Kearsley (1684–1772), a physician in Philadelphia. In 1746, prompted by Benjamin Franklin, Bard moved to New York City to replace a physician who had recently died in an epidemic of yellow fever. Bard became friendly with Peter Middleton, one of the founders of the medical department at King's College and, with his assistance, completed the first recorded human dissection for instructional purposes in North America (1750). Bard established a lucrative surgical practice, but he remains best known as the author of the first published scientific paper on a surgical topic to come from the American colonies. In 1759, he wrote a letter to John Fothergill (1712–1780), an English physician, describing a case of ectopic pregnancy: Bard had successfully performed a laparotomy to remove a nonviable fetus from a 28-year-old woman. In 1764, Fothergill had the letter published as a scientific contribution in the *Medical Observations and Enquiries* of the Society of Physicians of London. Among Bard's other contributions was the creation of an infirmary at New York City's house of correction, which would later become Bellevue Hospital. He was also first president of the New State York Medical Society.

James Lloyd (1728–1810) was born in Oyster Bay, Long Island, New York, and began his medical studies with Sylvester Gardiner of Boston. After five years, Lloyd sailed to London, where he spent two years as a "wound dresser" for Joseph Warner (1717–1801) at Guy's Hospital while also attending lectures by William Hunter and William Smellie (1697–1763). Returning to Boston in 1753, and having served as a "surgeon" at Castle William, a British military installation, Lloyd was able to build up a large clinical practice, primarily oriented around obstetrics and midwifery. It is claimed that Lloyd was the first surgeon in the colonies to "use ligatures instead of searing wounds with the actual cautery, and to use the double flap in amputation after the method of Cheselden." He also performed multiple lithotomies and was an influential advocate of smallpox inoculation. In 1781, Lloyd was an incorporator of the Massachusetts Medical Society, and nine years later he received an honorary degree of doctor of medicine from Harvard University. His son, James Lloyd, served as United States Senator from Massachusetts during the first half of the nineteenth century.

11. *(following page spread)* "The Death of General Warren" (circa 1786). Joseph Warren (1741–1775), older brother of John Warren, was an eminent physician-surgeon in Boston by the age of 23. Respected for his successful treatment of smallpox patients, Warren became a zealot in the cause of patriotism and democracy. John Trumbull (1756–1843), the renowned American painter of historical scenes, recreated Warren's death by a rifle ball to the head at the Battle of Bunker Hill (June 17, 1775). *(Yale University Art Gallery, Trumbull Collection)*

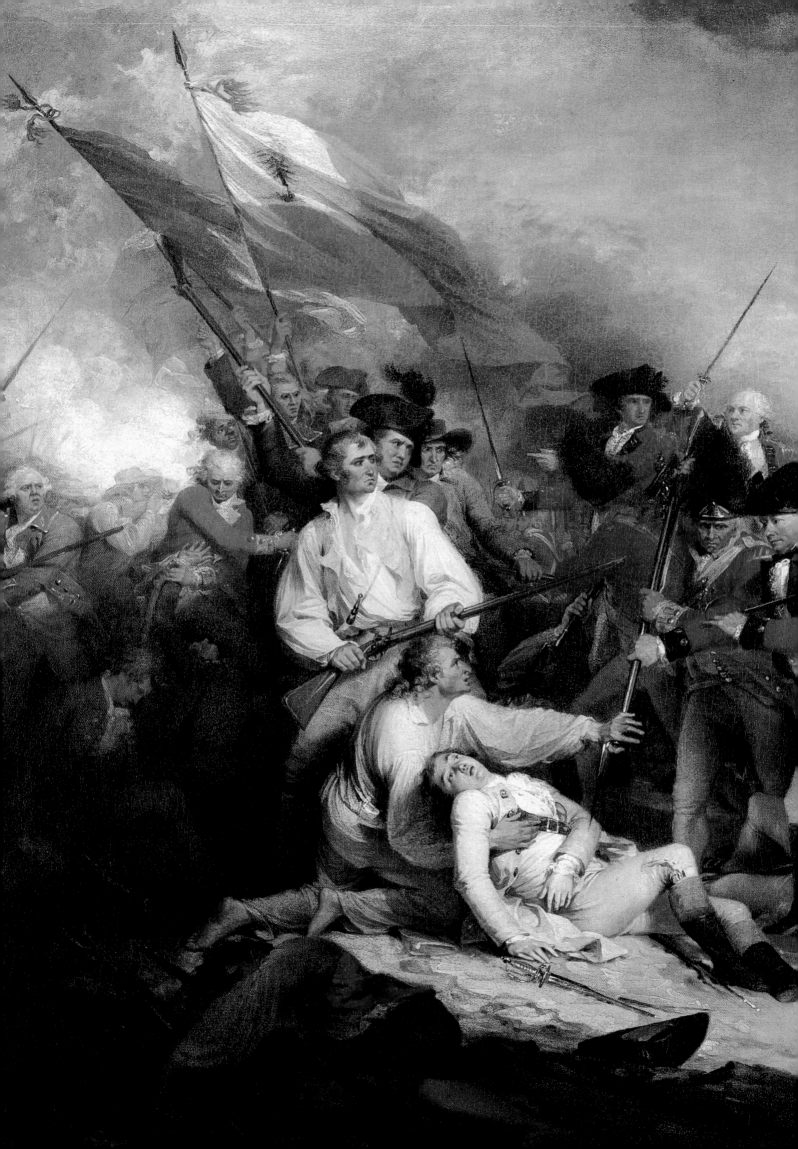

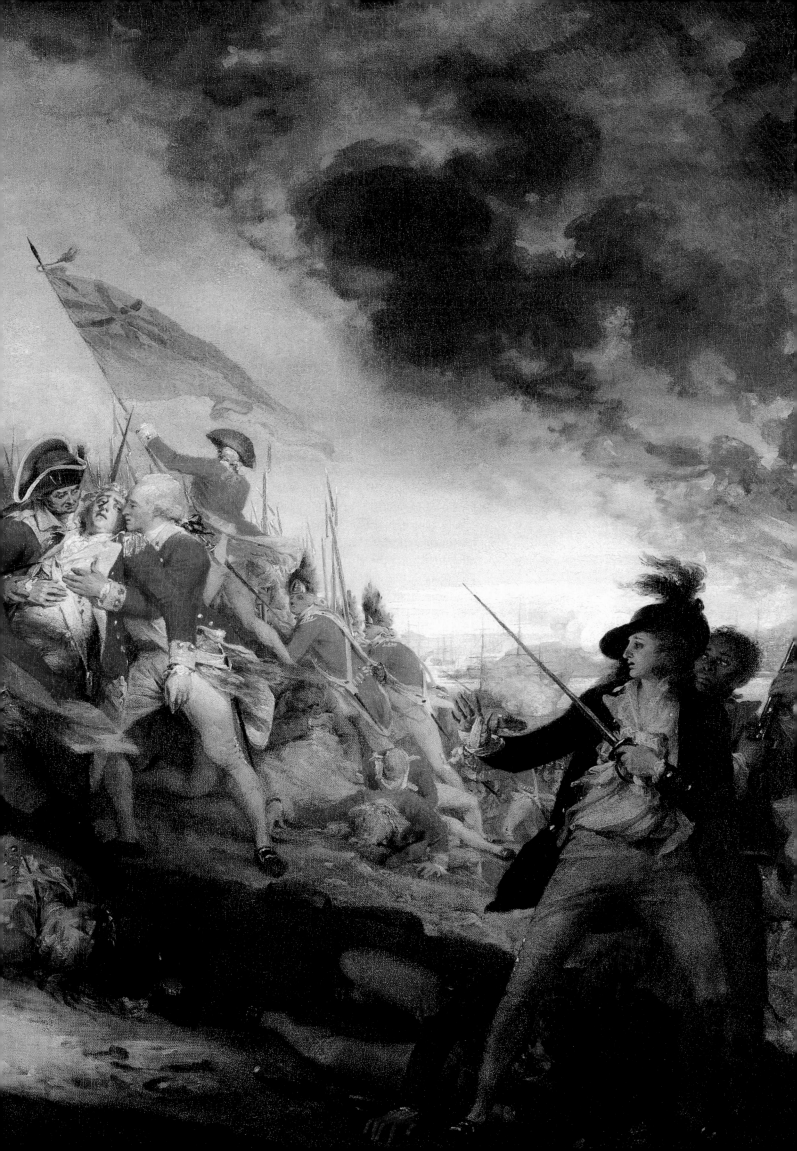

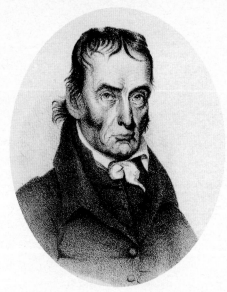

12. James Tilton *(Historical Collections, College of Physicians of Philadelphia)*

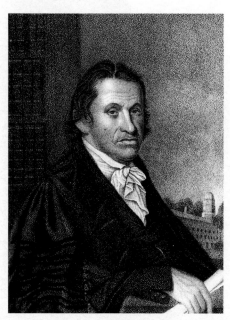

13. Samuel Bard *(Author's Collection)*

William Shippen (1736–1808) graduated from Princeton University (1754) and was apprenticed as a medical student to his father, William (1712–1801), in Philadelphia. Traveling to Europe, Shippen studied anatomy in London with John Hunter and midwifery with William Smellie, and he spent much time on the surgical service of John Pringle (1707–1782). Before returning to Philadelphia, Shippen obtained his formal medical degree from the University of Edinburgh (1761), having written, as a graduation thesis, *Dissertation Anatomico-Medica, de Placentae cum Utero Nexu.* The following year Shippen began teaching anatomy in his father's house, using anatomical pictures that John Fothergill had given to the Pennsylvania Hospital. In 1765, He was elected professor of anatomy and surgery at the College of Philadelphia, which would later become the University of Pennsylvania. At the outbreak of Revolutionary War hostilities, Shippen was named chief physician and director-general of hospitals for the Continental Army. He was soon involved in a bitter quarrel with John Morgan, and following the latter's dismissal from the corps, Shippen was named chief physician and director-general of the Medical Corps, Continental Army. Shippen served through 1781, when he was forced to resign as part of the Morgan scandal associated with financial improprieties. Among Shippen's most important academic accomplishments was his being the first in the colonies to lecture on midwifery and to establish a hospital for its teaching.

James Tilton (1745–1802) was born in Delaware and apprenticed to Charles Ridgely (1738–1785). Tilton did not study medicine in Europe, but instead matriculated at the College of Philadelphia, where he received his M.D. in 1771. He immediately established himself in private practice but in 1776 entered the Continental Army as surgeon to the Delaware Regiment. By 1778, Tilton had been promoted to the grade of hospital surgeon and was placed in charge of hospitals at Trenton and Princeton, New Jersey, and New Windsor, Maryland. Best known for his untiring efforts to secure army medical organizational reform, Tilton refused an offer to assume the chair of materia medica at the University of Pennsylvania. Following the war, he served one term as a member of the Continental Congress and later was often reelected to the Delaware state legislature. During the years 1802–1813, Tilton retired from active practice and simply farmed his land on the outskirts of Wilmington. The 1813 publication of his sixty-four page *Economical Observations on Military Hospitals and the Prevention and Cure of Diseases Incident to an Army* brought him to the attention of President James Madison (1751–1836). Remembered as an early pioneer in army sanitation and the prevention of the spread of disease, Tilton was appointed Surgeon General of the Army. By personal inspection and supervision, he greatly improved the sanitary conditions of the army and substantially reduced the sick rate. During his later years, Tilton developed a malignancy affecting one lower extremity. This necessitated the amputation of his leg, during the course of which he is said to have "supervised and directed the operation with unexampled fortitude."

Samuel Bard (1742–1821), son of John Bard, was born in Philadelphia. He received his early education at King's College in New York City and also spent five years (1760–1765) in London and Edinburgh. In the latter city, he received his M.D. after submitting a graduation thesis entitled *Tentamen Medicum Inaugurale, de Viribus Opii.* In 1765, Bard joined his father's practice in New York City and helped found the school of medicine affiliated with King's College, where he served as professor of the theory and practice of physick. Although known primarily as a general practitioner, Bard performed an operation on George Washington for a large abscess of the thigh. Among Bard's prominent written works are *A Discourse Upon the Duties of a Physician* (1769), the first American treatise on medical ethics; *An Enquiry into the Nature, Cause and Cure of the Angina Suffocative, or Sore Throat Distemper* (1771), one of the earliest accurate descriptions of diphtheria; and *A Compendium of the Theory and Practice of Midwifery* (1807), the first significant textbook on obstetrics written by an American. Bard served as dean and later president of the College of Physicians and Surgeons and helped establish the New York Dispensary, New York Hospital, and the New York City Library. A favorite pastime was sheep raising, and as president of the Agricultural Society of New York, Bard authored that era's best practical work on the subject, *A Guide for Young Sheperds* (1811).

William Baynham (1749–1814) was born in Virginia and initially took a five–year apprenticeship under Thomas Walker in his native colony. He followed the apprenticeship with several years of study at St. Thomas' Hospital in London, where he gained considerable knowledge of anatomy. From 1772 to 1775, Baynham taught anatomy under the guidance of Charles Collignon (1725–1785), professor of anatomy at Cambridge University. Baynham transferred positions in 1776, returning to St. Thomas' Hospital to instruct students in preparing anatomical specimens and to oversee the anatomical and dissecting rooms. In 1781, after failing to obtain election by St. Thomas' governors to the professorship of anatomy, Baynham became a member of London's Company of Surgeons. He returned to the United States in 1785 and entered private practice in Virginia. Despite the rural background of his patients, Baynham gained a national reputation as a surgeon and frequently traveled to other cities and states to perform surgical operations or provide consultation. He is best remembered for performing two operations for ectopic pregnancy, in 1791 and 1799. In both instances, the fetus had died, leaving the mother with a "tumor" of the abdomen. In the first case, the pregnancy had occurred five years earlier, and the woman had become progressively more ill. Baynham feared a fatal outcome and, realizing the need to extract the five years' dead fetus, he

> made a deep incision…into the cavity of the tumour, and with that as a director, cautiously extended the incision upwards and downwards on the left side, from nearly opposite to the umbilicus, obliquely across the rectus muscle towards its inner edge, and thence almost to the pubes, and in the direction of the linea alba, taking particular care…not to open the cavity of the peritoneum. Through this opening I happily succeeded in extracting the foetus, which, however, could not be done but in parts, in consequence of putrefaction.

The woman recovered uneventfully, although she never became pregnant again. Baynham did not report his two cases until 1809, when they were discussed in the *New York Medical and Philosophical Review*. This paper was the first important gynecological article published in an American medical periodical. Long regarded as the most renowned of early American anatomists, Baynham spent the remainder of his professional life in Essex County, Virginia.

John Warren (1753–1815) of Boston studied medicine with his brother Joseph (1741–1775), who later became a hero during the Revolutionary War and was killed at the battle of Bunker Hill. Unlike many of the prominent physician-surgeons of his era, John Warren did not complete his medical education in Europe. He possessed a lifelong passion for anatomy and was a member of the original faculty of Harvard Medical School, serving as its first Hersey professor of anatomy and surgery. Warren was the single most important figure in the early institutionalization of Boston medicine, being a founder of the Boston Medical Society and the Massachusetts Medical Society. Largely known for his surgical skills, Warren is said to have completed an amputation of the shoulder joint on a soldier during the Revolutionary War (1781), an abdominal laparotomy for a dermoid cyst of the left hypochondrium (1785), and an excision of the parotid gland (1804). Noted for his steely calm while performing surgical operations, Warren was also "stridently ambitious and disagreeably self-righteous." The father of seventeen children, John Warren was the immediate progenitor of what was to become the famous Warren medical family of Boston and Harvard.

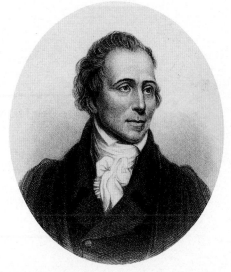

14. John Warren, first professor of anatomy and surgery at Harvard Medical School. Engraving after the painting by Rembrandt Peale (1778–1860). *(Historical Collections, College of Physicians of Philadelphia)*

ENGLISH AND FRENCH INFLUENCES, 1784–1845

DAILY LIFE

Bifocal glasses (1784)

Ice cream made commercially in New York City (1786)

Political buttons appear for the first time (1789)

The Farmer's Almanac (1792)

Union College (Schenectady, New York) first nondenominational college in the United States (1795)

America's first suspension bridge built in Westmoreland, Pennsylvania (1796)

John Chapman (a.k.a. Johnny Appleseed) visits settlements in the Ohio Valley (1800)

Lewis and Clark expedition (1803)

Gas street lighting introduced for the first time in Newport, Rhode Island (1806)

First Bible society established in Philadelphia (1808)

The Lawrenceville School (Lawrenceville, New Jersey) one of America's oldest college preparatory schools (1810)

Lead pencils (1812)

Rebuilding of the Capitol and White House following their burning by the British (1815)

American Society for the Return of Negroes to Africa (1817)

America's first tunnel opens near Auburn, Pennsylvania (1821)

Erie Canal (1825)

John James Audubon's The Birds of America (1827)

First modern hotel, the Tremont, with 170 rooms, opens in Boston (1829)

Horse-drawn streetcars appear on New York City streets (1832)

Tomatoes eaten for the first time (1834)

Colt revolver (1835)

Morse code (1838)

Steamboat Erie explodes on Lake Erie; 175 persons are killed (1841)

P. T. Barnum's American Museum opens in New York City (1842)

Scientific American magazine (1845)

U.S.A. POPULATION

1800 = 5.3 million

1820 = 9.6 million
(New York City 124,000;
Philadelphia 113,000;
Baltimore 63,000;
Boston 43,000;
New Orleans 27,000)

1840 = 17 million

HISTORY AND POLITICS

Land Ordinance of 1785 (1785)

Shays's Rebellion (1786)

Northwest Ordinance (1787)

George Washington elected president (1789)

Bill of Rights adopted (1791)

Whiskey Rebellion (1794)

Washington's "Farewell Address" warns against U.S. involvement in foreign affairs (1796)

XYZ Affair (1797)

Federal seat of government moves permanently to Washington, District of Columbia (1800)

Thomas Jefferson inaugurated as president (1801)

Louisiana Purchase (1803)

Peace treaty ends the Tripolitan War (1805)

Aaron Burr tried for treason and acquitted (1807)

James Madison elected president (1808)

Non-Intercourse Act replaces Embargo Act (1809)

United States declares war on Great Britain (1812)

United States troops under Andrew Jackson defeat British at the Battle of New Orleans (1815)

United States and Great Britain establish U.S.–Canadian boundary at the 49th parallel (1818)

Missouri Compromise (1820)

Monroe Doctrine (1823)

House of Representatives chooses John Quincy Adams as president (1825)

Democratic Party is formed (1828)

President Andrew Jackson introduces the spoils system into national politics (1829)

Webster–Hayne debate on the nature of the Union (1830)

African-American slave revolt led by Nat Turner (1831)

"Bank War" over rechartering Bank of the United States (1832)

ENGLISH AND FRENCH INFLUENCES, 1784–1845

	1780	1790	1800	1810	1820	1830	1840	1850	1860

HISTORY AND POLITICS

South Carolina legislature rescinds its Ordinance of Nullification *(1833)*

Unsuccessful attempt to assassinate Andrew Jackson is first attack on the life of a U.S. President *(1835)*

Supreme Court membership increased from seven to nine *(1837)*

Underground Railroad *(1838)*

Independent Treasury Act *(1840)*

Dorr's Rebellion *(1842)*

James Knox Polk defeats Henry Clay in "Manifest Destiny" presidential election *(1844)*

United States annexes Texas *(1845)*

FAMOUS AMERICANS

HEROES, POLITICIANS, AND STATESMEN

Zachary Taylor *(1784–1850)*
David Crockett *(1786–1836)*
Winfield Scott *(1786–1866)*
James Gadsen *(1788–1858)*
John Tyler *(1790–1862)*
James Buchanan *(1791–1868)*
James Knox Polk *(1795–1849)*
John Brown *(1800–1859)*
Millard Fillmore *(1800–1874)*
Nat Turner *(1800–1831)*
David Farragut *(1801–1870)*
William Seward *(1801–1872)*
Franklin Pierce *(1804–1869)*
Robert E. Lee *(1807–1870)*
Salmon Chase *(1808–1873)*
Jefferson Davis *(1808–1889)*
Hamilton Fish *(1808–1893)*
Andrew Johnson *(1808–1875)*
Kit Carson *(1809–1868)*
Abraham Lincoln *(1809-1865)*
Horace Greeley *(1811–1872)*
Charles Sumner *(1811–1874)*
Stephen Douglas *(1813–1861)*
John Fremont *(1813–1890)*
Edwin Stanton *(1814–1869)*
Samuel Tilden *(1814–1886)*
George Meade *(1815–1872)*
Frederick Douglas *(1817–1895)*
William Tecumseh Sherman *(1820–1891)*
Ulysses S. Grant *(1822–1885)*
Rutherford B. Hayes *(1822–1893)*
Schuyler Colfax *(1823–1885)*
William "Boss" Tweed *(1823–1878)*
Winfield Hancock *(1824–1886)*
Thomas "Stonewall" Jackson *(1824–1863)*
George McClellan *(1826–1885)*
Chester Alan Arthur *(1830–1886)*
James Garfield *(1831–1881)*
Benjamin Harrison *(1833–1901)*
George Armstrong Custer *(1836–1876)*
Grover Cleveland *(1837–1908)*
George Dewey *(1837–1917)*
James "Wild Bill" Hickock *(1837–1876)*
John Hay *(1838–1905)*
William McKinley *(1843–1901)*
Edward White *(1845–1921)*

1780	1790	1800	1810	1820	1830	1840	1850	1860

FAMOUS AMERICANS

SCIENTISTS AND INVENTORS

Samuel B. Morse (1791–1872)
Walter Hunt (1796–1859)
Charles Goodyear (1800–1860)
John Deere (1804–1886)
Cyrus McCormick (1809–1884)
Elisha Otis (1811–1861)
Isaac Singer (1811–1875)
Samuel Colt (1814–1862)
Richard Gatling (1818–1903)
Cyrus Field (1819–1892)
Elias Howe (1819–1867)
Linus Yale (1821–1868)
George Pullman (1831–1897)
Louis Waterman (1837–1901)

THEOLOGIANS AND PHILOSOPHERS

Peter Cartwright (1785–1872)
Charles Grandison Finney (1792–1875)
Brigham Young (1801–1877)
Joseph Smith (1805–1844)
Isaac Meyer Wise (1819–1900)
Mary Baker Eddy (1821–1910)
Henry Adams (1838–1919)
Charles Sanders Peirce (1839–1914)
John Fiske (1842–1901)
William James (1842–1910)

EDUCATORS, SCHOLARS, AND REFORMERS

Emma Willard (1787–1870)
George Ticknor (1791–1871)
Horace Mann (1796–1859)
William McGuffey (1800–1873)
Dorothea Dix (1802–1887)
William Lloyd Garrison (1805–1879)
Henry Ward Beecher (1813–1887)
Elizabeth Cady Stanton (1815–1902)
Julia Ward Howe (1819–1910)
Susan B. Anthony (1820–1906)
Clara Barton (1821–1912)
Francis Parkman (1823–1893)
Daniel Coit Gilman (1831–1908)
Edward Gallaudet (1837–1917)

AUTHORS

James Fenimore Cooper (1789–1851)
William Cullen Bryant (1794–1878)
Ralph Waldo Emerson (1803–1882)
Nathaniel Hawthorne (1804–1864)
Henry Wadsworth Longfellow (1807–1882)
John Greenleaf Whittier (1807–1892)
Oliver Wendell Holmes (1809–1894)
Edgar Allan Poe (1809–1849)
Harriet Beecher Stowe (1811–1896)
Henry David Thoreau (1817–1862)
Herman Melville (1819–1891)
James Russell Lowell (1819–1891)
Walt Whitman (1819–1892)
Emily Dickinson (1830–1886)
Louisa May Alcott (1832–1888)
Mark Twain (1835–1910)
Bret Harte (1836–1902)
Henry James (1843–1916)

ENGLISH AND FRENCH INFLUENCES, 1784–1845

	1780	1790	1800	1810	1820	1830	1840	1850	1860

FAMOUS AMERICANS

VISUAL ARTISTS

John James Audubon *(1785–1851)*
George Catlin *(1796–1872)*
Asher Durand *(1796–1886)*
Thomas Cole *(1801–1848)*
Fitz Hugh Lane *(1804–1865)*
George Caleb Bingham *(1811–1879)*
Eastman Johnson *(1824–1906)*
George Inness *(1825–1894)*
Frederic Church *(1826–1900)*
Albert Bierstadt *(1830–1902)*
James Whistler *(1834–1903)*
Winslow Homer *(1836–1910)*
Thomas Eakins *(1844–1916)*
Mary Cassatt *(1845–1926)*

PERFORMING ARTISTS

Thomas Rice (1808–1860)
Edwin Christy (1815–1862)
Daniel Emmett *(1815–1904)*
Stephen Collins Foster *(1826–1864)*
Carl Zerrahn *(1826–1909)*
Louis Gottschalk *(1829–1869)*
Adah Menken *(1835–1868)*
Theodore Thomas *(1835–1905)*
Tony Pastor *(1837–1908)*
Charles "Tom Thumb" Stratton
(1838–1883)

BUSINESSMEN AND INDUSTRIALISTS

Seth Thomas *(1785–1859)*
Peter Cooper *(1791–1883)*
Cornelius Vanderbilt *(1794–1877)*
Johns Hopkins *(1795–1873)*
P. T. Barnum *(1810–1891)*
Leland Stanford *(1824–1893)*
Andrew Carnegie *(1835–1919)*
Jay Gould *(1836–1892)*
Augustus Julliard *(1836–1919)*
J. Pierpont Morgan *(1837–1913)*
John Wanamaker *(1838–1922)*
John D. Rockefeller *(1839–1937)*

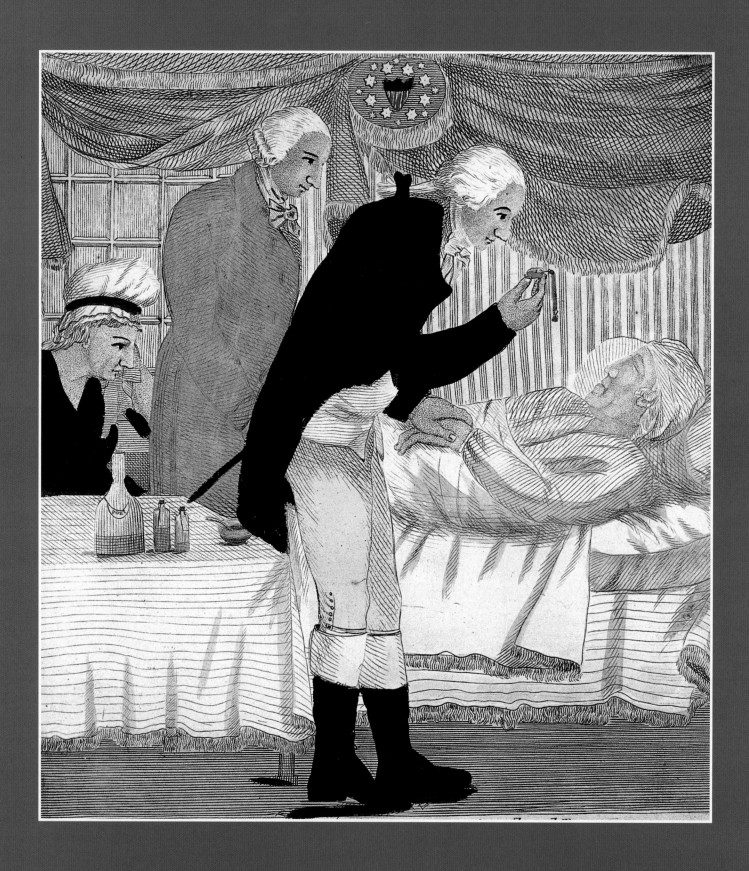

CHAPTER 3

ENGLISH AND FRENCH INFLUENCES
1784–1845

omanticism can be defined as a reaction against classic thought with its stress on reason and intellect. Romanticism emphasizes the imagination and emotions and their freely individualized expression or realization in all spheres of human activitiy. In America, the first half of the nineteenth century should be considered the Romantic era of medicine and surgery. Despite a general indifference to basic science, medicine was in a marked period of transition from ancient thinking to more modern methods of clinical practice. Individualism prevailed, and numerous examples of distinguished personal achievement were noted in the applied sciences, especially technology, inventions, and the practice of surgery.

Regardless of the problems caused by the general ignorance of antisepsis and anesthesia, surgery remained the most important medically valid therapy in the first half of the nineteenth century. This seeming paradox, in view of the terrifying nature of surgical intervention, is explained by the simple fact that operations were usually performed for external difficulties that required objective anatomical diagnoses. Surgeons saw what needed to be fixed (abscesses, breast lumps, hernias, etc.) and could treat the problem in as rational a manner as the times permitted. Conversely, physicians had to render care for disease processes that were not visible. It was difficult to treat the symptoms of illnesses such as asthma, congestive heart failure, and diabetes if the physician had no knowledge of what constituted their underlying etiology.

With the advances made in pathological anatomy and experimental physiology during the eighteenth and the first part of the nineteenth centuries, physicians would soon adopt a therapeutic viewpoint that had long been prevalent among surgeons. It was no longer a question of just treating symptoms; the actual pathological basis of illness could finally be understood. Disease processes were now being described physiologically or viewed pathologically through the lens of a microscope. Because this reorientation of internal medicine occurred within a relatively short time, and brought about such dramatic results in the classification, diagnosis, and treatment of diseases, the rapid ascent of mid-nineteenth century medicine seems more impressive than the agonizingly slow but steady advance of surgery. In a seeming contradiction of reality, medicine appears as the more progressive branch, with surgery lagging behind. The art and craft of surgery, for all its practical possibilities, would be restricted until the advent of antisepsis and anesthesia. Still, surgeons never needed a diagnostic and pathologic revolution in the manner of the physician. Despite the imperfections of their scientific knowledge, the early nineteenth-century American surgeons did cure with some technical confidence.

1. *(facing page)* "G. Washington in his Last Illness Attended by Doctors Craik and Brown." There is no more prototypical scene of late eighteenth- and early nineteenth-century American medicine than that of a dying George Washington surrounded by his attending physician-surgeons. Although there has been controversy over the exact cause of Washington's death, the diagnosis is now believed to have been a throat infection secondary to streptococcal pharyngitis (quinsy), diphtheria, or pharyngeal abscess. Washington's breathing was compromised, and one of his physicians urged a radical surgical maneuver, a tracheotomy, but was adamantly opposed by his professional peers. The death of "the father of our country" was hastened by excessive bloodletting, a fashionable medical therapy of that era. *(Collection of the New York Historical Society)*

2. A contemporary ink watercolor (circa 1827) showing the ill-fated Rutgers Medical College, designed by the famous New York architect Alexander Jackson Davis and located on Duane Street. The facility proved an instant success, numbering among its renowned faculty George Bushe, John Francis, John Godman, David Hosack, William McNeven, and Valentine Mott. Unfortunately, as was typical of the many proprietary institutions found in virtually every state, the school led a precarious legal existence. In this case, medical degrees were offered in New York State but under a New Jersey charter. By 1830, only a short four years after it opened its doors, and following intense political maneuvering, the college was forced to close permanently. *(Collection of the New York Historical Society)*

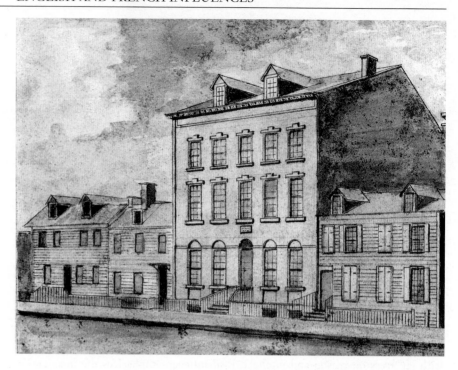

IMPROVEMENTS IN MEDICAL EDUCATION

The initial decades (1784–1825) of this surgical era were in most respects an extension of clinical practice as it had developed in the thirteen colonies. However, several forthcoming developments presaged progress toward the professionalizing of American surgery. Foremost was an attempt to upgrade the level of formal medical education. After 1800, medical colleges were founded wherever there seemed to be large enough populations to support them financially. By 1810, seven medical schools (University of Pennsylvania, Columbia, Harvard, Dartmouth [1797], College of Physicians and Surgeons of New York City [1807], University of Maryland [1807], and the short-lived medical department of Brown University [1807]) were providing course work. The total number of students in attendance was approximately 650, 406 of whom were at the University of Pennsylvania.

Following the War of 1812, the growth of new facilities continued unabated, especially in sparsely settled areas of the country. This demand for institutions in the frontier led to the establishment of the College of Physicians and Surgeons of the Western District at Fairfield, Herkimer County, New York (1813), the Medical Department of Transylvania University in Lexington, Kentucky (1818), Castleton Medical College in Castleton, Vermont (1818), and the Medical College of Ohio in Cincinnati, Ohio (1819). By 1845, almost forty medical schools were in existence, scattered from Maine down to Georgia, out to Louisiana and Missouri, and up to Illinois. Although many of these medical "colleges" were associated with academic institutions of higher standards than medical education itself could claim, the connection was largely nominal and in name only. Quite simply, a group of local practitioners who wished to start a medical school would approach a "name" academic institution and seek permission to grant degrees under its charter, or would obtain a license from the state as an independent educational institution authorized to award the medical degree.

By 1845, the typical American physician-surgeon had received his education at one of several dozen proprietary medical schools. Still, the opportunity to become a physician was so haphazard that not until Robley Dunglison (1798–1869) authored his *The Medical Student; or, Aids to the Study of Medicine* (1837) did Americans have a rudimentary, albeit practical, guide to the numerous schools, their requirements, the members of the faculty, and their physical facilities.

More often than not, these schools consisted of a single large room suitable for lectures, a small library containing books on loan from a local faculty member, and an adjoining space for anatomical or chemical demonstrations. Clinical instruction was by lecture and textbook. The standard curriculum consisted of seven courses (anatomy, physiology, and pathology; materia medica, therapeutics, and pharmacy; chemistry; medical jurisprudence; theory and practice of medicine; principles and practice of surgery; and obstetrics and the diseases of women and children). There was no consideration of scientific research or other nonpractical matters. Students endured six to eight hours daily of a humdrum existence. The entire student body would be assembled in a large amphitheater to sit and listen to one lecturer after another, and this routine would last from mid-October to the beginning of March. Following a second year of this monotonous existence, with the second term identical in course content to the first, the student became eligible to receive his degree. The other requirements varied from school to school, but the annual catalogue of the College of Physicians and Surgeons in the City of New York during the early 1840s summed up their state of affairs:

> Candidates for the degree of Doctor of Medicine must have attended two full courses of lectures, the last in this college; they must also have studied medicine three years, including the attendance upon lectures, under the direction of a regular physician, and have attained the age of twenty-one. Each candidate is required to write a thesis on some subject connected with the science of medicine.

For surgeons-to-be, the study of human anatomy is a fundamental requirement in their education and training. Important as dissection is for the proper education of medical students, there existed strong popular prejudice against it. In colonial America and well into the nineteenth century, societal indignation proved a constant deterrent to medical schools and the supply of cadavers. In 1765, to quiet public apprehension that graves were being robbed, William Shippen issued a statement testifying that only bodies of suicides, murderers, or those buried in paupers' graves were used for dissection. Human remains from church graveyards were considered sacrosanct and not to be disturbed.

With "dissection" riots occurring intermittently, including the trashing of surgeon John Beal Davidge's (1768–1829) anatomical theater in Baltimore, faculty members were often forced to calm public opinion. For instance, the physicians of the Vermont Medical School in Woodstock disseminated a proclamation stating somewhat dubiously that "bodies disinterred hereabouts would not be used in the department of practical anatomy." At the medical school in Herkimer, New York, the professor's annual report to the state's Regents included an announcement that "any attempt, proved on a student, to disinter the dead, is punished with expulsion."

Sadly, a community's fear that fresh graves were plundered for their anatomical booty was not that far from the truth. Many students were actively engaged in bodysnatching, or the American equivalent of European resurrectionism. The onerous task of obtaining cadavers for dissection required remarkable enthusiasm and enterprise. No less a future surgical notable than Valentine Mott, when he was only 25 years of age and a lecturer on surgery and demonstrator in anatomy in New York City, wrote of his experiences:

> Material for dissection was scarce.... I well remember on one occasion driving, in disguise, a cart containing eleven subjects, from the old Pottersfield Burying ground, sitting on the subjects, and proud enough of my trophies; but we were not always so fortunate, being on many occasion discovered and pursued and obliged to leave our spoils behind us...
>
> One little incident of the times occurs to me. A German who had been hung, was given to the College for dissection, and with the colored porter, I went in a carriage in the evening, to get the body. My other associate was a Doctor Buchanan, a Scotchman, and Professor of Obstetrics...
>
> On calling at his rooms to take him up, I found him arranging his pistols, and complaining of feeling very agueish, and with difficulty persuaded him to proceed. The night was cold, and on arriving on the ground, the Doctor's ague increased so rapidly, that he decided to return home, begging strongly for the use of the carriage, which I peremptorily refused him. With great difficulty we

exhumed the body, but then my colored associate also deserted me, declaring that he could not touch the subject, on account of his having been hung.

I had, therefore, to lug the body, attired in its white robes, by my own strength, to the carriage, and partly by force and partly by menaces, compelled the man to assist me in getting the body into the carriage, and what was still more difficult, to get in along with it, so thoroughly was he terrified. On arriving at the College, I found my valorous associate, slowly recovering from his ague fit, by the aid of a strong glass of brandy-toddy, and deeply lamenting his inability to assist me on the occasion...

Throughout the early part of the nineteenth century, the passage of numerous laws regarding "sepulcher disturbance" was testimony to the success of professional grave thieves and their competitiors and customers, the medical students. Yet by 1845, despite popular opposition, the movement for practical anatomy to be part of the requirements for a medical degree resulted in half of the country's medical schools incorporating such a course into their standard curriculum. No doubt this change in attitude was aided by laws enacted in Massachusetts (1831), Connecticut (1833), Illinois (1833), New Hampshire (1834), and Maine (1844) that provided for the ready access to executed criminals as dissection material. In addition, there was an obvious racial question: in the South, African Americans provided an easy and, unfortunately, "unembarrassing source of experimentation." Despite not being written into law, it was an acknowledged fact that a deceased slave could be dissected solely with the consent of the owner.

Although dependence on European textbooks was initially greater in anatomy than other subjects, it would be erroneous to assume that there were no well-known early nineteenth-century American anatomists. The relationship between anatomy and surgery was so close that America's earliest established anatomists, Caspar Wistar (1761–1818), who authored the country's first anatomical treatise, the two-

3. Medical students were admitted to clinical lecture series by showing individually purchased attendance cards. Some of the cards were quite ornate; others were ordinary in appearance. *(Historical Collections, College of Physicians of Philadelphia)*

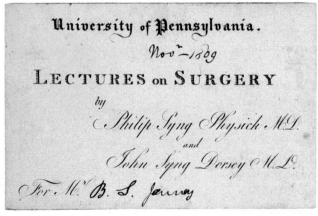

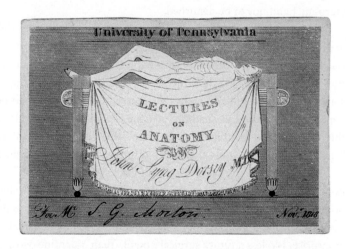

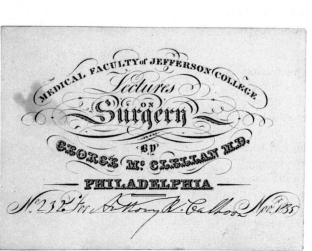

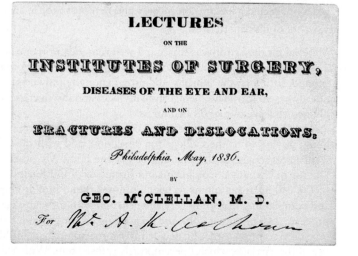

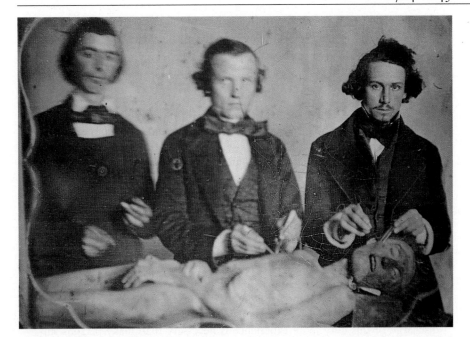

4. An extremely rare medical photograph showing physicians, or possibly medical students, dissecting a cadaver. This is the earliest extant American medical image depicting doctors at work, a type of occupational genre portrait. The original daguerreotype was taken in 1844 or 1845, and this photograph is from a full-plate tintype, which was made from the daguerreotype by Byron Reed of Kokomo, Indiana (circa 1866). It was extremely unusual for human dissection to be depicted in a posed photograph, since such anatomical studies were illegal in many sections of the United States. Where the photograph was taken remains unknown, although it is most likely somewhere in the East, where human dissection would not have been as legally hazardous as in the more rural areas of the South and West. *(Courtesy of Stanley B. Burns, M.D., and The Burns Collection and Archive)*

volume *A System of Anatomy* (1811–1814); William Horner (1793–1853), author of *Lessons in Practical Anatomy* (1823) and the two-volume *Treatise on Special and General Anatomy* (1826); and John Godman (1794–1830), who wrote *Anatomical Investigations* (1824) were all considered among the more renowned surgeons of their time. This dual function of the anatomist as surgeon became particularly evident during the 1820s and 1830s, when American surgical luminaries authored the first comprehensive works in the English language in the burgeoning field of pathological anatomy. They included Godman (*Contributions to Physiological and Pathological Anatomy*, 1825), Horner (*A Treatise on Pathological Anatomy*, 1829), and Samuel Gross (*Elements of Pathological Anatomy*, 1839).

Horner was also influential in establishing medical microscopy in antebellum America. He received his degree in medicine from the University of Pennsylvania in 1814 and served as prosector to Wistar, the university's first professor of anatomy. Horner later worked with John Syng Dorsey and Philip Syng Physick. When the latter resigned his position as professor of anatomy, Horner was named successor. Horner in turn was succeeded by Joseph Leidy (1823–1891). From 1831 until his death, Horner remained as professor of anatomy while also serving as dean of the medical school. He bequeathed his personal anatomical collection to the University of Pennsylvania, enlarging what became known as the Wistar-Horner Museum. Horner's surgical accomplishments included the treatment of ectropion of the lower eyelid (1837) and the first operation to be performed in which the maxilla was excised without an external incision in the cheek (1850). He is eponymically remembered for his description of the tensor tarsi muscle, anatomically known as the pars lacrimalis musculi orbicularis oculi. In 1835, Horner examined, under a microscope, samples of the digestive tract of cholera victims in order to discover which lesions were caused by the dread disease. What Horner learned about the alimentary tract, other American anatomists were also discovering about other parts of the body. By 1843, in the sixth edition of his authoritative anatomy text, Horner, the surgeon-anatomist, announced with both pride and justification that recent improvements in the microscope had led to a "well-marked and triumphant advance" in the science of anatomy and, by inferrence, its clinical twin, surgery.

As closely related to anatomy as surgery was, the reality was that clinical subjects were generally taught without the provision to the students of any practical experience. All too often, graduates became doctors without having ever seen or assisted at a surgical operation, let alone having examined a live patient. The need for clinical instruction was evident, but only the medical colleges located in larger cities had clinical resources, and even these were barely adequate. Writing in 1832, Daniel

Drake (1785–1852), a heroic figure in the history of Western frontier medicine, described many of the conditions then existing in medical education as well as how to solve some of the problems. Concerning the student who intended to make "operative surgery, his principal object" Drake observed that special attention should be given to the following subjects:

> The anatomy of the parts which are the seats of the greater operations... he should be perfectly familiar: -not merely able to enumerate the muscles, and fasciae, and nerves, and blood vessels... but to conceive accurately of the relative situation of those anatomical elements. He should, moreover, learn to know each part, not only by the eye but by the finger; as it will frequently happen, in deep and bloody operations, that the sense of touch is the only one he can employ.
>
> He should practice the various operations on the dead subject; for by practice only, can he become adroit or acquire that confidence which gives self-possession in moments of difficulty and doubt. In this stage of his practical studies, he will often find it advantageous to supply this deficiency of human subjects by a resort to dead animals...
>
> He should practice on the living or the dead subject the application of the various kinds of bandages and apparatus of surgery. For the neat and efficient discharge of this duty more experience is necessary than many persons suppose, until they come to the trial in cases of real injury when it is too late to prepare themselves.

Even knowing of Drake's lofty goals, there was little doubt that American medical education remained in a deplorable condition throughout most of the first half of the nineteenth century. The concern for profits on the part of the proprietary faculty (i.e., admission requirements consisted of little more than the ability to pay tuition) caused a natural increase in enrollments with a corresponding decrease in student preparedness. The profit motive became so strong that in some schools the candidate for graduation would undergo his final oral examination knowing beforehand that he would pay the professors for the examination only if he passed. If a failure should occur, then the professors refunded the money in full. Such a biased system did little to produce outstanding physicians but certainly helped augment faculty incomes.

In retrospect, it is easy to be overly harsh in evaluating mid-nineteenth-century American medical schools. However, the country was experiencing a growth spurt unparalleled in its existence, past or future. With an expanding populace, scattered over frontier territory, the little training that most physician-surgeons received was better than none at all. In truth, medical science had not yet substantively advanced in its ability to treat most diseases. Accordingly, American citizens still remained wary of what doctors could actually accomplish.

Despite these deplorable conditions, early to mid-nineteenth-century American medical education did manage to produce numerous medical and surgical luminaries. In most instances, such individuals pursued alternative paths of medical education and training that existed as supplements to the poor instruction provided at proprietary schools. Among these secondary opportunities were those at non–degree-granting schools that operated in loose connection with "regular" schools, but only during summer and winter vacations. The very existence of these "private" medical schools was a stark reminder of the inadequate education provided at most degree-granting medical colleges.

Among the more famous of these alternative schools were the Philadelphia school established in 1817 by Philip Syng Physick, the Tremont Street School founded in Boston in 1838 by members of the Harvard faculty, and its younger rival the Boylston Medical School started in 1847 by recent graduates of Harvard Medical School. The emphasis was on physical diagnosis and the use of new diagnostic equipment such as the ophthalmoscope and the otoscope. For the student interested in surgery, these extramural schools were particularly important, since they provided opportunities to observe surgical operations while receiving experience in assisting at minor operations and bandaging wounds.

PHILADELPHIA
Anatomical Rooms.
—❋❋❋✿❋❋❋—
PALMAM QUI MERUIT FERAT.
—❋❋❋✿❋❋❋—

THE following honours will be awarded on the 1st *of March next, to such Students as excel in the different parts of the science of Anatomy, below specified:*

To the best Practical Anatomist, a full case of Rorer's Dissecting Instruments, of the value of twenty dollars.

To the second best Practical Anatomist, a copy of Wistar's or Bell's Anatomy, at his option.

For the best examination on General Anatomy, a copy of Bichat's Anatomie Generale.

For the best examination on the vascular system, a copy of Bell's plates and of Haller's plates of the Arteries.

For the best examination on the Bones, Joints and Muscles, a copy of Bell's engravings of these parts.

For the best Anatomical preparation made by the candidate during the present session, a copy of Bell's Manual of Anatomy.

Gentlemen desirous of becoming Candidates are requested to signify their intentions before the 20th of February next, stating the length of time they have been engaged in the study. The examinations will be conducted so that none but the successful candidates shall be known. To each of these an honorary certificate will be given and their names, together with an account of the subjects on which they excelled, published in the Medical Journals. JOHN D. GODMAN.
Philadelphia, January 1, 1824.

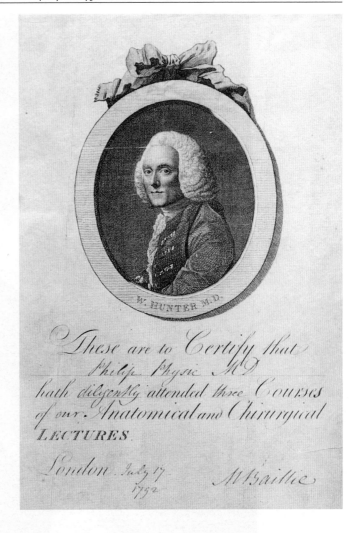

These are to Certify that Philip Physic MD hath diligently attended three Courses of our Anatomical and Chirurgical LECTURES

London July 17 1792 *M Baillie*

STUDY ABROAD

Young Americans with financial means and the ambition to further their careers were beginning to matriculate at leading European medical centers in increasing numbers. At the time of the Revolutionary War and up through 1810, European study in London and Edinburgh was an important adjunct to the well-established apprentice system of medical learning in the colonies. Those early Americans who managed to study abroad would come to form a considerable proportion of the leading surgeons in sparsely settled America. Among them were Wright Post (1766–1822), Valentine Mott (1785–1865), and J. Kearny Rodgers (1793–1851) of New York City. Post studied with John Sheldon (1752–1808) in London; Mott and Rodgers worked with Astley Cooper (1768–1841) and John Abernethy (1764–1831) in London. The Philadelphia surgeons Philip Syng Physick (1768–1837), his nephew John Syng Dorsey (1783–1918), and William Gibson (1768–1868) took lengthy periods of training in London and Edinburgh. Physick's training was of particular importance, since he was with John Hunter (1728–1793) for four years and became Hunter's most prominent American pupil. Both Ephraim McDowell (1771–1830) and Benjamin Winslow Dudley (1785–1870) returned, after studying in Edinburgh, to practice medicine and surgery in the wilds of Kentucky. The renowned John Collins Warren (1778–1856) of Boston received his medical degree from Edinburgh in 1802.

Following the War of 1812 and after cessation of the Napoleonic Wars, American students began to venture to Paris in search of their medical education. In contrast with the earlier American students, the majority of this second generation were already physicians, having obtained their basic education in the growing number of proprietary medical institutions. Between 1820 and the start of the Civil War, it is estimated that nearly 700 Americans furthered their medical education and training

5. *(left)* Numerous extramural facilities provided additional schooling beyond that available in formal medical colleges. John Godman supervised one such facility, the Philadelphia Anatomical Rooms. This 1824 broadside announces his intention to award prizes to the best student anatomists. *(Historical Collections, College of Physicians of Philadelphia)*

6. *(right)* Certificate given to Philip Syng Physick in July 1792, attesting to his attendance at three courses in anatomy and surgery at William Hunter's Great Windmill Street School in London. Hunter (1718–1783) is depicted in the cameo portrait, but it was his nephew, pupil, and successor Matthew Baillie (1760–1823) who signed Physick's testamur. *(Historical Collections, College of Physicians of Philadelphia)*

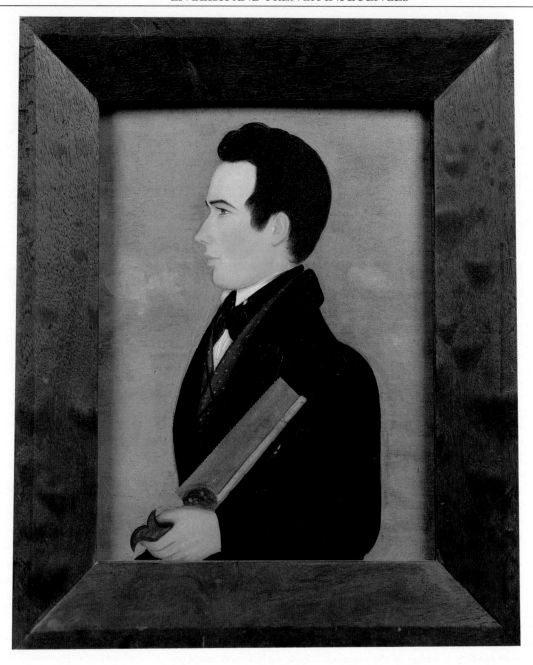

7. "Portrait of a Young Physician Holding a Surgical Saw." In this simple oil on poplar panel with a cherrywood frame (circa 1830–1840), the unknown artist, believed to be from the New York/Pennsylvania area, portrays an unidentified young American physician-surgeon proudly showing his most emblematic of surgical instruments, a Tenon-type amputation saw. *(From the Permanent Collection of the Museum of American Folk Art, New York City; Gift of Thomas R. Borek)*

in Paris. Ten percent of this number became professors in medical schools throughout the United States and constituted a mid-nineteenth-century elite cadre among American doctors.

As American surgical history evolved, it was virtually *de rigueur* for any surgeon who wished to be considered a leader within the profession to have lived and studied abroad. Because of this essentiality of overseas travel, there had long been a desperate need for practical information about educational opportunities and overall living conditions in Europe. In the first half of the nineteenth century, travel and study abroad constituted an enormous personal and financial undertaking, which had to be planned with a certain modicum of financial responsibility. Other than by word of mouth, little during this surgical era was available or published regarding the practicality of such travel for surgical education.

Finally, in 1843, there appeared for the first time in the United States a surgical travel guide, Ferdinand C. Stewart's (1815–1899) *The Hospitals and Surgeons of Paris.* Although additional treatises on the subject of European medical educational opportunities would be published during the latter half of the 1840s (i.e., David Yandell [1826–1898], *Notes on Medical Matters and Medical Men in London and Paris,* 1848, and L. J. Frazee [1819–1905] *The Medical Student in Europe,* 1849), the text by

Stewart represented the model for all future written information aimed at the American surgical traveler.

As a prominent New York City surgeon, Stewart provided a literary work that proved most important in encouraging young American physicians to travel to Paris in order to complete their medical and surgical education and training... Stewart's effort was informative, entertaining, gossipy, and, most importantly, overtly pragmatic in the advice it provided. Stewart received his medical degree from the University of Pennsylvania in 1837 and then went to Europe, where he studied in Paris until 1843. He returned to commence a practice in New York City but soon noticed a growing demand for information about opportunities for surgical study in Paris. Like the author of any modern travel book, Stewart furnished miscellaneous information on hotels, lodging houses, boarding houses, restaurants, and cafés in the city. He even detailed the anticipated expenses for a student wishing to remain in Paris for one year, noting that "this sum of three thousand francs... is only for such expenses as are absolutely necessary to enable a student to live comfortably and respectably. His extra expenses and clothing will cost whatever he can afford to spend on them."

The surgeons of Paris are the subjects of Stewart's most incisive and gossipy comments. Rarely can such provocative statements concerning foreign surgeons be found in the early American surgical literature:

> **Cloquet...** is one of the very few foreign surgeons who thinks highly enough of American authorities to quote them, which he frequently does-speaking, on such occasions, with the greatest respect and kindness of the distinguished scientific men of our country...

> **Lisfranc...** notwithstanding his many good qualities...is unpopular with a number of his fellow practitioners in Paris; he has made enemies of many by being too plain spoken, and overbearing in his manner towards them...his remarkable coolness and self-possession have acquired for him the unenviable reputation of being brutal in his operations, and wholly unmindful of the sufferings of his patients...

> **Marjolin...** no man is his enemy. His practice is the most extensive and lucrative in Paris.... One of the principal merits of Marjolin is his modesty, which induces him never to push himself forwards, or to arrogate more than he is justly entitled to, he has never been thought to be, and does not consider himself, a good operator...

> **Velpeau...** his clear and distinct enunciation renders him more easily understood by foreigners than most of the other surgeons. Hence, his hospital is a favourite resort of American and English students.... His manner towards his public patients, is sometimes inexcusable and harsh in the extreme, whilst his treatment of the young men placed under him, is occasionally such, as to give rise to a strong feeling of indignation on the part of the spectator...his personal appearance is difficult to describe, and probably dangerous to attempt.

Stewart's travel guide remains relatively unknown. However, to read it is to better understand the trials and tribulations endured by an entire generation of future leaders in American surgery during their study abroad. Two other texts by American surgeons concerning their travels throughout Europe were also published during the early 1840s: William Gibson's (1788–1868) *Rambles in Europe in 1839 with Sketches of Prominent Surgeons* (1841) and Valentine Mott's *Travel in Europe and the East* (1842). These lengthy texts provided information about surgical conditions throughout the Continent, but their diary-like form provided less practical information than Stewart's.

ALLOPATHIC PHYSICIANS VERSUS THE IRREGULARS

Having basked in the glory of British and French medicine, the returning physician was faced with the stark reality of having to practice in medically unsophisticated and increasingly unregulated America. Despite the rapid increase in the number of new medical schools in the United States and the quality of students returning from their

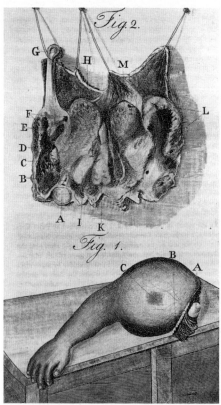

8. One of early America's surgical spectaculars. William Bowen (1785–1815), a graduate of Union College in Schenectady, New York, received his medical education in Edinburgh, Scotland. His paper in the *New England Journal of Medicine and Surgery* (vol. 3, pages 313–319, 1814) was the first published report of a shoulder amputation in the United States. The patient went back to his farm work in one month but succumbed to "fungus haematodes" (an obsolete term denoting a soft, fungating, easily bleeding malignancy) fourteen months later. *(Historical Collections, College of Physicians of Philadelphia)*

European experience, an obvious deterioration in the existing quality of medical care occurred during the 1830s and 1840s. In an era of Jacksonian democracy, the openess of American society subverted the efforts of elite physicians to promote professionalism within their ranks. Attempts to raise educational and licensing standards and to elevate the status of doctors were compromised when many legislatures withdrew the licensing privilege from state medical societies and medical schools and created gubernatorially appointed boards of medical examiners. Political beliefs soon became a major influence in directing the future of medical practice, especially once physician licensure began to be viewed as little more than the granting of a monopoly to a favored few as opposed to its intended purpose of promoting clinical competence.

Much of the skepticism concerning prior attempts to control medicine emanated from vociferous attacks by "irregular" or sectarian doctors upon "regular" or orthodox practices. The irregulars challenged the political justification for the privilege given to a favored few to practice under government-sanctioned monopolistic conditions. As a result, democratizing influences brought about the repeal of many state licensing laws as well as a lack of public support for even politically appointed examining boards. Quacks and cultists abounded, making the concept of professional regulation and licensing little more than a haphazard and essentially worthless process. For instance, in Philadelphia in the late 1840s it was reputed that two of every three physicians and surgeons were neither members of the local medical society nor graduates of a bona fide medical school.

Cultists attacked customary medical practices through highly organized professional political action committees. In tearing down the medical monopoly previously granted by state legislatures, cultists would eventually force "regular" doctors to defend their profession by developing more scientifically based and rational therapies. The demise of such old-fashioned and disagreeable clinical practices as blistering, bloodletting, emetics, purging, and sweating caused orthodox American medicine to undergo a long-needed therapeutic transformation.

Among the numerous cults that developed in the first half of the nineteenth century, the Thomsonians acquired many followers and for three decades were considered a serious threat to the survival of allopathic, or orthodox, medicine. Based on a "more gentler type of treatment," Thomsonians proclaimed that diseases were due to an excess of "cold" in the body. Their therapies consisted of hot baths and the administration of botanical preparations to eliminate or neutralize the body's "cold." When the Thomsonians began to lose momentum, what was left of their membership joined forces with the rising Eclectic cult. Combining what were considered the best features of allopathic medicine with the teaching of the Thomsonians, the Eclectics established their own medical schools, whose professors of surgery even authored textbooks on the American eclectic system of surgery. Other prominent cults advocating gentler methods of treatments included the Grahamites and the homeopaths. The Grahamites, founded by Sylvester Graham (1794–1851), believed that most forms of illness were iatrogenic and that calomel and other "poisonous drugs" then in common use were the catalyst for many problems. Graham preached hygienic measures, the avoidance of alcoholic drinks, vegetarianism, and the use of whole-wheat flour rather than refined flour in the daily diet. Graham's cracker, originally used among other things as a method to control sexual urges, specifically premarital and extramarital sex and masturbation, is the most enduring symbol of this long-defunct system of therapeutic behavior.

Although "popular" medicine began to engulf the entire United States, developments in health care delivery were little more than "scientific" expressions of much greater cultural, political, and socioeconomic upheavals in American society. The entire concept of exclusive privileges was an affront to Jacksonian ideology. As a consequence, orthodox physicians might have viewed the situation as a "we" (science) versus "they" (quackery) confrontation, but the citizenry couched it in capitalistic terms of free competition versus monopoly. Not until the rise of true scientific medicine and surgery in the last decades of the nineteenth century would the cultural and professional authority of allopathic medicine be formally established in America.

The fondness with which Americans embraced this populist healing philosophy was rapidly translated into examples of do-it-yourself surgery. Several texts were published in which physician-authors instructed laypersons in performing their own surgical operations. The titles alone bespeak the intent of the writers: Josiah Batchelder's *Every Seaman his Own Physician* (1817), William Hand's *The House Surgeon and Physician, Designed to Assist Heads of Families…in Discerning, Distinguishing, and Curing Diseases* (1818), and Ira Warren's (1806–1864) immensely popular *The Household Physician* (1859). Batchelder describes the technique of amputation and the dressing of the stump in a short half page while wryly noting, "It is not probable that even necessity will make the above operation necessary where no surgeon can be had; but through fear that it might, I quoted the aforegoing from a very short and imperfect statement; yet short and imperfect as it is, it may afford a few rays of light in a dark hour." Warren was not nearly as circumspect as Batchelder, since he advised excision of an exotosis with a hunting knife, ligation of aneurysms accompanied by an illustration and written instructions, repair of a depressed skull

9. "Doctor Operating." This simple watercolor, ink, and pencil work on paper originally served as the frontispiece to Silas Cummings' (1803–1882) book of medical notes, compiled when he was a student at Dartmouth Medical School in 1827. It is a unique piece of American surgical ephemera, as it represents the earliest known depiction of an actual operation in progress. Whether Cummings was the artist remains uncertain. The scene is of an assistant holding a rag or sponge while the tailcoated physician-surgeon closes a laceration in the patient's right forearm. Cummings spent most of his career in a rural New Hampshire-based practice. *(Abby Aldrich Rockefeller Folk Art Center, Williamsburg, Virginia)*

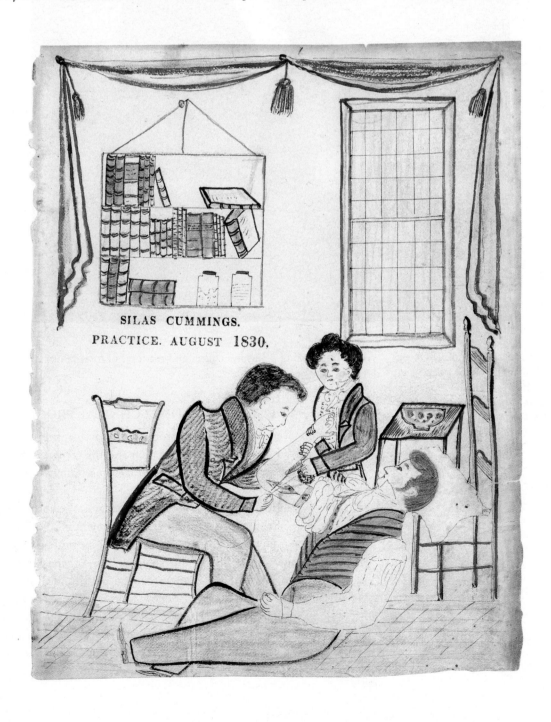

SILAS CUMMINGS.
PRACTICE. AUGUST 1830.

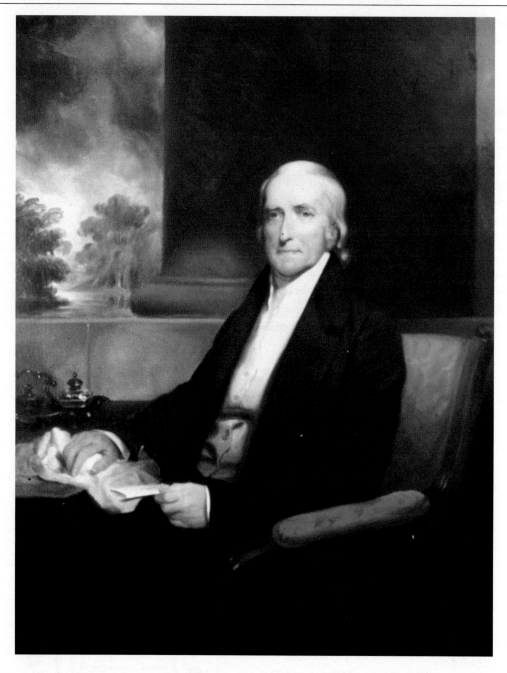

10. Philip Syng Physick as depicted by Robert Reynolds (circa 1840), who copied an earlier portrait (1836) of Physick by Henry Inman (1801–1846). *(Courtesy of the College of Physicians of Philadelphia)*

fracture utilizing a mason's chisel, and retrieval of foreign bodies in the nasal cavity with a knitting needle.

THE SLOW PACE OF TECHNICAL PROGRESS

Until the discovery of ether and chloroform, improvements in the art and craft of surgery occurred mainly in instrumentation and the technical intricacies of performing difficult or, as they were termed at the time, "capital" operations. From a scientific standpoint, the mid-1820s to the mid-1840s represented an era in which physicians were groping for more consistent standards of clinical practice. In every sense, these decades proved a pioneering era for American surgeons, who attempted to cut loose from past dogma and search for new surgical principles.

Up to this time, the ordinary American physician-surgeon, who depended more on the crops in his field for income than on performing surgical operations, undoubtedly would incise abscesses, remove foreign bodies, or amputate extremities with instruments of dubious merit and would base his incision and dissection strategies upon a meager knowledge of human anatomy. Yet, surgeons and their ancient craft were strangely exempt from the overwhelming suspicions and criticisms heaped on their nonoperating colleagues. The higher esteem in which the public viewed surgeons was painfully evident to many medical men. Some, such as Elisha Bartlett (1804–1855) in his *Inquiry Into the Degree of Certainty in Medicine* (1848), dealt with it in a forthright manner:

> Surgery has escaped almost entirely the charges of incompetence and uncertainty which have been so liberally bestowed upon practical medicine. The reasons of this are simple and obvious enough. Its processes are not only more showy than those of practical medicine, but they are more easily seen and apprehended; they appeal immediately and strongly to the senses; they are so manifest that they can be neither doubted nor mistaken. The restoration of a dislocated bone to its socket; the removal of a calculus from the bladder, either by the lithotriptor or by the knife and forceps; the closure of an aneurysm by a ligature on the diseased vessel; the instantaneous arrest of the spouting torrent of blood from a cut artery; the re-admission of the long-excluded light to the retina by the withdrawal, or the dropping down, of the darkened curtain of the crystalline lens are achievements so brilliant in their execution and so striking and positive in their results as not merely to leave no room for cavilling or for skepticism, but to excite in us at once, emotions both of wonder and delight.

It was generally believed that surgery's immunity from detractors was contingent on its use of "mechanical processes." In essence, this working with one's hands appealed directly to the common sense of America's vast unskilled work force. Alfred Stillé (1813–1900), a Philadelphia physician, complained even more pointedly, "The surgeon is commonly judged by his operation, i.e., his prescription.... The public form a notion of the comparative value of surgery and medicine, by contrasting the agents of the one with the results of the other. A comparison of nutritious food and strong men would be just about as rational."

Although it is true that on the whole, the competency level of surgeons in the United States lagged behind that of their counterparts in many of the larger urban centers of Europe in the 1830s and 1840s (clearly, American surgeons were not contributing as meaningfully to the larger community of world surgery as their European brethren), it is just as certain that in a large proportion of various types of operations (i.e., according to Samuel Gross, "surgery of the blood vessels...fractures...reduction of dislocations...affections of the joints...amputations...excision of the bones and joints...trephining of the skull...extirpations of the upper jaw...excision of the lower jaw...staphylorraphy...palatoplasty...thoracentesis...and lithotrity") American practice was the equal of European standards. American society could not support the growth of specialized surgical centers like those in Paris and Berlin, nor could scientific research centers exist in the still unsophisticated cities of the New World. But the clinical practice of surgery was and largely remains a hands-on event dependent on the mental and physical agility of the surgeon. Accordingly, when the technical wizardry of early American surgeons like McDowell, Mott, Physick, and Warren is fully appreciated, it seems reasonable to state that some surgical operations were being completed with about equal success on both sides of the Atlantic Ocean.

In 1835, a patient with urinary bladder stones, an aneurysm of the femoral artery, or a rapidly growing tumor of the lower jaw would have been in comparably competent clinical situations whether operated on by Valentine Mott in New York City, John Collins Warren in Boston, Philip Syng Physick in Philadelphia, Benjamin Collins Brodie in London, Johann Friedrich Dieffenbach in Berlin, or Guillaume Dupuytren in Paris. Perhaps Gross best summed up mid-nineteenth-century American surgical chauvinism when he wrote, "Let it not be supposed...that the American surgeon is a mere operator; if he ranks high in this particular, he ranks high also as a therapeutist. Nowhere, it may safely be asserted, are the great principles of surgery better taught, or better understood, than they are in this country.... The cultured and refined American [surgeon] is a prince among men. Let us be grateful for what we are and for what we have done...." A somewhat contrasting viewpoint was offered by members of the Indiana State Medical Society's

Committee on Surgery when, in 1853, they noted, "there is nothing in Indiana surgery entitling it to be regarded as especially beneficial or skillful."

Despite the American surgeon's occasional boldness, even when complemented by a European medical education, the fact remained that surgical operations were rarely performed. Students in medical colleges received little training in surgery and frequently complained about the lack of clinical surgical experience. Without the ability to alleviate pain, doctors were reluctant to resort to the surgeon's knife over less intrusive botanic preparations, and an operation was performed only in a case of absolute necessity. Elective surgery was virtually nonexistent; most patients consented to undergo surgery only when their suffering from the disease process outweighed what they anticipated the intraoperative and postoperative pain to be. According to one midwestern physician-surgeon writing in 1831, "I shall never forget the earnestness with which [the patient] employed me not to operate on him, and he so far worked on my feeling & sympathies that it was with much difficulty that I could man my self up to the operating point."

The strikingly small volume of operative surgery is best appreciated by a reading of the surgical casebook of Philip Syng Physick. Commonly regarded as the father of American surgery, Physick was among the most prominent American surgeons in the first three decades of the nineteenth century. It would seem, therefore, that if any surgeon had a busy operative schedule, it should have been Physick. Physick's daily clinical caseload for 1798 and 1799 was faithfully recorded by his nephew-apprentice John Syng Dorsey (1783–1818), who was himself to become a renowned surgeon. In this little-appreciated but classic handwritten document, Dorsey enumerated all of thirty-two surgical operations–stark testimony to how little operative surgery was actually performed:

1. Case of amputation.
2. Case of hydrocephalus.
3. Case of dissection of an ulcerated cancerous tumor from the eye of a person.
4. Case of dissection of a thick membrane from the eye.
5. Case of aneurism of the popliteal artery.
6. Case of fractured femur.
7. Case of dissection of an encysted tumor from beneath the eye.
8. Case of amputation of thigh.
9. Case of extraction of cataract.
10. Case of operation for the cure of hydrocele.
11. Case of excision of a cancerous underlip.
12. Case of extraction of cataract from each eye.
13. Case of extraction of cataract.
14. Case of operation for fistula lachrymalis.
15. Case of dissection of tumor from the breast.
16. Case of injury of the head.
17. Case of extraction of cataract.
18. Case of amputation of cancerous mass.
19. Case of operation for radical cure of hydrocele.
20. Case of dissecting off a large cancer from the cheek.
21. Case of amputation of the leg below the knee.
22. Case of polypus.
23. Lithotomy on a child.
24. Varicose veins secured by ligature.
25. Lithotomy.
26. Trepaning.
27. Hydrocele-cured.
28. Amputation of cancerous mamma and tumor in axilla.
29. Harelip.
30. Tumor from eyelid.
31. Case of divided radial artery secured by ligature.
32. Case of injured head which ended fatally after symptoms of compression.

Operating in the poorly lit, cramped home of a screaming individual, a surgeon was forced to be efficient with the knife but hardened to the patient's pleas for mercy. With a roughly hewn kitchen table serving as an operating bench, the surgeon frequently enjoined the patient's family and friends to assist in the procedure, particularly to hold down a caterwauling patient. Performing surgery in one's street clothes was the accepted practice, and after completing an operation, the surgeon simply wiped the bloodied instruments on his well-stained black frock coat and placed the still moist implements back in their case for the next operation. There was no sense of cleanliness, nor even close postoperative supervision. Most patients were simply left to fend for themselves in the privacy of their homes. In reality, surgery as a viable therapeutic modality was only a minor part of the general practice of medicine and would remain so for another four decades.

THE WAR OF 1812

Like most eras in the history of American surgery, the carnage of battle, in this case the War of 1812, provided surgeons with unique opportunities to treat injuries and observe wound pathology that might not otherwise have been encountered in civilian life. Not surprisingly, though, most of the written observations of the military physicians were directed at medical diseases and their treatment and the effects of climate and geography on the soldiers' overall health. Camp diseases and the medical sequelae of surgical injuries proved far more troublesome for the medical corps than the actual treatment of battlefield trauma. In fact, no important surgical breakthroughs came out of this conflict.

Few surgical operations were completed even in areas of major military activity, and those that were consisted mostly of extremity amputation for gunshot injury. Similarly, no surgical manuals were specifically written for American physicians serving in the War of 1812. However, James Mann (1759–1832), a respected surgical authority who described his wartime experiences in *Medical Sketches of the Campaigns of 1812, 13, 14, to which are Added, Surgical Cases…*(1816), urged his colleagues to pay particularly close attention to the work of the renowned French military surgeon Dominique Larrey (1766–1842).

11. During the early years of the nineteenth century there were few surgical instrument makers at work in America. By the 1820s, a growing number of British expatriate cutlers, specializing in surgical fabrications, had appeared in New York City. Among the most distinguished was Peter Rose, who hand-manufactured this exquisite and historically important (circa 1830) minor surgical set. Containing eleven knives, bistouries, suture guides, and other instruments, all with mother-of-pearl handles and highly ornate ferrules, the set originally belonged to Erasmus Darwin Hudson (1805–1880), a well-known orthopedic surgeon and designer of prosthetic appliances. The instrument set was passed down to Erasmus Darwin Hudson, Jr. (1843–1887), whose calling card is attached by spirit gum. *(Author's Collection)*

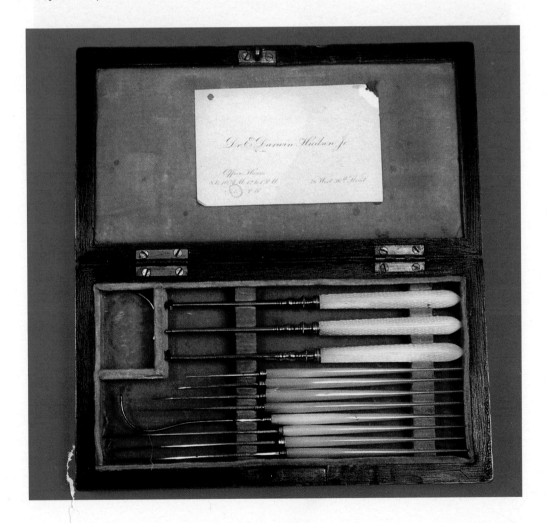

Mann graduated from Harvard College and was apprenticed to Samuel Danforth (1740–1827), a physician in Boston. Following military service during the Revolutionary War, when he was reported to have been a prisoner of war for two months, Mann commenced private practice in his native town of Wrentham, Massachusetts. However, he remained active in military affairs, including on-site visits to the militia camps involved with Shays' Rebellion in 1786. Until 1812, he remained in practice in upstate New York and western Massachusetts, but on the commencement of hostilities he formally joined the U.S. Army as a hospital surgeon. After the war, Mann was appointed consulting physician to the Massachusetts General Hospital in place of Danforth. There he performed the country's first successful amputation at the level of the elbow joint. For unknown reasons, Mann returned to public life and was stationed as a port physician at Governor's Island, New York City harbor, where he died. His chapter on surgery in the *Medical Sketches* is especially valuable for its first-hand description of the treatment of wounds during the War of 1812 and the vagaries of the surgical decision making process itself:

> In many cases it is difficult to determine, most correctly, whether it is best to amputate immediately, or defer it, to see if the limb may be saved-and if it cannot be saved, to operate at a future period. When an opinion is formed that the chance of saving a limb is greater than the risque of losing life by deferring an amputation until an experiment is made to save it-to defer the operation is proper. While taking this into consideration, due weight should be given to all the circumstance which may tend to promote, retard, or prevent a cure.

12. Ammi Phillips (1788–1865), one of the country's most celebrated folk artists, worked as an itinerant painter in the Hudson River Valley of New York State and in the border regions of Connecticut and Massachusetts. Among his many portraits in the primitive style were occasional ones of professional men, including physician-surgeons such as Levi King (1799–1878) (circa 1830). King, a graduate of the College of Physicians and Surgeons of the Western District at Fairfield, Herkimer County, New York, practiced in Cairo, in the Catskills region, from 1826 until his death. Although detailed biographical material about King is unavailable, the very fact that Phillips portrays him so proudly clutching volume one of London-based Samuel Cooper's (1780–1848) *Dictionary of Practical Surgery* points to a unabashed pride in his surgical skills. *(From the collection of Dr. King's great-great grandson)*

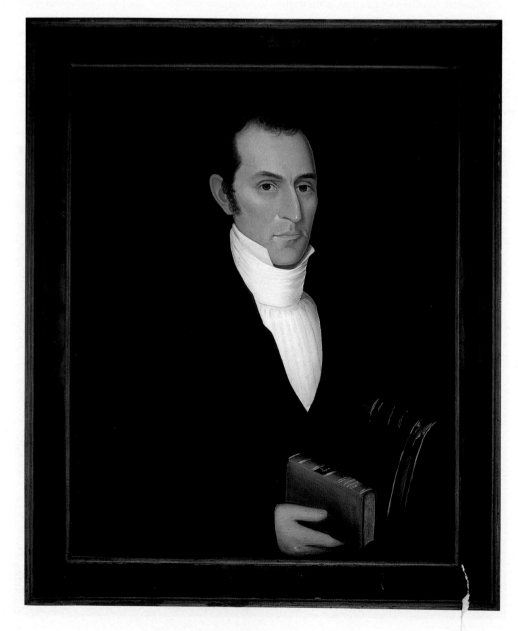

When a case is of such a nature as would render a cure dubious under the best attendance, and most eligible situation-if circumstances do not admit of these, the operation should not be deferred; because a case, which is doubtful in the first instance, becomes, from unfavourable circumstances, not only hazardous, but fatal, under their influence.

ATTITUDES TOWARD PAIN

The subject of pain during surgery was little discussed by American surgeons. Nowhere in the American surgical literature before 1846 can a substantive article, a chapter, or even a few discursive sentences be found on the alleviation of pain. This is not to suggest that the importance of minimizing pain during surgical operations and preparing the patient for the inevitable postoperative shock was not worth commenting upon. It simply signifies that little could be done or, oddly, that pain was sometimes perceived as a functional part of life and a necessary stimulant to the process of wound healing. In the preanesthetic era, pain was considered *pari passu* with being alive, and the harshness of day-to-day living had inured many individuals to it. Thus, techniques to suspend sensibility were often likened to nullifying life itself. Strangely, even surgeons were occasionally loath to lessen operative pain, as was noted by a New York Hospital physician in the mid-1830s, who remarked, following a leg amputation, "The sensibility of the nerves much impaired by his long continued disease, the man seeming to suffer comparatively little during the operation - a circumstance which is generally considered rather unfavorable..."

Among sectarian surgeons, Benjamin Hill (1813–1871), professor of surgery at the Eclectic Medical Institute in Cincinnati, was of an even more powerful persuasion. Hill contended that operative pain served as a "moral medication" in the treatment of cancer. There was a spiritual altruism or "compensation" inherent in undergoing such an experience:

> I have not unfrequently had patients, after submitting, perhaps for an hour, to this 'burning alive,' without flinching or groaning, open their mouths for the first time, after I had got through, to express their fears that the operation had not been carried far enough, because they had felt it so much less than I had given them reason to expect. I have told them beforehand that, unless they had fortitude enough to bear to have their arm chopped off, inch by inch, on a block, or to hold it out like the Roman youth of old, while it burnt off on the altar, they need not expect to have their cancer cured - that its moral 'final cause' was to develop such heroism in them!

Of the measures taken to prevent or decrease pain, the most common were brandy and wine, henbane and lettuce, laudanum, mesmerism or hypnotism, strapping above the point of the operation in order to decrease blood flow so as to numb the nerves, water of night shade, and noise as a diversion. Bleeding to the point of syncope was also attempted, albeit with limited success. Proselytism to the contrary, it was an absurd notion to deny a patient's suffering. As Valentine Mott wrote in the mid-1840s, "every day [we] see individuals praying in mercy that we would stop, that we would finish, thus imploring and menacing us, and who would not fail to escape if they were not firmly secured." But, he was realistic enough to understand that, "to avoid pain in operation is a chimera that we can no longer pursue in our times."

PROFESSIONALIZATION AND THE RISE OF MEDICAL PUBLISHING

To understand the history of American surgery is to be able to answer the question: When was the process of professionalization completed? It is not so readily apparent because there is controversy over what constitutes a profession, although few authorities would dispute medicine's claim to professional status. One fact is certain: in addition to the incorporation of scientific discipline into its essential content, there had to be a complex interaction of economic, political, and sociological changes within American society before the art, craft, and science of surgery could be transformed into a prototypal profession.

Most professions enjoy special power and prestige in society. To achieve this standing, a substantial number of individuals, united by membership with a common goal, are required, along with expert technical competence, standardized training, autonomy, monopoly over practice, and an undeniable "ethos of public service." Once these conditions are achieved, social prestige usually follows. The passage from a preindustrial, precapitalist, largely rural and tradition-based society to one in which American surgeons regarded themselves as a distinct class of practitioners within the overall hierarchy of medicine would not be completed until the beginning of the twentieth century. However, during the early nineteenth century, important preparatory steps were taking place. Among the most important was the appearance of a meaningful body of surgical literature indigenous to the American surgeon.

There emerged in the last years of the eighteenth century an important new source of medical information: the scientific journal. As John Shaw Billings (1838–1913), a surgeon and founder of the Index Medicus and director of the New York Public Library, noted in 1876:

> It is not in text-books or systematic treatises on special subjects that the greater part of the original contributions to the literature of medicine have been first made public during the last century...since the year 1800 medical journalism has become the principal means of recording and communicating the observations and ideas of those engaged in the practice of medicine, and has exercised a strong influence for the advancement of medical science and education...this country has contributed a noteworthy share...we find that one hundred and ninety-five medical journals have been commenced in this country...making in all one thousand six hundred and thirty-seven volumes, or a greater bulk than the textbooks and monographs.... The weekly and monthly periodicals are omnivorous and insatiable in their requests for contributions. Through the medical journals have been given to the world nearly all the discoveries which the science and art of medicine owes to American physicians.

In 1790, Thomas Kast (1755–1820) published an article entitled "An account of an aneurism in the thigh, perfectly cured by the operation, and the use of the limb preserved" in the *Medical Communications* of the Massachusetts Medical Society. Kast was born in Boston and graduated from Harvard College in 1769. He studied medicine as an apprentice to his father and also spent two years in London as a wound dresser at Guy's and St. Thomas' Hospitals. Kast returned to his native city in 1774, where he soon became a prominent practitioner and one of the founders of the Massachusetts Medical Society. His account of the ligation of a femoral aneurysm is the first article on a surgical topic to appear in the American medical periodical literature. Consequently, it is also the first known femoral ligation to be reported in the United States.

Although it is not usually recognized as the initial American periodical, publication of the first and only volume of the *Medical Communications* preceded the first printing of the more widely known *Medical Repository* by seven years. The appearance of the *Medical Repository* in July 1797 truly inaugurated the American medical journal. The new publication was edited by three New York physicians, Samuel Mitchill (1764–1831), Edward Miller (1760–1812), and Elihu Smith (1771–1798), and was met with an immediate, gratifying response from the medical community. It provided American physicians with their first native source of medical news and information and set the example for the many journals that would follow in the next century. Within its pages could be found meterologic observations, reviews of foreign medical literature, and numerous clinical articles. It also published some important "firsts," including John Otto's (1774–1844) account of hemophilia (1803).

With the beginning of meaningful American contributions to surgical literature, the many epic events that enliven our surgical past began to receive wide dissemination. During this era the first systematic treatise on surgery authored by an American surgeon, John Syng Dorsey's two-volume *Elements of Surgery* (1813), was published. Dorsey's effort was unique in many respects, although little of its contents were original to Dorsey. He merely organized the lectures of his uncle, Philip Syng Physick,

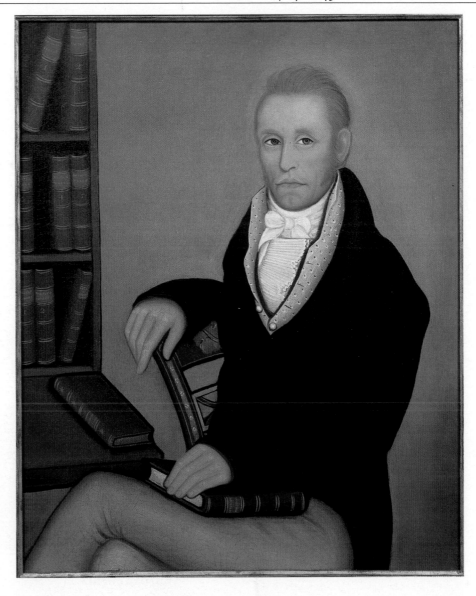

professor of surgery at the University of Pennsylvania, in the form of a surgical handbook. With seventy-two chapters ranging from "General remarks on accidental injuries and their effects" to "Of schirrus and cancer," the *Elements* was an important beginning in the professionalization process. Dorsey's comments on what he regarded as the essential difference between American and European surgeon-authors are most telling:

> An American, although he must labour under many disadvantages in the production of an elementary treatise, is in one respect better qualified for it than a European surgeon. He is, -at least he ought to be, -strictly impartial, and therefore adopts from all nations their respective improvements. Great Britain and France have been foremost in the cultivation of modern surgery, but their deficiency in philosophick courtesy and candour has in some instances greatly retarded its progress…. This spirit of hostile rivalship extending from the field of battle to that of science, cannot fail to exert a pernicious influence on practical surgery.

The only other systematic textbook of surgery authored by an American surgeon in the preanesthetic era was William Gibson's two-volume *Institutes and Practice of Surgery* (1824). Like Dorsey's work, Gibson's effort became one of the most popular medical-surgical texts of its time, passing through a total of eight editions. Gibson was Physick's successor to the chair of surgery at the University of Pennsylvania, and much of his information was gleaned from the latter's lectures. The eight chapters in the first volume include such topics as abscess, fractures, inflammation, ulcers, and wounds, while the sixteen chapters of the second volume present diseases of specific organs.

13. "Dr. Crane" by Ammi Phillips (circa 1814–1819). Although little is known about the life of Crane, this early folk piece is particularly important to the country's surgical iconography because of the presence of John Syng Dorsey's two-volume *Elements of Surgery* (first edition 1813, second edition 1818). As it was the first systematic treatise on surgery authored by an American, the very fact that Phillips included it in this portrait demonstrates the beginnings of a homespun influence on that era's physician-surgeons. *(The Alice M. Kaplan Collection, photograph courtesy of the Museum of American Folk Art, New York City. Photo by Gavin Ashworth)*

14. A water-stained and weathered title page from John Syng Dorsey's *Elements of Surgery* (1813), the first systematic treatise on surgery authored by an American surgeon. The cameo engraving is a view of Pennsylvania Hospital. *(Author's Collection)*

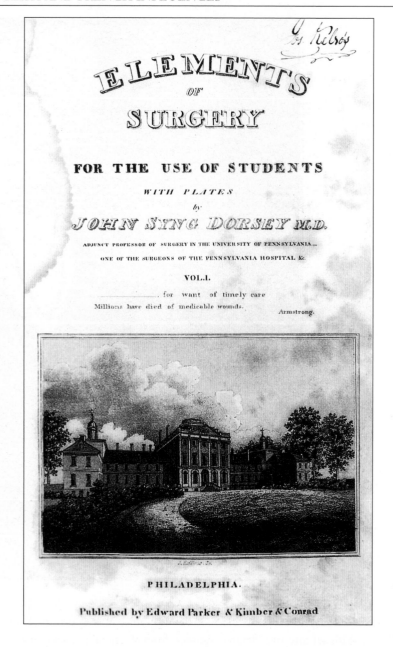

ELEMENTS
OF
SURGERY

FOR THE USE OF STUDENTS

WITH PLATES

by

JOHN SYNG DORSEY M.D.

ADJUNCT PROFESSOR OF SURGERY IN THE UNIVERSITY OF PENNSYLVANIA —
ONE OF THE SURGEONS OF THE PENNSYLVANIA HOSPITAL &c.

VOL. I.

———————— for want of timely care
Millions have died of medicable wounds.
Armstrong.

PHILADELPHIA.

Published by Edward Parker & Kimber & Conrad

Concurrent with the appearance of textbooks of surgery, monographs and treatises on more focused surgical topics were also being written. Examples include Heber Chase's *A Treatise on the Radical Cure of Hernia by Instruments* (1836), Joseph Parrish's (1779–1840) *Practical Observations on Strangulated Hernia* (1836), and John Collins Warren's *Surgical Observations on Tumours* (1837). The latter is regarded as one of the great classics in American surgery and is considered Warren's magnum opus. Divided into fourteen sections plus a glossary of the distinguishing characteristics of tumors, the work was especially prized because it contained sixteen hand-colored plates of "oncologic" surgical patients by the master engraver and caricaturist David Claypoole Johnston (1799–1865). Warren succinctly defined the essence of what was still missing in surgical oncology, an understanding of tissue physiology and pathology:

> The difficulties of diagnosis are not the greatest which attend this subject. We are in ignorance of the causes of these morbid changes; of their intimate texture and organization; and in many instances of their diversity from or identity with that of the textures in which they are situated. More facts are wanted. More histories of the origin, course, and results of such affections. More observations on their intimate structure at the different periods of their existence.

Samuel Gross set the tone for all future experimentation on animals when he authored the country's first full-length treatise on surgical research, *Experimental and*

Critical Inquiry Into the Nature and Treatment of Wounds of the Intestines (1843). Although Gross's work had been preceded by Thomas Smith's (1785–1831) short *Essay on Wounds of the Intestines* (1805), the *Inquiry* was more complete, having resulted from a full two years of experimentation on seventy dogs with the "wound made in the small bowel, not only because it is the more accessible portion of the alimentary tube, but because it is more liable, when thus injured, to become the seat of faecal effusion, and also, perhaps, of high inflammation." Describing the effort in his autobiography, Gross noted that

> The labor spent upon these experiments was very great, and the expense itself was not inconsiderable, as I was obliged to pay for nearly all the dogs, and to hire a man to watch and feed them…. The experiments besides, involved a great sacrifice of feeling on my part. I am naturally fond of dogs, and my sympathies were often wrought to the highest pitch, especially when I happened to get hold of an unusually clever specimen…if I were not thoroughly satisfied that the object had been most laudable, I should consider myself a most cruel, heartless man, deserving of the severest condemnation.

The book itself is among the rarest of surgical Americana. Virtually all copies were destroyed in a fire in the printer's office just after a handful had been distributed the day before. Gross allegedly never owned a copy and made it a point in his travels to attempt to locate one, with no success.

The most physically impressive of all American surgical texts in the preanesthetic period is Joseph Pancoast's (1805–1882) massive *Treatise on Operative Surgery* (1844). With eighty quarto plates comprising 486 separate illustrations, the book's most distinguishing characteristics are the wonderfully executed lithographs, including some by the renowned lithographer Nicolas Jacob (1782–1871). The *Treatise* was the country's first "atlas" of surgery, and the illustrations are so graphic that religious purists often removed the two plates depicting female genitalia. Pancoast was professor of surgery at Jefferson Medical College and was primarily known for his efforts in "reparative" or plastic and reconstructive surgery. The work contains four parts: "Elementary and minor operations," "General operations," "Special operations," and "Plastic and subcutaneous operations." The latter section is the earliest and most extensive chapter published on the state of plastic surgery in the United States. The *Treatise* went through three separate editions. Despite an original subscription price of ten dollars, almost 4,000 copies were sold within nine years. A limited number of copies of all three editions were issued with hand-colored plates printed on thicker and finer paper. The hand-colored copies are among the most magnificent of all American surgical works issued in the nineteenth century and are highly prized by present–day bibliophiles.

Although the concept of specialization in surgery did not yet have practical meaning in America, several texts were written that, in retrospect, can be regarded as the rudimentary beginnings of surgical specialization. For instance, William Dewees (1768–1841) was an adjunct professor of midwifery at the University of Pennsylvania when he authored *A Treatise on the Diseases of Females* (1826). Primarily concerned with medical gynecology, Dewees did write about "tumours and excrescences of the external parts," "displacements of the uterus," and even milk abscess of the breast, along with various surgical treatments, including puncturing and seton placement.

Samuel Gross was only 25 years old when he wrote the country's first major work on orthopedic surgery, *The Anatomy, Physiology, and Diseases of the Bones and Joints* (1839). Gross apologized that he did not have the "experience which was necessary to make the work what it should be. I need hardly add that, young as I was when the book was issued, I had to depend for the facts mainly upon the labors of others, though in the composition of it I used my own language…For this book I never received a cent of remuneration!" In 1823, George Frick (1793–1870) authored *A Treatise on the Diseases of the Eye*, the first American book on ophthalmology by the first American who is believed to have restricted his practice solely to diseases of the eye.

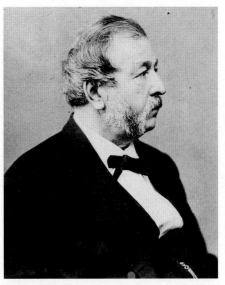

15. Joseph Pancoast *(Historical Collections, College of Physicians of Philadelphia)*

16. *(facing page)* Operation for cancer of the tongue, as drawn on stone by S. Chichowski for Joseph Pancoast's *Treatise on Operative Surgery*. It almost seems impossible in today's world to imagine that this surgical procedure was carried out without benefit of anesthesia. Following a long tradition of European surgical illustration, the idealized patient is depicted as being placid in demeanor while undergoing what must have been an unbearable therapeutic ordeal. Hand-colored versions of Pancoast's atlas, which are especially rare, help highlight the graphicness of mid-nineteenth-century surgical texts. *(Author's Collection)*

What distinguishes some of these early surgical texts is not only their clinical content but the abilities of the artists involved in their production. The most notable is Nathaniel Currier (1813–1888), later of Currier and Ives fame, who as a young lithographer produced many of the illustrative plates in Alfred Post's (1806–1886) *Observations on the Cure of Strabismus* (1841) and Augustus Doane's (1808–1852) *Surgery Illustrated* (1836).

NOTABLE SURGICAL OPERATIONS

Among the most renowned "general" surgical operations performed during this era (and the year in which it was reported in the American periodical literature) are Samuel White's small intestine enterotomy (1807) and ligation of the internal iliac artery (1828); Dorsey's ligation of the external iliac artery (1812); Physick's introduction of the stomach tube as a means of removing unwanted substances (1813) and surgical creation of a colocutaneous fistula secondary to a strangulated hernia (1826); Philip Wright Post's ligation of the common carotid artery (1814) and subclavian artery (1817); Mott's ligations of the innominate artery (1818), common carotid as prelude to performing a mandibular resection (1822), common iliac (1827), carotid artery distal to an aneurysm (1829), subclavian artery within the scaleni muscles (1833), and internal iliac artery (1837); Gibson's ligation of the common iliac artery (1820); Horatio Jameson's resection of the superior maxillary bone (1821); William Deaderick's (1773–1858) hemimandibulectomy (1823); Mason Cogswell's 1803 common carotid ligation (1824); David Rogers' (1799–1877) removal of "both superior maxillae as far back as the posterior external portion adjacent to the pterygoid processes" (1824); George McClellan's parotidectomy (1826); Zina Pitcher's (1797–1872) successful anastomosis of the small intestine (1832); Nathan Ryno Smith's hemithyroidectomy (1835); Amos Twitchell's 1807 ligation of the common carotid artery secondary to trauma (1842); and John Watson's (1807–1863) esophagotomy (1844).

Within the "specialties" there were also numerous famous surgical operations including: John King's (1774–1840) vaginotomy for abdominal pregnancy (1817); Nathan Smith's ovariotomy (1822), amputation at the knee joint (1825), and operative treatment of bone necrosis (1827); John Strachan's excision of the cervix (1829); George Hayward's and John Mettauer's repairs of vesicovaginal fistulae (1839) and (1840), respectively; John Atlee's bilateral oophorectomy (1843); Physick's use of a seton to treat nonunited fractures (1804), tonsillectomy (1828), and treatment of hip joint disease (1830); Mann's amputation at the elbow joint (1822); John Rhea Barton's osteotomy for ankylosis (1826) and description of wrist fractures (1838); Mott's amputation at the hip-joint (1827), resection of the clavicle (1828), and division of the nasal and maxillary bones to remove a fibrous growth (1843); John Rodgers' wiring of a nonunited humeral fracture (1827); John Ball Brown's tenotomies for clubfeet (1839); Josiah Nott's resection of the coccyx for coccydynia (1844); Gurdon Buck's treatment of joint ankylosis (1845); Benjamin Dudley's use of trephining to treat traumatic epilepsy (1828); John Collins Warren's repair of cleft palate (1828); Thomas Mütter's release of burn contractures for oral disfigurement (1837); and Jonathan Mason Warren's rhinoplasty (1837).

Of the many magnificent stories that make up American surgical lore, two of the most renowned occurred during the first half of the nineteenth century. Ephraim McDowell (1771–1830) was a native Virginian who studied medicine under Alexander Humphreys of Staunton. In 1793, McDowell traveled to Edinburgh, where he attended the academic sessions of 1793 and 1794, followed the anatomy lectures of Alexander Munro *secundus* (1733–1817) and studied surgery under John Bell (1763–1820). Returning to the United States in 1795, McDowell commenced practice in Danville, Kentucky, where he was a general practitioner and also acquired a reputation for his surgical skills. Among McDowell's more interesting surgical cases was the successful extraction of bladder stones in 1812 from James Knox Polk (1795–1849), who later became President of the United States. On Christmas Day

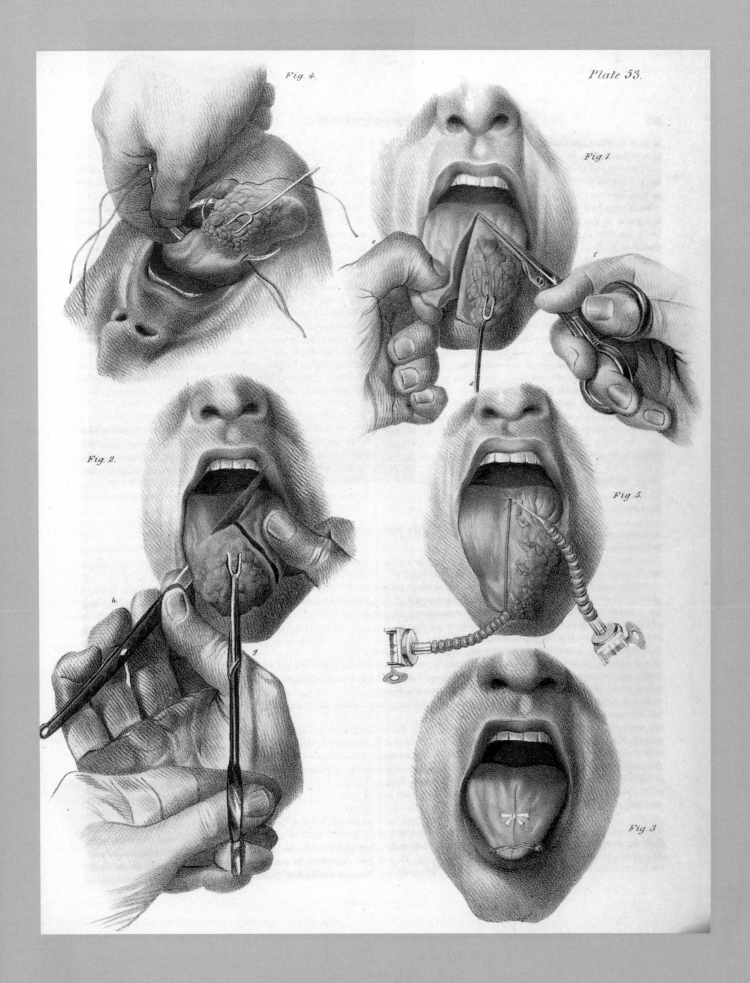

Fig. 4.

Plate 53.

Fig. 1.

Fig. 2.

Fig. 5.

Fig. 3.

17. Ephraim McDowell is known to have sat for one formal painting (circa 1822). The artist, Patrick Davenport (1803–1890), while still in his teens, almost certainly completed this oil in the library of McDowell's home in Danville, Kentucky. Symbolically noted on the bookshelves are copies of books by McDowell's Edinburgh-based mentor, John Bell, *Anatomy of the Human Body* and *Principles of Surgery*, as well as a volume by Hippocrates. *(McDowell House, Danville, Kentucky)*

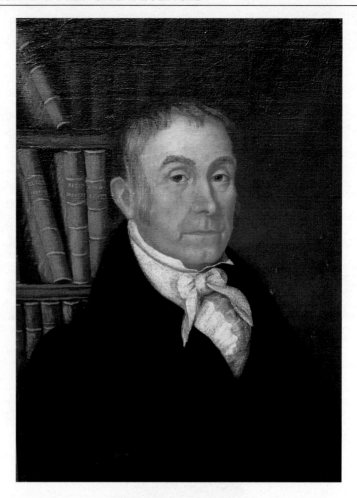

in 1809, McDowell introduced ovariotomy to the world as a successful operation for treatment of ovarian tumors. The story is best related in his own words:

> In December 1809, I was called to see a Mrs. Crawford, who had for several months thought herself pregnant.... The abdomen was considerably enlarged.... Upon examination, per vaginum, I found nothing in the uterus; which induced the conclusion that it must be an enlarged ovarium. Having never seen so large a substance extracted, nor heard of an attempt, or success attending any operation, such as this required, I gave to the unhappy woman information of her dangerous situation. She appeared willing to undergo an experiment, which I promised to perform if she would come to Danville...she performed the journey in a few days...I commenced the operation...I made an incision about three inches from the musculus rectus abdominis, on the left side, continuing the same nine inches in length.... The tumor...appeared full in view, but was so large that we could not take it away entire. We put a strong ligature around the fallopian tube near to the uterus; we then cut open the tumor, which was the ovarium and fimbrious part of the fallopian tube.... We took out fifteen pounds of a dirty, gelatinous looking substance. After which we cut through the fallopian tube, and extracted the sack, which weighed seven pounds and one half.... We closed the external opening with the interrupted suture, leaving out, at the lower end of the incision, the ligature which surrounded the fallopian tubes.... In five days I visited her, and much to my astonishment found her engaged in making up her bed...in twenty-five days, she returned home...in good health.

For twenty-five minutes and obviously without the benefit of anesthesia, Jane Todd Crawford (1763–1842), while repeating psalms and singing hymns, underwent the first successful elective exploratory laparotomy known in the world. McDowell disliked writing, and so this most famous of operations performed by an early nineteenth-century American physician was not reported in the periodical literature until 1817. It seems unlikely that McDowell was unaware of the significance of his clinical achievement, but for various reasons, he waited until he had completed two further successful ovariotomies in 1813 and 1816, both on African-American women, before finalizing his monumental report. Like many of the most influential contributions to surgery, McDowell's paper in the *Eclectic Repertory* was met with scattered criticisms and aroused little initial interest. Two years later, McDowell reported on another two cases, only one of which was successful. In this second paper he set the tone for what came to be a serious and potentially destructive problem in American surgery, the performance of operations by inexperienced individuals:

> I thought my statement sufficiently explicit to warrant any surgeon's performing the operation when necessary, without hazarding the odium of making an experiment; and I think my description of the mode of operating, and of the anatomy of the parts concerned, clear enough, to enable any good anatomist, possessing the judgment requisite for a surgeon, to operate with safety. I hope no operator, of any other description, may ever attempt it.

American surgery would be plagued for the next century with what McDowell elucidated as this most difficult of professional problems: the performance of surgical operations by individuals who were temperamentally unsuited, educationally ill-prepared, and technically unskilled. McDowell, however, went on to perform at least seven more ovariotomies. He authored no further papers on his "experiments," nor, for that matter, did he ever make any other contributions to the surgical literature. McDowell remained in Danville until his death from "an acute attack of inflammation of the stomach."

In contrast with William Beaumont's reception in North America and Europe, it took some time for McDowell's successes to be accepted in both the Old and New Worlds. A copy of the 1817 report was sent to both his old mentor, John Bell in Edinburgh, and the renowned Philip Syng Physick in Philadelphia. Unfortunately, Bell was in Rome, where he soon died, and McDowell's article ended up in the possession of John Lizars (1794–1860), an ambitious young surgeon who had charge of Bell's patients and correspondence. For seven years Lizars did nothing about the upstart American's offprint, but in 1825 he reported in the British literature his own four cases of "extraction of diseased ovaria." Lizars' paper played an important role in focusing the medical community's attention on the legitimacy of ovariotomy as a valid medical therapy. Other than for Lizars' brief mention of McDowell's achievements, the American received "as scant a courtesy and as shabby a treatment as it was possible to accord him, without resorting at once to his complete obliteration." To what extent McDowell's successes led to Lizars attempts at the "experimental" operation remains conjectural. As far as Physick was concerned, McDowell could hardly have made a worse selection. Unapproachable, unsympathetic, and mechanical in his everyday social graces, the "father of American surgery" must have been leery of the country doctor who was "doing impossible deeds under impossible circumstances." Physick, in his many professional roles, was never known to have mentioned McDowell's intrepidity.

In the United States, little experimental physiologic research was conducted before the Civil War. A scarcity of laboratories and the lack of a cadre of scientists able to perform basic research were the major difficulties. One individual, however, did attain worldwide recognition for a series of experiments conducted in an isolated military outpost in northern Michigan and the wilderness of upstate New York. William Beaumont (1785–1853) was the first to study the gastric juice *in situ*, through a permanent gastrocutaneous fistula. Beaumont was born in Lebanon, Connecticut, and from 1810 to 1812 apprenticed with Benjamin Chandler of St. Albans, Vermont. In December 1812, Beaumont enlisted as a surgeon's mate in the United States Army. After serving for three years as an assistant surgeon in the 6th Infantry Regiment, he entered private general practice near Plattsburgh, New York. Beaumont's experiences in private practice were unsatisfactory, and in late 1819 he reentered the army as a post surgeon and was assigned to Mackinac Island, Territory of Michigan.

On June 6, 1822, a 19-year-old French Canadian hunter, Alexis St. Martin (1803?–1880), was wounded in the upper abdomen by an accidental shotgun blast.

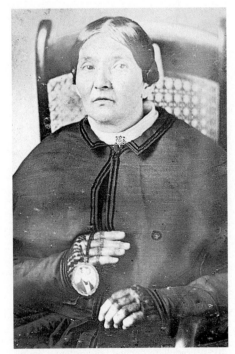

18. Print of a daguerreotype of Jane Crawford (circa 1840). She is holding a medallion portrait of Ephraim McDowell. (*McDowell House, Danville, Kentucky*)

19. In John Collins Warren's masterpiece, *Surgical Observations on Tumours* (1837), not all the cases related to malignant growths. In the chapter on "dermoid tumours" he described an "eiloides" (from the Greek, to coil) excrescence on a 15-year-old girl. Warren stated that no cause was known, "but a scrophulous habit seems to predispose to it." Astonished at its unsightly appearance, Warren "executed its removal." Eighteen months later, the girl suffered a complete recurrence of the neoplasm, and "she died dropsical." Postmortem examination of her body revealed that "the lymphatic glands in the abdomen were greatly increased, forming large tumours throughout the cavity." (*Author's Collection*)

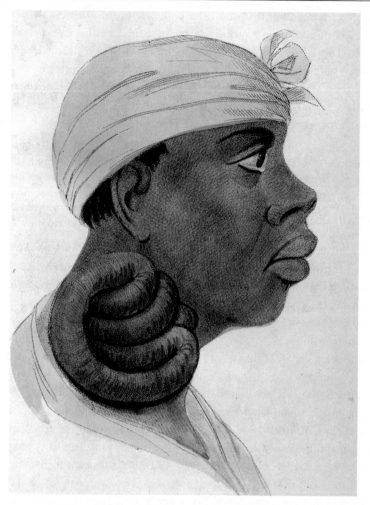

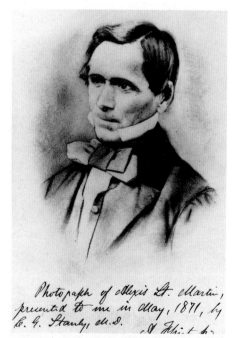

Photograph of Alexis St. Martin, presented to me in May, 1871, by C. G. Stanley, M.D.

20. A crudely retouched but authentic photograph of Alexis St. Martin (circa 1870). This particular image belonged to Austin Flint, Jr. (1836–1915). (*Archives, Washington University School of Medicine*)

The incident occurred just outside the fort where Beaumont was stationed, and his treatment of St. Martin's injury was to have a profound impact on the evolution of medicine and surgery:

> The charge...entered posteriorly, and in an oblique direction, forward and inward, literally blowing off integuments and muscles of the size of a man's hand, fracturing and carrying away the anterior half of the sixth rib, fracturing the fifth, lacerating the lower portion of the left lobe of the lungs, the diaphragm, and perforating the stomach...I saw him in twenty-five or thirty minutes after the accident occurred...a portion of the stomach was lacerated through all its coats, and pouring out the food he had taken for his breakfast, through an orifice large enough to admit the fore finger...
>
> By the 6th of June, 1823, one year from the time of the accident, the injured parts were all sound, and firmly cicatrized, with the exception of the aperture in the stomach and side.... The perforation was about two and a half inches in circumference, and the food and drinks constantly exuded, unless prevented by a tent, compress and bandage.... In the spring of 1824 he had perfectly recovered his natural health and strength; the aperture remained; and the surrounding wound was firmly cicatrized to its edges. In the month of May, 1825, I commenced my first series of gastric experiments on him...
>
> When he lies upon the opposite side, I can look directly into the cavity of the stomach, observe its motion, and almost see the process of digestion-I can pour in water with a funnel, or put in food with a spoon, and draw them out again with a syphon. I have frequently suspended flesh, raw and roasted, and other substances in the hole, to ascertain the length of time required to digest each; and at one time used a plug of raw beef, instead of lint, to stop the orifice, and found that in less than five hours it was completely digested off...

In the fall of 1824, Beaumont sent a complete account of St. Martin's case to Joseph Lovell (1788–1836), Surgeon-General of the United States Army, asking Lovell's opinion of the treatment plan and suggesting that the account be published in some reputable medical journal. Lovell's response was encouraging, and Lovell forwarded the report to the *Medical Recorder*, where it appeared in early 1825.

Through an unfortunate oversight, the article was credited to Lovell; Beaumont's name was not even mentioned. Later that year, a correction was placed in the "Medical Intelligence" section of the journal.

Emboldened by Lovell's interest, Beaumont went on to execute a series of experiments, which continued periodically through 1833. A second paper was published in the *Medical Recorder* in 1826, but it described little in the way of experimentation on gastric physiology. Not until the publication of Beaumont's classic *Experiments and Observations on the Gastric Juice, and the Physiology of Digestion* (1833) would the full extent of his scientific curiosity become known. In its time, Beaumont's work was the most important research ever conducted on the physiology of digestion. The primitive conditions, the lack of laboratory facilities, and the tenacity of Beaumont in completing his tasks made his experiments even more remarkable. In contrast with McDowell's report, which was cynically denied, Beaumont's published monograph was treated with relative indifference in the United States, because few experimental physiologists were able to appreciate the weightiness of his observations. In Europe, conversely, many of the leading scientists praised Beaumont's observations and even had *Experiments and Observations* translated into German (1834).

Beginning to feel isolated in the frontier wilderness, Beaumont requested a transfer and was eventually ordered to St. Louis, where he spent the remainder of his life. He continued as a member of the Army Medical Corps until 1840, when after a disagreement with Surgeon-General Thomas Lawson (1795–1861), Lovell's successor, Beaumont entered private practice. For the next thirteen years, Beaumont practiced general medicine until a fractured hip resulted in his death.

Surprisingly, the first cesarean section reported in the American periodical literature (1828) was performed by the patient herself. Samuel McClellen (1787–1855), a physician in Schodack, New York, was consulted in the case of a 14-year-old quadroon servant girl who had given birth to twins, the first vaginally and the second via a self-inflicted "irregular incision of about four inches in length, extending in a diagonal direction, as respects the abdomen, about two inches above the umbilicus, and an incision of about two inches in length at nearly a right angle with the for-

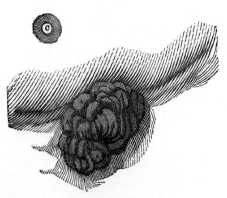

21. One of three engravings from William Beaumont's *Experiments and Observations on the Gastric Juice* (1833), considered the greatest surgical classic of pre-Civil War America. *(Author's Collection)*

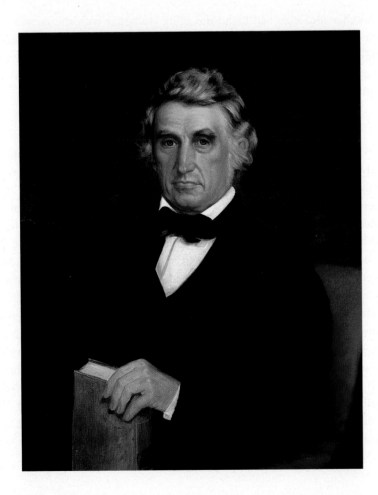

22. William Beaumont (circa 1850) by Chester Harding (1792–1866), one of the country's foremost portraitists of that era. The bulk of Harding's professional life was spent in Springfield, Massachusetts, although he traveled throughout the United States to paint such prominent citizens as John C. Calhoun, Daniel Webster, and William Tecumseh Sherman. The Civil War found Harding in a particularly tragic situation when two of his sons fought for the Union and two for the Confederacy. *(Archives, Washington University School of Medicine)*

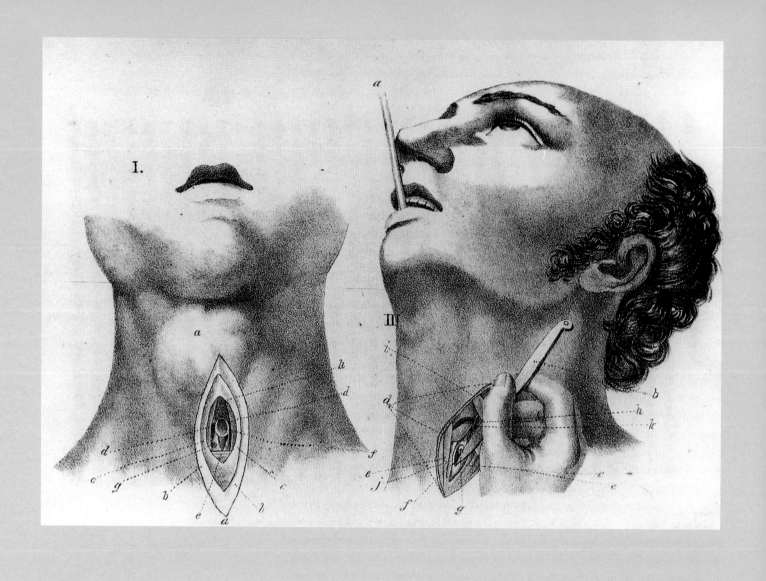

23. Nathaniel Currier (1813–1888), of Currier and Ives fame, was the lithographer for this demonstration of esophagotomy from Augustus Sidney Doane's (1808–1852) *Surgery Illustrated* (1836). *(Author's Collection)*

mer." Another physician had found the ailing youngster with the incision "from which he had extracted a full-grown foetus, that was in part protruded, together with a considerable portion of her intestines." McClellen, the surgeon, reduced the intestines, evacuated blood from the peritoneal cavity, and closed the incision. The young patient recovered without any difficulty.

BIOGRAPHIES OF EARLY FEDERAL-ERA SURGEONS

Ralph Waldo Emerson (1803–1882) contended "there is properly no history; only biography." Yet, biographies, even when combined with interesting case reports, cannot alone constitute an adequate history of American surgery. However, there is an understandable thrill in reading about the surgical exploits of earlier surgeons. Like their European counterparts, nineteenth-century American surgeons were great individual achievers, and it becomes impossible to fully understand the evolution of surgery without knowing something of the surgeons' personal lives. **Mason Cogswell** (1761–1830), valedictorian of Yale College (1780), studied medicine and surgery as an apprentice to his brother James in Stamford, Connecticut. In 1789, Cogswell moved to Hartford, where he remained for the rest of his professional life. The father of a mute child, Cogswell was actively involved in the education of the deaf; it was under his auspices that Thomas Gallaudet (1787–1851) traveled to Europe to acquire the necessary knowledge to found the first American school for the deaf. Known throughout Connecticut as an able surgeon and accoucheur, Cogswell reported the first ligation of the carotid artery in America (1803). When the Medical Institute of Yale College was established in 1812, Cogswell was invited to join the faculty as professor of surgery. He withdrew his name when Nathan

Smith became available for the position. Cogswell remained active in medical politics throughout his professional life and was a founder and later president of the Connecticut State Medical Society.

Nathan Smith (1762–1829), a native of Rehoboth, Massachusetts, studied at Harvard Medical School and graduated in 1790. From 1784 to 1787, Smith had been apprenticed to Joshua Goodhue (1759–1829) of Vermont. Quite early in his career, Smith became interested in medical education, and he convinced the trustees of Dartmouth College of the advisability of establishing a medical school on their campus. With his plans essentially approved, Smith traveled to Edinburgh and London to receive further medical and surgical training and better qualify himself for the task that lay ahead. He returned in the fall of 1797 and shortly thereafter commenced a course of medical lectures at Dartmouth. Smith, serving as the entire faculty, repeated his lecture series for many years. In 1813 he was invited to help organize a medical school at Yale University and become professor of physick, surgery, and obstetrics. Smith also founded the medical department of Bowdoin College in Maine in 1820. Similarly, he was involved with the early organization of the University of Vermont School of Medicine and Jefferson Medical College. He wrote little and left no great textbooks or treatises, although in his *Practical Essay on Typhous Fever* (1842) he did recognize the contagious nature of typhoid. As a surgeon, Smith ranks among the greatest that early America produced. He completed the second reported ovariotomy in America (1822) and the country's first amputation of a knee joint (1825). He published the first description of cleft palate closure in America (1826) and authored a classic account of osteomyelitis (1827). One of his children was the renowned surgeon Nathan Ryno Smith (1797–1877).

Wright Post (1766–1822) apprenticed under Richard Bayley (1745–1801), a physician in New York City. From 1784 to 1786, Post studied in London under John Sheldon (1752–1808). Returning to New York City, Post began to practice as partner with his now father-in-law, Bayley. In 1792, Post was named professor of surgery at Columbia College. A decade later, he transferred to the chair of anatomy in the newly organized College of Physicians and Surgeons, and from 1821 to 1826 served as its president. Post's reputation is largely based on his surgical prowess. As one of the first American students to study under John Hunter, Post was instrumental in introducing Hunterian methods and principles of surgery in the United States. Post was not a prolific writer, but he did provide a few accounts of his surgical cases, which included the country's first ligation of the common carotid artery for aneurysmal disease (1814); a description of the second ligation of the external iliac artery (1814), and the first successful ligation of the subclavian artery in the United States (1817).

John Davidge (1768–1829) studied medicine with James (1739–1819) and William (1751–?) Murray, brothers who practiced in Annapolis. He then attended lectures in Philadelphia, Edinburgh, and Glasgow and received his medical degree from the University of Glasgow in 1793. After practicing briefly in Birmingham, England, Davidge returned to the United States, where he became one of the first attending physicians to the Baltimore General Dispensary. From 1802 to 1807, Davidge offered private lectures in anatomy, surgery, obstetrics, and physiology. In that last year, Davidge, James Cocke (1780–1813) and John Shaw (1778–1809) obtained a state charter for the College of Medicine of Maryland, which the state formally recognized as the medical department of the University of Maryland in 1812. Davidge held the chair of anatomy and surgery from 1807 to 1829, and for many years he also served as dean. As a gift to the institution, he had an anatomical theater built that was subsequently demolished by an antivivisectionist mob. Respected for his surgical skills, Davidge performed an extirpation of the parotid gland (1823), which was the first American case published in the periodical literature. He also authored an important study on femoral fractures (1823).

Philip Syng Physick (1768–1837) was born in Philadelphia and received his college education at the University of Pennsylvania. He apprenticed in the office of

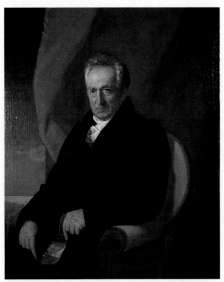

24. Nathan Smith, founder of numerous medical schools and widely recognized surgical innovator, as portrayed by Samuel Finley Breese Morse (1791–1872). Morse, best remembered for inventing the telegraph, was also one of the United States most prominent portrait painters and a photographic pioneer. In March 1839, Morse visited Louis J. M. Daguerre (1789–1851) in Paris and wrote back to his brothers in New York City of Daguerre's wonderful new invention. The brothers, who owned a newspaper, the *New York Observer*, published Morse's letter in their May 18th edition. The accounting represents one of the earliest notices of photography found in the American press. Morse soon opened the world's first photographic portrait studio in New York City in association with a dentist, Alexander Wolcott (1804–1844). Having learned about photography, Morse never painted a portrait again. This portrait of Nathan Smith was presented to Yale University School of Medicine by its class of 1826. *(Yale University, Harvey Cushing/John Hay Whitney Medical Library)*

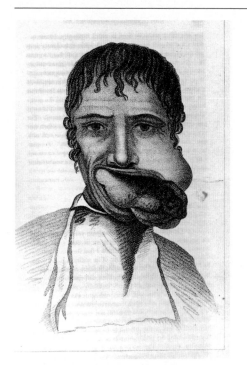

25. Horatio Jameson reported that his patient suffered from a "mouth stuffed in a wonderful manner with a tumour having three lobes...so as to render respiration and deglutition nearly impracticable." Fully described in the *American Medical Recorder* (vol. 4, pages 222–230, 1821), the operation was the first attempt in the country to resect the superior maxillary bone and involved Jameson's initially ligating the common carotid artery so as to reduce blood flow to the tumor. *(Historical Collections, College of Physicians of Philadelphia)*

Adam Kuhn (1741–1817) for three years. In 1789, Physick went to London, where he became a pupil of John Hunter and a house surgeon at St. George's Hospital. Three years later, after attending a year-long course of instruction at the University of Edinburgh, Physick received his medical degree (1792). Shortly after returning to his native city, Physick was appointed surgeon to the Pennsylvania Hospital (1794), and a decade later he was named to the newly established chair of surgery at the University of Pennsylvania. In 1819, he transferred to the professorship of anatomy, where he remained for twelve years until his retirement. In the operating room, his deftness and composure were said to be remarkable, and as a lithotomist, he was probably without equal. Among his most famous surgical cases was the removal of multiple bladder stones from Chief Justice John Marshall (1755–1835) in 1831. Described as a "cold, dyspeptic, pessimistic, unsociable man," Physick remained a creative and respected surgeon, although he never considered himself a competent writer. Often referred to as the father of American surgery, he was the first in the United States to introduce the use of a seton in the treatment of a nonunited fracture (1804) and as therapy for a fracture of the mandible (1822). He authored the first American report of the use of mechanical countertraction for the reduction of a dislocated femur (1805) and the first American report of the surgical repair of an arteriovenous fistula (1805). Physick was responsible for the introduction and popularization of the gastric tube as a means of removing unwanted substances from the stomach (1813), the development of dissolving buckskin and kid ligatures (1816), the surgical creation of a colocutaneous fistula to treat strangulated hernia (1826), and the development of an instrument that was the progenitor of all tonsil guillotines (1828). Physick is eponymically remembered for a proctitis with mucous discharge and burning pain that primarily involves the sacculations or pouches between the rectal valves, and for an iridectomy with the formation of a circular opening.

David Hosack (1769–1835) received his medical degree from the University of Pennsylvania in 1791 after having been a private pupil of both Richard Bayley (1745–1801) and Nicholas Romayne (1756–1817). In 1792 and 1793 Hosack attended medical lectures in Edinburgh, and the following year he traveled to London, where he studied botany under William Curtis and James Smith. Hosack returned to New York City, where he became a partner of Samuel Bard (1742–1821), and from 1796 to 1811 he also served as professor of botany and materia medica at the College of Physicians and Surgeons. During the last four of those years he lectured on surgery. In 1811 he transferred to the chair of theory and practice of physic and clinical medicine, where he remained until 1826, when he helped found the short-lived Rutgers Medical College in New York City. Hosack received an honorary degree in 1818 from Union College in Schenectady, New York, the nation's first nondenominational college. Although Hosack originated no new surgical procedures, he was considered an outstanding clinical surgeon. In 1798, he introduced to American surgeons the method of treating hydrocele by injection. A decade and a half later, Hosack authored an article describing the importance of leaving wounds open to the air to promote healing Contained within this paper was the first case report in an American medical periodical of a mastectomy (1814). He was the founder and first editor of *The Medical and Philosophical Register* (1810). Always involved in civic affairs, Hosack was a staunch supporter of the New York Public Library, the New York Historical Society, and the New York Horticultural Society. Among his many nonprofessional interests, Hosack was an internationally known botanist and founded the Elgin Botanic Garden in Hyde Park.

Valentine Seaman (1770–1817) was born in North Hempstead, New York, and apprenticed with Nicholas Romayne of New York City. Seaman served for a year as a resident physician at the city's almshouse and completed his education when he received his medical degree from the University of Pennsylvania (1792). From 1792 until his death, Seaman was in private practice in New York City and served on the staff at the New York Hospital. Among his numerous contributions to American medicine were the use of vaccination for smallpox, about which he wrote *A Discourse*

Upon Vaccination (1816), and authoring the first work on midwifery in the United States, *The Midwives Monitor, and Mothers Mirror* (1800). Seaman was well known for his surgical skills and wrote the earliest known surgical formulary for a civilian hospital in the United States, *Pharmacoepia Chirurgica in Usum Nosocomii Novi Eboracencis, Being An Account of the Applications and Formulae…Employed in the Clinical Practice of the Surgical Department of the New-York Hospital* (1811). Among his non-medical political interests was the liberation of all slaves.

Horatio Jameson (1778–1855) initially studied medicine with his father and went into practice at the age of 17. Not content with the level of his education, Jameson moved to Baltimore and attended lectures at the College of Medicine. He received his M.D. in 1811 after submitting a graduation thesis on "The supposed powers of the uterus." Jameson remained in Baltimore, where he became an influential member of the community and a respected surgeon. In 1827 he was one of the founders of Washington Medical College and then served as professor of surgery. Eight years later he accepted a professorship and the presidency of the Ohio Medical College at Cincinnati, but his wife's ill health caused their return to Baltimore less than a year later. Jameson is best remembered surgically for the first known report of a resection of the superior maxillary bone (1821); a ligation of the superior thyroid artery in an attempt to cure a pathologic process of the thyroid gland (1822); the first known attempt in America, albeit unsuccessful, to remove a cancerous uterus via the vagina (1824); a detailed report on the surgical treatment of urethral stricture (1824); and an important paper on various methods used to control hemorrhage (1827).

John Collins Warren (1778–1856) was the eldest son of John Warren. After receiving an undergraduate education at Harvard College, Warren served a short apprenticeship with his father. Warren studied further in London and Paris and received his formal medical degree from Edinburgh in 1802. In that year, he returned to Boston because of his father's illness and assumed his private practice. From 1806 to 1815, Warren served as adjunct professor in anatomy and surgery at Harvard Medical School. He was promoted to full professor in 1815 and remained

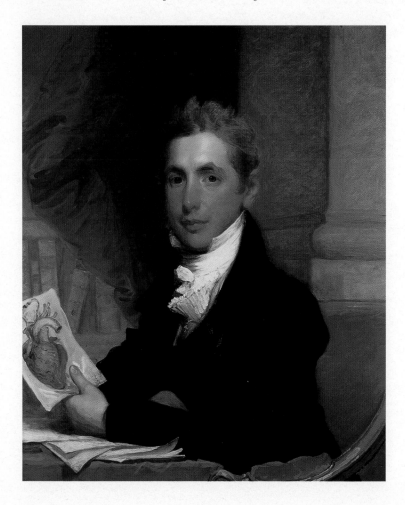

26. In 1805, Gilbert Stuart (1755–1828) moved to Boston, where he resided for the remainder of his distinguished career as one of the country's most respected portraitists. Two years later, he painted a youthful John Collins Warren, then 29 years of age. *(Private Collection, The Francis A. Countway Library of Medicine)*

inspiration of the said term which will be one year from the date hereof.

In Witness whereof as well the said William Beaumont as the said Alexis St. Martin have executed set their respective hands & seals the day & year first herein written in the presence of each other & of the subscribing witnesses hereto & in the presence of Jonathan Douglass Woodward Esquire the subscribing notary Public —

J. Douglas Woodward

Thomas Green —

Benj. J. Moores

Wm Beaumont —

his
Alexis X St. Martin
mark

United States of America
State of New York
Clinton County ss. I the Subscriber a Notary Public in and for said State duly Commissioned and sworn and authorised in all respects to act as such Notary Public do hereby Certify and attest that the said William Beaumont and Alexis St. Martin who are both personally known to me, executed signed Sealed and delivered the above instrument in writing in my presence, and in the presence of each other & in the presence of the above named subscribing Witnesses who also subscribed their names as Witnesses to the due execution of said instrument in my presence, & the presence of each other, and also in the presence of both of said parties. In testimony whereof & for the due manifestation whereof I have hereunto Signed my name and affixed my seal of office as Notary Public at Plattsburg aforesaid this nineteenth day of October in the year of our Lord one thousand Eight hundred and thirty two.

J Douglas Woodward
Notary Public

Rec'd on the above contract forty dollars being the amount advanced on the same by William Beaumont.

his
Alexis X St. Martin
mark

Witness J Douglas Woodward
Notary Public

Rec'd on the above, forty dollars April 23d 1833

his
Alexis X St. Martin
mark

Rec'd November 7th 1833. Sixty Seven dollars on The above Contract —

his
Alexis X St. Martin
mark

Witness
S. Beaumont

in that position until 1846, when he retired. Warren was a founder of the Massachusetts General Hospital (1821) and the *New England Journal of Medicine and Surgery* (1811), and he was instrumental in establishing the American Medical Association (1847). He will always be remembered as having performed the first surgical operation in which ether anesthesia was administered (1846) and for writing two monographs on the subject: *Etherization with Surgical Remarks* (1848) and *Effects of Chloroform and of Strong Chloric Ether, as Narcotic Agents* (1849). Among his other important surgical works were the country's first surgical textbook on surgical oncology, *Surgical Observations on Tumours* (1837), and a lengthy orthopedic treatise, *Dislocation of the Hip Joint* (1824). Warren authored several important case reports, including one on the third known ligation of the femoral artery in the United States (1806), the second report of repair of a strangulated hernia (1807), the first description of an accidental dislocation of the lens of the eye (1813), a report on the treatment of neuralgia by division of nerves (1817), an important paper on cleft palate repair (1828), the first published account of air embolism (1832), and a report on excision of the clavicle (1833). Warren devoted much time to studying comparative anatomy and paleontology. From these efforts he wrote three nonsurgical works: *A Comparative View of the Sensorial and Nervous Systems in Men and Animals* (1822), *The Mastodon Giganteus of North America* (1852), and *Remarks on Some Fossil Impressions in the Sandstone Rocks of the Connecticut River* (1854).

Joseph Parrish (1779–1840) was an apprentice to Caspar Wistar and also received his medical degree from the University of Pennsylvania in 1805. From 1806 to 1822, Parrish was a surgeon to the Philadelphia Almshouse, where he gave a series of lectures on surgical topics. In 1816 he succeeded Philip Syng Physick as surgeon at the Pennsylvania Hospital. Parrish was associated with the founding of Wills Eye Hospital and was an active member of the College of Physicians of Philadelphia. His major academic effort was the country's first full-length text on the treatment of hernias, *Practical Observations on Strangulated Hernia, and Some of the Diseases of the Urinary Organs* (1836), and he also served as editor for the first American edition of William Lawrence's (1783–1867) *Treatise on Ruptures* (1811). In addition, Parrish wrote a paper that was the earliest in American periodical literature to deal extensively with breast carcinoma (1828). Parrish's son, Isaac (1811–1852), became a well-known surgeon in his own right, and one of Joseph's great-grandsons was the renowned artist Maxfield Parrish (1870–1966).

Amos Twitchell (1781–1850) was born in Dublin, New Hampshire, and apprenticed with Nathan Smith. In addition, Twitchell received an M.D. from Dartmouth Medical School in 1811, after having been in practice for almost five years. In 1810, Twitchell settled in Keene, New Hampshire, and spent the remainder of his professional life there. Described as an "indefatigable worker, with a practice so extensive that he had an arrangement of post-horses at country inns," Twitchell was best known for his surgical skills. Although offered professorships in surgery at Dartmouth, Vermont, and Brunswick Medical Colleges, he declined them all. Twitchell is believed to have been the second surgeon in the world to ligate the common carotid artery successfully, for the victim of a gunshot accident in 1807. Since Twitchell was not interested in writing case reports, this technical feat was not reported until 1842. Twitchell was a founder of the American Medical Association and president of the New Hampshire Medical Society (1829), and he was elected to honorary membership in the Massachusetts Medical Society (1838).

John Syng Dorsey (1783–1818) was the nephew of Philip Syng Physick, with whom he apprenticed. While working in his uncle's office, Dorsey also attended medical lectures at the University of Pennsylvania, where he received his medical degree (1802). In 1803, he traveled to London, where he studied with John Hunter and Everard Home (1756–1832), and he later spent time in Paris. After returning to the United States, Dorsey commenced private practice in Philadelphia and in 1807 was named adjunct professor of surgery at his alma mater. Shortly thereafter, he was appointed surgeon at the Pennsylvania Hospital. He undertook his new duties with a

27. *(facing page)* One of the most intriguing pieces of surgical Americana: the last pages of a contract dated October 19, 1832, between William Beaumont and Alexis St. Martin (his "X" mark), granting the use of the latter's stomach for experimental purposes. At the bottom, are St. Martin's signed acknowledgments of payments, amounting to $107. This item of ephemera is unique because it represents the first documented instance in the United States when concern for patient welfare was demonstrated, and acknowledgment of human experimentation obtained, via formal written informed consent. *(Archives, Washington University School of Medicine)*

thoroughness and ability that soon made him popular among his students. In 1810, Dorsey edited the American edition of Samuel Cooper's (1780–1848) *Dictionary of Practical Surgery*. Two years later, Dorsey reported the country's first successful ligation of the external iliac artery for an expanding aneurysm. Physick was professor of surgery at the University of Pennsylvania, but he never became a competent writer. He therefore asked Dorsey to organize his lectures into the form of a surgical handbook, and in response to this request, Dorsey authored the two-volume *Elements of Surgery* (1813), the first systematic treatise on surgery to be written by an American surgeon. The *Elements* was a publishing success. This octavo-sized book went through three more editions and was even reprinted in Edinburgh and used as a surgical textbook at that university. In 1813, the medical faculty at the University of Pennsylvania was made up of six professorial chairs, which were occupied by Caspar Wistar (1761–1818) (anatomy); Benjamin Rush (1745–1813) (medicine); Benjamin Smith Barton (1766–1815) (materia medica); John Redman Coxe (1773–1864) (chemistry); Philip Syng Physick (surgery, with Dorsey as adjunct professor); and Thomas Chalkley James (1766–1835) (midwifery). In 1816, Dorsey occupied the chair of materia medica, succeeding Barton. Wistar died unexpectedly in January 1818. The chair of anatomy was suddenly vacated, and competition for Wistar's successor became keen. No doubt William Shippen and Wistar had made it famous, and the competition was partly due to the almost $10,000 a year it would bring its holder in addition to earnings from practice. After much discussion and many arguments between the medical faculty and the trustees over attempts by the university's administration to control professorial appointments, Dorsey was elected as a compromise candidate in May 1818. His success was short-lived: within a few days of delivering his inaugural anatomical lecture in November he succumbed to typhus.

George Bushe (1793–1836) was born in Ireland and received his medical and surgical training in Europe. He came to America in 1818, at the request of the recently formed faculty from Rutgers Medical College, to serve as professor of anatomy. Bushe was widely regarded as a surgeon and gave daily office lectures on various surgical topics for almost three years. Bushe's most impressive text was *A Treatise on the Malformations, Injuries, and Diseases of the Rectum and Anus* (1837), the first book to deal solely with rectal surgery in the United States. He also authored various case reports, including the country's third known common iliac ligation (1832), surgical treatment of phymosis and hypospadias (1831), and the treatment of cleft palate (1835). Bushe died of tuberculosis shortly after completing his rectal surgery text, but prior to its being published.

J. Kearny Rodgers (1793–1851) studied medicine with Wright Post and graduated from the College of Physicians and Surgeons in New York City in 1816. After serving as a house surgeon in the New York Hospital, Rodgers traveled to London to complete his medical training. On returning to New York City, he became one of the founders of the New York Eye Infirmary. In 1818, he was appointed demonstrator of anatomy at his alma mater, and four years later, surgeon to the New York Hospital. His most important paper presented the earliest successful wiring of a nonunited fracture of the humerus to be found in the American periodical literature (1827). Rodgers also reported the first attempt at ligation of the left subclavian artery within the scalenus muscle for treatment of an aneurysm (1846).

John Godman (1794–1830) was born at Annapolis and apprenticed with William Luckey of Elizabethtown, Pennsylvania, and John Davidge in Baltimore. While living in Baltimore, Godman attended lectures at the University of Maryland School of Medicine and received his medical degree in 1818. He began practice in New Holland, Pennsylvania, but soon moved to a small village near Baltimore in anticipation of obtaining an appointment at the University of Maryland. When the position did not materialize, Godman moved to Philadelphia, where he lectured on anatomy and physiology. In 1821 he was asked by Daniel Drake (1785–1852) to accept the chair of surgery in the Medical College of Ohio in Cincinnati. After the move to Ohio, political difficulties arose among the school's faculty and Godman was forced to resign. Subsequently, he established the *Western Quarterly Reporter of Medical, Surgical and Natural Science* (1822), the first medical journal west of the Alleghenies. Returning to Philadelphia, Godman assumed charge of the Philadelphia School of Anatomy and began elaborate anatomical investigations. From these studies two books were written: *Anatomical Investigations, Comprising Descriptions of Various Fasciae of the Human Body* (1824) and *Contributions to Physiological and Pathological Anatomy* (1825). The latter work was the first text written by an American surgeon to deal with pathological anatomy. The *Anatomical Investigations* contains his description of the extension of the pretracheal fascia into the thorax and on to the pericardium, now known as Godman's fascia. In 1826, Godman was offered the chair of anatomy at Rutgers Medical College, where he remained for two years. Miliary tuberculosis had taken its toll on Godman, and in 1828 he traveled to the West Indies to seek a cure. Having received minimal health benefits, Godman resettled in Germantown, Pennsylvania, where he finally completed work on his massive three-volume *American Natural History* (1826–1828) before succumbing to his disease. Godman was amazingly prolific, having translated Jacques Coster's (1795–1868) *Manual of Surgical Operations* (1825), and edited the American edition of Astley Cooper's (1768–1841) *Treatise on Dislocations and on Fractures of the Joints* as well as John (1763–1820) and Charles Bell's (1774–1842) fifth American edition of *The Anatomy and Physiology of the Human Body* (1826).

George McClellan (1796–1847) received his undergraduate education at Yale College (1816). He apprenticed with John Syng Dorsey and received his medical degree from the University of Pennsylvania (1819), having written a graduation thesis on the surgical anatomy of arteries. In 1821, McClellan founded and taught at the Institution for the Diseases of the Eye and Ear. Four years later, he and several fellow Philadelphia physicians founded the Jefferson Medical College. McClellan served as professor of surgery from 1826 until 1838, and in the process acquired a rather extensive private practice. Political machinations brought about the firing of the entire founding faculty of Jefferson Medical College, so that in 1839, McClellan was forced to obtain a charter for another school, the medical department of Pennsylvania College, having an affiliation with Gettysburg College. The school survived up to the time of the Civil War. McClellan was one of the country's pioneers in the extirpation of the parotid gland, which he reported for the first time in 1826. After his death, his son John (1823–1874) posthumously published McClellan's lectures, notes, and other material in the *Principles and Practice of Surgery* (1848), which, although an utter failure financially and professionally, contained an excellent description of shock.

Jacob Randolph (1796–1848) received his medical degree from the University of Pennsylvania (1817). He completed his medical education in Scotland and France and after returning home began his practice in Philadelphia. Randolph married Philip Syng Physick's eldest daughter and with his father-in-law's support was appointed surgeon to the Almshouse Infirmary (1830). From 1840 to 1842, Randolph lived in Europe and attended surgical operations at various Parisian hospitals. During this time he was offered the professorship of operative surgery at Jefferson Medical College but declined it, as it would have necessitated his immediate return. After holding the position of lecturer of clinical surgery, Randolph was eventually appointed to the professorship of clinical surgery at the University of Pennsylvania (1847). Highly regarded as an expert lithotomist, Randolph introduced the lithotrite into American surgery in 1831, and his 1834 article on lithotripsy set the tone for bladder surgery in the country during the mid-nineteenth century. His most extensive literary effort was the lengthy biography *A Memoir of the Life and Character of Philip Syng Physick* (1839).

1845	1850	1855	1860	1865	1870	1875	1880	1885

DAILY LIFE

First baseball game at Elysian Field in Hoboken, New Jersey *(1846)*
Adhesive postage stamps *(1847)*
Women's Rights convention at Seneca Falls, New York *(1848)*
California Gold Rush *(1849)*
Fugitive Slave Act *(1850)*
YMCA organized in Boston *(1851)*
Yale and Harvard hold first intercollegiate rowing race *(1852)*
Baltimore & Ohio Railroad *(1853)*
Paper collars for shirts are invented *(1854)*
First oil business in the United States, the Pennsylvania Rock Oil Company *(1855)*
Western Union Company *(1856)*
American Chess Association *(1857)*
Macy's department store *(1858)*
John Brown raids Harper's Ferry *(1859)*
Pony Express *(1860)*
Telegraph wires strung between New York City and San Francisco *(1861)*
Gatling gun patented *(1862)*
Roller skating introduced *(1863)*
Knights of Pythias *(1864)*
River steamer *Sultana* explodes at Memphis, killing
1,400 people *(1865)*

U.S.A. POPULATION

1850 = 23 million,
including 3.2 million
slaves
1860 = 31 million

HISTORY AND POLITICS

Mexican War commences *(1846)*
Battle of Buena Vista *(1847)*
Treaty of Guadalupe Hidalgo *(1848)*
U.S. Department of Interior created *(1849)*
Compromise of 1850 *(1850)*
Maine enacts prohibition law *(1851)*
Franklin Pierce elected President *(1852)*
Gadsen Purchase *(1853)*
Kansas–Nebraska Act *(1854)*
U.S. Court of Claims established *(1855)*
Pro-slavery legislature accepted in Kansas Territory *(1856)*
Dred Scott decision *(1857)*
Lincoln–Douglas debates *(1858)*
Kansas ratifies antislavery constitution *(1859)*
Abraham Lincoln elected President *(1860)*
Seven seceding states form the Confederate States of America *(1861)*
Battle between the *Monitor* and the *Merrimack* *(1862)*
Emancipation Proclamation *(1863)*
General William Tecumseh Sherman's march through
Georgia to the sea *(1864)*
Assassination of President Lincoln *(1865)*

FAMOUS AMERICANS

HEROES, POLITICIANS, AND STATESMEN

J. B. "Champ" Clark *(1850–1921)*
Charles Bonaparte *(1851–1921)*
Charles W. Fairbanks *(1852–1918)*
James P. Clarke *(1854–1916)*
Jacob S. Coxey *(1854–1951)*
Thomas R. Marshall *(1854–1925)*
Robert M. LaFollette *(1855–1925)*
James S. Sherman *(1855–1912)*
Thomas E. Watson *(1856–1922)*
Woodrow Wilson *(1856–1924)*
William Howard Taft *(1857–1930)*
George W. Goethals *(1858–1928)*
Theodore Roosevelt *(1858–1919)*
John L. Sullivan *(1858–1918)*
George W. Wickersham *(1858–1936)*
Billy the Kid *(1859–1881)*
Charles B. Aycock *(1859–1912)*
Walter C. Camp *(1859–1925)*
Charles Comiskey *(1859–1931)*
Victor L. Berger *(1860–1929)*
William Jennings Bryan *(1860–1925)*
Charles Curtis *(1860–1936)*
John J. Pershing *(1860–1948)*
Albert Beveridge *(1862–1927)*
Nicholas Butler *(1862–1947)*
Charles Evans Hughes *(1862–1948)*
Connie Mack *(1862–1956)*
William Borah *(1865–1940)*
Warren Harding *(1865–1923)*
Charles Dawes *(1865–1951)*

SCIENTISTS AND INVENTORS

George Westinghouse *(1846–1914)*
Alexander Graham Bell *(1847–1922)*
Thomas Alva Edison *(1847–1931)*
Luther Burbank *(1849–1926)*
Albert Michelson *(1852–1931)*
George Eastman *(1854–1932)*
Charles Tainter *(1854–1940)*
John H. Hammond *(1855–1936)*
Percivall Lowell *(1855–1916)*
William Burroughs *(1857–1898)*
Frank Sprague *(1857–1934)*
Nikola Tesla *(1857–1943)*
William Bayliss *(1860–1924)*
Leo H. Baekeland *(1863–1944)*

1845	1850	1855	1860	1865	1870	1875	1880	1885

FAMOUS AMERICANS

THEOLOGIANS AND PHILOSOPHERS

John Dowie *(1847–1907)*
Anna Shaw *(1847–1919)*
Charles Taze Russell *(1852–1916)*
William "Billy" Sunday *(1862–1935)*
George Santayana *(1863–1952)*
John Raleigh Mott *(1865–1955)*

EDUCATORS, SCHOLARS, AND REFORMERS

Carry Nation *(1846–1911)*
Jacob Riis *(1849–1914)*
Samuel Gompers *(1850–1924)*
Lafcadio Hearn *(1850–1904)*
Felix Adler *(1851–1933)*
Mary E. Lease *(1853–1933)*
Eugene Debs *(1855–1926)*
Louis Brandeis *(1856–1941)*
Booker T. Washington *(1856–1915)*
Ida Tarbell *(1857–1944)*
John Dewey *(1859–1952)*
Jane Addams *(1860–1935)*
Alfred North Whitehead *(1861–1947)*
Bernard Berenson *(1865–1959)*

AUTHORS

Joel Chandler Harris *(1848–1908)*
James Lane Allen *(1849–1925)*
Frances E. H. Burnett *(1849–1924)*
Sarah Orne Jewett *(1849–1909)*
Edward Bellamy *(1850–1898)*
Howard Pyle *(1853–1911)*
David Belasco *(1853–1931)*
L. Frank Baum *(1856–1919)*
Kate Douglas Wiggin *(1856–1923)*
Hamlin Garland *(1860–1940)*
Owen Wister *(1860–1938)*
Margaret Saunders *(1861–1947)*
Albert Paine *(1861–1937)*
Edith Wharton *(1862–1937)*

VISUAL ARTISTS

William Chase *(1846–1916)*
Ralph Blakelock *(1847–1919)*
Albert Pinkham Ryder *(1847–1917)*
William Michael Harnett *(1848–1892)*
William Merritt Chase *(1849–1916)*
Abbott Thayer *(1849–1921)*
John H. Twachtman *(1853–1902)*
Otto Bacher *(1856–1909)*
John Singer Sargent *(1856–1925)*
Childe Hassam *(1859–1935)*
Maurice Prendergast *(1859–1924)*
Joseph Pennell *(1860–1926)*
Anna Mary "Grandma" Moses *(1860–1961)*
Frederic Remington *(1861–1909)*
Arthur B. Davies *(1862–1928)*
Robert Henri *(1865–1929)*

PERFORMING ARTISTS

Clarence Eddy *(1851–1937)*
Arthur Foote *(1853–1937)*
George Chadwick *(1854–1931)*
John Philip Sousa *(1854–1932)*
Edgar Stillman Kelley *(1857–1944)*
Victor Herbert *(1859–1924)*
Edward MacDowell *(1861–1908)*
Harrison Fiske *(1861–1942)*
Loie Fuller *(1862–1962)*
Ethelbert Nevin *(1862–1901)*
Horatio Parker *(1863–1919)*
Clyde Fitch *(1865–1909)*

BUSINESSMEN AND INDUSTRIALISTS

Edward H. Harriman *(1848–1908)*
Nathan Strauss *(1848–1931)*
Louis Comfort Tiffany *(1848–1933)*
Henry Clay Frick *(1849–1919)*
Frank W. Woolworth *(1852–1919)*
King Gillette *(1855–1932)*
Andrew Mellon *(1855–1937)*
Elmer Sperry *(1860–1930)*
William Bausch *(1861–1944)*
Julius Rosenwald *(1862–1932)*
Charles Schwab *(1862–1939)*
Thomas C. Du Pont *(1863–1930)*
Henry Ford *(1863–1947)*
William Randolph Hearst *(1863–1951)*

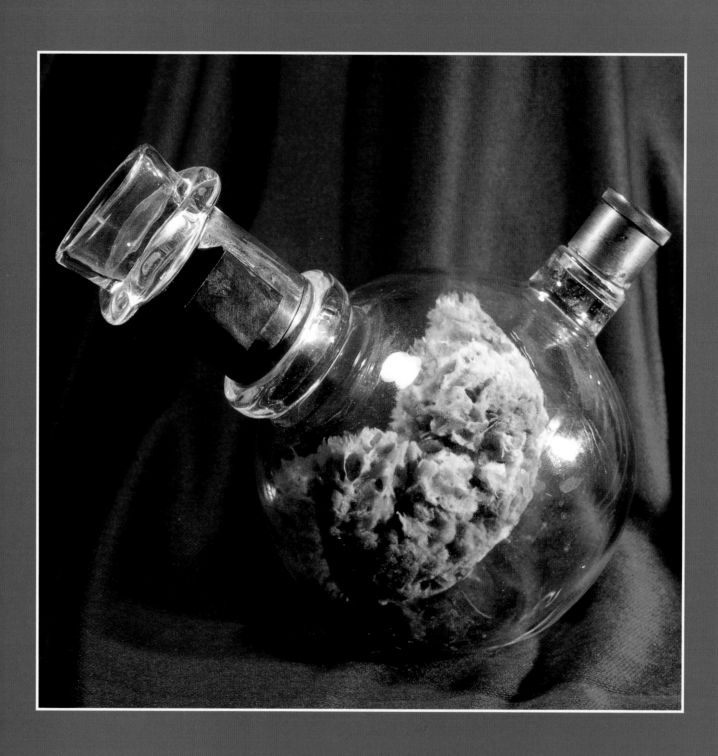

CHAPTER 4

SURGICAL ANESTHESIA
1846–1860

B y the mid-1840s, the "romantic" period of American medicine was coming to an end. Imagination and pseudoscientific hypotheses, spurred on by laissez-faire attitudes in socioeconomics and previously unassailable concepts of Jacksonian democracy and personal freedoms, were being replaced by a growing skepticism of old-fashioned medical remedies. A unique philosophy of therapeutic nihilism was slowly being incorporated into American medical beliefs as health care providers sought out new therapeutic cures. Patients were beginning to reject the older "heroic therapies" of bloodletting, diuretics, emetics, sweating, and physicking (i.e., cathartics, laxatives, and purgatives), and these ineffectual analeptics would no longer serve as the signposts of a sophisticated clinical practice.

With scientific progress seemingly assured, the question of implementing adequate professional standards became most pressing. There were virtually no legal restrictions on the delivery of health care in most states. Whether Americans had an inherent "natural" right to practice medicine, as exemplified by widespread medical cultism, was put into a more sober perspective when the physician-essayist Oliver Wendell Holmes (1809–1894) wrote in 1844, "good intentions constitute no ground for the privilege of endangering human life." Still, in the two decades prior to the Civil War, a wave of states repealed their licensing laws, causing the field of medical practice to be thrown open to virtually all citizens who wished to call themselves doctors.

THE AMERICAN MEDICAL ASSOCIATION AND
ITS COMMITTEE ON SURGERY

In 1845, alarmed at the growing societal acceptance of "quack" and "irregular" physicians in conjunction with the deteriorating situation of American medical education, the leadership of the Medical Society of the State of New York called for a national convention of medical societies and medical schools. In May 1847, delegates to this too long delayed meeting assembled at the Academy of Natural Sciences in Philadelphia, and the American Medical Association was founded. With so many individuals representing such a wide variety of allopathic health-care and related institutions, the American Medical Association was regarded as democratic in design and national in authority, albeit elitist in its membership. From its very inception, the association was viewed by its founders as the only possible mechanism for bringing about higher standards for preliminary medical education and improved clinical training. Within a few years, these goals would be supplemented by growing national dissatisfaction with lax medical standards, unrestricted licensing, and the vagaries of health-care sectarianism.

Much of this discontent was reflected in a growing spate of medical malpractice claims. Between 1846 and 1860, physicians became so alarmed at the increase in

1. (*facing page*) William Morton's original ether inhaler, which he can clearly be seen holding in Robert Hinckley's painting, "The First Operation Under Ether" (*pictured on pages 90 and 91*). (*Warren Museum, Harvard Medical School*)

malpractice suits that Alden March, professor of surgery at the Albany Medical College in upstate New York, declared, "legal prosecutions for malpractice in surgery occur so often that even a respectable surgeon may well fear for the results of his surgical practice." One Ohio-based "surgeon" told of four legal cases in four different Ohio counties in one week. It was a common assumption that some practitioners were closing the surgical side of their practices because of the legitimate possibility of malpractice inquiries. No less an authority than Daniel Drake, writing in his *Practical Essays on Medical Education and the Medical Profession in the United States*, alluded to the fact that fewer medical school graduates practiced surgery because of the perceived threat of legal penalties.

To a certain extent, this diminution of surgical services was not unwelcome. The technical expertise of many physician-surgeons was poor at best, and when this lack of skill was combined with an inadequate knowledge of surgical anatomy, postoperative results were too often disappointing. Of course, these horrendous clinical outcomes were also related to a lack of understanding of antisepsis and aseptic surgical techniques, compounded by a rudimentary knowledge of surgical anesthesia. On a practical side, realistic complaints were also being voiced regarding the legal inconsistency of expecting surgeons to be responsible for an accurate knowledge of human anatomy while withholding the means of obtaining that education. Partially in response to such difficulties, in the 1830s and 1840s various state legislatures began passing acts calling for an increased use of human dissection to be incorporated into the standard medical curriculum.

Among the dozen or so "organizing zealots" behind the founding of the American Medical Association, several individuals, regarded more as surgeon than as physician, were at the forefront. This bias was particularly evident in those men who held the position of president during the organization's first twenty years. In chronological order of their incumbency, they were Alexander Stevens (1789–1869), John Collins Warren (1778–1856), Reuben Mussey (1780–1866), Jonathan Knight (1780–1864), Charles Pope (1818–1870), Paul Eve (1806–1877), Alden March (1795–1869), and Samuel Gross (1805–1884). For American surgery, the founding of the association would prove to be a significant event in the evolution of profes-

2. Daguerreotypes of four American physician-surgeons (circa 1845–1847) holding surgical instruments and medical paraphernalia. By the mid- to late 1840s, the use of the daguerreotype was reaching its zenith in the United States, and occupational portraiture was not uncommon. One doctor *(this page, left)* poses with a saw and bones, illustrating the classic metaphor "sawbones," a slang term used to denote a physician or surgeon. The army surgeon, wearing a uniform of Mexican War vintage with plumed hat and officer's sword *(facing page right)*, demonstrates his soldierly work by having a field operating kit placed on the table beside him. *(Courtesy of Stanley B. Burns, M.D., and The Burns Collection and Archive)*

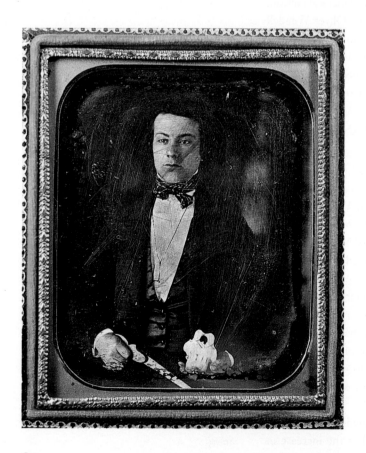
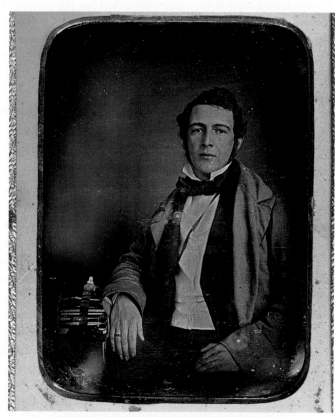

sionalization. This was especially evident when within a year of the American Medical Association's organization, standing committees were established on medical education, medical sciences, medical literature, obstetrics, practical medicine, publications, and surgery.

The Committee on Surgery, as the country's first nationally organized and recognized surgical council, was a necessary presence if surgeons were ever to be regarded as a professional class within American society. The committee was immediately assigned the task of preparing a report on all the important improvements in the management of surgical diseases in the country during the past year. In a bow to technical realities, the written report succinctly stated, "Neither brilliant discoveries nor any extraordinary improvements in surgery marked the past year."

The influence of the American Medical Association on the development of surgery became a steadying force, witnessed by an 1859 resolution calling for the "scientific sessions" to be divided into four sections so as to "facilitate the transaction of business: 1. Anatomy and Physiology. 2. Chemistry and Materia Medica. 3. Practical Medicine and Obstetrics. 4. Surgery." The Section on Surgery, which superseded the Committee on Surgery, underwent changes from time to time depending on the interests of the members and on scientific advances. Thus, both the Committee and the Section provided the earliest opportunities for the discussion of wide-ranging surgical topics before large groups of physicians from all areas of the country. Long before elite surgical societies of a nationwide scope (e.g., American Surgical Association, American Gynecological Association) were organized, the American Medical Association and its surgical forums demonstrated the importance of such yearly gatherings. Beginning in 1851, scientific contributions were sought by a special American Medical Association committee for the expressed purpose of awarding a yearly prize to the best report. The first paper on a surgical topic to garner this distinction was Washington Atlee's (1808–1878) ninety-nine-page monograph, *The Surgical Treatment of Certain Fibrous Tumours of the Uterus, Heretofore Considered Beyond the Resources of the Art* (1853).

In 1848, when the Committee on Surgery stated that there had been few improvements in the art of surgery over the past year, the members could easily be

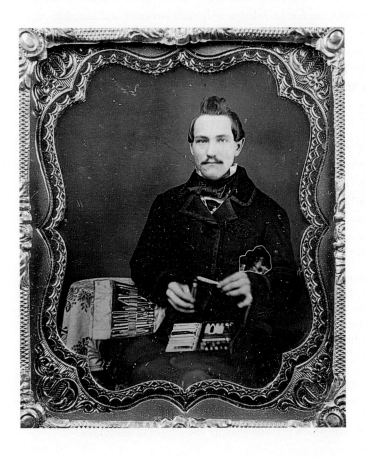

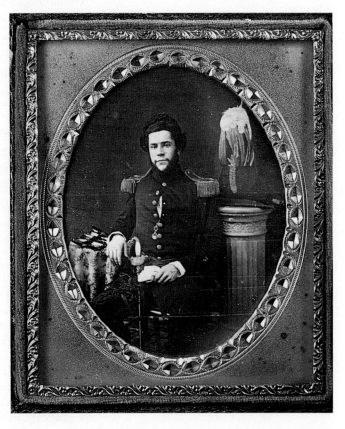

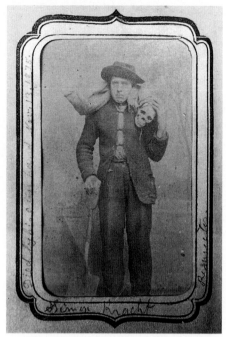

3. By the 1840s, various state legislatures had begun to pass acts allowing human dissection. Still, cadavers remained scarce, and clandestine exhumations of recently buried bodies continued as a thriving business. This photograph (circa 1850s) of Simon Kracht is from a medical class picture album of the Louisville Medical College. Handwritten notes label the gentleman as a "resurrector." In a bizarre final act to what must have been a disquieting existence, Kracht "died by his own hand, Nov. 13, 1875." *(Collection of Alex Peck, Antique Scientifica)*

accused of carrying out one of the more egregious oversights in the annals of American surgery. It had only been a short eighteen months since the introduction of the first fundamentally major contribution by American physicians to the world of medicine: the implementation of inhalational surgical anesthesia. Even a century and a half later, the introduction of general anesthesia remains our country's greatest gift to the healing arts. Perhaps the committee members should be excused for their omission because they could not be expected to understand the ultimate effect that "painless surgery" would have on establishing surgical operations as a valid therapeutic measure. Nor could the committee members be asked to comprehend the role that "surgery without pain" would come to have in the evolutionary process of professionalization. Strangely, a large and intelligent body of the medical community, including some of the country's most eminent surgeons, considered the "anesthesia question" unsettled for a number of years. Still, it would be incorrect to infer from the Committee's statement that surgical anesthesia had not already had a strong impact on the art and craft of surgery. Some three decades later, Henry J. Bigelow (1818–1890), professor of surgery at Harvard Medical School, placed the discovery in more proper perspective:

> What surgeons and patients needed was an inevitable, complete, and safe condition of insensibility; and this they were soon to have. The moment arrived. In three months from October, 1846, ether anaesthesia had spread all over the civilized world. No single announcement ever created so great and general excitement in so short a time. Surgeons, sufferers, scientific men, everybody, united in simultaneous demonstration of heartfelt mutual congratulation.

Since the end of the nineteenth century, it has been recognized that four fundamental prerequisites were required for the surgical operation to be regarded as a viable therapeutic procedure: first, a knowledge of human anatomy; second, a method for controlling hemorrhage and maintaining intraoperative hemostasis; third, anesthetics to permit pain-free procedures; and fourth, an understanding of the nature of infection and methods for achieving antiseptic and aseptic operating room conditions. The first two prerequisites were essentially solved in sixteenth-century Europe. The work of such individuals as the great anatomist Andreas Vesalius began to elucidate our knowledge of human structure and function, while Ambroise Paré showed that in performing an amputation it was more efficacious to ligate individual blood vessels than to attempt to control hemorrhage by means of mass cauterization. The third desideratum would not be settled until the mid-nineteenth century in America!

THE PREANESTHETIC ERA

Since time immemorial, the inability of surgeons to complete pain-free operations had been among the most terrifying of medical problems. In the preanesthetic era, surgeons were forced to be more concerned about the speed with which an operation was completed than the clinical efficaciousness of their dissection. In a similar vein, patients refused or delayed surgical operations for as long as possible in order to avoid the personal horror of experiencing the surgeon's knife. John Collins Warren (1842–1927) described an amputation of the preanesthetic era:

> It was the custom to bring the patient into the operating room and place him upon the table. The surgeon would stand with his hands behind his back and would say to the patient, "Will you have your leg off, or will you not have it off?" If the patient lost courage and said, "No," he had decided not to have the leg amputated, he was at once carried back to his bed in the ward. If, however, he said "Yes," he was immediately taken firmly in hand by a number of strong assistants and the operation went on regardless of whatever he might say thereafter. If his courage failed him after this crucial moment, it was too late and no attention was paid to his cries of protest. It was found to be the only practicable method by which an operation could be performed under the gruesome conditions which prevailed before the advent of anesthesia.

Numerous efforts had been made throughout the past to relieve the discomfort of surgical operations, and the ultimate conquest of pain is one of the most important and stirring accomplishments in the evolution of American surgery. Before the advent of inhalation anesthesia, various pain-reducing measures were proposed, one of the most important being mesmerism, a method of quasi-hypnosis named after the German physician Friedrich Mesmer (1734–1815). The possibility of using mesmerism for surgical anesthesia was actively fostered by several European surgeons. In the United States, Louis Dugas (1806–1884), professor of physiology and surgery at the Medical College of Georgia, was its most vociferous proponent. In 1845, he authored a report concerning a patient who was mesmerized twice, first for a simple mastectomy and again for the removal of a recurrent tumor of the chest wall. In some instances, mesmerism proved quite successful in reducing pain, but on the whole the method was a failure.

SULFURIC ETHER AND NITROUS OXIDE

By the early 1830s, both sulfuric ether and nitrous oxide had been discovered in Europe. In 1832, the American physician Samuel Guthrie (1782–1848) stumbled on the modern method of making chloroform by distilling alcohol with chlorinated lime. "Laughing gas" parties and "ether frolics" soon came into vogue, particularly in America. Young people were amusing themselves with the pleasant side effects of these new compounds. Throughout the 1830s and 1840s, itinerant "professors" of chemistry would travel to villages, towns, and cities to lecture on the new gases and demonstrate their exhilarating features. Often, the most important part of such presentations consisted of having members of the audience inhale sulfuric ether vapor

4. A rare "laughing gas" broadside advertising a public exhibition of the use of nitrous oxide (1845). *(Warsaw Collection of Business Americana, Archives Center, Smithsonian Institution, Museum of American History)*

5. This intriguing papier-mâche mannequin served American physician-surgeons as an anatomical model. At a time when human cadavers were scarce and European wax models were too expensive to import, such a crude educational aid became crucial in a physician-surgeon's training. Fully numbered, with an accompanying guide to identify specific body structures, this frightening figure was constructed in the region of Massillon, Ohio (circa 1848). *(Collection of Alex Peck, Antique Scientifica)*

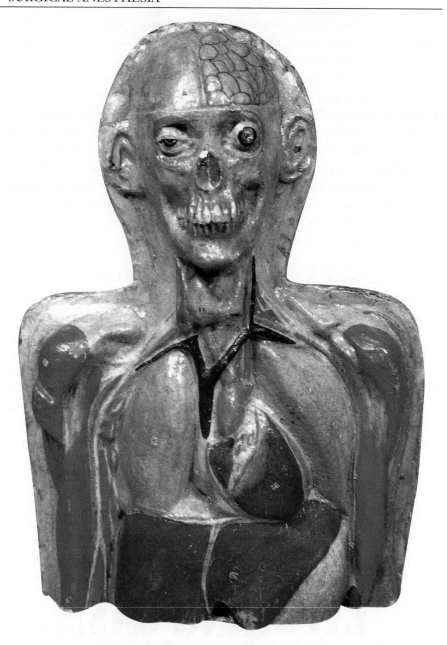

or nitrous oxide. These willing individuals lost their sense of equilibrium and acted with an apparent loss of inhibition.

It soon became evident to various American physician-surgeons and dentists that the mind-altering aspects of sulfuric ether and nitrous oxide might also reduce pain and that the gases could therefore be used in surgical operations and tooth extractions. By December 1844, a Connecticut dentist, Horace Wells (1815–1848), had evidently grasped the concept of inhalation anesthesia. Specifically, this occurred when Wells attended a public demonstration of the effects of "laughing gas" at Union Hall in Hartford. Sam Cooley, a drugstore clerk who was seated beside Wells, volunteered to breathe the gas. While under its influence Cooley injured his knee, but he seemed unaware of the accident until the effects of the nitrous oxide had worn off. Wells, as a perceptive observer, immediately understood the significance of Cooley's feeling no pain despite having a severe laceration. The following morning, Wells persuaded one of his dental colleagues to extract one of Wells' teeth while under the effects of nitrous oxide. On recovery, Wells supposedly exclaimed, "It is the greatest discovery ever made. I didn't feel as much as the prick of a pin."

Satisfied that nitrous oxide could be used safely, Wells traveled to Boston to demonstrate the finding to William Morton (1819–1868), his former student and partner. To further publicize his understanding of the effects of "laughing gas," Wells, through Morton's social and professional connections, met with John Collins

Warren (1778–1856), professor of surgery at the Massachusetts General Hospital, and asked for permission to demonstrate his claims. In January 1845, in front of a class at Harvard Medical School, Wells administered nitrous oxide to a schoolboy as an anesthetic for tooth extraction. Supposedly the level of anesthesia was too light, and the youngster screamed out. Wells was labeled a fake, and his career never recovered from the embarrassing episode. In an incident of history gone awry, Well's young patient would later admit that he actually suffered no conscious pain and did not know when the extraction occurred. Soon-to-be-learned scientific facts would show that his outcry was simply one of the common side effects of inhaling nitrous oxide gas. Individuals groaned, screamed, or exhibited agitated behavior while remaining insensible to pain. However, the skeptical Harvard audience could not know this, and in his confusion and panic, Wells did not realize it either.

Prior to Wells' discomfiting experience, Morton had become acquainted with Charles Jackson (1805–1880), one of the most eccentric and bizarre of all personalities connected with the discovery of surgical anesthesia. Jackson, an 1829 graduate of Harvard Medical School, was more mineralogist and geologist than physician. His involvement with surgical anesthesia dates as far back as 1841, when he inhaled nitrous oxide for the first time. In 1844, Jackson proposed to the areas' dentists that nitrous oxide be used to relieve an acute toothache. By September 1846, Jackson had become knowledgeable about sulfuric ether and suggested to Morton that sulfuric ether mixed with air might make a more suitable anesthetic agent than plain nitrous oxide. Morton proceeded to experiment with this new concept. He, in turn, persuaded John Collins Warren to let him administer the substance to another surgical patient. On October 16, 1846, Morton gave his first public demonstration of the effects of the then "anonymous" liquid on a patient from whom Warren removed a small, congenital vascular tumor of the neck. After the operation, Warren, greatly impressed with the new discovery, uttered the five most famous words in American surgery: "Gentlemen, this is no humbug." The following day, Morton repeated his demonstration, again successfully, on a patient for whom George Hayward (1791–1863) was removing a small lipoma of the upper arm.

Precisely because both demonstrations were such unqualified triumphs, Morton was initially unwilling to disclose the nature of his new agent. At the same time, because of his desire to obtain a patent, he decided to permit no more public trials for a period of three weeks. From several names suggested for the drug, Morton chose the descriptive designation "Letheon," a term derived from the title of the mythical river of forgetfulness (Lethe) in Greek mythology, which flowed through Hades and caused loss of memory in anyone who drank from it. In early November 1846, Henry Bigelow (1818–1890), a young entrepreneurial Boston surgeon, began to force the issue of further demonstrations by telling Morton that his achievement would have no meaning unless the compound was used during the performance of a "capital" or major operation. Bigelow already suspected that the preparation was sulfuric ether, and he so advised Morton. Subsequently, on November 6th, Morton again called on Hayward and asked if he might use his preparation on a patient for whom Hayward was preparing to perform an amputation of the thigh. Hayward agreed, but with the stipulation that Morton must tell the surgeons what the vapors were. Morton acquiesced, and the following day, after Morton had rendered the patient unconscious and insensitive to pain, Hayward successfully completed the amputation.

Elated at the course of events, Morton authorized Bigelow to make a detailed public announcement of his discovery, which the latter did in a paper read before the Boston Society of Medical Improvement on November 9th. A slightly revised version of Bigelow's report was then published in the *Boston Medical and Surgical Journal* on November 18th; it represents the first formal announcement of the discovery of surgical anesthesia to the medical profession.

Few discoveries have been so readily accepted as inhalation anesthesia. News of the momentous event spread rapidly throughout the United States and Europe: a

6. "The First Operation Under Ether." Robert Hinckley (1853–1941) was a little-recognized American artist who studied in Paris and even spent some time as the roommate of John Singer Sargent (1856–1925). This massive canvas (96 by 115 inches) is an authentic summary of the whole series of events that transpired between October 16 and November 7, 1846, when the world was introduced to sulfuric ether as a viable anesthetic agent. Hinckley went to great lengths to confirm the many individuals who claimed to be present during those dramatic days and to portray their faces accurately. Having taken more than ten years to finish the painting (1882–1893), Hinckley was personally devastated by the lack of critical acclaim following its completion. He was never able to sell it, nor was any reputable museum willing to accept it as part of a permanent collection. The disillusioned artist even contemplated cutting up the canvas. In 1903, after lengthy negotiations, the Executive Committee of the Boston Medical Library decided to acquire the painting as a gift from Hinckley. *(The Francis A. Countway Library of Medicine)*

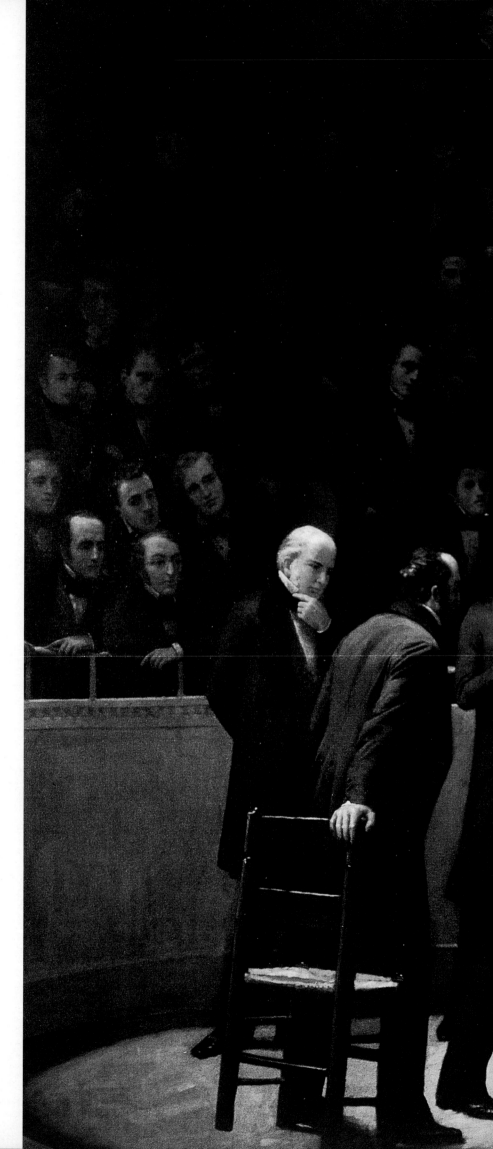

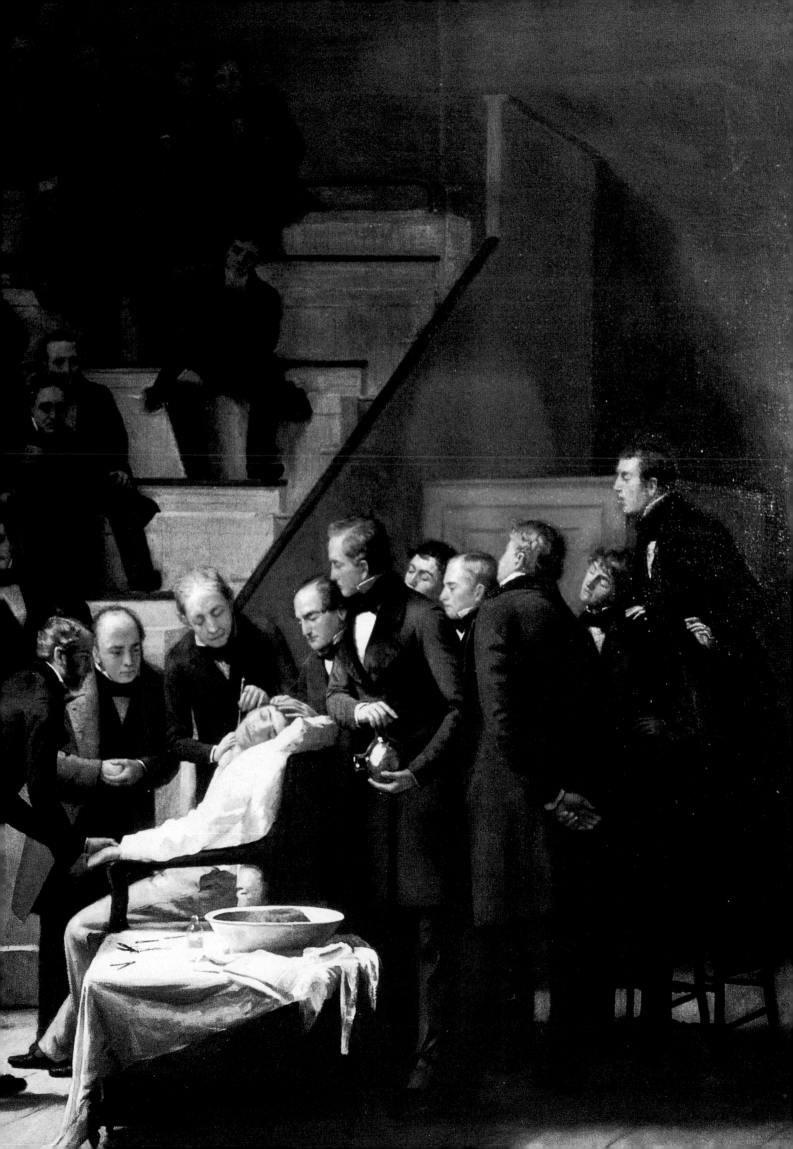

new era in the history of surgery had begun. Within a few months after the first public demonstration in Boston, ether was used in hospitals throughout the world. Yet, no matter how much it contributed to the relief of pain during surgical operations and decreased the surgeon's *angst*, the discovery did not immediately further the scope of elective surgery. Such technical triumphs awaited the recognition and acceptance of antisepsis and asepsis. Anesthesia helped make the illusion of surgical cures more seductive, but it could not bring forth the final prerequisite: the all-important hygienic reforms.

On December 8, 1846, Valentine Mott removed a "cluster of tumefied glands from the right axilla" of a woman after she had inhaled sulfuric ether. This first use of inhalation anesthesia in New York City was soon followed by a spate of reports from throughout the country. By mid-January 1847, Daniel Brainard (1812–1866), professor of surgery at Rush Medical College in Chicago, was presenting his series of "etherial vapor" patients, and in March of the same year Jonathan Allen (1787–1848) wrote about the use of sulfuric ether in the rural setting of Middlebury, Vermont.

Despite the apparent speed with which surgical anesthesia spread throughout the country, there were various pockets of resistance. For instance, the editor of the influential *Medical Examiner* commented, "We are persuaded that the surgeons of Philadelphia will not be seduced from the high professional path of duty into the quagmire of quackery by this will-o'-the-wisp. We...regret that the eminent men of...Boston should have...set so bad an example to their younger brethren." A writer in *The Annalist*, a New York City medical journal, declared in January 1847, "The last special wonder has already arrived at the natural term of its existence, and the interest created by its first advent has in a great measure subsided. It has descended to the bottom of that great abyss which has already engulfed so many of its predecessor novelties." In view of such comments, it is no wonder that the first use of sulfuric ether at the University of Pennsylvania did not occur until October 1847, a full year after its initial demonstration in Boston, and that the board of managers of Philadelphia's venerable Pennsylvania Hospital barred the utilization of surgical anesthesia for a full seven years.

7. The personal surgical kit of John Peter Mettauer, who is remembered for his use of metallic sutures in the first successful repair in America of a torn rectovaginal septum (1833) and perineum (1847). Examples of Mettauer's metallic sutures are visible on the piece of paper in the lower left. Also of note is the ivory-handled rectal and vaginal speculum of the Weiss type. *(Mütter Museum, College of Physicians of Philadelphia)*

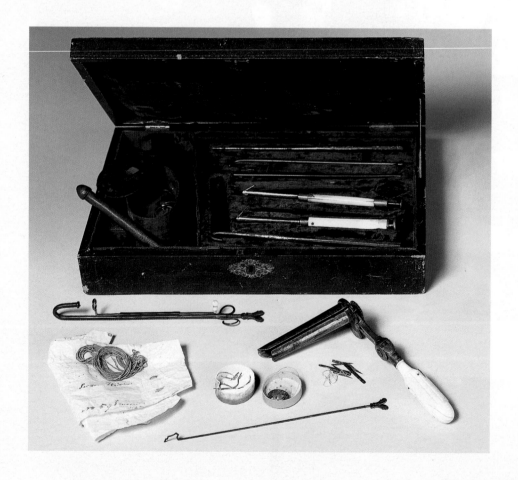

Although most physicians eventually incorporated inhalation anesthesia into their clinical practices, the frequency with which any particular provider employed the new pain-killer increased only gradually between 1846 and the mid-1870s. A doctor's demographics (i.e., age, location, education and training, professional associations, therapeutic sect) all influenced how frequently that physician decided to prescribe anesthesia. Accordingly, "irregular" doctors and other alternative healers, who generally prided themselves on the benignity of their botanical and other mild therapies, initially utilized anesthetics less often than did the more established allopathic practitioners.

Despite their differences with orthodox surgeons, practitioners of sectarian surgery, including the importunate Benjamin Hill, slowly became enamored with surgical anesthesia. Writing in his *American Eclectic System of Surgery* (1850), the first nonallopathic surgical work to be published in America, Hill noted that "surgical operations have, of late, been rendered much less formidable by the discovery that a state of insensibility to pain can be artifically induced." But Hill railed against calling the anesthetic agent "by the quack-like name of 'letheon,' for the purpose of making money" when "any one can prepare the article for himself from the common sulphuric ether of the shops." Socioeconomics, as the driving force of American medicine, was slowly and inevitably becoming a barrier between orthodox and sectarian surgeons.

THE CONTROVERSY OVER ANESTHESIA

Clearly, more than the simple fact of its newness caused initial concerns over the use of inhalation anesthesia. The first decade's reports of morbidities and mortalities associated with surgical anesthesia were truly fearsome. As early as mid-1848, Henry Bigelow wrote a series of articles detailing the supposed dangers of anesthetic agents, which were later reprinted as an influential monograph, *Ether and Chloroform; Their Discovery and Physiological Effects* (1848). He also prepared a report for presentation to members of the Committee on Surgery of the American Medical Association. Eighteen months had elapsed since Morton's electrifying event. Some physicians considered the question settled. These healers felt the dangers of anesthesia to be so inconsiderable, in contrast to its benefits, that this justified its use for any surgical operation. Other surgeons were of the opinion that anesthetic agents should be strictly limited to severe "capital" operations and their general employment should be discouraged. A small percentage of health care providers were adamant that anesthetics were dangerous and "harmful in their tendency." There can be no more colorful quote regarding the question of utilization than that of William Atkinson, a physician and first president of the American Dental Association:

> I think anesthesia is of the devil, and I cannot give my sanction to any Satanic influence which deprives a man of the capacity to recognize the law! I wish there were no such thing as anesthesia! I do not think men should be prevented from passing through what God intended them to endure.

Bigelow's report expressed pride in the fact that anesthesia was an American contribution. But the five committee members investigating the controversy, George Norris (1808–1875), Isaac Parrish (1811–1852), John Watson (1807–1863), Abel L. Peirson (1794–1853), and Hugh H. McGuire (1801–1875), refused to take a definite stand. Their findings were issued in the first volume of the *Transactions of the American Medical Association* (1848) and are especially valuable for the accompanying tables, which detail the initial use of inhaled sulfuric ether and chloroform at the Massachusetts General Hospital, the New York Hospital, the Clinic of the University of Pennsylvania, and Jefferson Medical College.

In defense of the new discovery, John Collins Warren authored the one-hundred-page *Etherization with Surgical Remarks* (1848), in which he provides a fascinating account of the initial use of sulfuric ether in surgery and proposes for the first time the employment of ether "in regard to animal vivisection." In his *Etherization,*

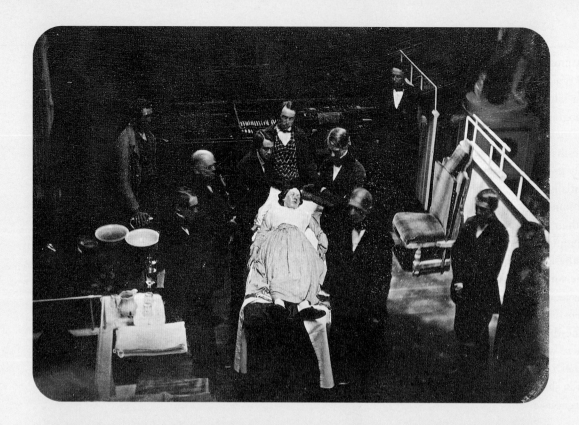

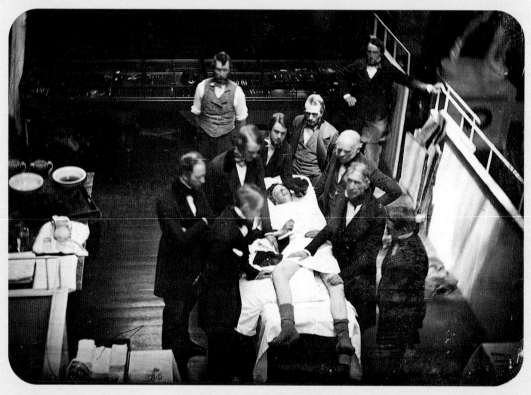

8. A few months after the value of sulfuric ether had been conclusively established, several whole-plate daguerreotypes (March 1847) of surgical operations were taken at the Massachusetts General Hospital by daguerreotypists Albert S. Southworth (1811–1894) and Josiah J. Hawes (1808–1901). Since operative surgery was a relatively rare event, and the taking of a daguerreotype required the setting up of photographic equipment, the occasion had to be scheduled in advance. These daguerreotypes (whether they were taken on the same day remains open to historical inquiry) show two different patients: one presumably before ether induction (the surgeons are milling about, the patient stares straight ahead, and the anesthesiologist has not approached the table) *(top left)*, the second following ether induction (an ether sponge is used rather than Morton's original glass inhaler, and the patient's head lies listlessly to the side) *(bottom left and right)*, and after his operation was completed (blood stains on the sheet, bandage on the posterior right leg, and the patient turned over to facilitate operative exposure) *(top right)*. Several of the surgeons are identifiable, although they move about from picture to picture. Using the bottom photographs as a frame of reference, the six surgeons standing three each on the side of the operating table are Samuel Parkman (1816–1854), Henry G. Clark (1804–1892), and Jonathan M. Warren *(left side, top to bottom)*, and Solomon D. Townsend (1793–1869), John C. Warren, and Henry J. Bigelow *(right side, top to bottom)*. Other individuals in the photographs are unidentified, although most are

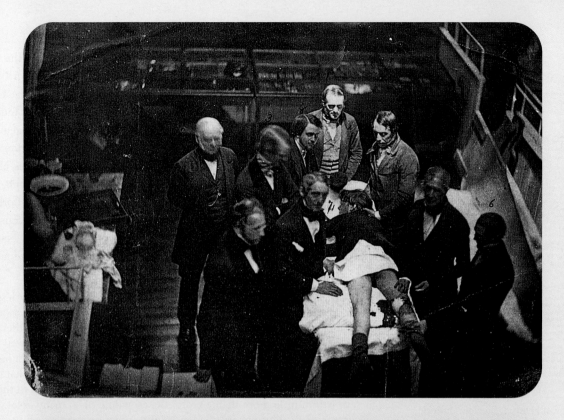

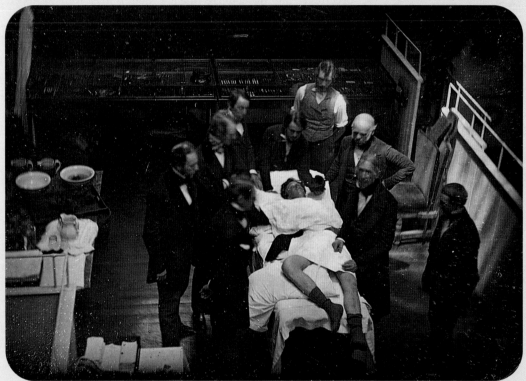

house surgeons, one of whom has acted as anesthesiologist, and one is a ward tender. At the back in all three photographs are glass cases containing surgical instruments. On the left side is a table with towels, basins, and ether equipment. The seats for spectators lie directly in the foreground and face the surgeons. The beginnings of the railing that surrounds the spectator section of the amphitheater can be seen in the lower left-hand corner. A stretcher for removing the unconscious patient is noted on the right side in the top right daguerreo-

type. It is assumed that the chair on the right side in all the photographs was the one in which Gilbert Abbott sat when he underwent his momentous excision of a small vascular tumor of the neck on October 16, 1846. In the extreme right upper corner is a large statue of the Greek god Apollo (a replica of the Apollo Belvedre from the Vatican Museum), the god of music, poetry, prophecy, and medicine. Contrary to what has been written in the past, these famous daguerreotypes of early "ether operations" are not reenactments or staged

recreations. They are actual surgical operations and represent some of the earliest uses of documentary photography in the United States. They are shown together for the first time. *(facing page, top and bottom: Courtesy of the Fogg Art Museum, Harvard University Art Museums, Loan from Massachusetts General Hospital Photo Collection) (this page, top: The Francis A. Countway Library of Medicine) (this page, bottom: Collection of the J. Paul Getty Museum, Malibu, California)*

THE

BOSTON MEDICAL AND SURGICAL JOURNAL.

Vol. XXXV.   Wednesday, November 18, 1846.   No. 16.

INSENSIBILITY DURING SURGICAL OPERATIONS PRODUCED BY
INHALATION.

Read before the Boston Society of Medical Improvement, Nov. 9th, 1846, an abstract having been
previously read before the American Academy of Arts and Sciences, Nov. 31, 1846.

By Henry Jacob Bigelow, M.D., one of the Surgeons of the Massachusetts General Hospital.

[Communicated for the Boston Medical and Surgical Journal.]

It has long been an important problem in medical science to devise some method of mitigating the pain of surgical operations. An efficient agent for this purpose has at length been discovered. A patient has been rendered completely insensible during an amputation of the thigh, regaining consciousness after a short interval. Other severe operations have been performed without the knowledge of the patients. So remarkable an occurrence will, it is believed, render the following details relating to the history and character of the process, not uninteresting.

On the 16th of Oct., 1846, an operation was performed at the hospital, upon a patient who had inhaled a preparation administered by Dr. Morton, a dentist of this city, with the alleged intention of producing insensibility to pain. Dr. Morton was understood to have extracted teeth under similar circumstances, without the knowledge of the patient. The present operation was performed by Dr. Warren, and though comparatively slight, involved an incision near the lower jaw of some inches in extent. During the operation the patient muttered, as in a semi-conscious state, and afterwards stated that the pain was considerable, though mitigated; in his own words, as though the skin had been scratched with a hoe. There was, probably, in this instance, some defect in the process of inhalation, for on the following day the vapor was administered to another patient with complete success. A fatty tumor of considerable size was removed, by Dr. Hayward, from the arm of a woman near the deltoid muscle. The operation lasted four or five minutes, during which time the patient betrayed occasional marks of uneasiness; but upon subsequently regaining her consciousness, professed not only to have felt no pain, but to have been insensible to surrounding objects, to have known nothing of the operation, being only uneasy about a child left at home. No doubt, I think, existed, in the minds of those who saw this operation, that the unconsciousness was real; nor could the imagination be accused of any share in the production of these remarkable phenomena.

I subsequently undertook a number of experiments, with the view of ascertaining the nature of this new agent, and shall briefly state them,
16

9. The first page of Henry J. Bigelow's historic paper, which announced to the professional world the discovery of sulfuric ether as a true anesthetic for surgery. It was published in the *Boston Medical and Surgical Journal* (vol. 35, pages 309–317, 1846), and Bigelow had an exact copy of the text reprinted in a local lay newssheet, the *Boston Daily Advertiser,* on the following day, November 19th. *(Historical Collections, College of Physicians of Philadelphia)*

Warren explicitly noted that "another year was necessary to give us the means of judging fully and definitively on the merits of the ether practice." In November 1847, James Young Simpson (1811–1870), professor of obstetrics at the University of Edinburgh, substituted chloroform for ether. American surgeons, intrigued by what were considered the lesser side-effects of the newer anesthetic agent, initially met Simpson's discovery with enthusiasm. But their eagerness to use chloroform was soon tempered by reports of intraoperative deaths. As surgical deaths blamed on anesthesia mounted, Warren was forced to write a second monograph, *Effects of Chloroform and of Strong Chloric Ether as Narcotic Agents* (1849), in an effort to make both the public and the surgical community better aware of what he considered to be the dire consequences of using chloroform as an inhalation agent. Nationalism aside, Warren, ever mindful of his status in the anesthesia debate, had an obvious bias toward ether:

> The introduction of chloroform produced an excitement scarcely less than that of the discovery of the narcotic effect of ether.... We were soon awakened from our dreams of the delightful influence of the new agent, by the occurrence of unfortunate and painful consequences, which had not followed in this country on the practice of etherization. The profession were led to hesitate, many of them to suspend the use of chloroform.... Now, it appears that no less then ten well-authenticated fatal cases have presented themselves to the public eye within little more than a year...the crowding of so many cases of rare occurrence into the compass of a few months must form an epoch in the history of this constitutional sympathy.

One indication of surgeons' reactions to the discovery of anesthesia is evidenced in the textbooks of the time. Because there was such bitter initial controversy over inhalation anesthesia, it is not surprising that chapters on "diminishing pain during operations" did not appear in print until mid-1848. Fitzwilliam Sargent (1820–1889), a Philadelphia surgeon and father of the painter John Singer Sargent (1856–1925), included a six-page discussion of anesthesia in his *On Bandaging and Other Operations of Minor Surgery,* the first American textbook on surgery to even broach the subject. Sargent was far from an accepting advocate:

> These agents have been employed to relieve pain in all sorts of operations...they have been administered by the ignorant as well as by the learned, and without any discrimination of cases. It is not at all surprising, therefore, that in many instances injurious, and sometimes fatal, consequences have ensued.... It should be recollected, that the mere performance of an operation, with comparative freedom from suffering to the patient and with satisfaction to the surgeon, is but one step towards the cure of the affection for which the operation is performed: the treatment of the patient subsequently is a matter of equal importance; and with reference to this part of the surgeon's duty, any cause which disturbs the healthy play of important functions, whether it be the impression of too intense pain, or of too powerful narcotic agents, is to be regarded as an evil.

Not until 1852 was a more sanguine viewpoint expressed by an orthodox surgeon, when Henry H. Smith (1815–1890), who in three years would be named William Gibson's successor as professor of surgery at the University of Pennsylvania, authored his massive *A System of Operative Surgery: Based Upon the Practice of Surgeons in the United States* (1852). This comprehensive volume would also prove important to the photographic history of American medicine because it was the first American surgical textbook to have illustrations based on daguerreotypes. In addition, Smith provided an extremely detailed introductory section describing the progress of American surgical history, a bibliographical index of American surgical writers with a list of their works by subject, and an extensive alphabetical list of American surgeons including the titles of their most important papers. No other mid-nineteenth-century textbooks by American surgeons present so much information about the era's technical advances in surgery. Smith writes of surgical operations, pain, and anesthesia:

In the majority of cases, the creation of pain by any operation can only be regarded, at the present time, as both unnecessary and injurious. The surgeon should therefore prevent it, and endeavor to save his patient the excitement arising from suffering, by resorting to the use of Anaesthetics.... Let him...blunt the nerves of sensation either by partial or entire Etherization; and as its safety has been widely tested, philanthropy and that desire to ameliorate the sufferings of mankind, which is the true basis of sound practice, demand that neither prejudice nor ignorance of its effects should longer prevent its employment by every operator.

Also, the same year that Smith penned this paean, a series of inflammatory articles on anesthesia appeared in the prestigious *American Journal of the Medical Sciences* by John Porter (?–1864), an army surgeon. He offered the opinion that "by the inhalation of ether, in the most cautious manner...the blood is poisoned, the nervous influence and muscular contractility is destroyed or diminished, and the wound is put in an unfavourable state for recovery...in consequence...hemorrhage is much

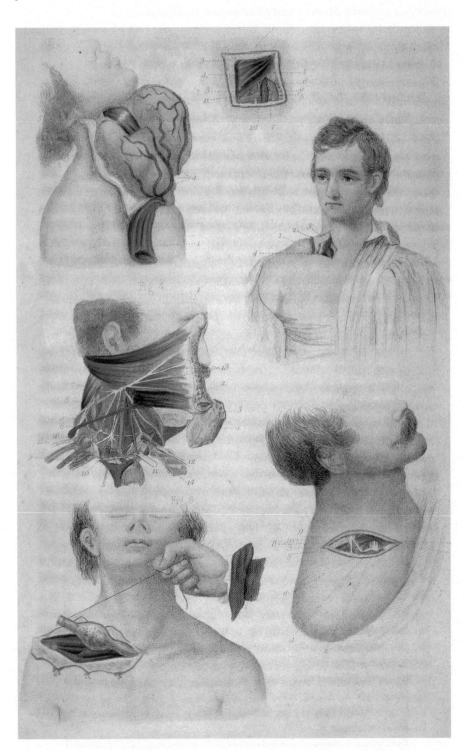

10. Henry Smith's *System of Operative Surgery* (1852) was a massive compendium of various surgical operations. Like Pancoast's *Treatise* of a decade earlier, a limited number of Smith's texts were produced with "colored to life" plates. The coloring helped highlight certain aspects of surgical technique, in this particular case "operations practiced at the lower portion of the neck." Dedicated to Charles Pope (1818–1870), professor of surgery at St. Louis University, Smith's volume is particularly important to the photographic history of American medicine because it was the country's first surgical textbook to have illustrations based on daguerreotypes. *(Author's Collection)*

more apt to occur, and union by adhesion is prevented." Medical journals became flooded with reports, and arguments continued for the next decade over the benefits of ether versus chloroform and the relative overall safety of anesthesia. As surgeon's experience with inhalation anesthesia increased, especially during the Civil War, many of those supposed dangers were disproved or found to be minimal.

THE GRADUAL ACCEPTANCE OF ANESTHESIA

The most important early advance in surgical anesthesia occurred in 1868, when Edmund Andrews (1824–1904), professor of the principles and practice of surgery at Chicago Medical College, reported on the concept of providing oxygen and an anesthetic agent simultaneously to a patient. Andrews stated that "the best proportion of oxygen will be found to be one-fifth volume, which is the same as in the atmospheric air…. The oxygen mixture will enable us to anaesthetize a patient for the longest as well as for the shortest surgical operations." This breakthrough idea set the stage for the further scientific advancement of inhalation anesthesia.

A decade later, Laurence Turnbull (1821–1900), an aural surgeon at Jefferson Medical College, authored the country's first full-length work to discuss anesthesia and its application in depth. Like most of the early monographs on anesthesia, the authors were usually physicians with an active interest in surgery. The concept of a physician who specialized solely in the administration of anesthesia would not come about until the beginning of the twentieth century. Turnbull's *Advantages and Accidents of Artificial Anaesthesia* (1878) and Henry Lyman's (1835–1904) *Artificial Anaesthesia and Anaesthetics* (1881) were of a practical nature and represent the first generation of true anesthesia textbooks in the United States.

The lives of many of the principals involved in the initial discovery of surgical anesthesia ended in tragedy. Morton and Jackson became embroiled in a dispute concerning each other's priority in the events of 1846. When Morton applied for a patent on ether anesthesia, he recognized his debt to Jackson by consenting to take the patent out under both their names. In January 1847, Morton was chagrined to find that Jackson had submitted to the French Academy of Sciences a claim in which the former's name was never mentioned. This was the beginning of a bitter feud that

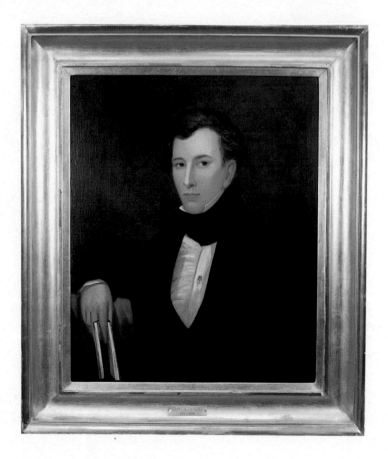

11. A recently identified portrait of Crawford Long (1815–1878). There are few authentic images of Long, and this painting is believed to have been completed soon after he completed his course work at the University of Pennsylvania School of Medicine in 1839. Long spent the first eighteen months following his graduation working in various hospitals in New York City. Therefore, it is more than likely that the unidentified American folk-artist was from that area of the country. *(The Francis A. Countway Library of Medicine)*

consumed both men for the remainder of their lives. Multiple lawsuits were filed and culminated in Morton's retirement from dental practice. He then became involved in one failed business venture after another and died in abject poverty, having suffered a fatal stroke while on the way to his lawyer to institute one final set of lawsuits against Jackson. Late in life, Morton was somewhat vindicated by the United States Congress, when House members investigated his claims and a committee composed of physicians reported, after hearing the evidence on both sides, that he was entitled to the merit of the discovery. Bills appropriating $100,000 for the discovery of practical anesthesia were introduced into Congress during three separate sessions but were never passed. Jackson continued his lifelong struggle to proclaim himself the inventor of surgical anesthesia. His efforts ended in mental instability, and he spent the last fifteen years of his life in the McLean Asylum for the Insane in Massachusetts. Following Bigelow's announcement, Wells unsuccessfully attempted to establish his priority in both the United States and France. In late 1847, he moved to New York City, where in January 1848, he was arrested and incarcerated for throwing sulfuric acid on a prostitute. That night, Wells, who had become mentally deranged, committed suicide after first inhaling some chloroform and then severing the femoral artery of his left thigh.

Crawford Long (1815–1878), an American physician-surgeon who practiced in the backwoods of Georgia, played a tangential role in the early history of surgical anesthesia. Long graduated from the University of Pennsylvania School of Medicine in 1839 and spent the next year in New York City continuing his medical education and training. Family committments caused him to return to his native state, where he began practice in the village of Jefferson. While a medical student, Long had become familiar with nitrous oxide frolics at which the chemical compound was inhaled to achieve a high. In January 1842 a group of his friends induced him to have a frolic in his home. Long could find no readily available nitrous oxide in the town and did not have the necessary equipment to prepare the compound. He suggested to his friends that sulphuric ether might produce similar mind-altering results. His acquaintances proceeded to inhale the ether and during their antics received various bruises and cuts. None of these injuries had been felt, and Long rightfully concluded that ether must also abolish pain. He promptly attempted to prove the value of his observation, and in March 1842 he successfully removed a small cyst from the neck of a patient who had been etherized. The gentleman underwent a second such procedure that June. By September 1846, Long had performed eight surgical operations involving the administration of ether. Only after he had become aware of the controversy surrounding the conflicting claims of Jackson, Morton, and Wells did Long publish his results in the *Southern Medical and Surgical Journal* (1849). Long's story was told modestly and with an apology for not having written about it earlier. Consequently, although Long's use of sulphuric ether for surgical anesthesia certainly antedates Morton's by more than four years, it is also true that his actions did not encourage other physician or surgeons to follow his example. Although it would be incorrect to withhold from Crawford Long the credit for independent observation and scientific experimentation, he cannot be assigned any distinctive influence on the historical development of surgical anesthesia.

The expanding use of ether and chloroform did not increase the relative safety of surgical operations. In fact, for the few decades following the introduction of anesthesia there was an unanticipated rise in operative mortality throughout the country. This is not as bewildering as it may first seem. Although the complexity of surgical operations had not manifestly changed (incisions into the abdomen, thorax, and cranium continued to remain taboo), the indications for procedures that were already being performed (e.g., arterial ligations, amputations, lithotomy) predictably expanded. As a consequence, individuals who might have succumbed naturally to a disease process in the preanesthetic era were left with the sometimes unhappy prospect of facing the surgeon's knife at an earlier stage of their illness. Since surgeons did not yet employ antiseptic or aseptic measures, it was inevitable that

THE SURGEON

I wish to portray to you tonight, the character of the True Surgeon for the present and the coming time. First, then:- What is demanded to constitute a good surgeon? I answer,- the primary requisite for a good surgeon, is to be a man,-a man of courage, a man of moral rectitude, a man of broad views and noble sentiments. Narrow minded, mean-souled, little brained men ought never to plunge into the learned professions. Their circumstances bewilder them; they become entangled in their learning like a fly in a cobweb; their language is barbarized by technical phrases; their mental vision is obscured by professional squints, and their hearts, cut off from the great life-current of humanity, dry up to nonentities. Such men never grasp the grand and inspiring truths at the core of their profession, but flounder bewildered among its accidental surroundings…

Among the particular traits which go to make up a manly character, one of the first, and one which is eminently necessary to a good surgeon, is courage. In battle, a portion of the surgeons go with the line and dress the wounded under fire…. Unless, therefore, a man can tie up an artery with a cool head and steady hand, while the bullets are singing past him, he will not do for a surgeon. Again, he must sometimes walk his hospital day by day, when it is filled with contagious and pestilential disease, breathing an air more deadly than that of the battlefield. If he cannot do this without flinching, he will not do for a surgeon.

Another requisite of high profession quality is breadth of knowledge, not only of the practical branches, but of those general and preliminary topics which are necessary to constitute a well-educated man. The intensely practical character of the American mind has unfortunately misled many students as to the real requisites of high success. Every year, medical teachers receive applications from men who desire the honors of a diploma, but wish to be excused from attention to, what they call, the non-practical branches…. One man who claimed to be eminent already in surgery, objected to pathology as not practical; it was not necessary to study the nature of the disease, the practical thing was to cure it. God help his patients; I think they had better send for a butcher, as being the more practical man of the two…

The first years of a practitioner's life are not usually fully occupied with business. Of the leisure hours on hand, let one-half be devoted, for six years, to general literature and science, and the other half to reading, writing, and hard thinking directly upon his profession…. Mathematics confers precision of reasoning, and accuracy in mechanical contrivance, which a surgeon especially requires…. But beware of becoming so entangled in the meshes of your studies that they become master of you and not you of them…. You should pursue them not as an end but as a means, in order that by self-culture you may bring to your professional duties a finer and more powerful mind-that you may become more perfect men, more splendid surgeons…

Among the qualities of a true surgeon, not the least important is his enthusiasm…and…his diligence in his work. You occasionally hear men say that the study of medicine and surgery is very interesting, but the practice is tedious and dull. Now I can assure you, that to a well trained mind this is an unmitigated lie. Practice is dull only to those who do not think, reason, and study about their cases; in short, who are routine practitioners…. Make your practice a perpetual study and it will be a perpetual enjoyment…

Among well-balanced minds there are, however, some which naturally give preference to medicine and others to surgery…. This preference depends on differences of the two positions and the relative mental qualities brought in play. Thus medicine requires more breadth and philosophical depth of thought than surgery, but less precision and mechanical ingenuity…. A good physician secures a warm, earnest attachment from his patrons. There is a circle of families who look on him as a permanent and confidential friend…. The surgeon, on the other hand, has a less warm but a more glittering reputation presented to his ambition. His patrons are transient. They come, perhaps, hundreds of miles for a single operation and, being relieved, return to their homes and disappear…. They look upon an eminent surgeon much as they do upon a renowned soldier. They yield the tribute of high admiration to one who dares to put his hand to the machinery of life and can, with impunity, take out its living wheels. If a surgeon's renown is less warm than a physician's, it is wider and more splendid…

Surgeons, on the average, are more clear and accurate in their ideas than physicians and less in danger of running away into obscure theories which neither are nor can be definitely proved…. But, on the other hand, these very advantages draw many inferior men to the surgical ranks. As surgery is easier to comprehend, too many of its votaries are superficial and narrow…. As its renown is glittering and brilliant, it attracts men, too often, who are more cold and selfish than physicians-men incapable of warm friendships, over eager for notoriety, and greedy of gain. So it has been in time past. I call upon you to take this stain away from the profession by bringing to it hearts full of generous emotions; hearts whose rich pulses of youth live on in riper age; hearts that love nobleness and despise meanness and that feel for the sufferings of the afflicted…

Edmund Andrews: Introductory lecture delivered before the Medical Department of Lind University. *Chicago Medical Examiner*, vol. 2, pages 589–598, 1861.

patients would continue to die secondary to the common postoperative problems of wound sepsis and shock. The result of this rise in rates of surgical operations was a concommittant increase in postoperative morbidity and mortality.

In 1864, Jonathan M. Warren (1811–1867), surgeon at the Massachusetts General Hospital, prepared a report to the Massachusetts Medical Society concerning "recent progress in surgery." Warren showed that the total number of limb amputations at his hospital for the three decades 1822 to 1850 was 173. After the introduction of anesthesia, for the single decade 1850 to 1860, the number of amputations was 207. Most glaring was that the percentage of amputations ending in a fatal result increased from 19 to 23 percent during the two study periods. William Halsted (1852–1922), professor of surgery at The Johns Hopkins Hospital, reiterated Warren's conclusion regarding the absolute numbers of operations when he reported in his classic 1904 paper "The Training of the Surgeon" that "in the entire decennium prior to the discovery of anaesthesia only 385 operations were performed in the [Massachusetts General Hospital], an average of 38.5 operations a year. In the first decade subsequent to the employment of ether 1893 operations were performed, an average of 189 per year."

The introduction of anesthesia deeply altered the practice of surgery. It allowed surgeons to have greater control over their patients, which was a most important step in the overall process of professionalization. The sheer availability of inhalation anesthesia promoted the development and eventual bureaucratization of hospitals and facilitated the medicalization of human suffering and healing. There can be little doubt that the discovery of surgical anesthesia was a great scientific achievement and an important milestone in the history of world humanitarianism.

The advent of anesthesia allowed surgeons to exploit the drama of the operating room. Painless surgery was considered bold therapy, and the intrinsic theatricality of the event was not lost on the increasing number of physicians who performed surgical operations. The devising of new and more technically complex surgical operations eventually became an accepted fact of American medical life. Unfortunately, these new procedures sometimes provided little more than a poor excuse to perform the sheer physical act of surgery.

"CONSERVATIVE" VERSUS "RADICAL" SURGERY

More thoughtful members of the surgical community were becoming alarmed with what was considered the exploitation of the manual art of surgery. As this seemingly boundless enthusiasm for questionably appropriate surgical intervention continued, the terms "conservative" and "radical" surgery crept into the jargon of American medical life. Both words took on different meanings at different times. The phrasal idioms became especially salient to the surgeon's world, where conservatives and radicals enunciated sharp philosophic differences over the indications for the performance of the then burgeoning number of surgical operations.

In 1859, Gross pointed out that conservative surgery had taken its rise from Philip Syng Physick. Gross had defined and would continue to use "conservative surgery" as a phrase solely applicable to the treatment of bone excision, dislocations, fractures, and the consequent preservation of limbs. However, a reading of that era's medical literature shows that by 1850, "conservative surgery" was being given another, more expansive meaning applicable to all branches of surgery. No longer was the phrase reserved solely for the preservation of limbs. It was felt that surgical procedures, particularly in view of the growing acceptance of inhalation anesthesia, should be devised solely within the context of the growing science of surgery, and not used indiscriminately on anyone who would hold still. As early as 1853, an anonymous editorial writer in New York City lamented:

> No department of our profession attracts so much eclat from the populace, nor awakens the ambition of the medical tyro to such an extent, as do the operations of surgery. By the former they are looked upon as evidences of bravery, daring, and skill, just in proportion to their desperate character, and without

the least reference to their necessity or propriety, or even to their fatal results. The more bloody, and even the more uniformly fatal, the higher is the huzza of the ignorant and vulgar multitude for the surgeon, so called, who figures in these "deeds of blood." Hence, students and junior practitioners will often run miles to witness a capital operation, and ransack neighborhoods and cities to find patients whose surgical diseases will furnish them opportunities to cut, or to witness cutting, performed by others. And they too become partakers in the popular idolatry of the mere operators, whose frenzy for the use of the scalpel and saw, mallet and chisel, and even the red hot iron, upon the living bodies of their victims, becomes a passion, which too often degrades surgery into human butchery. And the ambition to learn surgery upon the living body, instead of the dead subject, and thus share the ephemeral reputation of being called surgeons, too often seduces students from the diligent cultivation of the science of surgery, which includes the whole of among its principles, into the degrading pursuit of the mere art, which requires little study, and promises distinction among the ignorant multitude, though at the expense of self-respect and all professional character worthy of possession.

John Watson (1807–1863), a prominent New York City surgeon, expressed it even more emphatically, "Surgery…is a good thing, a useful, an excellent thing in its way; but too much of it is a great evil. And the sooner you find this out for yourselves, the better for your patients." By the time of the Civil War, a new sense of conservative medicine, sharply contrasted with the previous era's heroic practices, was becoming a dominant philosophic force. This fundamental change in the way American physician-surgeons viewed themselves presaged the soon-to-come ascent of scientific medicine and was a significant signboard in the inevitable process of surgical professionalization.

At the first meeting of the Section of Surgery of the American Medical Association, held in New Haven in June 1860, the assigned room was too small to contain all the physicians who wanted to attend. The meeting was adjourned to the larger chapel of Yale College so that all could participate in what was expected to be a momentous occasion. The first business before the Section was a report by Joseph McDowell (1805–1868), dean and professor of surgery at the Missouri Medical College in St. Louis, on the improvements in the "art and science of surgery," particularly American, during the previous fifty years. McDowell was a nephew of the famed Ephraim McDowell and brother-in-law to Daniel Drake. His remarks set the tone for what would become the self-championing of American surgery over that of European medicine during the remainder of the nineteenth century:

The obvious reason for the great success of American surgeons over the European is, that they follow less the dogmas of the schools, less the hyperborean practice of European schools, and are more governed by reason and common sense, and operate on a people of better constitution…. If some of our American authors…could not read French…and were less disposed to be led like an ape by a string, to the music of a…French hand organ, we should justly

12. The ancient tradition of sharing knowledge of healing helped transform medicine from superstition to science. The pristine condition and clarity of the image *(left)*, coupled with its unusual pose and props, makes it a valuable medical photograph. The man with the long pipe is Charles L. Allen (1820–1890), a physician in Vermont and professor at Castleton Medical College. To commemorate his teaching appointment, Allen had this picture taken of himself instructing medical student Charles Robbins. The dauguerreotype (circa 1855) is the earliest existing photograph depicting physicians in a didactic session. Surgical teaching was also beginning to occur at the bedside, as is noted in this photograph *(right)* of Gurdon Buck and his students (circa 1860s). *(Courtesy of Stanley B. Burns, M.D., and The Burns Collection and Archive)*

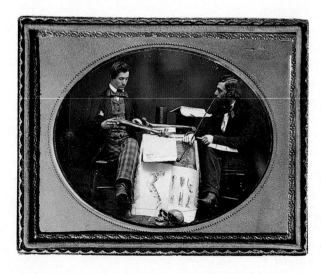

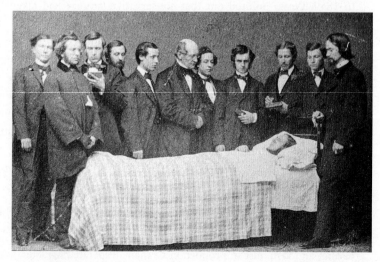

expect improvement at home...when anything that is either good or great is done by American surgeons, it is first denied in Europe, then claimed by them, and their claim admitted by us as just.... American teachers should feel that they are justified in the conclusion that they are most capable of giving instruction in their own country, to their own countrymen. Why should pupils be sent to Europe if they can be taught better on our own continent?

SURGICAL LITERATURE

As in earlier times, a very respectable amount of surgical literature appeared. Samuel Gross's massive two-volume *System of Surgery; Pathological, Diagnostic, Therapeutic, and Operative* (1859) is considered one of the most important surgical treatises of its time and was a truly herculean effort. Its forty-seven chapters, 936 illustrations, and 2,360 pages attest to its encyclopedic scope, while the six editions demonstrate how widely distributed it was. The authority with which Gross was quoted was justifiably matched by his prolificacy, as is witnessed by his 1854 *Practical Treatise on Foreign Bodies in the Air-Passages.* Gross's literary output was closely followed by Henry Smith's *System of Operative Surgery* (1852) and *Treatise on the Practice of Surgery* (1856). These two textbooks were combined into an exhaustive two-volume *The Principles and Practice of Surgery, Embracing Minor and Operative Surgery* (1863). With over 500 pages of additional material added, the *Principles* was especially valuable, since it contains a detailed history of surgery in the United States and a bibliography of American works on surgery from 1783 to 1860. The most engaging of surgical textbooks was Paul Eve's (1806–1877) *Collection of Remarkable Cases in Surgery* (1857). This volume, written when Eve was professor of surgery at the University of Nashville, presents unusual surgical problems grouped according to various divisions of the human body. From serious surgical dilemmas (e.g., "an immense ovarian tumor, in which the patient measured eight and a half feet around the body, and five feet from pubes to sternum") to oddities (e.g., "amputation of the head with the patient surviving thirty-six hours") to human misery (e.g., "extraordinary case of suicide; patient thrusting a red-hot poker into the abdomen, and subsequently pulling out and detaching a portion of the omentum and thirty-two inches of the colon") this book provides some of the most fascinating reading to be found in any nineteenth-century American surgical text.

Sectarian surgeons were also active in producing textbooks. Benjmain Hill authored his *Lectures on the American Eclectic System of Surgery* in 1850 and followed it with his two-volume *Homoeopathic Practice of Surgery, Together with Operative Surgery* in 1855. In the same year, William Helmuth (1833–1902), then only 22 years old, issued *Surgery and its Adaptation to Homoeopathic Practice.* Both Hill's and Helmuth's efforts reflect different schools within the homeopathic movement. In 1858, William Henry Cook (1832–1899), professor of surgery at the Physio-Medical College of Ohio, penned *A Treatise on the Principles and Practice of Physio-Medical Surgery.* As in most of the sectarians' textbooks, the technical aspects of completing a surgical operation were no different from those of their orthodox competitors. Disagreements were most often found in the pre- and postoperative care rendered to the patient. Botanical and herbal preparations were usually shunned by the "regulars," while sectarians incorporated them into most perioperative decisions.

OPERATIVE GYNECOLOGY

Of the many surgical *tours-de-force* that occurred during the mid-nineteenth century, the repair of vesicovaginal fistulae and the performance of ovariotomies were among the most notable. These procedures, which signalled the beginnings of operative gynecology, were largely performed by surgeons from the southern and western areas who were attempting to repair the errors and omissions of backwoods obstetrics and gynecology. John Atlee (1799–1885) was a graduate of the medical department of the University of Pennsylvania (1820). After completing his medical studies in Paris and Berlin, Atlee returned to his rural home town of Lancaster, Pennsylvania, where he was on the anatomy and physiology faculty of Franklin and

Marshall College. Atlee was the first to perform a successful removal of both ovaries (1843), and in so doing he helped revive the operation of ovariotomy in America. The surgical procedure had fallen into disfavor following the earlier limited successes of Joseph Gallup (1769–1849), Ephraim McDowell, Nathan Smith, and David Rogers (1799–1877). Washington Lemuel Atlee (1808–1878), John's younger sibling, graduated from Jefferson Medical College in 1829 and spent the early part of his professional career in Lancaster. After 1844, he practiced in Philadelphia, where he was on the medical chemistry faculty of the Medical College of Philadelphia. During his lifetime, Washington was reputed to have performed almost four hundred ovarian extirpations and, like his brother, established a stellar reputation as one of America's premier ovariotomists. A large measure of his prominence was garnered following the publication of his paper in the *Transactions of the American Medical Association* (1851), detailing all known operations of ovariotomy from 1701 to 1851.

In virtually all instances, massive enlargement of the ovaries was due to cyst formation. Since the surgical procedure of oophorectomy had found little favor because of its generally poor results, the only treatment that could be offered the hapless sufferer was palliation by "tapping" to withdraw the reaccumulating fluid. The frontier-based stories of the repeated removal of increasing amounts of "cyst material" are simply amazing. One physician reported a case in which paracentesis or tapping was completed eighty times on one patient over a twenty-five-year span, with an accumulated removal of 6,630 pints of fluid. Another surgeon told of an ovarian cyst from which 427 pounds of fluid were withdrawn over ten months. Although records were not kept, undoubtedly the most staggering amount was reported in 1825, when an ovarian cyst (or more likely the peritoneal cavity for recurring ascites) was tapped 299 times to remove the almost unbelievable total of 9,867 pounds of fluid. In view of these numbers and the uniformly poor operative results, it is easy to understand why surgeons were fearful of attempts at extirpation. Charles Meigs (1792–1869), a respected Philadelphia clinician and later to be named professor of obstetrics and diseases of women and children at Jefferson Medical College, even attempted to have ovariotomy prohibited by legal statute, insisting that it was immoral and not justified by any number of surgical successes.

In 1856, George Lyman (1819–1891) of Massachusetts, in his *History and Statistics of Ovariotomy and the Circumstances Under Which the Operation May be Regarded as Safe and Expedient*, summed up the collected American experience. Reviewing all aspects of the surgical removal of the diseased ovary, Lyman established the safety of the operation and the necessity for its performance. Following this formulation of precise indications for ovariotomy, the procedure became the first of a multitude of surgical operations that centered on opening the previously unexplorable abdominal cavity. This paved the "technical" way for the blossoming of all abdominal surgery and its importance in the maturation of the whole of surgery.

The grim plight of women afflicted with vesicovaginal fistula was among the era's most heart-wrenching surgical conditions. This abnormal opening between the bladder and vagina, almost always associated with the difficulties of childbirth, created victims who became social pariahs because of their uncontrollable urinary leakage. As described by Johann Dieffenbach (1792–1847), a German surgeon, no sadder situation could exist; the embarrassment was enough to drive some women to suicide:

> A source of disgust, even to herself, the woman…becomes…the object of bodily revulsion…everyone turns his back, repulsed by the intolerable, foul, uriniferous odor…The labia, perineum, lower part of the buttocks, and inner aspects of the thighs and calves are continually wet, to the very feet…Intolerable burning and itching torment the patients. The refreshment of a change of clothing provides no relief, because the clean undergarment, after being quickly saturated, slaps against the patients…sloshing in their wet shoes as though they were wading through a swamp…. Even the richest are usually condemned for life to a straw sack, whose straw must be renewed daily. One's breath is taken away by the bedroom air of these women…. Washing

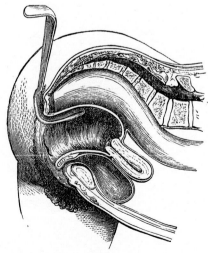

13. An illustration from J. Marion Sims's *Clinical Notes on Uterine Surgery* (1866) showing placement of his double duck-billed vaginal speculum. (*Author's Collection*)

and anointing do not help; perfume actually increases the repugnance of the odor.... This horrendous evil tears asunder every family bond.... Indifference overtakes some of these unfortunates; others give themselves over to quiet resignation and pious devotion.

Physicians had long struggled with the vesicovaginal fistula problem, including a host of hoped-for surgical cures involving cauterization, skin grafting, suturing, and even obliteration of the vagina. All invariably ended in failure, the result being an additional amount of suffering and inconvenience for the poor patient. Such despair came to an abrupt conclusion in 1852, when J. Marion Sims (1813–1883) of Alabama authored one of the most influential case reports ever presented by an American surgeon. "On the treatment of vesico-vaginal fistula" was published in the January issue of the *American Journal of the Medical Sciences*, the most respected of all mid-nineteenth-century American medical periodicals. With the stroke of a pen, it seemed, Sims initiated a new era in American gynecology by devising a successful and easily learned operation that allowed surgeons to permanently cure vesicovaginal fistula.

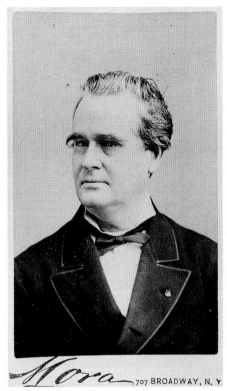

14. A *carte de visite* of James Marion Sims *(Courtesy The New York Academy of Medicine)*

The career and achievements of Sims are so extensive that his life's story alone provides a distinctive window into mid-nineteenth-century American surgery. His reputation in Europe during the 1860s, unlike that of nearly every other American surgeon, probably accounted for the increased respect accorded to our country's practitioners. Yet, through it all, Sims was plagued by chronic misfortune, unending disappointment, poor health, and the ill will of many of his surgical colleagues. Born in Lancaster, South Carolina, Sims graduated from South Carolina College in 1832. He chose medicine as a career not because he thought he would like it but because law and religion did not appeal to him. Sims initially apprenticed with a local physician in his home town, and then in 1833 attended a three-month course of lectures in Charleston at the new proprietary Medical College of South Carolina. He eventually matriculated at Jefferson Medical College, where he received his medical degree in 1835. Among the most memorable of all his teachers was the fiery and fiercely independent "surgeon," George McClellan. McClellan provided a strong example for Sims, who chose to emulate him. McClellan had a sense of bravado, which Sims would evince in his own surgical practice. McClellan was known for his hot temper and unending arguments with lay administrators; personality traits that Sims would rapidly acquire. Most of all, McClellan took early notice of Sims and encouraged the young man to pursue bold and innovative surgical operations by providing hands-on experience.

Purchasing instruments to pursue a surgical practice, Sims returned to Lancaster and hung out his shingle. Disaster was lurking, and his confidence soon sagged. In the first two months, Sims had only two patients; both were infants, and both died of cholera. In desperation, Sims packed his belongings and fled westward to Alabama, where he was able to establish a successful practice at Mount Meigs, a few miles east of Montgomery. Malaria was endemic, and after a few months, Sims was debilitated by recurrent malarial paroxysms of chills accompanied by a high fever. Seeking a "healthier climate," Sims finally settled in Montgomery in 1840, along with his wife of four years, Theresa Jones, daughter of the Lancaster physician who had been his original mentor.

By the mid-1840s, Sims had gained a reputation as a competent surgeon. His technical skills developed rapidly as he performed procedures for cataract, cleft lip and palate, clubfoot, strabismus, and tumors of the mandible and maxilla. In the spring of 1845, Sims first ventured into women's surgery and began his surgical experimentation on the now legendary African-American slaves Anarcha, Betsy, and Lucy, all victims of childbirth-induced vesicovaginal fistula. Prolonged labor, lasting days at a time, was not an unanticipated event. With the unborn infant's head pressing aginst the bony pelvic floor and cutting off blood circulation to the soft vaginal and bladder tissues covering the area, extensive sloughing of tissues often occurred, creating an abnormal opening between the vagina, the bladder, and sometimes the rectum.

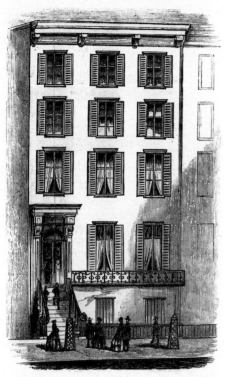

15. Building temporarily used as the Woman's Hospital at 83 Madison Avenue in New York City (circa 1855). *(Collection of the New-York Historical Society)*

Anarcha was only 17 years old when she suffered through three days of unremitting labor pains, finally delivering a stillborn infant. Five days after the birth, the gangrenous vaginal wall fell apart, and Anarcha lost her ability to control either urination or bowel function. By Sims's account, her "urine was running day and night...producing an inflammation of the external parts...almost similar to confluent small-pox, with constant pain and burning...the odor permeated everything...her life was one of suffering and disgust." Betsy and Lucy suffered similar fates, although their fistulae were not as onerous as Anarcha's.

In their zeal to cure vesicovaginal fistula, American surgeons would first have to improve on certain fundamental surgical techniques before success with the operation would be possible. As early as 1838, John Peter Mettauer (1787–1875), professor of surgery and surgical anatomy at Washington College in Baltimore, had utilized lead wire to repair a parturient laceration of the vesicovaginal septum. Metal sutures were found to cause less tissue reaction than organic-based sutures (e.g., buckskin, catgut, cotton, flax, parchment, silk). Mettauer's observation was an important contribution, but he did not report his case until 1840, following the country's first published record of surgical success by George Hayward (1839). Still, Hayward's triumph was accomplished by use of "old-fashioned" organic sutures.

Sims discovered that changing the examination posture of a female patient, placing her in a knee-chest position, and inserting a speculum of his own design–a bent pewter soup spoon–allowed visualization of the vaginal walls and cervix with a degree of thoroughness and clarity that had not previously been possible: "I saw everything, as no man had seen before." Despite his success in these preliminary steps, including the invention of a rubber catheter to keep the bladder emptied, Sims was plagued by repeated failures to close the fistulae of his patients. Writing in his 1884 autobiography, *The Story of My Life*, Sims recalls the next important advance:

> I have improved the operations till the mechanism seems to be as perfect as possible, and yet they fail. I wonder if it is in the kind of suture that is used? Can I get some substitute for the silk thread? Meltor [Mettauer], of Virginia, had used lead.... What can I do? Just in this time of tribulation...I was walking from my house to the office, and picked up a little bit of brass wire in the yard. It was very fine...I took it around to...my jeweler, and asked him if he could make me a little silver wire about the size of a piece of brass wire. He said yes...and made it of all pure silver. Anarcha was the subject of this experiment. The operation was performed on the fistula in the base of the bladder, that would admit of the end of my little finger.... The edges of the wounds were...neatly brought together with four of these fine silver wires.... This was the thirtieth operation performed on Anarcha. She was put to bed...and the next day the urine came from the bladder as clear and as limpid as spring water...

Over the next few months of experimentation, many Montgomery physicians attended Sims's operations. His surgical triumphs assured Sims's local reputation, but the publication of his 1852 paper made him nationally and internationally famous. To appreciate the fortitude and heroism of little-known Anarcha, Betsy, Lucy and other unnamed slaves is to understand that they endured the great majority of their operations and recovery periods without "bedstead, bed, mattress, or pillow, with no covering but the clothes they had on and some filthy rags of blanket" and without the benefit of anesthesia. Like other physician-surgeons of his locale, Sims was initially fearful of using inhalation anesthesia. In addition, he apparently subscribed to a belief, prevalent in his racial and socioeconomic group, that African Americans had a specific physiological tolerance to pain, whereas wealthy white women were exceptionally vulnerable to postoperative suffering. This hesitation to relieve surgical discomfort, compounded by what appears to be an exploitation of female slaves, has led to accusations that Sims was amoral, brutish, sexist, and unethical. Evidence does not support such a judgement, especially when it is viewed against the ethical, moral and social fabric of his time. Sims lived in an area where slavery, abhorrent as it is, was prevalent and where few individuals questioned its morality. There is no grounds for any belief that Sims ever participated in the random violence and mindless brutality that existed in the perverse relationship between slave and master. Like most doctors, he seems to have concentrated on the relief of suffering without questioning the *Zeitgeist* of the era in which he lived.

With fame in hand, and despite a severe form of chronic disabling diarrhea, Sims decided to again seek a healthier climate and exploit his new renown by moving to New York City. With his wife and six children in tow, Sims bought a large home at 79 Madison Avenue, in a newly developed area between 28th and 29th Streets. As his colitis slowly resolved, Sims resumed his clinical practice. Within a few months he was receiving numerous referrals for the evaluation of vesicovaginal fistula. Once his surgical successes were assured, Sims became enamored with the idea of establishing a special hospital for the treatment of women's diseases. He had a persuasive personality, and following appeals to prominent citizens, in particular their wives, Sims convinced several benefactors to financially assist him in founding the Woman's Hospital in the State of New York (1855). With forty beds, mostly occupied by indigent patients, Sims and his assistants, including Edmund Peaslee

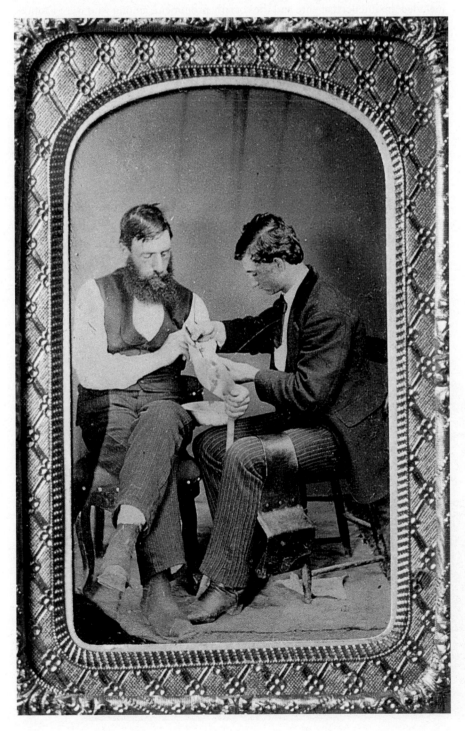

16. Up to the mid-nineteenth century, the bleeding lancet ruled the world of American medicine. Such a sanguinary spirit bordered on therapeutic nihilism as physicians transferred the applicability of bleeding from one disease entity to another with an enthusiasm that knew few limits. It was not uncommon to bleed thirty or more ounces at a sitting, and children were bled until their lips turned blue. In 1859 one doctor reminisced that he had drawn more than one hundred barrels of blood during his medical lifetime. This photograph (early 1860s) is a tintype (one-of-a-kind positive photograph on a thin sheet of iron) and is believed to be the earliest known American image of an actual bloodletting. The composition is intriguing, as it depicts a physician and patient conforming to the ancient positions of bleeding. The patient holds onto a stick, while a bleeding bowl is suspended between the knees of the two men. Other interesting details are the saddlebag over the physician's right thigh and the use of a tourniquet. The photograph was tinted red to show blood running from the arm into the basin. *(Courtesy of Stanley B. Burns, M.D., and The Burns Collection and Archive)*

(1814–1878), Thomas Addis Emmet (1828–1919), and Theodore Gaillard Thomas (1831–1903), eventually devised or improved on numerous gynecologic operations, including an important new method for cervical amputation in 1861.

In 1857, Sims was invited to give an anniversary discourse before the New York Academy of Medicine. He felt that this would be a propitious occasion to advocate his method for wound closure to prevent inflammation. He detailed the use of silver sutures, not only for gynecologic surgery but for plastic surgery of the face, cleft palate repair, and scalp wounds. Sims even spoke of suturing gunshot wounds of the large bowel with fine silver wire. His remarks were published in 1859 as a seventy-nine page monograph, *Silver Sutures in Surgery,* one of the most influential texts to come out of pre-Civil War America. With the outbreak of the country's internicine conflict, Sims found himself an alien Southerner living in the North. Disgusted with the growing political strife, and not feeling strongly about either side's positions, Sims took refuge in Europe. As he was already internationally known, his sojourn on the Continent amounted to a seven-year triumph of welcomes. He became an intinerant surgeon, practicing in England, France, Germany, and Italy. His patients included the intellectual elite and the socially prominent, among who were Empress Eugenie of France (1826–1920), wife of Napoleon III (1808–1873). There can be little doubt that Sims was America's first surgeon with a truly international reputation.

Sims continued his writing while in Europe, authoring an important paper describing the condition of vaginismus (1862), or painful spasm of the vagina preventing satisfactory sexual intercourse. During this time he also penned the most important textbook of his entire professional career: *Clinical Notes on Uterine Surgery; with Special Reference to the Management of the Sterile Condition* (1866). Written while Sims was in London, the work was originally serialized in *Lancet* in 1864–1865. It was published in London, with an American edition coming out a few months later, and was met with a storm of controversy. Sims's critics inveighed against his frank presentation of subjects previously considered *verboten.* Particularly distressing to European sensibilities was Sims's practice of visiting married sterile couples in their bedrooms and applying various treatments, including etherization of the wife, to overcome the obstacles preventing conception.

17. Surgeons and visiting surgeons of the Massachusetts General Hospital (circa 1858). This is the earliest known photograph of an assembled group of American surgeons, and Robert Hinckley used it to authenticate faces for his painting "The First Operation Under Ether." From left to right are Henry J. Bigelow, Samuel Cabot, Jonathan M. Warren, Solomon D. Townsend, George H. Gay, and Henry G. Clark. *(The Francis A. Countway Library of Medicine)*

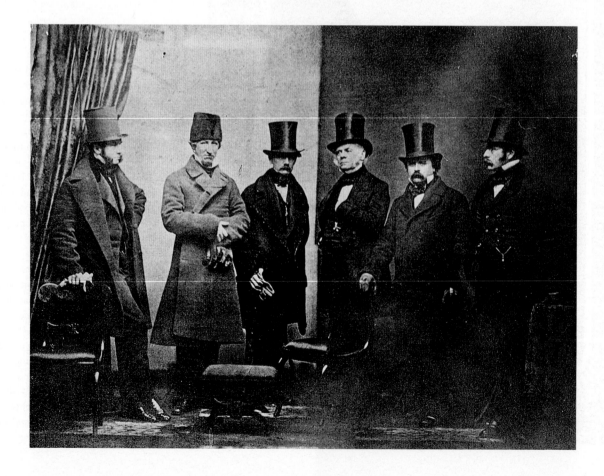

In 1868, Sims returned to New York City to celebrate the opening of a greatly expanded Woman's Hospital at 50th Street and 4th Avenue, now the site of the Waldorf-Astoria Hotel. Appointed chief consulting surgeon, Sims resumed some aspects of his old practice, but for the remainder of his life he alternated his clinical affairs between Europe and the United States. At the outbreak of the Franco-Prussian War in 1870, Sims organized the Anglo-American Ambulance Corps and served as surgeon-in-chief. At the Battle of Sedan, Sims' group served with distinction, and he subsequently received military decorations from both the Prussian and the French governments.

Sims returned once again to the United States, but his lengthy association with the Woman's Hospital came to an abrupt end in 1874. The institution's lay board of governors passed two rules that were unacceptable to his sense of self-importance. Most offensive was a regulation permitting no more than fifteen visitors to witness any surgical operation. Many physicians came to watch Sims perform surgery, and his operating amphitheater was always crowded with far more than fifteen observers. The kind-hearted but impulsive Sims declared his determination to disregard the new decrees and signaled his intention to resign from the staff. Politics overshadowed the whole affair, and Sims later regretted his intemperate outburst, but the psychological damage had been done and Sims was relieved of his surgical privileges.

Bitter recriminations followed between Sims and members of both the lay and medical boards. The effect of such an acrimonious dispute was a tarnishing of Sims's reputation in New York City. Nevertheless, he had many American followers and was shortly thereafter elected to the presidency of the American Medical Association (1876). In 1879 he became president of the American Gynecological Association, and in 1880 he was even reinstated at the Woman's Hospital. Defiant to a fault, Sims spent much of his later career in Europe. While in Paris, he performed and reported the last of his important surgical operations, an unsuccessful cholecystotomy (1878).

At the age of 70, Sims continued to perform surgical operations. On November 12, 1883, he completed a difficult procedure on a prominent New York woman, having postponed a trip to Europe to do so. Less than twelve hours later, he died of a coronary thrombosis. Even in death, Sims gained a measure of medical immortality, since he was only the second individual in this country upon whom a postmortem diagnosis of coronary occlusion was made. Sims was interred at the Greenwood Cemetery in Brooklyn, a burying ground that also holds the remains of William Halsted, Valentine Mott, Lewis Pilcher, and John Wyeth.

In modern times, Sims's name is linked with a double duck-billed vaginal speculum and with a position used to facilitate vaginal examination, in which a woman lies on her side with her lower arm behind her back, and the thighs flexed, the upper one more than the lower. Sims received adulation not only from surgeons and medical historians but also from the public. A statue of him stands in New York City, near Central Park at 5th Avenue and 103rd Street, opposite the building of the New York Academy of Medicine. Engraved in brass are the words of a fitting epitaph: "Surgeon, Philanthropist, Founder of the Woman's Hospital, State of New York. His Brilliant Achievement Carried the Name of American Surgery Throughout the Entire World."

BIOGRAPHIES OF MID-NINETEENTH-CENTURY SURGEONS

As in any other surgical era, numerous surgeons were involved in the expansion of medical progress during the mid-nineteenth century. The engrossing tales of their life's work are part of the grand tradition of surgical stories that echo through all operating rooms. **Reuben Mussey** (1780–1866) graduated from Dartmouth College in 1803, apprenticed with Nathan Smith, and received his medical degree from the University of Pennsylvania in 1809. In 1809, Mussey went into practice in Salem, Massachusetts, as a partner with Daniel Oliver (1787–1842). Having established his surgical skills, Mussey began the life of a peripatetic academician. From

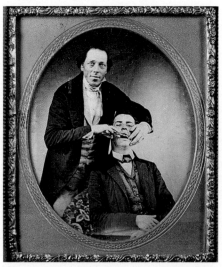

18. During the late 1830s and early 1840s, the triad of dental professionalism (education, organization, and literature) was established for the first time anywhere in the United States, and dentistry was soon acknowledged to be the country's only leading health care specialty in the world. One reason was that many prominent American dentists had also received a medical education. For instance, James Garretson (1828–1895), author of *A Treatise on the Diseases and Surgery of the Mouth, Jaws and Associate Parts* (1869), created oral surgery as a dental specialty, although he initially attempted to bring his activities into much closer relationship with medicine-based surgery. This daguerreotype shows an American dentist performing a tooth extraction (circa 1847), which for many physician-surgeons of that era was simply viewed as another form of operative surgery. *(Courtesy of Stanley B. Burns, M.D., and The Burns Collection and Archive)*

1814 to 1838, he served as professor of anatomy and surgery and of medical theory and practice at Dartmouth. For four of those years, 1831–1835, Mussey concurrently was professor of surgery at the medical department of Bowdoin College in Maine. Moving westward, Mussey was appointed professor of surgery at the Medical College of Ohio (1838–1852) and professor of surgery and anatomy at the Miami Medical College in Cincinnati (1852–1857). In 1857, he retired to Boston after having served as president of the American Medical Association (1850). Mussey was a diligent and perhaps obsessive scientist. In one of the most brazen examples of self-experimentation, Mussey was at issue with Benjamin Rush (1745–1813) concerning the latter's belief in the nonabsorptiveness of the skin. Mussey, to prove his theory, had himself immersed up to his neck in a strong solution of madder, a red vegetable dye, for three hours. Much to his satisfaction, he detected the red dye in his urine for the next two days. This concept of bold self-experimentation nearly caused Mussey's demise when he attempted to see whether he could pass ink by immersing himself in a solution of nutgall and subsequently in sulphate of iron. Mussey's only contributions to surgical literature were case reports published in various journals. The most prominent included the ligation of both common carotid arteries within a few days of each other as treatment for an ulcerated vascular tumor of the scalp (1829) and the earliest reported scapulectomy in America (1838). Mussey's son, William (1818–1882), became a well-known surgeon in his own right and similarly served as professor of operative and clinical surgery at the Miami Medical College (1865–1882).

John Batchelder (1784–1868) received his medical degree from Harvard Medical School in 1815. He initially practiced in Charlestown, New Hampshire, but his surgical renown resulted in his eventual appointment as professor of anatomy and surgery at Castleton Medical School in Vermont and Berkshire Medical Institution in Massachusetts. Considered an outstanding lithotomist, Batchelder was also regarded as something of a specialist in cataract extraction. He became most well known for his ligation of the carotid artery to cut off the blood supply to a large osteosarcoma of the mandible, which he later resected (1825). He wrote on many surgical topics and produced a detailed study of inflammation in 1848. It has been claimed that he was the first surgeon in America to successfully remove the head of the femur.

John Ball Brown (1784–1862) apprenticed under various general practitioners in New England. In 1812, he moved to Boston, where he soon married the daughter of John Collins Warren. At the urging of his father-in-law, Brown began to specialize in orthopedic operations. In 1838, he founded the Orthopedique Infirmary, eventually renamed the Boston Orthopedic Institution, the first such specialty hospital in America. He wrote little of consequence, his few reports being descriptions of cases performed at his institution. Brown was the first in America to perform a subcutaneous tenotomy for clubfoot (1839), and he enjoyed a wide reputation in the treatment of torticollis and spinal curvature. His son was the renowned orthopedic surgeon Buckminster Brown (1819–1891).

Benjamin Dudley (1785–1870) was born near Lexington, Kentucky, apprenticed with Frederick Ridgely (1757–1824), and matriculated at the University of Pennsylvania, where he received his medical degree in 1806. He spent the next few years in Europe studying at various clinical centers, including the Royal College of Surgeons of London, which admitted him by examination, and eventually returned to settle in his home town. In 1815, Dudley was appointed professor of anatomy and surgery in the medical department of Transylvania University. He held both chairs until 1844, after which he retained only that of surgery. Dudley established an enviable reputation as a physician throughout all of Kentucky and several adjoining states. He was a dynamic lecturer and prided himself on his independence from authoritative beliefs, but it was as a practicing surgeon that his clinical reputation was truly established. His fame as a lithotomist was based on 225 lithotomies with a mortality rate of only 2 percent. Dudley summarized his clinical cases in a short

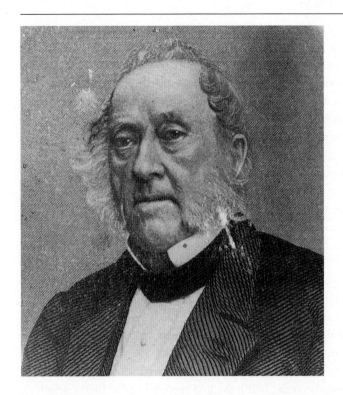

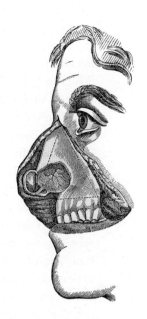
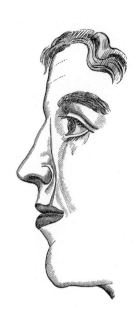

monograph, *Observations on the Nature and Treatment of Calculous Diseases* (1836). He also authored one of the preeminent early American papers on the treatment of traumatic head injuries (1828) and an important study on the use of the bandages in the care of contusions and lacerations (1829). Dudley's pioneering efforts in the surgical treatment of epilepsy by removing depressed skull fragments (1832) were regarded with modest success but paved the way for the beginnings of neurologic surgery in the United States. He spent the last twenty years of his life in retirement on his estate, "Fairlawn," outside Lexington, where he entertained visiting surgeons from throughout America and Europe.

Valentine Mott (1785–1865) was among the most prominent of early American surgeons. He initially apprenticed with a cousin, Valentine Seaman (1770–1817), a well-known New York City practitioner, who authored the unrecognized but important *Pharmacoepia Chirurgical In Usum Nosocomii Novi Eboracencis* (1811), an account of the clinical practices of the surgical department of New York Hospital. After Mott obtained his medical degree from Columbia College (1806), he decided to remain for another year under Seaman's tutelage. That year's experience persuaded Mott to become a surgeon and to seek further education in London and Edinburgh. Mott became a student under Astley Cooper (1768–1841) and was so well regarded that Cooper made him "dresser of wounds" for all of his patients. In 1808, Mott worked with John Thomson (1765–1846) and John Bell (1763–1820) in Edinburgh. Having received a great deal of technical experience, Mott returned to New York City in 1809. Almost at once he began to teach a course of private instruction in surgery, which attracted a large student following. An outstanding teacher of surgery, Mott was one of the first physicians in America to give formal clinical instruction, and in 1811 he was elected professor of surgery at his alma mater. In the following year the medical department of Columbia College was united with the College of Physicians and Surgeons of the University of New York. This new College of Physicians and Surgeons represented the major medical institution in New York City, and Wright Post nominated Mott to the first chair of surgery. For political reasons, Mott resigned from his position in 1826 and helped found the Rutgers Medical College in New York City. He occupied the chair of operative surgery until he resigned in 1834 because of poor health. In early 1835, Mott left for an extended stay in Europe that lasted seven years. During his travels, Mott was received by the most famous of European surgeons; he described his experience in *Travels to Europe and the East*

19. Valentine Mott, having sat for several photographic sessions in the early 1860s, was an outstanding surgical technician, who completed 138 ligations of major arteries. Extremely versatile in his approach to a variety of surgical diseases, he described many procedures, including one of the earliest removals of a fibrous growth from the nostril by dividing the nasal and maxillary bones *(American Journal of the Medical Sciences*, vol. 4, pages 87–91, 1843). *(Historical Collections, College of Physicians of Philadelphia)*

(1842). Before returning home in 1841, Mott was informed that he had been elected to the new chair of surgery at the recently established University Medical College, which was associated with New York University. The presence of Mott on the faculty guaranteed that the school would be an immediate success, and during the next ten years Mott enjoyed one of the busiest surgical practices in the United States. In 1850, ill health again forced him to retire, and he set out once more for Europe. After a year-long sojourn, Mott felt better and reaccepted his old position at the University Medical College. Although in good health, he decided to retire in 1853 and assumed an emeritus position. Mott's later years were spent in humanitarian pursuits. In 1862, at the request of the United States Sanitary Commission, a civilian body that aided Civil War soldiers, he prepared two papers on the use of anesthetics and the treatment of hemorrhage from gunshot wounds. Although Mott never authored a surgical textbook, he did edit the three-volume American edition of Alfred Velpeau's (1795–1867) *New Elements of Operative Surgery* (1847). Mott's numerous contributions to the advancement of clinical surgery are evidenced by his many journal articles, including the first reported attempt in the history of surgery to ligate the innominate artery for aneurysm (1818), an early case of common carotid artery ligation and mandibular resection (1822), the first successful ligation of the common iliac artery in the United States (1827), the first reported amputation at the hip joint in the United States (1827), the earliest resection of the clavicle in the United States for an osteosarcoma (1828), the first reported use of Pierre Brasdor's (1721–1797) technique of treatment of aneurysm by ligation of the artery immediately distal to the lesion (1829), a case of external iliac ligation (1831), the first attempt in the United States to ligate the subclavian artery within the scalenus muscle (1833), the second successful reported ligation of the internal iliac artery in the United States (1837), and an operation to remove a fibrous growth from the nostril by division of the nasal and maxillary bones (1843). Mott's reputation was such that Cooper said of his pupil, "he has performed more of the great operations than any man living." Gross considered Mott to be the leading American surgeon of the first half of the nineteenth century. Mott was so imbued with a deep sense of tradition that in the mid-1830s he surgically sacrificed a rooster at the Greek temple of Epidaurus in the valley of Peneus. He ligated both carotid arteries of the cock and then sacrificed the bird in the name of Aesculapius. Mott's demeanor was at times overbearing, and he was characterized as being somewhat egotistical, especially while lecturing. Fanatically neat in appearance, he always remained the courtly, kindly, polished, cultured, nineteenth-century gentleman. Among his children were the surgeons Valentine Mott, Jr. (1822–1854), and Alexander Brown Mott (1826–1889).

John Mettauer (1787–1875) received his medical degree from the University of Pennsylvania in 1809. He soon returned to his home state of Virginia, where he remained for most of his professional life. For one year, from 1835 to 1836, Mettauer was professor of surgery at Washington Medical College in Baltimore. In 1837 he opened his own medical institute, which became part of Randolph-Macon College a few years later. Mettauer was an outstanding clinical surgeon and reported the first successful repair of a lacerated perineum and rectovaginal septum in America (1833). This achievement assumed particular importance because he espoused the use of metallic sutures during such an operation. In 1838, Mettauer was the first in America to operate successfully for vesicovaginal fistula. Among his other case reports was the first paper on amputation of the penis to appear in the American periodical literature (1837) and the country's first repair of a cleft palate based on the method of Dieffenbach (1837).

William Gibson (1788–1868) studied in Edinburgh, where he received his medical degree in 1809. After returning to the United States, he was appointed to the chair of surgery at the University of Maryland. Following Physick's retirement, Gibson was appointed his successor at the University of Pennsylvania and remained there until his own voluntary resignation in 1855. In 1824, Gibson authored the two-volume *Institutes and Practice of Surgery*, the second systematic American text-book of surgery. Among his surgical accomplishments were the first known performance of a ligation of the common iliac artery (1820), the country's second known case of subclavian artery ligation (1828), the first published case of ligation of the internal jugular vein (1834), and the first recorded instance of two successful cesarean sections in the same woman (1835 and 1838). Gibson also wrote a popular travel book, *Rambles in Europe* (1841). Among his numerous community-oriented activities was his active participation in a crusade against the evils of tobacco. Gibson's son, Charles Bell Gibson (1816–1865) served as professor of surgery at the Medical College of Virginia in Richmond.

Usher Parsons (1788–1868) became a medical naval hero in the War of 1812 as a result of heroic and brilliant work in treating American wounded sailors at the Battle of Lake Erie under Captain (later Commodore) Oliver Hazard Perry (1785–1819). Parsons studied medicine with various physicians in New England and in 1812 was licensed to commence clinical practice by the Massachusetts Medical Society. From 1812 to 1823, Parsons served in the medical corps of the U.S. Navy, rising in rank from surgeon's mate to surgeon. His surgical deeds on the *Lawrence* were extraordinary and included six amputations of the thigh in the midst of continuous cannonading. Parson's military exploits were recounted in his paper published in the *Eclectic Repertory* (1819). For years afterward, it was said that Parsons, the surgeon war hero, was greeted by cheers whenever he attended a medical meeting. Following his retirement from military duty, Parsons moved to Providence, Rhode Island, and was appointed professor of anatomy and surgery at Dartmouth Medical School (1820–1822) and to the same position at the Brown University Medical School (1823–1828). He was one of the founders of the Rhode Island Hospital and played an active role in that state's medical affairs. Parsons was also a founder of the American Medical Association and served as its vice-president (1853). He was the winner of the Boylston Prize, awarded by Harvard University for dissertations on subjects connected to the medical sciences, four times. Those papers, three of which were on surgical topics, including cancer of the breast, were collectively published in 1839. Parson's other books were the popular *Sailor's Physician* (1820) and *Directions for Making Anatomical Preparations* (1831).

Jonathan Knight (1789–1864) attended medical lectures at the University of Pennsylvania but never received a formal medical degree. He was licensed to practice by the Connecticut Medical Society and at the founding of Yale Medical School was named professor of anatomy and physiology (1813–1838). Subsequently he was transferred to the chair of surgery (1838–1864). Knight's organizational capabilities were recognized when he was chosen president of the National Medical Convention, which formed the American Medical Association (1846). He served two terms as president of the latter organization in 1853 and 1854. Knight wrote sparingly; his most important paper presented the world's first reported cure of aneurysm by means of digital compression (1848).

Alexander Stevens (1789–1869) attended Yale College and received his medical degree from the University of Pennsylvania in 1811. He served on the surgical service of New York Hospital for seven months; then, in an attempt to travel to Europe to complete his education, he was captured by the British and detained as a prisoner of war. Following his release, Stevens visited London and Paris and studied with Alexis Boyer (1757–1833) in the latter city. In 1814, Stevens was appointed professor of surgery at the New York Medical Institute, and four years later he became one of the visiting surgeons to the New York Hospital. During this time he completed his translation from the French of Boyer's *Treatise on Surgical Diseases*. In 1826, Stevens succeeded Mott as professor of surgery at the College of Physicians and Surgeons of New York City. Among Steven's many accomplishments was founding the New York Academy of Medicine and serving as the second president of the American Medical Association (1848). Although Stevens was not a prolific medical author, he did write one of the earliest American treatises on urologic surgery,

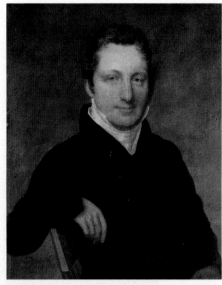

20. William Gibson as portrayed by Joseph Wood (1778–1830) (circa 1819). (*Courtesy of the College of Physicians of Philadelphia*)

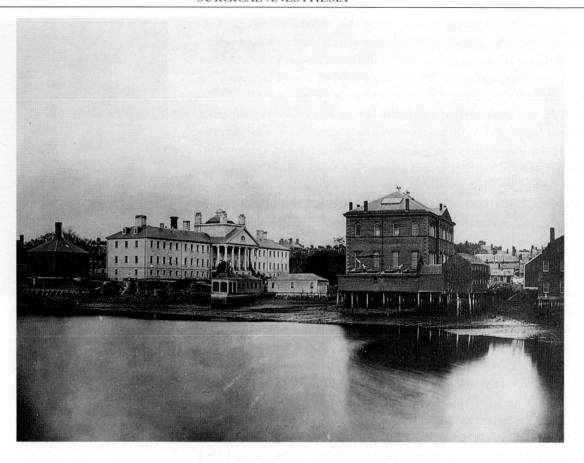

21. The Massachusetts General Hospital and Harvard Medical School, built on the tidal basin of the Charles River, were set on pilings to avoid flooding (circa 1853). *(The Francis A. Countway Library of Medicine)*

Lectures on Lithotomy (1838), and the first major paper on trauma in the United States surgical literature (1837). He also penned the second description of cleft palate closure (staphylorrhaphy) in America (1827) and was involved with the country's first report of cardiac tamponade (1826).

George Hayward (1791–1863) received undergraduate degrees from both Harvard and Yale in the same year (1809) and then matriculated in the medical department of the University of Pennsylvania, graduating in 1812. He spent time abroad, working with Astley Cooper, among others, but returned to his native Boston and founded a private medical school with John Collins Warren and Enoch Hale (1790–1848). In 1835, when Harvard University established a professorship of the principles of surgery and clinical surgery, Hayward was appointed to the position. He is most remembered for being the first American surgeon to perform a major surgical operation with ether anesthesia, an amputation of the thigh, on November 7, 1846. Hayward translated Xavier Bichat's (1771–1802) massive *General Anatomy* (1822) from the French, but his most important book was *Surgical Reports and Miscellaneous Papers* (1855). His most memorable contributions to the surgical literature were the report of a successful operative cure of vesicovaginal fistula (1839) and various papers on the use of inhalation anesthesia, including the short pamphlet, *Remarks on the Comparative Value of the Different Anaesthetic Agents* (1850).

George Frick (1793–1870) graduated from the University of Pennyslvania Medical School in 1815 and spent several years in Vienna studying under George Beer (1763–1821), a famed ophthalmologist. Frick later returned to his native city of Baltimore (1819), where he became ophthalmic surgeon at the Baltimore General Dispensary. He is best remembered for being the first in America to restrict his professional work to ophthalmology, and he authored the country's first ophthalmologic text, *A Treatise on the Diseases of the Eye* (1823). In 1840, Frick abandoned the practice of medicine and spent the rest of his life in Europe.

Alden March (1795–1869) attended medical lectures on anatomy and surgery while apprenticing with William Ingalls (1769–1851) of Boston (1813). Ingalls was renowned because five years earlier, while serving as professor of surgery at Brown

University, he had completed the country's first amputation at the shoulder joint for gunshot injury. In 1820, March received his medical degree from Brown University. From 1820 to 1838, March practiced medicine while managing a private school of anatomy near Albany, New York. There he became one of the first persons in the United States to teach anatomy by actual dissection. In 1839, March was the principal organizer of the Albany Medical College, which later became affiliated with Union College; he served as professor of surgery until his death. A founder of the American Medical Association, March served as its president in 1864. Widely traveled, he visited Europe in 1841, 1848, and 1856 to gain further experience with various operative techniques. March wrote no great texts, but he did author several case reports, including one on the use of a splint for hip disease (1853) and another on the invention of a forceps used in repairing cleft lip (1855).

Samuel Pomeroy White (1801–1867) matriculated at Union College in Schenectady, New York, as an undergraduate. He then spent two years attending lectures in the medical departments of the University of New York and the University of Pennsylvania. In 1823, the Medical Society of the County of Columbia, New York, granted White a license to practice. He joined his father Samuel (1777–1845) in practice in the mid-Hudson valley of New York. The father had previously described the first case of open intestinal surgery in America (1807). In 1828, the son reported the country's first successful ligation of the internal iliac artery. As his reputation grew, White was appointed to the chair of surgery and obstetrics in the Berkshire Medical Institution in Pittsfield, Massachusetts, and in 1830 he received the expanded title of professor of theoretical and operative surgery. For unknown reasons, White resigned from these positions in 1833 and moved to New York City, where it is said he was equally successful in pursuing his clinical endeavors.

Horace Green (1802–1866) is considered the father of American laryngology and was the first specialist in the United States to devote his practice exclusively to diseases of the throat. After serving an apprenticeship with his brother and brother-in-law, Green matriculated at the Castleton Medical College in Vermont and received his medical degree in 1824. After almost seven years of pursuing private practice in Rutland, Vermont, and in New York City, Green decided to advance his education by traveling to Europe. During a five-month visit to London and Paris (1838), Green acquired an interest in laryngology. From 1840 to 1843 he was connected with his alma mater as professor of medicine. In the 1840s, Green helped found the New York Medical College, and through 1860, when he became an invalid from tuberculosis, he served as professor of medicine and was elected president of the faculty and also of the board of trustees. Green was the recipient of an honorary degree from Union College in Schenectady, New York. He became a controversial and colorful figure in American surgery and excited an international medical uproar when he announced, in 1846, that he was able to pass a sponge-tipped probang into the larynx and thus directly apply medication to the laryngeal mucosa. For the next two decades, he was involved in stormy, often acrimonious debate concerning his research and claims. By 1854, the controversy had become so bitter that Green was summoned to defend his position before the New York Academy of Medicine. His talk caused so much heated discussion that the presiding officer was compelled to subdue the clamor by appointing a committee to investigate the truth of his claims. The committee came to no definitive conclusions, and this seems to have ended the bitter campaign waged against Green. In due time, his conclusions were found to be correct, and he assumed his rightful role in the pantheon of American surgeons. Despite the ill feelings, Green built up a very lucrative practice, which consisted mainly of the application of silver nitrate to the lining membrane of the larynx, and an occasional surgical operation. Green authored the first laryngology text in America, *A Treatise on Diseases of the Air Passages* (1846). He also wrote *Observations on the Pathology of Croup* (1849), *On the Surgical Treatment of Polypi of the Larynx, and Oedema of the Glottis* (1852), and *A Practical Treatise on Pulmonary Tuberculosis* (1864).

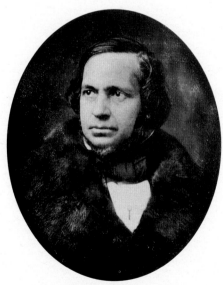

22. Horace Green. *(Courtesy of The New York Academy of Medicine)*

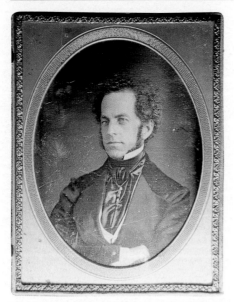

23. A daguerreotype of Thomas Dent Mütter (circa 1846), taken by M.P. Simmons of Philadelphia. Mütter lives on as the guiding force behind the medical museum, which bears his name, at the College of Physicians of Philadelphia. *(Courtesy of Stanley B. Burns, M.D., and The Burns Collection and Archive)*

Charles Stuart Tripler (1806–1866) was born in New York City and received his medical degree from the College of Physicians and Surgeons (1827). He immediately entered the army and was soon advanced in rank to full surgeon. During the Mexican War he served at various posts throughout the West. With the start of the Civil War, Tripler was appointed medical director of a corps serving in the Shenandoah Valley. When General George McClellan (1826–1885) assumed the chief command, Tripler was made general medical director of the Army of the Potomac. Political and organizational problems soon became evident, and following the battles of the Peninsula, Tripler was relieved of his command, appointed to duty in Michigan, and soon brevetted colonel for "meritorious service." Shortly before his death, he was promoted to brevet brigadier general. His best-known work was the Civil War surgical manual *Handbook for the Military Surgeon* (1861).

John Watson (1807–1863), a native of Ireland, was brought to America as a young child. He received his medical degree from the College of Physicians and Surgeons in New York City in 1832. In the following year, Watson was appointed to the staff of the New York Dispensary, where he served as attending surgeon from 1839 to 1862. In 1838, he also joined the staff of the New York Hospital, where he introduced regular clinical instruction in surgery. Watson remains best known for the first report of an esophagotomy in the American periodical literature (1844). In the mid-1850s, Watson became involved in a nasty public debate with Frank Hamilton (1813–1886) concerning priority over the use of plastic surgical operations to treat skin ulcers. Watson never authored a lengthy surgical text, but he did write an obscure but valuable historical monograph, *The Medical Profession in Ancient Times* (1856).

Thomas Dent Mütter (1811–1859) graduated from the University of Pennsylvania (1831) and then studied medicine in Paris. He eventually became professor of surgery at Jefferson Medical College (1841) and remained there for fifteen years until ill health forced his retirement. Mütter was well recognized for his surgical skills, particularly in the areas of plastic and reconstructive surgery. In 1837, he authored the country's first article in the periodical literature on surgery for disfigurement. His pamphlet *Cases of Deformity of Various Kinds Treated by Plastic Operations* (1843) is highly prized for containing the first description of a pedicle flap published in the American medical literature. By 1843, Mütter had completed over twenty cleft palate repairs. His only lengthy textbook was the loosely written *A Lecture on Loxarthrus or Clubfoot* (1839). In addition, as professor of surgery he had published a *Syllabus of the Course of Lectures on the Principles and Practice of Surgery* (1843). Mütter endowed a series of talks in his name at the College of Physicians of Philadelphia, and the present-day medical museum at that institution carries his appellation.

Jonathan Mason Warren (1811–1867) was the son of John Collins Warren. He studied with his father, graduated from Harvard Medical School in 1832, and received further education in both London and Paris. After a three-year stint abroad, Warren returned to the United States and immediately began to assist his father at the Massachusetts General Hospital. He aided his father in the performance of the first operation on a patient under ether, and a few weeks later he substituted for Morton's inhalation apparatus a cone-shaped ether sponge. A decade later he was elected a visiting surgeon to that institution and was eventually named senior surgeon. Warren's only major text was *Surgical Observations, with Cases and Operations* (1867). He is particularly remembered for his extensive experience with rhinoplastic operations (1837) and cleft palate repair (1843). Warren's son was John Collins Warren (1842–1927), professor of surgery at Harvard.

Daniel Brainard (1812–1866) graduated from Jefferson Medical College (1834). He spent the next few years in practice in Chicago, and then traveled to Paris in the hope of furthering his medical knowledge. On his return to America in 1841, Brainard again settled in Chicago, where he founded Rush Medical College and became its first professor of surgery. He also helped establish the Chicago Medical

Society (1850), the Illinois State Medical Society (1850), and the first general hospital in Chicago. Brainard reported on intravenous treatment of cancer (1852), did experimental work regarding snake bites (1854), and authored a short essay on the treatment of nonunited fractures (1854). He also performed the earliest recorded necropsy in Chicago (1844).

Horace Ackley (1813–1859) received his medical degree from the College of Physicians and Surgeons in Fairfield, New York in 1833. In 1836 he was appointed demonstrator of anatomy in the Willoughby Medical College in Ohio. When the Cleveland Medical College was organized in 1843, Ackley was appointed to the chair of surgery and remained in that position until 1858. He was considered the most renowned of surgeons in Northern Ohio and was recognized as an outstanding expert witness in medical malpractice cases. He authored few clinical reports but did describe an amputation of the entire lower jaw for osteosarcoma in 1853 and two ovariotomies in 1857. Ackley was president of the Ohio State Medical Society (1852). In his later years, Ackley became an alcoholic, which contributed to his premature demise.

24. With his elaborately staged office, Professor Palmer was typical of many mid-nineteenth-century quack physicians. They traveled from town to town, bringing with them phrenological and anatomical charts that helped mask their lack of medical and surgical education. In Palmer's milieu (late 1850s), medical practice merged with medical entertainment and provided a forum for itinerants and other charlatans to enter the profitable field of health care delivery. *(Courtesy of Stanley B. Burns, M.D., and The Burns Collection and Archive)*

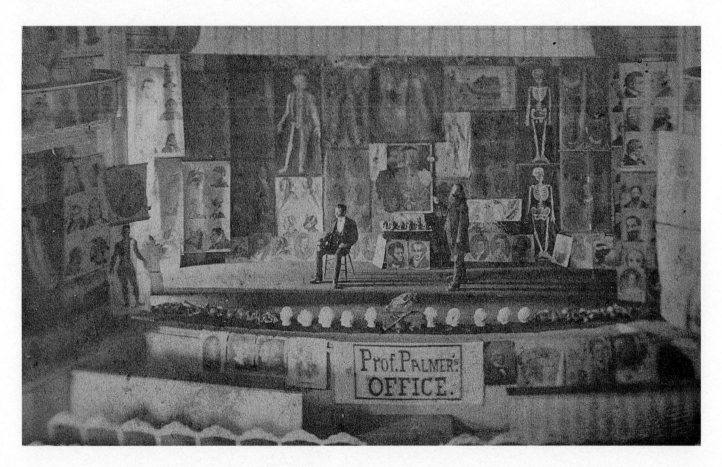

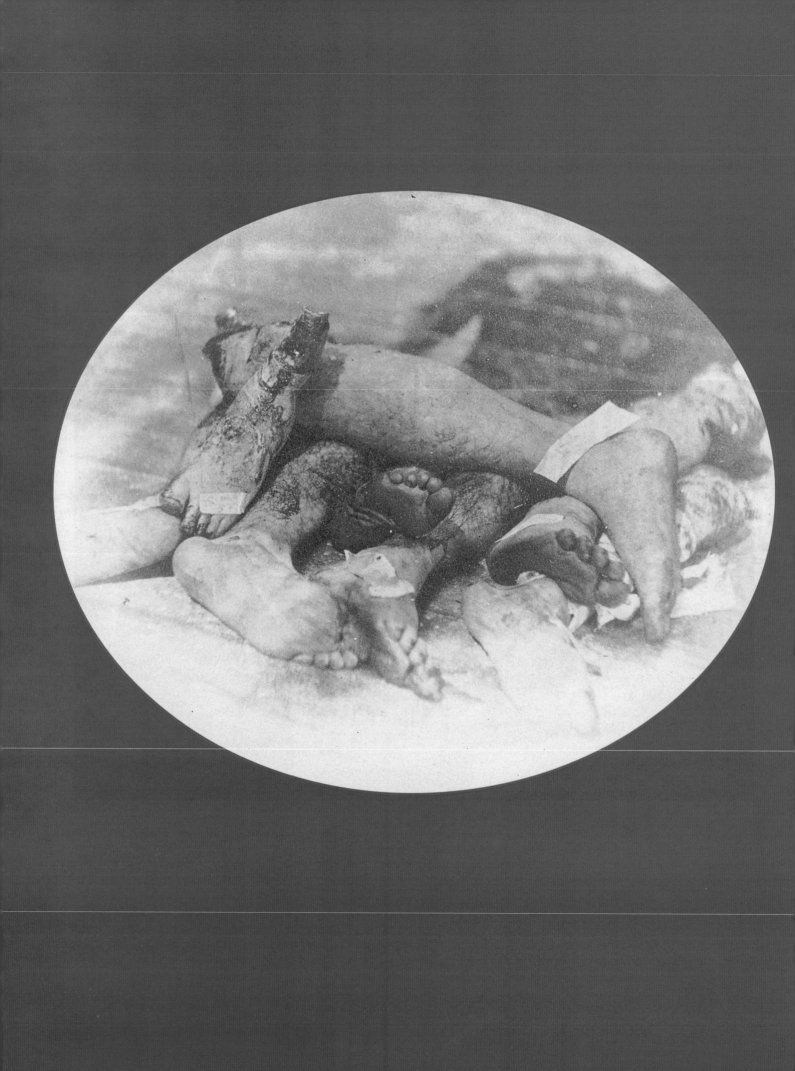

CHAPTER 5

CIVIL WAR SURGERY
1861–1865

Throughout the centuries the savagery of warfare has served surgeons well, as the battlefield proves fertile ground for the on-site training of young surgeons. The loss of life and limb that combatants must ruefully contemplate are viewed objectively by the surgeon as an invaluable learning experience. The Civil War proved no different. This tragic episode in our country's history had unquestioned importance in the development of an American profession of surgery.

Unlike the Revolutionary War and the War of 1812, the five-year internecine struggle was a "cut and carve" drama. Hundreds of amputated arms and legs lay outside makeshift field hospitals. The very size of the rebellion, with casualty counts not infrequently in the tens of thousands for a single day, dictated its surgical significance. Untold numbers of the most horrific surgical cases imaginable were cared for in a space of time that would have taken many years of peace to match. Physicians, whether they considered themselves surgically trained or not, had no choice but to become familiar with the surgical principles of caring for the war wounded and to develop an appreciation for surgical anesthesia.

In late 1862, Brigadier General Carl Schurz (1829–1906) marched his division past a Northern field hospital. Mud was all around, bloated corpses filled the scene, and severed limbs were thrown helter-skelter in a pile next to the tent. Schurz told of the surgeons with "their sleeves rolled up to their elbows, their bare arms as well as their linen aprons smeared with blood, their knives...held between their teeth...one operation accomplished, the surgeons would look around with a deep sigh, and then - 'Next!'" For the wounded soldier, the horrors of battle did not cease at the front. Evacuation plans were so ineffective that the seriously wounded often lay on the battlefield for several days. The rotting corpses of their dead comrades surrounded them, and little surgical assistance was in sight. In agony from wounds that were soon to be filled with pus, the injured crawled into the shelter of shaded groves or sought the comfort of running streams. There they would suffer from dehydration or suffocate in their own vomit.

In order to comprehend such a disquieting scene, we must understand that the Civil War resulted in the highest number of casualties of any war in our country's history. What began almost light-heartedly at the first battle of Bull Run soon turned into a national dance of the medical macabre. The exact number of deaths from battlefield injuries and its miserable twin, camp infection and disease, remains unknown. According to the estimates, however, 110,000 Union soldiers died directly or indirectly of their wounds and 250,000 perished from infection and disease. In the Confederate forces, there were approximately 95,000 deaths from fighting and 165,000 from infection and disease. By comparison, some 125,000 Americans perished in World War I and 405,000 in World War II. So intense was the fighting during the War of the Rebellion that in certain battles the dead and dying littered the battlefield as far as the eye could see. For example, at Antietam 5,510 were killed and

1. *(facing page)* Few pictures so utterly portray the human devastation and misery of Civil War surgery as "A Morning's Work." This dramatic scene shows a pile of lower extremity amputations, representing a few hours worth of surgery, at one Civil War hospital. Multiply this sorry spectacle by all the nonstop carnage that typified the American Civil War, and the enormity of just the surgical side of the hostilities becomes evident. This particular illustration is taken from the personal photographic album of Reed B. Bontecou (1824–1907), surgeon-in-charge of Harewood United States Army General Hospital, Washington, D.C. A great many wartime surgical photographs were taken at this medical facility, and it was Bontecou who personally directed the institution's numerous photographic projects. He pioneered the technique of close-up operative views to teach other surgeons various types of operations. Bontecou took preoperative and postoperative pictures of hundreds of wounded soldiers, and these images constitute the largest extant collection of actual Civil War surgical photographs. *(Courtesy of Stanley B. Burns, M.D., and The Burns Collection and Archive)*

25,815 wounded, at Chickamauga 4,033 were killed and 22,674 wounded, and at Gettysburg 6,334 were killed and 28,209 wounded. Such carnage was to become an enormous physical and emotional burden for the poorly educated, inadequately trained, and ineffectually organized physician-surgeons of 1860s America.

Sunday, July 21, 1861, was to be an exciting day for the elite of Washington society. The potential of an armed conflict twenty-seven miles south of the city at Manassas, Virginia, had been publicly announced the day before. Dressed in their holiday finest and transported by horse and carriage, a large segment of the city's residents left the capitol to observe the battle. Initially, the 30,000-strong Army of the Potomac appeared to be defeating the outnumbered rebels, who were led by Confederate General Pierre Beauregard (1818–1893). For the noncombatant spectators, it was a festive morning until noon, when suddenly some 9,000 Shenandoah Valley regulars under the command of Joseph Johnston (1807–1891) reinforced the collapsing Confederate line. With the addition of Thomas "Stonewall" Jackson's (1824–1863) First Brigade, the battle which had started so well for the Union troops, turned instead into a sustained rout. Forced back, the tired, hungry, and mostly untrained Northern troops panicked and fled from the field. The battlefield gogglers were similarly terrified, and soldiers and civilians en masse began a frightened flight back to Washington. All that saved Washington from Southern troops, Johnston noted, was that "our army was more disorganized by victory than that of the United States by defeat." The battle scene was aptly summed up by one war correspondent: "Bull Run, They Run, We Run."

Lost amid this chaotic exodus were the wounded and about-to-be-dead. According to official government statistics, 481 Union troops were killed outright and another 1,011 wounded. In addition, some 1,460 soldiers were missing in action. On the Confederate side, 269 were killed, 1,483 wounded, and an unknown number unaccounted for. The scene became one of profound confusion. There was no organized evacuation of the wounded, and no provisions had been made for field hospitals to handle casualties. The dying were left on the sun-scorched battlefield to end their life in tortured ignominy. Fleeing soldiers and their equipment blocked the path of the few horse-drawn carts, serving as makeshift ambulances, that were attempting to evacuate the injured. Most of those unable to walk were simply left to the clemency of the enemy. Those wounded soldiers fortunate enough to be able to walk without assistance filled the twenty-seven mile return route begging for assistance at every doorway they passed and similarly scouring the streets of Washington in search of any form of boarding.

2. By the time of the Civil War, surgical instrument fabricators were well established in Boston, New York City, and Philadelphia. Richard Satterlee (1798–1880), in his role as Medical Purveyor of the United States Army, placed contracts with numerous instrument makers for the fabrication of cased instrument sets and related military surgical equipment. During his tenure, Satterlee requisitioned over 4,900 amputating and general operating cases, 1,150 cases of trephining, exsecting, post-mortem, and "personal" instruments, and 12,700 minor surgery and pocket instrument sets. This staff surgeon's capital operating set, manufactured by Horatio B. Kern of Philadelphia, included everything from scalpels to urethral sounds. Such Civil War sets can be considered more conventional than innovative, as Civil War surgery did not produce any major advances in instrumentation. It did, however, prove quite lucrative to Kern and several other Philadelphia instrument makers, including Jacob H. Gemrig, Dietrich W. Kolbe, and Jacob J. Teufel. *(Collection of Alex Peck, Antique Scientifica)*

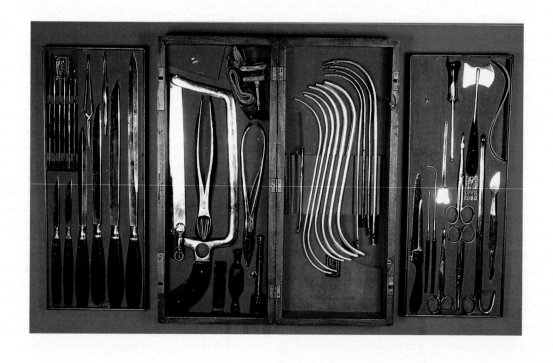

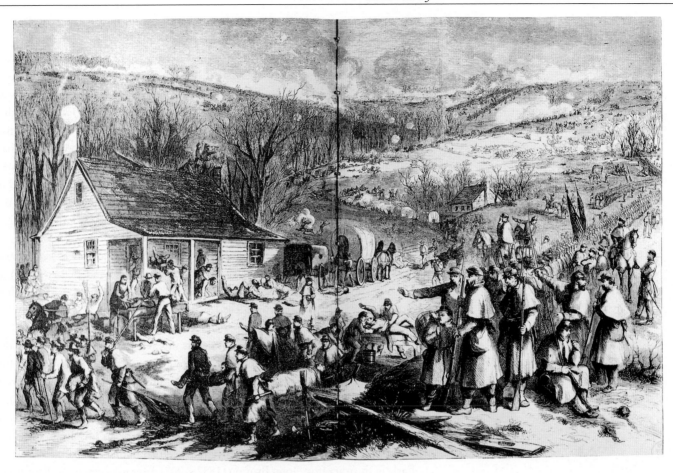

MEDICAL AND SURGICAL CARE IN THE
EARLY DAYS OF THE WAR

The rather cavalier attitude toward the necessity for post-battle treatment of the wounded at Bull Run was indicative of the general ineptitude of the military medical-surgical establishment as well as of an unprepared civilian physician and administrative population. The few military medical officers present at Bull Run had received no instruction about their duties, privileges, and powers. Consequently, they had no formal authority to organize battlefield relief efforts and to direct their subordinates and stretchermen of the various regiments. Even when military surgeons did issue orders, enlisted men were loath to receive orders from a stranger. As a result, each regimental surgeon assumed direct responsibility only for the men of his particular unit. Therefore, any soldier wounded at a distance from his regimental surgeon usually went untended. The physical and emotional devastation at Bull Run was summed up by assistant surgeon William Williams Keen (1837–1932):

> My first initiation into real warfare was at the First Bull Run.... Up to that time, and, in fact, during the entire engagement, I never received a single order from either colonel or other officer, Medical Inspector, the surgeon of my regiment, or any one else. It was like the days when there was no King in Israel, and every man did that which was right in his own eyes...I was as green as the grass around me as to my duties on the field...I was...dressing a man who had a fracture of the humerus from a Minie ball. I was applying a splint and an eight-yard bandage...when suddenly one hundred or more of the soldiers rushed pell-mell down the road from the battlefield screaming "the rebs are after us!" It did not take more than one positive assertion of this kind to convince the man whose arm I was bandaging that it was time for him to leave, and he broke away from me.... As he ran, four or five yards of the bandage unwound, and I last saw him disappearing in the distance with this fluttering bobtail bandage flying all abroad. My experience in this battle is a good illustration of the utter disorganization, or rather want of organization, of our entire army at the beginning of the war.

3. Of much historical accuracy is this dramatic wood-engraved scene recorded by the well-known illustrator Thomas Nast (1840–1902) while working for *Harper's Weekly* (1862). The reserves are lined up, waiting to be called into action, while a fierce battle is being waged just a short distance away. Many of the anxious soldiers focus their attention on the improvised field hospital, in front of which a surgeon is operating. Scattered about on the ground are amputated arms and legs. *(Collection Boston Public Library)*

The description of the battle of Bull Run and its confusing aftermath well illustrates the difficulties facing American surgery and its physician-surgeons at the time of the Civil War. The education, training, and day-to-day clinical skills of the average medical practitioner were hopelessly inadequate to cope with the rising tide of injured and maimed bodies. To the vast majority of soon-to-be conscripted American physicians, military medical mien was entirely unknown. Even more disillusioning was the fact that despite the past nine decades of state-of-the-art English and French influence on America's medical elite, such education and training had not adequately filtered down to the more common but less privileged class of ordinary rural practitioner. This latter group remained unsophisticated and unskilled in the basic surgical therapies. An even greater problem was that neither among the urban medical noblesse nor the inarticulate rural healers could be found a critical mass of full-time surgeons. Few American physicians in the 1860s could be considered career surgeons. Consequently, the vast number of army doctors lacked knowledge about operative techniques and were totally unqualified to practice surgery. Yet, the tens of thousands of medical men who served in the Civil War, whether they approved of it or not, were considered first and foremost surgeons and always referred to as such.

The semantic liberty of titling all physicians in Civil War army service with the sobriquet of surgeon greatly complicated future efforts to define and regulate the role of surgery within American medicine and overall society. The conscripts, while enjoying the title of surgeon, were still more physician than "scalpel handler." One thing was certain: there was no organized group of surgeons or other surgically related association to warrant any conclusion that American physician-surgeons would be able to mount a well-organized effort to treat military casualties.

Early in the war effort, John Brinton (1832–1907), later to become a well-respected Philadelphia surgeon, related how a fellow Civil War "surgeon" was treating a patient whose seriously wounded leg demanded amputation. Brinton had recently been appointed a Brigade Surgeon when this novice physician "begged me...to perform the operation for him." The conscripted medical officer confessed that he had never done an amputation, nor had he ever seen one. Moreover, the newly named "surgeon" had no idea how such an operation should be performed. Brinton explained that "this would never do; his position in the regiment demanded that he himself should remove the limb." After ceaseless coaxing, Brinton finally acquiesced and assisted the trembling recruit with the removal of the limb. Brinton was dumbfounded because within a few days' time, this amateurish affair somehow established the new "surgeon's" reputation so well that the troops quickly regarded him as an experienced surgeon.

A few months later, when Brinton was serving at the battle of Fort Donelson, he was informed that a "great surgeon was busy operating in one of the field hospitals." Brinton walked into the commandeered house, temporarily serving as a hospital, and found "bloodstained footmarks on the crooked stairs and in...the room stood my friend of memory; amputated arms and legs seemed almost to litter the floor; beneath the operating table was a pool of blood, the operator was smeared with it...'Ah, Doctor,' said the new-fledged surgeon, 'I am getting on, just look at these,' pointing to his trophies on the floor."

Conscripts and particularly volunteer "surgeons" were accused of performing needless surgical procedures, most notably amputation, as a way of perfecting their noticeably absent technical skills. In so doing, they would find their professional reputations enhanced on their return to private practice. Such individuals were there to "cut" and would condescendingly refuse other assignments, particularly those that might prove uninteresting. Distrust of the recruited "surgeon" was manifested by the countless stories of combatants who halted the surgeon's sharpened saw at gunpoint, only to be forcibly restrained, immediately anesthetized, and quickly relieved of their injured arms or legs. "Butcher" became a catchphrase intended to impugn the reputation of battlefield surgeons. In the most callous of situations, John

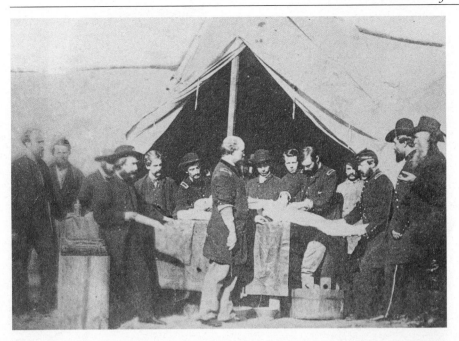

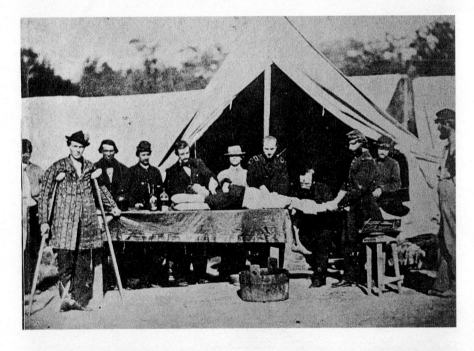

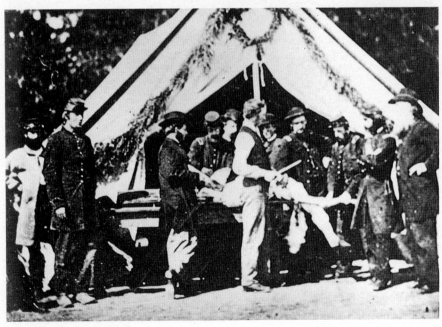

4. Scenes of surgical operations conducted in a field hospital during the Civil War are quite rare. These photographs, probably taken by either the Tyson Brothers or Peter Weaver (circa, October 1863), show surgery at an "operating tent" that was part of the General Hospital located in Camp Letterman near the Gettysburg battlefield. A bucket to catch the free-flowing blood is located on the ground, and already blood-saturated sheets are evident *(top and middle)*. In this environment, anyone could watch the operation, even wounded soldiers who knew they too could end up on that operating table. The garlanded tent *(bottom)* is not the same as the "operating tent," since the "operating tent" has attached "side areas" while the garlanded tent stands by itself. It is difficult to establish the identity of most of the individuals in view, although it has been claimed that the surgeon in front of the garlanded tent is James T. Calhoun (1838–1866) of Rahway, New Jersey. All three scenes were probably photographed on the same day, but whether they are staged recreations or genuine surgical operations remains open to historical inquiry. *(top and middle: Courtesy of Stanley B. Burns, M.D. and The Burns Collection and Archive) (bottom: Edward G. Miner Library, University of Rochester Medical Center)*

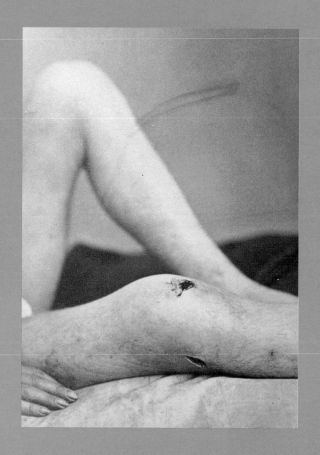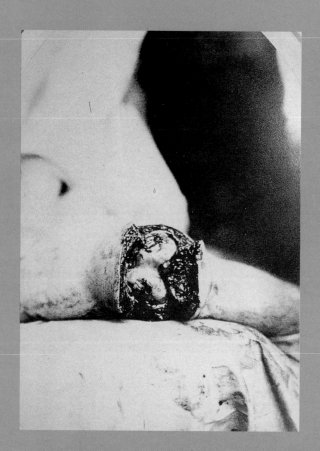

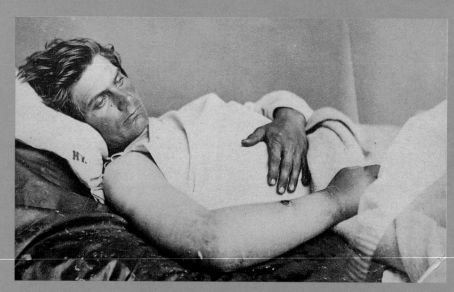

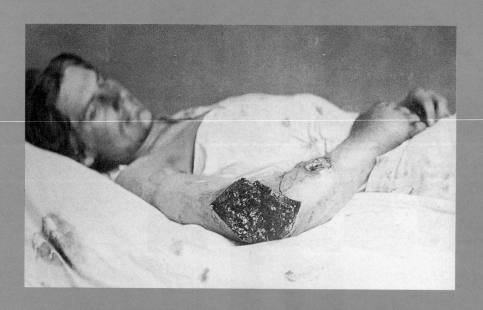

Claiborne (1828–1905), a Southern commissioned surgeon assigned to the 12th Virginia Infantry, observed a fellow "surgeon" in full view of the troops taking time off from the work of mutilation by refreshing his knowledge of "open anatomy" on a freshly killed corpse. A surgeon's disagreeable attitude was affirmed by nurse's aide Louisa May Alcott (1832–1888):

> [he] had acquired a somewhat trying habit of regarding a man and his wound as separate institutions, and seemed rather annoyed that the former should express any opinion on the latter, or claim any right in it, while under his care…. [He] seemed to regard a dilapidated body very much as I should have regarded a damaged garment…. The more intricate the wound, the better he liked it. A poor private, with both legs off, and shot through the lungs, possessed more attractions for him than a dozen generals, slightly scratched in some "masterly retreat;" and had any one appeared in small pieces, requesting to be put together again, he would have considered it a special dispensation.

Surgery during the War of the Rebellion was chaotic and horrifying. Thus, it was not unreasonable to expect that in the medically unsophisticated America of the 1860s, the hastily rearranged army medical departments would initially contain large numbers of backward and incompetent medical men. Yet, it must not be overlooked that by the end of the hostilities, an important cadre of earnest and intelligent surgeons had arisen. Numerous young men took the opportunity to compensate for their educational and training deficiencies by utilizing the unique clinical and scientific circumstances that were opened for them by the war. From their battlefield and hospital experiences, many individuals, including William Williams Keen and John Shaw Billings in the North and Hunter Holmes McGuire (1835–1900) in the South, began to forge national and international surgical reputations.

Some young men, like the 27-year-old Keen, achieved their prominence more from research endeavors than from actual clinical triumphs. For instance, Keen, along with his fellow authors S. Weir Mitchell (1829–1914) and George Morehouse (1829–1905) conducted wartime research into traumatic neuroses at the U.S. Army Hospital for Injuries and Diseases of the Nervous System in Philadelphia. Their investigations resulted in the publication of one of the acknowledged classics of nineteenth-century American surgery, *Gunshot Wounds and Other Injuries of Nerves* (1864). This treatise, now scarce, introduced for the first time the concept of causalgia and ways to treat the disabling condition. In response to such earnest efforts, it is perhaps easier to understand why by war's end, Walt Whitman (1819–1892), working as a wound dresser, presented a more sympathetic picture of surgeons when he wrote, "All but a few are excellent men."

Competent or incompetent, surgically skilled or not, vast numbers of doctors were needed to treat the army of injured. So great was the demand that more than 12,500 physicians for the North and 3,000 for the South, not including unknown numbers of volunteers, were called into service in either field or civilian hospitals. Most of these men served as regimental surgeons and assistant surgeons and were commissioned by state governors rather than by the Congress or President Abraham Lincoln (1809–1865). Full surgeons with commissions held the rank of major and received $169 per month. Assistant surgeons served as captains or first lieutenants and were paid $155 and $105 per month, respectively.

These "surgeons" were usually only capable of general medical practice. Being surgically inept, they frequently botched the simplest of surgical operations and often caused wounded soldiers more harm than good. Preenlistment examinations to determine a physician's clinical competence were perfunctory at best. The editor of one leading medical journal was particularly succinct in his denunciation of the examining process: "We may estimate by hundreds the number of unqualified persons who have received the endorsement of the medical examining bodies as capable surgeons. Indeed, these examinations have in some cases been so conducted as to prove the merest farce."

5. *(facing page)* The Bontecou picture album documents almost 600 clinical surgical cases, many of which did not involve amputation or bone excision. For instance, these two cases demonstrate how wound infections were often incised and débrided. It was hoped that "laying open" infected areas would enhance the healing process. Whether for a bullet to the knee *(top left and right)* or an injury to the forearm *(middle and bottom)*, following the débridement many surgeons used nitric acid on the wound to cleanse it. The pain was intolerable, and some soldiers had to be anesthetized in order to undergo the nitric acid treatment. In certain cases, the scarring from the nitric acid was so severe that while the limb itself was saved, it was little more than a disfigured and dysfunctional appendage. *(Courtesy of Stanley B. Burns, M.D., and The Burns Collection and Archive)*

One peculiar aspect of Civil War surgery was the untold numbers of civilian medical volunteers who flocked down South after any major engagement, supposedly to lend a hand with the operative workload. Whether their motives were entirely patriotic or stemmed more from opportunism remains unclear. Lewis Stimson (1844–1917), a young medical recruit, related the case of a Captain Graves, who was shot at Gettysburg in the thigh: "He was taken to the field hospital, a [volunteer] surgeon came by, glanced at his wounds, and said, 'Amputate.' While awaiting his turn, he saw a medical acquaintance passing and called to him, asking for at least an examination before condemnation. It proved to be simply a flesh wound and in a month he was back on duty."

Following the gory battle at Gettysburg in July 1863, this "civilian-auxillary" system was totally revamped. Each state formed a reserve surgeons corps, whose civilian recruits were certified and paid to supplement the enlisted medical officers. By 1864, operating surgeons, particularly those in the field hospitals, were being screened on the basis of actual performance, including "prudence, judgement, and skill." These new reserve surgeons were particularly evident in General Ulysses Grant's (1822–1885) spring campaign of 1864, during the great battles of the Wilderness (3,288 killed, 9,278 wounded, 6,784 missing), Spotsylvania (2,146 killed, 7,956 wounded, 2,577 missing), Cold Harbor (1,905 killed, 10,570 wounded, 2,456 missing), and Petersburg (1,298 killed, 7,474 wounded, 1,814 missing). Within one month of the commencement of action, some 194 reserve surgeons, 42 contract surgeons, and 775 nursing and medical students had gathered around Fredericksburg, Maryland, the medical base of Grant's Army of the Potomac.

The army surgeon often obtained the surgical lessons of the war at great personal sacrifice. There was an incorrect perception that the military surgeon was exposed to little danger during a battle. Nineteen officers of the medical staff of the regular and volunteer forces of the Union Army were killed outright in action, one by Sioux Indians. Thirteen officers were killed by partisan troops or assassinated by guerrillas or rioters. Eight officers died of wounds received in action, while nine succumbed through accidents occurring in the line of duty. Surgeon General Joseph Barnes (1817–1883) noted the Medical Department's losses were "proportionately larger than that of any other staff corps" and included eighty-three officers wounded in action. In addition to the battle casualties, the medical corps lost almost three hundred individuals to death by disease, four of them in Confederate prisons.

MANUALS OF MILITARY SERVICE

The military and clinical inexperience of the average Civil War "surgeon" soon made it evident that military surgical manuals were needed. Unfortunately, there had been little prior demand for works on military surgery, and no American texts were available. A greater problem was the general disinterest by the American army medical community regarding recent developments in the conduct of European military surgery. During the Crimean conflict, Florence Nightingale (1820–1910) had effected sanitary reforms in both military hospitals and campsites. Nightingale's measures brought about a drop in hospital mortality from 42 to 2 percent. The French, in their recently completed Italian campaign, had developed evacuation procedures for their wounded using horse-drawn ambulances. These covered carts brought the trauma victim to one of a multitude of small but clean lazarettes. But American indecision delayed the development of an efficient system of managing mass casualties until midway through the civil conflict.

At the outbreak of the war, Samuel Gross wrote a *Manual of Military Surgery* (1861). Designed to be a "kind of pocket companion for the young surgeons who were flocking into the army, and who for the most part were ill prepared for the prompt and efficient discharge of their duties," the work was composed in just nine days. The *Manual* was destined to become the most popular of the various Northern surgical manuals published during the Civil War, and an unauthorized edition was

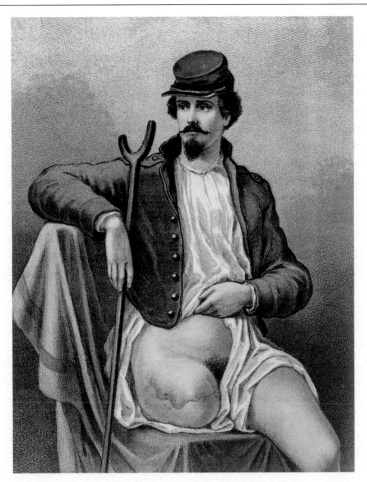

6. Private Woodford Longmore, a "rebel soldier, twenty-five years of age" was wounded on June 11, 1864, during a brief skirmish at Cynthiana, Kentucky (*A Report on Amputations at the Hip-Joint in Military Surgery*, 1867). Placed in a rebel field hospital, he was found to have suffered a complete shattering of the shaft of the femur. For six excrutiating weeks, extension and counter-extension were maintained, but with little evident healing. Confined to bed for almost nine months, Longmore was forced to tolerate intermittent bouts of thigh abscesses accompanied by an unrelenting elimination of necrotic bone fragments. By January 1866 he had undergone two minor operations to drain abscess sites, and his situation was deemed surgically hopeless. George Blackman was consulted, and it was decided to proceed with a secondary amputation at the hip joint. Pathological examination of the amputated limb revealed the entire femur to be affected by osteomyelitis. Eighteen months later, Blackman found his patient in excellent health and recently married. Longmore remained subject to occasional attacks of "neuralgia of extreme severity," which he relieved by "taking large doses of morphia." (*Author's Collection*)

even reprinted in Richmond. Extensively cited, particularly by Confederate surgeons, the thirteen chapters provide much in the way of clinical facts but little instruction in the actual performance of surgical procedures. Gross's manual was soon followed by Frank Hamilton's (1813–1886) *Practical Treatise on Military Surgery* (1861), Charles Tripler's and George Blackman's (1819–1871) *Handbook for the Military Surgeon* (1861), Stephen Smith's (1823–1922) *Hand-Book of Surgical Operations* (1862), and John Packard's (1832–1907) *Manual of Minor Surgery* (1863). All these later treatises were overtly pragmatic, some providing simplified instructions to complete an amputation, elevate a skull fracture, etc.

In the South there was a similar dearth of clinical surgical experience: only twenty-four of the almost three thousand surgeons who served in the Confederate army had received previous military medical training. To add to the woes of the Southern physicians, the government of the United States had developed an efficient blockade, which among other things prevented an adequate number of medical or surgical texts from reaching the front lines. Forced to fend for themselves, Southern physician-surgeons soon authored an impressive array of military medical literature and surgical manuals. In the fall of 1861, John Julian Chisholm (1830–1903), professor of surgery at the Medical College of South Carolina, prepared his *Manual of Military Surgery*. Based largely on the experience Chisholm had gained while observing the medical and surgical treatment of wounded soldiers in Italy in 1859, the *Manual* became widely used by Confederate surgeons. Considerable space was also given to the subjects of amusements, clothing, duties, food, and camp hygiene. In addition, the last fifty pages were devoted to the interminable certificates, forms, and reports that became the bureaucratic nightmare of all Southern surgeons. Although Chisholm's monograph was quite similar to Gross's effort, their attitudes toward surgical anesthesia differed widely. Gross believed that anesthetics should not be given as long as the "vital powers are depressed and the mind is bewildered by shock…their administration will hardly be safe…. Moreover, it is astonishing what little suffering the patient generally experiences, when in this condition, even from a severe wound or operation." Conversely, Chisholm was of the opinion that "whenever operations are to be performed…it should be administered. It is a remedy which the surgeon should never be without…. The effects of chloroform are wonderful in mitigating the suffering of the wounded."

An Epitome of Practical Surgery by Edward Warren (1828–1893) appeared in 1863. Warren was Surgeon General of the State of North Carolina and a former professor of surgery at two small proprietary medical schools in Baltimore. His treatise, a rare and important work, was used by virtually all Confederate medical officers, although Warren made no claim to clinical originality. The most ambitious of Southern surgical works is *A Manual of Military Surgery, Prepared for the Use of the Confederate States Army* (1863). This scarce monograph was put together by order of Samuel P. Moore (1813-1889), Surgeon General of the Confederacy. Although it was written anonymously, most of its authors are known to have been surgeons working in the Office of the Surgeon-General. For instance, Henry Fraser Campbell (1824–1891), professor of surgery at the Medical College of Georgia, authored the sixty-eight page section on ligation of arteries. The book has neither a table of contents nor an index, but within its five chapters ("Surgical diseases," "Gun-shot wounds," "On the arteries," "Amputations in general," and "On resections") are numerous illustrations of various operations. The Southern soldier must not have been altogether comforted to realize that the "outline lithographs" were intended to demonstrate how to perform "amputation and resection" by simplified line drawings. In other words, the mass of uninitiated Confederate military surgeons often could do little more than follow the dotted anatomical line drawings in performing surgical procedures.

The most ambitious medical work published in the South during the war period was the *Confederate States Medical and Surgical Journal.* Issued monthly from January 1864 to February 1865, it was the only medical periodical published under the

7. "The Surgeon at Work at the Rear During an Engagement." The celebrated artist Winslow Homer (1836–1910), in his role as a reportorial illustrator for *Harper's Weekly* (1862), sketched realistic war scenes throughout the hostilities. At the time of the Civil War, the depiction of wartime medical attention did not appear in formal easel paintings. Therefore, it was the function of artists, working for various newspapers and magazines, to provide the public with such visual information both during and immediately after a battle. *(Collection Library of Congress)*

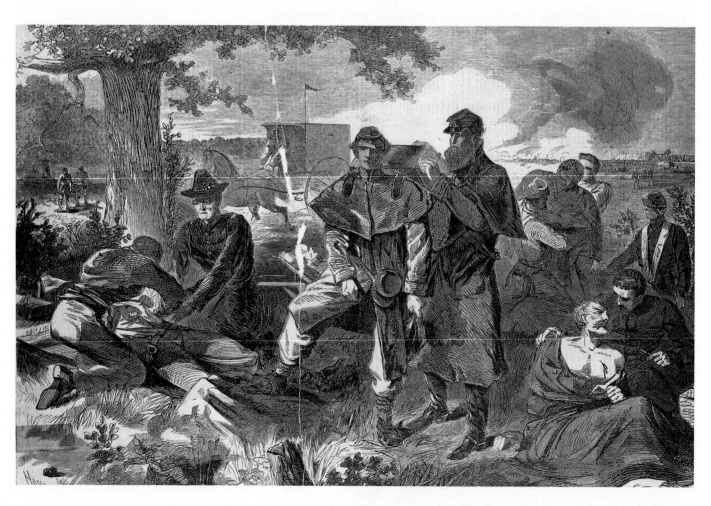

Confederacy. The *Journal* contained numerous editorials, articles by Confederate physicians and surgeons on their battlefield experiences, and analyses of reports from foreign journals. Many of the articles were on surgical topics, including such controversial opinions as G. M. B. Maugh's (?–1901) belief that it might be "well for the cause of humanity" if a "surgeon's case was left…bare of amputating knives." At a time when surgeons believed that suppuration (i.e., "laudable pus") and its attendant morbidity were natural events of the inflammation-healing cycle, William Michel's (1822–1894) report on the healing of gunshot injuries by first intention was highly unusual. For Michel to state that "a wound may present the phenomenon of spontaneous cure: that is, without suppurating…" showed that some Civil War surgeons were beginning to move away from the preconceived position that all injuries must have purulence present to heal satisfactorily.

SURGICAL CARE ON THE BATTLEFIELD

Dramatizations of Civil War battles notwithstanding, there was little hand-to-hand combat. Bayonet and saber wounds were rarely seen, and artillery shelling caused minimal human losses. The real killer was the rifle, along with its messenger of death, the Minie ball. Ninety-four percent of wounds suffered in the Civil War were inflicted by gunshot, and the .58-caliber cone-shaped Minie bullet was all too well known for the tremendous amount of tissue destruction it caused. Arms, legs, and even heads were literally blown away. Edward Warren related that "James Hawkins - the son of our village undertaker…could only be recognized by his body, as his head had been carried entirely away by a single shot." As the soldiers fired in volleys, frequently without bothering to aim, and the smoke was so thick that hitting a specific target was sometimes nothing more than happenstance, "the shattering, splintering, and splitting of a long bone by the impact of the Minie ball was…both remarkable and frightful."

When a battle began, the first stop for a wounded soldier was an aid station located in a protected or semiprotected position at the edge of the battlefield. If the individual was lucky, he walked; if not, he was carried by stretcher-bearers. Although it seems ludicrous to go into battle without some method of providing field evacuation, this was exactly the position in which the Union and Confederate forces initially found themselves. Even at the second battle of Bull Run (August 1862), knowing of the previous evacuation problems at the site, three thousand wounded lay on the field for three days, and an extraordinary six hundred soldiers remained for one week. Many of the generals were unsympathetic to the immediate needs of the wounded. None were more detested than Don Carlos Buell, General of the Army of the Ohio, who resolutely refused to assign men to evacuate the wounded or even so much as provide resources so that the Medical Corps could accomplish this task on their own. Buell was of the singular opinion that a soldier unfit for war had no priority in receiving medical assistance.

Such military nonsense reached its zenith when Henry Ingersoll Bowditch (1808–1892), professor of medicine at Harvard and one of the country's first physician-surgeons to specialize in diseases of the chest, experienced one of the cruelest of life's many hardships: the death of his oldest son on a battlefield. The young man was a lieutenant when he received an abdominal wound in the Peninsular Campaign in 1862. He lay on the field for at least two agonizing days without any medical attention. When a horse-drawn ambulance finally reached him, it carried no water. The driver refused to procure some, and young Bowditch died a pathetic death. Henry Bowditch was familiar with the shortcomings of military surgery, and his anger at the War Department's apathy in implementing an ambulance corps was born of personal grief. Bowditch's constant agitation and his nationwide appeals to rectify this error became a most potent factor in bringing about the desired change. His efforts did not cease until the Ambulance Corps Act of 1864 was passed by the United States Congress. By the time of the engagement at Cold Harbor in June

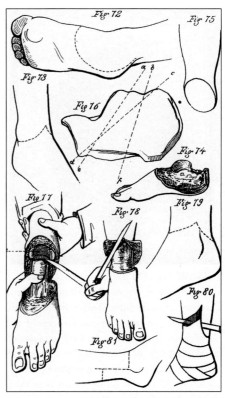

8. As seen in a *Manual of Military Surgery for the Use of the Confederate States Army* (1863), it was not uncommon that such simplified line drawings were all that inexperienced physician-surgeons had to guide them in their surgical endeavors. (*Author's Collection*)

129

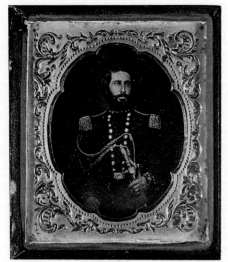

9. David Camden DeLeon (1816–1872), a Sephardic Jew from Charleston, South Carolina, organized the South's medical corps and became the first Surgeon-General of the Confederate States Army. An 1836 graduate of the University of Pennsylvania School of Medicine, and known as "the fighting doctor," a sobriquet he earned during the Mexican War, DeLeon had this daguerreotype taken of himself in full military regalia following the final battle to capture Mexico City (circa 1847). *(Courtesy of Stanley B. Burns, M.D., and The Burns Collection and Archive)*

1864, the ambulance system had been reorganized, and four-wheeled horse-drawn vehicles with professional drivers were ready to take the wounded to the aid station or the field hospital.

At the aid station, treatment was typically confined to the control of bleeding, the bandaging of wounds, and the administration of opiates and whiskey for pain and shock. Stabilizing lower-extremity fractures was a particularly difficult problem, especially in view of the rough, rutted dirt roads on which the horse-drawn carriages had to travel in order to transport the wounded to their next destination, a field hospital. Realistically, the field hospital was often little more than a barn, church, or private home hurriedly commandeered by the medical corps. Following the battle of Antietam, one surgeon was placed in charge of caring for some sixty wounded at a "hospital" installation that "comprised one small old farmhouse, without any furniture…two negro huts, and one cow stable, the earth floor covered to a depth of two feet with manure."

In 1862, Jonathan Letterman (1824–1872), Medical Director of the Army of the Potomac, reorganized the field system of care. By the time of Cold Harbor, the divisional field hospitals were grouped together by corps to form a large "hospital" complex. As part of this reorganization, the most clinically experienced medical officers were assigned to perform all major surgical operations. Less capable individuals were titled surgical assistants or wound dressers, while the clinically inept were assigned administrative responsibilities. Despite the new efficiencies, the situation of many field hospitals remained dreadful. All soldiers knew when they neared a hospital complex, since there was an "ineffable smell of gore which no man can fail to recognize."

The surgical activity around the field hospital became ever more grim, especially as the intensity of fighting increased. According to J. T. Calhoun, assistant surgeon in charge of a Depot Field Hospital for Colored Troops, "It would be difficult…to convey, in words, a truthful picture of the scenes attendant upon a field hospital where wounded are counted by thousands…. Day and night the operating surgeons plied the knife, performing a number of amputations which would appear to be enormous." At a field hospital near Petersburg, one soldier wrote, "the poor wounded fellows lie all about me, suffering intensely from heat and flies. The atmosphere is almost intolerable from the immense quantity of decomposing animal and vegetable matter upon the ground…. Many of the surgeons are ill…the decay…of human bodies in the trenches, causes malaria of the worst kind."

In the most terrible of situations, the surgeons were so overwhelmed that darkness fell before the day's surgical work was completed. Torches and candles provided illumination as another victim of the surgeon's amputation knife was strapped down. Groans and shrieks, maniacal ravings, bitter sobs, heavy sighs, piteous cries, despair, death rattles, darkness, and death: these were the sounds that filled the field hospital's air. Still, as one surgeon related by letter to his wife, he had been operating steadily for four days and three nights, "yet there are a hundred cases of amputation waiting for me. Poor fellows come and beg almost on their knees for the first chance to have an arm taken off. It is a scene of horror such as I never saw."

Once a battle began, the wounded initially arrived at the field hospital in manageable numbers. During the continuing carnage, however, the flow of injured increased so dramatically that these temporary hospitals were instantly transformed into scenes of great human suffering. It was always easy to recognize a busy field hospital, since enormous piles of severed limbs were tossed into a heap in the plain sight of everyone. Upon arrival, the less seriously wounded were attended by a "dressing surgeon." These slightly injured individuals were usually given a few opium pills or, rarely, a shot of morphine. After a sponging of the traumatized area, the walking wounded were set aside until further notice. They would never cross the path of an "operating surgeon." Even less of a surgical problem were the mortally wounded, those soon to die. Laid out in tidy rows, the nearly dead were given pain medicine and allowed to drift into never-ending unconsciousness. Unfortunately, it was often an unpleasant road to oblivion, punctuated by the excruciating pain of sepsis and other ungodly horrors.

As the seriously wounded arrived they were lifted from the stretcher and placed on an operating table for complete evaluation. In most cases the operating table was little more than wooden planks laid across two barrels. Be it a door or a splintery piece of wood, as long as it could withstand the weight of a man, it served its purpose. Congealed blood matted everything as the unperturbed surgeon went about his business. The injured underwent a cursory evaluation, which included the probing of wounds with dirty instruments and dirty fingers, followed by the removal of detritus and an attempt at debridement. Porcelain probes were utilized to distinguish between lead bullets, other foreign bodies, and splintered bone. More often than not, water was unavailable to wash the wounds because it was "snatched up and drunk by stragglers as they passed." Marine sponges, if available, were used to soak up the blood, the same sponge serving a multitude of patients.

INFECTION AND ITS CONSEQUENCES

Because of the lack of knowledge of antisepsis and the inability to control infection, gunshot wounds of the abdomen were fatal in over 90 percent of all cases. When the small intestine was injured, the mortality rate approached 100 percent. Injuries to the colon carried a 59 percent fatality rate. Such gruesome statistics were emphasized by George Otis (1830–1881), a surgeon and curator of the Army Medical Museum. In writing an introduction to the massive six-volume *Medical and Surgical History of the War of the Rebellion*, he matter-of-factly stated, "as to wounds of the abdomen, it may be that their extreme fatality and brevity of the period through which, commonly, they remain under observation, deprive them of the interest with which they would otherwise be regarded." In reality, surgeons in the mid-nineteenth century had not yet progressed to the point where opening an individual's abdomen to explore for injury or disease was a viable clinical option.

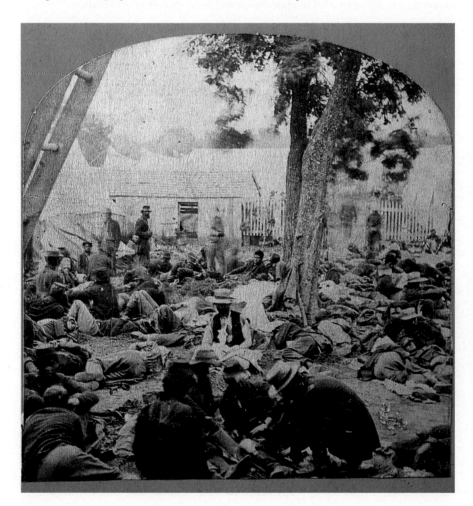

10. This dramatic image shows the true nature of triage and care of wounded after a typical battle. In this case the fighting took place at Maryland Heights, Virginia, in July 1864. The wounded in the foreground are being treated by surgeons. Lying in the dirt with open or temporarily dressed wounds proved a major cause of that era's enormous infection rate. *(Courtesy of Stanley B. Burns, M.D., and The Burns Collection and Archive)*

Penetrating gunshot wounds of the chest were fatal in almost two thirds of all cases. The ability to operate on a patient's heart, lungs, or aorta did not exist. Consequently, the Civil War surgeon could provide little to soldiers with gunshot injuries of the thoracic cavity. Yet, chest wounds inflicted by sabers or bayonets carried a mere 9 percent mortality. If death from a thoracic injury did not intervene, the resulting menace of accumulating pus in the chest cavity would create a tortured existence. Short of the surgical creation of a hole in the chest wall to allow the pus to drain out, or the insertion of a rudimentary drainage tube, there were no other therapeutic alternatives.

Eleven percent of all Civil War wounds were to the face and neck. Although obviously disfiguring, these injuries were not often fatal, and surgeons were subsequently confronted with considerable aesthetic challenges. As the war progressed, the ability to operate on the deformed face was among the more celebrated areas of American surgical successes. The case of private W. M. Wyatt of the 1st Virginia Artillery provides an apt example. Aged 46 years, he was wounded "by a fragment of shell: which carried away his "lower jaw…the soft tissues forming a portion of the cheeks…the whole lower lip and the…covering of the chin." His appearance was described as "frightful and most pitiable." Charles Bell Gibson, one of the South's most illustrious surgeons, thought the prognosis "most unfavorable." Fortunately, for Wyatt, the healing process "miraculously became fairly established:" and fifty-four days after having been injured he was sent home on furlough. Gibson suggested that an attempt "be made to improve his appearance by an operation." Some four months after being shot in the face, and without the use of surgical anesthesia, "it was determined to…make a new lower lip, by dissecting up the tissues of the throat and cheeks, sliding them to a level with the border of the upper lip, and securing them in position by sutures." Wyatt bore the operation and its "necessarily attendant, extreme suffering…with patience and courage rarely witnessed." On the tenth day the sutures were removed, and by March 1st, "the patient left the hospital…greatly improved in appearance and in his power of articulation."

AMPUTATIONS WITHOUT ANTISEPSIS

The most common location for wounds was the extremities, the upper and lower limbs being equally affected. Therefore, it is not difficult to understand why the trademark operation of Civil War surgery became the amputation. Such was the nature of the combat that more arms and legs were chopped off during these hostil-

11. Probably staged recreations of extremity amputations being performed in a tent at "Fortress Monroe, Virginia," as is written on the back of the original picture (circa 1862). In one photograph *(left)*, the wounded soldier is in the process of being anesthetized (note the surgical assistant's hand, near the left side of the patient's face, with the cloth in it). The upper extremity amputation begins with one surgeon holding a knife and the other a saw. In the second view within the same tent *(right)*, one assistant holds a Petit-type screw tourniquet in place on the soldier's thigh and another steadies the leg, while the surgeon has the amputating knife in hand. Sporting the North African style Zouave uniforms that were popular among some regiments of both North and South, curious soldiers stand about casually watching the operation. A metal catch basin is in place on the ground, an open medicine chest is in the background, and an open amputating set is in the foreground. Although possibly an actual operative photograph, the image is most important for the details its shows relative to the live event. *(left: Edward G. Miner Library, University of Rochester Medical Center) (right: Courtesy of Stanley B. Burns, M.D., and The Burns Collection and Archive)*

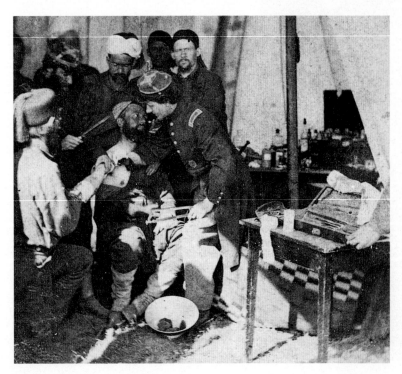

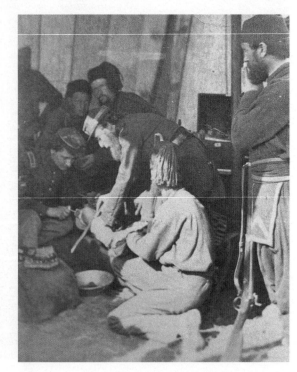

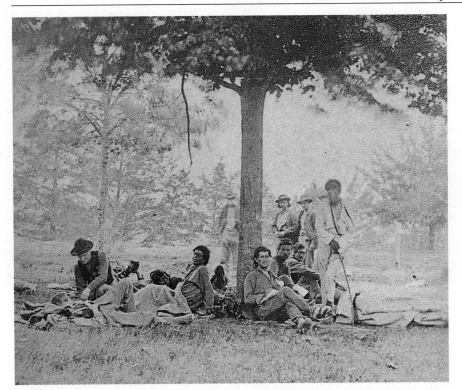

12. Just as Northerners fought Southerners in the Civil War, Native Americans were also pitted aginst each other. Members of the Cherokee, Chickasaw, Choctaw, Creek, and Seminole tribes frequently battled one another. Union and Confederate agents attempted to enlist Native Americans to their side by manipulating internal tribal dissension and utilizing frank exploitation to gain favor. This photograph, one of the few taken of Native Americans in the Civil War, shows a group of Indian soldiers wounded in the battle of Fredericksburg, Missouri (July 1864). A physician, possibly a contract surgeon, is kneeling while he ministers to one of the injured. (*Courtesy of Stanley B. Burns, M.D., and The Burns Collection and Archive*)

ities than in all other conflicts in which the United States has been engaged. Three out of four surgical operations by Northern physicians were amputations, and there is no reason to believe that the same statistics did not apply to the Confederacy. Within a short five years, veterans with amputations could be found in virtually every city, hamlet, and town in America. Enduring undeniable physical and social hardships, this army of amputees represented to the next generation of Americans the horror of mid-nineteenth century military surgery.

Numerous acts of surgical machismo relating to extremity amputation became part of Civil War lore. At Gettysburg, General Daniel Sickles was wounded by a cannon ball and underwent an amputation of his lower leg. Sickels so wished to memorialize his dismembered extremity that he presented the leg in a small coffin to the Army Medical Museum. There, his fractured bones went on permanent display (where they remain even today), and their previous owner made an annual pilgrimage to visit "his old friend." Mary Livermore (1820–1905), a well-known Union army nurse who served at the battle of Fair Oaks, related in *My Story of the War* (1889):

> General Howard's right arm was shattered by a ball, so that it had to be amputated above the elbow. Waving the mutilated arm aloft, he cheered on his men, and was borne from the field. While being carried on a litter, he passed General Kearney, who had lost his left arm…Rising on the litter, he called out gayly, "I want to make a bargain with you, General. Hereafter let's buy our gloves together!"

Amputation and its all too frequent aftermath of pus, pyemia, and paroxysms were the exemplars of Civil War surgery, and they were epitomized in one of the great surgical stories of the war: the wounding and death of Thomas "Stonewall" Jackson. Jackson, after attending a strategy meeting with Robert E. Lee (1807–1870) at Chancellorsville, was accidentally shot by his own troops at about 8 in the evening on Saturday, May 2, 1863. He was "struck by three balls," one of which went "through the left arm, three inches below the shoulder joint, shattering the bone and severing the chief artery." A handkerchief was applied as a tourniquet, but it did little to stanch the hemorrhage, which was "spraying those at his sides."

Jackson was transported for over an hour by hand-held litter, and the evacuation party was finally met by Hunter McGuire, medical director and chief surgeon of Jackson's corps. The general was placed into a horse-drawn ambulance, where McGuire quickly compressed the artery with his finger while the handkerchief was

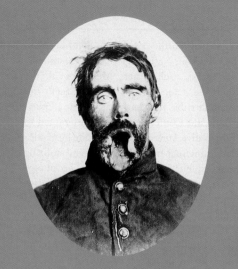
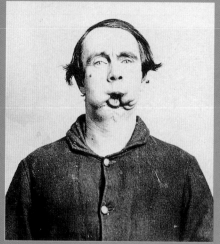
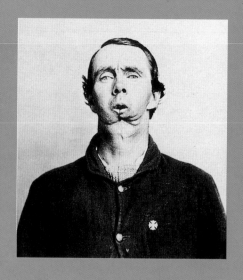

13. Roland Ward was a private in the 4th New York Heavy Artillery when he sustained this most horrible of injuries from an exploding cannon shell at the Battle of Weldon Rail Road. Ward was admitted to Lincoln General Hospital on August 28, 1864, three days after being wounded. His entire mandible had been shot off, destroying the muscles of his tongue and impairing his voice. By October he was considered completely recovered and ready to undergo reconstruction of his mouth and lips. Two procedures were performed, both in the first half of 1865. Ward was discharged in June of that year having an oral-cutaneous fistula. The secretion of saliva was controlled by the use of a rubber button, which was adjusted to the fistulous orifice. These prints, one of which is hand-tinted, are from the eight-volume *Photographs of Surgical Cases and Specimens: Taken at the Army Medical Museum* (1865–1881). *(Historical Collections, College of Physicians of Philadelphia)*

readjusted. McGuire's patient was in cardiovascular collapse: "His suffering...was intense; his hands were cold, his skin clammy, his face pale, and his lips compressed and bloodless." There was little immediate effective first aid that surgeon McGuire could provide other than to administer whiskey and morphine.

It was a long two hours before the ambulance finally arrived at a Southern field hospital. Jackson was given an additional drink of water and whiskey while McGuire waited for "sufficient reaction" to take place to warrant a complete examination. Not until 2 in the morning, some six hours after the original gunshot wound, was McGuire satisfied that Jackson had recovered from his initial "shock." The surgeon informed the general "that chloroform would be given...and his wounds examined." Under the flickering light of lamps fed by coal oil, McGuire proceeded to poke and probe the bullet holes with his unwashed fingers and unsterile instruments and became convinced that amputation was necessary: "the left arm was...amputated, about two inches below the shoulder, very rapidly, and with slight loss of blood, the ordinary circular operation having been made...Throughout the whole of the operation, and until all the dressings were applied, [Jackson] continued insensible."

That surgical operations were completed by unkempt surgeons with dirty knives was perfectly understandable. The concepts of antisepsis and asepsis were still two decades away from being accepted by American physicians, and the necessity for absolute cleanliness of surgical instrumentation was not recognized. Surgeons operated in blood-stained and pus-soiled frocks. Sponges that had already been used in pus cases and had been only rinsed in unsterile water were continually reemployed as if they were clean.

What self-respecting American surgeon of the 1860s would not think of using his own filth-encrusted fingers to explore the track of a bullet? After all, there was no better way to control acute hemorrhage than to place a facile finger on the severed surface of an injured artery. So unrecognized was the concept of surgical sterility that the appearance of "laudable pus" in a postoperative wound was viewed with satisfaction and welcomed as a harbinger of a successful surgical outcome. Such were the misunderstood efforts to promote healing in the form of this creamy, sweet-sour-smelling suppuration that the atmosphere of field and general hospitals was said to be "heavy and nauseating" with its stench.

Despite the fact that approximately 60,000 amputations were performed, the great surgical controversy of the Civil War concerned amputation versus nonamputation. The conservative surgeons and their overly concerned civilian supporters wished to save a wounded extremity at any price. The radical "cutters" believed only in prompt amputation. At the start of the hostilities, conservatism seemed to hold sway. As early as June 1861, the United States Sanitary Commission, a civilian-organized soldiers' relief society that set the structure for the later development of the American Red Cross, authorized an American edition of the British Surgeon General George Guthrie's (1785–1856) *Directions to Army Surgeons on the Field of Battle*. From his experiences at the Crimean front, Guthrie expounded the conservative viewpoint that "a leg should be seldom amputated for a fracture from a musket ball."

The distribution of Guthrie's pamphlet, which was brought out in multiple editions and given to all surgeons of the Northern army, did much to strengthen the resolve of conservative surgeons concerning extremity amputation. However, like most controversies in surgery, the question of the appropriateness of amputation was not so easily settled. In December 1861, in a move meant to provide some balance to ongoing discussions, members of the Sanitary Commission voted to distribute a dissenting report from a committee of associate medical members. This eight-page paper, written by Daniel Slade (1823–1896), a physician from Boston, contained more orthodox, or some would say radical, views regarding the necessity for battlefield amputation and seems to have been eventually accepted by a majority of the military surgeons. Slade and his supporters argued that when a limb's soft tissues were badly lacerated or the bone had been shattered and was penetrating the skin, it was best to amputate at once, particularly where joints were involved. This more orthodox viewpoint was promulgated because the rough conditions of wartime surgery precluded such attempts to conserve a limb as might be deemed proper in civilian clinical practice.

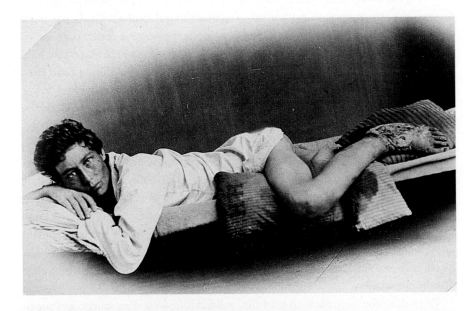

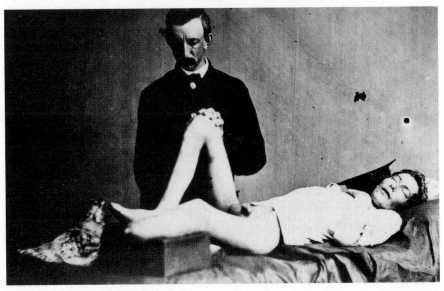

14. One of the most poignant sets of photographs to come out of Reed Bontecou's surgical album are the images of Private John Parmenter. Parmenter was wounded in the left lower extremity by a Minie ball on April 3, 1865, only six days before Robert E. Lee surrendered to Ulysses S. Grant. Two weeks later, Parmenter was admitted to Harewood Army Hospital with an infected ankle and foot, soon to become ulcerated. By mid-June, the private was losing weight and deteriorating rapidly when Bontecou decided to perform a mid-calf amputation. Parmenter's boyish good looks as he lies on his hospital bed *(top)* belie his upcoming date with the surgeon's amputation knife and saw. Several aspects of the postamputation photograph *(bottom)* are most unusual and indeed unique. First, the image was recorded with Parmenter still on the operating room table and unconcious from the effects of chloroform anesthesia. In addition, his amputated ankle and foot are displayed next to him while one of the surgeons poses at his side. Parmenter's youth seems stripped from him, as his face is distorted under the relaxation induced by the miraculous pain-killing agent. By July 30, the stump was healed and Parmenter was discharged from the United States Army. *(Courtesy of Stanley B. Burns, M.D., and The Burns Collection and Archive)*

Without knowledge of antisepsis and the inescapable fact that soldiers were treated in settings where cleanliness could not exist, it was only natural that the conservative treatment of splinting and simple excision of shattered bone soon led to universal disastrous results: infection, gangrene, and death. The few soldiers fortunate enough to avoid the Grim Reaper were left with deformed and often totally useless limbs. In retrospect, if the advocates of conservatism had taken their tenet to the length of letting the wound strictly alone matters might have been different. What they could not realize was that it was their own meddling fingers and the repeated exploration of wounds that helped disseminate bacteria throughout the tissues.

The more orthodox "cutters" argued that a decision to amputate promptly did not necessarily mean they were against the more politically correct conservative principles. In reality, their own brand of septic surgery, utilizing dirty instruments and sponges along with malodorous water, also involved a terrible risk of infection. As one surgeon writing in *United States Service Magazine* (1864) lamented:

> It seems but a sorry remedy to lop off a hand or a foot; and the public at large are apt to call amputation the opprobrium of surgery...it is not so, for an amputation is necessarily conservative. Life is better than limb; and too often mutilation is the only alternative to a rapid and painful death...delaying an operation until its necessity becomes unmistakeable...cannot be the rule in military surgery. Tetanus...gangrene, and worse than all, hemorrhage, lie in wait for the surgeon...like harpies to seize their victims, and shout back in derision, too late!

There was actually no right or wrong answer. It was a "damned if you do, damned if you don't" situation with neither side assuring survival. Samuel Gross was more eloquent in his indecision when he stated that "while the surgeon endeavors to avoid Scylla, he may not unwittingly run into Charybdis, mutilating a limb that might have been saved, and endangering life by the retention of one that should have been promptly amputated."

Although there was a general societal aversion to the concept of amputation, by mid-war it had become evident that more soldiers were surviving prompt amputation than those who became part of the "wait and see" contingent. By war's end, the accepted opinion was that if a limb were severely lacerated or had sustained a fracture where bone fragments pierced the skin, then the extremity should immediately come off. As ghastly as it sounds, in the surgical context of the Civil War era, such action was proper. In hindsight, many medical luminaries, including Jonathan Letterman, felt that "conservative surgery was practiced too much and the knife not used enough." Years later, William Keen proffered that "taking the army as a whole, I have no hesitation in saying that far more lives were lost from refusal to amputate than by amputation."

Worn down by daily physical hardship, malnutrition including scurvy, and rough handling during transportation that caused tortuous pain and, for compound fracture patients, the constant dread of often fatal secondary hemorrhage, it is not difficult to understand why the circumstance of Civil War battles compelled immediate amputation. Although one of the major contributions to medical care that developed during the Civil War was the accumulation for the first time of adequate medical records and detailed operative reports, the disorganization of the medical department during the first eighteen months of strife meant that few or no reports were sent in. Consequently, the 29,980 "official" amputations performed on Union soldiers, which Joseph Barnes reports in the *Medical and Surgical History of the War of the Rebellion*, is undoubtedly an underestimate. Likewise, the report of 25,000 total amputations performed on Confederate soldiers is a low figure. Of these known amputations, it is estimated that the overall mortality rate was 30 percent; ranging in the lower extremity from a high of 83 percent for amputations at the hip joint, 58 percent at the knee joint, and 25 percent at the ankle joint to a low of 6 percent for foot or toe amputation. In the upper extremity, amputations had a case fatality rate of 29 percent at the shoulder joint, 24 percent at the upper arm, and 10 percent at the wrist.

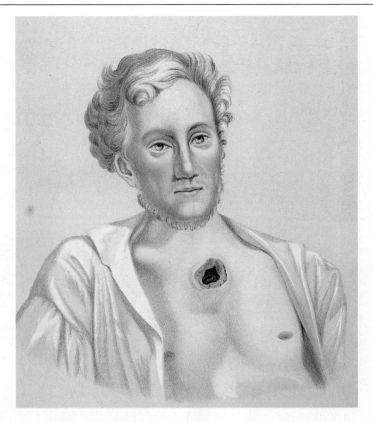

15. Private Charles Betts of the 26th New Jersey Volunteers was struck by a "three ounce grapeshot, on the morning of May 3d, 1863, in a charge upon the heights of Fredericksburg." A metal fragment shattered his sternum and tore through the "costal pleura," collapsing the left lung *(Medical and Surgical History of the War of the Rebellion,* part I, vol. II, page 486, 1875). Unbelievably, the arch of the aorta was visible through the wound and its pulsations could be counted. With little that could be done surgically, Betts was admitted to an army field hospital, and much to the surprise of his surgeons the wound began to granulate. By mid-June, he "ultimately recovered perfectly," and other than for occasional shortness of breath remained well. *(Author's Collection)*

Statistics concerning the time after injury when an amputation took place were similarly revealing. Of 23,762 amputations on Northern soldiers, where both date of injury and amputation were known, primary surgery (occurring within forty-eight hours of the injury except for hip-joint amputations, which were defined as primary if performed within the first twenty-four hours) had a mortality rate of 24 percent, intermediate surgery (occurring on the third to the thirtieth day) 35 percent, and secondary surgery (occurring after the thirtieth day or when the inflammation had abated or entirely subsided) 29 percent. In 1871, Stephen Smith (1823–1922) gave the Sanitary Commission a final report on the success of amputations performed during the war:

1. Immediate amputations, or those performed *before the shock*, give good results in military surgery.
2. Amputations performed between the first and sixth hour after the injury, or *during the shock* are more successful than when performed at a later period, but are not probably more successful than when performed immediately.
3. Amputations performed between the sixth and forty-eighth hour, or in the period of reaction, are more successful than at any subsequent period, but are not nearly as successful as amputations performed previously to the sixth hour.
4. Amputations performed between the forty-eighth hour and seventh day, or in the intermediary period, are more fatal than at any time prior to or subsequent to that period.
5. Amputations performed after the seventh day, or in the secondary period, are more fatal than amputations performed at any time prior to the forty-eighth hour after the receipt of the injury.

In a reversal of previously accepted terminology, Smith came to believe that immediate amputation was no longer radical. Instead, primary excision should be "considered conservative since with an artificial limb the person could have a 'better' limb than if the injured one were saved."

As post-Civil War experience would demonstrate, many lives and limbs could have been spared if better fracture splints had been available and if those which were available had been more widely used. Understandably, there was little concern about the protection of upper extremity fractures, since most of those patients could sit up

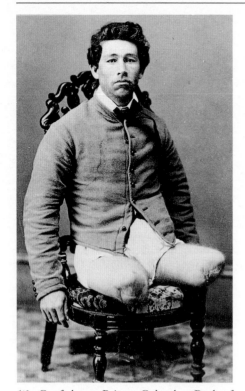

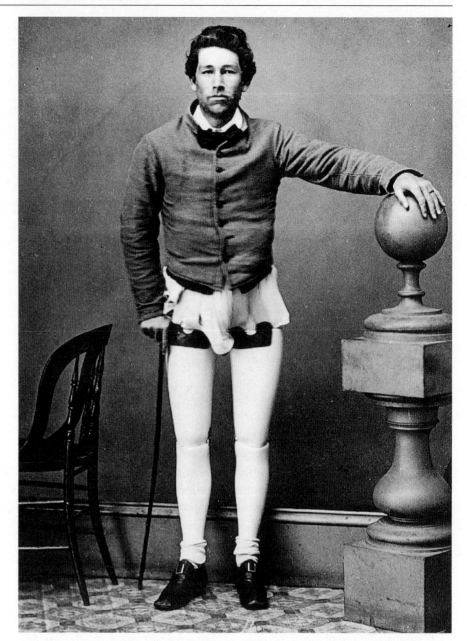

16. Confederate Private Columbus Rush of the 21st Georgia Regiment was wounded on March 25, 1865, by a shell fragment "which laid open the right knee-joint, and shattered the upper third of the left tibia, and produced great laceration of the soft parts of the left leg." He was made a prisoner of war and within four hours of his injury underwent amputation of both thighs by the surgeon Doctor Bliss (*Photographs of Surgical Cases and Specimens: Taken at the Army Medical Museum, 1865–1881*). Having survived that ordeal, Rush was moved to St. Luke's Hospital in New York City, where he was fitted with artificial limbs. (*Historical Collections, College of Physicians of Philadelphia*)

in an ambulance and help protect themselves. That was not the case, however, with lower limb fractures, particularly those of the femur. These patients suffered terribly, not only on the battlefield but after attempts at amputation. During the war years, the Army furnished Smith's anterior splint as an aid in the treatment of fractures of the leg. Nathan Ryno Smith had devised his suspensory splint while serving as professor of surgery at the University of Maryland. Originally described in the *Maryland and Virginia Medical Journal* (1860), Smith's apparatus was a clumsy affair, which could be suspended from the roof of an ambulance only with difficulty, and many surgeons never learned how to properly rig it.

John Swiburne (1820–1889), a surgeon from Albany, New York, believed that long bone fractures could be healed by simple extension, without splints and bandages. His concept was expanded upon by Gurdon Buck, who in 1862 described a new treatment for fractures of the femur in the *Bulletin of the New York Academy of Medicine*. Buck's traction device applied tensile force on the leg by means of a tape on the skin; friction between the tape and skin permitted the application of force, which was mediated through a cord over a pulley, suspending a weight. Perhaps the greatest contribution to orthopedics during the Civil War was the Hodgen splint, invented in 1863 by John Hodgen (1826–1882) a surgeon on the faculty of St. Louis Medical College. His splint was a wire suspension device for the treatment of fractures of the middle or lower segment of the femur. Writing in the *St. Louis Medical and Surgical Journal*, Hodgen claimed that his apparatus was a combination of the principles of Smith's anterior splint, Swinburne's extension, and Buck's strip bandage support. The use of Hodgen's splint assured complete extension of the limb while preventing contraction. It was able to accomplish this in such a way that "the limb is entirely free from compressing bandages...the limb may at any time be examined without disturbing the dressings...[and] the freedom with which the limb moves...allows the patient to sit up, to move to any part of the bed...without disturbing the fracture or causing the least pain."

Although many models of artificial limbs were available prior to the war, the tremendous increase in amputees caused a flowering in prosthetic technology. From 1861 to 1873, a period of just thirteen years, 133 patents were issued for various artificial limbs and assisting devices. Prosthesis manufacturers aimed to make their artificial limbs both strong and light but durable for comfort. The craftsmen attempted to give their products as realistic an appearance as possible. Among such efforts were the painting or covering of wood with varnished parchment so that it resembled skin and A. A. Mark's patenting of artificial limbs with india-rubber hands and feet so they would be more pleasant when viewed or touched.

B. Frank Palmer (?–1870) was among the best-known American prosthetists, and the Palmer arm and leg were considered to be superior. The various articulations consisted of detached ball-and-socket joints, which were meant to perform many months without need of oil or attention. The stump received no weight on the end and was covered to protect against undue friction and excoriation. Palmer was an outstanding businessman, and in a business decision rivaling that of any modern entrepreneur, he donated 7,000 limbs to the nation for its mutilated veterans. He described his "great national benefaction" in a thirty-two page self-promotional pamphlet in 1868. Of course, by donating the already popular Palmer arm and leg, the inventor realized that the recipients would sing their praises so highly that ever-increasing numbers of the device would be sought and bought by those who had not received them gratis. In the end, Palmer became quite wealthy through his Yankee ingenuity and savvy business sense.

In the middle of all the professional confusion between "conservatives" and "cutters" were the soldiers. Although they no doubt dreaded the surgeon's knife, their camp-fire humor seemed to indicate an understanding for the rationale behind prompt surgery:

> To amputate, or not to amputate? That is the question.
> Whether tis nobler in the mind to suffer the unsymmetry of one-armed men,
>   and draw a pension.
> Thereby, shuffling off a part of mortal coil.
> Or, trusting unhinged nature, take arms against a cruel surgeon's knife,
> And, by opposing rusty theories, risk a return to dust in the full shape of man.

Once amputation was decided on, it was performed with dispatch by a surgeon and three assistants. Notwithstanding the dearth of adequate surgical instrumentation on the Southern side, where the surgeons were known to have completed amputations with little more than a sharpened penknife and a carpenter's saw, battlefield surgery was conducted in the same manner and with the same results on both sides of the Mason-Dixon line.

With one aide acting as an impromptu anesthesiologist, another would compress the main artery with a tourniquet while maneuvering wooded tubs to catch any spurting blood. The surgeon made a deep incision, usually down to the bone. A third assistant awkwardly supported the limb to be dismembered, while the surgical operator completed his task by sawing the bone in two. Considering the haste of Civil War field surgery, precautions also had to be taken to assure that the surgeon did not inadvertently relieve his assistants of their own fingers.

Surgeons argued the relative merits of two fundamental amputation procedures: circular and flap variations. The circular method was older and involved incising the skin and folding it back into a type of cuff. The muscle was then cut and bone was sawed through. The cuff of skin was then brought back down over the stump and sutured closed. Military surgeons had long utilized this circular amputation because there was less soft tissue to suppurate, the wound healed quickly, and pain throughout the healing process seemed to be minimized. Most importantly, the circular method withstood the difficulties of nineteenth-century travel well and because of its simplicity seemed ideally suited for wartime conditions.

The flap operation had been devised by William Cheselden (1688–1752), an English surgeon, and consisted of skin and soft tissues being cut in a crescent shape in front, front to back, or side to side. In this manner, the soft tissue flaps could dip below the severed bone and, when folded over the bone's end, provided a considerable amount of soft tissue as well as skin coverage. The advantages of this method over the circular operation were that it supposedly left a better stump. The admitted disadvantages were that the flap operation required sacrificing more of the limb (i.e., bone) and created a larger wound. In this preantiseptic era, the presence of an excessive healing area could conceivably lead to increased risk of infection, sloughing of the soft tissues, and the dreaded complication of secondary hemorrhage.

Both methods had their advocates, and there were reports purporting to show that Confederate surgeons preferred the circular operation whereas Union physicians utilized the flap procedure. Both methods worked well in experienced hands, but neither could be recommended if the surgeon was a bungler. In the most common complication, the bone would push through the soft tissues and cause necrosis of the skin. Such a surgical nightmare could be resolved only with a second amputation and greater loss of tissue.

When amputation was considered unnecessary, surgical intervention not uncommonly consisted of resection, the excision or removal of joints with preservation of the extremity. Obviously it was more aesthetically successful when applied to the arms than to the legs, since such a radical operation often left a nonfunctional limb. Although there was little approbation for such procedures, and it came to be called reprehensible, Joseph Barnes reported that 4,656 known resections were completed by Union surgeons. Over 80 percent involved the upper extremity and carried a mortality rate of approximately 20 percent. Of the 815 lower extremity resections, case mortality rates hovered around 80 percent. The chief value of excision, despite its high death rate, was that occasionally some arm function was maintained, and when the periosteum was preserved, surgeons could anticipate a considerable amount of bone regeneration. Even without regeneration, the arm was sometimes surprisingly useful despite gaps in its bony continuity. Some surgeons regarded the

17. The relatively new invention of photography quickly became a medical and surgical teaching device during the Civil War. The prime private example is the Reed Bontecou surgical album, for which he arranged to have cases photographed so they could be shared with other physicians. For these two patients Bontecou sketched the line of the bullet's suspected pathway. Medical students and surgeons were thereby given an opportunity to match the wound with the location of the operation. Particularly intriguing is the technique of bone excision *(left)* in which shattered bone was removed in the vain hope that it would eventually lengthen and bridge the missing gap. As expected, Private Porubsky's limb was essentially useless. In many cases the impotent extremity eventually had to be amputated. *(Courtesy of Stanley B. Burns, M.D., and The Burns Collection and Archive)*

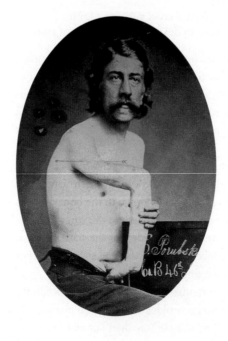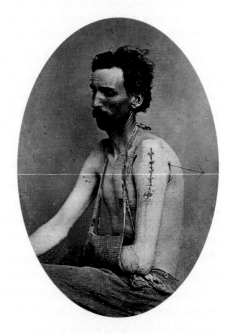

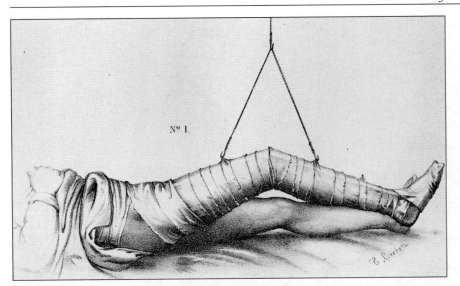

Nº 1.

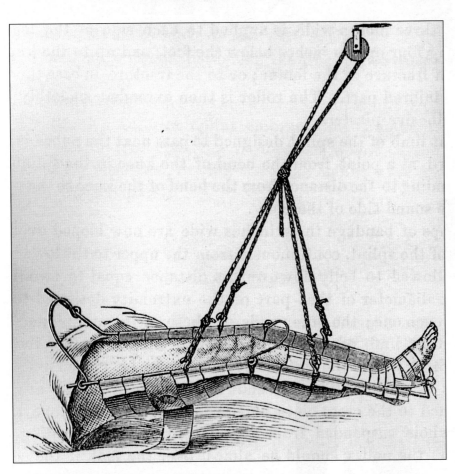

Nº 1.

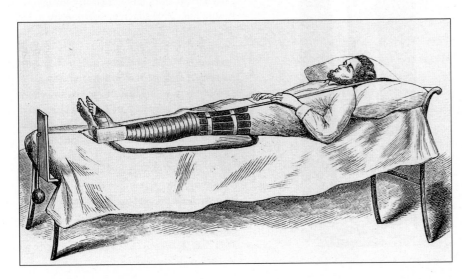

18. The three most common splints developed in the 1860s, Nathan Ryno Smith's anterior splint for the treatment of fractures of the lower extremity *(top)* *(Maryland and Virginia Medical Journal,* vol. 14, pages 1–5, 1860), John Hodgen's wire suspension device for fractures of the middle or lower segment of the femur *(middle)* *(St. Louis Medical and Surgical Journal,* vol. 1, pages 17–21, 1863), and Gordon Buck's extension apparatus, more commonly known as Buck's traction *(bottom)* *(Transactions of the New York Academy of Medicine,* vol. 2, pages 233–249, 1863). *(Historical Collections, College of Physicians of Philadelphia)*

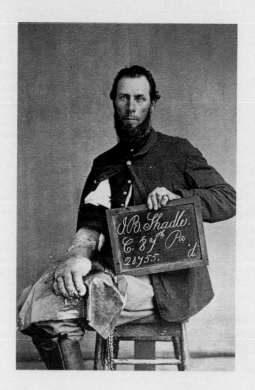

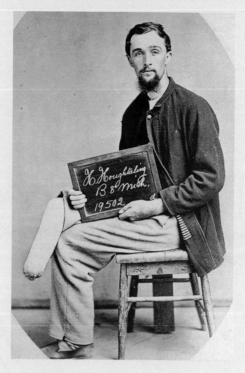

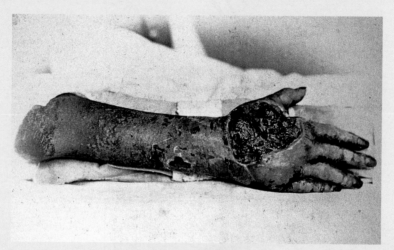

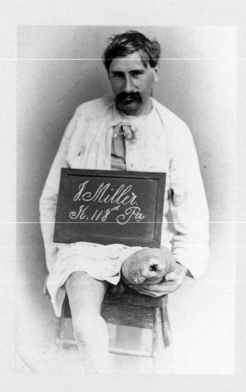

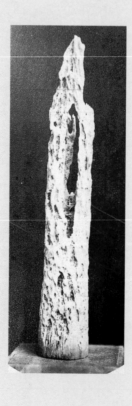

19. Four deadly infections of the Civil War killed more soldiers than actual battlefield injuries. Erysipelas *(upper left)*, pyemia affecting a soldier who was shot in the arm but lost his leg *(upper right)*, hospital gangrene *(middle)*, and osteomyelitis *(lower left)* are dramatically displayed. Two cases are particularly intriguing. Private John B. Shadle suffered an injury to his thumb, which was amputated at a field hospital. Ten days later, he was admitted to Harewood General Hospital, where he was stricken with erysipelas. Despite the obvious toxicity of his disease process, Shadle managed to sit calmly for the formal hospital portrait taken by surgeon Reed Bontecou in April 1865. Shadle was a lucky individual, who survived this infection and went on to receive his military discharge. The case of Private J. Miller and his osteomyelitis is interesting, the sequestrum of bone *(lower right)* represents a portion of his femur that fell out of his open thigh wound six months after his initial gunshot injury. *(Courtesy of Stanley B. Burns, M.D., and The Burns Collection and Archive)*

slightest function as being better than no limb. Conversely, many excisions resulted in an upper extremity that did little else than dangle loosely from the shoulder. In these instances, time and gravity would cause the arm to deteriorate and swell to immense proportions.

Operative surgery had always been a speed event, in which a surgeon's ego was intimately bound up with whether he could, for example, complete an amputation in less than one minute or remove urinary bladder stones in under three minutes. Such surgical expediency became especially consequential in view of the mushrooming workload that followed a battle. Since amputation was the Civil War's most common surgical operation, operative exigency meant that injured combatants did not have to undergo lengthy periods of anesthetization. Accordingly, chloroform was sprinkled onto a cloth or sponge and placed over a soldier's mouth and nose. Once he was unconscious, the anesthetic was immediately discontinued, in full knowledge that the operation would be over with before the patient could awaken. Only in the rare event of an exceedingly protracted case were additional applications of chloroform necessary. Unfortunately, the lack of adequate postoperative pain medicine meant that the intense suffering that followed the conclusion of surgical anesthesia could not be pharmacologically controlled.

To return to the account of Stonewall Jackson's injury and treatment, on Wednesday, May 6, Hunter McGuire found Jackson's amputation stump "covered with healthy granulations." However, on Thursday, Jackson began to suffer from persistent nausea, and "examination disclosed pleuro-pneumonia of the right side." The wound was dressed again on Friday, but "the quantity of the discharge [pus] had diminished…and [Jackson] breathed with difficulty and complained of a feeling of great exhaustion." By Saturday, Jackson "was evidently hourly growing weaker." On Sunday, slightly over seven days after being shot, Jackson's ordeal came to a delirious end.

In Jackson's demise can be found the *bete noire* of all Civil War surgeons. Sepsis, also known as pyemia or by its laymen's locution, "blood poisoning," could not be controlled. Such a vicious infection, now thought to have been transmitted by the bacteria *Staphylococcus aureus* and *Streptococcus pyogenes*, affected almost one-third of all reported amputation cases. With its 90 percent fatality rate, postsurgery recovery could be an unpleasant experience at best. As ligatures pulled away in infected amputation sites, severe bleeding inevitably occurred. Secondary hemorrhage three or four days after injury was quite frequent and carried a death rate of more than 60 percent. When stables were used as hospitals, tetanus was a major problem: "His teeth came together with a crash and the lad passed away in that struggle." Erysipelas occurred in epidemics in some hospitals and carried a mortality rate of 90 percent. William Keen described the situation in a nutshell:

> A poor fellow whose leg or arm I had amputated a few days before would be getting on as well as we then expected; that is to say, he had pain, high fever, was thirsty and restless, but was gradually improving, for he had what we looked on as a favorable symptom, an abundant discharge of pus from his wound. Suddenly, overnight, I would find that his fever had become markedly greater, his tongue dry, his pain and restlessness increased, sleep had deserted his eyelids, his cheeks were flushed, and on removing the dressings I would find the secretions from the wound almost dried up and…watery, thin, and foul-smelling…Pyemia was the verdict and death the usual result within a few days.

HOSPITAL GANGRENE

Pyemia might have killed, but "hospital gangrene" was the surgical disease soldiers feared most. What began as a small black spot on a healing wound would soon spread throughout the extremity to produce a "rotten, evil-smelling mass of dead flesh" on a still living patient. The condition occurred chiefly in hospitals and temporary shelters, where diseased and wounded individuals were crowded together with poor ventilation and inadequate nutrition.

The first epidemic of hospital gangrene was noted in late 1862 among the soldiers wounded at the battle of Antietam. The overwhelming majority of cases seem to have been bacterial in origin, but because hospital gangrene is an extinct pathologic entity, its specific bacterial genesis (*Streptococcus*, a synergistic combination of aerobes and anaerobes, or *Clostridium perfringens*) remains unclear. There was no standardization of treatment, and each surgeon seemed to have his own particular approach to the problem. Some surgeons utilized the knife and then applied corrosive chemicals; nitric acid was particularly favored but tortuous in its effect. Henry Campbell even instituted what he thought to be the common-sense approach of ligating large arteries of the extremities to check the spread of gangrene. Of course, these ligations were often the unsuspected cause of gangrene in their own right.

Eventually, Middleton Goldsmith (1818–1887), son of Alban Goldsmith, developed the bromine treatment for hospital gangrene while serving at the army hospital at Jeffersonville, Indiana. Bromine was closely related to other halogens—iodine and chlorine—and would prove more effective than the simple application of nitric acid to raw flesh. With the soldier under chloroform anesthesia, the surgeon removed all gangrenous tissue, causing the part beneath to bleed quite freely. Stripped of all dead flesh, the undermined edges of the wound were saturated with pure bromine, and the entire cavity was lined with lint moistened in a weak solution of bromine. In most instances, a period of about one week would be followed by the sudden healing of the wound.

If official government statistics are to be believed, Goldsmith's bromine therapy was an important surgical success. In one series of 334 cases, those treated with bromine had a mortality rate of less than 3 percent; when nitric acid was used the rate jumped to over 60 percent; and a hodge-podge of other methods accounted for a mortality rate of almost 40 percent. In a prelude to the coming of antisepsis, bromine solution was soon being touted for its prophylactic qualitites. It was sprayed into the air of hospitals to counteract what Goldsmith termed the "sewer effluvia." Additionally, physicians and nurses discovered that "dressing" minor lacerations and abrasions of their hands with liquid bromine reduced the likelihood that they would later contract hospital gangrene from their patients. The studies of Middleton Goldsmith in the North and Joseph Jones (1833–1896) in the South showed hospital gangrene to be closely linked to generalized conditions of filth. Consequently, by war's end, it was recognized that cleanliness of the hospital environment, in addition to adequate ventilation, were an absolute necessity if the incidence of infection was to be decreased.

ANESTHESIA

Initially, the general ignorance of the average Civil War "surgeon" regarding the use of chloroform and ether, combined with widely reported incidents of anesthetic mishaps, accounted for considerable controversy over whether anesthesia was appropriate in the military setting. This dispute led to romanticized tales of uncountable soldiers biting a bullet or getting rip-roaring drunk as a prelude to their confronting the surgeon's knife. Despite a tinge of truth, many of these surgical stories represent nothing more than imaginative folklore. The simple fact is that surgical anesthesia had been available for almost fifteen years and was extensively applied early in the war, and by the end of the conflict it was universally used. According to George Otis's account, anesthetics were employed on Civil War battlefields "as near as can be ascertained…in no less than eighty thousand (80,000) instances." It would soon be apparent that few lessons proved of greater value to the evolution of American surgery than this vast and positive experience with surgical anesthesia.

At the beginning of the war effort, opinion regarding anesthetic use was decidedly mixed. J. Julian Chisolm, in his *Manual of Military Surgery for Surgeons in the Confederate States Army*, offered the advice that "whenever operations are to be per-

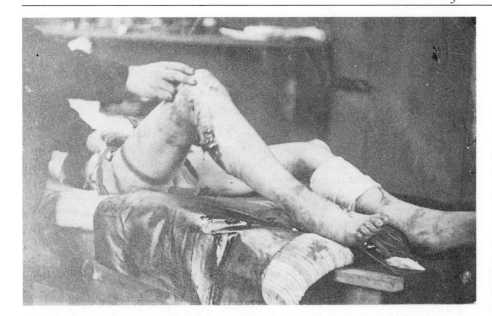
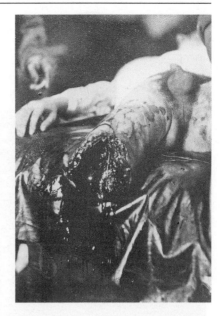

formed in military surgery, chloroform should be administered…[it is] wonderful in mitigating the suffering of the wounded." Frank Hamilton stated in his *Practical Treatise on Military Surgery* that he "preferred ether to chloroform, as being the least liable to destroy life," but that he would never employ either agent when the patient was suffering from a disease or was undergoing the "shock of a recent injury." The editor of the *New York Medical Journal*, in 1861, discussed the arguments against inhalation anesthesia by restating Guthrie's commonly accepted belief that the "excitement" of a wounded soldier would be sufficient to "carry him" safely through the severest operation. The editorial further suggested that shock after injury was aggravated by anesthetics because by obviating pain there would be no stimulant to counter the effects of physiologic depression. Similarly, surgical anesthesia was also stated to retard primary wound healing and predispose the patient to the twin horrors of secondary hemorrhage and pyemia. However, in the final analysis and despite dire predictions, the editorial writer did not hesitate to advise surgeons to anesthetize their patients before all surgical operations.

Regardless of the varied arguments, the anesthetic record of Civil War surgeons was quite remarkable. Of the 8,900 cases where the anesthetic agent was definitely known (76 percent chloroform, 15 per cent ether, and 9 per cent mixed agents), a total of just thirty-seven deaths from chloroform, four from ether, and two from a combination of both were reported. This is an extraordinary fact, largely attributable to the rapidity with which battlefield surgical procedures had to be completed.

By dispensing short-term doses of anesthetic agents, the surgeon inadvertently averted many complications, most noticeably sudden death from heart stoppage, which had plagued the worldwide use of inhalation anesthesia since its discovery. Chloroform rapidly became the anesthetic of choice because of its nonflammability and speed of action. The technique for administering it was a model of military efficiency, now colloquialized as the "open method." The sweetish-smelling liquid was liberally sprinkled onto a sponge, handkerchief, or cotton cloth, which was held in place over the soldier's nose and mouth. Ingeniously designed inhalers were sometimes used to protect the hands of the person who administered the corrosive chloroform and also to help prevent excessive evaporation. Chisholm preferred a common funnel into which chloroform was dripped through the funnel's neck onto a sponge that was supported on a metal bar or cribiform plate within the wide portion of the device. The bottom of the funnel was placed over the patient's face, and air, which entered through the funnel neck, mixed with the chloroform, providing an unsophisticated but effective means of providing anesthesia. The chloroform or ether was given until the patient became limp, which was a crude, but for that era

20. Previously unpublished photographs showing an injured soldier's leg just before and after surgeon Reed Bontecou performed an amputation. The first scene *(left)* is an exceptionally rare depiction of a preoperative setting with tourniquet in place and other paraphenalia such as the already blood-stained oilcloth covering the operating table. The wound involves the right knee; vascular compromise is already evident in the distal portion of the extremity. The graphic second image *(right)* is an uncommon closeup of the actual amputation stump immediately after the leg has been removed. Dynamic visualization of an amputation in progress is virtually unheard of in the annals of Civil War photodocumentation, and the Bontecou surgical album probably provides the only such pictures. *(Courtesy of Stanley B. Burns, M.D., and The Burns Collection and Archive)*

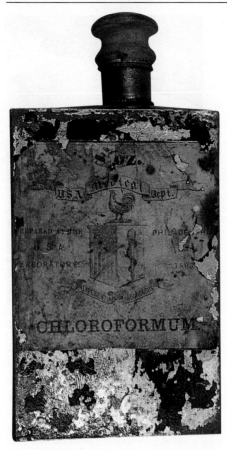

21. The use of chloroform in a battlefield setting was initially controversial. However, the colorless liquid soon became a wounded soldier's best friend. This rare extant example of bottled chloroform was prepared in 1863 at the United States Army Laboratory in Philadelphia. *(Collection of Alex Peck, Antique Scientifica)*

fairly accurate, way of determining adequate surgical anesthesia. Since the surgical procedure was usually so brief, inhalation of the agent was promptly suspended with little need to ever renew the dosage.

Of the thirty-seven deaths from chloroform, little can be learned about the actual cause of expiration. Still, Otis' description of each case provides a fascinating glimpse into the conduct of surgery during the Civil War:

> Case 1244. - Private Thomas Hamilton, Co. A, 1st Maryland Infantry, aged 31 years, admitted into Patterson Park Hospital, Baltimore, June 25, 1864, with a gunshot wound of the hand. September 3, 1864, patient placed on table to undergo an operation for necrosis of the carpal bones. A sponge wet with chloroform was carefully held at first some three or four inches from the face, and at no time less than two or three inches. The patient inhaled for about five minutes and still remained conscious, frequently making some remark. He soon, however, commenced muscular efforts, such as are quite common with patients inhaling chloroform, except that the muscular contractions were more violent than usual. Before the contractions ceased the pulse grew feeble and the chloroform was withdrawn for two or three minutes; the breathing continued regular, only that the patient occasionally took a deep inspiration and expired forcibly, then the muscles became relaxed; the operation was commenced; but the respiration soon commenced to fail, and the pulse became imperceptible; the operation was stopped. All known means for resuscitation were resorted to, but life had fled. The friends of the deceased could only be persuaded to allow an examination of the heart. The organ was found of normal size and appearance; both auricles were distended with venous blood, but the ventricles were empty. A clot of white fibrin, streaked in some places with coagula of blood, was found in each auricle.

Cruel as it may seem, chloroform and ether were not invariably available, especially for Southern troops, who were often without important supplies. Nor, for that matter, did surgical anesthesia always appear necessary. Phoebe Pember, a matron at the renowned Chimborazo Hospital in Richmond, observed that following the engagement at Crury's Bluff in May 1864, the men "were so exhausted by forced marches, lying in entrenchments and loss of sleep that few even awoke during the operations." Believable or not, that manner of behavior was similarly related by a Northern surgeon telling of how, during amputations, his patients "frequently lay and smoked their cigars, and kept up a conversation with their fellow sufferers."

CARE IN THE GENERAL HOSPITALS

Following definitive field surgery, the large volume of casualties dictated relatively swift transfer to a general hospital. These institutions were situated in major urban areas and provided a final health care facility for hundreds of thousands of injured and seriously wounded. In many instances, the wounded and postoperative patients were taken from the field hospitals and loaded onto the floors of railroad freight cars, which were covered with layer upon layer of straw. These trains were marked, in enormous red letters, **U.S. Hospital Train,** and the locomotive boiler and tender were painted red. After the dreadful horrors of the field hospital and the painful, lurching journey aboard a hospital train or steamboat, the general hospital proved to be a godsend to the wounded.

The general hospitals were designed in a pavilion style; interconnected buildings had excellent ventilation. This plan ensured the maximum amount of light and air, and separate areas were created for laundries, kitchens, dispensaries, operating rooms, and nurses' quarters. Each separate building was its own ward, with high vaulted ceilings and large air vents, and usually accommodated about sixty patients. Cross-contamination was minimized by the maintainance of adequate space between beds. The success of these large, airy institutions was evident: federal hospitals cared for more than a million men during the war, and less than 10 percent of them died.

Despite the overall crudity of many aspects of trauma therapy, some Civil War casualties received unusually modern forms of treatment. For instance, there were two known cases of blood transfusion as therapy for both primary and secondary wound hemorrhage. Both patients had undergone amputation of a lower extremity. In the first case, concerned that Private G. P. Cross did not seem "to rally," surgeon E. Bentley, U.S.V. decided to "test the method of transfusion of blood as recommended by Brown-Séquard." Blood was obtained from the temporal artery of a "strong healthy German," an opening was made into Cross' median basilic vein, and "about two ounces were transfused by means of a syringe." Bentley relates that "immediately after the injection a marked difference was noticed in the patient's pulse, which became stronger and firmer." The patient was eventually discharged and fitted with a prosthesis. Whether, in fact, two ounces of blood were enough to create such rapid clinical improvement remains highly questionable. Private J. Mott was not so fortunate. Although he received approximately sixteen ounces of blood, which resulted in a temporary improvement in his general condition, secondary stump hemorrhage began a week following the transfusion and caused his demise. There is no evidence to suggest that these two cases of blood transfusion were anything but a therapeutic aberration. Certainly, the mixed results were not sufficiently spectacular to initiate any type of surgical trend

Although surgical operations other than arterial ligation, extremity amputation, and bone resection played a minor role in Civil War medicine, additional complicated technical *tours-de-force* were becoming common place in the civilian population. J. Marion Sims and Thomas Emmet were beginning their work on various methods of cervical amputation and surgical treatment of procidentia uteri. Charles Fayette Taylor (1827–1899), a surgeon from New York City, traveled through Europe and brought back to America the "Swedish movement" system, or kinesitherapy, which played an integral role in the development of American orthopedic surgery; its remnants remain fixed in our culture as Swedish massage. Albert Walter (1811–1876) of Pittsburgh reported one of the country's earliest cases of deliberate exploratory laparotomy during which he repaired a rupture of the urinary bladder. Erastus Wolcott (1804–1880) performed the first recorded nephrectomy in America in 1862. Henry Sands (1830–1888), an attending surgeon at the New York Hospital, completed the first successful laryngotomy for papillomata described in the American medical literature in 1865.

THE WRITTEN RECORD

Of the many contributions to medical care that developed out of the horrors of the Civil War, one of the most significant, but least appreciated, was the accumulation of clinical records and detailed medical and surgical reports. For the first time in the history of the world, a complete profile of wartime medical activities was available. Many of these proceedings were published over a two-decade period (1870–1888) in the six-volume, fifty-five-pound *Medical and Surgical History of the War of the Rebellion, 1861–1865*. One of the most remarkable works ever written on military medicine and surgery, the text has been accurately called the earliest comprehensive American medical book. European physicians regarded the effort as the first major academic accomplishment by American medicine. These massive volumes, containing thousands of pages of densely printed text, present a detailed overview of the medical and surgical conditions encountered by the Civil War physician-surgeon and his patients. The introduction to the first surgical volume contains an extensive list of American books and papers on military surgery. The surgical topics covered include every imaginable wartime injury, with detailed summaries of virtually all known cases. An index of surgical "operators" appears at the end of the third surgical volume and allows the wartime activities of thousands of surgeons to be scrutinized. The set was prepared under the direction of Surgeon-General Barnes, but was actually written by Joseph Woodward (1833–1884), Charles Smart (1841–1905), George Otis, and David Huntington (1834–1899). The six volumes are illustrated with hundreds of tinted lithographs, made primarily by Julius Bien after photographs by William Bell, E. J. Ward, and others. Also noteworthy are the numerous chromolithographs by Bien of histologic and pathologic studies by Edward Stauch, and other chromolithographs after paintings by Herman Faber.

Otis's life was changed during the Civil War when in 1864 he was assigned as successor to John Brinton, then curator of the Army Medical Museum. Otis, who had previously been head of the surgical and photographic sections of the government's collation efforts, spent the remainder of his life expanding the wartime medical collection. Among his other published efforts were the remarkable eight-volume *Photographs of Surgical Cases and Specimens: Taken at the Army Medical Museum* (1865–1881). This enormous and remarkable collection of early photographs depicted wounded Civil War soldiers and pathologic specimens. Each volume consists of fifty tipped-in albumen photographs showing the soldier's mutilating injury and the postoperative results. All of the pictures were made from large glass plate negatives, mainly ten inches by twelve inches, and most were taken by Army photographer William Bell. The initial four volumes provide the earliest examples of actual tipped-in silver-print photographs found in any American surgical work.

Otis compiled other important surgical works. In 1867, the Government Printing Office brought out his eighty-seven-page *Report on Amputations at the Hip-Joint in Military Surgery* and two years later published a companion piece, *A Report on Excisions of the Head of the Femur for Gunshot Injury*. The strength of these monographs was the spectacular illustrative plates, many of which were chromolithographs. In 1871, Otis's 269-page *Report of Surgical Cases Treated in the Army of the United States from 1865 to 1871* was published. This report describes 1,037 surgical cases in detail and included a graphic twenty-page section on arrow wounds of the head and neck, chest, and abdomen sustained in clashes with Native Americans on the Western frontier.

THE UNITED STATES SANITARY COMMISSION

Of all the outstanding aspects of Civil War medicine, the most humane was the emergence and formal organization of a national civilian volunteer corps, the United States Sanitary Commission. Its general objective was to report information about the health, comfort, and morale of the troops to the U. S. Army's Medical Bureau and the federal government's War Department. The civilians hoped to supplement the work of the government as an agency similar to the modern-day Red Cross. Not unexpectedly, the volunteer organization was initially received without enthusiasm by both military and government officials as a group of bothersome and interfering interlopers. However, through an intensive lobbying campaign, both Secretary of War Simon Cameron and President Lincoln agreed in June 1861 to the formal establishment of such a commission.

At the insistence of the twelve original Commissioners, including the renowned New York surgeon William Holmes Van Buren (1819–1883), William Hammond (1828–1900) was appointed Surgeon-General of the Army in April 1862. Hammond immediately ordered that proper records be kept for the sick, wounded, and deceased, and he introduced a meaningful system for the classification of diseases. In addition, he founded the Army Medical Museum while embarking upon a massive government-directed building program of general hospital construction in large urban areas. Through Hammond's efforts the Sanitary Commission was instrumental in educating American society about the evils of bad water, bad sanitation, and bad food. Public health as an important medical issue was brought to the forefront of our national conscience.

All of the numerous activities of the Sanitary Commission were documented in an endless stream of official essays and, later, memoirs. For the surgeon, the official *Military Medical and Surgical Essays, Prepared for the United States Sanitary Commission* (1864) was a gold mine of clinical facts. Included in this group of essays, originally written between 1862 and 1864, were papers by several surgeons: Valentine Mott ("Pain and anaesthetics" and "Hemorrhage from wounds and the best means of

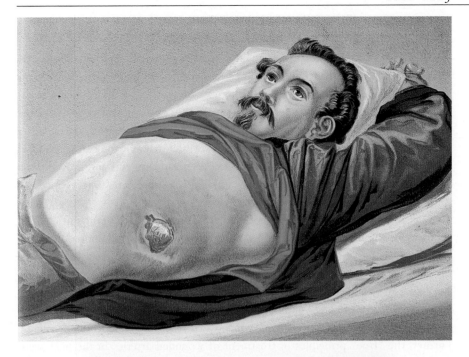

22. Captain Robert S. of the 29th New York Volunteers was wounded by a musket ball on May 2, 1863, at Chancellorsville *(Medical and Surgical History of the War of the Rebellion*, part I, vol. II, pages 514–515, 1875). Fired from a distance of 150 yards, the shot pierced his left thoracic cavity, fracturing the ninth rib, and without injuring the lung passed through the diaphragm and entered "some portion of the alimentary canal." The captain walked a mile and a half to a field hospital, where surgeons unsucessfully attempted to reduce a herniated lung. The following day, hostilities in the vicinity of the field facility necessitated evacuation of all patients, and Robert S. was forced to walk half a mile farther to the rear, where he was placed in a horse-drawn ambulance and brought to a base hospital. Seemingly in good health, the patient passed the musket ball in his stool on May 7th. Three days later the protruding portion of the lung was "carnified" and granulations began to appear *(top)*. After a two-month furlough, the wound was reexamined *(bottom)*, and other than for a slight hernia of the lung, Robert S. was pronounced healed. A four-year follow-up showed that the hernia had increased considerably in dimension and contained not only the lung but also portions of the alimentary tract, including the stomach. By 1872, the hernia had stabilized in size, measuring four and a half inches in diameter. Captain S. had little pain, some dyspnea, and "weighs about one hundred and sixty pounds, and enjoys good health." *(Author's Collection)*

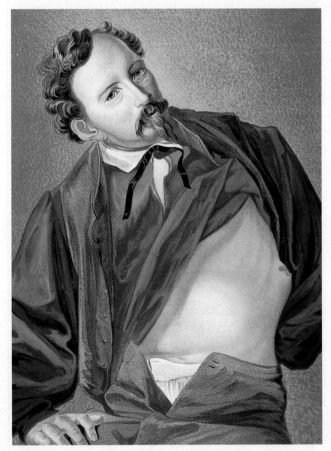

arresting it"), Alfred Charles Post (1805–1885) and William Holmes Van Buren ("Military hygiene and therapeutics"), Stephen Smith ("Amputations"), Richard M. Hodges (1827–1896) ("Excisions of joints for traumatic causes"), Freeman Bumstead (1826–1879) ("Venereal diseases"), and John Packard ("Treatment of fractures in military surgery"). In 1870 and 1871 the two-volume *Surgical Memoirs of the War of the Rebellion; Collected and Published by the United States Sanitary Commission* appeared. Edited by the well-known professor of the principles and practice of surgery at Bellevue Hospital Medical College, Frank Hamilton, the first volume contains three lengthy articles by John Lidell (1823–1883) on wounds of blood vessels, traumatic lesions of bone, and pyemia. The second volume has an analysis of lower extremity amputations by Stephen Smith and a treatise on hospital gangrene by Joseph Jones.

THE INFLUENCE OF THE CIVIL WAR
ON THE PROGRESS OF SURGERY

The Civil War's devastation proved an enormous physical and emotional burden on the poorly educated, inadequately trained, and ineffectually organized physician-surgeons of 1860s America. Even the American Medical Association's newly organized Section on Surgery was forced to cancel some of its annual sessions. In the evolution of American surgery, the years 1861 to 1865 might appear to have been a time of chaos and little growth. However, this was clearly not the case. The Civil War provided new direction and impetus for American surgeons and proved to be the greatest single influence in the development of American surgery since the founding of the nation.

A decade after Appomattox, George Otis was preparing the government's official summary of the medical and surgical aspects of the Civil War. He noted that "the experience acquired during the war should have added largely to every subject connected with military surgery was not to be anticipated." Otis reminded us that American surgeons learned something about head injuries. They had been "schooled to deal with the most ghastly injuries of the face without dismay" and to "accomplish favorably reparative operations from which, formerly, they would have recoiled." Further, the "true" principles of treatment of wounded arteries in the neck were "now generally understood" including the "futility of tying the great arterial trunks of the neck for haemorrhage from face-wounds." Before the war, Otis lamented that there were "few surgeons who chose to undertake operations on the great vessels, but now thousands of physicians knew "when and how a great artery should be tied." Information on injuries of the vertebral column had been "augmented," while the "theory and practice" of chest wounds had undergone a "complete revolution." In writing his summary of particular surgical cases, Otis stressed that he intended no "discourtesy to individual [surgeons], nor violation of the *homines amare, errores immolare* precept of St. Augustine." Otis finished by stating that the "additions to surgical knowledge acquired in the war are of real and practical value."

23. In the pavilion-style hospital, thousands of patients could be sheltered, and it was thought that the spread of "contaminated air" was limited by the division of sick and wounded into relatively small groupings, each kept separate from the others. Hospital designers believed that the ideal facility consisted of multiple one-story buildings, twelve to fourteen feet high, twenty-five feet wide, and up to two hundred feet long. These structures were set three to four feet above ground level with each patient theoretically enjoying 1,000 cubic feet of "fresh" air. The Satterlee facility comprised 34 wards and over 4,500 beds. Although it covered sixteen acres of ground, the compound was so inundated with casualties following the great battles of the Wilderness and Spotsylvania that several hundred auxiliary tents were erected outside the formal enclosure. Lincoln Hospital *(left). (Historical Collections, College of Physicians of Philadelphia)* Satterlee Hospital *(right). (Collection of Alex Peck, Antique Scientifica)*

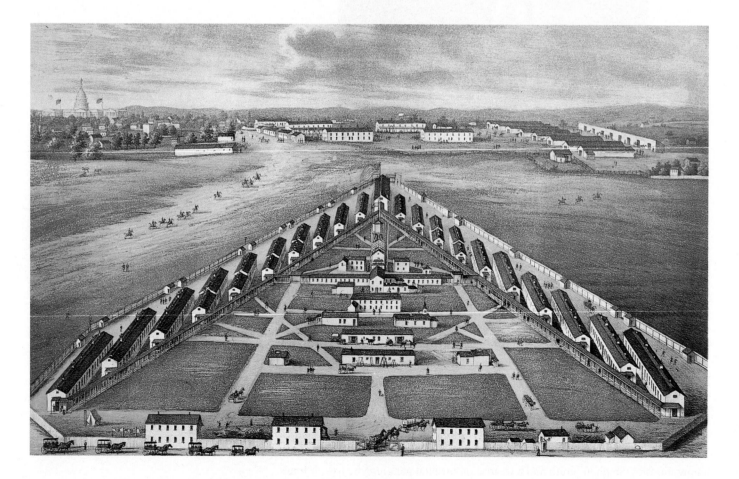

Otis's list was a compendium of dizzying clinical accomplishments, but his thinking was directed more toward military as contrasted with civilian advances. What he did not have was the luxury of time and historical reflection. It would be years before the many important contributions of the war to the evolution of surgery as a profession within American society and assorted allied health endeavors became apparent. For instance, in response to the tens of thousands of surgical specimens collected from both surgeons and soldiers, the Army Medical Museum was established. Today it exists within the organizational framework of the world-renowned Armed Forces Institute of Pathology.

The Civil War engendered the modern pavilion-style hospital with the important concepts of adequate lighting, wholesome food, and necessary ventilation. This model was replicated in the design of large civilian hospitals over the next century. American nursing was established, and the status of the female health care worker was elevated from that of the simple almshouse attendant to one of a professional directly involved in the caring for the sick and infirm. Finally, the Sanitary Commission set the pattern for the 1877 development of Clara Barton's (1821–1912) American National Committee, which was a direct precursor to the American Red Cross.

As worthwhile as these matters were, the events of the Civil War most profoundly brought the true meaning of public health to the American populace. The role of sanitation and hygiene in preventing infection, disease, and death was finally beginning to be understood. Hunter McGuire and Stephen Smith began a nationwide lobbying effort calling for a national department of health, which ultimately led to the founding of the American Public Health Association.

In matters of clinical surgery, a sophisticated system of managing mass casualties, including battlefield first-aid stations and field hospitals, was developed. The 1864 Ambulance Corps Act helped set a method of evacuating war wounded that persisted through the end of the Korean War. The first priority of immediate and definitive treatment of wounds and fractures, including the completion of surgical procedures within 24 hours after injury, was demonstrated. Anesthesia was no longer

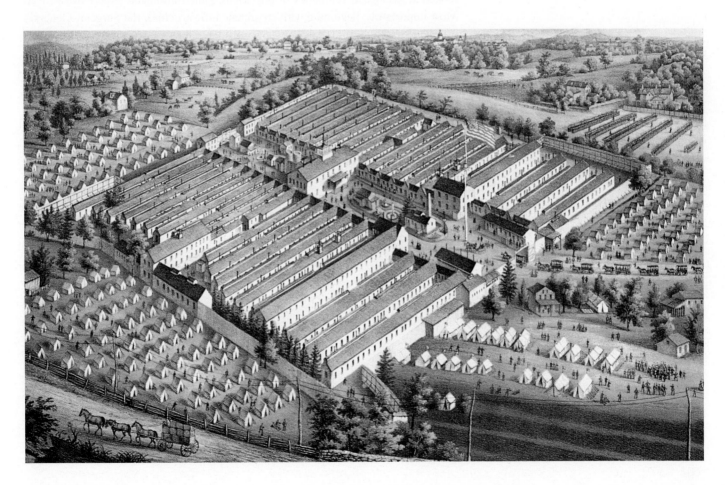

24. So many soldiers died during the Civil War that battlefield embalming of the deceased became a much-needed and lucrative business. "Embalming surgeons" followed the troops in order to ply their trade. Because many military units were composed of men from a single town or well-defined geographic district, when a soldier died his comrades willingly assumed the grim responsibility of arranging to embalm his body and ship it home. Fees for the service were not modest; they were often listed in local newspaper as $25 for enlisted men and $100 for officers. This image (circa 1864) is among the most famous likenesses of a Civil War embalmer. It was taken by a member of Matthew Brady's (1823–1896) photographic team and shows surgeon Richard Burr (1819–1885) of Philadelphia outside his work tent, utilizing an embalming pump-syringe on his latest client. Whether the image is a staged recreation or not remains opens to historical dispute. *(Courtesy of Stanley B Burns, M.D., and The Burns Collection and Archive)*

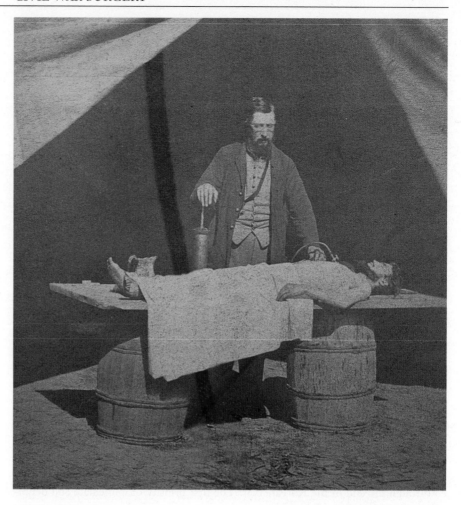

looked at askance as thousands of physicians gained invaluable experience with it. Most importantly, beginning with an archaic infrastructure, the Surgeon-General's office and its Medical Bureau was soon considered on a par with those of European armed forces and began to serve as a model of military medical efficiency.

The dramatic progress in care for the wounded was accompanied by a most important truth: all at once a generation of American physicians, who had previously regarded the craft of surgery as little more than a barbarous sideline of overall medicine, was imbued with a respect for their newly acquired technical skills. By returning in scores to their hamlets, towns, and villages, Civil War surgeons unwittingly set the stage for the blossoming of the American profession of surgery. Led by this rapid advance in the overall quality of surgical practice, American surgeons were finally beginning to approach clinical parity with their European counterparts.

1865	1870	1875	1880	1885	1890	1895	1900	1905

DAILY LIFE

Metropolitan Museum of Art in New York City *(1866)*

Ku Klux Klan *(1867)*

Transcontinental railroad completed at Promontory, Utah territory *(1869)*

Great Atlantic and Pacific Tea Company ("A & P") *(1870)*

National Rifle Association *(1871)*

Yellowstone National Park *(1872)*

Yale, Princeton, Columbia, and Rutgers Universities establish rules for college football *(1873)*

Philadelphia Zoological Garden, America's first zoo *(1874)*

Kentucky Derby held at Churchill Downs *(1875)*

National Baseball League *(1876)*

Electric street lights installed for first time in Newark, New Jersey *(1877)*

Thomas Edison patents the phonograph *(1878)*

Frank Woolworth opens his first 5-and-10-cent store in Lancaster, Pennsylvania *(1879)*

American branch of the Salvation Army established in Philadelphia *(1880)*

Barnum and Bailey's "The Greatest Show on Earth" *(1881)*

Knights of Columbus *(1882)*

Brooklyn Bridge *(1883)*

The Adventures of Huckleberry Finn (1884)

Washington Monument *(1885)*

American Federation of Labor *(1886)*

Mail is delivered to all communities with a population of at least 10,000 *(1887)*

Kodak hand camera *(1888)*

Walter Camp selects first all-American football team *(1889)*

> **U.S.A. POPULATION**
>
> 1870 = 39.8 million, of whom 4.9 million were freed African Americans
>
> 1880 = 50.1 million

HISTORY AND POLITICS

Congress passes Civil Rights Act over President Andrew Johnson's veto *(1866)*

Alaska bought from Russia for $7.2 million *(1867)*

President Johnson impeached and acquitted *(1868)*

Fifteenth Amendment guaranteeing voting rights for African-American men *(1869)*

Department of Justice created *(1870)*

Civil Service Commission *(1871)*

Ulysses S. Grant reelected president *(1872)*

Congress makes gold the U.S. monetary standard *(1873)*

Carpetbaggers seize control of the Arkansas government *(1874)*

Whiskey Ring investigation *(1875)*

Centennial Exposition held in Philadelphia to celebrate the 100th anniversary of the Declaration of Independence *(1876)*

Military reconstruction of the South officially ends *(1877)*

Bland-Allison Act requiring U.S. Treasury to buy from $2 to $4 million of silver bullion for coinage *(1878)*

James Garfield and Chester Arthur elected president and vice-president, respectively *(1880)*

Assassination of President Garfield *(1881)*

Chinese Immigration Restriction Act *(1882)*

Pendleton Act reforms the spoils system *(1883)*

Grover Cleveland and Thomas Hendricks elected president and vice-president, respectively *(1884)*

Contract Labor Act forbids the immigration of laborers under contract to work for cost of transit *(1885)*

Presidential Succession Act *(1886)*

Interstate Commerce Act and establishment of Interstate Commerce Commission *(1887)*

Department of Labor created *(1888)*

North Dakota, South Dakota, Montana, and Washington become the 39th through 42nd states *(1889)*

1865	1870	1875	1880	1885	1890	1895	1900	1905

FAMOUS AMERICANS

HEROES, POLITICIANS, AND STATESMEN

Henry Stimson *(1867–1950)*
John Nance Garner *(1868–1967)*
Cordell Hull *(1871–1955)*
Calvin Coolidge *(1872–1933)*
Al Smith *(1873–1944)*
Herbert Hoover *(1874–1964)*
Robert Wagner *(1877–1953)*
Herbert Lehman *(1878–1963)*
William "Billy" Mitchell *(1879–1936)*
Will Rogers *(1879–1935)*
Douglas MacArthur *(1880–1964)*
George C. Marshall *(1880–1959)*
Branch Rickey *(1881–1965)*
Felix Frankfurter *(1882–1965)*
Fiorello La Guardia *(1882–1947)*
Francis Perkins *(1882–1965)*
Sam Rayburn *(1882–1961)*
Franklin Roosevelt *(1882–1945)*
Jonathan Wainwright *(1883–1953)*
Harry Truman *(1884–1972)*
Chester Nimitz *(1885–1966)*
George Patton *(1885–1945)*
Tyrus "Ty" Cobb *(1886–1961)*
Harry Byrd *(1887–1966)*
Alvin York *(1887–1964)*
Richard Byrd *(1888–1957)*
John Foster Dulles *(1888–1959)*
Knute Rockne *(1888–1931)*
Henry Wallace *(1888–1965)*
Robert Taft *(1889–1953)*

SCIENTISTS AND INVENTORS

Frank Lloyd Wright *(1867–1959)*
Wilbur Wright *(1867–1912)*
Robert A. Millikan *(1868–1953)*
Orville Wright *(1871–1948)*
Willis Carrier *(1876–1950)*
Robert Yerkes *(1876–1956)*
Charles Beebe *(1877–1962)*
Glenn Curtiss *(1878–1930)*
Irving Langmuir *(1881–1957)*
Percy Bridgman *(1882–1961)*
Vincent Bendix *(1882–1945)*
Robert Goddard *(1882–1945)*
Clarence Birdseye *(1886–1956)*
Thomas Hunt Morgan *(1886–1945)*
Ruth Benedict *(1887–1948)*
Selman Waksman *(1888–1973)*
Edwin Hubble *(1889–1953)*
Igor Sikorsky *(1889–1972)*

THEOLOGIANS AND PHILOSOPHERS

Edgar Goodspeed *(1871–1962)*
Rabbi Stephen Wise *(1874–1949)*
Father Devine *(1877–1965)*
Joseph Fielding Smith *(1877–1972)*
Will Durant *(1885–1981)*
Paul Tillich *(1886–1965)*
Walter Lippmann *(1889–1974)*
Cardinal Francis Spellman *(1889–1967)*

EDUCATORS, SCHOLARS, AND REFORMERS

Lincoln Steffens *(1866–1936)*
Lillian Wald *(1867–1940)*
W. E. B. Du Bois *(1868–1963)*
Emma Goldman *(1869–1940)*
Charles Eliot *(1872–1948)*
Learned Hand *(1872–1961)*
Harlan Fiske Stone *(1872–1946)*
William Green *(1873–1952)*
Charles Beard *(1874–1948)*
Edward Thorndike *(1874–1949)*
Mary Bethune *(1875–1955)*
John Watson *(1878–1958)*
H. L. Mencken *(1880–1956)*
Helen Keller *(1880–1968)*
Margaret Sanger *(1883–1966)*
Norman Thomas *(1884–1968)*

1865	1870	1875	1880	1885	1890	1895	1900	1905

FAMOUS AMERICANS

AUTHORS

Edgar Lee Masters *(1869–1950)*
Stephen Crane *(1871–1900)*
Theodore Dreiser *(1871–1935)*
Zane Grey *(1872–1939)*
Willa Cather *(1873–1947)*
Robert Frost *(1874–1963)*
Amy Lowell *(1874–1925)*
Gertrude Stein *(1874–1946)*
Sherwood Anderson *(1876–1941)*
Carl Sandburg *(1878–1967)*
Upton Sinclair *(1878–1968)*
William Carlos Williams *(1883–1969)*
Edna Ferber *(1885–1968)*
Ring Lardner *(1885–1933)*
Sinclair Lewis *(1885–1951)*
Ezra Pound *(1885–1972)*
Louis Untermeyer *(1885–1977)*
Eugene O'Neill *(1888–1953)*
Conrad Aiken *(1889–1973)*
Marianne Moore *(1889–1972)*

VISUAL ARTISTS

George Luks *(1867-1933)*
Alfred Maurer *(1868–1932*
William Glackens *(1870-1938)*
John Marin *(1870–1953)*
John Sloan *(1871–1951)*
Lyonel Feininger *(1871–1956)*
Ernest Lawson *(1873–1939)*
Everett Shinn *(1876–1953)*
Marsden Hartley *(1877–1943)*
Joseph Stella *(1877–1946)*
Arthur Dove *(1880–1946)*
Hans Hofmann *(1880–1966)*
Morton Schamberg *(1881–1918)*
George Bellows *(1882–1925)*
Edward Hopper *(1882–1967)*
Charles Demuth *(1883–1935)*
Georgia O'Keefe *(1887–1986)*
Thomas Hart Benton *(1889–1975)*

PERFORMING ARTISTS

Scott Joplin *(1868–1917)*
Florenz Ziegfeld *(1869–1932)*
W. C. Handy *(1873–1958)*
Charles Ives *(1874–1954)*
D. W. Griffith *(1875–1948)*
Lee Shubert *(1875–1953)*
Lionel Barrymore *(1878–1954)*
George M Cohan *(1878–1942)*
Ethel Barrymore *(1879–1959)*
W. C. Fields *(1880–1946)*
Mack Sennett *(1880–1960)*
Cecil B. DeMille *(1881–1959)*
John Barrymore *(1882–1943)*
Douglas Fairbanks *(1883–1939)*
Billie Burke *(1886–1970)*
Al Jolson *(1886–1950)*
Ed Wynn *(1887–1966)*
Huddie "Leadbelly" Ledbetter *(1888–1951)*
Sophie Tucker *(1888–1966)*
Monty Woolley *(1888–1963)*

BUSINESSMEN AND INDUSTRIALISTS

Herbert Dow *(1866–1930)*
Sebastian Kresge *(1867–1966)*
Harvey Firestone *(1868–1938)*
Bernard Baruch *(1870–1965)*
Charles H. Swift *(1872–1948)*
John D. Rockefeller, Jr. *(1874–1960)*
Owen Young *(1874–1962)*
Walter Chrysler *(1875–1940)*
James C. Penney *(1875–1971)*
Alfred P. Sloan *(1875–1966)*
Eugene Grace *(1876–1960)*
Duncan Hines *(1880–1959)*
William Boeing *(1881–1956)*
Samuel Goldwyn *(1882–1974)*
Henry Kaiser *(1882–1967)*
Elizabeth Arden *(1884–1966)*
Bernard Gimbel *(1885–1966)*
Harold Swift *(1885–1962)*

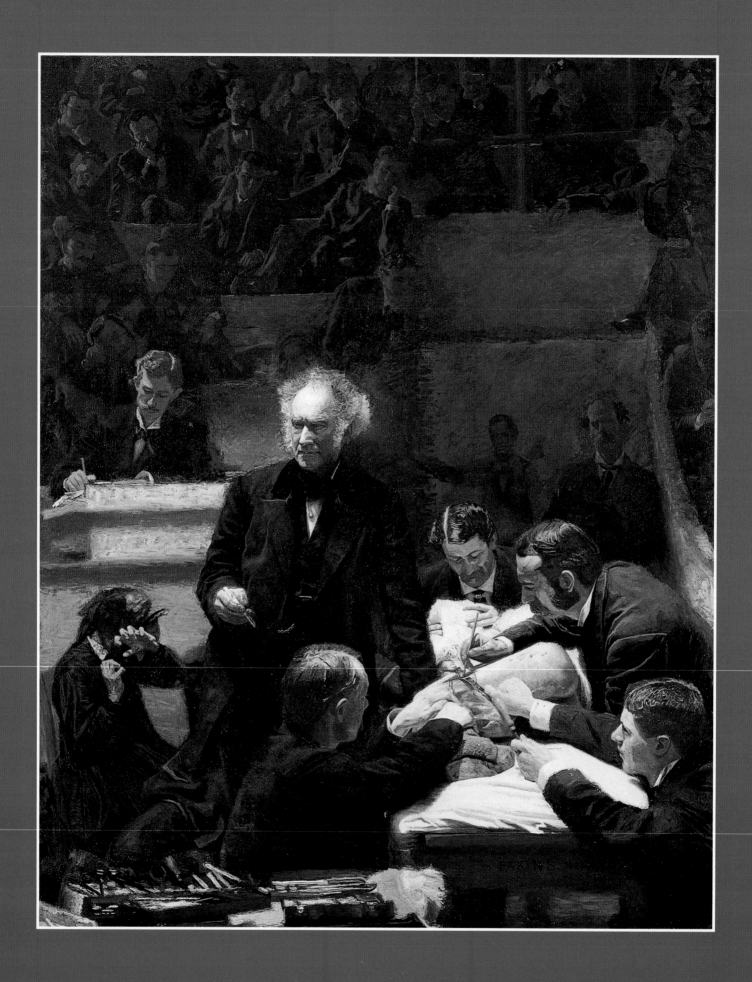

CHAPTER 6

PROFESSIONALIZATION AND ANTISEPSIS
1866–1889

or the American public, the years following the Civil War became what Mark Twain (1835–1910) termed the Golden Age: an era of unbridled optimism and showy wealth. The psychological burdens of our great internecine struggle were beginning to heal. Citizens moved to the cities, waves of immigrants rushed to our shores, and the industrial development of the North, the taming of the West, and the rise of a new South proved the cultural, political, and socioeconomic focal points of the beginning of our second century. The routine of American life was being affected by massive expansion in virtually all areas of daily existence. Capitalism, industrialization, and immigration, along with their resulting conflicts, inevitably influenced the practice of medicine.

For American physician-surgeons, it was a time of reorganization and transformation, which by the 1890s led to a consolidation of their professional authority. What made this post-Civil War era so important to the evolution of American medicine was that doctors were finally showing a demonstrable appreciation of basic scientific research and its practical effects on everyday living. In addition, the activities of medical societies changed from a focus on licensing and membership restriction to a more confident attitude of open membership, albeit controlled, through tighter regulation of their members' professional conduct. In essence, doctors were beginning to understand that if medicine in the United States was ever going to be considered a learned profession, then the necessity for adequate education and training, along with legal licensure and appropriate discipline, was paramount.

Over the next quarter of a century, American medicine became stratified internally as wealthier physicians increased in number and as medical and surgical specialization emerged. Affluent physicians and specialists, especially in urban areas, joined together to form elite medical and surgical organizations so as to politically further their own ambitions and interests. For surgeons in particular, as a consequence of the multiple interactions of societal and scientific circumstances, powerful cultural and political forces were unleashed that made this era one of the most influential in the inevitable progression toward professionalization and specialization.

For too long there had been an American indifference to basic science. Alexis de Tocqueville (1805–1859) postulated that Americans found it easier to "borrow" science from European countries than to provide it for themselves. Tocqueville believed that the fermenting combination of an immature democracy with burgeoning economic opportunities inevitably led to the wholesale neglect of theoretical sciences in favor of more practical and economically viable technological advances. For this simple reason, the greatest achievements in American medicine, at least through the mid-nineteenth century, seemed to be the clinical accomplishments of such sur-

1. *(facing page)* "The Gross Clinic." Painted in 1875, this work (8 by 6½ feet) is considered the crowning achievement of Thomas Eakins (1844–1916), who studied medicine at Jefferson Medical College for one year (1864). It is probable that Eakins, whose artistic endeavors won out over a surgical career, had the upcoming Centennial Exhibition, which was held in Philadelphia in the summer of 1876, in mind when he decided to paint his first large medical scene. It was an entirely private decision, since the work was not commissioned by Samuel Gross or by Jefferson Medical College. The dramatic effect of surgery is heightened by Eakins' choice to depict not merely the physical presence of a surgeon and his team about to operate, but the actual procedure in progress, including an open wound, dripping blood, and retractors being held. Assisting the gray-haired Gross are W. Joseph Hearn, in the rear of the group administering anesthesia, and James M. Barton, Daniel Apple, and Charles S. Briggs in the front. A fifth unidentified assistant is immediately behind Gross, unseen except for a portion of his arm and hand. Other identified figures are the clinic clerk, Franklin West; Gross's son, Samuel Weissell Gross, at the entrance to the amphitheater; and the school's janitor next to the son. Below West is a woman, presumably the patient's mother, who is shielding her eyes in horror. There has been much speculation about why Eakins included her in the scene, ranging from the creation of a dramatic aura to a suggestion of parental consent, but her presence remains a mystery. As for the actual operative procedure, contemporary sources claim that Gross was about to remove a sequestrum of the femur from a male patient. Apart from the event's emotionality, what is most striking is that the surgeons are operating in their business suits with bare hands and no masks or caps. (*Jefferson Medical College of Thomas Jefferson University, Philadelphia, Pennsylvania*)

gical geniuses as Valentine Mott, Philip Syng Physick, and Wright Post and their complicated but technically stupefying vascular ligations and bone resections.

What Tocqueville had witnessed in America in the early 1830s underwent dramatic alteration by the late 1880s. In 1850, less than 15 percent of the nation's populace resided in cities. Yet, by 1890, 35 percent of some 60 million Americans resided in an urban environment. Utilizing this rapidly expanding and urbanized labor pool, visionary businessmen such as Cornelius Vanderbilt (1794–1877), Andrew Carnegie (1835–1919), and John D. Rockefeller (1839–1937) helped transform the United States into a great industrial power. Concurrently, leaders of the labor movement, including Samuel Gompers (1850–1924), directed efforts to improve conditions for the common laborer.

SOCIAL AND LEGAL ASPECTS OF MEDICINE AND SURGERY

A little appreciated but intriguing example of industry, labor, and medicine joining together in the 1870s and 1880s to produce an organized surgical specialty was railway surgery. During the heyday of railroad expansion, enormous construction projects created employment opportunities for more than one million railroad workers. Not unexpectedly, there were numerous injuries, often disabling if not fatal, to both employees and passengers. Railroad companies were forced to retain part-time private medical practitioners along the proposed routes to treat accident victims. However, as rapid growth took the railways farther into the undeveloped areas of the West, it became necessary to provide medical services under full-time chief surgeons. Thus, the specialty of railway surgery arose and a new breed of physician, the railway surgeon, emerged.

As the number of railway surgeons increased and expertise regarding the management of trauma cases evolved, the necessity for some form of focused organizational activity became apparent. Accordingly, in 1882, twenty-five physicians in Illinois formed the Surgical Society of the Wabash, St. Louis, and Pacific Railway. This was the forerunner to the National Association of Railway Surgeons, founded in Chicago in June 1888. From this society there grew a well-orchestrated specialty movement, which supported its own journal, *The Railway Surgeon*, and treatises by bonafide railway surgeons: Christian Stemen (1838–1915) (*Railway Surgery...for Railway Surgeons; and Practitioners in the General Practice of Surgery*, 1890), and Clinton Herrick (1859–1915) (*Railway Surgery, A Handbook on the Management of Injuries*, 1894).

As railway surgeons increased in number, there was growing resentment on the part of organized medicine (i.e., national, state, county, and city medical societies) toward all forms of contract practice. It was regarded as a method of evil exploitation because companies were placed in the enviable position of having physicians bid against each other's services. Thus, the price of medical care was driven down while higher profits were realized for the company. Railway surgeons, and virtually all doctors who worked for companies, were generally regarded with suspicion by their professional peers who were not employed by companies.

In reality, though, railway surgeons, like other practitioners, were quite concerned about corporate capitalism creeping into their medical practices. Railway surgeons did not wish to be dominated by private corporations any more than by government bureaucracies. However, the vast majority of railway surgeons were physician-surgeons who had neither the educational nor financial wherewithal to limit their practice to noncorporate medicine. More importantly, many of these individuals had served in the Civil War and obtained crude but competent surgical skills on the battlefield. The need for their clinical expertise, especially in trauma care, was evident when the Interstate Commerce Commission reported in 1900 that one of every twenty-nine railroad employees was injured and one of every 399 was killed on the job. The reality was that the Civil War surgical training of many thousands of physician-surgeons was ideally suited for corporate America's need.

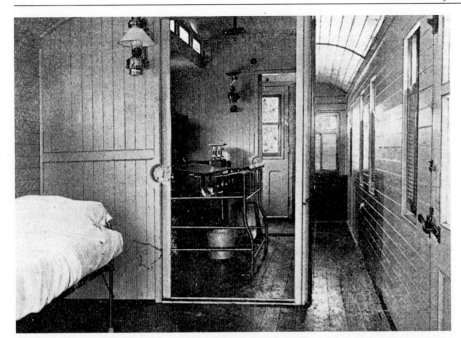

2. From Christian Stemen's *Railway Surgery* (1890), a hospital railroad car as seen from the transportation room looking into the operating room, including an always available operating table. (*Author's Collection*)

Ultimately, vast numbers of America's physicians became dependent on corporate medicine and the livelihood it provided.

By the time of World War I, corporate involvement in health care delivery was becoming a thing of the past. The enactment of legal protections for collective bargaining and the growing strength of labor unions in heavy industry signified the abandonment of company-controlled medical and surgical services. The legion of railway surgeons soon faded from the active scene of health care provision, and their affairs now exist as little more than a long-forgotten chapter in American surgery. Still, railway surgeons, although regarded with contempt by their fellow physicians, fostered such revolutionary concepts in American health care delivery as private inpatient hospitals and elementary managed care plans. Most importantly, railway surgery showed that specialization within the profession could benefit many aspects of American culture.

In 1876, a heralded series of five articles celebrating one hundred years of American medicine appeared in the prestigious *American Journal of the Medical Sciences*. Among the physician authors was Samuel Gross, professor of surgery at Jefferson Medical College and the leading surgical authority of his day. Gross chauvinistically pointed out that:

> the medical profession has kept steady pace with the general progress of the arts and sciences on this continent; and not the least gratifying circumstance connected with it is the knowledge that it occupies a position in the social circle not accorded to it in any other part of the world...The cultured and refined American physician is a prince among men.

Gross's perceptions of the socioeconomic and political structure of pre-1880s American medical practice, particularly those relative to surgical practice, were seconded by John Erichsen (1818–1896), professor of surgery at University College in London, England. Erichsen was a leading voice in European surgery, and after visiting the United States in 1874, he authored an account of his impressions concerning American medicine:

> As to the profession, I may at once say that it appears to me to occupy in America, relatively to the rest of the community, a far higher social status than it does in this country. The reason for this seems tolerably obvious. In the absence of an exalted hierarchy in an established church and of great dignitaries of the law, these professions do not offer sufficient inducement for men of the highest intellectual caliber to enter them. Medicine, therefore, stands prominent as probably the best-educated, certainly the most scientific, and,

consequently, in a country where education is so widedly diffused and so much regarded, the most respected of the professions. Perhaps, also, the high position that medicine occupies is owing…to the greater uniformity of practice that prevails amongst medical men in America than with us. For, just as in the law there is no division into barristers and solicitors, so in medicine there is none into physicians, surgeons, and general practitioners.

It was true that American medicine had made definite progress during the first century of the country's existence. Still, few clinical improvements were perceptible to the average layman other than the steadying decline in "heroic therapies" and the utilization of inhalation anesthesia for surgical operations. The demise of bleeding, emetics, and purging as the three mainstays of a physician's practice signified a distinct break from past Galenic and Paracelsian traditions. With a growing appreciation of developments in biochemistry, microbiology, pharmacology, and physiology, American physicians were pursuing the use of less harmful drugs. Accordingly, analgesics, antipyretics, and tonics became the mainstay of the late-nineteenth-century physician.

Despite improvements in clinical acumen and therapeutics, epidemics still raged and the same old infectious diseases of cholera, diphtheria, malaria, tuberculosis, typhoid fever, and yellow fever continued to exact a heavy toll. Regardless of the glowing praises of Gross and Erichsen, the unvarnished reality was far less favorable. Arthur Hertzler (1870–1946) grew up in Kansas and later started the Hertzler Clinic in Halstead, Kansas. Renowned for his surgical skills, Hertzler depicted in his autobiography, *The Horse and Buggy Doctor* (1938), a far less glowing portrayal of frontier doctors:

3. A fascinating broadside of American surgical ephemera. Indian cancer doctors and other quacks flooded the American medical scene in the late nineteenth century. These charlatans claimed to be jacks of all trades but served up little more than false hopes based on empty promises. (*From the Collection of Andrew L. Warshaw, M.D.*)

Most of the doctors had never attended a medical school. Most of them had "read medicine" with some active doctor but many just bought a book.... Most of the doctors of that day had drug stores and they examined patients as they were seated beside the counter in view of other customers.... It was generally believed by the laity in our community that...two-thirds of the doctors went to hell.... Most of the doctors of that day were addicted to liquor, smoked pipes and did not go to church.... My father believed...that approximately all doctors were parasites of society.

Hertzler may have caricatured the situation, but a serious dichotomy did exist. Physicians were often the only men boasting any kind of education in most communities. Therefore, it was inevitable that they frequently stood out in civic and social life. Still, William Pepper (1843–1898), professor of clinical medicine at the University of Pennsylvania, summed up the truth by pointing out that despite their esteem, "there are but few classes of the community of which a larger proportion are not earning a living than of the medical profession."

The number of medical schools grew rapidly after the Civil War, and the many institutions became noticeably stratified in their educational quality and cost. Quacks and irregular physicians abounded, which added to the overcrowding of American medicine. If the professionalization of surgery and its evolution as a specialty were to succeed, then various government and other societal institutions, including educational, organizational, and regulatory reform within medicine, needed substantive transformation. True changes in American medical education began in the 1870s and paralleled developments in undergraduate colleges and universities. Charles Eliot (1834–1926) of Harvard University and Daniel Coit Gilman (1844–1901) of The Johns Hopkins University instituted dramatic innovations in collegiate education that led to the inevitable reform of medical education.

As college students became better educated, it was easier to insist that requirements for medical school admission be similarly upgraded. Prior to the 1870s, there was little in the way of effective state licensing boards. Any attempt at utilizing federal or state powers as a method of governing the medical profession was met by apathy and the public's unwillingness to recognize such authority. However, the country's socioeconomic environment after the Civil War placed greater demands on government to regulate many aspects of American society. For instance, in 1886, the United States Supreme Court ruled that interstate commerce could be regulated only by the federal government. Congress responded to this challenge and within one year had passed the Interstate Commerce Act, setting up the Interstate Commerce Commission. Four years later, the Sherman Antitrust Act was legislatively enacted.

Within this increasingly regulated environment, it was inevitable that the practice of medicine would be similarly affected. Much as laborers and farmers wanted railroad abuses to be curbed, the public and physicians themselves were beginning to demand protection against incompetent practitioners. This became especially critical because the quarter century following the Civil War was the heyday of proprietary medical schools and bogus diploma mills. In 1880, there were innumerable "regular" medical schools, homeopathic institutions, and eclectic or other facilities attended by almost 12,000 students. Huge numbers of "doctors of medicine" were being graduated; almost 20,000 new individuals titled themselves "doctor" during the decade of the 1870s. John Shaw Billings spoke of the situation:

There is another large class [of physicians], whose defects in general culture and in knowledge of the latest improvements in medicine, have been much dwelt upon by those disposed to take gloomy views of the condition of medical education in this country...their work in medical school was confined to so much memorizing of text-books as was necessary to secure a diploma.... Certainly, the standard for admission and for graduation at almost all our medical schools is too low, and one-half, at least, of these schools have no sufficient reason for existence.

Key reforms in medical licensing and regulation led to the adoption of graded curricula by numerous medical schools. These licensing laws required applicants to have graduation certificates from medical schools that met minimum entrance, term length, and course complexity requirements. The advent of state licensing boards contributed to the standardization of medical practice by requiring the same medical knowledge of all applicants. In 1877, following much deliberative hesitation, the Illinois Board of Health became the country's first agency authorized to maintain a statewide register of recognized physicians and the medical schools from which they graduated. Within twelve years, the Board had learned of 179 "regular" schools, twenty-six homeopathic colleges, twenty-six eclectic institutions, and thirteen other sectarian schools throughout the nation many of which were considered to be totally fraudulent. By finally regulating and focusing both the scientific and organizational aspects of the medical profession, licensing boards helped foster professionalization and specialization.

In addition to the problem of poorly educated allopathic, or regular, physicians, there was growing financial competition with so-called irregular dispensers of medical care (botanics, eclectics, homeopaths, phrenologists, quacks, water-cure men, etc.). These numerous unorthodox healers and their alternative therapies posed a serious threat to the professional and financial survival of late-nineteenth-century allopathic physicians. Not unexpectedly, the sectarian movements attempted to professionalize their own status by seeking federal and state regulation of their particular methods of health care practice.

In a bit of historical irony, it was only with the cooperation of homeopaths and eclectics that the regular profession was finally able to secure adequate medical licensing legislation in most states. Such collaboration was encouraged by both political and social pragmatism as well as the convergence of forms of practice. By the mid-1890s, significant therapeutic distinctions between allopaths, eclectics, and homeopaths had begun to disappear. In point of fact, the technical aspects of surgery had never differed substantively among the three groups.

THE SURGEON AS MEDICAL SPECIALIST

As surgeons became more narrowly focused, especially with regard to scientific dogma, it was inevitable that differences in "thinking and doing" would also disappear. The coming of age of the surgeon as a specialist within the whole of medicine served to lessen all dissimilarities between regular and sectarian surgeons. John B. Roberts (1852–1924), professor of surgery at the Woman's Medical College of Pennsylvania and a leading figure in organized medicine, provided proper perspective to the entire question of sectarian surgery and discrimination in general:

> This society should be liberal enough to accept as a member any physician whose education and personal character make him a fit associate for intelligent men. I state my belief that the test of qualification for membership should not be the college from which the applicant received his diploma; but an education enabling him to understand and appreciate the science of medicine, and an honest purpose to treat his patients by all means and methods which experience, investigation and research show to be serviceable. It seems to me...that such a physician's political, religious or social beliefs and affiliations should not disqualify him...

By the late 1880s, specialists in surgery had assumed influential standing within all of medicine. They controlled the burgeoning elite medical societies and held politically powerful medical faculty positions. Most important, surgical specialists were beginning to rule the staffs of hospitals while gaining ever more wealthy and socially prominent patients. To fully appreciate the phoenix-like rise of the American surgeon, an analysis of individuals who held the presidency of the American Medical Association during the last three decades of the nineteenth century is quite revealing. During the 1870s, three practitioners who were recognized more as surgeons than physicians served as president: David Yandell (1826–1898), J. Marion Sims

4. (*facing page*) Following the Civil War, it was accepted that human dissection was to be a standard part of the modern medical school curriculum. Thomas Anshutz (1851–1912) was Thomas Eakins' assistant at the many courses in artistic anatomy given by the latter at the Pennsylvania Academy of the Fine Arts. Anshutz's "Dissecting Room" (circa 1879) (*top*) shows a group of male students examining a skeleton and a cadaver. Charles Stephens's "Anatomical Lectures by Dr. Keen" (circa 1879), portrays the surgeon engaged in a presentation using a male student model with a cadaver, skeletons, and other demonstration pieces strewn about the room (*bottom*). Keen had been in charge of the Philadelphia School of Anatomy for many years, but closed its doors in 1875, when a financial crisis was brought about by the decreasing numbers of students who left because they could obtain better anatomical instruction in formal medical schools. Both of these paintings were completed in monochrome and served as illustrations in a scholarly article (*Scribner's Monthly Magazine*, September 1879) by William Brownell, a leading art critic of that time, regarding Eakins' teaching methodology. (*Courtesy of the Museum of American Art of the Pennsylvania Academy of the Fine Arts, Philadelphia. Gift of the artist.*)

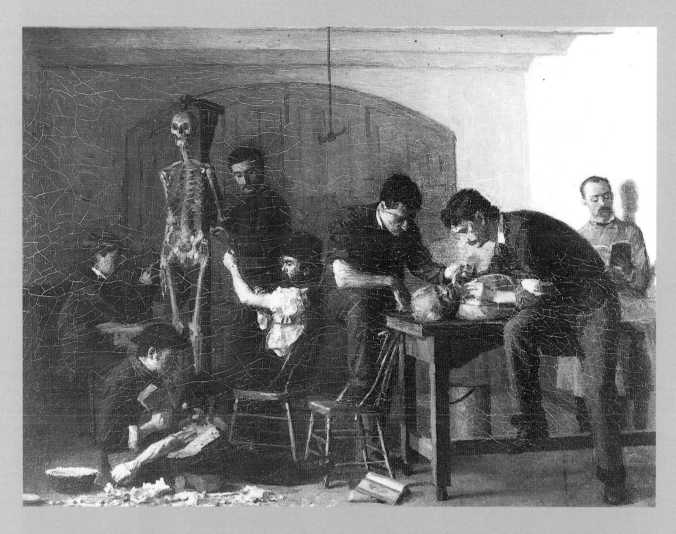

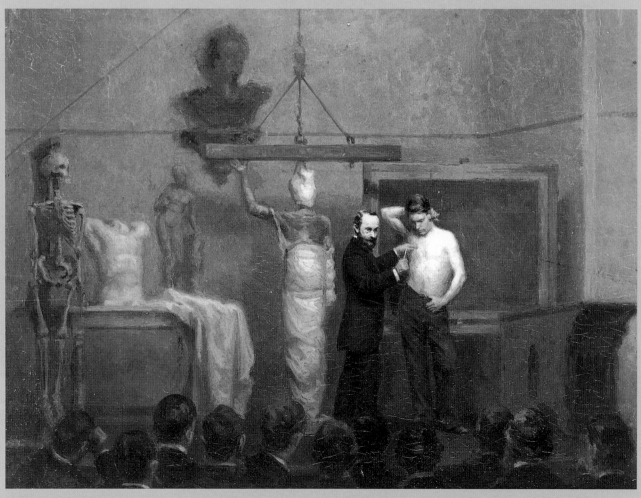

(1813–1883), and Tobias Richardson (1827–1892). Over the next ten years, the number increased to six: Lewis Sayre (1820–1900), John Hodgen (1826–1882), John Atlee (1799–1885), Henry Campbell (1824–1891), Elisha Gregory (1824–1906) and William Dawson (1828–1893). In the 1890s, eight specialists in surgery served as president: Edward Moore (1814–1902), William Briggs (1829–1894), Henry Marcy (1837–1924), Hunter McGuire (1835–1900), Donald MacLean (1839–1903), Richard Cole (1829–1901), Nicholas Senn (1844–1908), and Joseph Mathews (1847–1928).

Both in a professional sense and in the view of the lay public, American surgeons were finally separating themselves from physicians. Surgery enjoyed a spectacular rise in prestige and accomplishment in the late 1800s, although it would not undergo its most dramatic makeover until the 1890s and early 1900s. Surgery as a respected specialty within medicine had come of age, and surgical practitioners enjoyed social prestige and cultural acceptance. The fact that a young medical school graduate finally had a legitimate opportunity to pursue diverse professional choices within both medicine and surgery would have an enormous impact on the future direction of American medicine.

Writing in *Harper's Magazine* in 1889, William Keen waxed enthusiastically that "In no department of medicine has there been more rapid and in many respects more astonishing progress in recent years than in surgery." Keen attributed this advance "to two things-the introduction of antiseptic methods, and to...laboratory work and experiments upon animals." There is certainly no disputing Keen's comments, but to more fully appreciate this scientific

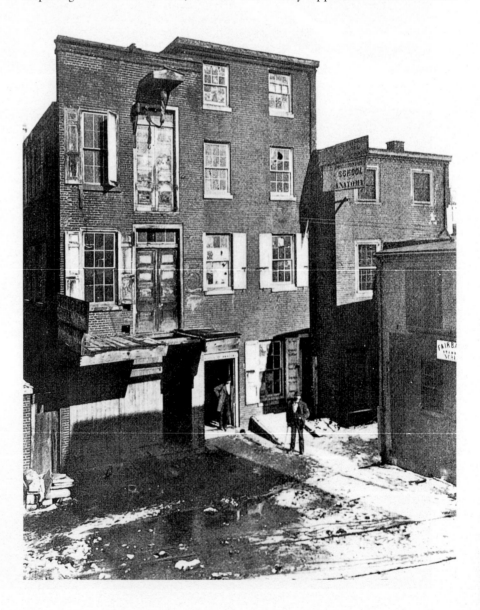

5. The Philadelphia School of Anatomy (1820–1875) was among the best known of the American extramural medical schools. The summer months proved particularly busy for such institutions, as they filled the long educational hiatus between April and November, when proprietary and university-affiliated medical schools were closed. (*Author's Collection*)

progress, it is important to understand the respective positions of surgery and medicine in the mid-part of the century. While nineteenth-century physicians favored general remedies for whole-body symptoms, surgeons had long ago made the assumption that ablating local lesions in specific organs could cure specific diseases. By 1865, American doctors and patients were coming to hold surgery in relatively high regard for its pragmatic appeal, technological virtuosity, and "unambiguously measurable results." Surgery might have seemed a mystical craft to both doctor and patient. To be allowed to consensually cut into another human being's body, to gaze at the depth of that person's suffering, and to excise the demon of disease seemed an awesome responsibility. Yet, it was this very mysticism, long associated with religious overtones, that so fascinated the public and their own feared but inevitable date with a surgeon's knife. Henry Bigelow captured the essence of this surgical *gestalt* when he wrote:

> Why is the amphitheatre crowded to the roof…on the occasion of some great operation, while the silent working of some drug excites little comment? Mark the hushed breath, the fearful intensity of silence, when the blade pierces the tissues, and the blood of the sufferer wells up to the surface. Animal sense is always fascinated by the presence of animal suffering.

Surgeons began to view themselves as combining art and nature, essentially assisting nature in its continual process of destruction and rebuilding. This regard for the natural sprang from the eventual, though preternaturally slow, understanding and use of Lister's techniques. Concurrent with the advent of surgical antisepsis and asepsis was the appearance of other elements fundamental to the professionalization and specialization process. Most notable was the establishment in 1880 of the first nationally recognized elite surgical organization, the American Surgical Association; the founding in 1885 of the first journal devoted exclusively to the surgical sciences, the *Annals of Surgery*; and the beginning of the surgeon's understanding of the value of science to his craft, as is evidenced by Reginald Fitz's (1843–1913) enunciation in 1886 of the natural history of the quintessential American surgical disease, appendicitis.

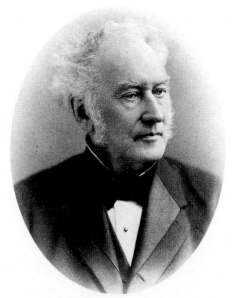

6. Samuel Gross. (*Historical Collections, College of Physicians of Philadelphia*)

THE INFLUENCE OF SAMUEL GROSS

Many of these changes can be appreciated through an understanding of the life of Samuel Gross, who must be ranked among the most important surgeons that the United States has produced. The range of his intellectual work, his prodigious literary output, and his outstanding clinical acumen explain his enormous influence on the practice of medicine and surgery at this critical juncture in American history. Gross was born on July 8, 1805, in the Pennsylvania Dutch country near Easton, Pennsylvania, of German ancestry. As a child he spoke only the Americanized German indigenous to his native region. He first learned English after the age of 12, and he carried a slight foreign accent for the remainder of his life.

Gross was the fifth of six children. His father died in 1813, and Gross developed an especially strong attachment to his mother. She was a devout Lutheran, who lived to be 85 years old, and he later attributed much of his strength of character to her influence and religious training. Gross's childhood was typical of the time and place; he started public school at the age of 7 in a log cabin near his home. In his posthumously published two-volume *Autobiography* (1887), Gross noted that he first decided to become a doctor at the age of 6: "If I was not born a doctor, I was determined from my earliest boyhood to study medicine; and, although I have sometimes thought that I had mistaken my calling, I am not sure that I have not done well in being a doctor, and living by men's diseases."

As was common then, Gross began to study medicine as the private pupil of various country practitioners. He found their assistance inadequate and complained that they never examined him on the material he was studying or provided any encouragement. As a result, Gross attempted to learn anatomy essentially on his own, primarily using the massive compendium of Andrew Fyfe (1754–1824), an English anatomist. However, Gross soon realized that his Latin was insufficient for medical study and that a knowledge of Greek would also be necessary. Accordingly, in 1821 he asked his rural-based preceptor to release him from his contractual obligations. Gross considered this act one of the turning points in his life, since it required courage—not only to face up to his teacher but to admit his own lack of education.

Gross immediately enrolled in an academy at Wilkes-Barre, Pennsylvania, in order to gain the classical education that he needed. After completing a year of study there, he transferred in the winter of 1822–1823 to a classical school on the Bowery in New York City. Within six months he returned to Easton to take private instruction in Latin and Greek. In less than five months, he again became restless and enrolled at the then well known "High School at Lawrenceville, New Jersey." Gross spent six months at what is now The Lawrenceville School, one of the country's elite secondary boarding schools, there completing his rather desultory secondary education.

Gross recommenced his study of medicine in 1824 under the tutelage of Joseph Swift, a country practitioner who was a graduate of the medical department of the University of Pennsylvania. Gross was a precocious student and within two months had mastered Wistar's 2 volume textbook of anatomy. Although his health was at times precarious, he agreed to remain with Swift for three years, including two lecture terms. By the fall of 1826, Gross had gained as much knowledge as Swift could offer, and Swift urged Gross to move to Philadelphia and attend the University of Pennsylvania. However, Gross had heard so much about the achievements of George McClellan, professor of surgery at Jefferson Medical College, that he disregarded Swift's wishes and matriculated at Jefferson, at the same time becoming a private office pupil of McClellan.

Gross flourished in medical school, with anatomy and surgery being his favorite subjects. He received his M.D. in 1828 after writing a thesis on the nature and treatment of cataract. Gross decided to remain in Philadelphia and opened an office on the corner of Library and Fifth streets. However, his practice was meager at best, and he earned less than three hundred dollars during the first year.

At this stage in his professional career, Gross's talent as a medical writer first became apparent. In 1828–1829, he undertook the translation of several European works: the *General Anatomy* of Antoine Bayle (1799–1858) and Henri Hollard (1801–1866), the *Manual of Practical Obstetrics* by Jules Hatin (1800–1839), a work on typhus fever by Johann von Hildenbrand (1763–1818), and the *Elements of Operative Surgery* by Alphonse Tavernier (?–1850). Although Gross completed these translations in less than eighteen months, he never undertook another one, having become convinced that the United States should have its own medical texts and that this would occur only if potential authors stopped doing translations.

Gross's practice continued to be quite limited, and he therefore had the leisure time to author the first systematic American work on bones and joints. His *Anatomy, Physiology, and Diseases of the Bones and Joints* (1830) was completed when he was only 25 years of age. It was published in Easton, where Gross had moved meanwhile, having decided that he could not earn a living in Philadelphia.

Gross did not enjoy his stay in Easton because of what he considered to be the general mediocrity of medical practice in the town. He became demonstrator of anatomy at the newly founded Medical College of Ohio at Cincinnati in the spring of 1833, but remained there for only two sessions because he did not like the internal political conflicts that plagued the institution. However, during his short stay at the school he became joint editor of the *Western Medical Gazette* with John Eberle (1787–1838), Alban Gilpin Smith (1795–1876) and Gamaliel Bailey. He subsequently contributed a paper to the journal on intrauterine respirations in relation to infant mortality, but his connection with the periodical ended when he left the school in the summer of 1835.

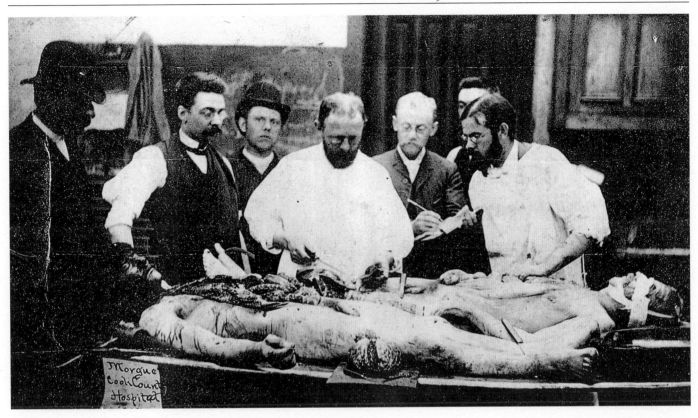

The medical department of Cincinnati College was then being organized, and the chair of pathological anatomy was open. Gross was appointed to the position by unanimous vote. Among his faculty colleagues were Daniel Drake, Joseph Nash McDowell (1805–1868), and Willard Parker (1800–1884). There he delivered the first systematic course of lectures on pathological anatomy ever given in the United States. Gross prepared large numbers of pathologic specimens, and these dissections, an elaborate course of reading, and numerous visits to the slaughterhouses of Cincinnati constituted the research for his two-volume *Elements of Pathological Anatomy* (1839). With his *Elements*, Gross produced the first English language textbook to exhaustively and systematically analyze the new science of pathological anatomy.

Following the Civil War, there was a growing emphasis on the correlation of clinical manifestations of illness with specific pathological findings in organs. As surgery became increasingly sophisticated, the importance of pathology became paramount. Gross's monograph paved the way for the anatomist-surgeon of earlier times to be replaced by the pathologist-surgeon of the late nineteenth century. Gross recognized that surgical pathology would be a fundamental force in the rational empiricism that was reshaping nineteenth-century medical therapy, and that his own pathology studies would have to embrace the fundamental principals of scholarship that had been defined a century earlier by the "father of pathology," Giovanni Morgagni. Gross was especially proud that in the *Elements* "the description of the morbid anatomy of every organ in the body was preceded by an account of its healthy color, weight, size, and consistency, founded upon original investigation, a plan until then unknown in such works." By setting an early and exemplary model, Gross paved the way when other American surgeon-pathologists, in particular David Gilliam (1844–1923) (*The Essentials of Pathology*, 1883) and John Collins Warren (1842–1927) (*Surgical Pathology and Therapeutics*, 1895), authored their texts.

Cincinnati College closed in 1839, leaving Gross free to devote himself to his expanding and lucrative practice. During the spring of 1840, the chair of surgery at the University of Louisville became vacant. Gross gladly accepted it after having previously turned down the chair of anatomy at the University of Louisiana as well as a professorship of medicine at the University of Virginia. For various political rea-

7. In this 1888 photograph of the morgue at Chicago's Cook County Hospital, Christian Fenger conducts an autopsy on one of two male victims. Fenger served as pathologist to the institution from 1878 to 1893 and became recognized as the "father of modern pathological surgery." Among his assistants are Ludvig Hektoen (1863–1951) (*second from the left*), later to become director of the McCormick Institute for Infectious Diseases in Chicago and founder and editor of the *Archives of Pathology* and *Journal of Infectious Diseases*, and James Herrick (1861–1954) (*third from the right with pen in hand*), the first physician to describe and diagnose coronary thrombosis in a living person. (*Historical Collections, College of Physicians of Philadelphia*)

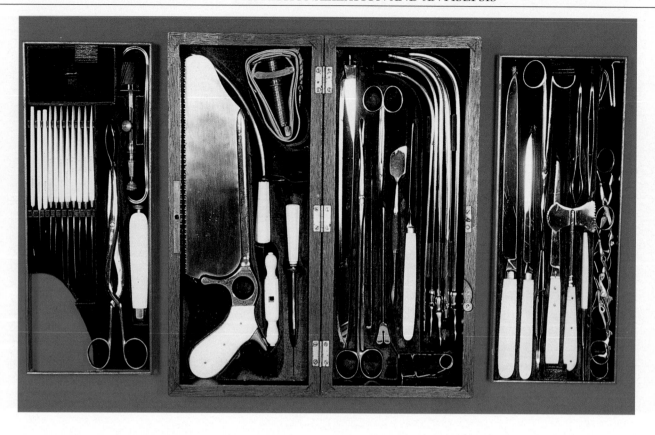

8. By 1889, the firm of George Tiemann & Co. of New York City reached a degree of international renown unmatched by any other American surgical instrument manufacturer. That year, the company's 846-page trade catalogue *The American Armamentarium Chirurgicum* proudly displayed in its introduction two silver medals awarded by the Paris Exposition of 1867, one bronze medal from an International Exhibiton in Paris that same year, and two first medals and an honorable mention obtained at a trade festival in Santiago, Chile, in 1875. Tiemann & Co. offered any number of different general operating sets, all carrying the eponyms of famous American surgeons. This set (circa 1870s) was named after Willard Parker, cost $104.90, and contained over one hundred surgical implements housed in a rosewood case, brass bound, lined with silk velvet. The ivory handles on the instruments, although beautiful to look at, could not be sterilized, and confirm that this particular surgical set dates from a period before antisepsis was widely accepted in America. (*Collection of Alex Peck, Antique Scientifica*)

sons Gross's reception in Kentucky was less than cordial, but the strength of his personality and his teaching abilities eventually won over his reluctant colleagues. Austin Flint, Gross's friend in later life and a distinguished New York City physician in his own right, described Gross in the lecture room:

> His tall commanding figure, his clear voice, his features beaming with intelligence and animation, his zealous manner - all contributed to render his teaching effective. He had that magnetism which is a gift invaluable to a speaker.

The education of medical students was a priority for Gross. He had little use for incompetent professors whose only interest was a pecuniary one: the lecture fee. Gross knew that he was a good teacher and attributed his success to enthusiasm, proper preparation including wide reading, and an obsessive-compulsive attitude toward personal organization. His lectures were delivered with such authority and vigor that David Yandell (1826–1898), who succeeded Gross as professor of surgery at the University of Louisville, recalled his predecessor as being a "sometimes excited, even boisterous lecturer who looked his students in the eye, shook his fist, stamped his foot and swore 'by the Eternal'."

Shortly after his arrival in Louisville, Gross began a series of surgical experiments on dogs. His specific goal was to determine techniques that could be used to successfully treat patients with stab wounds to the abdomen through which injured bowel had eviscerated. Within three years, he had completed the research for and had written his *Experimental and Critical Inquiry into the Nature and Treatment of Wounds of the Intestines* (1843), the first American book of experimental animal physiology. Because most of the copies were destroyed in a fire at the printer's warehouse, the monograph never received wide distribution, and its lack of literary success and surgical influence was a bitter disappointment for Gross.

Gross related in his Autobiography that he "had an ardent desire in my professional youth to become an experimentalist, both with a view of throwing light upon certain obscure points in physiology, and of earning some reputation." Once again, he was percipient in his understanding of what was important to the evolution of American surgery. Gross realized that pure research in the surgical sciences was a fundamental aspect of any surgical scholar's career. Experimental procedures on animals would have to become part of the standard for all future surgical research. The rise of such practices during the 1870s and 1880s necessarily paralleled the growth of laboratories and the physician's acceptance of basic science research as an integral part of the whole of clinical practice.

Gross's *Experimental and Critical Inquiry* was an immediate precursor to the organized advancement of further experimental research within American surgery. In 1888, Hal Wyman (1852–1908), professor of surgery and operative surgery at the Michigan College of Medicine and Surgery, authored a surgical text devoted to experimental animal surgery, *Abdominal Surgery*. The following year, Nicholas Senn (1844–1908), professor of the principles of surgery and surgical pathology at Rush Medical College, wrote his *Experimental Surgery*, which established the experimental foundation on which future American surgical successes would occur. Senn, like Gross, was of the opinion that "experimental surgical work…is a necessary complement to clinical observations, it tends to purify science from the sterile *a priori* reasons and theories with which medical science has in former times been heavily loaded down."

The fifteen years Gross spent in Louisville were among the happiest and most fruitful of his life. He cultivated many close relationships, and his home provided true Southern hospitality for distinguished guests from all over the world. In 1850 there was a political controversy over the governing of the medical school. Gross was particularly unhappy with the chain of events, and during this crisis he received the offer of the chair of surgery at the University of the City of New York. Uncertain about the Louisville school's future, Gross decided to accept the New York appointment, which had been vacated following the retirement of the well-known Valentine Mott.

Gross spent the winter of 1850–1851 in New York City. Although he greatly enjoyed his teaching responsibilities, he found the school to be mismanaged and unpopular with many of his professional associates in that city. In addition, he felt that the rents and living conditions in urban New York were intolerable. Since Gross considered the overall prospects of the institution to be bleak, upon hearing that the political problems in Louisville had been rectified, and having been solicited by his old colleagues to return, Gross moved back West. On the way, the workaholic Gross left with his publisher, Blanchard and Lea in Philadelphia, the text for his next book, *A Practical Treatise on the Diseases, Injuries and Malformations of the Urinary Bladder, the Prostate Gland, and the Urethra* (1851). In this, the first comprehensive American textbook on urology, Gross managed to "present in a systematic and connected form, a full and comprehensive account of the diseases and injuries of the organs in question." Gross's innovative scholarship is possibly best exemplified in his next book, *A Practical Treatise on Foreign Bodies in the Air-Passages* (1854). Using over one hundred case reports, Gross presented principles concerning symptoms that even now remain fundamental to the care of pulmonary patients.

Gross's stature in American medicine grew rapidly with the publication of his many texts, and he proudly boasted of having "a more commanding surgical practice than any man in the Southwest." Although he had planned on spending the remainder of his professional life in Louisville, this was not to be the case. In 1855, Gross was solicited by a member of the board of trustees of the University of Pennsylvania to allow his name to be nominated for the recently vacated chair of surgery. Gross refused the offer. However, when in the following year his alma mater asked him to assume the vacated professorship of surgery, he hesitantly accepted.

In September 1856, Gross and his family departed for his new position at Jefferson Medical College. There he would spend the remaining years of his professional life, resigning from the chair of surgery in 1882 at the age of 78. Upon his arrival in Philadelphia, Gross found himself partially relieved of the demands of a busy clinical practice. As had been his custom in the past, his response was to write.

He began work on an encyclopedic textbook of surgery, a compilation of all his clinical knowledge. Considered among the most important surgical treatises of its time, the two-volume, 2,360-page *A System of Surgery; Pathological, Diagnostic, Therapeutic, and Operative* (1859) was a truly herculean effort, which went through six editions by 1882. Gross described his writing efforts and detailed the life of the surgeon-author thus:

> I had determined to do my best to make it...the most elaborate, if not the most complete, treatise in the English language...I generally spent from five to eight hours a day upon my manuscript, subject of course to frequent and sometimes annoying interruptions by patients. In the winter I commonly sat up till eleven and half past eleven o'clock at night.... Unless I was greatly interrupted, I seldom wrote less than from ten to fifteen pages of foolscap in the twenty-four hours, and I rarely retired until they were carefully correct-ed.... What compensation does the reader think I obtained for this hard work, this excessive toil of my brain...and the proof-reading, in itself a horrible task, death to brain and eyes.... Eighty-five cents a copy. All told, and no extra div-idends.... No wonder authors are poor and publishers are rich!

During the Civil War, Gross served in several different capacities, although he participated little in actual battlefield surgery. Three days after the battle of Shiloh (April 6–7, 1862), Gross toured the battlefield and gave several extemporaneous lectures on amputations and gunshot wounds. In the spring of 1862, Surgeon-General William Hammond offered him the post of surgeon-in-chief of the George Street Hospital in Philadelphia. Gross turned down the appointment because he believed he was ill-suited for the position. In the summer of that year, Hammond prevailed upon him to become a member of a board of commissioners to examine how mutilated soldiers could be expeditiously fitted with artificial limbs.

Gross's career at Jefferson was one of complete involvement in the medical affairs of the day. His interest in the politics of medicine was incomparable. Gross was one of the founders and early president of the Kentucky State Medical Society, and he was a founder of the Philadelphia Pathological Society, in conjunction with Jacob Mendez Dacosta (1833–1900), and served as its president. He was also a founder of the Medical Jurisprudence Society of Philadelphia, president in 1870 of the Pennsylvania State Medical Society, and founder and first president of the Philadelphia Academy of Surgery (1879).

On a national level, Gross was the twentieth president of the American Medical Association (1868) and founder and first president (1880) of the American Surgical Association. Gross also served as president of the American Philosophical Society, the American Academy of Sciences, and, in 1870, as presiding chairman of the Teacher's Medical Convention in Washington, D.C. Furthermore, he belonged to such international societies as the World Medical Congress (president, 1876); the Imperial Medical Society of Vienna, and numerous similar organizations in the British Isles.

Among Gross's other honors are the inscription of his name in mosaic in the ceiling of the east corridor of the main building of the Library of Congress. A statue was erected in his honor in 1897, for which the U.S. Congress donated the granite base. Originally situated opposite the Army Medical Museum, the statue now stands in the courtyard of Jefferson Medical College. Among the universities that granted Gross honorary degrees were Cambridge, Edinburgh, and Oxford.

Besides his clinical activities, Gross was widely acclaimed as one of the country's preeminent medical historians. For the centennial celebration of the founding of the United States, Gross authored an important paper detailing the history of the first century of American surgery. In 1861, the same year that Gross brought out his *Manual of Military Surgery*, he also authored the nearly 800-page *Lives of Eminent American Physicians and Surgeons*. Among his other historical contributions are a 200-page report on the history of surgery in Kentucky (1853), a full-length biography of Daniel Drake (1853), a sketch of the life of Ambrose Paré (1861), an extensive memoir of Valentine Mott (1868), a lengthy memorial oration in honor of Ephraim McDowell (1879), and a 106-page account of John Hunter and his pupils (1881).

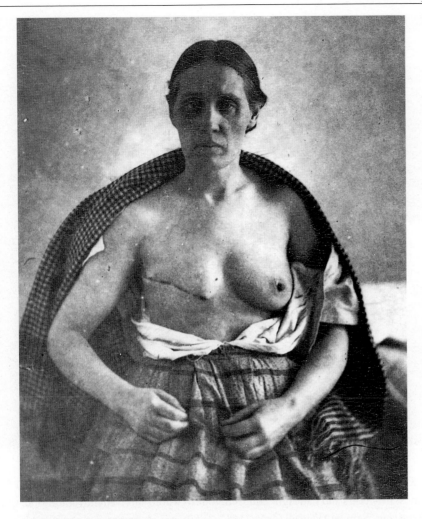

9. In 1872, Addinell Hewsen (1828–1889), surgeon to the Pennsylvania Hospital, authored one of the most intriguing yet bizarre nineteenth-century American treatises on surgery, *Earth as a Topical Application in Surgery*. In an era when the spurious notion that suppuration in a wound favored healing, as expressed by the term "laudable pus," Hewson's earth dressings resulted in faster healing and less painful wounds. It must be assumed that the "earth" used by Hewson contained a type of mold that had an antibiotic effect. If more inquisitive and less disdainful minds had paid attention to Hewson's results, the development of antibiotics might have occurred earlier. The book itself is also significant, being one of the first American medical texts to have photomechanical prints-in this case, Woodburytypes, within the actual volume. Shown is Hannah C., (*top*) aged 41, ten days after undergoing a right mastectomy in February 1869. On completion of the procedure, "dry earth was spread over the site of the breast, and retained by some pieces of white unglazed paper and a roller around the chest." The earth dressing was then renewed every morning. J. F., (*bottom*) a 26-year-old man, underwent forearm amputation for osteomyelitis of an unhealed fracture of the wrist. According to Hewsen, the "whole stump was well covered by the dry garden earth, which was retained by the Scultetus of dry paper, a rectangular splint, and bandage of muslin." This dramatic photograph was taken on the fifteenth postoperative day. (*Courtesy of Stanley B. Burns, M.D., and The Burns Collection and Archive*)

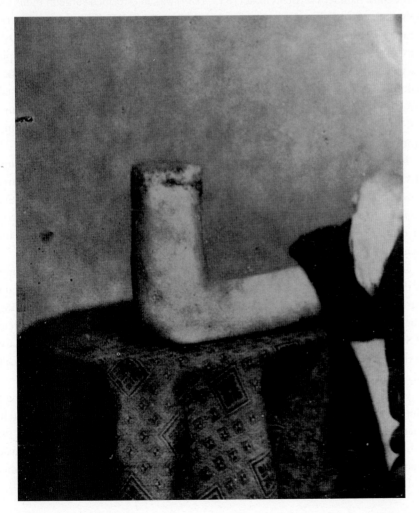

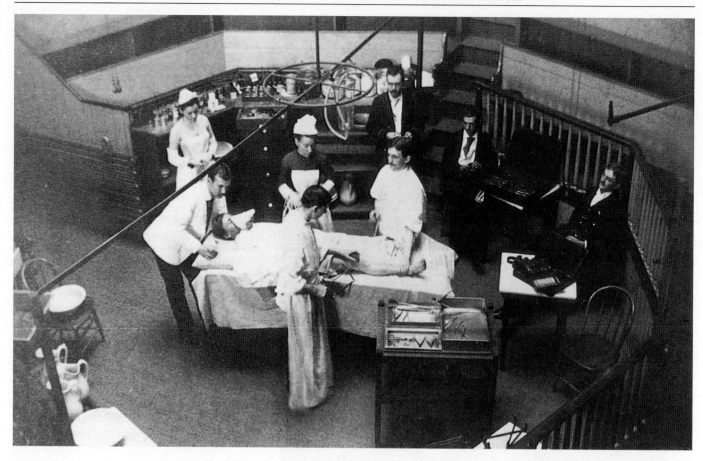

10. An 1888 view of the surgical amphitheater at Old Blockley Hospital in Philadelphia. The picture is unique because photographic images of entire operating rooms were rare prior to the 1890s. Electric lights had not yet been installed in this particular facility, although such a convenience had been available by the mid-1880s. With the patient receiving anesthesia via an ether cone, a boxed amputation set is laid open and John Bower, the surgeon, has a Satterlee-type saw in his right hand. (*Historical Collections, College of Physicians of Philadelphia*)

Gross married Louisa Ann Weisell (1807–1876) in 1828. They were together for almost fifty years and had eight children, four of whom survived into adulthood. One of the sons, Samuel Weissell Gross (1837–1889) was an esteemed surgeon in his own right and succeeded his father in the chair of surgery at Jefferson. Samuel married Grace Revere Linzee, who, following his death, was married to William Osler (1849–1919). A. Haller Gross, the other son, became a prominent Philadelphia lawyer. The eldest daughter, Maria Rives Gross, married Orville Horwitz, a Baltimore lawyer. She was a distinguished linguist and musician. In 1910, she established the Samuel D. Gross chair of surgery, the first endowed professorial chair at Jefferson Medical College. Her younger sister, Louisa Gross, married Benjamin Horwitz, the brother of Orville, also a Baltimore lawyer.

In the autumn of 1883, Gross began to develop signs of congestive heart failure. His condition worsened, and on May 6, 1884, he died. A postmortem examination was completed by Jacob DaCosta and disclosed marked gastric mucosal inflammation, a fatty heart, and a large cyst of the right kidney. Gross was always a strong advocate of cremation, and his ashes were placed in the family vault at Woodlands Cemetery in West Philadelphia.

In his will, Gross left his extensive medical library (approximately 4,000 volumes) to the Philadelphia Academy of Surgery, with the stipulation that they be housed in the library of the College of Physicians of Philadelphia. A special room was created, where they remain today. In addition, Gross provided a $5,000 gift to the Academy of Surgery as a permanent fund so that an award could be presented every five years to the writer of the best original essay on a surgical subject. This prize continues to be awarded.

Gross's most widely appreciated and long-lasting project is the famous painting of him by Thomas Eakins (1844–1916). This renowned work of art depicts Gross in his operative amphitheater prior to the days of antisepsis. Completed in 1875 and first publically exhibited at the Philadelphia Centennial Exhibition in 1876, it is considered one of the masterpieces of American art. It remains on view at Jefferson Medical College and attests to the continuing influence of Gross on American surgery.

In 1876, the apparent slowness of the surgeons' professionalization and specialization process was brought into national focus when Gross wrote in his centennial survey of American surgery:

> Although this paper is designed to record the achievements of American surgeons, there are, strange to say, as a separate and distinct class, no such persons among us. It is safe to affirm that there is not a medical man on this continent who devotes himself exclusively to the practice of surgery. On the other hand, there are few physicians, even in our larger cities, who do not treat the more common surgical diseases and injuries...or who do not even occasionally perform the more common surgical operations. In short, American medical men are general practitioners, ready...to meet any and every emergency, whether in medicine, surgery, or midwifery.

Gross's comments, although widely read and respected, were somewhat self-serving. It would be misleading to suggest that he was unaware of a growing sentiment among certain of his fellow physician-surgeons to devote their professional skills solely to the emerging science of surgery. Conservative in his political viewpoints, Gross consistently sounded a cautionary note against all manner of specialization, and when given the opportunity (e.g., the 1876 paper) would typically speak disparagingly of it:

> Of late, the specialists have seriously encroached upon the province of the general practitioner, and, while they are undoubtedly doing much good, it is questionable whether the arrangement is not also productive of much harm. The soundest, and, therefore, the safest, practitioner is, by all odds, the general practitioner, provided he is thoroughly educated, and fully up to his work.

THE CONTROVERSY OVER SPECIALIZATION

Pejorative comments aside, Gross's attitude represented the viewpoint of an older generation of American physicians. The Committee on Medical Ethics of the American Medical Association had issued a report in 1866 outlining the advantages versus the disadvantages of specialization in medicine. The committee considered the advantages to be minuteness of observation, acuteness in study, wideness of observation, skill in diagnosis, multiplicity of invention, and superior skill in manipulation, and the disadvantages to be narrowness of view, a tendency to magnify unduly the diseases covered by the specialty, a tendency to undervalue the treatment of special diseases by general practitioners, some temptation to employ undue measures for gaining a popular reputation, and a tendency to increased fees. The majority of committee members believed that the advantages far outweighed disadvantages from the point of view of the patient and of the advancement of American medicine and surgery as a profession. However, the committee's report stressed that these disadvantages could be overcome only if the specialist were to begin his career as a general physician-surgeon and slowly adopt his new specialty.

In reality, there were practical reasons why American physicians were so slow in separating surgery from general medical practice. Foremost was that before the 1880s, operative surgery was rarely performed. Despite the discovery of anesthesia in 1846, without a knowledge and acceptance of the nature of postoperative infection and methods for its prevention, the performance of surgical operations remained a risky business for both physician and patient. There really did not appear to be a need for American physicians to act as surgical specialists within the whole of medicine until surgery was considered a more valid therapeutic endeavor. Consequently, in the United States, the rise of surgery as both a scientific and well-regulated profession, whiich included an attendant cadre of specialists, would not begin in earnest until the late 1880s.

Of course, this is not to suggest that a select few eighteenth- and nineteenth-century American practitioners had not managed to develop local and regional reputations as surgeons. Contemporary written histories of American medicine are rife with the technical operative feats of such early "surgical" luminaries as John Collins

Warren, William Gibson, and Nathan Ryno Smith. Valentine Mott was said to be financially successful as a surgical practitioner; in the 1820s, he requested the then enormous sum of $239 from a lawyer for treatment of his son's fractured femur. Even Gross was impressed enough to write that at the time of Mott's death, his estate "was valued at nearly one million dollars, an immense sum for a professional man who was the architect of his own fortune, although it is indisputable that great surgeons make more money by their practice than great physicians."

Despite Gross's earlier protest over specialization, just six years later (1882), in his role as founder and president of the American Surgical Association, he did welcome twenty-four members to their second annual meeting by stating:

> We have in the United States according to a reasonable estimate, not fewer than sixty thousand medical men. Among these are large numbers of surgeons, who, in point of culture, practical skill, and reputation, as writers and teachers, would be an honor to any country, however high its standard of excellence.... The surgical profession was never so busy as it is at the present moment; never so fruitful in great and beneficent results, or in bold and daring exploits.

John Brooks Wheeler (1853–1942), Vermont's most prominent surgeon for over fifty years, described in his autobiography *Memoirs of a Small Town Surgeon* (1935) the dilemma of wanting to specialize in surgery at a time when such professional stratification did not exist:

> When I began to practice in Burlington (1881), I did not suppose...that it would be possible to make a living there by the exclusive practice of surgery...I did not realize the power of the 'boost' that 'Listerism' would give to the practice of surgery, but it is shown by the fact that now...nine men are practicing general or special surgery exclusively.

Wheeler's recollections were echoed by Arpad Gerster, an 1873 immigrant from Hungary and author of the country's first surgical text based on Listerian principles:

> Since 1877 great changes have taken place both in the personnel and the character of medical endeavor in New York. Specialists in the modern sense were then few.... With few exceptions, the men who practiced these specialties were more or less still in general practice, and though not a few called themselves surgeons, the venerable 'Jimmie' Wood was perhaps the only one who confined himself strictly to surgery. This he could well afford because of independent means. His office practice was enormous, for it was free to all. Willard Parker, Thomas Markoe, Robert Weir, Henry Sands, Frank Hamilton, Buck, Little, Detmold, Briddon, Lewis Stimson, and some others whom I do not recall, were all general practitioners at first, and surgeons only in an accessory way. Up to the eighties, or thereabouts, no one could have supported himself by the exclusive practice of surgery; there was not enough of it.

Although the physician-surgeon, vis-a-vis the family doctor, would remain an integral part of American health care delivery well into the 1960s, the groundwork for surgical specialization within American medicine was first evidenced a century before. In particular, the founding of national specialty societies, such as the American Ophthalmological Society (1864), the American Otological Society (1868), the American Gynecological Society (1876), the American Laryngological Association (1879), the American Surgical Association (1880), the American Association of Genito-Urinary Surgeons (1886), and the American Orthopedic Association (1887), presaged the emergence of the surgeon as a specialist.

It is now evident that American medicine could not become specialized until certain scientific and social conditions were present. First, a scientifically based and authoritative body of medical knowledge and clinical techniques had to be available within the given specialty. For instance, in surgery certain discoveries and clinical inventions with immediate practical applications needed to be conceived. The use of inhalation anesthesia in the late 1840s was of major consequence in allowing physicians to place less emphasis on operative speed and more on developing technical skill. The acceptance of listerism in the 1880s finalized the therapeutic revolution for surgeons by assuring that operative surgery would not likely end in a fatal septic episode. The development of the ophthalmoscope (1851) and the laryngoscope (1855) were examples of instrumentation needed by surgeons to increase the body of scientific knowledge within their field.

In addition to needing a medically valid body of knowledge, specialists were totally dependent on urban populations that were large enough to support their more narrowly focused practice goals. The surgeon had to have sufficient numbers of diverse surgical cases available to obtain adequate operative skills and to observe how postoperative patients fared. Such a situation existed only in major cities, and the sociological phenomenon of moving from a rural, agrarian-based society to an urban economy dominated by manufacturing did not occur in the United States until the 1880s.

Once urbanization took place, institutions could then be developed that provided a "patient gathering function" for the specialist. The rise of America's hospital system is one potent example of these late-nineteenth-century socioeconomic forces that helped promote clinical specialization. By the mid-1870s, many directors of urban hospitals recognized the growing importance of specialists by organizing outpatient dispensaries along specialty lines. For example, the managers of Boston City Hospital established an outpatient ophthalmic department in 1864 and similar divisions for skin (1868), ear (1869), neurological (1877), and throat (1879) conditions. As specialists became more prominent and their clinical practices flourished, they were naturally placed on ever greater numbers of hospital's boards of trustees. Such practitioners were then able to gain invaluable administrative experience while ultimately obtaining the necessary social and financial backing to establish their own specialty institutions.

By the late 1880s, specialty hospitals had become a fixture in urban America. They included such well-known clinics as the Boston Eye and Ear Infirmary, the Manhattan Eye and Ear Hospital, the New York Ophthalmic and Aural Institute, New York City's Hospital for the Relief of the Ruptured and Crippled, New York's Woman's Hospital, and Philadelphia's Will's Eye Hospital. Equally important as the establishment of specialty institutions were the decisions made by administrators of large city hospitals to assure that beds were available for newly created specialty wards.

One final condition had to be met before physicians could be induced to limit their clinical skills to a specialty. Specialization had to become financially rewarding. Many physicians in the mid-nineteenth century had already obtained specialty skills that they were applying to their general medical practice. However, it was a far different financial matter to narrow one's entire practice to a single specialty and refuse all unrelated cases. Economics, just as in modern medicine, would have to be the driving force behind any major alterations in the delivery of health care services. Accordingly, various institutions within the rapidly emerging profession of medicine had to undergo sometimes difficult transformations to assure the specialist's financial survival. It was certain that patients would go to the new breed of specialist only when general practitioners could no longer supply the sophisticated and effective therapies that knowledge of the specialties provided.

Specialists and specialties multiplied rapidly during the final decades of the century. At last, the physician who wished to specialize in surgery had available a growing body of valid scientific surgical knowledge, which led directly to a repertoire of acceptable manual techniques. In America, this scientific authority first became apparent with the introduction of surgical anesthesia, gathered momentum with the development of surgical pathology, and culminated in an understanding of bacteriology and antisepsis and asepsis.

THE GERM THEORY AND RESISTANCE TO IT

Unlike anesthesia and pathology, the acceptance in America of the germ theory of disease and its natural medical endpoints, antisepsis and asepsis, was a slow and often contentious process requiring almost two decades. The simple fact was that surgery could not evolve smoothly until the grave problem of postoperative infection was resolved. Infectious diseases such as fulminating gas gangrene, erysipelas,

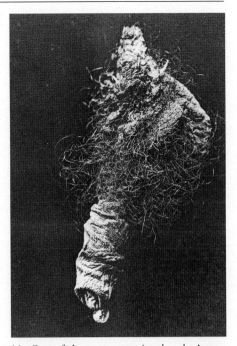

11. One of the most sensational early American surgical photographs from Charles Brigham's (1845–1903) 110-page *Surgical Cases with Illustrations* (1876). Brigham was professor of orthopedic and military surgery at the University of California in San Francisco. In his chapter on "A remarkable injury of the perinaeum, scrotum, and penis. - recovery," he describes the unfortunate circumstance of Emile B., a 17-year-old farm boy. The youngster was assisting at a threshing machine when his clothing was caught in the apparatus and his pants and skin from his genital region were torn away. The denuded raw surface of the body of the penis and testicles was subsequently covered with pedicle grafts and the transplantation of "eight bits of skin." The patient recovered and the pathologic specimen was preserved and sent to Brigham, who had this heliotype mechanical photograph made. (*Courtesy of Stanley B. Burns, M.D., and The Burns Collection and Collection*)

septicemia, and tetanus were of paramount concern in the health of any surgical patient. Without a clear understanding of bacteriology and the sources of surgical infection, however, most surgeons could do little more than provide high standards of generally ineffectual surgical cleanliness, adequate hemostasis, and open wound management.

Historically, most of the deadly postoperative diseases had been viewed as the result of some form of "contagion." For a millenium, it had been incorrectly believed that these various infections were generated spontaneously in wounds, or, alternatively, that air itself was the etiological agent in the formation of pus. The spurious notion that suppuration in a wound favored healing, expressed by the salutary cognomen "laudable pus," would plague surgeons until the pathogenic character of bacteria was completely understood and accepted.

In many respects, the recognition of antisepsis and asepsis was a more important event in the evolution of surgical history than the advent of inhalation anesthesia. There was no arguing that the deadening of pain permitted a surgical operation to be conducted in a more efficacious manner. Haste was no longer of prime concern. However, if anesthesia had never been conceived, a surgical operation could still have been performed, albeit with much difficulty. Such was not the case with listerism. Without antisepsis and asepsis, major surgical procedures more than likely ended in death rather than just pain. Clearly, surgery needed both anesthesia and antisepsis, but in terms of overall importance, antisepsis proved of greater singular impact.

In the long evolution of world surgery, the contributions of several individuals stand out as being preeminent. Joseph Lister (1827–1912), an English surgeon, can be placed on such an elite list because of his monumental efforts to introduce systematic, scientifically based antisepsis in the treatment of wounds and the performance of surgical operations. Lister pragmatically applied Louis Pasteur's (1822–1895) research into fermentation and microorganisms to the world of surgery by devising a means of preventing surgical infection and securing its adoption by a skeptical profession.

It was evident to Lister that Pasteur's method of destroying bacteria by excessive heat could not be applied to a surgical patient. Lister turned instead to chemical antisepsis and, after experimenting with zinc chloride and the sulfites, decided on carbolic acid. By 1865 he was instilling pure carbolic acid into wounds and onto dressings. Lister made numerous modifications in the technique of the dressings, the manner of applying and retaining them, and the choice of antiseptic solutions of varying concentrations. Although the carbolic acid spray remains the best remembered of his many contributions, it was eventually abandoned in favor of other germicidal substances. Lister not only used carbolic acid in the wound and on dressings but also went so far as to spray it in the atmosphere around the operative field and table. He did not emphasize hand scrubbing but merely dipped his fingers into a solution of phenol and corrosive sublimate. Lister was incorrectly convinced that scrubbing created crevices in the palms of the hands where bacteria would proliferate.

A second important advance by Lister was the development of sterile absorbable sutures. He believed that much of the deep suppuration found in wounds was created by previously contaminated silk ligatures. Lister evolved a carbolized catgut suture (1869), which was better than any previously produced. He was able to cut short the ends of the ligature, thereby closing the wound tightly and eliminating the necessity of bringing the ends of the suture out through the wound.

As early as 1869, various American surgeons who had visited with Lister in Glasgow brought back materials and directions on how to implement antiseptic surgery. Their reception was far from overwhelming. John Collins Warren was told by the likes of Henry J. Bigelow and Richard Hodges at the Massachusetts General Hospital that the "carbolic acid treatment" had already been tried and permanently discarded. Faneuil Weisse (1842–1915), of New York City, worked with Lister in the summer of 1868. In March of the following year, Weisse addressed the New York County Medical Society on "Lister's antiseptic treatment in surgery." The young surgeon was met with immediate and vociferous opposition by several prominent medical personalities in the audience, including Edward R. Squibb (1819–1900) and Abraham Jacobi (1830–1919).

Much has been written about the reasons why Americans delayed adopting the principles of antiseptic surgery. Discussing the situation in 1877, Robert Weir (1838–1927), a respected New York City surgeon, analyzed his colleagues' reluctance. First, the many procedural changes Lister had made during the evolution of his methodology "created confusion." Second, listerism as a technical exercise was "too complicated." Third, various early attempts to use antisepsis in surgery—for example, those at the Massachusetts General Hospital—had proved "utter failures." Finally, and most important, the acceptance of listerism depended entirely on an understanding and ultimate recognition of the veracity of the germ theory—a hypothesis that practical-minded Americans were loathe to accept.

Other problems aggravated these difficulties and caused even further reluctance to adopt Lister's system. "Hospitalism," a term coined in England and popularized by John Erichsen, described the high incidence of surgical infection caused by cross-seeding from one patient to another in the large open charitable wards that characterized European hospitals. In America, the urban hospital system was just being developed, and hospitalism was not recognized as a serious problem. As late as 1884, according to Hunter McGuire, it was considered unnecessary to use Lister's system because of "the pure country air in Virginia being in itself aseptic." In a naive sort of way, McGuire was absolutely correct. Hospitals in America experienced their epidemics, but in general, the country's hospitals were smaller and less crowded than their European counterparts. The United States was a physically immense country, and a greater percentage of surgery was conducted by rural-based practitioners than in Europe, where most patients needing surgery went to the specialist surgeons of the cities. American physicians believed that hospitalism was of greater concern in Europe than in America and that antiseptic methods were consequently less necessary here. Because they did not view cleanliness in the context of the germ theory, the more conservative American surgeons remained unconvinced of antiseptic principles. It was easier for them to regard Lister's techniques as an obsessive ritual than as part of the burgeoning science of surgery.

There was little disputing the diverse opinions of American surgeons. In 1871, John Ashhurst, surgeon at the Episcopal Hospital in Philadelphia, noted in his textbook, *The Principles and Practice of Surgery*:

> Under the name of the "antiseptic method," Prof. Lister, of Edinburgh, has urged the employment of carbolic or phenic acid as a dressing in surgical cases, and the practice has, both in his hands and those of others, certainly met with a large measure of success. At the same time, other surgeons equally competent and careful, and who have endeavored conscientiously to carry out Prof. Lister's instructions, have utterly failed in obtaining the promised results, so that the merits of the antiseptic plan must as yet be considered as undetermined. The theory of the method is founded on the observations of Pasteur, and supposes that animal decomposition is due to the presence of organic germs floating in the atmosphere, and carbolic acid is used on account of its known destructive effects upon low forms of organic life.

Five years later, Gross caustically commented:

> Little, if any faith, is placed by any enlightened or experienced surgeon on this side of the Atlantic in the so-called carbolic acid treatment of Professor Lister, apart from the care which is taken in applying the dressing, or, what is the same thing, in clearing away clots and excluding air from the wound...

Certain events are seminal. Such was the visit of Lister to the International Medical Congress held in conjunction with the Centennial Exhibition in Philadelphia in 1876. His speech on antisepsis, to a gathering of hundreds of distinguished physicians from all over the world presided over by the section chairman Samuel Gross, was a milestone in the slow process of acceptance by American physicians. Lister was evangelical in his appeal, and his enthusiasm was evident when his talk went far beyond its allotted time of three hours. Undoubtedly, some in the audience of over five hundred persons were convinced, particularly the younger surgeons. Still, ambivalence ruled the day, and neither Lister's visit nor any other single event can be pointed to as having greater influence than any other.

Lister's trip to the United States did not end in Philadelphia. He and his entourage traveled west through the Rockies to Salt Lake City and beyond to San Francisco, ending in New York City after Lister had lectured in Chicago and Boston. In the latter city, at Harvard Medical School, Lister spoke to a group of Henry Bigelow's students and is said to have convinced them of the appropriateness of antisepsis.

The literature on surgical infections and the debates over the pros and cons of listerism grew markedly during the late 1870s. Still, because only a few surgeons followed Lister's exact ritual, it remains difficult even with historical hindsight to estimate how widely antiseptic surgery was in general use throughout the country. Such impediments to historical research are manifested in Gross's further comments concerning Lister. In the preface to the sixth and final edition of his surgical textbook, Gross writes:

> To Professor Lister must be accorded not a little praise for the part he has played in this wonderful work.... It was he who first taught surgeons the importance and value of thorough cleanliness in their operations and dressings, before his time so little understood.

Yet, in the very same book, in the chapter on wounds and contusions, Gross provides an antithetical message:

> I have never found any appreciable benefit in such a case from the use of antiseptic dressings, although they are regarded by many surgeons as most valuable accessories.

The rationale for Gross's conservatism in this matter is evidenced throughout his textbook. Gross only grudgingly accepted the very foundation of Lister's thoughts: the germ theory. He halfheartedly agreed that Pasteur and Lister had established the existence of microorganisms in the atmosphere, but he rejoined, "the demonstration of living, disease-producing germs is wanting." Perhaps Gross's true feelings about Lister can be found in the former's *Autobiography*. Describing the 1876 International Medical Congress, Gross barely mentions the presence of Lister other than to remark that at the public dinner of the Congress, "I occupied the chair, with Professor Lister...on my right." In his only other utterance about Lister, Gross relates that in 1879 he visited England and, at a dinner given by the British Medical Association, was seated directly opposite "Mr. Lister, the famous reformer of the surgical treatment of wounds and other injuries." So much for Lister in the mind of Gross!

The 1880s saw an increasing acceptance of the germ theory in America. Along with this growing appreciation of the pathogenicity of microorganisms came the introduction of crude aseptic techniques into many of the country's operating rooms. Lewis Pilcher (1845–1934), the first editor of the *Annals of Surgery*, wrote a monograph, *The Treatment of Wounds* (1883), which demonstrated the appreciation for Lister felt by the younger generation of American surgeons. Pilcher's text included three lengthy chapters based largely on the research of Lister and others: "The relations of micro-organisms to wound-disturbances", "Asepsis and antisepsis - wound-cleanliness", and "Wound-disinfection - antiseptics." In that same year, a young Chicago surgeon, Henry Gradle (1855–1911), authored *Bacteria and the Germ Theory of Disease*, a work credited with being the first book in the English language on the topic of the germ theory. This 219-page treatise, consisting of eight lectures delivered at the Chicago Medical College, is quite remarkable because it convincingly shows that a tremendous body of bacteriological knowledge had entered mainstream American medical education. Although it is not primarily a surgical text, Gradle discusses surgical bacteriology, including Lister's work and even Robert Koch's (1843–1910) contributions to microbiology.

Despite appearances, there still remained an underlying suspicion of listerism at the highest levels of American surgery. At the Cincinnati meeting of the American Surgical Association in 1883, Beriah Watson (1836–1892), a respected surgical researcher from Jersey City, New Jersey, commented favorably on his results after applying Lister's techniques. Conservative surgeons in the audience were aghast and immediately took Watson to task. What was said that day is worth quoting from the meeting's official transcripts because it portrays the state of emotion that still blocked American acceptance of antisepsis sixteen years after Lister's first publication on the subject. John Packard opened the verbal assault by telling Watson that on "behalf of the surgeons of Philadelphia, I feel warranted in saying that it has not in their hands yielded such results as to induce them to adhere to it." Alfred Post (1805–1885) followed: "the surgeons of New York [City]; I do not think that any of them now use the method." Albert Vanderveer (1841–1929) of Albany, New York, chimed in: "I can say the same with regard to the surgeons of Albany and vicinity...I desire also to call attention...with regard to the value of carbolic acid...that it occupies one of the lowest positions in the list of antiseptic agents.... It is the thorough drainage that is the important factor in the treatment of wounds." From the South, Tobias Richardson (1827–1892) of New Orleans and Claudius Mastin (1826–1898) of Mobile unanimously declared that "not a surgeon" in Louisiana or Alabama "uses the Lister method." Theodore McGraw (1839–1921) of Detroit was even more venomous in his denunciation: "I had the misfortune some time ago to lose a patient from following out the Lister system; a loss which I ascribed to the poisonous effect of the carbolic acid." The attack was completed when Henry Campbell showed his general ignorance and basic indifference to scientific research by stating, "I believe that the action of the carbolic acid spray has the effect of retarding the suppuration...but I do not think that it is due to the influence of carbolic acid upon germs. I think that it arises from its effect on the reflex relations between the blood-vessels and the sensitive nerves."

To Watson's and Lister's defense came the likes of David Prince (1816–1889) of Illinois, who said, "If Listerism means the detail of the dressing of wounds, doubtless it is short-lived, but if Listerism means the principles which are involved in antisepsis, Listerism is immortal." Charles Nancrede (1847–1921) of Philadelphia added: "I have seen indisputable proof of the superiority of Listerism...I think that Dr. Packard is under some misapprehension when stating that no one in Philadelphia believed in the principles or adhered to the methods of Lister. Besides myself, there are a number of surgeons who...are Listerians." Watson concluded the stormy session:

> It seems to me that the gentlemen have mistaken entirely the tenor of my paper, as they do everything that relates to Listerism.... Although carbolic acid may be condemned, yet the system which was introduced by him must be saved...I know that Listerism in America has made but little progress; but, nevertheless, the present system of surgical practice has been modified to a very great extent by the introduction of the Lister treatment, and we find scarcely a wound treated in the United States to-day but what some part of Listerism is adopted.

THE ASSASSINATION OF PRESIDENT GARFIELD

Insinuating itself into the middle of this national medical debate on antisepsis came one of the most frightening and tragic events in the history of our country, the assassination of President James Garfield (1831–1881). Garfield was a man well suited for the presidency. He had served his country well as a teacher; successful lawyer; and notable military leader, having achieved the rank of major-general in the Union

Army; United States Congressman; and Senator, and as the Republican presidential victor in 1880. Garfield's abbreviated presidency was marred at the outset by intra-party squabbles over patronage. On the day that he was shot (July 2, 1881), Garfield was leaving Washington to deliver the commencement address at Williams College, his alma mater, in Williamstown, Massachusetts. Walking through the Baltimore and Potomac Railroad depot in Washington, Garfield was approached by Charles Guiteau (1841–1882), a disgruntled amd mentally disturbed lawyer, who had worked for the Republican victory and then been denied a political appointment under the spoils system. Approaching from behind, Guiteau fired twice with his handgun, an English .44 caliber centerfire Bulldog revolver. One shot missed, and the second struck the president in the mid-back, immediately causing his collapse. Shortly thereafter, a physician-surgeon from the District of Columbia Health Department arrived at the scene. D. W. Bliss (1825–1889), whose initials actually stood for Doctor Williard, was a prominent Washington surgeon and was the first of many to probe the wound with his unwashed fingers.

Bliss's private practice and personal life were about to be dramatically changed when he found the president lying on a mattress near the scene of the shooting.

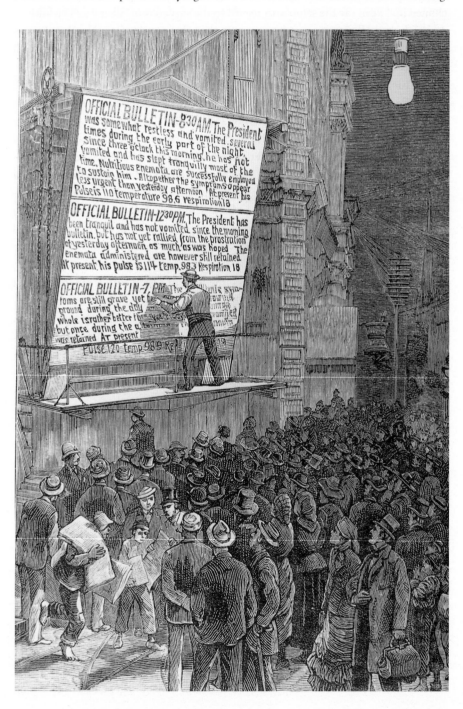

12. Crowds gathered on a daily basis outside the offices of the *New York Herald* to receive the latest information on President Garfield's medical condition. (*Collection of the Library of Congress*)

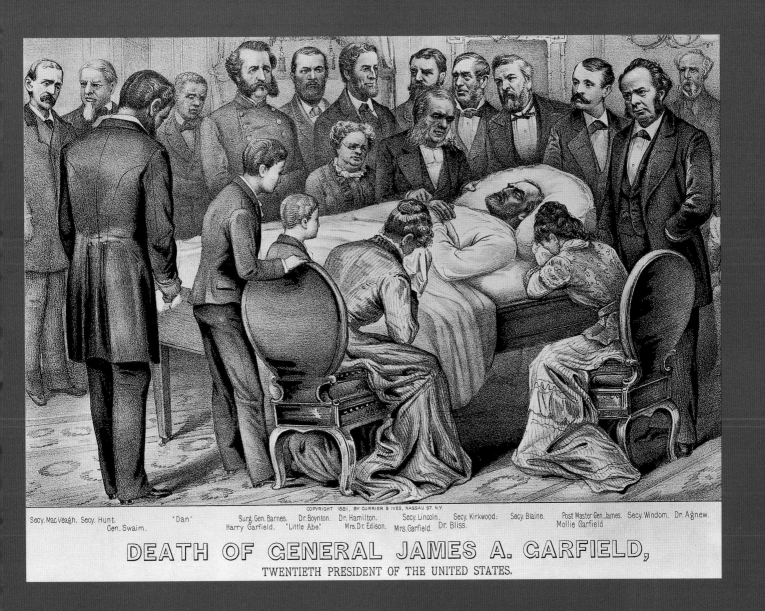

COPYRIGHT 1881, BY CURRIER & IVES, NASSAU ST. N.Y.

| Secy. Mac Veagh. | Secy. Hunt. | | "Dan" | | Surg. Gen. Barnes. | Dr. Boynton. | Dr. Hamilton. | | Secy. Lincoln. | Secy. Kirkwood: | Secy. Blaine. | | Post Master Gen. James. | Secy. Windom. | Dr. Agnew. |
| Gen. Swaim. | | | Harry Garfield. | "Little Abe." | | Mrs. Dr. Edison. | | Mrs. Garfield. | Dr. Bliss. | | | | Mollie Garfield | |

DEATH OF GENERAL JAMES A. GARFIELD,

TWENTIETH PRESIDENT OF THE UNITED STATES.

Garfield's lingering illness and his death two and a half months later in Elberon, New Jersey, occasioned a massive outpouring of surgical opinion, acrimonious debate, and unrelenting criticism, all pertaining to the care the president received. At a time when surgery in America was taking its first tentative steps towards professionalization and specialization, the events and discussions surrounding the assassination forced the medical profession to take a genuinely introspective look at surgery as it was then being practiced.

Bliss remained at Garfield's side until the latter's death on September 19th. In response to mounting controversy, Bliss was ultimately forced to author a lengthy explanation of his actions in a prominent periodical, *The Medical Record* (1881). When Bliss first encountered the president, he noted a feeble but rapid pulse and "ingesta lying upon the mattress" indicating that he had recently vomited and "large beads of perspiration stood upon his face, forehead, hands, and forearms." The president was in evident circulatory collapse. Bliss decided to manually explore "the wound to ascertain in the course of the ball the organs involved in its passage." Using a ceramic-tipped Nélaton probe, so it would be marked if it came in contact with a lead bullet, Bliss "was unable to detect any foreign substance beyond the rib to indicate the presence of fragments of bone or the missile." Concerned with the

13. The death of Garfield as portrayed in a Currier & Ives lithograph (circa 1881). The fictitious bedside gathering is significant from a surgical standpoint, in that surgeons Frank H. Hamilton, Doctor W. Bliss, and D. Hayes Agnew are included in the scene. (*Collection of the Library of Congress*)

14. Doctor W. Bliss wrote an extensive report on the case of President Garfield (*Medical Record*, vol. 20, pages 393–402, 1881). Included in his account were engravings of the actual specimens obtained at autopsy. Vigorously defending his treatment of the president, Bliss showed that the immediate cause of death had been rupture of a traumatic, and presumably septic, splenic artery aneurysm. (*Historical Collections, College of Physicians of Philadelphia*)

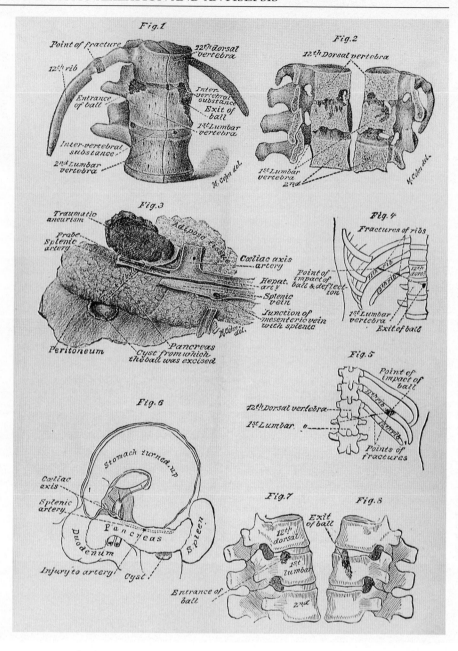

worsening condition of his patient, Bliss proceeded to do what most well-intentioned American surgeons of this era would have done: "I passed the little finger of my left hand to its full extent into the wound."

With these physical acts, Bliss began a chain reaction of contaminated events that culminated in Garfield's torturous demise. The morning after the shooting, ten physicians were summoned to the White House, most of whom further contaminated the wound by passing their fingers into the ragged opening. Over the course of weeks, some of the country's most prominent surgeons, including Philip Wales (1837–1906), Robert Reyburn (1833–1909), David Hayes Agnew (1818–1892), and Frank Hamilton (1813–1886), would be further consulted, all adding to the contamination. Three weeks after being shot, and with little evidence that he was improving, Garfield underwent an incision and drainage of a "pus-sac" in his back. The president did not improve as much as the physicians had hoped for, and they remained unable to locate the bullet. Alexander Graham Bell (1847–1922) was called upon to use "an induction device that he had constructed" for the purpose of locating metallic objects deep within the body. Unsuccessful in his efforts, Bell was forced to admit defeat and desisted in further efforts to find the bullet. On August 8th, with ether anesthesia in use, "another incision was made into the president's flank." This uncovered a "long sinus tract that extended from the first incision, deep under the muscles of the right flank, and into the pelvis."

By this juncture, it was obvious to all that Garfield was not going to improve. Not only that, but it was becoming increasingly difficult to care for him in the heat of a Washington summer. In fact, an air conditioning unit, possibly the first ever made, was built in the Executive Mansion. Created from an ice-cooled chamber with electrically driven fans, it was capable of cooling air at 99° F down to 54° F. On August 18th, Garfield experienced a "tumefaction of the right parotid gland," which soon led to facial paralysis, vomiting, mental disturbance, and jactitation. By the end of August, the president had lost over eighty pounds and suffered from massive sacral bedsores. His physicians discussed the possibility of moving him to the New Jersey shore in the hope that the sea air would improve his condition. A special section of railroad track was built from the main line in New Jersey to the coastal resort of Elberon. On September 6th, the President was transferred without any untoward events. In fact, it was believed that there was even some improvement in his condition, and the number of attending physicians was reduced.

Eleven days later, a "severe rigor occurred of half an hours duration, followed by a sharp rise in temperature." The president had a pulse of 120, a temperature of 102° F, and respirations of 24. As Bliss later wrote, this "chill was accompanied by severe pain over the anterior mediastinum, and the President said to me that it was similar to what he understood as angina pectoris." At 10:10 in the evening, Bliss was summoned hastily back to the president's bedside and found him in an "unconscious and dying condition, pulseless at the wrist…and respiration…gasping." Twenty-five minutes later, Bliss noted that "the brave and heroic sufferer, the nation's patient, for whom all had labored so cheerfully and unceasingly, had passed away." The detailed autopsy report that accompanied Bliss's article showed the immediate cause of death to have been rupture of a traumatic and presumably septic aneurysm of the splenic artery.

Engulfed in controversy, Garfield's death must have been a blessed relief for the overworked Bliss. Under the watchful but critical eye of a nation, Bliss had been in constant attendance, day and night, on a patient in chronic sepsis, without any means at his disposal to alter the seemingly preordained course of events. When Bliss was called upon by Congress to present a bill for services, claims were submitted for almost $25,000, a great deal of money for that day. How reasonable it was in view of all the time rendered remains impossible to evaluate. However, Bliss was awarded just $6,500 by the Congressional comptroller. Outraged by this action, Bliss refused his apportioned share, claiming with some justification that his private practice had been ruined and his health seriously impaired by "the close attention to the President that the exigencies of the case demanded." At the time of Bliss's death, a special bill was pending in Congress to compensate him for his services in this extraordinary case.

At once a maelstrom of indignant questioning swept the nation. The drama of the assassination, the stature of the patient, and the lingering course of illness ending in a torturous death all gave rise to endless arguments about President Garfield's care. Every newspaper had carried daily press briefings as well as speculation on the president's condition and the medical attention he was receiving. In the end, it was the rare surgeon who did not express an opinion, suggestion, or criticism. In America, J. Marion Sims and William Hammond were among the most prominent critics of the surgical treatment afforded to Garfield. In a set of papers written for the *North American Review*, Sims and Hammond were scathing in their denunciation of the failure of Garfield's surgeons to perform an exploratory laparotomy following the shooting.

Surgeons in Europe watched the drama unfold with similar interest. Among them, Johann Friedrich von Esmarch (1823–1908), the renowned German military surgeon, provided a blistering attack against the Americans for not utilizing antisep-

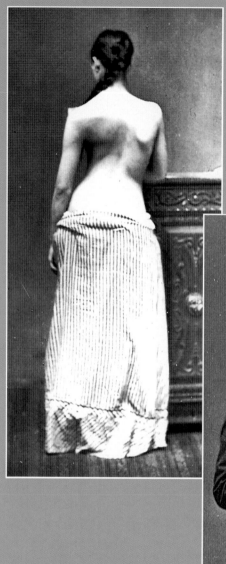

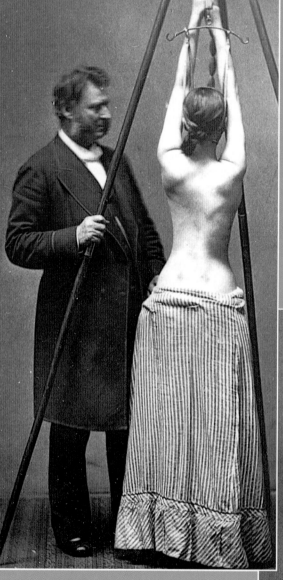

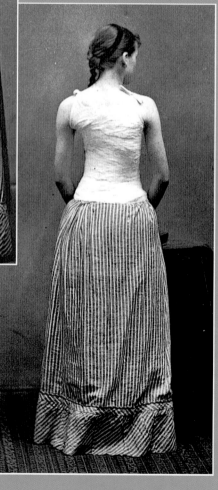

tic methods in caring for the wounded president. Esmarch argued with particular authority that the "physicians were under the pressure of the public opinion that they were doing far too little. But according to my opinion they have not done too little but far too much." Esmarch went on to state that if the physicians had "entirely omitted the search after the bullet, and immediately after the injury dressed the wound in a real antiseptic way, the President might perhaps be still alive."

THE SLOW ACCEPTANCE OF ANTISEPTIC SURGERY

It is not surprising that Esmarch was so critical of his transatlantic colleagues. German-speaking surgeons had grasped the importance of bacteriology and the germ theory some ten years before their American colleagues. Consequently, they were among the first to expand on Lister's message of antisepsis. Led by Ernst von Bergmann (1836–1907) and Curt Schimmelbusch (1860–1895), German surgeons began to develop newer "aseptic methods." Lister's spray was discarded in favor of boiling and the autoclave. The availability of heat sterilization engendered sterile drapes, aprons, sutures, and instruments. By the end of the 1880s, the less clumsy aseptic techniques were finding their way into American surgical amphitheaters.

Following the Garfield affair, textbooks began to hesitatingly trumpet the new techniques of antiseptic surgery. Robert Morris (1857–1945), of New York City, wrote *How We Treat Wounds Today; A Treatise on the Subject of Antiseptic Surgery Which Can Be Understood by Beginners* (1886). Although little known, this work was the first of a fresh onslaught of texts by surgeons on the value of antisepsis. Controversial because of what others described as a supercilious attitude and sarcastic writing style, Morris nevertheless understood the importance of surgeons as specialists, especially within the context of antiseptic surgery. One reviewer in the *Medical Bulletin* stated:

> The author of this bombastic book is fully imbued with his own importance and the importance of dressing wounds according to his method or the method of his friends. He announces "that the time has come when it is best for the general practitioner to have as little as possible to do with surgery." In our opinion the time has come when the general practitioner should have as little as possible to do with all such egotistical specialists, or would-be specialists.

Having obviously struck a raw nerve in the approaching economic battles between surgeon as specialist and general physician-surgeon, Morris's book was well received and went through three more editions. However, it was up to a Hungarian immigrant living in New York City, Arpad Gerster, to write the most important American publication pertaining to the new techniques of surgery. Gerster's 322-page *The Rules of Aseptic and Antiseptic Surgery* (1888) was the first systematic American surgical text based on listerian principles. Since an illustrated manual was needed to show surgeons how to go about performing "clean" surgery, Gerster's work proved immensely popular. It passed through two more editions within three years, selling almost 12,000 copies and finding its way, as one reviewer noted, "into every town, village, and hamlet in our broad land." However, what made the monograph truly outstanding was not only its content but also the efforts that were expended in its production. It was printed on heavy calendered paper with many halftone illustrations, which were then rare in scientific books. Gerster had mastered the technique of photography and made his own plates, using the slow film of that day, at a time when photography by an amateur was highly unusual. For the first time, a surgeon took numerous pictures of actual operations and surgical dressings, often including himself in the scenes.

In the last year of the decade of the 1880s, the first American textbook devoted solely to bacteriology made its appearance. Authored by Nicholas Senn, who borrowed heavily from German sources, *Surgical Bacteriology* (1889) provided a very thorough and exhaustive review of the current literature on bacteriology as it related to surgery. The volume was indispensible to the surgeon, but its chief value was its compilation, which made it possible for the busy practitioner to become conver-

15. *(facing page)* Among the first albumen photographic prints used to illustrate an American surgical text, this series of images appeared in Lewis Sayre's *Spinal Disease and Spinal Curvature, Their Treatment by Suspension and the Use of the Plaster of Paris Bandage* (1877). It shows the case of Jessie Brown, a 20-year-old woman, who had "an ordinary case of lateral curvature." Sayre demonstrates treatment by suspension and fitting with a "plaster of paris bandage." There is a subtle degree of eroticism in the way the young female patient is posed prior to her "suspension." Sayre relates that she had an increase in height of "one inch and one eighth, by accurate measurement." This book is a landmark in American medical photography, since it was among the earliest texts to contain actual mounted photographs. The illustrations are remarkable for their artistic qualities and were taken in both New York City and London. The photographer at Bellevue Hospital and at the New York Academy of Medicine sessions was O. G. Mason, who later became one of the most noted medical photographers of his time. In London, where this series was taken, many of the pictures were completed by J. R. Mayall, a transplanted Philadelphian, at Guy's, University, and Royal Orthopaedic Hospitals. *(Courtesy of Stanley B. Burns, M.D., and the Burns Collection and Archive)*

sant with the most advanced ideas of surgical pathology and bacteriology. Strangely, even with the excellent discussions of surgical wound infections, Senn mentioned Pasteur but once and Lister not at all! Still, the fact that American surgery was undergoing a complete and seemingly rapid transformation relative to antisepsis and asepsis is echoed in Senn's words:

> Within a few years bacteriology has revolutionized surgical pathology. All wound complications and most of the acute and chronic inflammatory lesions which come under the treatment of the surgeon are caused by microorganisms; hence the necessity of a proper recognition of the importance of bacteriology as an integral part of the science and practice of modern surgery.

By 1890, the interactions of socioeconomic, political, scientific, and technical factors set the stage for what would become a spectacular showcasing of surgery's new-found prestige and accomplishments. Surgeons were finally wearing aseptic-looking white coats. Patients and tables were draped in white, and basins for bathing instruments in bichloride solution abounded. Gowns, masks, and gloves were still not in the picture, but at least all was clean and tidy. John Wheeler wrote of doing antiseptic surgery in the countryside, more specifically in the very homes of his rural patients. Surgery was no longer a haphazard affair. For somebody like Wheeler, antisepsis "is nothing more nor less than surgical cleanliness - cleanliness of operator, assistants, patient, instruments and dressings. By surgical cleanliness is meant the complete absence of what we commonly understand by dirt, and, moreover, the complete absence of the germs whose development produces suppuration and the various diseases which may result from wound infection."

It was obvious to the medical and lay community at large that a new era in American surgery had arrived. Surgeons began to operate on the head, chest, and abdomen for the first time without fear that their patient would succumb to poorly understood infectious diseases. Concurrently, the increasing demand for surgery induced many urban general practitioners, who were honing their basic surgical skills obtained during the Civil War, to become full-time specialists in surgery. In rural America, the turn toward specialization in surgery would not occur until well into the twentieth century. Without large urban population centers, the rural physician was obliged to remain both general practitioner and surgeon.

16. Arpad Gerster was one of America's earliest amateur surgeon photographers. He took negatives for his classic text, *The Rules of Aseptic and Antiseptic Surgery* (1888), and had William Kurtz of New York City reproduce them using a halftone phototypographic process. This photograph shows Gerster (*on the left*) performing a change of dressing after amputation of the thigh. (*Author's Collection*)

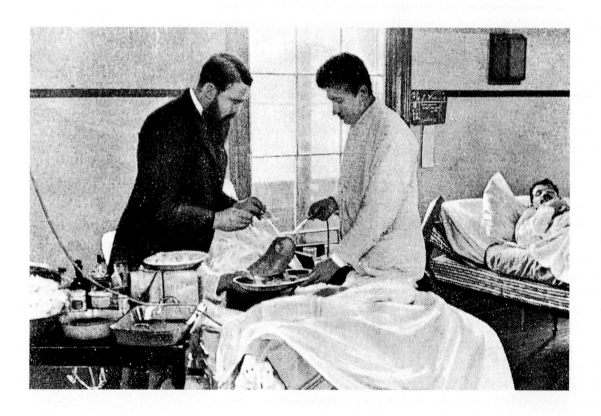

PROFESSIONAL ASSOCIATIONS AND PUBLICATIONS

Medicine was now approaching the point in American culture where it could be considered to have achieved the status of a profession, as defined in *Webster's Third New Unabridged Dictionary*:

> A calling requiring specialized knowledge and often long and intensive preparation including instruction in skills and methods as well as in the scientific, historical, or scholarly principles underlying such skills and methods, maintaining by force or organization or concerted opinion high standards of achievement and conduct, and committing its members to continued study and to a kind of work which has for its prime purpose the rendering of a public service.

According to this multidimensional definition, it becomes difficult for the historian to state with any precision the exact year when surgery in America could be considered a profession. Even if a profession is more simply thought of as "the ability to earn a livelihood through use of authoritative knowledge within a select set of institutions for the public good," it still remains a cumbersome undertaking. The reality is that so many disparate elements must be present for a profession to function properly that it develops over a long time, not in the course of a year. Although American medicine as a whole might have been regarded as a profession by the mid- to late 1880s, that was not the case with surgery. Surgery still needed several organizational elements to be operational before the terms "professional" and "specialist" could be accurately applied to the surgeon.

Members of any profession must demonstrate some inherent or instinctive fraternal propensity to organize themselves. Professional societies provide their members with two valuable and commercially desirable commodities: prestige and a degree of self-control. American physicians had accomplished a good deal of this task with the founding of the American Medical Association; the flourishing of state, county, and city medical societies; the establishment of licensure and discipline, and the strength of the periodical and textbook literature. Although surgeons had begun to open this pathway during the 1880s, much remained to be achieved, including the formation of a relatively exclusive, but not elitist, national fraternal organization (the American College of Surgeons) and the proper education and regulation of the members (residency training and various boards of surgery).

In 1878, the Brooklyn Anatomical and Surgical Club was founded, with Lewis Pilcher serving as President and George Fowler as secretary. This oldest surgical society in the United States had as its *raison d'être* "the promotion of the practical study of Anatomy and Surgery by the maintenance of proper rooms for the pursuit of such studies; by the formation of a museum; by the accumulation of a library; by lectures and demonstrations, and by stated meetings for the discussion of subjects pertaining to that special field." In forming such an organization, it was hoped that the boundary between the club's members (those wishing to specialize in surgery) and lay physicians would be better delineated. In article I, section 2 of the club's by-laws, it was explicitly stated that "candidates for membership must be physicians...and must accompany their application for membership by such written contribution to the knowledge of Anatomy, Surgery, or Pathology, as shall be deemed by the Council worthy of publication in the Transactions of the Society." By forming these exclusive societies, physicians were able to derive such benefits from mutual association as appointments to medical school faculties and hospitals, referrals and consultations with affluent patients, and political influence.

The Brooklyn club was soon defunct, but it was not long before Samuel Gross founded the Philadelphia Academy of Surgery (1879), which remains the oldest functioning surgical society in the United States. One year later, Gross originated the prestigious American Surgical Association. As he relates in his autobiography:

> I had myself long seen the necessity for two such associations, one of a local and the other of a national character.... The object of both these societies, as

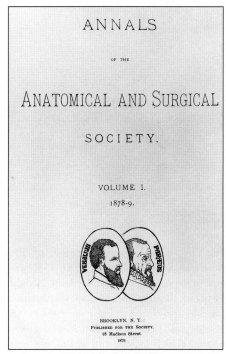

ANNALS

OF THE

ANATOMICAL AND SURGICAL

SOCIETY.

VOLUME I.
1878-9.

BROOKLYN, N. Y. :
PUBLISHED FOR THE SOCIETY.
28 Madison Street.
1879.

17. The title page from the annals of the oldest surgical society in the United States. The influence of Vesalius and Pare on the evolution of Western-oriented surgery is noted in their cameo engravings. *(Author's Collection)*

expressed in their respective constitutions, prepared by myself…is the cultivation and improvement of the art and science of Surgery, and the promotion of the interest, not only of their Fellows but of the Medical profession at large. Both societies…if judiciously conducted, cannot fail to contribute materially to the advancement and dignity of Surgical Science in the United States, which has already produced so many able and distinguished surgeons.

The need for camaraderie and social exchange is an important factor in the development of any profession, and until the founding of the American Surgical Association such fundamental attributes were not available to surgeons in this country. Yet, there was little disguising the fact that the American Surgical Association was intentionally designed to be an elite and exclusive surgical society. Membership was limited to one hundred individuals who "shall be at least thirty years of age, and…earned a reputation as a practitioner, author, teacher, or original observer." From a historical perspective, the importance of the American Surgical Association was that it represented the first attempt to bring together on a national level, admittedly in a small number, men of great professional stature whose names and deeds marked them as surgeons. The organization made certain that a record of its meetings were published in the form of bound transactions that could be easily disseminated.

Since separations between surgical specialities did not yet exist, the only criterion for membership was simply that a physician have a reputation as a surgeon: not an orthopedic surgeon, not a urologic surgeon, not a gynecologic surgeon, but simply, in 1880s America, a surgeon. Not surprisingly, the formation of the nation's first surgical organization was adamantly opposed by the American Medical Association on the grounds that the new society would detract from its Section on Surgery. When Gross welcomed the members to their second annual meeting in 1882, he commented:

If it be said that we are striking a blow at the American Medical Association, we deny the soft impeachment. On the contrary, we shall strengthen that body

18. The seventh annual session of the American Surgical Association in 1886 was held in the reading room of the Army Medical Museum (Ford's Theater, where Abraham Lincoln was assassinated in 1865) in Washington, D.C. Thirty-four members were registered as being present, and for the first time in the organization's short existence a photograph of the attendees was arranged by John Shaw Billings, chairman of the committee of arrangements. For unknown reasons, nine of the fellows (John Brinton, Samuel Weissell Gross, Christopher Johnston, Robert Kinloch, William Pancoast, John Roberts, Alan Smith, Stephen Smith, and Albert Vander Veer) were not available for the historic photograph. (*Historical Collections, College of Physicians of Philadelphia*)

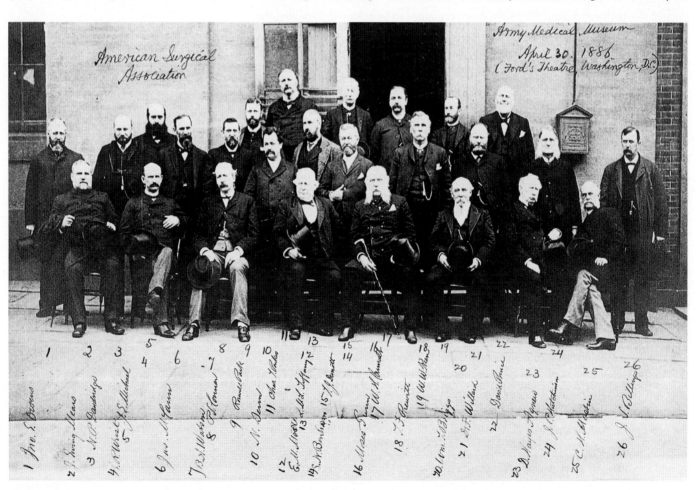

by rousing it from its Rip Van Winkle slumbers, and infusing new life into it. We can hurt no society now in existence, or likely to come into existence. We can hurt only ourselves, if we fail to do our duty…to…show the world that we are earnest and zealous laborers in the interest of human progress and human suffering.

The American Surgical Association held yearly meetings, and its membership list included all the important figures in American surgery. From every region of the nation, men gathered to better understand the great scientific surgical advances of the day. The discussions of the 1880s included an 1882 debate on bloodletting, the 1883 argument over listerism, an 1885 lecture on "operative surgery of the human brain" (the first time that this topic was ever discussed at a national level), a contentious examination in 1886 of "diagnostitial laparotomy," and, in 1889, an explanation by John Collins Warren of needle biopsy and frozen section—for which he was promptly rebuked by Frederic Dennis (1850–1934) of New York City. Dennis rose "to protest against the use of this instrument" for he had never been able to find a pathologist who would commit himself on the basis "of a few shreds of tissue."

The successful incorporation of scientific research and innovations into the clinical practice of surgery, along with critical discussions of pertinent socioeconomic and political movements is dependent on a periodical or journal to disseminate such information effectively. For American surgeons, this did not come about until the *Annals of Surgery* began publication in 1885. The *Annals* was the earliest important American medical periodical devoted solely to the practice of surgery, and the most influential and important of all periodicals for the specialist surgeon. By having their own surgical society and monthly journal, American surgeons were achieving some measure of the social and political organization that European surgeons had had for almost a century.

It can be noted, as a historical footnote, that the *Annals of Surgery* did have one American predecessor: the *Archives of Clinical Surgery*, found in 1877 by Edward Bermingham (1853–?) of New York City. Intended to be "a monthly periodical devoted to surgery in all its special departments," the *Archives* survived for only two volumes. One other American surgical journal of importance was founded in the 1880s: the *International Journal of Surgery and Antiseptics*, a quarterly publication beginning in 1888. Its editor was Milton Josiah Roberts (1850–1893), a New York City surgeon, who specialized in orthopedic surgery. This journal continued publication well into the twentieth century.

The *Annals of Surgery* became intimately involved with the advancement of the surgical sciences in the United States, and its pages record the history of American surgery during that time more accurately than any other written source. The first editor was Lewis Pilcher, who, while serving as president of the Brooklyn Anatomical and Surgical Society, arranged for the publication of its monthly meetings in the form of a journal under the name *Annals of the Anatomical and Surgical Society*. By the end of 1880, the Society had decided that as a corporation it should not be responsible for the expenses of such a publication, and the journal was taken over as a property by Pilcher and Fowler. They changed the name to the *Annals of Anatomy and Surgery* and it lasted so until the beginning of 1884. In May of that year, as Pilcher relates in his autobiography, *A Surgical Pilgrim's Progress* (1925), he was approached by a publisher from St. Louis who wished to discuss the "practicability of the founding in America of a strictly surgical journal, of a high class." In January 1885, the first issue of the *Annals* was published with Pilcher as editor-in-chief. Initially, Pilcher did not believe that such a national surgical journal would be very popular. At that early date, "the number of surgeons, as distinguished from general practitioners, was not very great, although their number was constantly increasing." Pilcher remained the editor of the *Annals* for over thirty years, during which time he developed a unique understanding of the journal and its role in the fostering of American surgery:

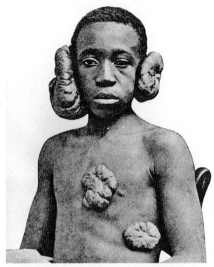

19. When Louis Tiffany authored a paper comparing "surgical diseases of the white and colored races" it included the first published photograph to appear in the *Transactions of the American Surgical Association* [vol. 5, pages 261–273, 1887]. The spectacular case of keloid in a young African-American child highlighted some of Tiffany's scientific findings, including his opinion that "surgical injuries and operations are better borne by negroes than whites." (*Historical Collections, College of Physicians of Philadelphia*)

The establishment of such a publication as the *Annals of Surgery* was the natural outcome of the new conditions in surgery that had begun to engage the attention of surgeons in the seventies and eighties of the nineteenth century. The whole field of surgery was undergoing revision; new avenues were constantly being opened; what was to be the end did not yet appear, but it was important that special media for the presentation and diffusion of knowledge as to the progress of events should be created.... When the first number of the *Annals of Surgery* was put in the mails in the last week of December, 1884, there was no other purely surgical journal printed in the English language. German surgery had for years been represented by able and important periodicals...France had only a short time before made a beginning to worthily chronicle the work of its surgeons.... Surely, surgery has come into its own...

Within a few years time, three great surgical societies of the United States, the American Surgical Association, the New York Surgical Society, and the Philadelphia Academy of Surgery, were using the *Annals of Surgery* as a vehicle for publishing the scientific proceedings of their respective organizations. In essence, the *Annals* served as the chronicler of this new national phenomenon, the surgeon as specialist.

As significant as periodicals were to the dissemination of scientific knowledge, American surgeons also began to communicate their surgical expertise to their medical colleagues and the lay public via lengthy treatises. Written by the likes of John Ashhurst, Frank Hamilton, David Hayes Agnew, Lewis Stimson, Stephen Smith, Joseph Bryant (1845–1914), William Van Buren, and John Wyeth (1845–1922), these individually authored works were massive in size and covered almost every conceivable surgical topic. In effect, American surgeons were saying to society that they finally had something to write about and were ready to stand behind their words.

Agnew's *Principles and Practice of Surgery* (1878–1883) was a three-volume "monument to his life-work." As explained by J. Howe Adams in his biography, *Life of D. Hayes Agnew* (1892), all 2,912 pages were written "with his own pen...doing it at odd times, such as working late into the night and getting up early in the morning, working before his early breakfast...it is a medical diary of his professional life for fifty-one years." The treatise was even translated into Japanese and published in Tokyo in 1888. At almost the same time, John Ashhurst was editing his-six volume *International Encyclopedia of Surgery* (1881–1886). This tome played an important role in American surgery because it introduced the concept of a multiauthored surgical textbook. Previously, surgical texts had been based on the cumulative experience of one individual. However, Ashhurst's *Encyclopedia* demonstrated that a

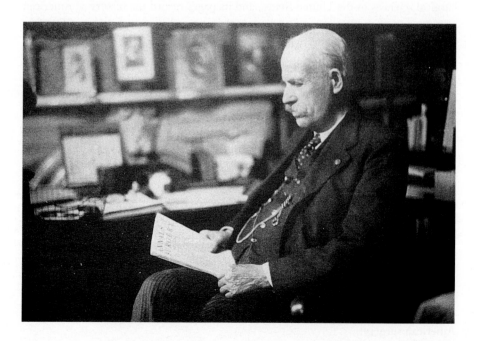

20. Although this photograph of Lewis Pilcher is from 1928, it shows the famous surgeon-author reading the *Annals of Surgery*, the country's first surgical journal, which he served as editor-in-chief for half a century (1885–1935). (*Courtesy of Stanley B. Burns, M.D., and The Burns Collection and Archive*)

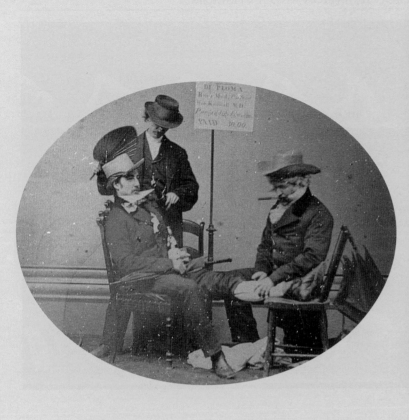 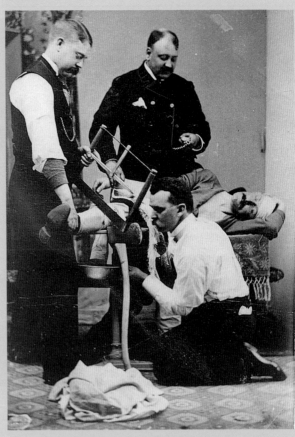

textbook written by many surgeons could be a publishing success. Not only did prominent American surgeons author various chapters, but foreign experts, including William Allingham (1829–1908), William Watson Cheyne (1852–1932), Christopher Heath (1835–1905), and Frederick Treves (1853–1923), added to the allure. So respected was Ashhurst as a result of this effort that he became recognized as the greatest authority in the world on surgical bibliography and, in 1888, was named John Rhea Barton professor of surgery at the University of Pennsylvania.

Appearing on the surgical literary scene for the first time in significant numbers were monographs on more narrowly focused surgical topics. Examples include Eugene Peugnet's (1836–1879) *The Nature of Gunshot Wounds of the Abdomen, and their Treatment* (1874); Homer Ostrom's (1852–?) *Treatise on the Breast and Its Surgical Diseases* (1877), the first surgical work written in the United States dedicated solely to breast disease; Samuel Weissell Gross' *A Practical Treatise on Tumors of the Mammary Glands…*(1880); John Butler's (1844–1885) *Electricity in Surgery* (1882), and Nicholas Senn's *Intestinal Surgery* (1889). The care of trauma victims received increasing attention by surgeons, as is demonstrated by Joseph Howe's (1843–1890) *Emergencies and How to Treat Them* (1871), Charles Dulles' (1850–1921) *What to do First in Accidents and Emergencies* (1883), James Gilchrist's (1842–1906) *Surgical Emergencies and Accidents* (1884), and George Fowler's *Syllabus of a Course of Lectures on First Aid to the Injured* (1887).

Of course, these texts were additional to monographs by surgeons performing what was already being euphemistically termed sub-specialty work (e.g., ophthalmology, gynecology, urology, orthopedics), for example, Henry Angell's (1829–1911) *Treatise on Diseases of the Eye* (1870), Jacob DaSilva Solis-Cohen's (1838–1927) *Diseases of the Throat* (1872), Gurdon Buck's *Contributions to Reparative*

21. As in prior eras, the surgical profession was the target of satirical barbs throughout the nineteenth century. Posed just for laughs are these leg "amputation" scenes. In one done at Rush Medical College (*left*) (circa late 1860s) the assistant fans the patient while holding a bottle of whiskey to his mouth, and the surgeon readies himself by clasping the amputating knife in his mouth. In a later photograph (*right*) (circa 1875) the surgical instrument is a giant hacksaw and the patient's leg rests on an axe. The "physician" looks at his watch and in so doing mocks the entire concept of speed by which some surgeons judged their technical competency. Such photographs were often sold commercially, and physicians sometimes posed for their own satirical purposes. (*Courtesy of Stanley B. Burns, M.D., and The Burns Collection and Archive*)

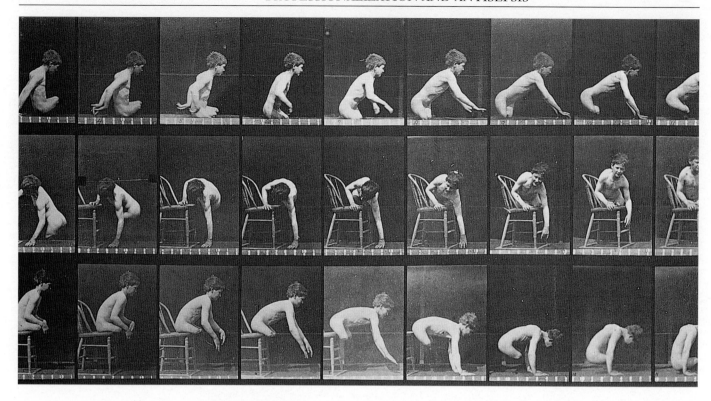

22. Physicians of the nineteenth century were fascinated by the movements of the human body. They studied crawling, walking, running, and other types of motion in order to improve artificial limbs for the tens of thousands of Civil War amputees. Edward Muybridge (1830–1904), an English-born photographer who emigrated to Philadelphia, became interested in capturing the mechanics of human motion and made use of individual cameras connected to trip wires. In 1887, he published *Animal Locomotion... Electro Photographic Investigations of Consecutive Phases of Animal Movements*, in which over 20,000 photographs in eleven volumes documented almost every detail of animal movement. But it was photographs of humans, particularly those of handicapped subjects, that proved invaluable to generations of physicians and surgeons. This photograph shows a boy with bilateral lower extremity amputations ambulating on his hands (circa 1887). *(Courtesy of Stanley B. Burns, M.D., and The Burns Collection and Archive)*

Surgery (1876), Charles Burnett's (1842–1902) *The Ear* (1877), Lewis Sayre's (1820–1900) *Lectures on Orthopedic Surgery and Diseases of the Joints* (1876), Edmund Peaslee's (1814–1878) *Ovarian Tumors*, John Gouley's (1838–1920) *Diseases of the Urinary Organs* (1873), and William Van Buren's *Lectures Upon Diseases of the Rectum* (1870).

As in any other surgical era, innovative surgical operations were also being performed. Among the most renowned were E. L. Marshall's first known successful extirpation of the entire thyroid gland (1867); John Bobbs's (1809–1870) case report, the first one published in the world, of cholecystotomy (1868); Frank Maury's (1840–1879) paper on gastrotomy for obstruction of the esophagus (1870); William Halsted's experimental research describing the importance of the submucosal layer in completing an intestinal anastomosis (1887); and Rudolph Matas's (1860–1957) report of the world's first known aneurysmorrhaphy (1888).

THE WILD WEST AND FRONTIER SURGERY

Of the many aspects of American life during the post-Civil War era, the Western frontier with its images of cowboys and Indians, cattle barons, and gunslingers remains one of the most exciting. The Western expansion produced many colorful figures, not the least of whom were the physician-surgeons who patched up scalped craniums, removed arrowheads, and cared for the victims of trauma suffered in a vast wilderness. Surgical skills were especially valued because the ruthless repression of Native Americans inevitably led to carnage. Typical of these traumatic injuries were penetrating injuries caused by arrows. Joseph Bill (1835–1885) was an assistant surgeon in the United States Army serving on the Arizona-New Mexico frontier when he authored the classic report "Notes on arrow wounds" in the *American Journal of the Medical Sciences* (1862). His sensationalized account of the brutal nature of frontier warfare, between Southwestern Indian tribes and the troops and settlers who were appropriating Indian lands, caused the paper to be read with more than passing interest. Warfare with the bow and arrow would soon be relegated to history, but for the young army surgeon, nothing in the medical textbooks prepared him for this type of specialized surgery. Bill was prescient in his understanding of what, unfortunately, was going to happen to the Native American:

"Sooner or later the government must undertake some great expedition against all the Indians of the plains. It may be possible to civilize Creeks, Choctaws, Cherokees, etc, but with a Cheyenne or Camanche or Apache the attempt will surely fail.... They are the professed exponents and great advocates of barbarism and universal ignorance."

Considering that an expert Indian bowman could discharge six accurate arrows per minute, arrow injuries were the bane of the cavalryman and settler in the 1870s. Bill realized the danger peculiar to all arrow wounds: the "shaft becoming detached from the head of an implanted arrow, leaves this so deeply embedded in a bone that it cannot be withdrawn, and that, remaining, it kills." According to Bill's statistics, of eighty cases reported, twenty-nine victims died. When the intestine was wounded, the mortality figure was a gruesome 100 percent. Bill's comments on how to conduct a surgical operation for extremity wounds, when an arrowhead was lodged in the bone, typifies a "wild west" attitude:

> It is not possible to lay down any fixed rules for such an operation. The incisions should be large and free-boldness rather than prudence governing our actions. We might as well cut the patient's limb up until we do find the arrow-head, for if it is left, amputation will be necessary, and worse than this can hardly ensue from the "cutting up" we have advised. We would, if we undertook such an operation, make up our mind to find the arrow-head, even if it were necessary to tear up every fasciculus of every muscle of the injured member. It is just in such cases as this that the motto, "Operative surgery is the art of cutting and tying what you cut," finds its best exemplification.

General George Armstrong Custer (1836–1876) and his aides, Major Marcus Reno and Captain Fred Benteen, led the approximately six hundred men of the Seventh Cavalry onto the banks of the Little Big Horn River in Montana in June 1876. This expeditionary force was accompanied by three army surgeons. George Lord (1846–1876) and James DeWolf (1843–1876), along with over two hundred men, would not survive the Battle of the Little Big Horn. Henry Porter (1848–1903) was left by himself to attend to all the surgical needs of the survivors of that military disaster. In writing home to his parents, Porter described the hellish conditions under which he performed his surgical duties while trapped on a hilltop with Reno and Benteen surrounded by Indians:

> The Indians keeping up a constant fire and picking off our men at a fearful rate. We were thus surrounded and our little squad of men being killed and wounded by twenty times their number of Indians...expecting every moment to be murdered and, perhaps, tortured and burned...you will imagine how thankful we felt when we saw them running on the evening of the second day and what a shout went up when we heard that Gen. Terry was within a few miles.... I established a hospital in the center of the mules and horses, where

23. Joseph Bill's forcep for the extraction of arrowheads as it appeared in the *Medical Record* (vol. 11, page 245, 1876). (*Historical Collections, College of Physicians of Philadelphia*)

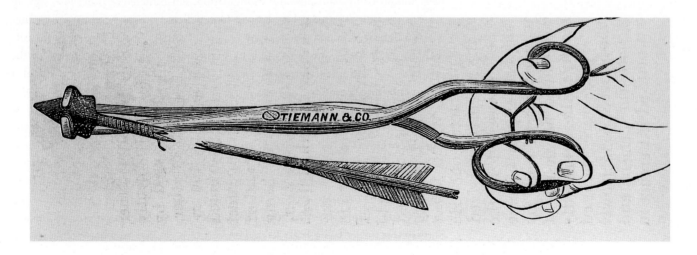

the wounded were brought faster than I could attend them. Men and animals were killed and wounded all around me, and the horses fell over on my wounded men…. My wounded were suffering terribly for water - they needed it for their wounds as well as their thirst. Some soldiers were ordered to get water, but some were killed and others wounded…. Volunteers were called for to get it for the wounded…. One man who volunteered was shot through the leg, both knees crushed and the fleshy parts lacerated so that I had to amputate the leg below the knee. He is doing well, although the operation was performed under many difficulties.

When soldiers and settlers were not battling Native Americans, they were frequently fighting among themselves. In October 1881, the most infamous gun battle of the Wild West took place in Tombstone, Arizona Territory. By the time the shooting stopped at the O. K. Corral, three individuals lay dead or dying. George Goodfellow (1855–1910), a graduate in medicine from Wooster University, Ohio, was practicing in Tombstone at that time. Known for his ability with surgeon's knife, playing cards, and guns, and also his love for the bottle, Goodfellow was a caricature of frontier medicine. Unlike the better-recognized John Henry "Doc" Holliday, who was not a physician but was little more than an inveterate gambler and gunman, Goodfellow was well respected for his surgical skills. In the late 1880s, he authored two journal articles detailing the surgical treatment, including several exploratory laparotomies, of the wounded and dying victims of a violent era.

Two months after the three Earp brothers took part in the O. K. Corral shootout, Virgil Earp was seriously wounded in the left upper extremity during a gunfight in front of the Eagle Brewery Saloon. Goodfellow was called on to control the hemorrhage and then proceeded to excise four inches of shattered bone from the area of Virgil's elbow. Earp survived the surgical operation but never regained functional use of the arm. In March 1882, Wyatt Earp (1848–1929) was observing his younger brother, Morgan, shoot billards. Shots rang out and Morgan collapsed on the floor. He was carried to Goodfellow's office, where his injury was ascertained to include a severing of the lumbar spine: in the words of Goodfellow to Wyatt, "His spine is broken, he's done for."

There was little medical work that the flamboyant Goodfellow did not perform. For example, serving as Tombstone's coroner, he had to authorize a death report on the mob lynching of a suspected horse thief. The robber had been unceremoniously taken from the town's jail after a crowd of almost two hundred men disarmed the sheriff and stormed the cell. The lynching party was led by the respected superintendent of the local copper mine, and there is even some evidence that Goodfellow himself was an active participant in the throng. Having to issue their findings, Goodfellow and other members of the jury of inquest matter-of-factly stated that "after viewing the body and hearing the testimony, find that the name of the deceased was John Heath, thirty-two years old, a native of Texas, and that he came to his death from emphysema of the lungs which might have been and probably was caused by strangulation, self-inflicted or otherwise, as is in accordance with the medical evidence." Goodfellow facetiously, but with a somewhat straight face, added that "emphysema was a swelling caused by air in the cellular tissue and was sometimes due to strangulation and sometimes due to the effects of high altitude (failure to keep your feet on the ground). All agreed that it was an uplifting ceremony."

Personalities such as the "older" Gross and the "younger" Goodfellow show how a jaunty, indomitable spirit was beginning to grip American surgery. Through the cumulative efforts of many individuals, surgery was transformed from an act of medical desperation to a more scientifically based method of dealing with human illness. The craft of surgery had risen from a menial and sometimes despised aspect of American culture to one of greatly increased prestige. Practitioners of medicine and surgery were benefitting from professional esteem and wide-ranging influence. Surgery was finally being regarded, albeit hesistatingly, as a true profession, having

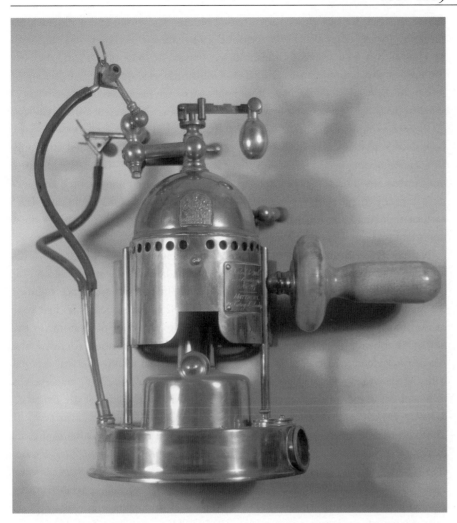

24. Lister-type carbolizer used for spraying a fine mist of disinfectant carbolic acid over the operative field, its immediate area, and the members of the surgical team (circa late 1880s). *(Warren Museum, Harvard Medical School)*

its own organizational and hierarchal structure and recognized specialty societies. The transformation of American surgery was almost complete, although it would take the next surgical era to finalize the ascent and provide the true imprimatur for its scientific underpinnings.

BIOGRAPHIES OF LATE-NINETEENTH-CENTURY SURGEONS

John Collins Warren wrote of the 1870s and 1880s that "no other generation of physicians in the history of medicine has seen such extraordinary changes in the practice of medicine and surgery." Warren was very close to the historical truth. As is noted in the biographies of some of the dominant surgical personalities who passed away during that time, it was clearly an era when the older generation of physician-surgeons gave way to the newer surgeon as specialist. **John Rhea Barton** (1794–1871) was an 1818 graduate of the University of Pennsylvania. Shortly thereafter, he became surgeon to the Pennsylvania Hospital. He is best known as the originator of osteotomy for joint ankylosis (1826). Barton's name is also associated with a figure-of-eight bandage that provides support below and anterior to the lower jaw; an obstetrics forceps with one fixed, curved blade and a lunged anterior blade for application to a high transverse position of a baby's head; and a fracture of the lower articular extremity of the radius. Following his death, Barton's widow gave $50,000 to the University of Pennsylvania to endow the professorship of the principles and practice of surgery in his name.

Alban Goldsmith (1795–1876), one of the most interesting personalities in American surgical history, had his name legally changed from Smith by an act of the New York State legislature in 1839. Goldsmith never received a formal medical degree. Instead, he apprenticed with both Ephraim McDowell and a Philadelphia surgeon, Joseph Parrish (1779–1840). Because of his early association with McDowell, it is believed that Goldsmith was present at some of the earliest ovariotomies in the United States. In 1833, Goldsmith was appointed professor of surgery at the Medical College of Ohio. Four years later, because of his irascible personality, his contract was not renewed. Shortly thereafter, the regents of the College of Physicians and Surgeons in New York City offered him the chair of surgery. Goldsmith's academic career in New York was short-lived. He resigned after only two years and remained in private practice for the rest of his life. Among Goldsmith's most important clinical contributions were the country's first documented laminectomy for relief of paralysis secondary to fracture of a vertebra (1829) and one of the earliest reported cases of lithotrity for bladder stone (1831). Goldsmith's most important text was *Diseases of the Genitourinary Organs* (1857).

Nathan Ryno Smith (1797–1877) studied medicine under the direction of his father, Nathan Smith, and in 1823 received his medical degree from Yale. Smith began practicing in Burlington, Vermont, and with his father's assistance founded the medical school at the University of Vermont (1825). He served as its first professor of anatomy and surgery but was soon called to the chair of anatomy at the newly established Jefferson Medical College. In 1827, Smith founded the *Philadelphia Monthly Journal of Medicine and Surgery*, which within one year merged with the *American Journal of the Medical Sciences*. From 1827 to 1838, he served as professor of surgery at the University of Maryland and was editor of the *Baltimore Monthly Journal of Medicine and Surgery*. Except for a three-year interval at Transylvania University in Lexington, Kentucky, Smith remained in Baltimore for forty years. Smith's surgical textbooks included *Surgical Anatomy of the Arteries* (1830) and *Treatment of Fractures of the Lower Extremities by the Use of the Anterior Suspensory Apparatus* (1867). He was the inventor of the lithotome, an instrument used to perform vesical lithotomy (1831). Among his most important case reports were the first thyroidectomy in America (1835) and his invention of the anterior or suspensory splint for the treatment of lower-extremity fracture (1860).

John Atlee (1799–1885) was a native of Lancaster, Pennsylvania, and graduated from the University of Pennsylvania in 1820. His entire professional life was spent in private practice in his native city, where he was on the faculty of anatomy and physiology at Franklin and Marshall College. In 1843, Atlee's widely noted report of a successful bilateral oophorectomy helped revive the operation in America. He played an active role in medical organizations and was a founder and president of the Lancaster County Medical Society, the Pennsylvania Medical Society, and the American Medical Association.

Dixi Crosby (1800–1873) received his medical degree from Dartmouth in 1824. He was professor of surgery at his alma mater from 1838 to 1870. In 1836, Crosby resected the entire arm and scapula and three-fourths of the clavicle for a reported osteosarcoma. This monumental operation, performed in preanesthetic America, was not reported in the literature until 1875 by Crosby's son, Alpheus (1832–1877). Dixi Crosby remains best known in the United States as the defendant in the first malpractice suit brought against a consulting surgeon. Crosby lost the initial suit and the plaintiff was awarded $800 in damages (1845). Almost a decade later, the decision was reversed on appeal. Crosby served two terms as president of the New Hampshire Medical Society.

Willard Parker (1800–1884) was a private pupil of John Collins Warren and graduated from Harvard (1830). After serving for one year as house surgeon to the Massachusetts General Hospital, Parker was appointed professor of anatomy at the Berkshire Medical College in Pittsfield, Massachusetts. In 1836, he transferred to the chair of surgery at the Medical College of Ohio, and three years later he accepted the professorship of surgery at the College of Physicians and Surgeons in New York City. He remained there until his retirement and also joined the staffs of

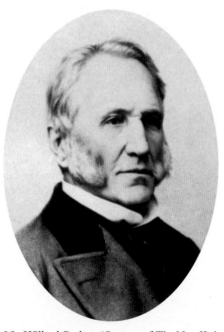

25. Willard Parker. (*Courtesy of The New York Academy of Medicine*)

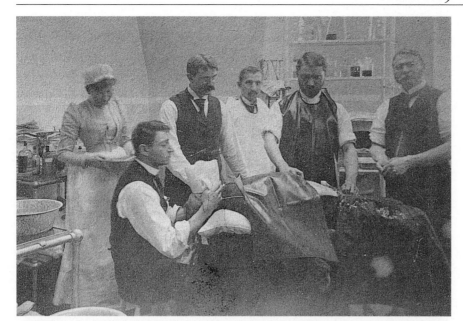

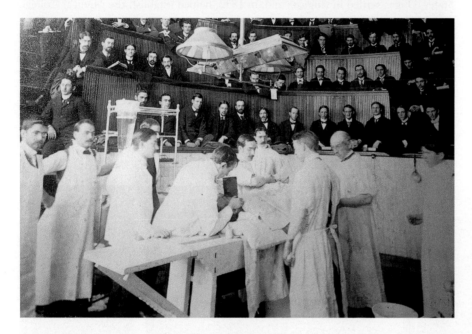

26. Surgery in the Bellevue Hospital operating room (circa mid–1880s) (*top*). No hats, no gloves, and few members of the operating room team wear a gown. Just half a decade later (*bottom*), the surgeons remain without gloves or hats, but they now don white operating gowns. Also note the appearance of electric lights above the operating room table. (*Courtesy of Stanley B. Burns, M.D., and The Burns Collection and Archive*)

Bellevue Hospital (1845) and New York Hospital (1856). In 1866, Parker served as commissioner of the New York Metropolitan Board of Health. Parker never wrote a true textbook of surgery, although after his death, his son compiled manuscript notes and had them published as *Cancer: A Study of Three Hundred and Ninety-Seven Cases of Cancer of the Female Breast* (1885). Parker remains well known for several clinical surgical triumphs. In 1851, he initiated cystotomy as a treatment for irritable bladder. Parker reported the simultaneous ligature of the left subclavian, the common carotid, and the vertebral arteries (1864) and advocated the opening of appendicular abscesses at an early stage (1867). Active in the public health and temperance movements, Parker is eponymically remembered for an oblique incision nearly parallel with the inguinal ligament over the area of dullness in an appendiceal abscess.

Joseph Pancoast (1805–1882) was a native of New Jersey and an 1827 graduate of the University of Pennsylvania. He began teaching practical anatomy and surgery in Philadelphia in 1831 and seven years later was elected professor of surgery at Jefferson Medical College. In 1841, he was reassigned to the chair of general, descriptive, and surgical anatomy, where he remained until his retirement in 1874. Pancoast authored the outstanding *A Treatise on Operative Surgery* (1844), which became one of the most popular surgical atlases in mid-nineteenth-century America. He is distinguished for his repair of an exstrophy of the bladder (1859) and for his procedure of sectioning the second and third branches of the fifth pair of cranial nerves as they emerge from the base of the brain (1872). Pancoast's name is linked with a suture that provides for the union of two edges in plastic repair by means of a tongue-and-groove arrangement.

Alfred Post (1805–1885), the nephew of Wright Post, graduated from the College of Physicians and Surgeons in New York City in 1827. He continued his studies in Berlin, Edinburgh, and Paris and returned to New York in 1829 to begin the practice of surgery. He was one of the founders of the medical department of the University of the City of New York and held its chair of surgery from 1851 to 1875. Post's only treatise was *Observations on the Cure of Strabismus* (1841). He was the first in America to successfully perform and report on plastic operations to correct eyelid deformities (1842).

Louis Dugas (1806–1884) was one of the leading surgeons of the South. An 1827 graduate of the University of Maryland, he soon traveled to Europe, where he continued his medical training for another four years. After returning to the United States, Dugas settled in Augusta and, in 1832, helped establish the Medical College of Georgia. From 1855 to 1883, he served there as professor of principles and practice of surgery. Dugas was dean of the medical college from 1861 to 1876 and was decisive in mandating that the institution would survive the hostilities of the Civil War—a struggle that Dugas, as a foe of secession, had adamantly opposed. His most noteworthy contribution to surgery came in an 1856 report in which he described a clinical test to determine shoulder dislocation: if the elbow cannot be made to touch the chest while the hand rests on the opposite shoulder, the injury is a dislocation, not a fracture of the humerus.

27. With a cadaver hanging from a support mechanism, a professor of anatomy at an unidentified medical school (circa late 1880s) provides instruction to an amphitheater full of medical students. Of the 250 fledgling doctors there are no visible women, but surprisingly, one African-American student was in attendance (*front row between the anatomist and cadaver*). (*Edward G. Miner Library, University of Rochester Medical Center*)

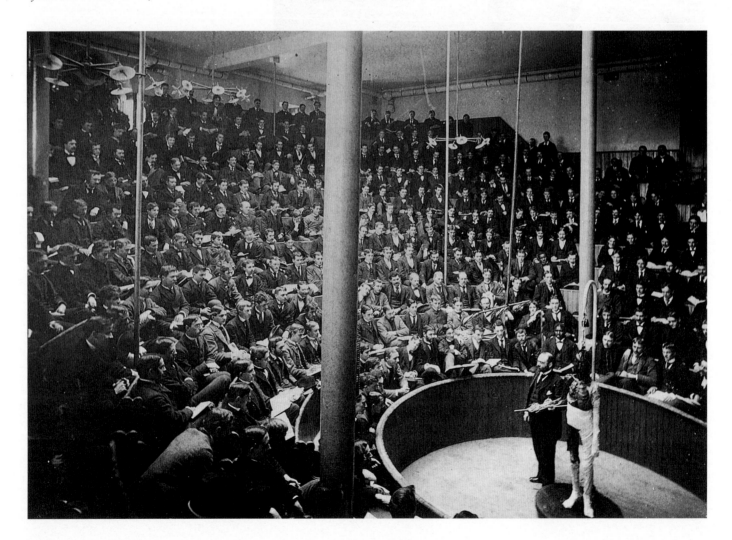

Paul Eve (1806–1878), a native of Augusta, Georgia, received his medical education at the University of Pennsylvania (1828). While continuing his studies in Europe, Eve served as a field surgeon in the Polish Army when the Polish people were revolting against Russian domination (1831). For his exploits, including thirty days as a Russian prisoner of war, Eve was awarded the Golden Cross of Honor by the Polish government. After two years in Europe, Eve returned home and was appointed professor of surgery at the newly founded Medical College of Georgia. In 1850, he transferred to the chair of surgery at the University of Louisville, but he left after one session to accept the professorship of surgery at the University of Nashville. In 1857, Eve served as the eleventh president of the American Medical Association. During the Civil War, he was chief surgeon to General J. E. Johnston's army and president of the Confederate Army Medical Board, which examined the qualifications of "surgeons" seeking appointment to the army. Eve was a prolific writer of journal articles, but his only textbook was the wonderfully interesting *Collection of Remarkable Cases in Surgery* (1857).

Gurdon Buck (1807–1877), a native of New York City, graduated from the College of Physicians and Surgeons in 1830. He served as a house surgeon at the New York Hospital for one year and then left for two years to study in Berlin, Paris, and Vienna. On his return to the United States, Buck was appointed attending surgeon to the New York Hospital, where he remained until his death. Buck was considered an outstanding clinical surgeon and authored the important *Contributions to Reparative Surgery* (1876), the first American text on plastic and reconstructive surgery. In addition, Buck wrote numerous case reports, including those in which ligatures were simultaneously applied to the common and internal carotid arteries (1855) and to the femoral, profunda, external, and common iliac arteries (1858). His most spectacular surgical feats include the restoration of an ankylosed right-angled knee joint to a straight position (1845) and the first known operation in America for a cancer of the larynx to be treated by an external incision (1853). He is eponymically remembered for the fascial sheath of the penis (1848) and for a traction device that applies tensile force on the leg by means of tape on the skin; friction between the tape and skin permits the application of force, which is mediated through a cord over a pulley, suspending a weight (1862). Among his children was the renowned surgeon Albert Henry Buck (1842–1922).

Washington Atlee (1808–1878), younger brother of John Atlee, graduated from Jefferson Medical College in 1829. The early part of his professional career was spent in Lancaster, Pennsylvania. After 1844, he practiced in Philadelphia, where he was on the medical chemistry faculty of the Medical College of Pennsylvania. He was a founder and president of the American Gynecological Society, and with his brother helped reestablish the operation of ovariotomy in the United States. In 1873, Atlee summarized his life's clinical work in *General and Differential Diagnosis of Ovarian Tumors*. Atlee was also a prolific contributor to the periodical literature; his articles included one in 1851 that detailed all known operations of ovariotomy from 1710 to 1851, a study of the surgical removal of uterine fibroids in 1853, and the description of an operation for vesicovaginal fistula 1860. In 1874, Atlee was president of the Pennsylvania State Medical Society, and the following year he was vice-president of the American Medical Association.

George Norris (1808–1875) was a graduate of the University of Pennsylvania (1830). After two years' service at the Pennsylvania Hospital, he went to Paris and studied with Dupuytren, Roux, and Velpeau. After returning to the United States, Norris succeeded John Rhea Barton as one of the surgeons in the Pennsylvania Hospital, serving from 1836 until 1863. In 1848, Norris was named professor of clinical surgery at his alma mater. Norris's sole full-length clinical text was *Contributions to Practical Surgery* (1873). His only other book of note, *The Early History of Medicine in Philadelphia* (1886), was published posthumously. Norris remains most remembered for the numerous statistical compilations of data about surgical operations that he authored in the 1830s and 1840s. His son was William Fisher Norris (1839–1901), a renowned ophthalmologist.

Warren Stone (1808–1872) was an 1831 graduate of the Berkshire Medical Institute in Massachusetts and also studied with Amos Twitchell (1781–1850). Twitchell, a general practitioner in Vermont and a well-respected surgeon, had performed the first ligation of the common carotid artery for traumatic injury in America (1807). Stone had difficulty establishing a practice in New England and resettled in New Orleans. There he became associated with the medical department of the University of Louisiana. In 1836, Stone was appointed lecturer on surgery and within a few years, professor of surgery. He served on the staff of Charity Hospital from 1834 to 1872. During the Civil War, Stone was surgeon-general of Louisiana and was imprisoned by federal authorities. Stone was a co-editor of the *New Orleans Medical and Surgical Journal* from 1857 to 1868. Although he wrote little, Stone did report the earliest use of metallic sutures in the ligation of an artery (1859), and he was among the first to resect part of a rib to secure drainage in empyema.

John Bobbs (1809–1870) received his medical degree from Jefferson Medical College in 1836. After settling in Indianapolis, he helped establish Indiana Central Medical College (1849), serving as its dean and professor of surgery. Two decades later, Bobbs became the founder of the Medical College of Indiana. Active in political affairs, Bobbs served in the Indiana state senate from 1856 to 1860. During the Civil War, he was medical director of the district of Indiana. Bobbs wrote sparingly and was typical of that era's surgeon in that he was both a general practitioner and, occasionally, a surgical operator. A principal figure in Indiana medicine during its pioneer period, Bobbs was instrumental in founding the Indiana State Medical Society. In 1868, he reported the world's first known account of a cholecystotomy for the removal of gallstones.

Benjamin Lord Hill (1813–1871) was professor of surgery and later professor of anatomy at the Eclectic Medical Institute in Cincinnati. Eclecticism was a botanical movement that first flourished in the 1840s and was strongest in the Midwest. Hill's important *Lectures on the American Eclectic System of Surgery* (1850) was the first textbook of surgery to come out of this movement and the first nonallopathic surgical work to be published in the United States. By the early 1850s, like many other eclectic physicians, Hill had turned his attention to homeopathic medicine. He became professor of obstetrics and diseases of women and, later, professor of surgery at Western Homeopathic College in Cleveland, where he authored *The Homeopathic Practice of Surgery, Together with Operative Surgery* (1855).

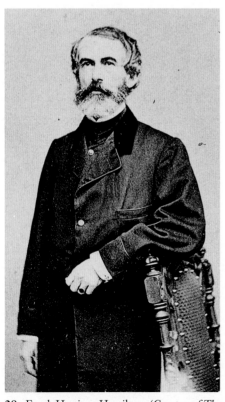

28. Frank Hastings Hamilton. (*Courtesy of The New York Academy of Medicine*)

Frank Hasting Hamilton (1813–1886) received a classical undergraduate education at Union College in Schenectady, New York, and later graduated with a degree in medicine from the medical department of the University of Pennsylvania in 1833. Hamilton served in several chairs of surgery, including the medical institute in Geneva, New York (1840), Buffalo Medical College (1846), Long Island College Hospital (1860), and Bellevue Hospital Medical College (1868). Hamilton was one of mid-nineteenth-century America's most versatile surgeons and produced an influential body of written work. His major texts include *Monograph on Strabismus* (1845), *A Practical Treatise on Fractures and Dislocations* (1860), *A Practical Treatise on Military Surgery* (1861), *A Treatise on Military Surgery and Hygiene* (1865), *The Principles and Practice of Surgery* (1872), and *Fracture of the Patella* (1880). He also edited the important two-volume *Surgical Memoirs of the War of the Rebellion* (1870–1871) published by the United States Sanitary Commission. Among Hamilton's most important contributions to the periodical literature were the earliest description of a crossleg pedicle flap as a treatment for chronic ulcer (1854) and a description of deformities after fractures (1855). His name is eponymically linked with a trophic affection of the subcutaneous connective tissue marked by a circumscribed swelling that may become indurated and red but never suppurates, and with a clinical orthopedic test whereby, in an axillary dislocation of the shoulder, a rod touches both the acromion process and the outer condyle of the humerus.

James Rushmore Wood (1813–1882) initially apprenticed with David Rogers (1799–1877), a little-known surgeon from New York City. Rogers is best remembered for performing an early excision of the superior maxillary bone (1824) and authoring *Surgical Essays and Cases in Surgery* (1849). Wood received his medical degree from Castleton Medical College in Vermont in 1834. He soon established a private practice in New York City and, in 1847, was appointed to the medical board of Bellevue Hospital. Fourteen years later, he was instrumental in establishing the Bellevue Hospital Medical College and eventually its school of nursing. Wood served as the first professor of operative surgery and surgical pathology at the new medical institute. Although recognized as one of America's most notable surgeons, Wood wrote little. Among his important contributions, however, were those on phosphorus poisoning (1856) and carotid ligation (1859). Wood was influential in the passage of the New York law (1857) permitting the unclaimed bodies of vagrants to be used for anatomical education.

Edward Mott Moore (1814–1902) attended the Rensselaer School in Troy, New York (1833–1835) and received his medical degree from the College of Physicians and Surgeons in New York City in 1835. He held chairs of surgery at several institutions, including the Vermont Medical College (1842–1853), Starling Medical College in Columbus Ohio (1853–1856), and the University of Buffalo (1856–1882). A well-known medical educator, Moore served as president of the American Medical Association (1890), the American Surgical Association (1884), and the New York State Medical Society (1874) and was first president of the New York State Board of Health. He is best remembered for describing Moore's fracture of the distal end of the radius with luxation of the distal end of the ulna.

Henry Hollingsworth Smith (1815–1890) graduated from the University of Pennsylvania in 1837, after which he studied in London and Paris. Smith was the son-in-law of William Horner and eventually succeeded William Gibson as professor of surgery at the University of Pennsylvania. Among Smith's many texts were *Minor Surgery* (1843), *Anatomical Atlas* (1844), *A System of Operative Surgery, Based Upon the Practice of Surgeons in the United States* (1852), *A Treatise on the Practice of Surgery* (1856), and the two-volume *Principles and Practice of Surgery, Embracing Minor and Operative Surgery* (1863). The latter work is especially important to surgical historians, since it contains a detailed history of surgery in the United States and a bibliography of American works on surgery from 1783 to 1860. Smith served as president of the Pennsylvania State Medical Society in 1883.

Henry Bigelow (1818–1890), a native of Boston, obtained his medical degree from Harvard in 1841 and then spent three years in Europe, mostly in Paris. Upon his return to America, Bigelow and Henry Bryant (1820–1867), who had also studied surgery in Paris, opened a "Charitable Institution for Outdoor Patients in Boston". Both physicians ran into strong criticism for advertising the fact that their school existed. In 1845, he was appointed instructor of surgery at the Tremont Street Medical School in his native city. The following year, he was elected surgeon to the Massachusetts General Hospital. In 1849, the two Harvard chairs of surgery and clinical surgery that had been previously held by Warren and Hayward were united, and Bigelow was named professor of surgery. Bigelow was a major contributor to the advancement of American medicine, especially orthopedic surgery. In 1844, he won the Boylston Prize for his *Manual of Orthopedic Surgery*, the first comprehensive treatment of the subject in America and a superb summary of the French orthopedic surgery of the day. Eight years later, Bigelow became the first American surgeon to excise the head of the femur. In his classic treatise *The Mechanism of Dislocation and Fracture of the Hip with the Reduction of the Dislocation by the Flexion Method* (1869), he described in detail the structure and function of the accessory Y (iliofemoral) ligament of the acetabulum, which clarified the pathology of disloca-

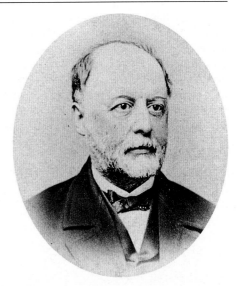

29. Henry Hollingsworth Smith. (*Historical Collections, College of Physicians of Philadelphia*)

30. Henry Bigelow as painted by Frederick Vinton (1876–1911). Vinton's work is little appreciated, but he was an outstanding portrait painter, who portrayed many well-known Bostonian medical figures. Bigelow's reputation as a surgeon are emphasized by the surgical implements placed on the table and the anatomical drawings of the bones of the hip joint. (*The Francis A. Countway Library of Medicine*)

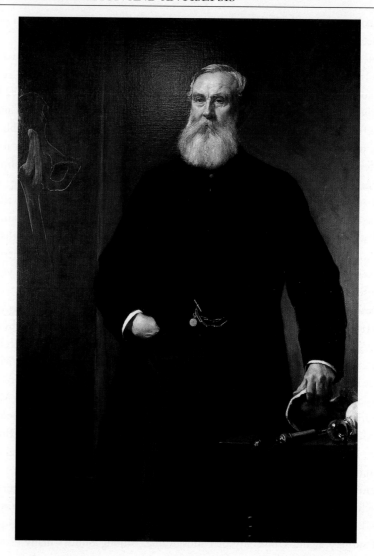

tion of the hip. In an 1875 report, he identified the calcar femorale, a bony spur springing from the underside of the neck of the femur above and anterior to the lesser trochanter, which adds strength to this portion of the bone. Bigelow provided the world with its first detailed understanding of inhalation anesthesia in his important papers on insensibility during surgical operations produced by sulfuric ether (1846). He followed these with another group of articles discussing the discovery of ether and chloroform and their physiological effects (1848). Of Bigelow's many contributions to American surgery, his improvement of the lithotrite used for crushing bladder stones and the development of a large-caliber evacuation tube to effectively remove bladder debris during the operation were considered major advances (1878). Bigelow was conservative in his viewpoints and was a bitter opponent of the admission of African Americans and women to Harvard Medical School. He was slow to accept any of the modernizing educational reforms of the president of Harvard, Charles Eliot.

David Prince (1816–1889) received his medical education at the Medical College of Ohio (1838), where his mentor was Reuben Mussey. From 1840 to 1843, Prince practiced in Illinois, but he eventually left to accept the chair of anatomy and surgery at the newly created medical department of Illinois College. After five years, he was appointed to the professorship of surgery at the St. Louis Medical College in Missouri. Prince resigned this professorship in 1852 and settled in Jacksonville, Illinois, where he spent the remainder of his life in the practice of general medicine and surgery. Prince's most important works were *Orthopedics: A Systematic Treatise Upon the Prevention and Correction of Deformities* (1866) and *Plastics and Orthopedics* (1871).

John Carnochan (1817–1887), a student of Valentine Mott, graduated from the College of Physicians and Surgeons in New York City in 1836. He spent most of his professional career in New York, where he was surgeon-in-chief to the State Emigrant Hospital on Ward's Island, then the largest hospital in the United States. He also served as professor of surgery at the New York Medical College. Carnochan was a daring operator, who excised an entire mandible in 1852 and reported the first excision of the superior maxillary nerve for the treatment of facial neuralgia in 1858. His book-length works were *A Treatise on the Etiology, Pathology and Treatment of Congenital Dislocations of the Head of the Femur* (1850) and *Contributions to Operative Surgery and Surgical Pathology* (1877).

David Hayes Agnew (1818–1892) was a graduate of the University of Pennsylvania (1838). After establishing a general medical and surgical practice, he became head of the Philadelphia School of Anatomy (1852). In 1863, Agnew left that position to become demonstrator of anatomy at his alma mater. Eight years later, he was named professor of surgery. Agnew was a highly skilled anatomist and an unusually dexterous surgeon, who acquired immense practical experience in all forms of surgical diseases. His life's work was embodied in his massive three-volume *Principles and Practice of Surgery* (1878–1883). His other important text was *Lacerations of the Female Perineum; and Vesico-Vaginal Fistula; Their History and Treatment* (1873). Agnew also authored the lengthy *History and Reminiscences of the Philadelphia Almshouse and Philadelphia Hospital* (1890).

Charles Pope (1818–1870) was a graduate of the University of Pennsylvania (1839). For the next year and a half he studied in Paris. Upon his return to the United States, Pope was named professor of anatomy and physiology in the medical department of St. Louis University (1843). From 1846 to 1867, he served as professor of surgery at St. Louis Medical College. Pope was a dynamic force behind the St. Louis Medical College, the second medical school established west of the Mississippi. With family money, he supplied the institution with its physical plant and built a free dispensary to provide care for the indigent and clinical experience for the students. Pope was president of the American Medical Association (1854), but he wrote little of importance.

George Blackman (1819–1871) graduated with a degree in medicine from the College of Physicians and Surgeons in New York City in 1840. He spent many years studying in London and Paris and, on his return to America, was appointed professor of surgery at the Medical College of Ohio. He made voluminous contributions to the periodical literature, but his only monograph, jointly authored with Charles Tripler (1806–1866) was *Handbook for the Military Surgeon* (1861).

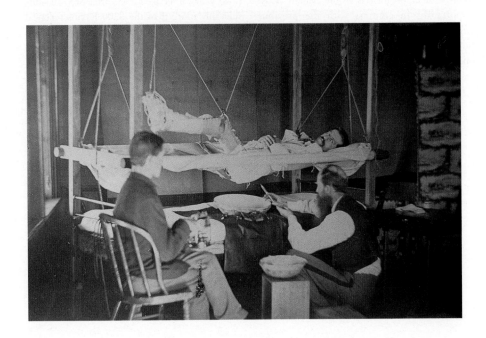

31. Osteomyelitis and other orthopedic conditions often resulted in lengthy hospital stays. This patient (circa 1885) was being treated for an apparent fracture or dislocation of the left leg when he developed a sacral pressure ulcer. Using the latest in hospital bedding and traction, the patient is held aloft while the physician syringes necrotic material off his decubitus ulcer. (*Courtesy of Stanley B. Burns, M.D., and The Burns Collection and Archive*)

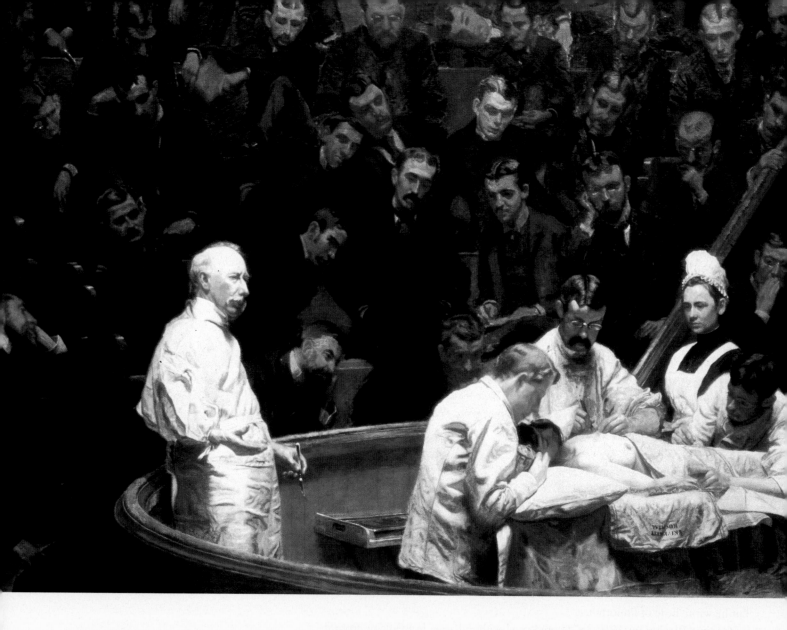

32. "The Agnew Clinic." It is only fitting that this surgical era concludes with the other celebrated surgical painting by Thomas Eakins, a portrait of David Hayes Agnew, which is physically larger (11 x 6 1/2 feet) than "The Gross Clinic." Eakins must have been a great admirer of Agnew as an individual, because on the frame of the painting, the artist inscribed: *D. Hayes Agnew, M.D. Chirurgus Peritissimus. Scriptor et Doctor Clarissimus. Vir Veneratus et Carissimus* (the most experienced surgeon, the clearest writer and teacher, the most venerated and beloved man). Several striking contrasts to "The Gross Clinic" are immediately evident. Agnew and his assistants are in operating gowns, not business suits. They are using instruments that could be sterilized, and a can to dispense chloroform is visibly evident. Most importantly, in contrast with the previous effort, where the only woman shown is an emotionally overwrought relative of the patient, an operating room nurse with a serious expression is now prominently portrayed as a member of Agnew's operating team. Finally, there is no evidence of blood anywhere in this operation on a young woman's breast. "The Agnew Clinic" was commissioned by Agnew's students on the resignation of their beloved teacher after twenty-six years of service for the price of $750, considerably more than the $200 Eakins received when he eventually sold "The Gross Clinic" to Jefferson Medical College. (*Courtesy of the University of Pennsylvania School of Medicine*)

William Van Buren (1819–1883) was a graduate of the University of Pennsylvania (1840). While studying in Paris, he made the acquaintance of Valentine Mott, who was then on an extended sojourn in Europe. In 1845, after having served as an assistant surgeon in the United States Army, Van Buren joined Mott in New York City as his prosector. With his surgical skills well honed at the side of Mott, who had since become his father-in-law, Van Buren was named to the chair of anatomy at the University of New York. In 1866, he was elected professor of surgery for the newly established department of diseases of the genitourinary system at the Bellevue Hospital Medical College. Van Buren was an extremely versatile surgeon and wrote *Contributions to Practical Surgery* (1865), *Lectures Upon Diseases of the Rectum* (1870), *A Practical Treatise on the Surgical Diseases of the Genito-Urinary Organs* (1874), and *Lectures on the Principles of Surgery* (1884). Van Buren is eponymically linked with fibrous cavernitis of the penis. During the Civil War, Van Buren was highly active in the daily management of the United States Sanitary Commission.

Edward Franklin (1822–1885) was one of the least known but most versatile and prolific of nineteenth-century American surgeons. Although trained by Valentine Mott, he became an adherent of homeopathic medicine and was appointed professor of surgery at Hahnemann Medical College in Chicago in 1862. Three years later, he was nominated professor of surgery at the Homeopathic Medical College of Missouri. There, he authored his two-volume *The Science and Art of Surgery, Embracing Minor and Operative Surgery* (1867–1873). The volumes were massive in size and contained an interesting general descriptive history of surgery, with a specific section on surgery in the United States. Franklin soon transferred to the surgical chair at the Homeopathic College of the University of Michigan, where he wrote *The Homoeopathic Treatment of Spinal Curvatures According to the New Principle* (1878), *A Complete Minor Surgery* (1882), *The Practitioner's and Student's Manual of the Science of Surgery* (1882), and *A Manual of Venereal Diseases* (1883).

Moses Gunn (1822–1887) received his medical degree from the Geneva Medical College in upstate New York in 1846. He immediately moved to Ann Arbor, Michigan, where he established a private practice and began to lecture on anatomy. Within ten years, he held the chair of anatomy and surgery at the University of Michigan. In 1867, Gunn accepted the professorship of surgery at Rush Medical College. Gunn's most important written work was a short pamphlet, *Luxations of the Hip and Shoulder Joints, and the Agents Which Oppose Their Reduction* (1859). He demonstrated that in dislocation of the shoulder or hip, the untorn portion of the capsule causes the characteristic attitude assumed by the limbs, and forms the true hindrance to easy reduction.

John Hodgen (1826–1882) received his medical degree in 1848 from Missouri Medical College, where he was a protegé of Joseph Nash McDowell. Hodgen began his career at his alma mater as a demonstrator of anatomy. He accepted a position as professor of anatomy at the St. Louis Medical College in 1854. Hodgen spent the remainder of his professional life at that institution and eventually served as both professor of surgical anatomy and dean. Among his most memorable accomplishments was the invention of a wire suspension device that offered a supportive role for traction in fractures of the middle or lower end of the femur. Hodgen was an organizer of the Association of American Medical Colleges (1876), although the St. Louis Medical College decided not to join.

Robert Kinloch (1826–1891) was a native of Charleston, South Carolina, and graduated with a degree in medicine from the University of Pennsylvania in 1848. He pursued further education in Edinburgh, London, and Paris. After the Civil War, Kinloch became professor of surgery at the Medical College of South Carolina, and in 1888 he was elected dean of the faculty. He was among the most prominent surgeons in the South, although he authored no major textbooks. Kinloch's claim to distinction concerned numerous surgical feats, including being the first to treat fractures of the jaw by wiring the fragments together (1859) and the first to resect the knee joint for chronic disease.

Henry Sands (1830–1888) received his medical degree from the College of Physicians and Surgeons in New York City in 1854. After further studies in Paris, Sands became professor of anatomy and then surgery at his alma mater. He was also on the staff of the Bellevue, New York, and Roosevelt Hospitals. From 1867 to 1870, his professional partner was Willard Parker. Sands was a major proponent in America for more aggressive surgical treatment of appendicitis. An 1880 paper detailed plans for opening appendiceal abscesses earlier than had been previously advocated. Eight years later, his clinical acumen became even more apparent when he reported a diagnosis of acute appendicitis made within forty-eight hours of symptom onset. His other important contributions to the periodical literature concerned the first successful laryngotomy for papillomata (1865) and the earliest report of trephining for a brain tumor (1883).

Beriah Watson (1836–1892) received his medical degree from New York University in 1861. Following the Civil War, he settled in Jersey City, New Jersey, where he was instrumental in the formation of the Jersey City, St. Francis, and Christ Hospitals. Although Watson is little known, he was one of the earliest advocates of Lister's techniques in the United States. His massive *Treatise on Amputations of the Extremities and Their Complications* (1882) was even dedicated to Lister and actually predated Gerster's textbook on antiseptic surgery. Watson performed some of the most unique and important surgical experiments undertaken by any nineteenth-century American surgeons. Using the results obtained in this basic science research, Watson authored a paper on cardiac sensitivity to chloroform anesthesia (1887) and a monograph, *An Experimental Study of Lesions Arising from Severe Concussions* (1890). Although Watson was minimally involved in organized medicine, he did provide the initial stimulus for the New Jersey legislature to legalize the dissection of human cadavers (1895).

Samuel Weissell Gross (1837–1889), the son of Samuel Gross, was an important Philadelphia surgeon in his own right. Gross graduated from Jefferson Medical College in 1857. He served most of his professional life on the faculty of his alma mater, where he eventually was named professor of the principles of surgery. In his first major text, *A Practical Treatise on Tumors of the Mammary Glands* (1880), Gross argued that breast tumors could be operated on successfully if the disease had not metastasized. His other textbook was *A Practical Treatise on Impotence, Sterility, and Allied Disorders of the Male Sexual Organs* (1881). As the result of his experiences in the Civil War, Gross espoused the idea that instead of relying on pressure alone to control hemorrhage, as was the accepted practice, veins should be ligated, as arteries were. In 1879, he authored the first comprehensive study of bone sarcoma and broadened and solidified the concept of giant-cell sarcoma. After Gross's early death, his widow married William Osler.

Charles Parkes (1842–1891) was born in Troy, New York, and graduated from Rush Medical College (1868). He was immediately appointed demonstrator of anatomy, a position he held until his elevation to professor of anatomy in 1875. Twelve years later, Parkes was nominated to succeed Moses Gunn, who was professor of surgery at Rush. Parkes was a pioneer in abdominal surgery and one of the most active proponents of animal experimentation as an integral part of basic surgical research. In 1884, he wrote a monograph, *Gun-Shot Wounds of the Small Intestine*, which was influential in establishing new lines of clinical treatment for gunshot injuries. For several years before his premature death, Parkes had begun to compile material for a textbook on general and abdominal surgery. His wife had the unfinished manuscript published as *Clinical Lectures on Abdominal Surgery and Other Subjects* (1896), with Albert Ochsner (1858–1925) serving as editor.

SCIENTIFIC ADVANCEMENT, 1890–1918

1890	1895	1900	1905	1910	1915	1920	1925	1930

DAILY LIFE

Sequoia and Yosemite National Parks *(1890)*

Boston Marathon *(1891)*

James Corbett knocks out John L. Sullivan to become first heavyweight champion *(1892)*

World's Columbian Exposition in Chicago *(1893)*

United States Golf Association *(1894)*

Sears, Roebuck and Company opens mail-order business *(1895)*

Rural free mail delivery is established *(1896)*

Library of Congress *(1897)*

First Food and Drug Act is passed *(1898)*

The Gideons, Christian Commercial Men's Association of America *(1899)*

International Ladies' Garment Worker's Union *(1900)*

U.S. Steel Corporation *(1901)*

First post-season football game is held at the Tournament of Roses in California *(1902)*

First annual World Series *(1903)*

New York City subway *(1904)*

Rotary Club *(1905)*

San Francisco earthquake *(1906)*

Mother's Day *(1907)*

Ford Motor company introduces the Model T *(1908)*

National Association for the Advancement of Colored People formed *(1909)*

Father's Day *(1910)*

Triangle Shirtwaist Factory fire *(1911)*

Jim Thorpe wins both decathlon and pentathlon at the Olympics in Sweden *(1912)*

Army–Notre Dame football game *(1913)*

Federal Trade Commission *(1914)*

First transatlantic radiotelephone communication *(1915)*

First birth control clinic opened in Brooklyn *(1916)*

Congress adopts the Fourteenth Amendment, prohibiting manufacture or sale of alcoholic drinks *(1917)*

Influenza epidemic *(1918)*

U.S.A. POPULATION

1890	=	62 million
1900	=	76 million
1910	=	92 million

HISTORY AND POLITICS

Sherman Antitrust Act *(1890)*

Circuit Courts of Appeals created *(1891)*

Grover Cleveland elected President for a second term *(1892)*

Supreme Court declares Chinese Exclusion Act constitutional *(1893)*

Pullman Railway strike *(1894)*

Income tax declared unconstitutional *(1895)*

William McKinley and Garret Hobart elected President and Vice-President, respectively *(1896)*

Dingley Tariff Bill *(1897)*

U.S. battleship *Maine* blown up in Havana, Cuba *(1898)*

U.S. annexes Wake Island *(1899)*

Congress enacts Gold Standard Act *(1900)*

Assassination of President McKinley; Theodore Roosevelt becomes 26th U.S. President *(1901)*

Philippine Islands declared an unorganized U.S. territory *(1902)*

Departments of Commerce and Labor *(1903)*

Roosevelt Corollary to the Monroe Doctrine of 1823 *(1904)*

United States assumes charge of finances of Dominican Republic *(1905)*

Meat Inspection Act *(1906)*

Oklahoma becomes 46th state *(1907)*

Root-Takahira Agreement *(1908)*

Payne-Aldrich Tariff *(1909)*

Ballinger-Pinchot affair *(1910)*

Supreme Court orders dissolution of Standard Oil Company and American Tobacco Company *(1911)*

Woodrow Wilson elected President *(1912)*

Sixteenth Amendment (income tax) to the U.S. Constitution is ratified *(1913)*

U.S. occupation of Vera Cruz, Mexico *(1914)*

Sinking of the Lusitania *(1915)*

Pancho Villa raids New Mexico *(1916)*

Diplomatic relations severed with Germany *(1917)*

President Wilson's Fourteen Points are accepted by Germany, and an armistice is signed *(1918)*

SCIENTIFIC ADVANCEMENT, 1890–1918

1890	1895	1900	1905	1910	1915	1920	1925

FAMOUS AMERICANS

HEROES, POLITICIANS, AND STATESMEN

Dwight D. Eisenhower *(1890–1969)*
Averell Harriman *(1891–1986)*
John McCormack *(1891–1980)*
Henry Morgenthau, Jr. *(1891–1967)*
Edward "Eddie" Rickenbacker *(1891–1973)*
Casey Stengel *(1891–1975)*
Dean Acheson *(1893–1971)*
Charles Atlas *(1893–1972)*
Omar Bradley *(1893–1981)*
J. Edgar Hoover *(1895–1972)*
George Herman "Babe" Ruth *(1895–1948)*
Christian Herter *(1895–1966)*
Roger Hornsby *(1896–1963)*
Paul Robeson *(1898–1976)*
Adlai Stevenson *(1900–1965)*
Ernie Pyle *(1900–1945)*
Richard Daley *(1902–1976)*
Charles Lindbergh *(1902–1974)*
Henry Cabot Lodge *(1902–1985)*
Thomas Dewey *(1903–1971)*
Estes Kefauver *(1903–1963)*
Ivy Baker Priest *(1905–1975)*
Lyndon Baines Johnson *(1908–1973)*
Thurgood Marshall *(1908–1993)*
Adam Clayton Powell, Jr. *(1908–1972)*
Nelson Rockefeller *(1908–1979)*
Barney Ross *(1909–1967)*
Dizzy Dean *(1911–1974)*
Hubert Humphrey *(1911–1978)*
Richard M. Nixon *(1913–1994)*
Jesse Owens *(1913–1980)*
Joe Louis *(1914–1981)*
John F. Kennedy *(1917–1963)*

SCIENTISTS AND INVENTORS

H. J. Muller *(1890–1967)*
Vannevar Bush *(1890–1974)*
Arthur Compton *(1892–1962)*
Harold Urey *(1893–1981)*
Norbert Wiener *(1894–1964)*
Alfred Kinsey *(1894–1956)*
Theodore Dobzhansky *(1900–1975)*
Charles Richter *(1900–1985)*
Margaret Mead *(1901–1978)*
Ernest O. Lawrence *(1901–1958)*
Linus Pauling *(1901–1994)*
Robert Van de Graaf *(1901–1967)*
Edward Condon *(1902–1974)*
Lars Onsager *(1903–1976)*
Robert Oppenheimer *(1904–1967)*
Chester Carlson *(1906–1968)*
Peter Goldmark *(1906–1977)*
Edward Tatum *(1909–1975)*

THEOLOGIANS AND PHILOSOPHERS

Sister Aimee Semple McPherson *(1890–1944)*
Rudolph Carnap *(1891–1970)*
Nima Adlerblum *(1892–1974)*
Cardinal Joseph Ritter *(1892–1967)*
Cardinal Richard Cushing *(1895–1970)*
R. Buckminster Fuller *(1895–1983)*
Lewis Mumford *(1895–1990)*
Elijah Muhammad *(1897–1975)*
Herbert Marcuse *(1898–1979)*
Harold Lee *(1899–1973)*
Eric Hoffer *(1902–1983)*
Hannah Arendt *(1906–1975)*
Rabbi Abraham Joshua Heschel *(1907–1972)*
Kathryn Kuhlman *(1910–1976)*
Paul Ramsey *(1913–1988)*
Thomas Merton *(1915–1968)*

EDUCATORS, SCHOLARS, AND REFORMERS

Arthur Schlesinger *(1888–1965)*
Pearl Buck *(1892–1973)*
James Conant *(1893–1978)*
John Wood Krutch *(1893–1970)*
Mark Van Doren *(1895–1972)*
Edmund Wilson *(1895–1972)*
William Langer *(1896–1977)*
Isador Lubin *(1896–1978)*
Catherine Drinker Bowen *(1897–1973)*
Jacob Marschak *(1898–1977)*
Bruce Catton *(1899–1978)*
John Marshall Harlan *(1899–1971)*
John Gunther *(1901–1970)*
Talcott Parsons *(1903–1979)*
Bergen Evans *(1904–1978)*
Lionel Trilling *(1905–1975)*
Rachel Carson *(1907–1964)*
Walter Reuther *(1907–1970)*

1890	1895	1900	1905	1910	1915	1920	1925

FAMOUS AMERICANS

AUTHORS

Edna St. Vincent Millay *(1892–1950)*
Dorothy Parker *(1893–1967)*
Ben Hecht *(1894–1964)*
Dorothy Thompson *(1894–1961)*
James Thurber *(1894–1961)*
John Dos Passos *(1896–1970)*
F. Scott Fitzgerald *(1896–1940)*
William Faulkner *(1897–1962)*
Thornton Wilder *(1897–1975)*
Bennett Cerf *(1898–1971)*
Hart Crane *(1899–1932)*
Ernest Hemingway *(1899–1961)*
Thomas Wolfe *(1900–1938)*
John Steinbeck *(1902–968)*
Langston Hughes *(1902–1967)*
Isaac Bashevis Singer *(1904-1993)*
Clifford Odets *(1906–1963)*
W. H. Auden *(1907–1973)*
L. Ron Hubbard *(1911–1986)*
Robert Lowell *(1917–1977)*

VISUAL ARTISTS

Man Ray *(1890–1976)*
Mark Tobey *(1890–1976)*
Jacques Lipchitz *(1892–1973)*
Grant Wood *(1892–1942)*
Milton Avery *(1893–1965)*
Charles Burchfield *(1893–1967)*
Stuart Davis *(1894–1964)*
Norman Rockwell *(1894–1978)*
William Gropper *(1897–1977)*
Reginald Marsh *(1898–1954)*
Ben Shahn *(1898–1969)*
Bradley Walker Tomlin *(1899–1953)*
Louise Nevelson *(1900–1988)*
Ansel Adams *(1902–1984)*
Edward Durell Stone *(1902–1978)*
Mark Rothko *(1903–1970)*
Arshile Gorky *(1904–1948)*
Clyfford Still *(1904–1980)*
Barnett Newman *(1905–1970)*
Franz Kline *(1910–1962)*
Jackson Pollock *(1912–1956)*
Ad Reinhardt *(1913–1967)*

PERFORMING ARTISTS

Groucho Marx *(1890–1977)*
Eddie Cantor *(1892–1964)*
Cole Porter *(1893–1964)*
Harold Lloyd *(1894–1971)*
Oscar Hammerstein II *(1895–1960)*
Francis "Buster" Keaton *(1895–1966)*
Bert Lahr *(1895–1967)*
George Gershwin *(1898–1937)*
Dorothy Gish *(1898–1968)*
Billy Rose *(1899–1966)*
Louis Armstrong *(1900–1971)*
Spencer Tracy *(1900–1967)*
Gary Cooper *(1901–1961)*
Nelson Eddy *(1901–1967)*
Clark Gable *(1901–1960)*
David O. Selznick *(1902–1965)*
Tallulah Bankhead *(1903–1968)*
Woodrow "Woody" Guthrie *(1912–1967)*
Mahalia Jackson *(1912–1972)*
Billie Holiday *(1915–1959)*

BUSINESSMEN AND INDUSTRIALISTS

Colonel Harland Sanders *(1890–1980)*
J. Paul Getty *(1892–1976)*
Howard Johnson *(1897–1972)*
John D. MacArthur *(1897–1978)*
Henry Luce *(1898–1967)*
Walter "Walt" Disney *(1901–1966)*
Meyer Lansky *(1902–1983)*
John Ringling North *(1903–1985)*
Bernard "Toots" Shor *(1903–1977)*
Howard Hughes *(1905–1976)*

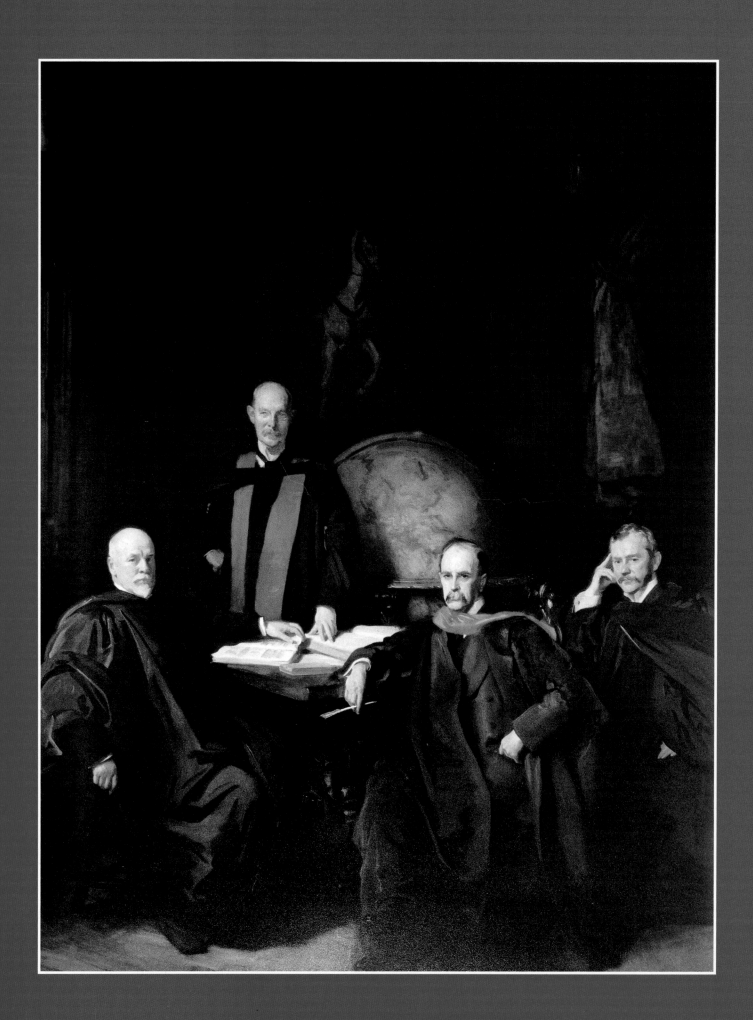

CHAPTER 7

GERMAN AUTHORITY AND SCIENTIFIC ADVANCEMENT *1890–1916*

n 1893, John Shaw Billings (1838–1913) prepared a report for the Board of Regents of the Smithsonian Institution on the achievements of American medicine. Billings, who began his medical career as a surgeon and statistician during the Civil War, had become one of the country's most respected physicians. He was a guiding light to the Surgeon-General's Library (precursor to the National Library of Medicine), originator of the *Index Medicus*, renowned hospital administrator and architect, president of the American Public Health Association, and soon-to-be-named director of the New York Public Library, and when Billings spoke the power-brokers of American society tended to listen. Asked to delineate the advances in medicine that highlighted the nineteenth century, Billings showed no hesitation in declaring:

> The most important improvements in practical medicine made in the United States have been chiefly in surgery, in its various branches. We have led the way in the ligation of some of the larger arteries, in the removal of abdominal tumors, in the treatment of diseases and injuries peculiar to women, in the treatment of spinal affections and of deformities of various kinds. Above all, we were the first to show the uses of anaesthetics - the most important advance in medicine made during the century. In our late war we taught Europe how to build, organize and manage military hospitals, and we formed the best museum in existence illustrating modern military...surgery.

Billings intentionally used an adjective that had broadly characterized American medicine since the time of Jamestown. "Practical" had long defined the American psyche and the development of its cultural and social institutions, particularly clinical medicine. However, this representation was about to undergo an astonishing reform and to resurface for the medical professional under the *raison d'être* of scientific medicine. Great changes in American medicine and surgery were soon to coincide with the sociopolitical realities of the early twentieth century. Not unexpectedly, these societal and scientific shifts were impelled by similar forces: a better and more widely educated population, bold political leadership, a compelling need to repudiate entrenched and obviously outmoded traditions, and breathtaking advances in the sciences that had previously been unimaginable.

This reformation would be successful not because physicians had fundamentally changed but because medicine and its relationship to scientific inquiry had been irrevocably altered. Sectarianism and quackery, the consequences of medical dogmatism in the United States, would no longer be tenable within the confines of scientific truth. By the time of World War I, the foundations of clinical medicine and surgery rested on demonstrable scientific proof and its attendant need for technical

1. *(facing page)* "The Four Doctors." Painted in London by the American expatriate John Singer Sargent, this monumental work (11 by 9½ feet) is considered among the highlights of formal medical portraiture in American art. Mary Garrett, a Baltimorean and benefactor of The Johns Hopkins University School of Medicine, commissioned Sargent to paint the school's first four clinical departmental chairmen and persuaded the men to meet in London to pose for the artist. Begun in the summer of 1905, the painting was not completed until the following year. It was first exhibited at London's Royal Academy. Formally presented to The Johns Hopkins University in 1907, the painting depicts William Welch, William Halsted, William Osler, and Howard Kelly gathered around a table on which rare folio volumes are strewn, and in the background is a giant Venetian globe. Welch's arm rests on a work by Petrarch. Also in the dim shadows is El Greco's painting "Saint Martin of Tours Dividing His Cloak with the Beggar." Intended to commemorate the clear success of the new medical school, actually the four physicians did not pose together more than a few times, and individual tales surround each man's likeness. For instance, legend has it that Halsted pointedly questioned Sargent's use of a blue pigment to paint the shadows under his eyes. In turn, Sargent took a strong disliking to Halsted and, in finishing his portrait, deliberately used materials that he knew would cause the likeness to inevitably fade. This tale is apparently without foundation, for restoration experts can detect no decrease in surgeon Halsted's painted luster. *(The Alan Mason Chesney Medical Archives of The Johns Hopkins Medical Institutions)*

expertise. In contrast with previously unexplainable doctrine, scientific research won out as the final arbiter between valid and invalid surgical therapies.

By the mid-1890s, surgeons had basically explored all the cavities of the body. Nevertheless, they retained a lingering sense of professional and social discomfort and continued to be perjoratively described by *nouveau* "scientific" physicians as "nonthinkers," who worked in little more than an inferior and crude manual craft. It was evident that research models, theoretical concepts, and valid clinical applications would be necessary to demonstrate the scientific basis of surgery to the public. The effort to devise new operative methods called for an even greater reliance on experimental surgery and an encouragement of it. Most importantly, a scientific basis for therapeutic surgical recommendations, consisting of empirical data, collected and analyzed according to nationally accepted rules and set apart from individual authoritative assumptions, would have to be developed.

Surgeons had to allay society's fear of the surgical unknown by presenting surgery as an accepted part of a newly established medical armamentarium. This would not be such an easy task. The immediate consequences of surgical operations, such as discomfort and associated complications, were often of more concern to patients than the positive knowledge that an operation could eliminate potentially devastating disease processes. Accordingly, the most consequential achievement by American surgeons during the late nineteenth and early twentieth century was assuring the social acceptability of surgery as a legitimate scientific endeavor and the surgical operation as a therapeutic necessity.

This ascent of scientific surgery would unify the profession and allow what had always been an art and craft to become a learned vocation for many Americans. It would finally be possible to objectively evaluate the curricula and facilities of medical schools and to determine how well surgery was taught to medical students. Standardized postgraduate surgical education and training programs could be established to help produce a cadre of scientifically knowledgable residents. In addition, the clinical competency of practicing surgeons themselves could be adequately measured, and this led to the establishment of surgical practice standards. And, in a final snub to an unscientific past, newly established basic surgical research laboratories offered the means of proving or disproving latest theories while providing a testing ground for exciting clinical breakthroughs. The era would shape American surgery for the next hundred years.

As Samuel Gross had epitomized American surgery of the past, its present and future were to be inextricably linked with the career of William Halsted (1852–1922), first professor of surgery at the recently opened Johns Hopkins Hospital. Although other surgeons of this era had greater national and even international reputations, it was Halsted, more than any other individual, who set the scientific tone for this most important period in surgical history. His work introduced a "new" American surgery, based as much on pathology and physiology as on anatomy. Halsted moved surgery from the heroics of the operating *theater* to the relative sterility of the operating *room* and the privacy of the research laboratory. American surgery was becoming a true science, and recognition of this fact and of surgery's therapeutic powers would shortly follow.

THE JOHNS HOPKINS HOSPITAL AND WILLIAM HALSTED

In May 1889, The Johns Hopkins Hospital in Baltimore opened its doors. Four years later, with the establishment of its sister institution, The Johns Hopkins School of Medicine, there was formalized a scientific center of the first rank in America and with it the beginning of organized medical research. Although it now seems axiomatic that basic scientific research is the living source from which the clinical practice of medicine derives daily sustenance, that was not always true in American medicine. It took the opening of the Johns Hopkins medical institutions to provide the necessary impetus to the logical advancement of therapeutic endeavors.

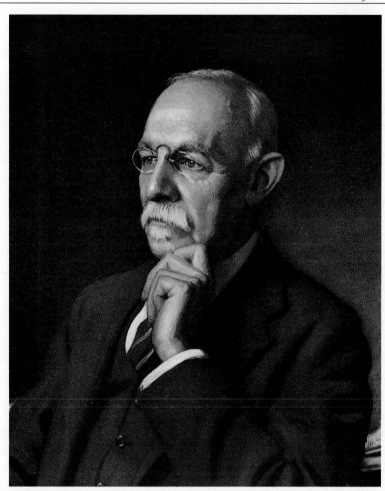

2. William Stewart Halsted, in an oil painting copy of John H. Stockdale's photograph from the winter of 1922. (*Author's Collection*)

Accordingly, from the moment that Halsted and other physicians breathed scientific life into the halls and walls of Hopkins, the United States ceased to be merely a passive recipient of European medical knowledge. From this time on, America began to collaborate fully in the worldwide solution of medical problems.

William Stewart Halsted was born in New York City on September 23, 1852, the son of a prosperous importer of wholesale dry goods. Parish registers from seventeenth-century England show that Halsted's direct family line can be reliably traced back nine generations to an Abraham Halstead (1570?–1612?), from the village of Northowram in the parish of Halifax in the western part of Yorkshire. Abraham Halstead's son Jonas Halstead (1611–1683) emigrated to what would become Stamford, Connecticut, in the early 1640s. A century later, one of Abraham's great-great grandsons, Caleb Halsted (1721–1784), for reasons that remain unknown, dropped the a in Halstead. Caleb was to become one of the paternal great-great grandfathers of William Halsted.

By the mid-eighteenth century, various members of the Halsted clan had moved to New Jersey, where they acquired approximately four hundred acres in Elizabethtown, now Elizabeth. This land, to become known as the Halsted Point Farm, later played an important role in the Revolutionary War. (It is now a site for heavy industry and consists of the land surrounding Exit 13 of the New Jersey Turnpike, near where the Goethals Bridge connects New Jersey with Staten Island.) As the closest location between Elizabethtown and Staten Island, the farm was often the site of military happenings. It was frequented by Patriot soldiers as a lookout against British marauders, but it was also easy prey to the forays of the Tories encamped on Staten Island. Such was the case in April 1779, when Caleb was taken prisoner of war, only to escape within a few days' time. Regardless of the constant plundering and chronic terrorist activities, the Halsted family remained liberal supporters of the Patriots' cause.

Caleb's eldest son, Robert (1746–1825), chose medicine as his profession and, like most physicians of that era, took all of his medical education under private preceptors, in this case in New York City. Thus, Robert Halsted became the first direct ancestor of his great-grandson William Halsted to practice medicine and surgery. The members of the Halsted clan became well known for their patriotic endeavors, and these actions were acknowledged by George Washington (1732–1799), who is said to have toasted the family at a public dinner, and by the visit of General Marquis de Lafayette (1757–1834) to one of the family homes.

In the 1820s, William Halsted's paternal grandfather, William Mills Halsted, Sr. (1788–1863), formed a business partnership with a boyhood acquaintance, Richard Townley Haines (1795–1870), who would become William's maternal grandfather. The Manhattan-based firm of Halsted, Haines & Co. proved quite successful and became a leading wholesaler of European dry goods. In 1810, William Mills Halsted, Sr., married Sarah Johnson (1791–1862), sister of Mariah Ward Johnson (1793–1840). Nine years later, Richard Townley Haines married Mariah Ward Johnson.

A curious strengthening of business ties as well as a blending of family genes occurred in 1851, when William Mills Halsted, Jr. (1825–1895), son of William Mills Halsted, Sr., married Mary Louise Haines (1829–1883), daughter of Richard Townley Haines. Not only were the bride and groom offspring of business partners, they were the children of sisters, and in 1852 this consanguineous union produced their first child, William Stewart Halsted.

Halsted enjoyed a princely youth and early adulthood, including the finest educational opportunities that the mid-nineteenth century could proffer its Anglo-Saxon upper class. Young Halsted had private elementary school tutors, attended boarding school at Phillips Andover Academy in Massachusetts, and matriculated at Yale College in 1870. He was an indifferent student at best, receiving disappointing grade point averages of 2.45, 2.35, 2.12, and 2.36 during his four years. His college years appear to have been devoted mainly to social activities, including athletics, where he excelled in football, baseball, and crew. Why Halsted decided to pursue the study of medicine remains conjectural. He never provided any definitive statements on this subject, but he did write once that during his senior year he "purchased Gray's *Anatomy* and a Dalton's *Physiology* and studied them with interest; attended a few clinics at the Yale Medical School." It should be noted, however, that Halsted's father was on the board of trustees of the College of Physicians and Surgeons in New York City and that his father's brother, Thaddeus Mills Halsted (1816–1870), was an attending physician-surgeon to the New York Hospital. Thaddeus Halsted had a childless marriage, suffered from severe rheumatism, and died of complications of diabetes. What effect this death had in later influencing Halsted to enter the College of Physicians and Surgeons is unknown, but it may have played some role.

Once in medical school, Halsted transformed his academic lifestyle completely. He became an excellent student and ranked among the top ten members of his medical school's graduating class in 1877. According to the rules of the college, each entering student was assigned as a preceptee to a faculty member. Halsted's preceptor was Henry Sands, who was professor of anatomy and a highly regarded surgeon. In addition, Halsted became student assistant to John Dalton (1825–1889), a pioneer experimental physiologist. These two men would have an important and recurring influence on Halsted's later role as an experimental surgeon. Halsted served an eighteen-month internship at Bellevue Hospital and by the summer of 1878 had completed a short stint as house surgeon to the New York Hospital.

Coming from a well-to-do New York family, Halsted had the financial means to travel to Europe to further his education. The year 1878 was the middle of the age of medical renaissance in Europe. The basic sciences of embryology, histology, and physiology and the new field of bacteriology were growing prodigiously. The German clinicians were the first to grasp the importance of the discoveries of Koch, Lister, Pasteur, and Virchow to the medical revolution. Because of this understanding, they were able to further the integration of the basic sciences with the clinical faculties that the French had begun earlier.

As the German-speaking empire grew, a great scholastic achievement was coming to fruition in the form of the richly endowed state university—highly organized, academically-free, crowded with laboratories, and ever growing. The university system was marked by certain distinctive features: freedom of teaching; the absence of any compulsion in the order, choice, and duration of studies other than those imposed by examinations; release from the division of students into classes according to fixed annual courses; academic wandering of students from one university to another; the outside lecturer system; and academic competition between teachers of similar subjects in the same and different institutions.

The national accomplishments of German universities soon became international, and from 1870 through the turn of the century their educational system became a mecca for aspiring students from all over the world. The education of any American or English scientist or physician was not considered complete until he had spent some time in a German-speaking university. So great was the attraction that it is estimated that almost 15,000 American medical personnel undertook some kind of serious study in a German university between the years 1870 and 1914.

This academic atmosphere of intense scholasticism was what Halsted encountered when he arrived on the Continent. In a letter he wrote to William Welch (1850–1934), professor of pathology at Johns Hopkins and his lifelong confidant, Halsted provided some idea of the depth and variety of his contacts and experiences during his European stay:

> In the Fall of 1878 I sailed for Europe…anatomy was my chief work…took a train arriving in Vienna…attended the clinics of Billroth…. My work with the embryologist Schenck was chiefly valuable because it led to friendly relations with Wölfler, Billroth's first assistant. We dined together not infrequently, and he gave me unrestricted entrée to the surgical wards…. What impressed me chiefly was the magnitude of the operations, the skill of Billroth and his assistants, particularly Mikulicz, and the great number of artery forceps used…leaving Vienna in the Spring of 1879 I went to Würzburg and attended the clinics of von Bergmann regularly…returned to Vienna in the Autumn…soon after Easter I deserted Vienna for Leipzig…I enjoyed the clinics of Thiersch although his operations were generally minor ones…traveled to Halle where with Volkmann I spent several profitable weeks…Volkmann invited me to his house several times…from Halle I went to Berlin, Hamburg (Schede), and I think, Kiel (Esmarch)…returned, via Paris and London, to New York early in September 1880.

The two years in Europe had a profound impression on Halsted. He could not help but notice the stark contrast between the American and German standards of surgical training. For the American surgeon of previous eras, any attempts at formal education and training were a matter of personal will with little practical opportunity. Although there were a few so-called teaching hospitals, their approach to surgical education consisted mainly of operating room work but essentially no integration of the fundamental sciences with clinical diagnosis and treatment. This inevitably meant that most surgeons were self-taught—and the self-made surgeon was not eager to hand down his hard-earned and valuable skills to younger men wishing to learn but certain to become financial competitors. The lesser material rewards of true academic life did not induce many men with a more pragmatic outlook to become the future teachers.

Conversely, the German system of surgical training had several outstanding features: a highly successful integration of the basic sciences with practical clinical teaching by full-time teachers, and unending competitive spirit among the young surgeons in training, only the brightest and most strong-willed of whom were rewarded. In this third or fourth year of medical school, the talented German student would make a choice of the field in which his interests lay. If it was surgery, he would petition for a position as demonstrator or voluntary technician in the basic

3. One of the most famous operating room scenes from all of American surgery, Halsted's "all-star operation." In October 1904, a separate surgical building was dedicated at The Johns Hopkins Hospital. To commemorate the event. Halsted gathered his senior team for a well publicized and much photographed event. John Finney describes the scene: "The Professor is operating on a patient with osteomyelitis of the upper end of the femur...He was performing a resection... [and] is holding a wooden hammer bound with metal. Jim Mitchell was giving the anesthetic, I was the first assistant, Cushing the second, Joe Bloodgood the third. Hugh Young was the instrument man." What is photographically significant about these scenes, some of which have never before been published, is the casual snapshot style of the images. They depict a table level view of the day's events and disregard sink placement and ancillary personnel, providing the viewer a feeling of being in the operating amphitheater. Several photo albums were produced to record the event, each different and containing between thirty and fifty photographs. The albums were given as souvenirs to the participants and other important hospital personnel. *(Courtesy of Stanley B. Burns, M.D., and the Burns Collection and Archive)*

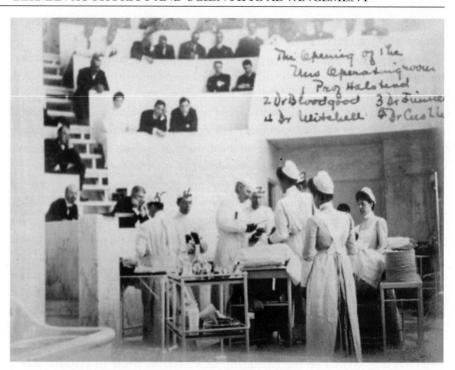

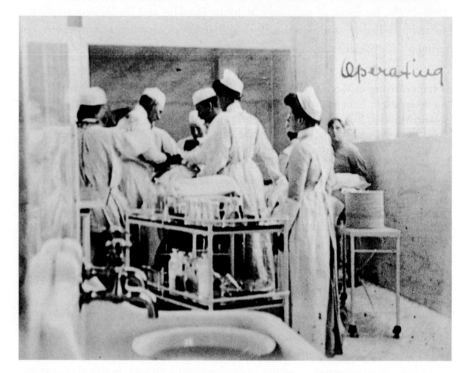

science laboratory. He would perform simple research assignments and hope to establish a reputation with the head of the institute of the specialty in which he wished to obtain his assistantship. Upon graduation and at the end of internship, which was considered an integral part of the overall medical curriculum, the young doctor would, if fortunate, be asked to become an assistant. At this point, the new doctor was thrust into the thick of an intense competition to become the first assistant. The first assistant, known as house surgeon in America at that time and called chief resident today, was selected after several years from a number of well-tried assistants. There was no regular advancement from the bottom to the top of the staff of the assistant residents, and only a small proportion of them ever ventured to entertain the hope of becoming the first assistant. Great German surgeons bred more great German surgeons, and it was these men and their schools of surgery who offered Halsted the inspiration and philosophies he needed to establish an American system of education and training in surgery.

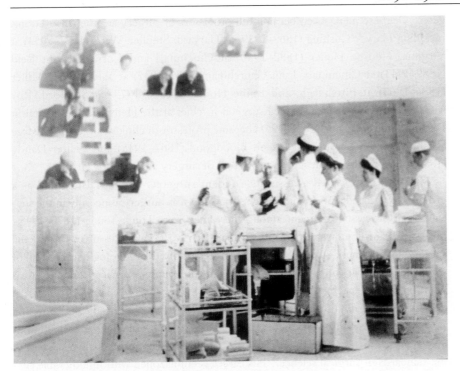

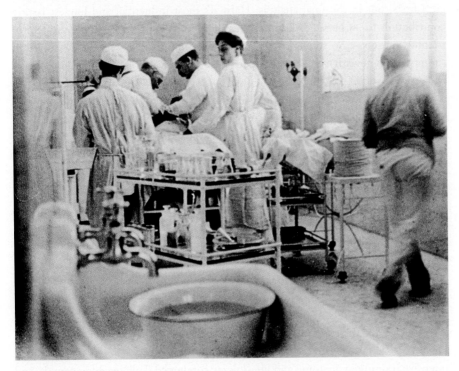

The surgical residency system that Halsted would implement at The Johns Hopkins Hospital was not an exact duplicate of the German approach but a close compromise. He insisted on a more clearly defined pattern of organization and division of duties. The residents had a larger volume of operative material at their disposal, a more intimate contact with practical clinical problems, less preoccupation with the pure basic sciences, and a concentration of responsibility and authority in them rather than the teacher.

Halsted's residency system of training surgeons was not merely the first program of its kind in America; it was unique in its primary purpose. Above all other concerns, Halsted desired to establish a school of surgery that would eventually disseminate throughout the surgical world the principles and attributes he considered sound and proper. His aim was to train surgical teachers, not merely competent operating surgeons. During the thirty-three years he spent as director of his system of surgical education and training, Halsted appointed seventeen chief resident surgeons. Of these men, seven became full professors of surgery at other institutions, including Harvey Cushing (1869–1939) at Harvard, Stephen Watts (1877–1953) at Virginia, George Heuer (1882–1950) at Cincinnati and Cornell, Mont Reid (1889–1943) at Cincinnati, John Churchman (1877–1937) at Yale, Robert Miller (1886–1960) at Pittsburgh, and Emile Holman (1890–1977) at Stanford. Roy McClure (1882–1951) was named surgeon-in-chief at the Henry Ford Hospital in Detroit, James Mitchell (1871–1961) became professor of clinical surgery at George Washington University, and Joseph Bloodgood (1867–1935) and Walter Dandy (1886–1946) remained on staff as professors of surgery at the Johns Hopkins.

Fifty-five men served as assistant resident surgeons under Halsted, and as a group, they exerted a profound influence on American surgery, especially in the specialization process. Prominent among these men were Hugh Young (1870–1945), professor of urologic surgery; William Baer (1872–1931), professor of orthopedic surgery, and Samuel Crowe (1883–1955), professor of otolaryngologic surgery, all of whom remained at Johns Hopkins and began the country's earliest residency programs in their respective specialties.

There is little doubt that Halsted achieved his stated goal of producing "not only surgeons but surgeons of the highest type, men who will stimulate the first youth of our country to study surgery and to devote their energies and their lives to raising the standards of surgical science." His career is emblazoned with innumerable surgical firsts, but in the final analysis, Halsted's most influential and longest-lasting contribution to surgery's evolution is his development of the residency system of training surgeons. So fundamental is this contribution that without it, American surgery could never have fully developed and would have remained mired in a quasi-professional state.

Halsted's many academic accomplishments were directly dependent upon his earlier European educational experiences. So much so that when he returned to New York City in September 1880, he was already imbued with a command of scientific methods, a broader educational foundation, an engaging spirit of intellectual inquiry, and a more sophisticated outlook on medicine, which was by no means limited to surgery. Halsted was immediately appointed demonstrator of anatomy at his alma mater and two years later accepted an offer by Henry Sands to become his associate in surgical practice at the Roosevelt Hospital. There, Halsted established an outpatient department, began his lifelong fascination with surgical research, and stepped onto the precipice of drug addiction.

The early 1880s were wondrous years for the young surgeon. He became attending physician to several institutions, including Bellevue, Charity, Emigrant's, and Presbyterian Hospitals. Halsted conducted extracurricular quizzes to prepare medical students for their graduation examinations. He and his associates at Roosevelt Hospital, Richard Hall (1856–1897) and Frank Hartley (1856–1913), provided intensive training in anatomy and physiology, conducted daily teaching rounds, and arranged for students to attend courses in pathology and bacteriology in William Welch's laboratory at Bellevue Hospital. From a clinical and technical standpoint, Halsted was known as a bold and original surgeon. His career was on the fast track, and he counted among his close friends some of the most eminent names in New York surgery, including William Bull and Lewis Stimson.

In September 1884, an event took place in Heidelberg, Germany, that would have a profound effect on both the professional and the personal life of William Halsted. A young German surgeon, Carl Koller (1857–1944), reported on the use of cocaine to anesthetize the cornea and conjunctiva. Koller's momentous discovery was reported back to American physicians by Henry Noyes (1832–1900) in a short letter published in the New York *Medical Record*. The letter excited great interest in that city's professional community, and demand for the alkaloid derivative of the coca leaf skyrocketed. Halsted, Hall, and James Corning (1855–1923) began performing experiments with the drug and demonstrated that it could be used to anesthetize deeper structures via injection into all parts of the body. This local infiltration anesthesia gained rapid popularity, since it was simple and required minimal amounts of cocaine. Hall wrote the first article of this research group in December 1884. He noted that "in a number of experiments made by Dr. Halsted and myself, we have found that, injected subcutaneously into the leg or forearm…it will cause anaesthesia for a distance of two or three inches below the point of injection…it is obvious that, when the limits of safety have been determined, it may find very wide application." The Roosevelt group went on to demonstrate the superiority of intradermal as opposed to hypodermal injection, the efficacy of dilute solutions of the analgesic drug when administered in large quantities, and the prolongation of effect of the drug when the circulation of the part is reduced. Most importantly, they demonstrated that sectional infiltration of a sensory or mixed nerve dulls sensation throughout the peripheral distribution of the nerve—the neuroregional method of anesthesia.

Despite having accumulated reams of experimental data on local cocaine anesthesia, Halsted himself would write only one short article on the subject. Yet, from January 1882 through March 1885 he had already authored or presented twenty-one scientific papers. There was a simple explanation for this sudden apparent lack of writing ethic. It is a poignant irony of surgical progress that after repeated self-experimentation, both Halsted and Hall had unwittingly become addicted to cocaine. "Practical Comments on the Use and Abuse of Cocaine" (1885) is so poorly written and almost incoherent that it contrasts markedly with the clarity and precision of Halsted's other writings.

As the effects of addiction became worse, Halsted was threatened with professional extinction. In periods of agitation engendered by the drug, he turned to morphine and alcohol. His attendance at meetings declined, and by April 1885, Halsted could no longer deliver a series of lectures in competition for the chair of surgery at his alma mater. His health continued its downward spiral, and in February 1886, he took an extended sailing trip to the Windward Islands in the hope of restoring his former self. With virtually no information available about cocaine addiction and little in the way of effective interventional treatment, the effort was to no avail. In May, with the encouragement of his friends and family, he voluntarily committed himself to the Butler Hospital in Providence, Rhode Island, a leading mental hospital that included alcoholics and drug addicts on its patient lists.

Halsted was discharged in November 1886 after seven months of inconclusive treatment. It is likely that during this time he was weaned from cocaine but became dependent on morphine—a dependency that would last for the rest of his life. Aware

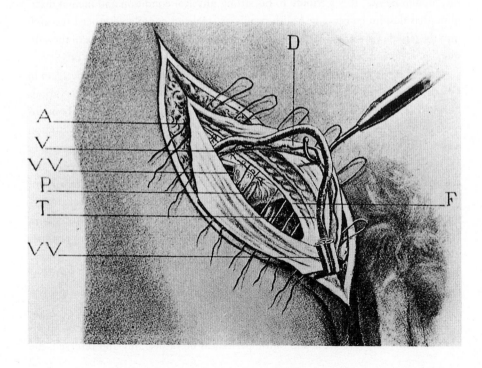

4. Halsted's "radical cure of inguinal hernia" remains among the most misunderstood of the surgical operations he devised. This drawing (*The Johns Hopkins Hospital Bulletin*, vol. 4, pages 17–24, 1893) shows the aponeurosis of the external oblique muscle being readied for reapproximation with interrupted silk sutures. The remaining blood vessels of the "skeletonized" spermatic cord (retracted by the curved instrument) are then transposed (i.e., placed above the external oblique layer), forming the Halsted I repair. (*Author's Collection*)

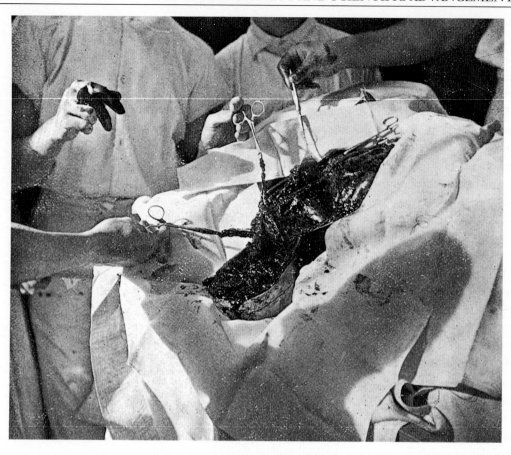

5. The first published photograph (*Johns Hopkins Hospital Reports*, vol. 4, pages 297–350, 1894–1895) of an actual Halsted radical mastectomy, taken just prior to the final severance of the breast, pectoral muscles, and axillary contents. The illustration is also significant because it is the earliest visual confirmation that members of Halsted's operating team were utilizing two finger rubber cots during the conduct of a surgical procedure. (*Author's Collection*)

of his family's recent financial reversals, cognizant of his poor health, and realizing that his career in New York City was over, Halsted accepted an invitation by his old friend William Welch to come to Baltimore to work in his newly established medical research laboratory at The Johns Hopkins University. It is interesting, in view of Halsted's later prominence and surgical accolades, that when he first went to Baltimore, it was neither to accept a professorship nor to assume chairmanship of a department. It was simply in response to the offer of a friend who wished to help him in dire times. All was not well, however, and in April 1887, Halsted reentered Butler Hospital and remained at the institution for nine months, until the last day of 1887. His problems having supposedly been treated, Halsted was listed as recovering from the "opium habit." It is a tribute to his strong physical condition and mental discipline that despite continuing health problems, Halsted completed crucial research into the circular suturing of intestines, which emphasized the importance of the submucosal layer to the integrity of an anastomosis, during the first months of 1887.

Halsted returned to Baltimore in January 1888 and began working once again in Welch's laboratory. He even began to treat patients and perform surgery at various hospitals around the city. It was his hope to become a staff member of the about-to-open Johns Hopkins Hospital. Finding a professor of surgery for the new institution was difficult, and finally in February 1889, in response to the unyielding urgings of Welch, Halsted was appointed surgeon-in-chief to the outpatient dispensary and acting surgeon to the hospital. Later that year, he was made associate professor, but he was not named professor of surgery until 1892. Regardless of historical conjecture and innuendo, it is a fact that Halsted continued to use morphine throughout his life. Other than the definite change from the former *joie de vivre* of his personality, there was no apparent physical or mental deterioration despite his forty-year drug addiction. From 1889 until his death in 1922, Halsted directed a department that produced an impressive array of surgical talent, which in turn brought his own philosophy to chairs of surgery throughout the United States.

Halsted never authored a textbook of surgery, a monograph, or a treatise. All his written contributions were made to the periodical literature. Shy and reserved, the introverted surgeon had little in-depth contact with his professional colleagues. Visitors to his clinic were greeted with utmost "European" courtesy, but Halsted remained reticent and aloof. He always appeared lost in thought, and he studiously avoided personal contact. Despite his demeanor as a professional recluse, Halsted's achievements were overwhelming in number and scope. By 1889, he had devised a new operation for the treatment of inguinal hernia. During the 1890s, he wrote a series of papers describing a method of radical mastectomy as treatment for breast cancer and also performed the first successful operation for a primary cancer of the ampulla of Vater. Concurrent with his investigations into breast cancer, Halsted showed that optimum healing in large wounds such as mastectomy dissections was most easily obtained by avoiding hematoma formation. In 1892, he completed the first successful ligation of the left subclavian artery. A decade and a half later, Halsted introduced a metal band in place of a ligature for the occlusion of arterial aneurysms. In 1909, he performed some of the earliest work on the autotransplantation and iso-transplantation of parathyroid glands. He is also credited with being one of the first surgeons in the world to introduce the use of rubber gloves during surgical operations. His name is eponymically associated with many things, including Halsted's law (transplanted tissue will grow only if there is a lack of that tissue in the host) and Halsted's suture (a stitch placed through the subcuticular fascia, used for exact skin approximation).

Halsted's search for perfection in his surgical work was mirrored in many aspects of his personal life. In matters of dress he was especially fastidious. Shoes, boots, shirts, and suits were all hand-made by tailors in Europe. Halsted was known to have been a true gourmet, and a typical dinner at his home might include caviar, roast oysters, terrapin stew, and quail. He married Caroline Hampton, one of his operating room nurses, in 1890. They remained childless and were said to have spent much time apart, each having separate apartments within their large three-story house at 1201 Eutaw Place in Baltimore. Lengthy summer vacations (up to four and five months) were enjoyed either at a second home in Cashiers in the mountains of North Carolina or, for Halsted alone, by making trips to Europe to visit the continent's great surgical centers and their renowned surgeons such as Theodor Kocher (1841–1917), Anton von Eiselsberg (1860–1939), Erwin Payr (1871–1946), Hermann Küttner (1870–1932), and Eugen Enderlen (1865–1940).

In the latter years of his life, Halsted suffered through repeated attacks of severe chest and abdominal pain, initially thought to be angina pectoris but eventually diagnosed as cholecystitis. In September 1919, Richard Follis, one of his former chief residents, performed a cholecystectomy and choledocholithotomy. Halsted obtained considerable relief for a period of time, but in the fall of 1921, pain began anew and within ten months was associated with unrelenting jaundice. In August 1922,

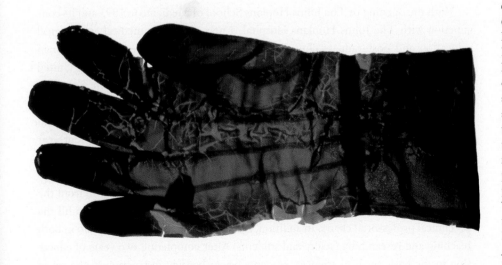

6. One of the original rubber surgical gloves (preserved in lucite) designed by William Halsted and fabricated by the Goodyear Rubber Company of New York City. Although Halsted neither invented rubber gloves nor originated their employment in surgery, he was among the first to promote their widespread application. Halsted became interested in the use of rubber gloves as a method of protecting the hands of his favorite surgical nurse ("the nurse in charge of my operating room complained that the solutions of mercuric chloride produced a dermatitis of her arms and hands"). This nurse, Caroline Hampton ("she was an unusually efficient woman"), later became Mrs. Halsted. (*The Alan Mason Chesney Medical Archives of The Johns Hopkins Medical Institutions*)

Halsted required additional surgery, this time by George Heuer and Mont Reid, who were summoned back from Cincinnati. Another common duct stone was removed, but the postoperative course was marked by hematemesis and Vincent's disease of the oral cavity and pharynx. Pneumococcal pneumonia developed, and Halsted expired on September 7, 1922. Following cremation, his ashes were placed in the family crypt in the Greenwood Cemetery in Brooklyn, New York.

William Halsted was a complex personality and remains the best-known historical personage in all of American surgery. The impact of this remarkable man, the new hospital and medical school in Baltimore, and his surgical residents was widespread. Halsted's influence, while constant, was most keenly felt in the years 1910 to 1945, when his former residents were at the peak of their influence, spreading change, raising standards, and increasing the flow of highly trained surgeons to communities throughout the United States.

Halsted showed that research based on anatomical and physiological principles, and often employing animal experimentation, made it possible to develop new operative procedures and perform them clinically with outstanding results. He proved, to an often leery profession and public, that an unamibiguous sequence could be constructed from the laboratories of basic surgical research to the clinical operating room. Most importantly, for American surgery's own self-respect, Halsted demonstrated during the turn-of-the-century renaissance in American medical education that departments of surgery could command a faculty whose stature was equal in importance and prestige to those of the other more academic or research-oriented fields, such as anatomy, bacteriology, biochemistry, internal medicine, pathology, and physiology. As a single individual, Halsted developed and disseminated a new system of surgery so characteristic that it is dignified with the phrase "school of surgery." More to the point, Halsted's methods revolutionized the world of surgery and earned his work the epithet "Halstedian principles," which remains a widely acknowledged and accepted scientific imprimatur. Halsted subordinated technical brilliance and speed of dissection to a meticulous and safe, although sometimes slow, performance. As a direct result, Halsted's efforts did much to bring about American surgery's self-sustaining transformation from therapeutic subservience to clinical necessity. With a bit of literary license, H. L. Mencken (1880–1956), the Baltimore-based critic of standards of taste and culture in the United States, wrote of Halsted:

> He was one of the first surgeons to employ courtesy in surgery, to show any consideration for the insides of a man.... The old method was to slit a man from the chin down, take out his bowels and spread them on a towel while you sorted them. Halsted held that if you touched an intestine with your finger you injured it and the patient suffered the effects of the injury. That was new doctrine when he began.... He was gentle - and a little inhuman. He had to be because he was so sensitive.

With the opening of The Johns Hopkins School of Medicine in 1893 and its conjunction with The Johns Hopkins Hospital, a new model for medical and surgical education and postgraduate clinical training emerged. Patterned after a German prototype, The Hopkins, more than any other medical institution in the United States, represented the *sine qua non* for further efforts at medical reform. From the outset, the new medical school required of its matriculants a baccalaureate degree or its equivalent, with emphasis on preliminary education in the basic sciences and modern languages. Both men and women students were accepted, and a four-year graded curriculum was provided. The faculty in the preclinical or basic medical sciences (anatomy, pathology, pharmacology, physiological chemistry, and physiology) were employed on a full-time salaried basis. This was a distinct departure from the American tradition of employing local practitioners on a part-time basis to fill the preclinical professorial chairs. In addition, there was an emphasis on freedom in both teaching and research by faculty and students. After completing two years of education in the basic medical sciences, students began bedside instruction in the art of

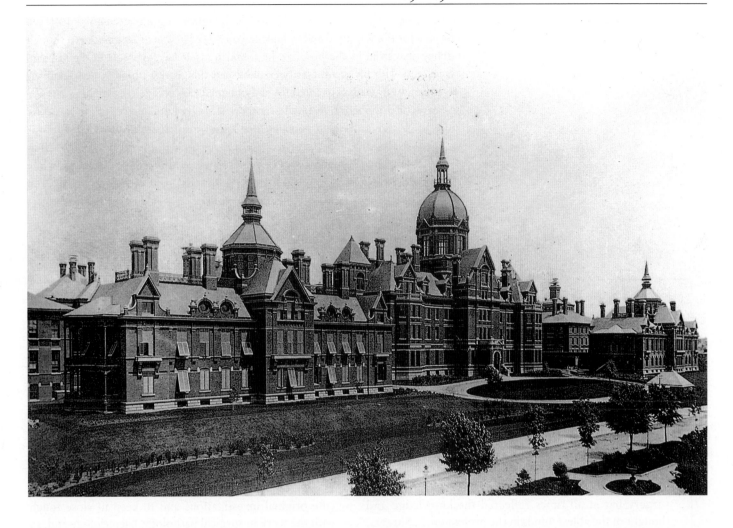

medicine and were given close daily contact with numerous patients. By their senior year, all students were spending considerable time, including nights, working the wards of The Johns Hopkins Hospital, thereby taking an active role in the decision making process of patient care.

Thus, it was from among the best medical students in the country that William Halsted was able to build his residency program. Exceptional young men were being brought to his attention, particularly those who wished to pursue a career in surgical research. The world of surgical possibilities had changed dramatically and the stakes were high for these ambitious young clinicians. Surgery now represented an activist or "intrusive" style of practice, with decreasing emphasis on old-time conservative or "expectant" management techniques.

This new surgical philosophy was exemplified by changing styles of practice at the country's first permanent orthopedic institution, New York's Hospital for the Ruptured and Crippled, presently known as the Hospital for Special Surgery. James Knight (1810–1887) founded the hospital and was its surgeon-in-chief from 1863 to 1887. A graduate of the Washington Medical College in Baltimore (1832), Knight studied with Valentine Mott and decided to devote himself to the emerging surgical specialty of orthopedic surgery. Knight was a physician-surgeon who assumed a paternalistic attitude toward his patients and their stay in his institution. He even went so far as to live in the hospital and serve as "father" to an extended health care family. Knight placed minor emphasis on operative procedures but a great deal on health reform, including diet, exercise, fresh air, bandages, and mechanical devices. In Knight's only textbook, *Orthopaedia or a Practical Treatise on the Aberrations of the Human Form* (1874), he advocates using the so-called conservative or expectant plan of treatment for joint lesions, as contrasted with surgical intervention. In a rather extensive description of lateral curvature of the spine, there is little in the way of operative therapy; instead, only the Knight spinal brace.

7. When The Johns Hopkins Hospital was opened in 1889, the trustees hired Frederick Gutekunst (1831–1917), a well-known Philadelphia photographer, to document the new buildings. Gutekunst took many of the pictures before the structures were occupied, so there is a certain lifeless quality to his work despite the fact that the heart of any health care complex is its patients and workers. This wide-angle view shows the hospital, taken from Broadway looking southeast. (*The Alan Mason Chesney Medical Archives of The Johns Hopkins Medical Institutions*)

In 1884, Virgil Gibney (1847–1927), Knight's second-in-command at the Hospital for the Ruptured and Crippled, wrote *The Hip and its Diseases*. Even though Gibney also lived in the hospital, he found himself having frequent clinical disagreements with his mentor. Gibney published this work without Knight's knowledge. Knight immediately asked for and obtained his protégé's resignation. Gibney an energetic orthopedist, believed ever more strongly in the power of the surgeon's knife to change a diseased person's life. Following Knight's death, Gibney was implored to return to the hospital as its surgeon-in-chief. He accepted, and within five years, the annual numbers of surgical operations dramatically increased while lengths of stay decreased. The old regimen of hospital stays lasting months or even years, as part of the "expectant" treatment of diseases, would never again be toler-

THE TRAINING OF THE SURGEON

Pain, haemorrhage, infection, the three great evils which had always embittered the practice of surgery and checked its progress, were, in a moment, in a quarter of a century (1846–1873) robbed of their terrors. A new era had dawned; and in the 30 years which have elapsed since...probably more has been accomplished to place surgery on a truly scientific basis than in all the centuries which had preceded this wondrous period.... Tempted to belittle by comparisons the performance of our progenitors, we should remember that the condition of surgery has at all times reflected the knowledge and thought of the ablest minds in the profession.... Surgery, like other branches of the healing art, has followed in its progress zigzag paths, often difficult to trace. Now it has seemed to advance by orderly steps or through the influence of some master mind even by bounds...

The times are changing, and we have learned in our own time, indeed within a decade, how superior in all respects is the endowed university medical school to the old-time proprietary school.... Although we now have in the United States several (five or six) moderately well-endowed medical schools with a university connection, the problem of the education of our surgeons is still unresolved. Our present methods do not by any means suffice for their training.... Do we require stronger proof of the inadequacy of these methods in producing young surgeons than is presented by the so-called sacrifices which our young men today are willing, nay, most eager, to make in order to obtain a training which seems even to them not only desirable but absolutely essential for success of a high order?

Here I may be permitted to instance conditions which have evolved in a natural way at The Johns Hopkins Hospital, where the plan of organization of the staff differs from that which obtains elsewhere in this country. The surgical staff consists of nine men, eight internes and one externe. The externe is an assistant in surgical pathology.... Four of the internes serve for one year, only the honor men of each class at graduation being entitled to these positions; but the permanent, so-called, consists of four men, the house surgeon and three in line of preferment.... Great care is exercised in the filling of the vacancy on the permanent staff, which occurs once in two or three years, and advancement is not guaranteed to the appointee. The House Surgeon's term of service is still optional. He receives a salary: the other assistants are not paid. The assistants are expected in addition to their ward and operating duties, to prosecute original investigations and to keep in close touch with the work in surgical pathology, bacteriology and, so far as possible physiology...

The average term of service in this hospital is at present eight years - six years as assistant, in preparation for the position, and two years of service as actual house surgeon. Adding to these the four years in the medical school and the junior and senior years in college...the prospective house surgeon has to contemplate 12 or 14 years of hard work, very hard work, in order to secure this prize to which in this country of necessity only a very few at present attain. Thus far the success of the three or four men who have received this training is so convincing that the very best graduates of our own and other schools are eager for the opportunity to be tested as to their fitness to rise to the position; and I know from applications which have been made to me this year that men of the desired quality would gladly serve 10 years on the surgical staff in order to obtain the experience which the house surgeonship and the training leading to it affords...

It will be objected that this is too long an apprenticeship, that the young surgeon will be stale, his enthusiasm gone before he has completed his arduous term of service. These positions are not for those who so soon weary of the study of their profession, and it is a fact that the zeal and industry of these young assistants seem to increase as they advance in years and as their knowledge

ated. To formally demonstrate his disavowal of past practices, Gibney refused to take up permanent residence in the hospital.

Halsted, the surgical scientist, and Gibney, the surgical clinician, were no longer content to only guide and monitor a patient along a multidimensional path to mental, physical, and social health. Surgery, by its very nature, was meant to be interventional. This surgical era would finally prove that point. Painless, aseptic surgery had far more to offer patients than the simple bandages and braces of times past. Consequently, the results of scientific surgery were being noticeably redefined by increasingly narrow but technically more forbidding operations. This meant that technology would play an ever more important role in the advancement of the surgical sciences.

---

and responsibilities become greater. Nowhere certainly can a surgeon in a given period acquire so much, mature so rapidly, as in a hospital with an active and properly-conducted service. The time devoted to the training in surgery of those who hope to be teachers should not be curtailed, but young men contemplating the study of surgery should as early in life as possible seek to acquire knowledge of the subjects fundamental to the study of their profession.

It was our intention originally to adopt as closely as feasible the German plan, which, in the main, is the same for all the principal clinics of the German universities.... It is a matter of great satisfaction and pride to a professor of surgery to have supplied from his staff one or more university chairs.... The professor of surgery in Germany is usually a man of great influence and power. His affiliations, his responsibilities, his knowledge of surgery and the allied sciences, and often of art, of music, of literature and of the world's affairs, produce a type of man which his country may well contemplate with pride.

America, too, in spite of discouraging circumstances has produced great surgeons, but it is to be deplored that here conditions prevail which hitherto have not encouraged, if they have not actually prohibited, special development [of surgery]. I have known professional chairs in some of the principal medical schools of this country to go actually a-begging - a-begging, of course, only of men who would adorn the position.... The faults of our own system of educating surgeons begin almost at the bottom and continue to the very top. I am considering only the training of the very best men, those who aspire to the higher career in surgery. On graduation they become hospital internes, but their term in the hospital is only one and a half, occasionally two years, only a little longer than the term of hospital service required in Germany of every applicant for the medical degree...the internes suffer not only from inexperience, but also from over-experience. He has in his short term of service responsibilities which are too great for him; he becomes accustomed to act without preparation, and he acquires

a confidence in himself and a self-complacency which may be useful in a time of emergency, but which tend to blind him to his inadequacy and to warp his career.... But much as the interne suffers from the brevity of his hospital experience, the hospital suffers more and the surgeon most. Every important hospital should have on its resident staff of surgeons at least one who is well able to deal not only with any emergency that may arise and to perform any operation known to surgery, but also to recognize the gross appearances of all the ordinary pathological tissues and lesions...

Reforms, the need of which must be apparent to every teacher of surgery in this country, must come on the side both of the hospital and of the university.... It is eminently desirable, if not absolutely essential, that the medical school should control a hospital of its own. There should be an organization of the hospital staff...providing the requisite opportunities for the prolonged and thorough training of those preparing for the higher careers in medicine and surgery, and permitting the establishment of close and mutually stimulating relations between chief and assistants...

While it has been my main purpose to call attention to certain defects in the existing methods of medical education, especially in the opportunities for the advanced training of surgeons in this country, I would not be understood to minimize or to decry the great achievements of American surgery. Courage, ingenuity, dexterity, resourcefulness are such prominent characteristics of our countrymen that it would have been surprising if from the labors of her many earnest and devoted teachers and practitioners there had not resulted contributions to the science and art of surgery which have carried the fame of American surgery throughout the civilized world.

William Halsted: The annual address in medicine delivered at the commencement exercises of the Yale University School of Medicine. *The Johns Hopkins Hospital Bulletin*, vol. 15, pages 267–275, 1904.

TECHNOLOGICAL PROGRESS AND
THE RISE OF HOSPITAL-BASED SURGERY

These years witnessed an enormous increase in the amount, scope, and technical daring of surgery. Improvements in diagnostic skills, led by development of the technology-based x-ray, spurred the advance. In early November 1895, Wilhelm Roentgen (1845–1922), professor of physics at Würzburg, Germany discovered what he termed x-rays. Roentgen noted the amazing property of x-rays to penetrate virtually all substances and the particularly intriguing fact that they were able to detail the bones of the human hand. His findings were so startling, and their expected value so great, that within two months a verbatim translation of Roentgen's paper was reprinted in the United States.

The discovery of x-rays must have seemed like a godsend to the American surgeon. After the assassination of President Garfield, much of the controversy surrounding his surgical care centered on the inability of the President's surgeons to physically locate the bullet. Although numerous electrical and magnetic devices were subsequently developed to help locate foreign objects in the human body, all proved technically unreliable. Since Roentgen's initial x-ray plate showed the bones of his wife's hand and the metal ring she was wearing, it is not surprising that surgeons were the first group of clinicians to appreciate the clinical value of x-rays. They correctly believed that x-rays could be useful in demonstrating pathologic problems of the skeleton and the localization of metal objects in the body. So great had the fas-

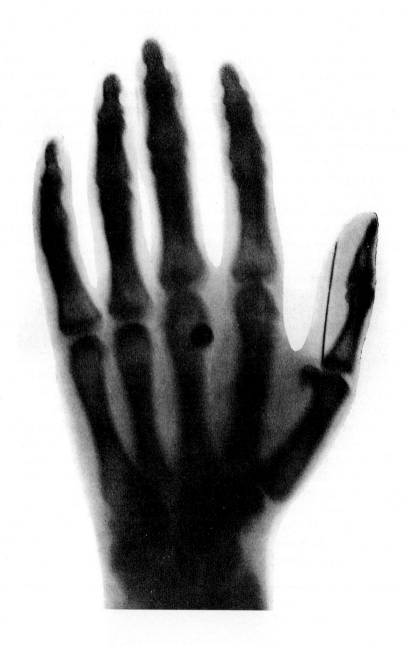

8. In March 1896, the first detailed contributions regarding the use of roentgenography in the practice of United States medicine appeared in the *American Journal of the Medical Sciences*. Writing on the surgical aspects of the new discovery, William Keen presented this fuzzy, but nonetheless distinct, roentgenogram of a "hand and wrist of a cadaver, into the palmar aspect of which a needle and two buckshot were thrust." (*Author's Collection*)

cination with radiographs become that as early as the March 6, 1896, edition of *Science*, Henry Cattell (1862–1936), of the medical faculty of the University of Pennsylvania, editorially invoked:

> The manifold uses to which Roentgen's discovery may be applied in medicine are so obvious that it is even now questionable whether a surgeon would be morally justified in performing a certain class of operation without having first seen pictured by these rays the field of his work, a map, as it were, of the unknown country he is to explore.... Our large hospitals where numerous accident cases are brought should have in the near future a plant sufficient to prepare skiagraphic reproductions at short notice.

Surgeons were so involved with the early experimentation and utilization of x-rays that the sole heading under "Roentgen Rays" in the 1896 *Index Medicus* is "See also Surgery (Diagnosis)." By March of that year the first detailed contributions regarding the use of roentgenography in the practice of American medicine were presented in print. Of these initial reports, a chapter by William Keen in Frederick Dennis's (1850–1934) four-volume *System of Surgery* had the greatest impact on the introduction of roentgenography into clinical diagnosis and therapeutics. Dennis, professor of the principles and practice of surgery at Bellevue Hospital Medical College, had asked Keen to contribute a chapter on the newly discovered x-ray and its use in surgery. Keen's contribution constitutes the concluding chapter in the final volume. Published in July 1896, the work represents the first American medical or surgical textbook to contain an account of x-rays, including actual roentgenograms. Keen was ecstatic with what he believed to be the potential for this new technology:

> It is very possible that we may hereafter be able...to skiagraph the viscera, and if so to determine the presence of calculi and of foreign bodies.... I think it not unlikely that we shall be able to determine the existence, size, and other facts in relation to abdominal tumors...we may be able during pregnancy to determine the position of the foetus and any abnormalities should they exist...thus far, all attempts to skiagraph the brain have been unavailing, and I fear may always prove to be such.... I think it not unlikely that the thoracic viscera may be skiagraphed.... The most important and useful applications of the x-rays, thus far, has been in the diagnosis both of diseases and injuries of the bones.... Gall-stones are quite permeable to the rays, and therefore their presence cannot be determined either in the gallbladder or in the ducts, but I think it probable that this difficulty may be overcome.... It is very greatly to be regretted that the new rays have, apparently, no deleterious influences upon the growth of bacteria.

During late spring of 1896, the most active American proselyte for x-rays was the Philadelphia surgeon De Forest Willard (1846–1910). Willard was a pioneering orthopedic surgeon who served as professor at the University of Pennsylvania. He provided the fellows of both the American Surgical Association and the American Orthopedic Association with their first demonstrations of roentgenograms in May. That summer another detailed report on x-rays was authored by James William White (1850–1916), also of the surgical faculty at the University of Pennsylvania, who concluded that roentgenography "will be an essential part of the surgical outfit of all hospitals."

By mid-fall 1896, it was becoming evident that the usefulness of x-rays for clinical purposes would extend far beyond just surgical conditions and include the treatment of various other disease processes. This is most obvious in the continuing work of White, who commenced in October 1896 the earliest recorded trial of x-ray therapy for treatment of cancer in the United States. His findings were incorporated into a lengthy paper presented at the 1897 session of the American Surgical Association. With the coming of the 1896–1897 winter season, Maurice Richardson (1851–1912), visiting surgeon to the Massachusetts General Hospital, writing in the influential *Medical News*, concluded that "no surgical consulting-room is fully equipped without an apparatus for X-ray investigation...it is as essential to the surgeon as the mirror to the laryngologist, or the stethoscope to the general practitioner."

In a matter of one year's time, the clinical use of x-rays had passed beyond simple demonstrations of skeletal abnormalities or the detection of metal objects in the body. Although American surgeons would no longer remain in the forefront of roentgenologic advances, the advent of technologies applicable to surgical practice had begun to affect the surgeon's *modus operandi* in ways previously thought unimaginable. Science and technology helped change physician's expectations as much as they did those of the public. Accordingly, many general practitioners were becoming just as impressed as their patients with the achievements of modern surgery. Surgery, which had always played a disproportionately dramatic role in the world of medicine, could finally and legitimately claim a potential for healing that overshadowed the tentative and many times inconclusive efforts of internal medicine. Surgery represented the spirit of the new century, and before long, surgical admissions far outnumbered medical admissions to the nation's rapidly expanding hospital system.

The heroic and dangerous nature of surgery might have been seemed appealing in less scientifically sophisticated times. But now, surgeons were to be courted for personal attributes beyond their unmitigated technical boldness. With the turn of the century, surgeons found themselves reigning supreme in the new health care delivery environment. A trend toward hospital-based surgery was increasingly evident, due in equal parts to new technically demanding operations and to modern hospital physical structures within which surgeons could work more effectively. The increasing complexity and effectiveness of aseptic surgery, the diagnostic necessity of the x-ray and clinical laboratory, the convenience of twenty-four-hour nursing, and the availability of capable surgical residents living within a hospital were making the hospital operating room the most plausible and convenient place for a surgical operation to be completed.

The rise of America's hospital system is closely related to growth in volume of surgical work of the late nineteenth and early twentieth centuries. The staggering surgical workload allowed the basis for expansion and profit in hospital care. At the Pennsylvania Hospital, for example, over 850 operations were performed in the year between May 1899 and May 1900. This was more than the total number of operations completed at that institution during the entire first half of the nineteenth century. Before 1900, most American hospitals held no special advantages over the home setting. Infections, which periodically swept through a hospital, made many surgeons nervous about sending their patients to such a place. Even after asepsis had been accepted and the concept of cleanliness had become part of routine hospital life, the lingering image of the hospital as a place to die, especially for the indigent, remained part of American culture. All this would have to change as surgical proce-

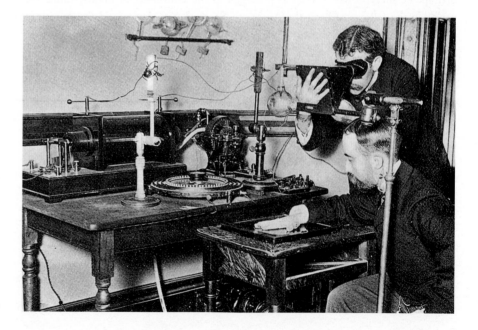

9. At the end of the nineteenth century it was not uncommon to find authors including photographs of themselves in their books. In this halftone photograph William Morton (1846–1920) and Edwin Hammer are shown in their laboratory conducting a roentgenologic experiment. Their text, *The X Ray or Photography of the Invisible and its Value in Surgery* (1896) was the first American treatise to describe and evaluate Wilhelm Roentgen's momentous discovery. *(Courtesy of Stanley B. Burns, M.D., and The Burns Collection and Archive)*

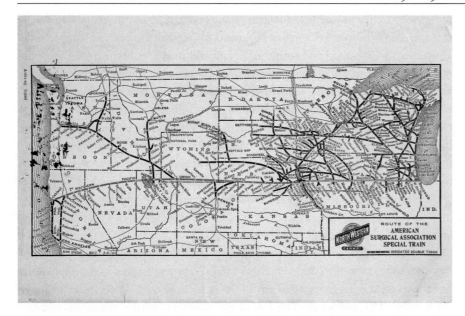

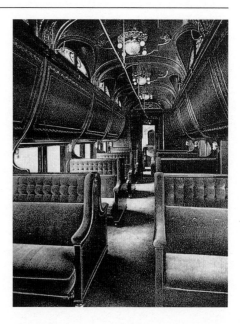

dures became technically more demanding. Thus, the hospital setting became central to the therapeutic successes of the early twentieth-century surgeon.

The "kitchen surgery" of the nineteenth century gave way to hospital-based surgery. Busy practitioners found it too inefficient and too costly in lost work time to travel to patients' homes. At first, to accommodate desires for privacy and fears of the hospital, more well-to-do surgeons built their own "medical boarding houses." It was not unusual in large urban areas for numerous such structures to dot the city landscape. Well-known surgeons, exemplified by Henry Marcy in Boston, Howard Kelly in Baltimore, and John Murphy in Chicago, owned their own facilities and completed much of their private operative work there. In rural America, groups of physicians joined together to build small community hospitals under private ownership. This socioeconomic phenomenon of proprietary hospitals was directly related to the emerging profitablity of institutional care that resulted from increasing numbers of surgical cases. In 1870, just under two hundred hospitals existed in the United States; by 1910, the number of acute care facilities topped 4,000.

It was obvious to both hospital superintendents and the whole of medicine that acute-care institutions were becoming a necessity more for the surgeon than for the physician. As a consequence, increasing numbers of hospitals went to great lengths to supply their surgical staffs with the very finest facilities in which to complete operations. For centuries, surgical operations had been performed under the illumination of sunlight and/or candles. Now, however, electric lights installed in operating rooms offered a far more reliable and unwavering source of illumination. Surgery became more efficient because operations could be completed on cloudy summer mornings as well as cold winter afternoons. Spring and autumn were no longer the seasons of the surgeon. There was no further need for an Addinell Hewson (1828–1889), surgeon to the Pennsylvania Hospital, to author a pamphlet *On the Influences of the Weather Over the Results of Surgical Operations* (1868). The simple fact was that major hospitals could afford complicated electric wiring and power generators before most private homeowners or even medical boarding houses could. In addition, the complicated and expensive equipment that permitted visualization of hard-to-see body parts could only be found in well-funded institutions.

The wooing of the surgeon based on his need for new technologies is evident in the era's surgical textbooks. Beginning with Albert Ochsner's (1858–1925) *The Organization, Construction and Management of Hospitals* (1907), it seemed as if surgeons were at the forefront of the hospital planning and construction business. In their eight–volume *American Practice of Surgery* (1906–1911), Joseph Bryant (1845–1914) and Albert Buck (1842–1922) included a chapter more than 200 pages long on administrative surgical work. Surgical texts no longer solely described clin-

10. The 1905 meeting of the American Surgical Association took place on July 5, 6, and 7 at the Hotel St. Francis in San Francisco. This was to be the organization's first meeting west of St. Louis, and since the annual session of the American Medical Association was to be held a few days later in Portland, Oregon, the many surgeon and physician members of both organizations decided to reserve a "Special Overland Limited Train" to transport them from Chicago to San Francisco. It was the height of sumptuous rail travel, and a colored brochure *(left)* and itinerary was specially issued by the Chicago, Union Pacific, and North-Western Line for the occasion. Among the surgical travelers were Arthur Bevan, Edward Martin, John Murphy, and Albert Ochsner, all scheduled to leave Chicago on the evening of June 29, with stops in such cities as Cedar Rapids, Des Moines, Omaha, Cheyenne, Laramie, and Sacramento and an anticipated arrival "less than seventy hours" later in San Francisco. Full details of the "exclusively first class" train, including pictures of the sleeping, dining, library, observation, and parlor cars *(right)*, were provided. The round-trip rate, inclusive of the stopover in Portland was $67.50. A sleeping car was an additional $14 for a double berth, $39.50 for a compartment, and $53 for a drawing room. *(Historical Collections, College of Physicians of Philadelphia)*

ical problems. They were now involved with commenting on the actual day-to-day management of hospitals. Christian Holmes (1857–1920), professor of surgery at the University of Cincinnati and author of Bryant and Buck's "Administrative" chapter, thought nothing of discussing such bureaucratic topics as "light," "window shades, screens, etc.," "heating and ventilating," "chapel, morgue, and pathological laboratories," and "the kitchen and service building." Holmes was so concerned that his chapter might be perceived as inadequate that in a beginning footnote he cautioned the reader to realize that "the writer has found it impracticable...to discuss more than a few of the aspects of the broad subject of hospitals and their management...it was not possible...to develop as fully...those aspects of the problem which are of special importance to the surgeon." One thing stands out in Holmes's presentation: he was adamant that the largest and best hospitals of the country, including those of "municipal foundation and those erected and maintained by private charity" be under the care of "medical superintendents" and furthermore that "there is no further discussion as to the relative merits of physicians and laymen as hospital superintendents and no suggestion that any of the latter be chosen as successors to any of the former." Throughout the first half of the twentieth century, physicians and surgeons ran American hospitals with marginal outside interference from boards of trustees and lay administrators.

Holmes described the proper surgical pavilion as "wellnigh perfectly adapted to the present status of operative surgery." The operating room, including an amphitheater if the "hospital in question conducts a clinical school of surgery," needed to be constructed with simplicity of "lines and surfaces." This would allow the thorough cleansing by "flushing with water - possibly with antiseptic solutions - and, if necessary, by disinfection effected through the generation or liberation of antiseptic gases." There should be abundant window space with skylights and a northern exposure. In addition to the operating amphitheater, it was necessary to have smaller operating rooms, at least one of which should be reserved for "pus cases." Another area was needed for "orthopedic surgeons, where, after tenotomies, transplantations, or osteoclasis, they may apply plaster of Paris bandages." Conveniently located near the main operating rooms should be "etherizing rooms." Holmes also discussed the necessity for recovery rooms so that patients did not have to be returned to their ward beds in a condition which would "disturb those seriously ill or terrify those yet to undergo operations." Locker rooms were needed, for both visiting staff and house staff, which should be spacious and contain the type of bathroom that can be "thoroughly flushed and cleaned." The surgical light fixture, called an "illuminator," had to be precisely designed so that both shadows and the adverse effects on the surgeon's eye from the bright glare of the lights could be avoided.

An additional reason why hospitals had become so important for the surgeon's work was the increasing availability of surgical instruments designed to withstand the high heat necessary to destroy bacteria. During this surgical era, a new breed of machined tools made the old hand-fashioned instruments less important. Wooden or ivory handles could not stand up to the rigors of the modern sterilizer. These new surgical implements were often expensive, and surgeons found it both convenient and financially sensible to use a hospital's instruments as well as its sophisticated sterilizing facilities.

The history of the American surgical instrument trade reveals that in the 1820s, an indigenous, albeit small, industry came into being in Boston, New York, and Philadelphia. At that time various artisans, most of them recent immigrants from Europe, began to style themselves as cutlers and surgical instrument makers. Despite the emergence of a fledgling domestic industry, medical practitioners influenced by English and French traditions still preferred foreign-made instruments, deeming them better in workmanship and design. This preference for foreign surgical implements waned only when American firms demonstrated their ability to produce instruments of equal quality. This occurred in the mid-1840s, when individuals such as George Tiemann (1795–1868) of New York were at the height of their creative skills. The Civil War era brought traditional instrument makers their most productive and profitable years, led by such items as a Tiemann amputating set, which sold for as little as thirty dollars.

Tiemann's company published a trade catalogue yearly, and by 1889 it had become the 846-page *American Armamentarium*. The *Armamentarium* not only gave descriptions of all the instruments the company sold but provided analyses of every surgical procedure for which its implements were used, with quotations taken from the surgical textbook or periodical article that most accurately described the equipment in question. With 4,412 black-and-white illustrations, the catalogue was indispensable to both surgeon and hospital. Unfortunately, it was also the company's final publication of that size.

Changes in surgical instrument design and manufacture after 1890, instigated by the acceptance of asepsis in surgical operating rooms, facilitated the rise of the large retail house and brought about the demise of the small artisanal instrument makers, including Tiemann and Company. The machine age of surgical instrument manufacturing came about partly because of the need for "aseptible" instruments. Even though final finishing still entailed much detail work, the simpler instruments that proved more compatible with the dictates of antisepsis and aseptic surgical practices were more easily produced by die-forging techniques and stamping presses. The one-piece alloy steel instrument, devoid of superfluous ornamentation, supplanted the gleaming, highly polished English cast steel instrument fitted into a carefully constructed ebony or ivory handle. The elegance and quality of implements would henceforth be defined strictly in terms of functionality and simplicity of design, characteristics paralleling the virtues of asepsis and machine age production.

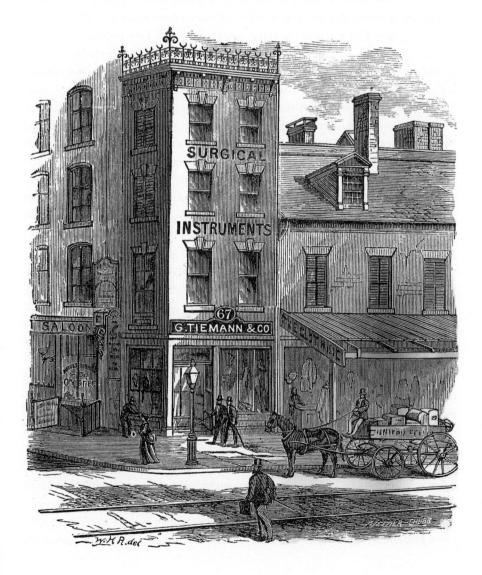

11. George Tiemann established his first surgical instrument shop at 35 Chatham Street in Manhattan in 1826. Seven years later he relocated to No. 63 and remained there until after the Civil War, when Tiemann & Co. settled at No. 67. In the 1870s the company also organized manufacturing operations in a factory in Brooklyn. At the new manufacturing facility, steam power, more sophisticated machinery, and an expanding work force enabled Tiemann & Co. to substantially increase its surgical instrument output throughout the last quarter of the nineteenth century. With showrooms located in Manhattan, and nationwide distribution capabilities, Tiemann & Co. was the acknowledged leader in the manufacture of American surgical implements. (*Jeremy Norman & Co., Inc.*)

12. As clinical teaching improved, the use of surgical grand rounds became an important part of every surgeon's training and continued education. In this view (circa 1892) of such a setting, a patient proudly displays his abdominal incision as members of his operating team look on. (*Courtesy of Stanley B. Burns, M.D., and The Burns Collection and Archive*)

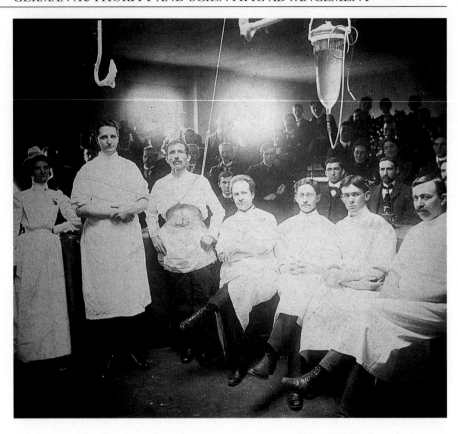

The decisive blow to many of the older artisanal firms, starting in the mid-1890s, was a steady and increasing influx of instruments made abroad, chiefly in countries where German was the major spoken language. Low production costs in foreign instrument factories, a depressed economy in the United States in the early to mid-1890s, and a lowering of the American tariff on foreign surgical instruments led to an alarming increase of foreign-made surgical instruments in the United States market. Of course, this fascination with German goods was also stimulated by the large numbers of American surgeons who had studied in Berlin, Munich, and Vienna and were enthralled with the quality of instruments they found there. Even the Chicago firm of Truax, Greene and Company, one of the major suppliers and fabricators of surgical equipment in the United States, was unable to stave off foreign competition despite publication of its *Mechanics of Surgery* (1899), the most comprehensive and authoritative catalogue ever published on nineteenth-century American surgical instruments and their usage. Surprisingly, Charles Truax's (1852–1918) publishing effort is still authoritative in the 1990s because no equally comprehensive compilation of this sort has been attempted in recent times and because many of the models and patterns of modern surgical instruments actually date back to the 1890s and earlier.

By 1901, continued inroads by German surgical instrument makers into the American market compelled manufacturers and dealers to form the American Surgical Trade Association. That domestic manufacturers and importers were represented by the same lobbying organization was highly unusual but underscored the extent to which all firms in the American surgical instrument trade relied upon foreign sources of supply. Simply described, the American side of the business had succumbed to German competition. Then, in September 1914, the Imperial German government placed an embargo on the export of surgical instruments. This unanticipated turn of events meant that the American surgical instrument industry was in the precarious quandary of having to meet unprecedented demand at home but with no potential to fulfil the requests without having to resort to foreign imports. Although it might seem that American surgical instrument makers would have benefited from such events, this was not the reality of the situation. The only companies to profit were those such as Pilling in Philadelphia and Sklar and Haslam in New York City that had retained some manufacturing capabilities despite German competition. Bankruptcy, leading to the loss of numerous family-owned businesses, affected those who had largely abandoned manufacturing in favor of importing and selling German surgical goods.

THE NEW MEANINGS OF "CONSERVATIVE" AND "RADICAL"

With all the newly emerging surgical technologies and the growing application of scientific principles to basic surgical research, the types of operations that could be performed reflected an emboldened medical ethos. Surgeons were truly able to view themselves as more than just highly skilled technicians. Now they could be thought of as courageous and progressive scientists who were practicing among the most exciting form of therapeutics then available. Not only had the complexity of the operations changed; there was a dramatic increase in the absolute number of procedures being performed. During all of the year 1900 at the Pennsylvania Hospital, the total number of operations was 870. Two and a half decades later, the number of surgical procedures increased to almost 4,200. This 380 percent increase far exceeded the 50 percent increase in the number of ward patients treated during the same time period in the hospital. By the first decade of the twentieth century, critics of so-called surgical euphoria were already issuing stern warnings against excessive and even unnecessary surgery. In 1897, William Keen summarized the state of American surgery and in so doing exposed a growing dichotomy in surgical thought:

> Two dramatically opposing tendencies are prominent…radical interference with disease so that there is now scarcely an organ or portion of the body not within our reach; yet on the other hand, a remarkably conservative tendency in cultivating remedial rather than radical surgery.

The terms "conservative" and "radical" crept into the jargon of American medicine and surgery during the first half of the nineteenth century. Both words took on different meanings at different times. They were alternatively used by physician, surgeon, specialist, and nonspecialist to connote particular types of therapeutic behavior. However, the terms became especially salient in the surgeon's world, where conservatives and radicals enunciated sharp philosophical differences relative to indications for the performance of the burgeoning number of surgical operations. This "surgical schizophrenia" was to play an instrumental role in shaping late nineteenth- and early twentieth-century surgical practices, as witnessed by Halsted's development of numerous innovative operations, including the radical mastectomy and radical hernia repair and the complaint in 1922 by William Haggard (1872–1940), professor of clinical surgery at Vanderbilt University, that "there are regrettably some unconscionable pothunters who will operate on anybody that will hold still. Every hospital should eliminate that kind of man."

When and why "conservative" and "radical" were first applied to surgical intervention in the United States is difficult to state with certainty. Samuel Gross wrote in 1876 that the concept of conservative surgery was initially introduced by Philip Syng Physick and "nowhere more thoroughly appreciated than it is in this country." Gross, ever the surgical disclaimant, noted that Physick "refrained from the employment of the knife whenever it was possible" and that such conduct was always a "prominent trait in the conduct of every enlightened American practitioner." Gross had defined and apparently continued to narrowly use "conservative surgery" as a phrase solely applicable to the treatment of bone excision, dislocations, fractures, and the consequent preservation of limbs. However, by the time of the Civil War, it was apparent that "conservative surgery" had taken on a more expansive meaning applicable to all branches of surgery. No longer was the phrase reserved solely for the surgeon who wished to preserve an extremity. More thoughtful members of the surgical community began to use it to signal a need for a tightening of indications for all operations.

During the Civil War, Austin Flint had begun to describe a new form of conservative medicine as contrasted with that era's heroic medical practices. Influenced directly by surgeons and their interest in conservative surgery, Flint's essays were an important signpost in the evolution of American surgery:

> A change has taken place in medical sentiment as regards surgical operations. New and grand achievements in surgery seemed formerly to be the leading objects of personal ambition...Boldness in the use of the knife was the trait in the character of the surgeon which was most highly admired...The change that has taken place is marked...What would once have been considered as a degree of courage to be admired is now stigmatized as rashness. It is an equivocal compliment to say of a practitioner that he is a bold surgeon...in a word, conservatism has become the ruling principle in surgery.

The concept of conservatism in surgery would remain a dominant force throughout the first decades of the present century. However, an ambiguity in meaning had become established that made it sometimes difficult to determine exactly what was implied. For instance, Halsted wrote in 1904 that "conservative surgery was made possible by general anaesthesia." What should be inferred? Is Halsted describing the surgical philosophy of limb salvage at any cost, or is he characterizing the hallmark of his approach to surgery (i.e., gentle handling of tissues, absolute hemostasis, coaptation of all wound edges without tissue tension, sterile technique, and a general reluctance to perform an operation which was not based on sound scientific principles)?

By 1900, following the beginnings of specialization, the term "conservative surgery" had taken on an additional denotation. It had become a catch phrase intended to signify a routing out of surgical incompetency. There was growing public and private debate as to who should be allowed to perform surgical operations. Would the minimally trained physician-surgeon of the past be permitted to continue his activities in the operating room, or should it be limited to the increasingly experienced specialist in surgery?

Maurice Richardson was a staunch believer in the specialist in surgery and felt that most medical practitioners were no longer skilled enough to act as surgeons. Speaking to members of the State Medical Society of Wisconsin in 1900, he articulated what the term "conservative surgery" had finally come to represent:

> Who is the physician and who the surgeon with whose proposed performance these remarks deal? Is he the general practitioner in a small community, who sees a gall-stone case once a year and an appendix twice? If he is, let him follow in every case the most conservative course possible, for to the dangers of operation will be added in his hands those of inexperience.... Is he the physician of large experience in medical cases, but small in surgical, who wishes now and then to perform a surgical operation? He too had better follow the line of his greatest experience and leave the patient to nature and to palliation.... The dangers in many of the diseases considered are not great if the patient is left to medical treatment. They will be exceeded, perhaps, by those of a clumsy dissection and a faulty asepsis.

Much as "conservative" underwent a change of definition over the course of the nineteenth century, so too, did the term "radical." What began as an adjective to describe nonsurgical treatment of certain disease processes would eventually signify the late 1890's, surgeon's willingness to perform extensive operations. How could conservatism in surgery be concurrently reconciled with a growing sentiment for radical operations?

Although by the turn of the century the term "radical surgery" had taken on the negative connotation of an unreasonable eagerness or aggressiveness to perform surgical operations, such was not the case when it first entered the lexicon of American surgeons. As early as 1836, Heber Chase, a Philadelphia physician, authored a treatise on the radical cure of hernia by instruments. Even Gross, in the first edition of his *System of Surgery*, utilized the phrase "radical cure" in discussing treatment of a reducible hernia by either a truss or operative methods. What was evident in these early usages of the word "radical" is the implied intent of providing a "complete" or long-lasting cure. Whether by surgeon's knife or mechanical device, "radical" meant permanent.

This usage remained essentially unchanged through the 1870s as varying surgical procedures were brought under the rubric of a "radical cure." The decade of the 1880s was an especially creative period in the history of surgery. During this time operations such as aneurysmorrhaphy, appendectomy, cholecystectomy, colectomy, duodenocholecystostomy, esophagotomy, exploratory laparotomy, gastrostomy, and gastroenterostomy first came into use by American surgeons. A major reason for this immense flowering of surgical skills was the growing appreciation of the value of science to the surgeon's craft. With this came a new-found ability to perform scientifically based procedures, involving extensive tissue dissection with removal of a wide variety of "offending" organs. This new style of surgery forced an alteration in the implied meaning of "radical surgery."

"Radical" no longer signified only "permanent." It took on a more expansive meaning intended to express an optimism that by undergoing a surgical operation that incorporated a large area of dissection, a patient could be expected to live. Without such treatment, the individual faced certain death! Unlike the change in definition for "conservative surgery," "radical surgery" was no opprobrium. Surgeons and their growing enthusiasm for the operating theater were going to remove all disease at its root and provide permanent surgical cures.

Although it is tempting to state that late nineteenth- and early twentieth-century American surgeons followed an obvious pathway from conservative to radical philosophies, that was not the case. Radical surgery was never a logical outgrowth from the conservative past. Instead, radical surgery represented a gathering of the many socioeconomic, organizational, political, and scientific forces that together helped create a "new" American profession of surgery. Without this professionaliza-

13. Although meant to be satirical in nature, these two posed tintypes (circa 1883) demonstrate the assumed potential lucrativeness of a career in medicine and surgery. *(Courtesy of Stanley B. Burns, M.D., and The Burns Collection and Archive)*

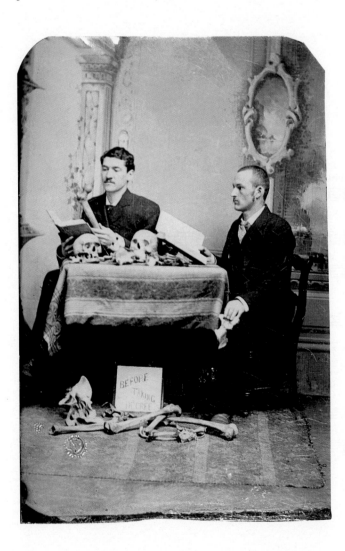

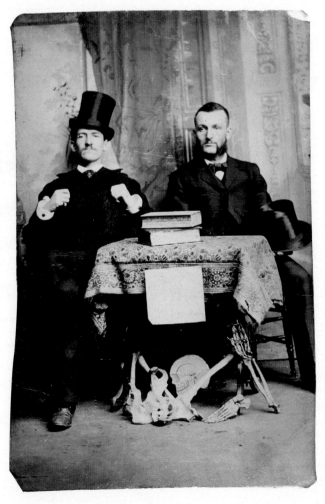

tion process, radical surgery would never have occurred. Conversely, conservative surgery had long been in place and would continue to exist regardless of the direction of American medicine,

Following the turn of the century, radical surgery was being juxtaposed with conservative surgery and the notion of a "radical conservative," or vice versa, was an intriguing possibility. Surgical authorities were beginning to define certain pathological situations where so-called conservatism was the first step in the radical approach to a disease process, for example, the treatment of appendicitis. If ever there was a single pathological condition that represented the quintessential American surgical disease, appendicitis filled all available criteria. Starting with Oliver Prescott's (1762–1827) and Wolcott Richards' early nineteenth-century accounts of death consequent to a perforated appendix, appendiceal abscesses had long been treated without surgical intervention. Not until George Lewis (1823–1863) authored the first major review on appendicitis in the American periodical literature in 1858 was the theoretical necessity for early incision of an appendiceal abscess ever mentioned. Willard Parker put Lewis's suggestion into clinical reality in 1867 when he became the first American surgeon to operate for appendicitis, albeit unsuccessfully, by incising an appendicular abscess at an early stage (i.e., prior to its spontaneous drainage through the skin).

As other surgeons joined Parker in the early opening of appendiceal abscesses, there continued to be numerous deaths of the disease. It was apparent that the surgeon's acumen was not ameliorating an already dangerous clinical situation. If anything, operative intervention was sometimes seen as enhancing the septic process and bringing about a speedier demise. These postsurgical difficulties became part of the clamor for conservative surgery that occurred during the 1860s and 1870s. Clearly, surgical intervention as treatment for appendicitis would require further knowledge of what seemed to be a simple but misunderstood intestinal inflammation.

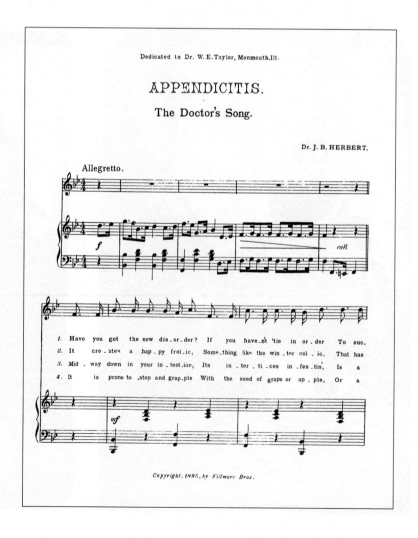

14. In 1895 the diagnosis and treatment of appendicitis was becoming all the rage. J. B. Herbert, a physician/surgeon from Illinois, composed this little ditty, perhaps to poke good-natured fun at the admittedly instant ubiquitousness of the "new" disease. *(Sam DeVincent Collection of Illustrated Sheet Music, Archives Center, Smithsonian Institution, Museum of American History)*

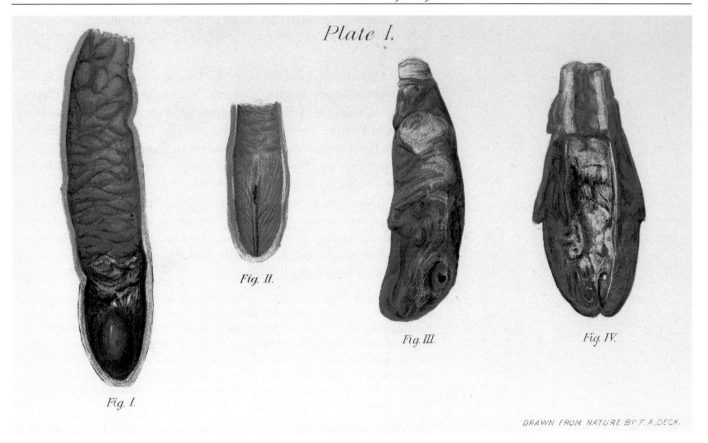

Plate I.

Fig. II.

Fig. III.

Fig. IV.

Fig. I.

DRAWN FROM NATURE BY F. A. DECK.

Such a possibility arose in 1886, when Reginald Fitz (1843–1913), not a surgeon but rather professor of pathological anatomy at Harvard Medical School, presented to the Association of American Physicians his now classic paper, "Perforating Inflammation of the Vermiform Appendix; with Special Reference to its Early Diagnosis and Treatment." Fitz stated that perforating inflammation of the appendix frequently caused death by peritonitis and declared the absolute surgical necessity of removing the appendix immediately if threatening symptoms did not subside within twenty-four hours. That same year, Richard Hall, Halsted's co-worker on local anesthesia from Roosevelt Hospital, reported the first case of survival after removal of a perforated appendix.

In 1887, Thomas Morton (1835–1903), a Philadelphia surgeon, deliberately operated for and removed an inflammed but nonperforated appendix after first correctly diagnosing appendicitis. Henry Sands suggested that an even more aggressive, or what was perceived to be radical, surgical approach to appendicitis be adopted. He realized that a physician's delay in attempting to treat appendicitis nonsurgically would bring about a clinical disaster:

> surgeons alone are competent to decide whether operations are expedient, and to perform them, when necessary, at the right time and in the right manner. A man who devotes his attention to internal medicine alone is generally ignorant of the resources of surgery, and is apt to put off sending for a surgeon until drugs have failed to cure.

This increasingly aggressive surgical posture in the treatment of appendicts was being widely promulgated by such renowned American specialists in surgery as Charles McBurney (1845–1913), George Fowler, William Keen, Robert Morris (1857–1945), and John Deaver (1855–1931). Five textbooks alone were written on the subject of appendicitis during the 1890s. In a treatise by Herman Mynter (1845–1903), professor of operative and clinical surgery in Niagara University in Buffalo, the terms "conservative" and "radical" took on new meaning:

> The surgical treatment, therefore, must be considered the conservative treatment, the quickly healing and least dangerous method, and it is radical in so

15. For the first full-length American treatise on appendicitis, George Fowler had F. A. Deck sketch specimens immediately after their removal. This lithographic plate, which served as the frontispiece in Fowler's *Treatise on Appendicitis* (1894), depicts four differing stages of the disease. *(Author's Collection)*

far as a relapse is impossible. The medical treatment is a makeshift, uncertain in its results, unable to prevent the often fatal complications, and therefore dangerous.

The boldness of radical surgery had finally become recognized as the gold standard of treatment for appendicitis. However, definitional roles changed. By being radical, that is, operating earlier and removing all of the disease, the surgeon was truly pursuing a more "conservative" course of action in the overall treatment of appendicitis. It was medical treatment, instead, and its slowness of action, which was perceived as being "nonconservative" and fraught with complications. Radical surgery actually gave the patient an increased chance of survival!

Clearly, American surgery as it entered the twentieth century had room for both conservative as well as radical surgeons. When viewed in the appropriate surgical setting, both conservative and radical cures could be regarded as progressive and benevolent. Finishing his talk in Wisconsin, Richardson placed "conservative" and "radical" within a proper surgical perspective:

> What does conservatism mean.... The word as commonly used in connection with surgery is synonymous with medical treatment, palliation; or in case two or more surgical methods are proposed, the least extensive and dangerous. But the word may be used in quite a different way to express a line of surgical treatment commonly called radical; when by operation under the most favorable circumstance the patient is subjected to a slight risk that he may avoid the possibilities of much greater dangers in the future. Such a line of treatment is true conservatism, -a conservatism of life at the least possible risk.

One thing was certain: the debates about conservative and radical surgery went *pari passu* with the idea of creating a more competent American profession of surgery. Understandably, by the end of World War I, citizens saw the surgical treatment of appendicitis as one of the most glorious triumphs of modern medicine. More importantly, the lay public viewed surgeons as playing the dominant role in these ongoing successes, and the crucial relation of science (e.g., bacteriology) and technology (e.g., white blood cell counts) to appendiceal surgery was becoming self-evident

At virtually all hospitals in the United States, the number of cases of appendicitis and the number of appendectomies rose steadily. In 1895, the most frequently performed operation at the Pennsylvania Hospital was excision of cervical adenitis, usually tuberculous, which was completed only twenty-five times. Thirty years later, in 1925, surgeons at the same institution performed 1,356 tonsillectomies and/or adenoidectomies, 234 appendectomies, 98 inguinal herniorrhaphies, and 39 thyroidectomies. So relevant had the role of surgery come into American medicine that at the New York Hospital in the same year, 95 per cent of patients who were diagnosed with even the slightest question of appendictis underwent exploratory laparotomy.

Who should make the diagnosis of appendicitis became part of an ongoing and growing battle between general physician-surgeons and specialists in surgery. It was a widely held belief that general practitioners were considered to have less surgical training, experience, and know-how in recognizing appendicitis than surgeons. They lacked what John Deaver called the "light touch" of a skilled surgeon. Paradoxically, these general practitioners were precisely the ones who most needed to be able to make the early diagnosis. Surgeons could always be called to the bedside when the diagnosis of appendicitis and the need for an emergency operation were clear. What happened, however, when a general physician saw the patient earlier in the course of the disease, when the abdominal pain could have been caused by various other processes, most less serious than acute appendicitis? The general practitioners were more accustomed to waiting and observing and less inclined to call in the services of their friendly competitors, the specialists in surgery.

Political battles between the general practitioner-surgeon and the specialist in surgery would haunt American surgery through the first half of the twentieth century. The growth of American surgery from general practice toward specialization proved to be both a strength and a weakness. Spurred on by the large number of physicians who obtained basic surgical skills during the Civil War, two generations of physician-surgeons, who knew their communities and patients well, were already practicing medicine in the United States as effectively as could be expected. Many of them became leaders in their field and, in some cases, professors in the hundreds of proprietary medical schools that proliferated so rapidly around the turn of the century. From this practical type of clinical background rose many of the era's leading specialists in surgery or, as they were termed, career surgeons. However, a major problem was that this type of unstructured evolution also produced large numbers of occasional surgeons. Rarely found in an operating room, the occasional surgeon was untutored and unskilled in the emerging technologies and basic science research that went into the making of modern surgery. Frequently accused of performing complex operations beyond his capabilities, the nonspecialist in surgery was too often beset with surgical disasters that required later referral to the emerging surgical centers for difficult and costly "redo" operations.

At a time when American surgery was struggling to be accepted as a profession and therefore needed to present itself as consisting of a well-educated and adequately controlled cadre of specialists in surgery, the occasional surgeon was a political liability. No one epitomized the acidity of this ongoing debate more than Arthur Hertzler, the Kansas "horse-and-buggy-doctor." His autobiography, published in 1938, describing events of the past fifty years, caught the imagination of the reading public. Hertzler portrayed an aspect of American surgery that was as much a part of the pioneering spirit of the frontier as were the building of the railroads across the Western plains.

In fairness to Hertzler, he was not the run-of-the-mill general practitioner engaged in occasional surgery but rather a self-described generalist committed to

16. An intriguing scene (early 1890s) from Bellevue Hospital, where a surgical operation is in progress, but not in the institution's main surgical amphitheater or the smaller Crane operating room. Instead, the patient is receiving ether anesthesia in her bed in a large open ward. Other individuals look on, thereby robbing the patient of any privacy. *(Bellevue Hospital Center Archives - Board of Managers' Collection)*

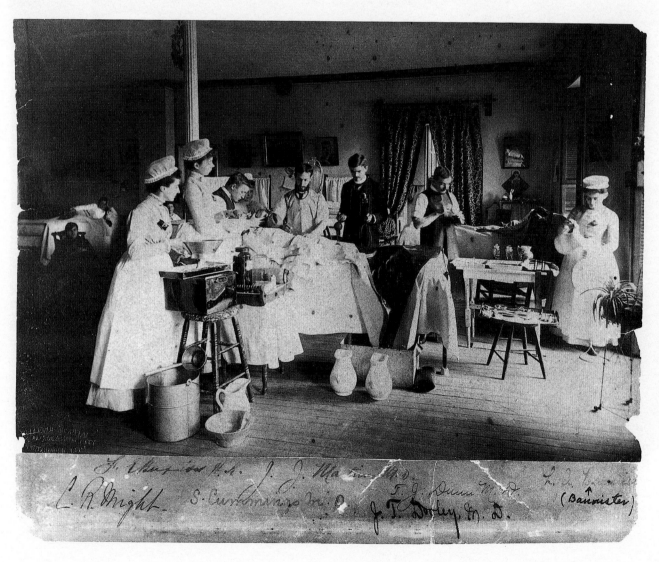

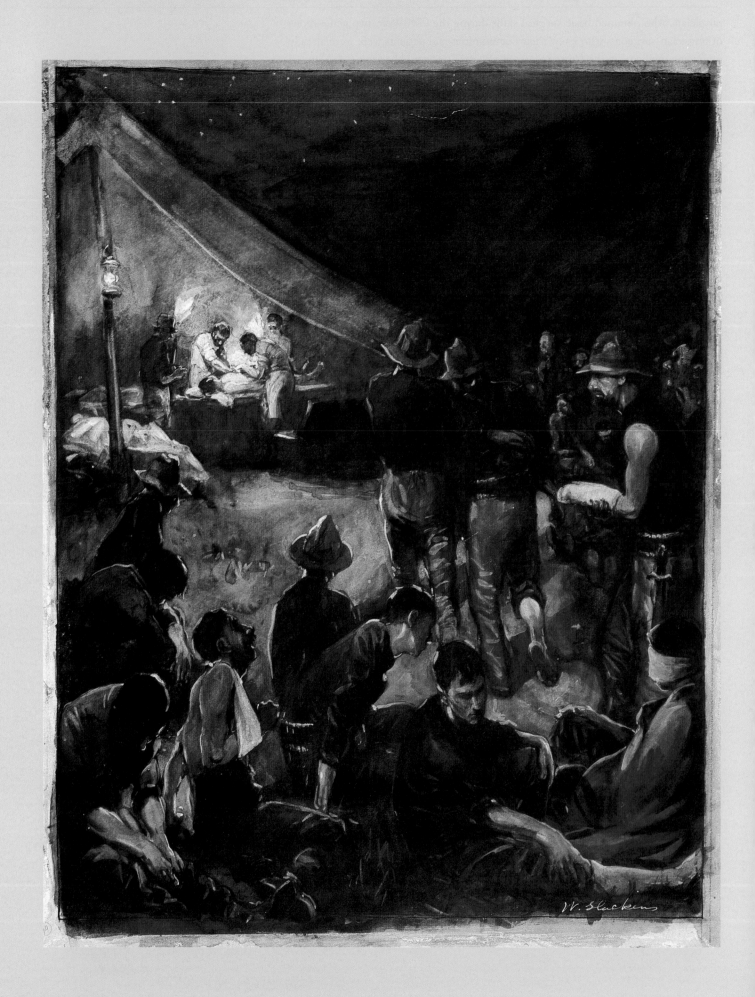

providing excellent surgical care within the framework of overall medicine. Known for his sharp pen and scalpel, Hertzler was given to pungent and corrosive statements about career surgeons. His down-to-earth attitude reflected, in part, Midwestern frustrations with "fancy" Eastern ideas, particularly the development of full-time medical faculty at places like The Johns Hopkins Hospital. Hertzler had started his own hospital in Halstead, Kansas, where he conducted a large volume of surgery for many years. Nonetheless, he was of the opinion that "specialism has become an avenue of escape for hard labor, a harbor for a one-cell brain rather than an opportunity to develop great skill or advance knowledge."

While few nonspecialists in surgery were as successful as Hertzler in pursuing a "nonsurgical" surgical career, the difficulties intrinsic in this type of surgical self-education were becoming painfully evident. The tradition of grass-roots origin for surgical work, as well as other emerging specialties such as radiology, anesthesia, and pediatrics, produced a lingering legacy of half-taught and sometimes half-capable nonspecialists in surgery well into the 1960s. It should be realized, however, that the frequency of appendectomies was partly responsible for the widespread development of the general practitioner-surgeon between 1890 and the end of World War I. Increasingly regarded as an easy-to-complete surgical operation, appendectomy enticed the general practitioner-surgeon to embark on intraperitoneal surgery, sometimes taking him far beyond the limits of his training or skills. As scientific advances rendered the care of surgical patients less troublesome, other seemingly "simple" operations, typified by cholecystectomy, hemorrhoidectomy, simple mastectomy, open reduction of fractures, ovariotomy, tonsillectomy and/or adenoidectomy, and varicose vein stripping, were taken up by the general practitioner. Although this generation of men was reaching retirement in the 1940s and 1950s, a time when formally structured surgical residency programs were finally able to provide increasing numbers of well-trained specialists in surgery to American communities, no history of surgery in the United States would be complete without an admiring understanding of those self-taught and conscientious country surgical practitioners of the first half of the twentieth century.

MEDICAL AND SURGICAL SECTARIANISM

Late nineteenth- and early twentieth-century American society not only was prone to the surgical vagaries of the nonspecialist in surgery but also was forced to contend with the political and economic strength of medical and surgical sectariansim. At a time when popular health reform movements led by John Harvey Kellogg (1852–1943), of cereal flakes and crispies fame, Horace Fletcher (1849–1919), the "Great Masticator," and Bernarr Macfadden (1868–1955) and his "Healthatoriums" were sweeping the nation, nontraditional practitioners of surgery were also finding a place of their own. Kellogg was typical of these surgeons and deserves a rightful place in the pantheon of American surgery. He received his medical degree from Bellevue Hospital Medical College in 1875. Always considering himself a surgeon first, Kellogg was appointed to the staff of the Battle Creek Sanitarium in Battle Creek, Michigan. Converted to the health reform ideas of Ellen White (1827–1915), founder of the Seventh-Day Adventist Church, he was soon made physician-in-chief and became editor of the Adventist *Health Reformer.* Despite writing numerous papers on surgical topics, including abdominal and gynecologic surgery, Kellogg remained a fringe figure within allopathic surgery because of his additional reliance on "natural" therapies such as botanics, hydrotherapy, and "biologic living."

Kellogg authored a succession of hygiene treatises, such as *Plain Facts for Old and Young* (1881), *The Stomach; its Disorders and How to Cure Them* (1896), *The Home Handbook of Domestic Hygiene and Rational Medicine* (1897), *Rational Hydrotherapy* (1900), *Man the Masterpiece, or Plain Truths Plainly Told About Boyhood, Youth, and Manhood* (1900), *The New Dietetics* (1921), *How to Have Good Health Through Biologic Living* (1932), that dominated the field in the late nineteenth and early twentieth centuries. His volumes constituted elaborate defenses of vegetarianism, scathing

17. The Spanish-American War marked the emergence of the United States as a world power. Fought between April and August, 1898, the hostilities ended with Spain granting Cuba its freedom and ceding Guam, Puerto Rico, and the Philippines to the United States. During this war, the army was less in need of surgeons than of sanitarians and physicians. Only 289 soldiers were killed or mortally wounded in battle, while over 3,700 succumbed to infectious diseases, primarily typhoid fever. William Glacken's (1870–1938) *Night After San Juan: Field Hospital* (1898) depicts the performance of a surgical operation in a field hospital. The artist dramatizes the event by arranging wounded soldiers, who are in need of obvious surgical attention, in front of the open tent, thereby forcing them to observe their intended fate. This inkwash on paper was one of a series of illustrations resulting from the commissioning of Glackens by *McClure's Magazine* to cover the war's events. *(Collection Library of Congress)*

denunciations of alcohol, and merciless attacks on sexual misconduct, complete with advice to parents that they make unannounced nighttime raids into their children's rooms to catch youthful masturbators in the act and cure their beastly urging with cauterization of the clitoris or circumcision without anesthesia. *Good Health*, one of Kellogg's monthly hygiene publications, attained a paid circulation of twenty thousand subscribers at its peak and was published continuously until 1955.

So popular were Kellogg and his concept of "biologic living" (avoiding stimulants and condiments, eating fruits and grains, obtaining rest, exercise, sunlight, bathing, and the wearing of proper clothes) that more than 30,000 patients during his sixty-seven year tenure, including such luminaries as President William Howard Taft (1857–1930), John D. Rockefeller, Jr. (1839–1937), Alfred I. DuPont (1864–1935), J. C. Penney (1875–1971), Montgomery Ward (1843–1913) and grape juice magnate Edgar Welch (1872–1956), stayed at the comfortable and attractive quarters of the Battle Creek Sanitarium. Meanwhile, at the Sanitarium Health Food Company's laboratory, several new foods intended to decrease constipation and the evils of autointoxication from a protein-engorged intestinal tract, including the first flaked cereals, were developed, were widely promoted and eventually became America's most popular breakfast foods. Ever the orthodox surgeon, Kellogg was an early member of the fledgling American College of Surgeons (1914) and readily admitted that he derived much of his health reform beliefs about digestive processes from observing at the operating room table and caring for postoperative patients.

Medical and surgical sectarianism represented the most serious threat to the professional survival of the turn-of-the-century allopathic physician. But the biggest concern was not over health care reformers like Kellogg. It was the homeopathic sect that caused grave financial problems. American homeopathy grew out of a system of experimental pharmacology originated by the German physician Samuel Hahnemann (1755–1843). He propagated a method of medical treatment based on the theory that large doses of a drug given to a healthy person will produce certain conditions that, when occurring spontaneously as symptoms of a disease, are relieved by the same drug in massively diluted doses. This was called the "law of similars" or "like is cured by like." Although its appeal was not readily apparent, by the time of the Civil War, homeopathy had won over converts, primarily in the urban middle and upper classes.

In the 1850s, growing numbers of surgically oriented articles were being published in the numerous homeopathic journals found throughout the country. One such article in the *North American Homoeopathic Journal* of February 1851 set the standard for what the homeopathic profession would expect of their surgeons for decades to come:

> So far as the manual operations of surgery are concerned, the homeopath most cheerfully records his approval and admiration of the perfection to which they have been brought by the scientific investigation, ingenuity, and untiring industry of the profession, and on all necessary occasions will promptly resort to them.... But while we award due credit to the mechanical portions of this branch of the healing art, as usually practiced by the allopath, we beg leave to enter an entire dissent from the accompanying medical treatment which he so often deems necessary...for numerous and well authenticated facts have only conclusively demonstrated, that, in many diseases which are denominated surgical, from the circumstances their requiring, for the most part, the manual aid of the surgeon, there are specific drugs, belonging to the homoeopathic Materia Medica, capable of curing the morbid action, and thus, of rendering surgical operations unnecessary.

Despite the many pitched political battles between allopaths and homeopaths, the latter grew in strength and reached their zenith as a medical sect during the 1890s. Their wealthy and influential patients provided the financial means to establish homeopathic hospitals in various cities and towns. Concurrently, homeopathic colleges were established across the nation, permitting the sect to increase in numbers through the education of students as well as the continued conversion

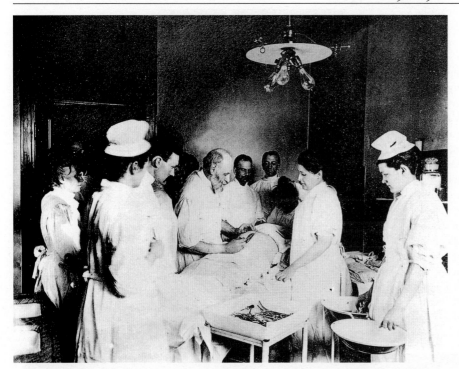

18. Reuben Ludlam (1831–1899) was professor of obstetrics and diseases of women at Hahnemann Medical College of Chicago. Although it was a homeopathic institution, Ludlam still performed many surgical procedures, as shown in this photograph (mid-1890s) of his gynecological clinic. *(Courtesy of the International Museum of Surgical Science, Chicago)*

of allopaths. The talent of William Helmuth (1833–1902) brought homeopathic surgery to its highest levels. An 1853 graduate of the Homoeopathic Medical College of Pennsylvania, two years later Helmuth was named professor of anatomy at his alma mater. That same year, he authored his influential textbook, *Surgery and Its Adaptation to Homoeopathic Practice*. Having taught for a few years in St. Louis and having spent 1868 in Europe touring various medical centers, Helmuth accepted an offer to assume the chair of surgery in the New York Homoeopathic Medical College and Flower Hospital (1870). His success as a surgeon, writer, and teacher was outstanding, and in 1893, he was named dean of the New York City institution.

By 1895, homeopathic surgery was so highly organized that three separate bureaus—of gynecology; surgery; and otology, ophthalmology, and laryngology—were active within the American Institute of Homoeopathy. Particularly intriguing was the emergence of "orificial surgery" as a side branch of homeopathy. This surgical specialty, based on the hypothesis that many disease processes were a direct consequence of abnormalities associated solely with the cervix, nares, rectum, urethra, or vagina, was founded by Edwin Hartley Pratt (1849–1930). He believed that both acute and chronic diseases could be treated by operating on virtually any orifice in the human body. For asthma out of control, a hemorrhoidectomy or vaginal scraping might just be the cure! Through his salesmanship skills, Pratt was able to establish a field of surgery that maintained its own national society in addition to publishing a widely distributed specialty journal.

The rise and demise of orificial surgery is among the interesting minor footnotes in the history of American surgery. The orificial philosophy attracted a large number of followers who were, in every sense of the word, surgeons. Their technical skills allowed them to perform many formidable types of surgical operations, including hysterectomy, repair of complicated cervical and perineal lacerations, and radical hemorrhoidectomy. Although it is impossible to state definitively how many Americans were victims of this unorthodox surgical philosophy, it would not be an understatement, based on the number of physician-surgeons who subscribed to it, to estimate they numbered in the tens of thousands. Like much that occurred in American medicine of this era, the long-forgotten, short-lived, and appropriately discredited movement of orificial surgery was more a symptom of the times than a well-organized effort to undo the parallel scientific evolution of surgery.

19. It was no wonder that the Spanish-American conflict became known as the splendid little war. It lasted only three months, fewer than three hundred American soldiers were killed, and important land acquisitions were achieved. Battlefield action photography, virtually impossible during the Civil War because of the slow speed of the film and the necessity of developing and printing the wet plates as soon as possible, finally became a reality. For the first time, unposed subjects could be candidly photographed with portable cameras, using the new roll film manufactured by Kodak. Views of field hospitals and the wounded were mass produced, sometimes on stereocards, to be sold to the American public. Both of these scenes are from the Philippine Islands and show a "wounded Filipino on the operating table" *(top)* and "one of the 20th Kansas Boys" *(bottom). (Courtesy of Stanley B. Burns, M.D., and The Burns Collection and Archive)*

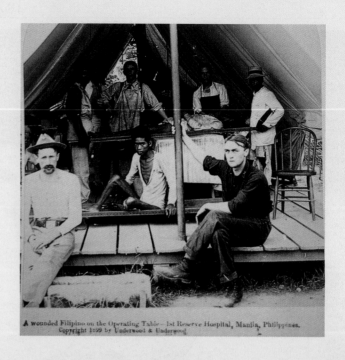

A wounded Filipino on the Operating Table—1st Reserve Hospital, Manila, Philippines. Copyright 1899 by Underwood & Underwood

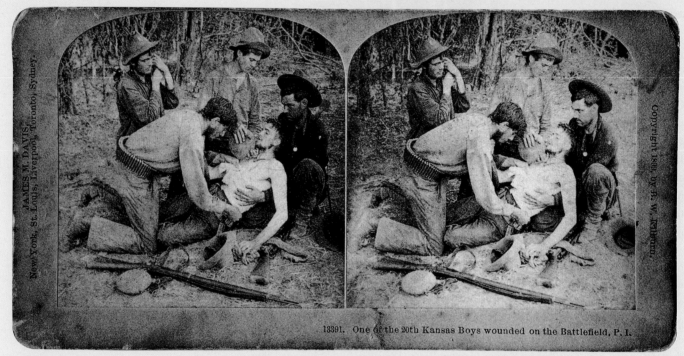

13391. One of the 20th Kansas Boys wounded on the Battlefield, P. I.

By the turn of the century, a revolution was occurring in American medical education. Attempts to set standards for all medical schools, both orthodox and sectarian, had begun. It was Abraham Flexner's (1866–1959) 1910 report on medical education that brought about the ultimate demise of homeopathic medical colleges. The conditions Flexner found in the vast majority of both regular and sectarian schools were simply appalling. Laboratory facilities were totally inadequate, while clinical material was not available to most students. Within ten years after the Flexner report, only four homeopathic medical colleges remained: Boston University, Hahnemann Medical College of Philadelphia, New York Homeopathic Medical College, and the homeopathic department of the University of Michigan. By 1920, Boston University had converted to a completely allopathic institution. Two years later, the homeopathic department at the University of Michigan disappeared. In 1936, the trustees of the New York Homeopathic Medical College voted to change its name to the New York Medical College. Hahnemann Medical College remained the sole holdout, but by the end of World War II, it had become an allo-pathic-dominated institution.

It is not difficult to understand why homeopathic surgeons met their ultimate demise. By the beginning of the twentieth century, true therapeutic distinctions between allopaths and homeopaths had essentially disappeared. The real value of homeopathy was to demonstrate the healing powers of nature and the therapeutic virtue of placebos. In point of fact, the technical aspects of surgery had never sub-stantively differed among surgeons in the three groups. In addition, the establish-ment of surgical specialization served to lessen all dissimilarities. As the scientific dogma and technical skills of surgeons became more narrowly focused, it was inevitable that essentially all differences in their approach to patients would disap-pear. For homeopathic surgeons, any pretense at sectariansim ended by the time of the Great Depression.

IMPROVEMENTS IN MEDICAL AND SURGICAL EDUCATION

By 1910, American medical education had progressed greatly, but further improve-ments were needed to elevate the average school to a minimum standard of excel-lence. In addition, the leadership of medicine realized that it would never be a respected profession until it was able to shed itself of what was commonly regarded as "coarse and common elements" who entered medicine through proprietary med-ical schools and weaker medical departments of universities. Only with such a deter-mined goal could medical students of the highest capabilities be adequately prepared to enter demanding surgical residencies similar to those of Halsted at The Johns Hopkins. The American Medical Association itself had undergone its own reorgani-zation and made the reform of medical education one of its top priorities. In 1904, the Association established a Council on Medical Education with a permanent sec-retary, a regular budget, and a mandate to elevate and standardize the requirements for medical education.

This was the setting for Flexner's famous report, now considered part of that era's genre of classic muckraking journalism. Issued in June 1910, under the auspices of the Carnegie Foundation for the Advancement of Teaching, the report with its mat-ter-of-fact style of presentation exposed the scandalous conditions and outright fraud that existed in half of the country's medical schools. To the author, only one type of medical school was acceptable: university-affiliated institutions, with large full-time faculties and a genuine committment to basic medical research (i.e., The Johns Hopkins School of Medicine and The Johns Hopkins Hospital). As a result of Flexner's critique, more than seventy-five medical schools, most of them proprietary, were closed during the decade of the 1910s. New medical school curricula were established and included such basic changes as the requirement of a baccalaureate degree for admission and the institution of a four-year program. Although Flexner's report was primarily concerned with undergraduate medical education, it does pro-vide some glimmerings of his attitude toward the teaching of surgery:

> The backbone of clinical training must be internal medicine. But it is precise-ly here that the schools are in general weakest.... The "additional facilities" of the larger schools are mainly surgical in character; and in general, the less a school has to offer in the way of clinical facilities, the more heavily is surgery overweighted. Its pedagogical value is relatively slight; for operations are per-formed in large amphitheaters in which the surgeon and his assistants sur-round the patient, to whom they give their whole mind, in practical disregard of the students, who loll in their seats without an inkling of what is happening below.... Inadequacy in general is thus aggravated by increasing predomi-nance of surgical over medical clinics.

Much as the Flexner report left an indelible mark on progressive medical edu-cation in the United States, the founding of the American College of Surgeons and its subsequent successes were a reaction to the one major void that still faced

American surgeons in their drive toward professional status. There remained the need for a national organization that would unite surgeons by membership in common sociopolitical and educational causes. The American Surgical Association, because it was composed of a small and elite group of senior surgeons mostly from the cities of the East Coast and the South, was never capable of serving as a national lobbying front. Despite the establishment of various regional surgical societies with less restrictive membership guidelines, including the Southern Surgical Association (1887) and the Western Surgical Association (1891), their geographical differences never allowed for countrywide unity. As a result, by the conclusion of the first decade of the twentieth century, all the elements needed to fulfill the definition of a profession (i.e., technical competence, standardized education and training, subspecialization, literature, autonomy, monopoly over practice, and an ethos of public service) were in place except a national organization to provide a proper sense of professional purpose.

Shortly after the turn of the century, various "surgeon" members of the profession of medicine demonstrated a change in their attitude toward surgical associations and their allied specialties. There was growing dissatisfaction with the routine but monotonous presentation of dry and uninformative academic-type papers. As surgical operations increased in complexity, the technical and mechanical problems inherent in such procedures impelled surgeons to seek actual demonstrations in the operating theaters of their confrères. Only in this way could the growing mass of specialists in surgery differentiate between worthwhile operations and those deemed unacceptable.

In July 1903, the Society of Clinical Surgery was organized by a select group of young surgeons, including John Munro (1858–1910), George Brewer (1861–1939), James Mumford (1863–1914), George Crile (1864–1943), Harvey Cushing (1869–1939), and Charles Frazier (1870–1936). This first travel club of men engaged in clinical surgical work was the expression of a brilliant impulse with far-reaching influence. There had been a growing resentment over control of the American Surgical Association by senior surgeons and the fact that it represented a staid aristocracy of American surgery. In an innovative precedent, twice a year the young surgeons visited one of the larger surgical centers in America and saw their colleagues actually at work in a clinical setting. The presentation of papers was never countenanced. Instead, the members engaged in informal discussions dominated by lengthy give-and-take. In this process, capable clinical surgeons were soon segregated from individuals with literary and theoretical talents alone.

By 1910, most of the major American surgical centers and their respective surgeons had been visited. This was easily accomplished, because in the opinion of the early members of the Society there were only seven cities worth visiting: Baltimore, Boston, Chicago, Cleveland, New York, Philadelphia, and Rochester (Minnesota). A certain wanderlust had set in, and at the instigation of Edward Martin (1859–1938) of Philadelphia, it was decided that members of the Society would visit Great Britain. The trip took them to surgical centers in Edinburgh, Leeds, Liverpool, London, and Newcastle. As American surgery grew in stature, overseas visits by organizations such as the Society of Clinical Surgery helped form essential international bonds.

As much as the membership of the Society rallied against the apparent snobbery of the American Surgical Association, in reality Cushing and his fellow travelers were overtly elitist in their own actions. The constitution of the Society of Clinical Surgery virtually assured that all members were expected to hold a teaching position in a medical school or hospital, to be connected with an institution of such a character as to make it a desirable place to visit and potentially in which to hold a meeting, to be involved in investigative work, and to have published worthwhile reports. More than anything else, membership remained restricted to a resolutely small number of individuals. Despite stated appearances, the Society served as little more than a springboard for a younger generation of American surgeons to ultimately become members of the surgical establishment. There was a certain irony in the fact that all but one of the original thirty-six members of the Society of Clinical Surgery became fellows of the American Surgical Association. Perhaps even more remarkable is that fifteen of the thirty-six became president of it!

Debates over membership restrictions of the early American surgical societies proved to be harbingers of town–gown disputes that have periodically marred the sociopolitical environment of surgery's growth. As the full-time professor of surgery gained acceptance in America and proprietary professorships were phased out, tensions with already practicing surgeons came to the surface. Many surgical educators, exemplified by the early members of the Society of Clinical Surgery and the American Surgical Association, looked upon practitioners with an air of professional superiority, while practitioners viewed the professors as impractical and lacking in clinical skills. Arguments continued to flare, and both sides were at extreme loggerheads by the time of World War I.

At the same time that the Society of Clinical Surgery was being established, a change was occurring in medical school and postgraduate surgical education. The oratorical, didactic mode of teaching was being replaced with practical demonstrations. Large classrooms served by one lecturer, who would drone on for hours at a time, were being separated into smaller groups taught at the bedside and in the clinical laboratory. Surgeons began to seek out technical masters in their field by visiting them and observing their clinical prowess. It was as if suddenly "show-me" had become more convincing than "tell-me."

In partial response to this "show-me" attitude, a new surgical journal was founded in 1905. *Surgery, Gynecology and Obstetrics* was the brainchild of Franklin Martin (1857–1935), a Chicago gynecologist, who was going to have a profound effect on the social and educational organizing of American surgeons. He believed there was a need for a different type of surgical periodical, namely, one edited by surgeons for practical surgeons, "instead of *littérateurs* only remotely connected with clinical

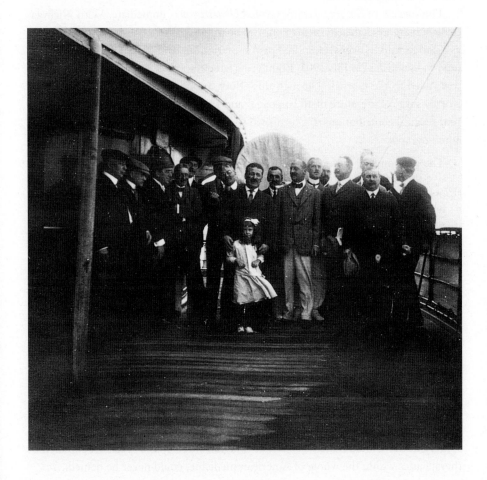

20. In June 1912, the Society of Clinical Surgery held its eighteenth meeting by arranging a *Rundreise* of several renowned Austrian and German surgical centers. Standing on the deck of the "S. S. Kronprinzessin Cecilie" in New York City harbor, Harvey Cushing himself took this previously unpublished photograph of the assembled members (among those identified are George Crile *[head tilted in the middle]* and John Finney *[holding the young girl]*) and incorporated it into his diary of the excursion. As Cushing wrote, the exhaustive trip included stops in "Hamburg (Kümmell), Berlin (Bier, Körte, et. al.), Leipzig (Payr), Jena (Lexer), Vienna (von Eiselsberg, Hochenegg, etc.), Munich.... From there by train to Tübingen where after a morning with Perthes we proceeded by motor to Stuttgart (Hofmeister), to Heidelberg (Wilms), to Würzburg (Enderlen), Frankfurt (Rehn).... From Frankfurt we motored down the picturesque Valley of the Rhine to Wiesbaden...and thus on to Coblenz and finally Bonn to visit Garrès' clinic." *(Yale University, Harvey Cushing/John Hay Whitney Medical Library)*

work." The new enterprise was to include articles in all special fields of surgery, but even more important to Martin was that the "caldron of old-style medical journalism" be "liberated from commercialism." He believed that profits should be used to strengthen the influence and worth of the periodical rather than accrue to individuals or commercial publishing companies.

Martin was born in Ixonia, Wisconsin, and obtained his medical degree from the Chicago Medical College (1880), now the Northwestern University School of Medicine. He was a general physician who initially served on the surgery staff of the South Side Dispensary and Polyclinic Hospital Medical School where he "specialized" in surgical gynecology. Martin eventually joined the gynecological staff at Chicago's Woman's Hospital, where he spent most of his later career years, as well as at the Charity Hospital, which he founded in 1887. Long involved in the politics of American medicine, Martin served from 1916 to 1921 on the Council of National Defense and during two of those years was chairman of the country's General Medical Board, which oversaw the mobilization of physicians, surgeons, and dentists during World War I. In 1919 he was honored with the presidency of the American Gynecological Society and ten years later with the presidency of the American College of Surgeons. Interestingly, Martin was never asked to join the American Surgical Association nor the Society for Clinical Surgery and provides little in his autobiography concerning his feelings about these obvious slights. One of the first Americans to practice aseptic gynecologic surgery, Martin reduced the mortality in operations for uterine fibroid by devising a procedure for ligating the uterine arteries to cause atrophy of the fibroid (1892). He also pioneered the surgical removal of the bladder by transplanting the ureters in the colon (1899). His major textbooks include *Electricity in Diseases of Women and Obstetrics* (1893), *Lectures On the Treatment of Fibroid Tumors of the Uterus* (1897), and *A Treatise on Gynecology* (1903). Besides his role in founding *Surgery, Gynecology and Obstetrics*, Martin helped edit the *American Journal of Obstetrics and Gynecology* and the Chicago *Medical Recorder.* In 1921 he established the Gorgas Memorial Institute of Tropical and Preventive Medicine.

The success of *Surgery, Gynecology and Obstetrics* was immediate. With Nicholas Senn serving as chairman of the editorial board and Allen B. Kanavel (1874–1938) as associate editor, over six hundred paid subscriptions were registered when the volume was published in July 1905. Eight years later, the *International Abstract of Surgery* was added to the journal. Through this effort, accurately prepared abstracts of the worthy surgical literature of all languages and a comprehensive bibliography of current surgical contributions was furnished to each subscriber. As Martin relates in his autobiography:

> The phenomenal acceptance of *Surgery, Gynecology and Obstetrics* was conclusive proof that the profession preferred to receive information directly from practicing surgeons rather than from non-practicing editors who acted merely as interpreters. And it was far better to have a practicing surgeon demonstrate his work than to have him tell about it.

Incisive comments from members of the Society of Clinical Surgery demonstrated to Martin how much more knowledge could be gained by actually witnessing operations in well-recognized surgical centers than by hearing or reading surgical papers. Somehow, Martin had to devise a method whereby the advantages of the cliquish Society could be extended to all "practical...progressive specialists." In 1910, Martin's thoughts became focused toward inaugurating a clinical meeting at which surgeons from throughout the United States could visit Chicago hospitals and their "master-surgeons" and observe operations from 8 in the morning to 5 in the afternoon each day during a two-week period. It was decided to invite all *Surgery, Gynecology and Obstetrics* subscribers to such a gathering. In September 1910, an editorial announcement appeared that crowned the process of professionalization for surgery in the United States. From that time on, surgery, as a specialized branch of therapeutics within the whole of American medicine, could never be denied:

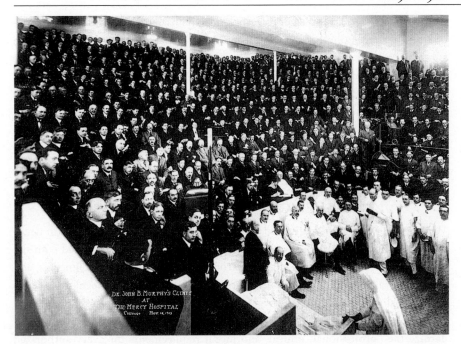

DR. JOHN B. MURPHY'S CLINIC
AT
THE MERCY HOSPITAL
Chicago   Nov. 14, 1913

21. In November 1913, the fourth annual Clinical Congress of Surgeons of North America was held in Chicago. John Murphy's "wet clinics" were given at Mercy Hospital and became the outstanding surgical event of the meeting. A list of cases operated on and demonstrated by the renowned Chicago surgeon during that week of November 10–15 totaled 149 patients and included more than twenty major operations. *(Collection of Mercy Hospital, Chicago)*

The tendency to learn by watching the actual work of the masters has become more and more popular, and the demand of the spirit this has engendered is for greater opportunities for clinical observation. If the technical skill of American surgeons, or those of any other community, is especially excellent it is because these surgeons are willing and anxious to learn by observing and being observed while actually at work in the operating room. This sort of training and observing has without doubt unhorsed a few literary and oratorical clinicians, but on the other hand it has brought to their proper perspective the hard-working, painstaking surgeons who make good.

A recognition of the above facts, after duly considering their purport and the tendency of the times, has led the editors of Surgery, Gynecology and Obstetrics, in an endeavor to still further amplify the clinical idea, to invite to a clinical meeting, not a limited number to see the work of a few surgeons, but, as far as practicable, every man in the United States and Canada who is particularly interested in surgery, to observe the principal clinics in one of the large medical centers.

Several thousand invitations were issued to all types of practitioners as long as they had the slightest interest in surgery. An attendance of two hundred was expected. Surprisingly, between November 7th and 19th, over 1,300 physicians and surgeons from almost every state in the Union traveled to Chicago. The registration booths in the LaSalle Hotel were underserved, the large clinics were overcrowded, and many of the smaller surgical centers were obliged to expand temporarily. The men in attendance, however, were discriminating. They went to see many "modest" operators whose work had attracted them but who were not prominent in the elite society meetings. These were practicing surgeons who would prove themselves in action, as opposed to the written page. Martin realized that while there were many surgical societies, there had never been a meeting like the one then in progress with the twin objectives of inclusivity of attendees and nationwide appeal. A business session was held, and the attendees urged perpetuation of the clinical meeting through some type of organization that would insure a yearly opportunity to observe the work of master-surgeons in one of several key clinical centers. So, with little fanfare but much enthusiasm, the Clinical Congress of Surgeons of North America was established.

The second Clinical Congress was held in Philadelphia in November 1911, and despite asking for a registration fee of five dollars (the first Congress in Chicago had been totally underwritten by the financial success of *Surgery, Gynecology and Obstetrics*), over 1,500 doctors enrolled, and it was estimated that fully as many more witnessed the clinics without registering. By the time of the third Congress in New

York City (1912), Martin began to realize that the basic structure of the event was too loosely knit. Surgical politics had reared its ugly head in that certain well-known surgeons, whose clinics were well organized, refused to be scheduled in the Congress's program with clinics they regarded as inferior. Of course, the latter group continued to insist on being included. There had to be some way to limit attendance to the registered surgeons and a means of controlling onlookers at each surgical clinic. If only "acceptable" clinics and clinicians were to be part of the Congress, then clinical standards, ethics, and the general acceptability of all members were acute problems that had to be resolved.

THE AMERICAN COLLEGE OF SURGEONS

With over 2,600 doctors registered for the New York City Congress, Martin needed little convincing of the necessity for a new organization, closely allied with the Clinical Congress, that would aid in controlling its members and its clinicians, and enforce moral and ethical guidelines. The idea of an American College of Surgeons patterned along the lines of the Royal Colleges of Surgeons of England, Ireland, and Scotland became the working prototype. Martin proposed a society that would standardize the "professional, ethical, and moral requirements for every authorized graduate in medicine who practices general surgery or any of its specialties" and would additionally provide formal recognition of their qualifications.

Martin spent the next year laying the groundwork for such an organization by visiting groups of the most prominent surgeons in every major city in the country. Opposition and skepticism were great. The formation of a "college" of surgeons was opposed by various political factions within American medicine, most notably the American Medical Association. At the Association's 1914 annual meeting held in Atlantic City, there came before its House of Delegates a resolution regarding the establishment of the American College of Surgeons. The Illinois delegation promptly deprecated the Chicago-based society, and although the question of endorsement lay unresolved, the House of Delegates encouraged its own Council on Health and Public Instruction to correlate any existing national health organizations in a manner favorable to control by the American Medical Association. The Association's opposition to the College was particularly goaded on by the sarcastic and demeaning Philip Mills Jones, editor of the *California State Journal of Medicine*. Jones published numerous vituperative editorials against the College, both before and for several years after the organization became a reality:

> Here it is at last, a full-blown attempt by would be conspicuous members of the home profession to engraft upon the democratic tree of free American medicine a royal sprout of would be aristrocracy from Old London Town.... But the great American profession has a temper all its own...and a dislike for all counterfeits. How well this latest attempt to build up an oriental oligarchy for the purpose of controlling honors, titles, offices and, incidentally, business is to be received by this progressive profession in the West, remain to be seen. There is more than an intimation in the air that many a man with the label of F.A.C.S. on him will be ready eventually to sell it very cheap.

Although plagued with initial growing pains and unavoidable opposition, the American College of Surgeons became a reality when in November 1913, 1,059 surgeons were admitted to fellowship (i.e., F.A.C.S.) at the first convocation in Chicago. According to its by-laws, the object of the new College was to "elevate the standard of surgery, to establish a standard of competency and of character for practitioners of surgery, to provide a method of granting fellowships in the organization, and to educate the public and the profession to understand that the practice of surgery calls for special training, and that the surgeon elected to fellowship in this College has had such training and is properly qualified to practice surgery."

In attempting to be a democratic and nationally representative society, the College formed a fifty-person board of governors to serve as one of its governing bodies. Fifteen national societies (e.g., American Surgical Association; Surgical Section on Obstetrics, Gynecology, and Abdominal Surgery of the American Medical Association; General Surgical Division and Division of Surgical Specialities of the Clinical Congress of Surgeons of North America; American Institute of Homeopathy; American Gynecological Society; American Orthopedic Association; American Otological Society; and one each from the United States Army and United States Navy) were given authority to nominate each year thirty of the fifty governors. The board of governors in turn elected members of a board of regents, who would be responsible for operation of the College between annual meetings. The regents were further authorized to employ a full-time director to administer the College.

From the outset, the primary aim of the College was the continuing education of surgical practitioners. Accordingly, the requirements for fellowship were always related to the educational opportunities of the period. In 1914, an applicant had to be a licensed graduate of medicine, receive the backing of three fellows, and be endorsed by his local credentials committee. In view of the stipulated peer recommendations, many practitioners, realistically or not, viewed the American College of Surgeons as just another elitist organization. Hertzler was more to the point:

> I am supposed to be a surgeon, but that is a mistake. I am just a general practitioner who operates. Don't let Franklin Martin get hold of this. He says that unless at least half of one's work is in surgery he can't be F.A.C.S. Though I have done a couple of thousand operations a year for a long time, that is only a small part of my work. My long suit is asthma, hyperacidity and ringworm.

In view of the obvious "blackball" system built into the membership requirements, there was a difficult to deny belief that surgeons who were immigrants, females, or members of particular religious and racial minorities were granted fellowships sparingly. Arguments such as Hertzler's, and feelings of exclusivity tinged with traces of bigotry, would continue for years and plague many of the positive results that came from the founding of the College.

It is significant that at the initial meeting of the American College of Surgeons a declaration against the division of surgical fees, the paying of commissions for clinical work, and the buying and selling of patients was adopted as a cardinal principle. It was a dramatic moment. So strong was the feeling that the College should fight what was regarded as an "abomination in the economics of medicine" that Martin had to urge this battle be conducted as part of the positive purpose of elevating the clinical standard of surgery without dominating it. The Clinical Congress itself continued more or less independently until 1917, when it was merged with the College, which has since controlled it as a self-contained activity. By the end of the College's sixth convocation or clinical congress (1918), a total of 3,795 candidates were received into fellowship. During these years, two main developments stand out as important activities in the College's campaign against unworthy financial practices and the development of science-based surgery. Beginning in 1916, Martin sensed increasing difficulties in determining which candidates should be recommended for fellowship. This occurred because of discrepancies in the standards of management among hospitals in which surgeons worked, a wide variation in the surgical training received by interns and house officers in hospitals with comparable equipment, the lack of a standardized system of presenting case histories through which the merit of work as submitted by candidates to the committee on examinations might be estimated, and, finally, little uniformity among graduate courses in surgery as offered by the educational institutions that controlled the great clinical centers and widely distributed polyclinics .

Martin was disheartened to learn that surgical case records submitted by applicants clearly showed that much day-to-day clinical work was being completed in hospitals that lacked even the most simple of facilities essential to the scientific care of patients. Cases were unsystematically recorded, laboratory facilities were woefully deficient, medical staffs were unorganized, and surgical work was generally without supervision. Only when increasing numbers of candidates were refused fellowship because of their unacceptable case records did hospitals begin to show an interest in the College's requirements and request that an example of acceptable record forms and suggested standards for laboratories and staff organizations and privileges be made available. Thus, quite early on, the American College of Surgeons became inextricably linked with the rise of modern America's hospital system.

This growing clamor led to a two-year analysis of hospital management conducted by the College. By 1917, the board of regents had decided that the time had come for the College to take a proactive position and publicly furnish a "minimum standard" for hospital activities. These standards would safeguard the care of every patient within an institution by insisting on competence on the part of the doctors and adequate clinical and pathological laboratory facilities to ensure correct clinical diagnoses. By demanding a thorough study and understanding of each admission, a monthly audit of the medical and surgical work conducted in the hospital during the preceding interval, the holding of weekly morbidity and mortality conferences and by prohibiting the practice of the division of fees under any guise whatsoever, the College launched a standardization program that became to the American hospital system what the Flexner report was to American medical education.

As concerned as College officials were about the quality of the nation's hospitals, there was similar distress over an apparent lack of concerted action on the part of medical societies, medical schools, hospitals, and government agencies to assure that safe and experienced surgeons were being educated and trained. There were no true scientifically grounded training programs for surgeons outside of a handful of conspicuous exceptions (e.g., Halsted's residency at The Johns Hopkins Hospital). The men who completed these sophisticated residency programs were admittedly skilled diagnosticians, pathologists, and technical operators, but they were so few that they could never realistically fill the teaching positions in the country's large population centers.

Martin was of the opinion that corrective action was necessary to standardize surgical competency, much like a movement to standardize hospitals. In October 1916, a Committee on Standards was authorized to consider ways and means to create supplementary training programs for surgeons. In addition, the Committee was to suggest ways to bring about legislative enactment and other methods to prevent dishonest practices, thereby protecting the public against untrained and unscrupulous surgeons. This deliberative body was the first to formally consider the matter of graduate education in surgery on a national scale, although it had admitted purposes beyond just the standardization of surgical residency and postresidency programs.

THE RISE OF THE POLYCLINICS

For surgeons, the reform of education and training had previously taken a unique American twist when in the early 1880s "polyclinic medical schools" began to open. These institutions were an amalgam of the German short clinical course and the ubiquitous urban dispensary. For a fee, professors in the polyclinics offered a practitioner courses, usually of six weeks duration, mostly in surgery. The three earliest and politically strongest schools were the New York Polyclinic, the New York Post-Graduate Medical School, and the Philadelphia Polyclinic, found by the surgeons John Wyeth (1845–1922), Daniel St. John Roosa (1838–1908), and John Roberts (1852–1924), respectively. The concept of postgraduate education was so well received that by the late 1880s, virtually every major city in the United States could boast of its own polyclinic school.

What made these schools so influential was that the wide variety of courses offered to surgical practitioners helped to make up for the dearth of other clinical educational opportunities. At the Philadelphia Polyclinic, for instance, the faculty

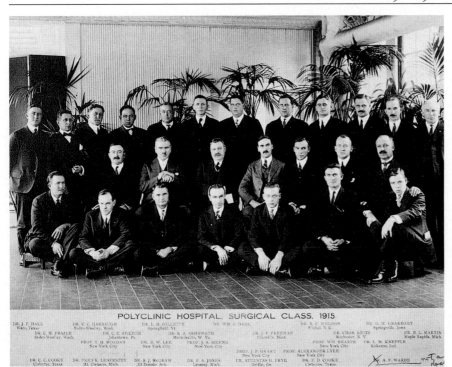

offered courses in operative surgery, general and orthopedic surgery, diseases of the throat and nose, diseases of the ear, diseases of the eye, and genitourinary and vene-real diseases, among other subjects. Although most of the polyclinics started out as dispensary-based schools, eventually surgical instruction required inpatient services, and the institutions were forced to fit up rooms as wards and operating areas. So popular had this mode of training become that the two New York City schools were enrolling over four hundred pupils annually by the early 1890s. Within just a few years, the polyclinics matured into true hospitals. The Philadelphia Polyclinic completed a new hospital in 1890, the New York Post-Graduate in 1893, and the New York Polyclinic in 1897 and again fifteen years later when it moved from Manhattan's East Side to 50th Street on the West Side. But they still continued the large dispensary services that supplied ward patients.

Not unlike what was occurring in the whole of American health care, surgery dominated medicine in the polyclinic setting. The schools usually employed several "professors" of surgery and initially listed two or three distinct surgical courses under slightly different headings. By 1888, the New York Post-Graduate offered five separate surgical options. Didactic lectures were forbidden, patient contact was kept to a maximum, and everything was thoroughly practical but crowded. Because so much of the course work at postgraduate schools was in surgical specialties, the poly-clinic phenomenon helped focus the process of specialization within American surgery. Arpad Gerster, who taught at the New York Polyclinic, discussed in his autobiography how the school's noisy operating amphitheater seemed "anything but sweet or clean," and how he "preferred to operate at [other] hospitals, where matters were under better control." Still, there was little doubt that the polyclinic setting was useful for knowledgeable students who desired specific types of training. However, to enroll at a polyclinic under the assumption that its faculty could take a recent medical school graduate and produce a mature surgeon in a few months was little more than an illusory pipedream. It was only when a student like William or Charles Mayo came to work with a specific affiliated surgeon like Gerster, Robert Abbe, or Robert Weir that the polyclinic was best able to fulfill its mission.

Despite large student enrollments (Wyeth mentions in his autobiography, *With Sabre and Scalpel*, that by 1914 "approximately twenty-five thousand graduates of medicine and surgery…attended the clinics and courses of study"), most polyclinics were not to have lengthy independent existences. As the Flexner report and the establishment of the residency system spurred on reforms in medical education and training, polyclinics were slowly closing their doors. The Philadelphia Polyclinic joined the Medico-Chirurgical College in a merger with the University of Pennsylvania in 1917, forming the University's clinical postgraduate appendage and Graduate Hospital. The New York Polyclinic continued as a totally independent hospital, minus course offerings, until a merger with the French Hospital in 1972 preceded its bankruptcy and demise in 1976. The New York Post-Graduate School and Hospital became the University Hospital of New York University–Bellevue Medical Center in 1948.

GROUP SURGICAL PRACTICES

The all-purpose polyclinics of America served an important but interim role in the schooling of American surgeons. However, another far-reaching development was occurring in the Middle West, which would have an enormously powerful influence on the evolution of American surgical education. The establishment on the upper Mississippi River of the Mayo Clinic, the earliest example of group surgical practice in the United States and one of the era's largest centers for graduate and postgraduate surgical training, provided geographic balance to those events taking place on the shores of the Chesapeake, Schuylkill, Hudson, and Charles Rivers.

William Worrall Mayo (1819–1911) was born in Manchester, England, and emigrated to America in 1845. Nine years later, he received his medical degree from the University of Missouri. After practicing in various places in the Midwest, he finally settled in Rochester, Minnesota, in 1863. Mayo was provost surgeon for southern Minnesota during the Civil War and, being recognized as among the most competent physician-surgeons in the area, was soon involved in local and state politics. A founder of the Minnesota State Medical Society (1868), he served as its president in 1873 and was instrumental in giving the ethical practice of medicine a legal standing in the state. Mayo married Louise Abigail Wright in 1851, and from this union were born William James Mayo (1861–1939) and Charles Horace Mayo (1865–1939). The elder Mayo had a strong influence on his two sons, imparting to them not only a love of medicine but a strong sense of social commitment.

William J. Mayo attended the University of Michigan School of Medicine (1883) and also received a certificate of competence from the New York Post-Graduate Medical School in 1884. The following year, he obtained another medical degree from the New York Polyclinic Medical School. His entire professional life was spent in practice with his father and brother, and together they made the Mayo Clinic one of the world's foremost centers for surgical care, training, and research. Mayo's professional career included close associations with numerous medical organizations, including the presidencies of the American Medical Association (1906), the Society of Clinical Surgery (1911), the American Surgical Association (1913), and the American College of Surgeons (1925). His name is linked with several surgical operations, including an excision of the pylorus and exclusion of the duodenum with posterior gastrojejunostomy, the cure of umbilical hernia, and the excision of the rectum with removal of the neighboring lymph glands for cancer. Mayo is eponymically associated with the prepyloric vein. He never authored a textbook of surgery, but he contributed more than six hundred papers to the periodical literature.

Charles Mayo received his medical education at the Chicago Medical College (1888). After a period of postgraduate study at the New York Polyclinic and New York Post-Graduate medical schools, he went into practice with his brother and father. Although not as prolific or as surgically innovative as his older brother, Mayo did serve as president of the Society of Clinical Surgery (1912), the Clinical Congress of Surgeons of North America (1914), the American Medical Association (1924), and the American College of Surgeons (1924). His name is associated with an operative treatment of tic douloureux, in which the affected nerve branch is exsected and the foramen of exit in the skull is plugged by a silver screw to prevent reunion, and also with a bunionectomy, the principal feature of which is the resection of the first metatarsal head.

Both brothers manifested a persistent intellectual curiosity and desire to improve their clinical skills. They traveled widely, working and studying in various surgical centers but particularly with Christian Fenger and Nicholas Senn in Chicago. Interspersed with their trips throughout the United States were numerous excursions to European hospitals. Like their father, the two brothers increasingly oriented their practice toward surgery, adopting the newest techniques and devising their own surgical cures. By the early 1890s, when their father retired, as a group they were completing hundreds of operations a year. The Mayo family's surgical practice attracted patients from all over the Midwest, and at the turn of the century the numbers were up to almost three thousand procedures annually.

The growth of the Mayos' surgical practice was simply phenomenal. Virtually free of competition or political interference, and inheriting the organizational ability of their father, the Mayos established not only an international reputation but a private multispecialty clinic that was to become a trademark of American medicine throughout the remainder of the twentieth century. In 1897, the brothers began to hire interns at their hospital. Many physicians also came to observe the Mayos at work, and these visits were soon organized into formal courses in graduate surgery. The clinic grew rapidly and by 1907 was treating almost seventy-five hundred patients yearly, of whom five thousand were surgical. In 1915, having accumulated a substantial fortune, the Mayos gave $1.5 million to endow the Mayo Foundation for Medical Education and Research in affiliation with the graduate school of the University of Minnesota. Thus, the Mayo clinic provided one of the first degree programs in graduate medical education and became a center for surgical training.

What made the Mayo Clinic so uniquely American was that through the excellence of its clinical work the idea of a cooperative, private, multispecialty medical practice was popularized. The Mayos were able to take in numerous associates who were given the opportunity to travel, study, and do their own surgical research. From Rochester, these young followers spread out and began multispecialty practices of their own, such as the Guthrie Clinic (1910) in Sayre, Pennsylvania, and the Menninger Clinic (1908) in Topeka, Kansas. During the 1920s, the Mayo Clinic served as a surgical role model for the Crile Clinic in Cleveland, the Lahey Clinic in Boston, and the Ochsner Clinic in New Orleans. The Mayo Clinic was visited by the surgical greats of Europe, and a whole generation of European surgeons did a postgraduate year there. In the end, the Mayo Clinic became the most renowned and atypically successful of small-town health care enterprises (Rochester was somewhat unique in having a railroad stop so that patients could easily get to this out-of-the-way hamlet). It owed much of its success to the unparalleled growth of scientific surgery and the active enthusiasm of surgeons and their willingness to solve diagnostic problems with the scalpel.

WOMEN SURGEONS

One of the many overlooked areas of American surgical history concerns the involvement of women and African Americans. Women's options for obtaining advanced surgical training were severely restricted during this surgical era. The major reason was that through the 1890s, only a handful of women had performed enough surgery to become skilled mentors. Without role models and with limited access to hospital positions, the ability of the few practicing female physicians to specialize in surgery seemed an impossibility. Consequently, women surgeons were forced to utilize different career strategies than men and to have more divergent goals of personal success in order to achieve professional satisfaction. Among the female surgeons of this era, most were known as ovariotomists with an expected interest in obstetrical surgery. Through determination and the aid of several enlightened male surgeons, most notably William Byford (1817–1890) of Chicago and

23. An unusual scene of a Philadelphia operating amphitheater (circa 1890) in that both male and female student observers are seated together. *(Courtesy of Stanley B. Burns, M.D., and The Burns Collection and Archive)*

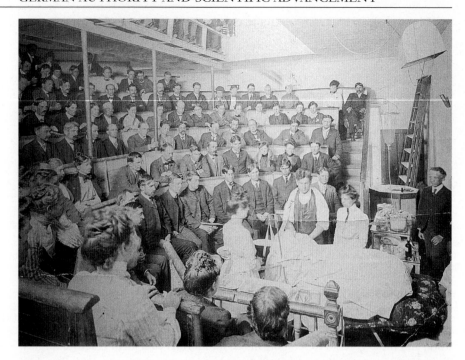

24. At the Woman's Medical College of Pennsylvania, Harry Deaver, the surgeon and only man in the photograph, stands in stark contrast to the seventy-two women gathered around him. Even though the medical school was for women, male surgeons still ruled the operating amphitheater. *(Historical Collections, College of Physicians of Philadelphia*

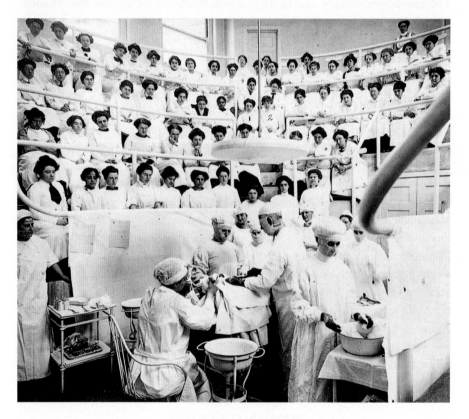

William Keen of Philadelphia, a small cadre of female surgeons did exist in late nineteenth-century America.

Mary Dixon Jones (1828–1908) originally studied medicine as an apprentice to two established Maryland practitioners: Henry Askew (1805–1876), later to become nineteenth president of the American Medical Association (1867) and Thomas Bond, professor of materia medica in Baltimore's Washington University Medical College. She later attended the New York Hygeio-Therapeutic College, an irregular, coeducational medical school, from which she received a medical degree in 1862. Dixon Jones practiced medicine in Brooklyn, but performed little in the way of surgical operations, for almost a decade. For unknown reasons, she decided to obtain a more formal medical background and entered the Woman's Medical College of Pennsylvania for a three-year course (1872). There, Dixon Jones learned the principles and practice of surgery from Benjamin Wilson and attended lectures by Emmeline Horton Cleveland, a Paris-educated professor of obstetrics and diseases of women, who eventually became dean of the school. Seeking additional training, Dixon Jones returned to New York City and enrolled for postgraduate training at John Wyeth's Post-Graduate Medical School and Hospital. Practicing once again in Brooklyn at the Woman's Hospital, and with her interest in surgery and pathology piqued, Dixon Jones completed her first laparotomy in 1883, assisted by her son Charles N. Dixon Jones, a recent graduate of Long Island Medical College Hospital. Three years later, both Dixon Joneses toured European surgical centers, including those in Dresden, Freiberg, Munich, and Vienna. Over the next decade, Mary Dixon Jones performed almost three hundred laparotomies, mostly of a gynecologic nature. Her most renowned case was the country's first panhysterectomy for fibroids (1888).

In many respects, Dixon Jones was an anomaly in that few other women were able to duplicate her professional accomplishments. At a time when women tended to be demure and subservient to men, Dixon Jones was pushy and aggressive, and had an amazing talent for self-promotion. Emmeline Horton Cleveland (1829–1878) seemed the exact opposite of the brash Dixon Jones. She graduated in 1855 from the Woman's Medical College of Pennsylvania and in 1875 became the first woman in world surgery to perform an ovariotomy and one of the first women in America to complete a laparotomy. Widowed, with a son, just two years after completing medical school, Cleveland sought postgraduate training abroad specifically to bring increased professional skills and knowledge of hospital management to the newly chartered Woman's Hospital of Philadelphia (1861). From 1862 to1878 she was professor of obstetrics and diseases of women and children at her alma mater and from 1872 to 1874 she served as its dean. Considered a warm and supportive teacher, Cleveland's career was cut short by tuberculosis.

Three other nineteenth-century female surgeons also deserve mention. Mary Harris Thompson (1829–1895) was known as the first woman in the United States to specialize in surgery. In 1863, she received her first medical degree from the New England Female Medical College in Boston. Seven years later, she followed it with another from Chicago Medical College. In 1865, Thompson founded the Hospital for Women and Children in Chicago and served as its head physician and surgeon. This small building was destroyed by fire in 1871, and a nationwide appeal raised funds to erect a new institution, which bore her name. Considered to have been the first woman to perform major surgery in Chicago, Thompson devised a widely used needle for abdominal surgery. Known as a staunch suffragist and philanthropist, she never married. Like all women physicians of this era, Thompson was denied membership in the American Medical Association and was forced instead to gain admittance to the less respected International Medical Association (1887).

Anna Elizabeth Broomall (1847–1931) graduated from the Woman's Medical College of Pennsylvania in 1871 and spent the next four years in Vienna studying obstetrics and gynecology. From 1875 to 1883 she was chief resident physician at the Woman's Hospital of Philadelphia and was eventually named professor of obstetrics at her alma mater. In 1892 she was among the first women admitted to the Philadelphia Obstetrical Society, and she was the first female physician to have a paper published in that society's *Transactions*. Noted for her extensive reading of French, German, and Italian medical literature, Broomall brought to women students in Philadelphia the most advanced European methods of obstetrical and gynecological care then available. She was among the first American obstetricians to emphasize thorough prenatal care, including pelvimetry, and remained a firm advocate of episiotomy. Cleveland strongly championed symphysiotomy, rather than cesarean section, as the treatment of choice for feto-pelvic disproportion. In 1878, she authored an article on encapsulated round fibroid tumors of the uterus in the *American Journal of Obstetrics and Diseases of Women and Children*. This was the earliest gynecological report in an American medical periodical to include a photograph, in this case a heliograph of a fibroid uterus. Broomall was never married.

25. Dr. Reifsnyder, a graduate of the Woman's Medical College of Philadelphia, performing a successful ovariotomy in Shanghai, as depicted on a Chinese handbill (circa 1885). Reifsnyder was a medical missionary surgeon, and in performing this surgical operation in male-dominated China she must have created quite a sensation. *(The Francis A. Countway Library of Medicine)*

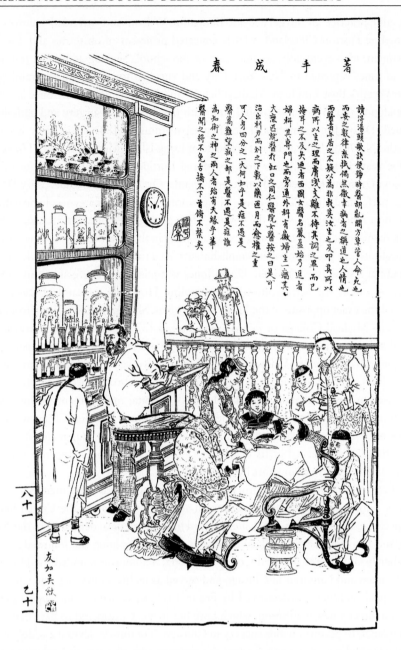

Marie Mergler (1851–1901) was born in Bavaria, Germany, and emigrated to the United States with her family in 1853. Her father, a physician, settled in Cook County, Illinois, where he established a general medical practice. Marie Mergler attended the Cook County Normal School and, after completing her course in 1869, entered the State Normal School at Oswego, New York, graduating in 1872. She subsequently matriculated at the Woman's Medical College in Chicago and graduated as valedictorian in 1879. Two years later she became assistant to William Byford at the Woman's Hospital of Chicago. In 1882 Mergler was appointed professor of materia medica at her alma mater and served until 1890, when she succeeded her mentor Byford to the chair of gynecology. Nine years later she was named dean of the faculty. Mergler also served as an editor of the *Medical Woman's Journal.* In 1893, she authored *A Guide to the Study of Gynecology.* This 160-page privately printed effort was one of only two textbooks written by American women surgeons in the nineteenth century. The other, by Gertrude Annie Walker (1863–?), clinical instructor in diseases of the eye at the Woman's Medical College of Pennsylvania, was *Students' Aid in Ophthalmology* (1895).

AFRICAN-AMERICAN SURGEONS

There is little disputing the fact that both gender and racial bias have affected the evolution of American surgery. Every aspect of American society is affected by such discrimination, and African Americans, like women, were innocent victims of injustices that forced them into never-ending struggles to attain competency in surgery. As early as 1868, a department of surgery was established at Howard University. However, the first three chairmen, Robert Reyburn (1833–1909), Neil Graham (1840–1904), and Edward Balloch, were all white Anglo-Saxon Protestants. Not until Austin Curtis was appointed professor of surgery in 1928 did the department have its first African-American head. Curtis received his medical degree from Northwestern in 1891, but like all black physicians he was forced to train at "Negro" hospitals. He spent two years at Provident Hospital, where he came under the tutelage of Daniel Hale Williams (1858–1931), the most influential and highly regarded of early African-American surgeons.

Williams was a graduate of Chicago Medical College (1883) and became a founder of the Provident Hospital in Chicago, the first hospital in the United States opened by African Americans. From 1893 to 1898, he was surgeon-in-chief at the Freedmen's Hospital in Washington, D.C. He was a charter member of the American College of Surgeons and later a founder of the National Medical Association. Williams received considerable notoriety when he reported in the *Medical Record* a successful suturing of the pericardium for a stab wound of the heart (1897). His patient, a 19-year-old man, was stabbed in the left side of the chest in 1893 and taken to Provident Hospital, where he was observed overnight. However, there was "such persistent hemorrhage, pain over the cardiac area...and such pronounced symptoms of shock" that the following morning, Williams decided to perform an operation. He found a small puncture wound of the heart and a laceration of the pericardium about an inch and a quarter long. Using all his technical skills on this beating heart, Williams proceeded to hold the edges of the pericardium together and close the wound using a "continuous suture of fine catgut." Williams' claim that this was "the first successful or unsuccessful case of suture of the pericardium that has ever been recorded" is incorrect, as he had been preceded by Henry C. Dalton (1847–?) in 1891. However, Williams' paper had the greater impact on the future course of American thoracic surgery by opening up new vistas in cardiac surgery. Daniel Williams was a complex personality, who made the Freedmen's Hospital into an important source of postgraduate training for black physicians. He promoted medical education for persons of color by many trips and educational programs, including the inauguration of annual surgical teaching clinics at Meharry Medical College (1899). In the 1890s he was so bold as to open the operating theater of Freedmen's Hospital to the general public to demonstrate the technical skills

26. *(left)* Daniel Hale Williams in his study at Freedmen's Hospital (circa 1896) *(Moorland-Spingarn Research Center, Howard University)*

27. *(right)* James Cornish shown after an operation for a stab wound of the heart. As described in Daniel Hale Williams's report *(Medical Record*, vol. 51, pages 437–439, 1897) a small puncture in the myocardium was left alone, but the one and one-quarter inch laceration of the pericardium was closed with catgut ligatures. *(Historical Collections, College of Physicians of Philadelphia)*

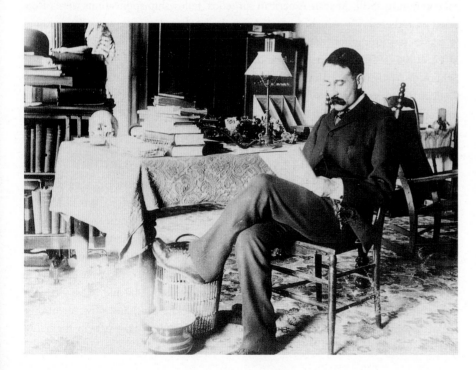

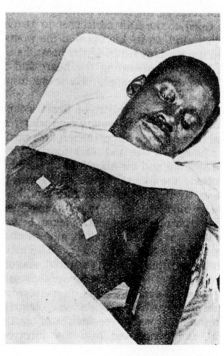

of black surgeons. Williams was also the first African-American physician to serve on the faculty of a medical school other than Meharry or Howard.

With little likelihood of obtaining membership in the American Medical Association or its related societies, particularly its Section on Surgery, in 1895, African-American physicians joined together to form the National Medical Association. Black surgeons identified an even more specific need when the Surgical Section of the National Medical Association was opened in 1906, with John Hunter of Lexington, Kentucky, as chairman. At the same time, surgical clinics were inaugurated at "Negro" hospitals and offered section members the opportunity to develop their surgical decision making abilities as well as technical skills under the direct supervision of renowned African-American surgeons. These National Medical Association surgical clinics, which preceded the Clinical Congress of Surgeons of North America by almost half a decade, represent the earliest instances of organized "show-me" surgical education in the United States.

The clinics sites were in predominantly black communities in the South, East, and Midwest, although hotel reservations in the face of "Jim Crow" barriers made the events logistical nightmares. Among the clinics utilized for such hands-on presentations, (including the St. Joseph and Presbyterian Hospitals in Lexington, Kentucky; Lincoln Hospital in Durham, North Carolina; and the Wheatley-Provident Hospital in Kansas City, Kansas), those held at the John A. Andrew Hospital in Tuskegee, Alabama, proved most popular. Conducted from 1912 to 1944, the Andrew "wet" clinic became the basic activity of the well-known John A. Andrew Clinical Society, which offered the first intensive postgraduate course in medicine and surgery for African-American physicians in the South in 1921. In virtually every respect, the historic evolution of African-American surgery through the 1960s, regardless of the organizational and scientific advances achieved by the American profession of surgery, depended entirely on the presence of the "Negro" hospital. These facilities evolved out of medical necessity because of the unavailability of care for black patients in white-dominated hospitals. Despite limited economic resources, reflected in generally inadequate buildings and equipment, the African-American–managed hospitals created a pride in the professional community that united black health care workers in a common effort.

Admittance to surgical societies and attainment of specialty certification were important social and psychological accomplishments for early African-American surgeons. When Daniel Williams was named a Fellow of the American College of Surgeons in 1913, the news spread rapidly throughout the African-American surgical community. Still, African-American surgeons' fellowship applications were often acted on rather slowly, which suggested that denials based on race were clandestinely conducted throughout much of the country. As late as the mid-1940s, Charles Drew (1904–1950), chairman of the department of surgery at Howard University School of Medicine, acknowledged that he refused membership in the American College of Surgeons because this "nationally representative" surgical society had, in his opinion, not yet begun to freely accept capable and well-qualified African-American surgeons.

INTERNATIONALIZATION OF AMERICAN SURGERY

Internationalization became an underlying theme of the many stories that demonstrate the remarkable transformation of American surgery before World War I. Whereas once streams of American physicians had traveled to the great German centers of medical learning, the trend was beginning to reverse in the decade and a half before the war. It became very clear by the increasing number of European surgeons who were visiting America that our state of dependence on European surgical know-how was fast changing to one of autonomy. Between 1900 and 1914, virtually every outstanding figure in German surgery made the long and now seemingly obligatory trip to America to observe, encourage, envy, and take part in the great surgical debates of the day.

The United States was a wondrous country, and many of the foreign visitors left colorful written impressions of their stay. The German ophthalmologic surgeon Julius Hirschberg (1843–1925) made three trips to the New World between 1888 and 1905. In his *Von New York Nach San Francisco; Tagebuchblätter* (1888), Hirschberg wrote of the phenomenal growth of American cities, the size and influence of the German immigrant group, and the changes in the quality of medical institutions and education that were beginning throughout the country. America might have seemed culturally backward, but the people exuded a sense of personal potential not found anywhere in Europe.

By the mid-1890s, European opinions about America, and especially the status of its medical and surgical institutions, were no longer in doubt. Adam Politzer (1835–1920), a Viennese otolaryngologist, after inspecting newly erected hospitals in Boston, Chicago, and New York, wrote in 1893, "We must ungrudgingly acknowledge that America has already surpassed Europe in its ideal aspiration to attain the highest fruits of knowledge and culture and simultaneously to alleviate the suffering of the poor." What most impressed visitors was that unlike the situation in European hospitals, which were largely dependent on government funding, scientific research and construction of hospitals in America was increasingly accomplished through private philanthropy. The industrial wealth of the United States was coming of age and creating change in medicine and surgery.

The most renowned of European surgeons traveled to America. And, in a measure of respect, letters from American physicians were increasingly featured in the leading medical publications in Germany. German orthopedic surgeons like Fritz Lange (1866–1952), Adolf Lorenz (1854–1946), and Albert Hoffa (1859–1908) were impressed with what they saw. Lorenz visited the United States in 1902 as the guest of a Chicago industrialist who wanted the discoverer of the nonoperative reduction of hip dislocations to treat his daughter. When asked what impressed him the most about the country, Lorenz unhesitatingly answered, "American beneficence and hospitality" and "in a technical-mechanical respect we can learn quite a bit from the Americans." Hoffa and Lange reported back to German readers how surprised they were with the quality of orthopedic facilities in New York City. Hoffa remarked that he only wished Berlin might some day have comparable equipment. Lange discussed the difference between orthopedic institutions in Boston and Munich and their environs. Both cities had approximately the same population, but in the Boston area, over three hundred beds for orthopedic cases were available, compared with less than fifty in Munich. What fascinated Lange more than anything else was the practicality of American surgical training. Writing in 1911 about his "Amerikanische Reiseerinnerungen," he expressed doubts about the vaunted wisdom of the oft-praised university training system in Germany and its object of training great research scientists. Lange believed that America produced medical graduates who "can do more and know more" than their German counterparts, particularly in surgery and orthopedics.

The academic surgeons Anton von Eiselsberg (1860–1939), Paul Clairmont (1875–1942), and Ernst Sauerbruch (1875–1951) made the requisite American tour, but it was the lesser-known Munich-based surgeon N. Guleke who provided the most cogent remarks. Guleke visited the States in 1909, and in a three-part report published in a Munich medical weekly he told of an American surgery that "scarcely existed twenty years ago" and had been heavily dependent on European traditions, but was now totally autonomous and actually superior in some fields. Visiting cities on the East Coast, Guleke could not believe the "astounding luxury" of such institutions as Mount Sinai Hospital in New York City. Like all European visitors, he was amazed at the purely private basis of support that many hospitals received. The physical size of operating rooms was impressive as well as the frequency with which visiting American physicians themselves were found at operations. Guleke believed that the American surgeon was more of a self-learner than his European colleague. Most importantly, operative techniques, especially those he observed at The Johns Hopkins

28. The internationalization of American surgery is evident in these three historically important photographs. In the summer of 1911, Halsted visited Theodor Kocher at the latter's clinic in Bern, Switzerland *(facing page)*. Although Halsted always felt ill at ease about performing surgical procedures while in Europe, he was asked to operate on a patient with an abdominal aortic aneurysm during his Swiss sojourn, and did so. Halsted *(the bald-headed figure, fourth from the left)* is standing directly across from the sitting and bearded Kocher. Three of Halsted's accompanying assistants (Arthur Fisher, Richard Follis, and William Sowers) form a triangle, the center of which is filled in by the nurse at Kocher's back. In October 1901, the renowned Heidelberg surgeon Vincenz Czerny performed a surgical operation before the faculty and students of Cooper Medical College in San Francisco *(top)*. In this photograph taken by Vaughan and Keith in that city's Lane Hospital surgical amphitheater, Czerny *(wearing an operating gown in center of the picture)* is posing next to Levi Cooper Lane *(dressed in street clothes)*. Nicholas Grattan, the first Irish surgeon to specialize full-time in orthopedic surgery, visited the Bellevue Hospital clinic of Lewis Sayre (circa 1892) *(bottom)* and demonstrated an osteoclasis for knock-knee. *(this page: Courtesy of Stanley B. Burns, M.D., and The Burns Collection and Archive) (facing page: The Alan Mason Chesney Medical Archives of The Johns Hopkins Medical Institutions)*

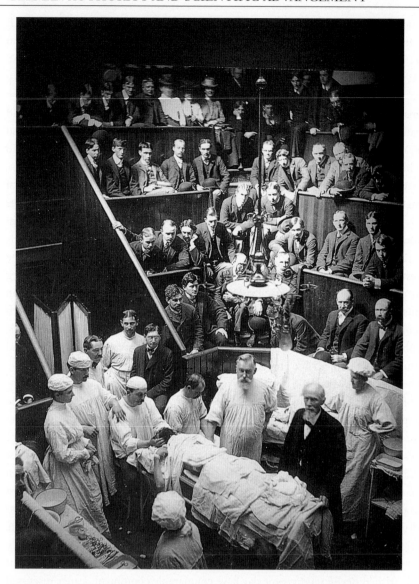

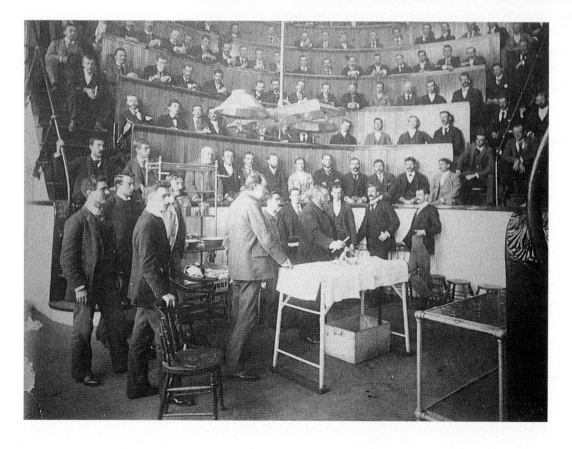

Hospital, were painstakingly methodical and involved minimal blood loss—admirable traits not noted in his German peers. What left the most lasting impression was the seeming respect with which patients regarded their surgeon. Guleke felt that Americans were more likely to risk an operation in the hope of ultimate recovery than the lay person in the Germanic countries. With this simple but meaningful observation, Guleke, the foreigner, confirmed that the social acceptability of surgery as a legitimate scientific endeavor and the surgical operation as a therapeutic necessity had finally been achieved within the context of American culture and society.

It was at the Mayo Clinic that Sauerbruch, von Eiselsberg, and Clairmont were best able to understand all the dimensions of American surgery. Not only was their visit intended to have them observe technical advances, but the new economics of surgical health care delivery were also to be studied. The multispecialty group medical practice, something unheard of in Europe, seemed appealing. All of the surgeons were quick to note that the social position of surgeons in America seemed more highly esteemed and, consequently, their practices more lucrative than in Europe. The wonderfully equipped private hospitals of such surgeons as Murphy and Marcy amazed Europeans. The visitors also saw the palatial homes of some surgeons, particularly the Mayos, which "betrayed the huge incomes from their practice." To the foreign guests, it seemed as if American surgery had grown up overnight and was threatening to quickly overshadow its European exemplar. American surgery was fast becoming fully autonomous, and the need for New World surgeons to seek out education and training in the Old World was drawing to a close.

Though distinguished German visitors continued to come to the United States after 1910, their numbers lessened as war threatened. In 1914, Halsted attempted a formal exchange of residents between The Johns Hopkins Hospital and Hermann Küttner's clinic in Breslau, Germany (now known as Wroclaw and located in southwestern Poland). Halsted was of the opinion that young physicians achieved greater surgical maturity by observing the practice of surgery in countries other than their own. To promote this belief, Halsted initiated the concept of exchanging residents between training programs in different lands. George Heuer was sent to Germany, while Felix Landois (1879–1945) came to Baltimore. Owing to the outbreak of

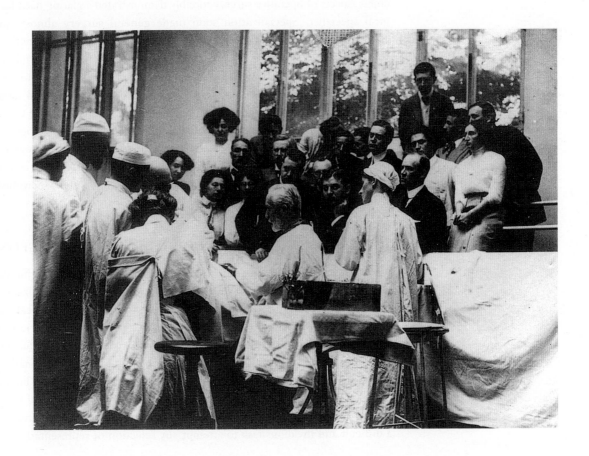

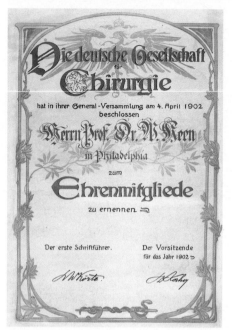

29. *Die Deutsche Gesellschaft für Chirurgie* is Germany's equivalent of the American College of Surgeons. Before World War I, the German society was the largest and considered the most distinguished surgical association in the world. In 1902 William W. Keen was bestowed an *Ehrenmitgliede* (Honororary Fellowship) in the organization. This proved an important event in the history of American surgery, not only because he was the first American so honored and the seventh foreigner but because it provided Germany's imprimatur to the many surgical achievements coming from nineteenth-century America. *(Historical Collections, College of Physicians of Philadelphia)*

World War I, Heuer's stay lasted slightly over six weeks. Despite the brevity of Halsted's resident exchange, the very fact that academic German surgeons were now attentive to American surgical work demonstrates the self-respect vis-à-vis Europe that was beginning to encompass our nation's surgeons.

The Europeans could hardly deny the truth of the matter. American surgeons were beginning to "flex" their growing nationalistic fervor. The W. B. Saunders Company published The American Text-Book Series, one of the company's most successful publishing ventures. Surgical titles included William Keen's and James White's *American Text-Book of Surgery* (1892), John Baldy's *American Text-Book of Gynecology, Medical and Surgical* (1894), Lemuel Bangs' and William Hardaway's *American Text-Book of Genito-Urinary Diseases, Syphilis and Diseases of the Skin* (1898), and George DeSchweinitz's and Burton Randall's *American Text-Book of Diseases of the Eye, Ear, Nose and Throat* (1899). For the first time in the country's history, numerous periodical articles were appearing that extolled the achievements of American surgery. Frederic Dennis (1850–1934), James Pilcher (1857–1911), George Shrady (1837–1907), and Martin Tinker (1869–?) gladly detailed all our surgical successes. Edmund Souchon's (1841–1924) article in the 1917 *Transactions of the American Surgical Association* was so effusive that it required over one hundred pages to list all the "original contributions of America to medical sciences." It was as if Americans could not receive information fast enough about the exploits of their newest professionals, the surgeons.

American surgery had come of age, and this era was its great turning point. After three centuries of dependence on European science and clinical expertise, American surgical research had attained a status equal to that of the best European centers. Following an equally long period of inferior training, surgical education was at a level similar to that available on the Continent. Last, but not least, the technical abilities of the average American surgeons were as reliable as those of their counterparts in Western Europe. Surgery was at the pinnacle of professional esteem and influence, as was demonstrated by the continued succession of specialists in surgery to the presidency of the American Medical Association.

It was also during the first two decades of the twentieth century that the broadening aspects of operative surgery forcibly demonstrated a glaring need for the surgical specialist. Specialization soon made general surgery almost completely abdominal surgery, and surgery involving other organs was delegated to surgical subspecialists. It had become impossible for any single surgeon to master all the manual skills, combined with other knowledge, required to perform every known surgical operation. For this reason, the evolution of the well-defined surgical subspecialty, with numerous individuals restricting their surgical practice to one highly structured field (e.g., gynecology, orthopedics, urology, otolaryngology), is one of the important by-products of the years leading up to World War I. It was also a time when the evolution of American surgery was beginning to be affected more by socioeconomic events and technological advances than by unique individual clinical achievements.

BIOGRAPHIES OF TURN-OF-THE-CENTURY SURGEONS

The United States had increasing numbers of specialists in surgery, but the future greatness of American surgery lay in expanding the role of specialization within surgery as basic science research opened up multiple new clinical pathways. Accordingly, this surgical era contained the last generation of American surgeons who were equally at ease performing an exploratory laparotomy, reducing a dislocated hip, extracting bladder stones, and completing a cranial trephination. These men were all-around surgeons in every sense of the clinical meaning, but they were part of a rapidly disappearing breed. Although by the conclusion of this surgical era the abundance of famous names and important written contributions makes it a difficult and invidious task to attempt any selection of representative personalities, hagiographic homage needs to be given to some of the country's original specialists in surgery.

Thomas Markoe (1819–1901) graduated from Princeton University in 1836 and from the College of Physicians and Surgeons in New York City in 1841. Always interested in pathological anatomy, Markoe was attending surgeon to the New York Hospital from 1852 to 1892. He was elected adjunct professor of surgery at his alma mater in 1860 and ten years later was promoted to full professor. In 1879, when the professorship was divided into various divisions, Markoe assumed the title of professor of the principles of surgery. Although his writings were limited, he did author the authoritative *A Treatise on Diseases of the Bones* (1872). His son, James Wright Markoe (1862–1920) was a well-known gynecologic surgeon in New York City. James Markoe was murdered in St. George's Church, where he was serving as a lay advisor, by a mentally deranged parishioner who fired a pistol point blank at his forehead.

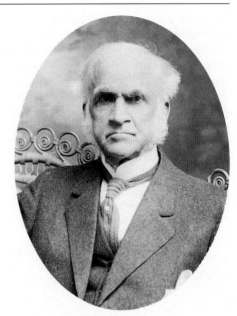

30. Stephen Smith. *(Courtesy of The New York Academy of Medicine)*

Stephen Smith (1823–1922), a native of upstate New York, received his medical education at the College of Physicians and Surgeons in New York City in 1850. He served on the resident staff of Bellevue Hospital and by 1855 had been elected one of the attending surgeons at that institution. In 1861 Smith helped found the Bellevue Hospital Medical College, where he served as professor of surgery from 1861 to 1865. He eventually transferred to the chair of anatomy, where he remained until 1874, when he became professor of clinical surgery in the medical department of New York University. Although a leading late nineteenth-century American surgeon and active in promulgating the doctrine of antisepsis in surgery, Smith did not gain his place in American medical history because of his career as a surgeon. Instead, he is remembered as a pioneer public health reformer who organized efforts for passage of the Metropolitan Health Bill in New York City (1866). From 1868 to 1875 he was a member and president of New York City's Board of Health. Through this position, Smith became a principal founder of the American Public Health Association (1872), serving as its first president. As commissioner of lunacy for the State of New York, Smith introduced training schools for hospital attendants and was responsible for the State Care Act of 1890 that brought responsibility for the mentally ill to state hospitals and out of county and city almshouses. Among his books are *The City That Was* (1911) and *Who Is Insane?* (1916), which describe long efforts to improve the sanitary and mental health conditions of New Yorkers. An authority on hospital construction, Smith designed the Roosevelt Hospital in New York City (1866), actively promoted improvements at Bellevue Hospital, and was one of five individuals invited to submit plans for The Johns Hopkins Hospital in 1875. Among Smith's major surgical texts were the *Hand-Book of Surgical Operations* (1862) and the *Manual of the Principles and Practice of Operative Surgery* (1879). In addition to his clinical contributions, including improved techniques for extremity amputation, Smith is also known for his remarkable historical essay on the evolution of American surgery, which appeared in 1906 as the first chapter in the eight-volume *American Practice of Surgery* edited by Joseph Bryant and Albert Buck. In 1872, Smith brought out *Doctor in Medicine*, a collection of his writings from his tenure as editor of the *American Medical Times* (1860–1864).

Edmund Andrews (1824–1904) was a graduate of the University of Michigan (1852). One year later, he founded the *Peninsular Journal of Medical and Collateral Sciences*. Most of his professional career was spent at either Chicago Medical College or Northwestern University, where he was professor of clinical surgery (1859–1901). Andrews was the first to report on the use of an oxygen–nitrous oxide mixture as an anesthetic agent (1868). He was among the earliest in the Midwest to use and promote Lister's antiseptic methods, which he brought over after a trip to England in 1867, and he pioneered blood transfusion in that area of the country. Along with his son Edward Wyllys Andrews (1856–1927), he wrote *Rectal and Anal Surgery, with a Description of the Secret Methods of the Itinerants* (1888).

Andrew Howe (1825–1892) was considered the foremost surgeon of eclectic medicine in nineteenth-century America. He received his medical education from

31. It was unusual for a colored illustration to be found in a surgical periodical of this era. However, this chromolithograph (*Annals of Surgery*, April 1904) vividly depicts a case of traumatic asphyxia following compression of the thorax by a moving freight elevator. The 30-year-old "large, muscular German" was held in position from "three to five minutes," during which time his "face became black and blood ran from his nose and mouths, and his eyes protruded." Brought to the West Surgical Service of the Massachusetts General Hospital, the patient made a slow but uneventful recovery. (*Author's Collection*)

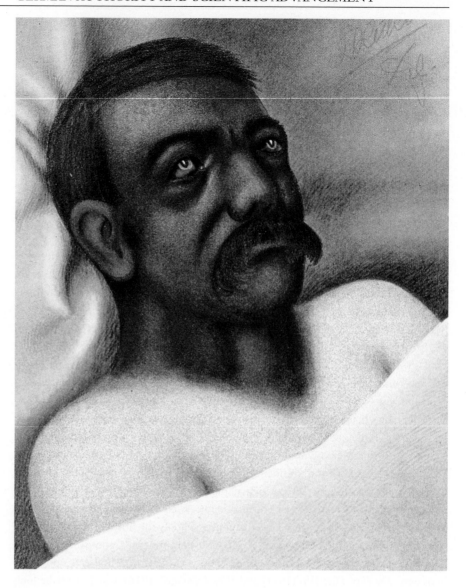

Worcester Medical Institute in Massachusetts (1855). In 1861, Howe was appointed to the chair of surgery at the Eclectic Medical Institute in Cincinnati and held that position until his death. His reputation became widespread, and he traveled extensively, to more than twenty states, to perform itinerant surgical operations. This frequency of travel probably contributed to his distaste for travel for pleasure. Throughout a rather active professional life, Howe would make only one trip to Europe, in 1886. His periodical contributions were voluminous, and his articles and editorials were a long-standing feature of the *Eclectic Medical Journal*. Howe authored several textbooks, including *A Practical and Systematic Treatise on Fractures and Dislocations* (1870), *Manual of Eye Surgery* (1874), *The Art and Science of Surgery* (1876), and *Operative Gynecology* (1890). He was always underrated and unacknowledged, primarily because of his affiliation with eclecticism. However, Howe is the only nineteenth-century American surgeon to have written texts in four different specialty areas.

Robert Kinloch (1826–1891) was a native of Charleston, South Carolina, and graduated with a degree in medicine from the University of Pennsylvania in 1848. He pursued further education in Edinburgh, London, and Paris. After the Civil War, Kinloch became professor of surgery at the Medical College of South Carolina. He was among the most prominent surgeons in the South, although he wrote no major surgical textbooks. His claim to distinction concerned numerous surgical feats, including the first treatment of fractures of the jaw by wiring the fragments together and the first resection of the knee joint for chronic disease (1859). Kinloch was a founding member of the American Surgical Association.

Claudius Mastin (1826–1898) spent most of his professional life in Mobile, Alabama, after his graduation from the University of Pennsylvania in 1849. He founded the American Association of Genito-Urinary Surgeons and served as president of the American Surgical Association (1890). He wrote only for the periodical literature; his most important paper described the use of metallic sutures to ligate aneurysmal arteries (1866). Mastin was the nephew of Henry Levert, who performed America's first published series of experiments on the use of metallic sutures in surgery as part of his medical graduation thesis for the University of Pennsylvania (1829).

David Yandell (1826–1898) was the son of the renowned Lunsford Pitts Yandell (1805–1878), a leading physician, editor, and educator in the Kentucky and Tennessee area. David Yandell received his medical degree from the University of Louisville in 1846. He spent two years in Europe completing his education and training. In 1850, Yandell was made demonstrator of anatomy in his alma mater. Following the Civil War, he was promoted to professor of surgery, a position he held for the rest of his professional career. Yandell served as president of the American Medical Association (1872) and the American Surgical Association (1890). Although he never wrote a surgical textbook, he founded the monthly medical periodical *Amercan Practitioner* and devoted a large portion of his writing efforts to this journal.

Richard Hodges (1827–1896) graduated from Harvard College in 1847 and from Harvard Medical School in 1850. Beginning in 1853, he was demonstrator in anatomy at his alma mater, working under Oliver Wendell Holmes (1809–1894). Hodges' dissecting ability was reputed to be second to none, and he authored the authoritative *Practical Dissections* (1858). Hodges was with Holmes for eight years and then was appointed visiting surgeon to the Massachusetts General Hospital, where he remained in that position until his retirement in 1885. His writings on joints, spiroidal fractures, and various other surgical conditions were widely respected, and his 204-page *Excision of Joints* was awarded the 1861 Boylston Prize. Hodges was the first to point out the frequency of a sinus in the sacrococcygeal region, to which he gave the name "pilo-nidal," from its hairy contents and nest-like shape. Among his other books is *A Narrative of Events Connected with the Introduction of Sulphuric Ether into Surgical Use* (1891).

Tobias Richardson (1827–1892) graduated in 1848 from the medical department of the University of Louisville, where he had studied with Samuel Gross. Initially made demonstrator of anatomy at his alma mater, Richardson later assumed the professorship of surgery. He had a peripatetic academic career, serving as professor of surgery in New Orleans at Tulane University as well as at one of the schools in Philadelphia. Richardson is best remembered for being the thirtieth president of the American Medical Association and also a founding member of the American Surgical Association. In 1854 he wrote *Elements of Human Anatomy*, the first systematic anatomical treatise of its kind to be published in the Mississippi Valley. The *Elements* was unusual in that it substituted English for Latin terms whenever possible.

Edward Warren (1828–1893) was one of the most flamboyant of nineteenth-century American surgeons. In 1850, Warren received his first medical degree from the University of Virginia. He followed this with a second degree from Jefferson Medical College in 1851 and immediately traveled to Paris, where he completed his medical education over the next two years. During the Civil War, Warren served as a member of the Confederate States Medical Examining Board and as surgeon-general of North Carolina. His surgical manual, *An Epitome of Practical Surgery for Field and Hospital* (1863) was used by virtually every Confederate medical officer. From 1867 to 1871 he was professor of surgery and director of the Washington University Medical School in Baltimore, and he followed this with a short stint as professor of surgery at the College of Physicians and Surgeons of Baltimore. In 1873, Warren left the United States for the Middle East, where he became chief surgeon of the general staff of the Khedive of Egypt. From 1875 to 1893 he practiced medicine and surgery in Paris. His life's adventures are wonderfully described in his autobiography, *A Doctor's Experiences in Three Continents* (1885).

William Briggs (1828–1894) completed a medical preceptorship under his father and received a medical degree from Transylvania University in 1849. He served as professor of surgery at the University of Nashville and Vanderbilt University from 1868 to 1894. Briggs was well respected for his technical surgical expertise and devised several new types of operations. He made important contributions to organized medicine in his capacities as a founder and president (1885) of the American Surgical Association, chairman of the Section on Surgery of the International Medical Congress (1887), and forty-third president of the American Medical Association (1890).

John Julian Chisolm (1830–1903) was a key figure in the surgical hierarchy of the Confederate Army. He studied at the Medical College of South Carolina (1850) and then spent two years in Paris and London. Most of his early career was devoted to general surgery, and before the Civil War he served as professor of surgery at his alma mater. During the conflict he authored *A Manual of Military Surgery* (1861), the first surgical treatise written expressly for the Confederate medical officer. At the conclusion of hostilities, Chisolm resumed practice in Charleston, South Carolina. However, in 1869, financial difficulties forced him to move to Baltimore, where he was appointed professor of operative surgery and diseases of the eye and ear at the University of Maryland. Chisolm was instrumental in establishing the Baltimore Eye and Ear Institute (1870) and the Presbyterian Eye and Ear and Throat Hospital in Baltimore (1877).

David Cheever (1831–1915) was a graduate of Harvard Medical School (1854) and also obtained additional medical training in Europe. He was made visiting surgeon of the Boston City Hospital in 1864 and concurrently joined the faculty of his alma mater. In 1875 Cheever was elected professor of clinical surgery, and seven years later he succeeded Henry Bigelow as professor of surgery, a position he held until his voluntary resignation in 1893. Cheever was the dominant medical figure at Boston City Hospital and its Harvard-based service, and he fought a long and ultimately unsuccessful battle against municipal politicians to maintain the institution's aristocratic traditions. His only textbook was the little known *Lectures on Surgery* (1894), but he authored numerous papers and pamphlets, including the first description of an esophagotomy in 1867. He was president of the American Surgical Association in 1889.

John Brinton (1832–1907) received his medical education at Jefferson Medical College (1852) and then spent two years in Paris and Vienna. From 1853 to 1861 Brinton was in general medical and surgical practice in Philadelphia. During the Civil War he served as a brigade surgeon, was named first curator of the Army Medical Museum (now the Armed Forces Institute of Pathology), and was inspector and director of patient evacuations after the battles of Antietam, Fredericksburg, Gettysburg, and Chancellorsville. Following the hostilities, Brinton went into full-time surgical practice in Philadelphia and eventually (1882–1906) succeeded Samuel Gross as professor of surgery at Jefferson Medical College. It was also during these years that he established a collection of war-related pathology and laid the groundwork for what later became a great public medical museum. Brinton was instrumental in planning and editing the three-volume *Surgical History of the War of the Rebellion*. His later years of active teaching and writing established him as a preeminent academic surgeon in this country. He authored an autobiography, *Personal Memoirs of John H. Brinton* (1914), which was published posthumously.

John Packard (1832–1907) was an 1853 graduate of the University of Pennsylvania. He never held an academic position but was on the surgical staff of the Episcopal Hospital and other Philadelphia institutions. Packard was the father of the well-known surgical historian Francis R. Packard (1870–1950). Among Packard's writings were *A Manual of Minor Surgery* (1863), *Lectures on Inflammation* (1865), and *A Handbook of Operative Surgery* (1870).

William Tod Helmuth (1833–1902) was the most prominent homeopathic surgeon of the nineteenth century. Because homeopathic medicine vanished from the

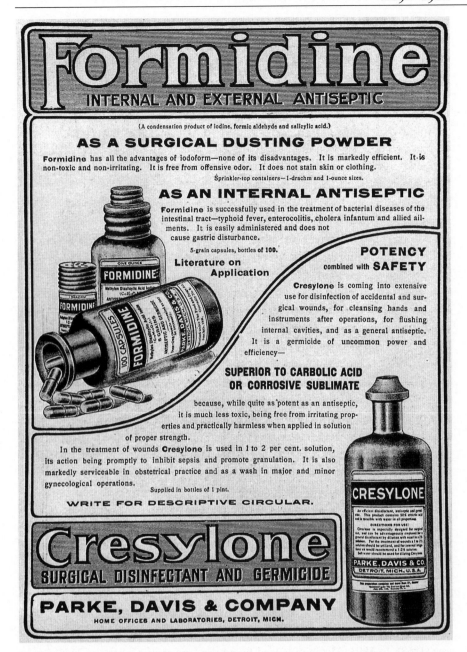

American scene almost a century ago, Helmuth remains relatively unknown. At the age of 22, after studying with his uncle William S. Helmuth (1801–1888), professor of the theory and practice of medicine in the Homoeopathic Medical College of Pennsylvania, Helmuth was made professor of anatomy at his alma mater. At that early stage of his career he authored his first textbook, *Surgery and Its Adaptation into Homeopathic Practice* (1855). In 1858, Helmuth moved to St. Louis, where he founded the Homeopathic Medical College of Missouri, served as professor of surgery, and completed *A Treatise on Diphtheria* (1862). In 1870, Helmuth accepted an offer to assume the chair of surgery at the New York Homoeopathic Medical College and Flower Hospital. Three years later, he authored *A System of Surgery* (1873). Helmuth was a vigorous defender of antiseptic and aseptic surgical procedures; as early as 1875 he was performing operations using antiseptic technique. He was president of the American Institute of Homeopathy in 1867.

Levi Cooper Lane (1833–1902) received his undergraduate education at Union College in Schenectady, New York. In 1851, he obtained his medical degree from Jefferson Medical College. His uncle was the renowned San Francisco surgeon Elias Cooper (1822–1862), who founded the first medical college on the Pacific Coast. Lane joined his uncle at the Toland Medical College and served on the anatomy and physiology faculty. In 1870, Cooper led a seceding group that established a rival medical school in San Francisco, where he became professor of surgery. In 1882 he set up new quarters for the school under the name Cooper Medical College. Subsequent discussions led to a merger with another institution and the creation of the Stanford University School of Medicine. His most important written work was *The Surgery of the Head and Neck* (1896), the first American treatise on this topic. Cooper was also editor of the *San Francisco Medical Press* and served as president in 1883 of the California State Medical Society.

Robert Reyburn (1833–1909) was born in Scotland but received his medical degree from the Philadelphia College of Medicine (1856). After serving in the Civil War, Reyburn was instrumental in founding the Freedmen's Hospital in Washington, D.C., where he served as surgeon in charge. From 1880 to 1892 he was professor of surgery at Howard Medical School, and later he served as dean. Reyburn was noted for his work with freed African Americans and fought unsuccessfully to have black physicians admitted to the Medical Society of the District of Columbia. Reyburn was one of several surgeons who attended President Garfield at the time of his assassination.

Frederick Bancroft (1834–1903) received his medical degree from the University of Buffalo in 1861. He was typical of many American physicians who received basic surgical training during battlefield experiences in the Civil War. Moving to Colorado, Bancroft served as surgeon for the Ben Holliday Overland Mail Express Company and the Wells Fargo Stage Line. In addition, Bancroft was the railway surgeon for every carrier serving Denver. Active in local and state politics, Bancroft was president of the Denver School Board (1872–1876), city physician of Denver, and first president of the Colorado State Board of Health. In 1881 he served as president of the Colorado Medical Society In the same year he organized the medical department of the University of Denver, where he served as professor of clinical surgery and fractures and dislocations from 1881 to 1894. He wrote little on surgical matters, although he was esteemed as the area's most respected surgical technician.

Hunter Holmes McGuire (1835–1900) achieved most of his fame quite early in life as medical director of the Army of the Shenandoah under the command of Stonewall Jackson. McGuire received his medical degree from the Medical College of Virginia in 1860 and from 1865 to 1878 was professor of surgery at the Virginia Medical College. Among his many honors were the presidencies of the American Surgical Association (1886) and the American Medical Association (1893). McGuire wrote no major texts but authored many articles in the periodical literature, including the first known attempt in America to ligate the abdominal aorta for aneurysmal disease (1868). In 1893, McGuire helped found the University College of Medicine in Richmond, the only medical school in the South with a three-year graded curriculum.

Thomas Morton (1835–1903) graduated from the University of Pennsylvania in 1856 and became professor of clinical and operative surgery at the Philadelphia Polyclinic. He was also on staff at the Pennsylvania Hospital and authored an authoritative historical review, *Surgery in the Pennsylvania Hospital* (1880). This lengthy text remains unique in American surgical history because it provides an in-depth look at the demographics of nineteenth-century surgical practices. Morton is also remembered for several important clinical contributions, including a description of neuralgia of an interdigital nerve of the foot (1876) and one of the earliest correct preoperative diagnoses of appendicitis (1887).

Oscar Allis (1836–1931) received his medical degree from Jefferson Medical College in 1866. He soon became one of the original staff surgeons at the Presbyterian Hospital in Philadelphia. Allis is eponymically remembered for a clinical sign in fracture of the neck of the femur in which the trochanter rides up and relaxes the fascia lata so that a finger can be sunk deeply between the great trochanter and the iliac crest. Allis's interest in hip disease was further evidenced when he won the Samuel Gross prize from the Philadelphia Academy of Surgery for *An Inquiry into the Difficulties Encountered in the Reduction of Dislocations of the Hip* (1896). Allis is most remembered for his description of a surgical clamp that remains part of modern surgical equipment.

William Carmalt (1836–1929) apprenticed with the brothers Morrill (1812–1903) and Jeffries Wyman (1814–1874) and received his medical degree from the College of Physicians and Surgeons in New York City in 1861. For four years (1870–1874), Carmalt studied in various European cities, including Breslau, Paris, Strassburg, and Vienna. In 1876 he began practice as an ophthalmologist in New Haven, Connecticut. From 1881 to 1907 Carmalt was professor of the principles and practice of surgery at Yale Medical School and attending surgeon at New Haven Hospital. He greatly influenced the course of medical education at the Yale Medical School, most notably by bringing about the union of the school and New Haven Hospital. Carmalt was well respected in the field of surgery and authored multiple case reports on his wide variety of interests. He was among the first to call attention to the epithelial origin of cancer and the connective tissue origin of sarcoma. A charter member of both the New York and American Ophthalmological Societies, he also served as president of the American Surgical Association in 1907.

John Homans (1836–1903) was a pioneer ovariotomist who graduated from Harvard Medical School in 1862. After serving in the Civil War, he returned to Boston and began to practice at several hospitals. Homan's only academic appointment was as clinical instructor in the diagnosis and treatment of ovarian tumors at his alma mater. He did little writing; his most important work was a monograph, *Three Hundred and Eighty-Four Laparotomies for Various Diseases* (1887). His son was the renowned surgeon John Homans (1877–1954), who described a clinical sign of slight pain at the back of the knee or calf when the ankle is forcibly dorsiflexed, indicating an incipient or established thrombosis in the veins of the leg.

William Williams Keen (1837–1932), a brilliant, innovative surgeon, gained worldwide recognition for several formidable surgical operations. He received his undergraduate degree from Brown University, where he was class valedictorian, and his medical education at Jefferson Medical College, graduating in 1862. He then

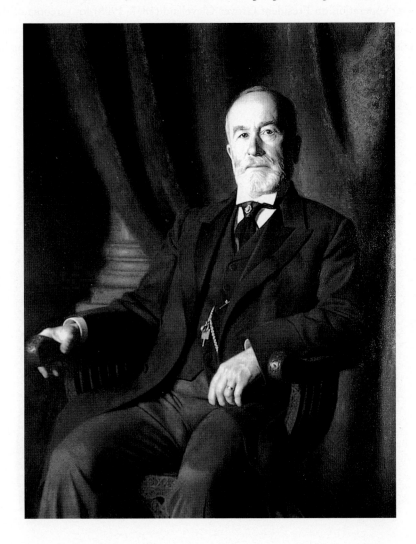

33. William Williams Keen, as painted by James Wood (1867–1938) in 1901. *(Courtesy of the College of Physicians of Philadelphia)*

undertook postgraduate studies in Berlin and Paris. During the Civil War, Keen was an assistant surgeon in the United States Army and worked with Silas Weir Mitchell (1829–1914) at a special hospital for neurological casualties in Philadelphia. A classic monograph, *Gunshot Wounds and Other Injuries of Nerves* (1864), was derived from their collaborative efforts. This work provided the first detailed study of traumatic neuroses and introduced the concept of causalgia. From 1866 to 1875, Keen taught pathological anatomy at his alma mater. He eventually was appointed professor of surgery at Woman's Medical College (1884), and five years later he succeeded Samuel Weissel Gross as professor of surgery at Jefferson. In 1892, Keen and James White jointly edited the impressive *American Text-Book of Surgery*, an important work because of its strong advocacy of listerian principles and because it was the first surgical text written by multiple contributors in which only American surgeons were involved. Keen, an exceptionally prolific writer, also authored *The Surgical Complications and Sequels of Typhoid Fever* (1898) and jointly edited, with John Chalmers DaCosta, the eight-volume *Surgery, Its Principles and Practice* (1906–1921). The latter work became the clinical bible of American surgeons in the first few decades of the twentieth century. Keen's contributions to the periodical literature were also legendary and included the description of a clinical sign of increased width at the malleoli in Pott's fracture of the fibula (1872). Keen remains particularly renowned as one of the major contributors to early neurological surgery. He performed an early successful resection of a brain tumor (1888) and the first tapping of the lateral cerebral ventricles (1888). He used a linear craniotomy incision (1891) and removed the trigeminal ganglion for the treatment of tic douloureux (1894). Among his many other operative accomplishments, Keen will long be eponymically linked with a procedure for the treatment of torticollis in which sections of the posterior branches of the spinal nerves to the affected muscles and the spinal accessory nerve itself are removed. Keen assisted Joseph Bryant in the performance of a "secret" operation on President Grover Cleveland (1837–1908) for sarcoma of the left upper jaw in 1893. Keen is also recognized as a medical historian, having written the well-known *Sketch of the Early History of Practical Anatomy* (1874). Among his

34. In the summer of 1893 the United States was passing through a severe financial crisis partially brought about by attempts to establish a silver standard. In the midst of all this political turmoil, President Grover Cleveland (1837–1908), a champion of the then existing gold standard, became ill from an ulcerating malignancy of the left upper jaw. To prevent panic in the financial markets, Cleveland's condition was concealed from all but his closest advisers. Surgical excision was advised, and a "secret" operation was performed on July 1 by Joseph Bryant, assisted by W. W. Keen, on board a yacht sailing in Long Island Sound. Not until many years later was the public informed of all the surgical particulars. Pictured are a cloth carrying case, hand-sewn by one of Keen's daughters, and two of the instruments used in the case, including a cheek retractor bought in Paris in 1866 by Keen. The operation, consisting of the removal of most of the sarcomatous left maxilla, was completed wholly within the mouth, thus avoiding any external scar. The president was later fitted with an artificial jaw of vulcanized rubber. This supported the cheek in its natural position and prevented it from falling in. In addition, when the prosthesis was in place, the quality of the president's voice was almost unaltered. Not only was this an important surgical triumph, carried out under the most difficult of circumstances on an extremely corpulent patient, it was the first major elective operation performed on a sitting president of the United States. *(Mütter Museum, College of Physicians of Philadelphia)*

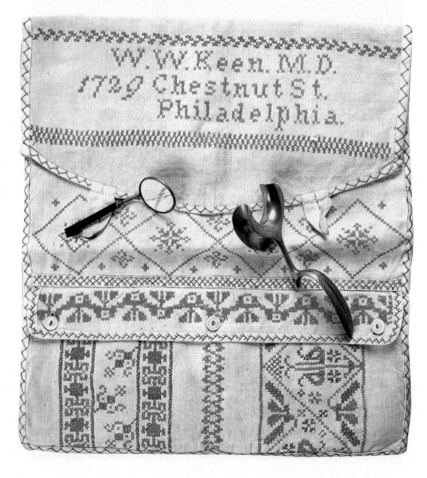

many honors were the presidencies of the American Surgical Association (1899) and the American Medical Association (1900). In the latter year, he was in the first group of American surgeons to be elected to honorary fellowship in the Royal College of Surgeons of England. Although Keen retired from active practice in 1907, he remained intellectually vigorous. In 1917, he wrote a monograph, *The Treatment of War Wounds*, which detailed the development and progress of surgery during World War I. In addition, he was an effective spokesman for various causes, advocating, for example, the theory of evolution and the importance of animal experimentation in the progress of biomedical research. During his later years, Keen authored *Animal Experimentation and Medical Progress* (1914), *Medical Research and Human Welfare* (1917), *I Believe in God and Evolution* (1922), and *Everlasting Life: A Creed and a Speculation* (1924). A kind, compassionate person with deep spiritual beliefs, Keen wrote a 511-page history of the Baptist church entitled *The Bicentennial Celebration of the Founding of the First Baptist Church of the City of Philadelphia* (1899). Widowed at an early age, Keen raised four daughters as a single parent.

Henry Orlando Marcy (1837–1924) graduated from Harvard Medical School in 1864 and soon traveled to Europe, where he became Lister's first American pupil. Upon his return to the United States, Marcy was among the first to introduce antiseptic methods in surgery. He practiced in Massachusetts, where he established a private hospital in Cambridge for the treatment of surgical diseases of women. In 1892, Marcy served as president of the American Medical Association. He authored two major texts, *A Treatise on Hernia, the Radical Cure by the Use of the Buried Antiseptic Animal Suture* (1889) and the monumental *Anatomy and Surgical Treatment of Hernia* (1892). He also wrote numerous journal articles, including several on the use of carbolized catgut ligatures (1878).

George Shrady (1837–1907) received his medical degree from the College of Physicians and Surgeons in New York City in 1858. He later became a surgeon at St. Francis Hospital and a consulting surgeon at both the New York Cancer Hospital and the Hospitals of the Health Department of the City of New York. He was best known as the editor of the *American Medical Times* (1860–1864) and the *Medical Record* (1866–1904). Shrady was a crusader for the reform of medical education and public health, and he vociferously opposed medical quackery. Highly regarded as a pioneer in plastic surgery, Shrady was the first in the United States to suggest using the finger as a medium of transplanting skin flaps from one part of the body to another, particularly in the restoration of a portion of a cheek.

James Ewing Mears (1838–1919) was a graduate of Jefferson Medical College (1865) and later served as professor of anatomy and surgery at the Pennsylvania College of Dental Surgery. Mears was a charter member of the American Surgical Association and served as its president in 1894. He was the first surgeon to suggest trigeminal ganglionectomy as treatment for trigeminal neuralgia (1884). His only textbook was *Practical Surgery* (1878).

Robert Weir (1838–1927) was a prominent New York City surgeon who received his medical degree from that city's College of Physicians and Surgeons in 1859. He was on the staff of numerous city hospitals and served as professor of surgery at his alma mater. All his written contributions were to the periodical literature, including articles on his technique for sterilization of the hands by scrubbing for five minutes with green soap, creating friction with calx chlorinata for five minutes, and rinsing with carbonate of soda and running water (1878); a method of appendicostomy (1887); and a logical, step-by-step rhinoplasty (1892).

John Ashhurst (1839–1900) completed his medical studies at the University of Pennsylvania in 1860. In 1863, he was appointed a surgeon to the Episcopal Hospital, and from that time on, he began to write voluminously. Ashhurst became professor of surgery at his alma mater in 1888 and held the John Rhea Barton chair until his death. Among Ashhurst's textbooks and monographs were *Injuries of the Spine* (1867), *The Principles and Practical of Surgery* (1871), and the six-volume *International Encyclopedia of Surgery* (1881–1886). The latter played an important role in the evolution of American surgery because it introduced the concept of a multi-authored surgical textbook. Previously, all surgical texts had been based on the cumulative experience of one individual. As a result of his efforts in this project, Ashhurst became recognized as one of the nineteenth century's greatest authorities on surgical bibliography.

Phineas Conner (1839–1909) attended Dartmouth College and received his medical education at Jefferson Medical College in 1861. Having been a surgeon during the Civil War, Conner was appointed professor of surgery at the Cincinnati College of Medicine (1866). The following year, he transferred to the Medical College of Ohio, where he held the chair of surgery from 1879 to 1902. He never published any lengthy surgical works, but he contributed numerous reports to the periodical literature, including the country's first report of a total gastrectomy. Unfortunately, Conner's patient was moribund prior to surgery and succumbed during the procedure, which makes it difficult to understand how the gastrectomy was ever completed! He served as president of the American Surgical Association in 1892.

Theodore McGraw (1839–1921) graduated from New York City's College of Physicians and Surgeons in 1863. Following his service during the Civil War as an assistant surgeon, McGraw moved to Detroit, where he helped found the Detroit Medical College and served as its long-time professor of surgery (1868–1914). In 1887 he was president of the Michigan State Medical Society and vice-president of both the American Medical Association and the American Surgical Association. McGraw was a pioneer in thyroid surgery, but his most important contribution to surgery was the development of a rubber ligature for use in intestinal anastomosis (1891).

Christian Fenger (1840–1902) was born in Denmark and received all of his education and training in his native country. In the late 1870s he emigrated to Chicago, where he became a pathologist at the Cook County Hospital. From 1893 to 1899 he taught surgery at Northwestern University Medical School, and from 1899 until his death, at Rush Medical College. Fenger was a versatile surgeon and reported many types of cases. His most important paper detailed an operation for stenosis of the ureter at the ureteropelvic junction (1894). He was considered the father of modern pathological surgery, and many of Chicago's later renowned surgeons received much of their clinical savvy from studying with Fenger.

Washington Peck (1841–1891) was unique because while studying at Bellevue Hospital Medical College (1863), he became the first medical student to combine lecture courses with hospital experience, serving as the first-ever undergraduate house surgeon at Bellevue Hospital. Having gained much-needed surgical skills during the Civil War, Peck moved to Davenport, Iowa, where he was instrumental in the establishment of a medical school (1868) and became first dean of the faculty and professor of surgery at the State University of Iowa department of medicine (1870–1891). In 1876 Peck was president of the Iowa State Medical Society, and fourteen years later he was a delegate to both the International Medical Congress in Berlin and the International Surgical Congress in Birmingham, England. Among his many honors were serving as vice-president of the American Medical Association (1885) and the American Surgical Association (1885). In addition, Peck was chairman of the American Medical Association's Section on Surgery and Anatomy (1882). Considered a superb surgical technician, Peck was well known for his abdominal and pelvic operations.

James Gilchrist (1842–1906) was an 1863 graduate of Hahnemann Medical College in Philadelphia. As a homeopathic surgeon, Gilchrist was quite influential within the sectarian movement because of his myriad writings. In 1873, while working as editor of the surgical department of *The Medical Investigator*, he wrote his first textbook, *The Homoeopathic Treatment of Surgical Diseases*. Gilchrist authored his second treatise, *Surgical Principles and Minor Surgery* (1881), while serving as lecturer on surgery at the Homeopathic Medical College of the University of Michigan. That year, Gilchrist was appointed professor of surgical pathology and therapeutics at the homeopathic division of the State University of Iowa. His last two important works were *Surgical Emergencies and Accidents* (1884) and *The Elements of Surgical Pathology with Therapeutic Hints* (1895).

Berthold Hadra (1842–1908) was born in Germany and received his medical education at the University of Berlin (1866). He soon emigrated to Texas (1872) and eventually settled in Galveston, where he held the chair of surgery at the Texas Medical College and Hospital. His only lengthy treatise was the detailed *Lesions of the Vagina and Pelvic Floor* (1888). Hadra remains best remembered as the first surgeon to plan and successfully complete spinal immobilization through the wiring of the vertebrae in cervical fracture (1891).

Charles Purvis (1842–1929) took his undergraduate education at Oberlin College (1863) and his medical degree from Wooster Medical College (now Case Western Reserve University) in 1865. After serving time in the U.S. Army as an acting assistant surgeon, Purvis eventually joined the staff of the Freedmen's Hospital in Washington, D.C., where he became surgeon in chief (1881–1894). As the second African American to join the faculty at Howard University Medical College, Purvis served as professor of obstetrics and gynecology from 1873 to1906. From 1906 until the time of his death, he was in the private practice of medicine and surgery in Boston. Purvis was a major force in keeping Howard Medical School open during the financial crisis of 1873 and also prevented the closing of Freedmen's Hospital three decades later. He was the first and remains the only African-American physician to attend an injured American president: James Garfield, following the assassination attack in 1881.

John Collins Warren (1842–1927), son of Jonathan Mason Warren, received his medical degree from Harvard Medical School in 1866. Having pursued postgraduate studies in Europe, Warren returned to Boston to begin surgical practice and served on the faculty of his alma mater for his entire professional career (professor of surgery, 1893–1907). In 1869 he performed one of the earliest operations according to listerian precepts in the United States, a mastectomy. An active member of the Harvard faculty, Warren was a driving force behind the decision to locate the medical school at its present location on Longwood Avenue. He was an editor of the *Boston Medical and Surgical Journal* (1873–1880) and served as president of the American Surgical Association in 1896. Largely through his efforts, the Collis P. Huntington Hospital for Cancer Research was built (1913). Among his textbooks are *The Anatomy and Development of Rodent Ulcer* (1872), *The Healing of Arteries After Ligature in Man and Animals* (1886), and *Surgical Pathology and Therapeutics* (1895).

Henry Walker (1843–1912) graduated from Albion College and received his medical degree from Bellevue Hospital Medical College in 1867. He returned to his native city of Detroit, where he was appointed demonstrator of anatomy in the newly organized Detroit Medical College and successively held several higher ranking teaching positions. Among them were lecturer on genitourinary diseases, professor of orthopedic surgery, and professor of surgery and clinical surgery (1881–1912). Although not a prolific writer, Walker authored *The Treatment of Diseases of the Bladder, Prostate, and Urethra* (1887). In addition, he edited the *Detroit Review of Medicine* and the *Detroit Clinic*. Among his honors was serving as vice-president of the American Medical Association and being chairman of its Section on Surgery.

Nicholas Senn (1844–1908) was born in Switzerland and emigrated to the United States in 1852. He was an 1868 graduate of the Chicago Medical College and initially practiced in Wisconsin. By 1878, Senn was so unhappy with his medical training that he decided to travel to Germany for further studies. He returned to Chicago in 1880 and was named professor of surgery at his alma mater. In 1888, Senn was appointed professor of surgery and surgical pathology at Rush Medical College, occupying the chair of surgery formerly held by Charles Parkes. At about this time he was also elected professor of surgery and military surgery at the University of Chicago. Senn was a pioneer in intestinal surgery and did much animal experimentation in this field. He was one of the most prolific of nineteenth-

35. Nicholas Senn had himself photographed while performing renal palpation. This particular illustration is from his *Tuberculosis of the Genito-Urinary Organs, Male and Female* (1897). *(Author's Collection)*

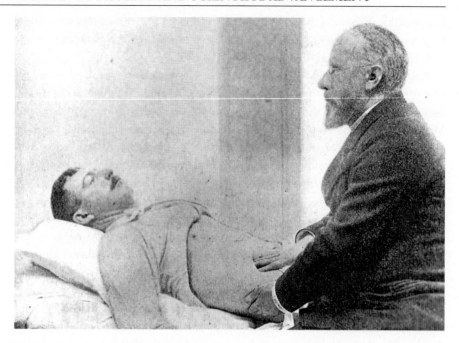

century surgeon-authors, and his texts included *Experimental Surgery* (1889), *Intestinal Surgery* (1889), *Surgical Bacteriology* (1889), *Principles of Surgery* (1890), *Tuberculosis of Bones and Joints* (1892), *The Pathology and Surgical Treatment of Tumors* (1895), *Tuberculosis of the Genito-Urinary Organs, Males and Females* (1897), *Practical Surgery for the General Practitioner* (1902), and *A Nurses's Guide for the Operating Room* (1902). Among Senn's most important papers were one on surgery of the pancreas (1886), one on the use of rectal insufflation to test for colonic perforation (1888), and a historical review of intestinal sutures and anastomoses (1893). Senn was president of the American Surgical Association in 1893 and the American Medical Association in 1897. In 1898 he served in Cuba during the Spanish-American War as chief surgeon. Senn did much to improve military surgery and founded the Association of Military Surgeons of the United States in 1891. He wrote about his military experiences in two texts, *War Correspondence* (1899) and *Medico-Surgical Aspects of the Spanish American War* (1900). In his later years, Senn became an indefatigable world traveler and documented his journeys in a series of books entitled *Around the World Via Siberia* (1902), *Surgical Notes from Four Continents and the West Indies* (1903), *Around the World Via India, a Medical Tour* (1905), *Tahiti, the Island Paradise* (1906), and *In the Heart of the Arctics* (1907). Senn was also a major bibliophile and collected one of the best private medical and surgical libraries in the United States, which was given to the Newberry Library and later transferred to John Crerar Library, both in Chicago.

Lewis Stimson (1844–1917) graduated from Bellevue Hospital Medical College in 1874. He occupied numerous academic positions in New York City medical schools but was most closely affiliated with New York Hospital. When Cornell University Medical Center was organized in 1898, Stimson became its first professor of surgery. Stimson's son, Henry L. Stimson (1867–1950), was secretary of state under President Herbert Hoover. Lewis Stimson's book-length works include *A Manual of Operative Surgery* (1878), *A Treatise on Fractures* (1883), *A Treatise on Dislocations* (1888), and *A Practical Treatise on Fractures and Dislocations* (1899).

Louis Tiffany (1844–1916) graduated in medicine from the University of Maryland in 1868. He remained at his alma mater, where he was demonstrator of anatomy (1869), professor of operative surgery (1875), and professor of surgery (1881). He resigned the chair of surgery in 1902 because of ill health. For fifteen years, Tiffany was also surgeon-in-chief of the Baltimore and Ohio Railroad. He held many local and national offices, including the presidency of the American Surgical Association (1896). His surgical achievements were varied, and he authored numerous papers for the periodical literature, including a widely read statistical report on the differences in the surgical diseases of the Caucasian and Negro races (1897).

Joseph Bryant (1845–1914) rose to prominence not only as a surgeon but also as sanitary inspector and health commissioner of New York City and commissioner of the New York State Board of Health. He graduated from Bellevue Hospital Medical College in 1868 and later became professor of anatomy and clinical surgery at his alma mater. Bryant is best remembered for having performed a "secret" operation on President Grover Cleveland for sarcoma of the left upper jaw in 1893. His assistant in this operation was William Keen, who wrote about the famous case in *The Surgical Operations on President Cleveland in 1893* (1917). Bryant's textbooks include the two-volume *Manual of Operative Surgery* (1884) and the massive eight-volume *American Practice of Surgery* (1906–1911), of which he was editor. He was the first American surgeon to report on a surgical approach to the posterior mediastinum (1895).

Frederic Gerrish (1845–1920) received his undergraduate education (1866) and medical education (1869) at Bowdoin College. From 1873 to 1882 he was professor of therapeutics at his alma mater. Gerrish was promoted to professor of anatomy in 1882, and from 1904 to 1911 he served as professor of surgery. An early member of the American Surgical Association, he was also a charter member of the American College of Surgeons. Gerrish's most memorable work was the *Textbook of Anatomy by American Authors* (1899). A leader in the movement to establish a public health service in Maine, Gerrish was a lecturer on medical ethics and director and consulting surgeon to Maine General Hospital from 1911 to 1915.

Charles McBurney (1845–1913) was born in Massachusetts and graduated from the College of Physicians and Surgeons in New York City in 1870. He then went abroad for further study in Berlin, London, Paris, and Vienna. When McBurney returned to the United States in 1873, he became demonstrator of anatomy at his alma mater. He progressed through the academic ranks to serve as professor of surgery (1889–1894) and professor of clinical surgery (1894–1907). Most of his clinical work was completed at Roosevelt Hospital, where, with the aid of a donation by a grateful patient, he had an elaborate private operating pavilion built. Roosevelt Hospital itself was to subsequently become nationally recognized as a center for surgical research and teaching. McBurney was the era's foremost authority on the diagnosis and treatment of appendicitis. He showed that a diseased appendix could readily be detected by applying pressure on a tender point, known thereafter as McBurney's point, located an inch and a half to two inches from the anterior spinous process of the ilium on a straight line drawn from that landmark to the umbilicus (1889). Five years later, McBurney detailed, in another paper, the incision that he used in cases of appendicitis, which parallels the course of the external oblique muscle, one or two inches from the anterior superior spine of the ilium. McBurney became a fellow of the American Surgical Association in 1892, but for unknown reasons he resigned five years later.

Lewis Pilcher (1845–1934) was an 1866 graduate of the University of Michigan Medical School. Beginning in 1872, Pilcher entered private practice in Brooklyn, where he was on the staff of various local hospitals. From 1885 to 1895 he served as professor of clinical surgery in the New York Post-Graduate Medical School. Pilcher was the first editor of the *Annals of Surgery* (1885–1934), which made him one of the most influential surgeons in the United States. His most important texts were *The Treatment of Wounds; Its Principles and Practice* (1883), *Clinical Studies of the Surgical Diseases of the Female Generative Organs* (1898), and *Fractures of the Lower Extremity or Base of the Radius* (1917). Pilcher was also a well-known surgical bibliophile; in 1918 he authored a lengthy annotated bibliography of his own collection of rare books, *A List of Books By Some of the Old Masters of Medicine and Surgery Together With Books on the History of Medicine and on Medical Biography*. Active in many areas of organized medicine, Pilcher was president of the Medical Society of the State of

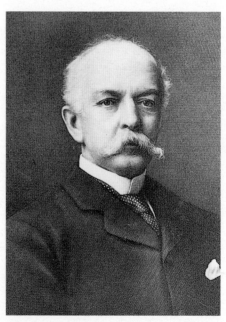

36. Charles McBurney. *(Courtesy of The New York Academy of Medicine)*

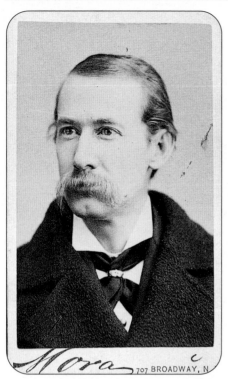

37. Visiting card of John Wyeth. *(Courtesy of The New York Academy of Medicine)*

New York (1892) and served on the state's Board of Medical Examiners (1913–1928). His life was richly described in his autobiography, *A Surgical Pilgrim's Progress* (1925), and many of his addresses and studies in medical life and affairs were published in *Odium Medicum* (1911).

John Wyeth (1845–1922) is little remembered, but his contributions relative to the founding of the New York Polyclinic Hospital and Medical College (1882) were extremely important in the evolution of the education and training of American surgeons. Wyeth was born in Alabama and graduated from the medical department of the University of Louisville in 1869. After spending a few years in private practice, he traveled to New York City in the hope of securing further medical training. Much to his consternation, Wyeth discovered that there were few formal courses for graduate students (i.e., practicing physicians) in medicine. After two years of study in Europe, Wyeth returned to New York City in 1878 and began to promote his plans for a postgraduate school of medicine. The concept received wide support, and the Polyclinic Hospital and College was opened. Wyeth devoted most of his professional life to the Polyclinic, serving first as surgeon in chief and later as president. He made several original contributions to clinical surgery, including a "bloodless" amputation of the hip in which hemorrhage was controlled by a strong elastic tube held in place by long needles transfixing the tissues above the joint (1892). Wyeth wrote extensively and authored four texts, *Essays in Surgical Anatomy and Surgery* (1897), *Handbook of Medical and Surgical References* (1873), *Textbook on Surgery: General, Operative and Mechanical* (1887), and *Surgery* (1908). He was active in numerous medical organizations and served as president of the American Medical Assoication in 1901. Despite all he accomplished, Wyeth was never recommended for membership in the American Surgical Association because of his lack of a true academic title.

Nathaniel Dandridge (1846–1910) graduated from Kenyon College in 1866 and received his medical education from the College of Physicians and Surgeons in New York City (1870). He had previously spent two years (1867–1869) studying medicine in Paris and Vienna. Returning to his hometown of Cincinnati, he was appointed pathologist to the Cincinnati Hospital (1872). Eight years later, he was named surgeon to the hospital, a position he held until 1909. Concurrently, Dandridge was nominated professor of surgery at the Miami Medical College. He never wrote any lengthy works, but he was well known for his numerous case reports in the periodical literature. Dandridge was president of the American Surgical Association in 1904. He never married but spent considerable time donating his services to the Episcopal Free Hospital for Children.

Charles Beylard Guerard de Nancrede (1847–1921) was an 1869 graduate of the University of Pennsylvania School of Medicine and for thirteen years was an assistant demonstrator of anatomy at his alma mater. Moving up the academic hierarchy, he eventually became professor of surgery and clinical surgery. In 1889, the trustees of the University of Michigan nominated Nancrede to the chair of surgery, which he held until his retirement in 1917. Every summer from 1900 to 1913, he also served as professor of clinical surgery at Dartmouth Medical College. Nancrede held positions in many national organizations, including the presidency of the American Surgical Association (1908). Among Nancrede's textbooks are *Essentials of Anatomy* (1887), *Lectures Upon the Principles of Surgery* (1899), and *Surgical Disease, Certain Abnormities and Wounds of the Face* (1908).

John Hamilton (1847–1898) graduated from Rush Medical College in 1869. He joined the staff of the U.S. Marine Hospital Service and rose to the rank of supervising surgeon-general. His surgical skills were widely respected, and he was also on the surgical faculty of Georgetown University from 1883 to 1891. In 1892 Hamilton returned to Chicago, where he was appointed professor of the principles of surgery and clinical surgery at his alma mater. He remained there until his early death of typhoid fever. Hamilton, always involved in the politics of medicine, induced members of Congress to place the Marine Hospital Service on an equal footing with the medical corps of the Army and the Navy. He helped establish the National Laboratory of Hygiene, a bacteriological laboratory devoted to research on communicable diseases (later to become the National Institutes of Health), within the Marine Hospital Service in 1887. Hamilton served as editor of the *Journal of the American Medical Association* from 1893 to 1898.

George Fowler (1848–1906) was an 1871 graduate of Bellevue Hospital Medical College. He practiced in Brooklyn and New York City and became professor of surgery at the New York Polyclinic Hospital and surgeon in chief of the Brooklyn Hospital. Fowler was a founder and first president of the Brooklyn Red Cross (1884) and introduced first-aid instruction to the New York National Guard. He is best remembered for completing the first known thoracoplasty (1893) and for describing an inclined patient position obtained by raising the head of the bed by as much as two to two and a half feet to ensure better dependent drainage after an abdominal operation (1900). Among his textbooks were the first American work to deal exclusively with appendicitis, *A Treatise on Appendicitis* (1894), the two-volume *A Treatise on Surgery* (1906), and *The Operating Room and the Patient* (1906).

Arpad Gerster (1848–1923) was born in Hungary and graduated in 1872 from the University of Vienna. He immediately left for the United States and settled in Brooklyn. In 1878 Gerster was made surgeon to the German Hospital (now the Lenox Hill Hospital), and in the following year he joined the staff of the Mount Sinai Hospital. Gerster accepted the professorship of clinical surgery at the College of Physicians and Surgeons of Columbia University in 1910. From 1882 to 1895 he also held the chair of surgery at the New York Polyclinic Medical School. In 1896 Gerster was president of the American Surgical Association. He was an outstanding pioneer of listerian surgery and one of the first American surgeons to actively use antisepsis for all his operations. His *Rules of Aseptic and Antiseptic Surgery* (1888) was the first American surgical text based on listerian principles. Gerster also authored a little-known paper that occupies an influential place in the history of oncological surgery in the United Sates. His description of the promotion of metastases by surgical incision of tumors constitutes the earliest discussion of the concept of surgically induced metastases found in the country's surgical literature (1885).

William Bull (1849–1909) was one of New York City's leading surgeons. He received his medical education at the College of Physicians and Surgeons (1872). After completing an internship at Bellevue Hospital and traveling throughout Europe, Bull was placed in charge of the New York Dispensary. Afterward, he worked at numerous institutions throughout the city, including Chambers Street Hospital, where he reported a case of gunshot wound of the intestine that had a profound effect on the evolution of American surgery. In 1884, Bull intentionally opened the peritoneal cavity of an individual who had just been shot in the abdomen, and repaired seven perforations in the small intestine and one in the sigmoid colon. The patient survived, and this widely reported surgical triumph electrified American surgeons and provided a major impetus for further emergency laprotomies for intestinal injuries. Bull was appointed professor of the practice of surgery and clinical surgery at his alma mater in 1888.

Frederic Dennis (1850–1934) was a native of Newark, New Jersey, and a graduate of Bellevue Hospital Medical College (1874). In 1876 and 1877 he traveled with his friend William Welch to Europe to study in the universities of France, Germany, and Scotland. Dennis practiced in New York City and was named professor of the principles and practice of surgery at his alma mater. Dennis served as president of the American Surgical Association in 1895. His most important text was the four-volume *System of Surgery* (1895), the first multivolume American surgical textbook in which various authors received credit for each individual chapter. The most prominent section was that by John Shaw Billings (1838–1913) on the history and literature of surgery. Dennis was widely respected for his clinical work with suprapubic cystotomy (1887) and breast cancer (1891). He persuaded Andrew Carnegie to endow a laboratory of medical research bearing Carnegie's name at Bellevue Hospital Medical School in an unsuccessful attempt to keep Welch from leaving Bellevue to accept an appointment at The Johns Hopkins Hospital. Dennis was a founder of Harlem Hospital.

James William White (1850–1916) was an 1871 graduate of the medical department of the University of Pennsylvania. Within a few years he became assistant to David Hayes Agnew and was appointed professor of genitourinary diseases at the school in 1886. White was elected to the chair of clinical surgery in 1889, and from 1900 to 1910 he held the John Rhea Barton professorship of surgery. He will be long remembered in the annals of urological surgery for his concept of orchiectomy as a means of bringing about atrophy of the prostate (1893). White's texts included *An American Text-Book of Surgery* (1892), co-edited with William Keen, and *Genito-Urinary Surgery and Venereal Diseases* (1897).

Robert Abbe (1851–1928) was an attending surgeon to St. Luke's Hospital, consulting surgeon to the Hospital for the Ruptured and Crippled, and professor of surgery in the Post-Graduate School and Hospital in New York City. He was an extremely versatile specialist in surgery who performed a widely acclaimed posterior root section (rhizotomy) for brachial neuralgia (1889), introduced the use of catgut rings for supporting the ends of intestine during an anastomosis (1892), and described a lip-switch operation for treatment of bilateral cleft lip (1898). Abbe was vice-president of the American Surgical Association in 1902.

Maurice Richardson (1851–1912) was a graduate of both Harvard College (1873) and Harvard Medical School (1877). He worked under Oliver Wendell Holmes in the department of anatomy of his alma mater and soon rose to the rank of assistant professor of anatomy. From 1895 to 1907 Richardson held the position of assistant professor of clinical surgery, and in 1907 he was named Moseley Professor of Surgery. All of his clinical work was done at the Massachusetts General Hospital, where he was surgeon in chief (1911–1912). Richardson reported numerous cases to the surgical literature, including the first exploration of the distal esophagus via a transgastric approach (1886) and the second successful total gastrectomy in America (1898). As a well-known abdominal surgeon, he was a vocal supporter of Fitz's concept of early removal of an infected appendix. Richardson was president of the American Surgical Association (1902) and chairman of the American Medical Association's Section on Surgery (1904).

Peter Dudley Allen (1852–1915) received his medical degree from Harvard Medical School in 1879 and spent a year as surgical house officer at the Massachusetts General Hospital. For the next twenty-four months he was engaged in postgraduate education in Berlin, London, Paris, and Vienna. In 1883 Allen settled in Cleveland, where he was appointed to the department of surgery at the Western Reserve University. He eventually rose to the rank of professor of principles and practice of surgery (1893–1911) and first surgeon in chief of Lakeside Hospital. Allen was president of the American Surgical Association in 1907. Three years later he resigned all his medical positions and, with his wife, made a year–long tour around the world.

Roswell Park (1852–1914) graduated from the Northwestern University Medical School in 1876. He became instrumental in promulgating listerian techniques to American surgeons and served as professor of surgery at the University of Buffalo from 1884 to 1914. Park was also a founder of the Gratwick Laboratory, which later became the New York State Institute for the Study of Malignant Diseases. Among his textbooks were *The Mütter Lectures on Surgical Pathology* (1892), the two-volume *A Treatise on Surgery by American Authors* (1896), and *The Principles and Practice of Modern Surgery* (1907). Park was highly regarded as a medical historian, having written *An Epitome of the History of Medicine* (1897) and *The Evil Eye*

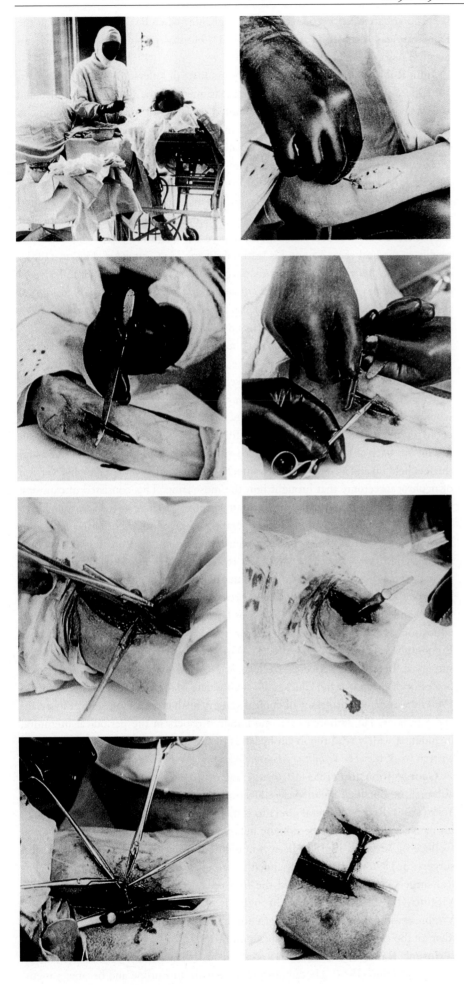

38. In 1904 George Crile began the experimental transfusion of blood between animals. Convinced of the relative safety of the procedure, he cautiously applied the technique to humans in 1906. Having devised a short cannula to facilitate what was then considered a formidable surgical operation, within three years Crile had completed sixty transfusions. Despite his successes, he described the technique as exacting and difficult. This was an appropriate choice of words in an era when surgery on blood vessels was in its infancy. As this series of previously unpublished photographs of Crile at work demonstrates (circa 1910), the procedure required an operating room; two teams of surgeons, one to isolate the donor's artery and the other to prepare the recipient's vein; and some delicate maneuvering around the patients' forearms. *(Courtesy of Stanley B. Burns, M.D., and The Burns Collection and Archive)*

(1912). Park attended President William McKinley when he was assassinated at the Pan-American Exposition in Buffalo (1901). He was president of the American Surgical Association in 1901.

John Roberts (1852–1924) was an 1874 graduate of Jefferson Medical College. In 1882, he proposed and assisted in the establishment of the Philadelphia Polyclinic and Medical College. He later was appointed professor of surgery at the Women's Medical College of Pennsylvania. Active in many organizations, Roberts served as president of the American Surgical Association in 1921. Of his clinical achievements, those concerning cardiac surgery are his least known but most important. In 1880 he authored the important monograph *Paracentesis of the Pericardium, A Consideration of the Surgical Treatment of Pericardial Effusions.* His major conclusion, which contributed to the advancement of cardiac surgery in the United States, was that paracentesis of the pericardium is indicated in every case of pericardial effusion that does not respond readily to medical care. Among his textbooks were *The Compend of Anatomy* (1881), *The Field and Limitation of the Operative Surgery of the Human Brain* (1885), *A Manual of Modern Surgery* (1890), *A Clinical, Pathological, and Experimental Study of Fracture of the Lower End of the Radius* (1897), *Notes on the Modern Treatment of Fractures* (1899), *Surgery of Deformities of the Face* (1912), and *A Treatise on Fractures* (1916).

George Edebohls (1853–1908) was born in New York City and attended the College of Physicians and Surgeons there, graduating in 1875. After postgraduate studies in Europe he returned to his native city and was appointed visiting gynecologist to St. Francis Hospital. Edebohls was later named professor of the diseases of women at the New York Post-Graduate Hospital and Medical College. He is eponymically remembered for a position for vaginal operations in which the woman lies on her back at the edge of the table, with her hips and knees partly flexed and the feet held up and apart by supports attached to the table. It was Edebohls' version of nephrocapsectomy that brought him the most fame. This consisted of exposing the diseased kidneys and stripping off their fibrous coverings to treat various forms of glomerulonephritis. Although the operation received much negative comment, Edebohls persisted in its use. His most renowned papers were on "floating" kidney and his nephropexy procedure (1893 and 1899). Edebohls also introduced the operation of renal decortication for the treatment of chronic nephritis (1901). His most important textbook was *The Surgical Treatment of Bright's Disease* (1904).

Alexander Ferguson (1853–1912) was born in Canada and received his medical education at Trinity University in Toronto (1881). After studying in Berlin, Edinburgh, and London, he settled in Winnipeg, where he served as professor of surgery at the Manitoba Medical College. In 1894 Ferguson relocated to Chicago as professor of surgery at the Chicago Post-Graduate Medical School and Hospital. In 1900 he was named professor of clinical surgery at that city's College of Physicians and Surgeons. He authored over one hundred papers in the periodical literature, including a widely read report on hydatids of the liver (1893). His most renowned written work was *The Technic of Modern Operation For Hernia* (1907).

George Johnston (1853–1916) was one of the leading surgeons of the South, although he obtained his medical education at the University of the City of New York (1876). Refusing several offers to settle in New York, Johnston moved back to his native Virginia, where he initially held minor teaching positions at the Medical College of Virginia. In 1884 he was appointed professor of didactic and clinical surgery; in 1896 the chair was changed to professor of practice of surgery and clinical surgery. Johnston completed the first operation using listerian principles in Virginia (1879). It was mostly through his efforts that the Medical College of Virginia was brought into the modern era of medical education. Johnston was president of the American Surgical Association in 1905.

Joseph Ransohoff (1853–1921) received his medical education at the Medical College of Ohio (1874). He did postgraduate work in Europe and became a member of the Royal College of Surgeons of England (1877). Returning to the United States, Ransohoff joined the surgical faculty of his alma mater, where he remained until his death, ultimately serving as professor of surgery from 1905 to 1921. Among his most important clinical contributions was one of the earliest successful gastroenterostomies performed in America (1884) as well as the country's first successful hindquarter amputation. Ransohoff served as vice-president of the American Surgical Association in 1912.

John Wheeler (1853–1942) received his medical degree from Harvard Medical School (1878). From 1879 to 1881 he studied in Berlin, Strasbourg, and Vienna. Returning to the United States, Wheeler set up practice in Burlington, Vermont, where he remained until his death. Appointed to the surgical faculty of the University of Vermont, he served as professor of clinical and minor surgery (1892–1900) and professor of surgery (1900–1924). Wheeler was the most prominent surgeon in the Vermont area for most of his sixty years of practice. He was among the first surgeons in his state to use listerian methods and was responsible for most of the surgical instruction of generations of medical students. Wheeler was a member of the founders' group of the American College of Surgeons and president (1917) of the New England Surgical Society. He discussed his life's work in his autobiography, *Memoirs of a Small Town Surgeon* (1935).

Augustus Bernays (1854–1907) was born in Germany and received his medical degree from the University of Heidelberg in 1876. He soon emigrated to the United States and settled in St. Louis, where he was appointed professor of anatomy at the St. Louis College of Physicians and Surgeons. Bernays was prolific in his contributions to the periodical literature, including his claim to have performed the country's first total gastrectomy (1898), but his only major textbook was *Golden Rules of Surgery* (1906).

Fred Robinson (1854–1910) was one of the least known but most important surgeon-anatomists of his time. His medical education was received at Rush Medical College (1882). Owing to lack of finances, he was not able to immediately pursue postgraduate education. Having entered practice, Robinson was able to save enough money over the next decade to attend postgraduate courses and also travel to Europe. In 1891 he moved to Chicago and was appointed professor of gynecology at the Chicago Post-Graduate Medical College. Later he became associated with the Illinois Medical College as professor of gynecology and abdominal surgery. While Robinson had a large clinical practice, his fame rested on his innumerable studies in anatomy, gross pathology, and basic surgical research. Among his texts were the two-volume *Practical Intestinal Surgery* (1891), *Landmarks in Gynecology* (1894), *The Peritoneum, Histology and Physiology* (1897), *The Abdominal Brain and Automatic Visceral Ganglia* (1899), *Arteria Uterina Ovarica; the Utero-Ovarian Artery, or the Genital Vascular Circle* (1903), and *The Arteries of the Gastrointestinal Tract with Inoscultation Circle, Anatomy and Physiology with Application in Treatment* (1908).

John Deaver (1855–1931) was an 1878 graduate of the University of Pennsylvania. He later was appointed professor of the practice of surgery at his alma mater and eventually filled the John Rhea Barton chair of surgery (1911). In 1886 he became a surgeon to the German Hospital of Philadelphia and chief of the department ten years later. At this institution, he made many contributions to American surgery and helped bring the profession of surgery to the forefront of medical practice. Among his surgical texts are *A Treatise on Appendicitis* (1896), the three-volume *Surgical Anatomy* (1899-1903), *Surgical Anatomy of the Head and Neck* (1904), *Enlargement of the Prostate* (1905), the two-volume *Surgery of the Upper Abdomen* (1913), and *The Breast, Its Anomalies, Its Diseases, and Their Treatment* (1917). Deaver is eponymically remembered for a technique used for appendectomy in which a vertical incision is made in the right lower abdominal quadrant with medial retraction of the rectus muscle, and also for a retractor used in abdominal operations. Deaver was president of the American College of Surgeons in 1921 and the Inter-State Post Graduate Medical Association of North America in 1928.

Samuel Mixter (1855–1926) graduated from the Massachusetts Institute of Technology in 1875 and the Harvard Medical School in 1879. After serving a year as surgical intern at the Massachusetts General Hospital, he traveled to Europe to complete his postgraduate training in Vienna. Upon his return to Boston, Mixter began a long association with his alma mater, which culminated in his being appointed chief of the West Surgical Service at the Massachusetts General Hospital (1911–1919). He received many honors, including being the first president of the New England Surgical Society and the president of the American Surgical Association (1917). He reported the country's first successful resection of a congenital esophogeal pouch in 1895. Mixter was said to have been a technical genius, and his name has long been associated with the Mixter tube, the Mixter punch, the Mixter scissors, and the Mixter incision for colostomy.

Edward Wyllys Andrews (1856–1927), son of Edmund Andrews, received his medical degree from Chicago Medical College in 1881. He studied at the University of Vienna (1884–1885) and on his return to Chicago joined the surgical faculty of Northwestern University Medical School. He was also on the staff of numerous other institutions, including Cook County, St. Luke's, Michael Reese, and Wesley Hospitals. His most important surgical contributions were the principle of imbrication of tissue flaps in hernia repairs (1895) and the utilization of glass tubes for subdural drainage in hydrocephalus (1911). As an associate editor of *Surgery, Gynecology and Obstetrics*, Andrews was instrumental in transforming it into one of the world's premier surgical journals. He helped establish the American College of Surgeons and the Association for Thoracic Surgery.

Frank Hartley (1856–1913) was a native of Washington, D.C., and received his medical degree from the College of Physicians and Surgeons in New York City in 1880. He interned for two years at Bellevue, afterward doing postgraduate work in Berlin, Heidelberg, and Vienna. On his return to New York City, Hartley was named demonstrator of anatomy at his alma mater. He later became clinical professor of surgery. Hartley is best known for his operation of intracranial neurectomy for facial neuralgia (1892).

Carl Beck (1856–1911) was born in Germany and obtained his medical degree from the University of Jena (1878). Four years later, he emigrated to the United States and gained here a reputation as a skilled surgeon. Beck was extremely prolific, but despite his intellectual prowess he was never afforded the opportunity to have a true academic title. Consequently, he was never given membership in any of the era's elite surgical organizations. For the last twenty years of his life, he was "professor" of surgery at the New York Post-Graduate Hospital and Medical College. Among his texts are *A Manual of the Modern Theory and Technique of Surgical Asepsis* (1895), *Fractures* (1900), *Röntgen Ray Diagnosis and Therapy* (1904), *Principles of Surgical Pathology* (1905), and *Surgical Diseases of the Chest* (1907).

John Benjamin Murphy (1857–1916), an enigmatic, colorful personality, was one of the most prominent nineteenth-century American surgeons. He received his medical education from Rush Medical College in 1879. After serving eighteen months as an intern at Cook County Hospital, he went into private practice until 1882, when he traveled to Europe. He pursued two years of postgraduate studies in Berlin, Heidelberg, Munich, and Vienna. On his return to the United States, he reestablished his office in Chicago for the practice of surgery. Murphy's brilliant, indomitable spirit allowed him to pioneer in many fields. His career as a surgical teacher began with his appointment in 1884 as lecturer in surgery at his alma mater. In 1892 Murphy was appointed professor of clinical surgery at the College of Physicians and Surgeons in Chicago. He remained there for a decade and in 1901 was elected professor of surgery at Northwestern University Medical School. Murphy stayed at Northwestern through 1905, when he moved to Rush Medical College as professor of surgery. Three years later, Murphy made his last career transfer and returned to Northwestern. He was also chief of the surgical staff at Mercy Hospital in Chicago, where he accomplished most of his clinical feats. Murphy served as president of the American Medical Association in 1911 and was a fellow of the American Surgical Association. In 1892, he startled the surgical world

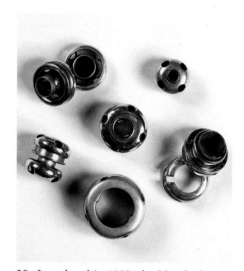

39. Introduced in 1892, the Murphy button revolutionized surgery by demonstrating that portions of the intestine and adjacent structures could be joined without sutures and that this technique was within the scope of any competent surgeon. In its time, Murphy's "anastomosis button" was considered the greatest mechanical aid in surgery. As improved suturing techniques were introduced, the device fell into disuse, but it was an important forerunner to twentieth-century anastomotic plates and stapling devices. *(Mütter Museum, College of Physicians of Philadelphia)*

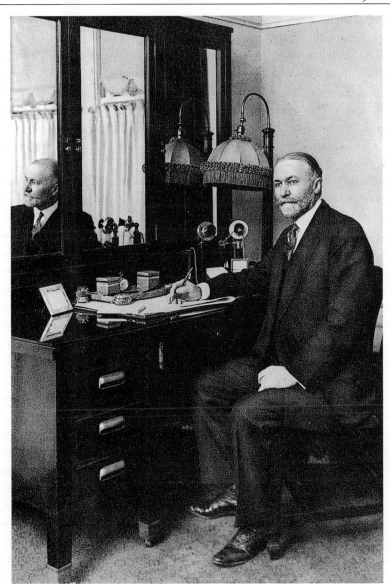

40. John Benjamin Murphy in 1914. Note the double telephone, which was quite an unusual addition to a physician's office of that era. *(Author's Collection)*

by introducing a mechanical device or "button" that allowed the approximation of hollow viscera without sutures. Four years later he published a report on research and clinical work in sutures of arteries and veins, including a description of one of the earliest repairs of a lacerated femoral artery. Although Murphy never authored a general textbook of surgery, he did edit the first *Year Book of General Surgery* (1901), and he served as editor-in-chief of *Surgery, Gynecology and Obstetrics*. Murphy was considered an outstanding teacher of surgery, especially in the operating room, where his clinical presentations were exceedingly popular. The demand for publication of his weekly conferences led to the organization of *The Surgical Clinics of John B. Murphy* (1912–1916). These volumes were the direct forerunner of the *Surgical Clinics of North America*.

Willy Meyer (1858–1932) was born in Germany and received his medical education at the universities of Bonn and Erlangen (1880). From 1880 to 1883 he was an assistant in the surgical clinic of Friedrich Trendelenburg. Meyer emigrated to America in 1884 and immediately began to practice medicine in New York City. From 1886 to 1893 he served on the clinical surgery faculty of the Woman's Medical College, and during those years he was also on the staff of the New York Skin and Cancer Hospital, the German Hospital, and the Post-Graduate Hospital. Meyer made many seminal contributions to clinical surgery, including the first published description of Trendelenburg's elevated pelvic position as an aid to the performance of certain pelvic and abdominal operations (1884). Simultaneously, but independently of William Halsted, Meyer originated a radical operation for breast cancer

(1894). He also helped introduce into the United States the concept of cystoscopy (1887) and the catheterization of the male ureters with the aid of the electric cystoscope (1896). An early advocate of the controlled pressure chamber for thoracotomy, Meyer had his own such facility built at the German Hospital. A pioneer of thoracic surgical operations, he helped found the New York Society for Thoracic Surgery and the American Association for Thoracic Surgery. His name is eponymically linked with Meyer's reagent, a solution of phenolphthalein, sodium hydroxide, and distilled water, which detects minute traces of blood when the solution turns purple or blue-red.

Albert Ochsner (1858–1925) was an 1886 graduate of Rush Medical College, and occupied the chair of clinical surgery at the University of Illinois College of Medicine from 1900 to 1925. He accomplished much in the world of American surgical politics, including the presidencies of the Clinical Congress of Surgeons of North America (1911), the American College of Surgeons (1923), and the American Surgical Association (1924). His most important journal article concerned peritonitis as a complication of appendicitis (1901). In that paper he proposed a treatment of appendicitis with which his name remains linked: when operation is not advisable, treatment should consist of intestinal rest obtained by abstention from cathartics and oral intake while gastric lavage and rectal irrigation are administered. Among Ochsner's textbooks were *Clinical Surgery* (1902), *A Handbook of Appendicitis* (1902), *The Surgery and Pathology of the Thyroid and Parathyroid Glands* (1910), and the four-volume *Surgical Diagnosis and Treatment by American Authors* (1920). He also wrote *The Organization, Construction and Management of Hospitals* (1907).

William Rodman (1858–1916) received his medical education at Jefferson Medical College (1879). From 1885 to 1893 he served as demonstrator of surgery in the medical department of the University of Louisville. In 1893 Rodman was named to the chair of surgery at the Kentucky School of Medicine. Five years later he moved to Philadelphia, where he assumed the professorship of surgery at the Medico-Chirurgical College of Philadelphia. Among his many accomplishments were the founding of the National Board of Medical Examiners (1915) and his service as president of the Association of American Medical Colleges (1902) and the American Medical Association (1915). His major written work was *Diseases of the Breast with Special Reference to Cancer* (1908). Rodman's name is linked with a surgical technique for radical mastectomy, and he was among the earliest to oppose the use of radium alone in cancer therapy.

Edward Martin (1859–1938), a native of Philadelphia, graduated from the University of Pennsylvania in 1883. He became an office assistant to David Hayes Agnew and James White, and after practicing medicine for a few years, he decided to specialize in urological diseases and general surgery. Martin was named professor of clinical surgery at his alma mater (1903) and John Rhea Barton professor of surgery (1910–1918). A founding member of the American College of Surgeons, he is remembered for being the first to perform a cordotomy for relief of intractable pain (1912). Among his many texts are *Questions and Answers of the Essentials of Surgery* (1888), *Essentials of Minor Surgery and Bandaging* (1890), *The Surgical Treatment of Wounds and Obstruction of the Intestines* (1891), *Impotence and Sexual Weakness in the Male and Female* (1895), *Genito-Urinary Surgery and Venereal Diseases* (1897), co-written with James White, and *Surgical Diagnosis* (1909).

Richard Douglas (1860–1908) received part of his formal medical education at the University of Nashville (1881) but received his medical degree from Jefferson Medical College (1882). He held the professorship of gynecology and obstetrics and later that of abdominal surgery at Vanderbilt University. He is best remembered as one of the founders of the Southern Surgical and Gynecological Society. Although he made many contributions to the periodical literature, his only book-length work was *Surgical Diseases of the Abdomen* (1903).

Clayton Parkhill (1860–1902) was a graduate of Jefferson Medical College (1883). After initial postgraduate training, he returned to his native city of Denver, where he eventually assumed the position of professor of surgery at the University of Colorado. Parkhill remains best known to American surgeons for his introduction of external fixation in fractures (1898). He was vice-president of the American Surgical Association in 1901.

William Davis (1863–1902) received his undergraduate education at the University of Alabama and took his medical degree at Bellevue Hospital Medical College in 1884. Returning to his native state, Davis entered practice with his older brother. From the outset he devoted himself to gynecologic and abdominal surgery, and he became actively involved in the politics of organized medicine. The Davis brothers organized the Alabama Surgical and Gynecological Society, and shortly thereafter William Davis helped found the Southern Surgical and Gynecological Society, of which he was president in 1901. He died in a railway accident.

It is a fitting tribute to **James Mumford** (1863–1914) that he is the final surgeon to be listed in this surgical era. Only 51 years old when he died, Mumford bridged the old and the new American surgery. As a humanist and man of letters, he was a model of the Renaissance scholar. As a superb surgical technician and organizer of socioeducational surgical societies, Mumford helped shepherd American surgery into the modern era. Born in Rochester, New York, and a graduate of Harvard College (1885) and Harvard Medical School (1890), he became a house pupil at the Massachusetts General Hospital and for some years was a junior associate to Maurice Richardson. Mumford was an assistant in surgery at his alma mater (1894), instructor (1903), and visiting surgeon (1904). In 1912 he resigned his Massachusetts General Hospital appointment and became physician in chief at the Clifton Springs Sanitarium in New York. Mumford had long been plagued by chronic heart disease, and the move to Clifton Springs was partially intended to ease his health problems. Unfortunately, his ambitious plans to upgrade the medical and surgical care of the sanitarium were not in harmony with the wishes of the board of directors. Mumford's connections with the institution were severed only a few weeks before his tragic death. Mumford was, in every sense of the word, a surgical scholar with broad interests in the humanities. He was highly regarded as a historian and possessed an interesting literary style, which was said to make his clinical writings "read almost like a novel." Among his historical texts and those about the lighter side of medicine are the introductory chapter on the history of surgery in Keen's *Surgery, its Principles and Practice* (1909), *A Narrative of Medicine in America* (1903), *Surgical Memoirs and Other Essays* (1908), *A Doctor's Table Talk* (1912), and *Harvard Medical School: a History* (1905), which he edited. His clinical texts include *Clinical Talks on Minor Surgery* (1903), *Surgical Aspects of Digestive Disorders* (1905), *The Practice of Surgery* (1910), and *One Hundred Surgical Problems: the Experiences of Daily Practice Dissected and Explained* (1911). Mumford was a founding member of the American College of Surgeons and a fellow of the American Surgical Association. In addition, he was an organizer, first secretary (1903–1913), and president (1914) of the Society of Clinical Surgery.

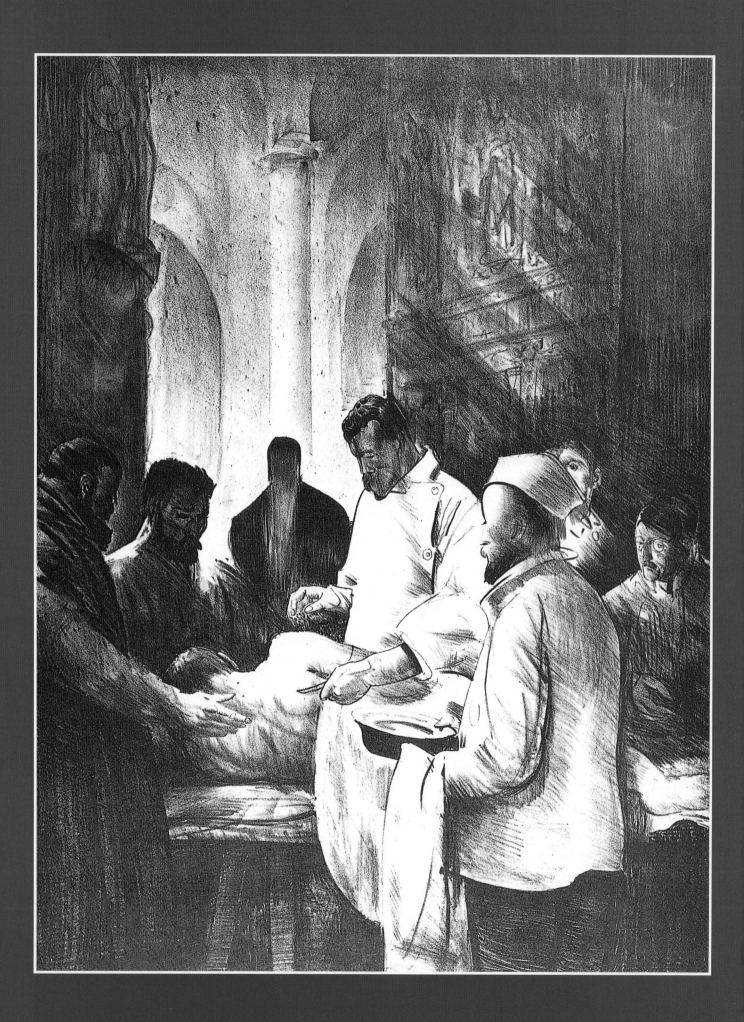

CHAPTER 8

WORLD WAR ONE SURGERY
1917–1918

he whole of American medicine was far better prepared to deal with the exigencies of the battlefield in World War I than it had been in the Civil War and the Spanish-American War. This came about because of better organization within the medical branches of the armed forces, which permitted a more realistic anticipation of the problems soon to arise. In addition, the maturation of scientific surgery assured the fact that operative intervention was to be regarded as an invaluable and integral aspect of total medical care. World War I began in the summer of 1914, following the assassination of Archduke Francis Ferdinand, heir to the throne of Austria-Hungary, and his wife Sophia, in Sarajevo, the capital of the Austrian province of Bosnia. Within one month of the murder, Austria-Hungary declared war on Serbia; Russia ordered a general mobilization of its populace; Germany declared war on Belgium, France, and Russia; and Great Britain declared war on Germany. Europe would soon be aflame, and for the first time in history, the mortality from battlefield casualties would almost exceed that from communicable diseases.

News of the war's outbreak astonished most Americans. President Woodrow Wilson (1856–1924) even went so far as to declare that the United States would be "neutral in fact as well as in name." His sentiments lasted for about two years. In January 1917, Germany began unrestricted submarine warfare, and two months later, three unarmed American merchant ships were sunk without warning and with heavy loss of life. On April 6th, the United States declared war on Germany. A year earlier, foreseeing the possibility of American involvement in the hostilities, the Committee of American Physicians for Medical Preparedness was created. Acting on behalf of five national societies (American Surgical Association, American College of Surgeons, Clinical Congress of Surgeons of North America, American Medical Association, and Congress of American Physicians and Surgeons), chaired by William Mayo, and dominated by surgeons, the committee tendered its professional services to the federal government.

In the opinion of Mayo and other members of the committee (e.g., George Crile, Edward Martin, Rudolph Matas, John Murphy, Albert Ochsner, and George de Schweinitz) , the profession of medicine had for too long been relegated to a position of minor activity in governmental affairs. They reasoned that the medical profession had failed to gain recognition in the past because its rank and file had been indifferent to the potential of political influence and had never fully understood the importance of effective lobbying efforts. This concern seemed warranted when, in the summer of 1916, Congress decided to activate a Council of National Defense with an auxiliary civilian advisory commission. Medicine, although deemed an important arm of defense in time of war, again

1. *(facing page)* "Base Hospital" (circa, 1918) by George Bellows (1882–1925). Bellows' lithographs were highly regarded for their expressive draftsmanship. (*Philadelphia Museum of Art: SmithKline Beecham Corp. Fund for the Ars Medica Collection*)

2. Motorized ambulances permitted more rapid evacuation of casualties. This particular vehicle was attached to Base Hospital No. 34, affiliated with the Episcopal Hospital in Philadelphia. Directed by Astley Ashhurst (1876–1932), a well-known surgeon from that city, the unit was stationed in Nantes, Loire Inférieure, France. (*Historical Collections, College of Physicians of Philadelphia*)

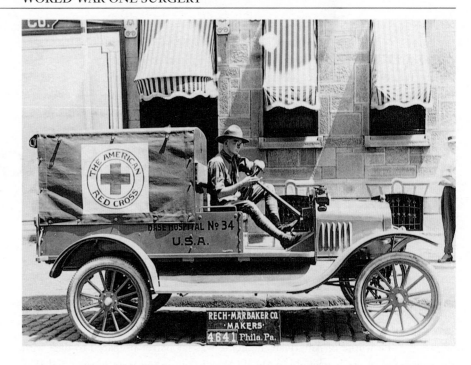

seemed likely to be denied a leading position and would not be represented on any influential policy-making body.

Persistent diplomacy was called for, as Mayo and other officials of the Committee of American Physicians urged federal officials and legislators to give proper recognition to medicine. Their lobbying efforts were richly rewarded when, in October, President Wilson announced the formation of the Council of National Defense, consisting of six members of the cabinet and chaired by Newton Baker, Secretary of War, and an adjunctive Advisory Commission, composed of seven civilians, including Bernard Baruch, Samuel Gompers, and Julius Rosenwald. Franklin Martin, then serving as Secretary-General of the American College of Surgeons, was presented as a member of the Advisory Commission with specific instructions to head its Committee on Medical Preparedness. Martin would prove extremely effective in bringing together all the disparate elements of the American health care system into a workable wartime effort.

Once war had been formally declared, much of the work of Martin's medical division was planned and controlled by its General Medical Board, which had among its members the surgeons John Finney and Stuart McGuire. Although American involvement in World War I was not long, lasting slightly less than eighteen months, approximately 1.4 million United States soldiers and sailors saw active combat service. Over 53,000 American soldiers were killed in action or died as a result of wounds, and another 204,000 were wounded. Yet, as in previous wars, the deaths from infectious diseases, of which there were 63,000, exceeded those from battlefield injuries. The high mortality from communicable diseases occurred mainly in the armed forces' camps stateside and was largely attributable to the influenza epidemic of 1918. In fact, if the influenza virus had not created such worldwide havoc, the death rate from diseases in the military forces during World War I would have been extremely low.

For surgeons, war has always posed a moral dilemma: they gain greater clinical experience while being surrounded by ever-mounting human suffering. Once again, it appeared as if the only human activity to benefit from hostilities was the surgical care of injury and the resultant on-site training of surgeons. It was a war of attrition that over the course of forty-eight months managed to move an intricate system of underground trenches little more than a few miles in either direction. On the battlefield, sepsis was inevitable. The soil of Belgium and France had been cultivated for over twenty centuries. The fields had been crossed by every imaginable farm animal and the soil fertilized thousands of times. As a result, trench warfare, conducted in soil thoroughly contaminated with fecal bacteria in addition to the ordinary pyogenic variety, made every soldier a potential carrier of infection. The aseptic ritual, which had finally become entrenched in the conduct of all surgical operations, became impossible to perform. The result was a revival of listerism: the treatment of wounds by antisepsis.

During the course of the hostilities, antiseptic methods grew in sophistication. Almroth Wright (1861–1947), a London pathologist, advocated the continuous irrigation of dirty wounds with a hypertonic salt solution and sodium citrate; this supposedly stimulated the effects of leukocytes and the "drawing" of lymph with opsonic power into the wounds. Finally there evolved a physico-chemical principle of wound irrigation by a solution of gas in a liquid, the Carrel-Dakin treatment. In addition, Henry Gray (1870–1938), an English surgeon, revived the mechanical precept of *débridement* or wound excision with *épluchage* and primary sutures. Admittedly, the treatment of combat injuries entailed various other sophisticated surgical methods, including x-rays, tetanus antitoxin, blood transfusions, and the more rapid evacuation of the wounded by motorized ambulances to hospitals where they could receive definitive surgery. As a result of all these measures, it is not an understatement to say that the greatest surgical achievement of World War I was a better understanding of the pathophysiology of traumatic injuries and refinements in the treatment of wounds and their infectious sequalae. From a technical standpoint, there were other far-reaching innovations, including previously unimaginable ingenuity in reconstructive maxillofacial surgery, and remarkable developments in the orthopedic treatment of gunshot fractures. Finally, there were the classic research studies of Walter Cannon (1871–1945) and George Crile (1864–1943) on "wound shock" as a physiological by-product of severe injury.

Technical neutrality might have been the official government position, but there were many who preached loudly against the continuing lack of military preparations. Such protestations proved prophetic; through mid-1915, only 330 physicians were registered in the United States Army Medical Corps, compared with 30,000 gathered within a few months after the country declared war. But even as early as August 1914, American citizens residing in Paris, under the leadership of the American ambassador, were concerned enough to organize a "military" hospital and motor ambulance service in connection with the American Hospital at Neuilly-sur-Seine. Although American in name, the existing hospital had been largely staffed by French physicians and surgeons. The expenses of this new *Ambulance Américaine* were met by voluntary subscriptions, and fund raising became so successful that a subsidiary

3. An Esmarch Bandage, the type that was supplied to surgical teams during World War I. Even in the hands of an inexperienced physician, the bandage was made useful by having illustrations of how it should be used printed on its front. (*Mütter Museum, College of Physicians of Philadelphia*)

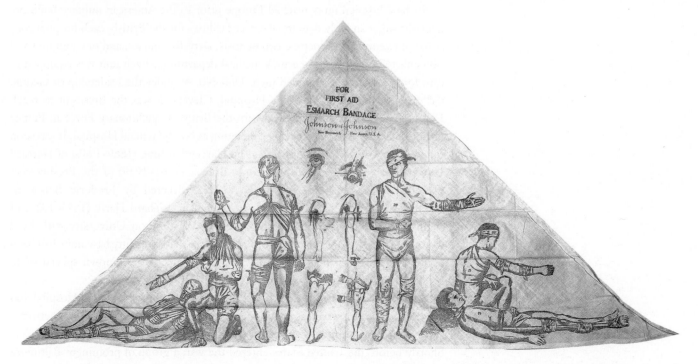

4. Numerous voluntary organizations were established as part of the government's war effort. One such group was the Committee of Women Physicians, chaired by Rosalie Slaughter Morton (1876–1968), chief of a gynecological clinic at the New York Polyclinic Hospital and Post–Graduate Medical School. Among the committee's many activites was setting up a network of American Women's Hospitals both in the United States and Europe to serve not only acutely injured soldiers but also the civilian population. In October 1917, the first complete unit of women physician and surgeons was sent to northern France, and this photograph (circa 1917–1918) shows an all–female operating room team at one of the French facilities. (*Courtesy of Stanley B. Burns, M.D., and The Burns Collection and Archive*)

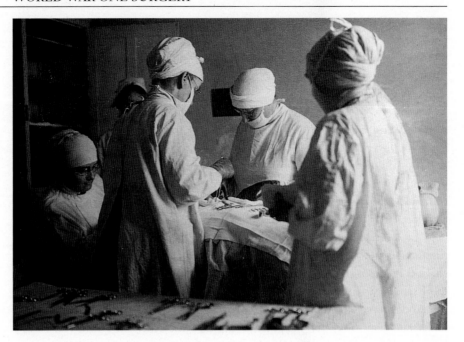

hospital at Juilly was also organized. Certain American universities were asked to participate in the project by supplying professional personnel capable of caring for ward patients in this *Ambulance Américaine* at Neuilly for three months. The first of these "military medical units" was led by Crile and arrived in January 1915. A Harvard unit organized by Harvey Cushing followed in April 1915.

The success of the *Ambulance Américaine* proved a temporary solution to the rapidly approaching crisis situation. Consequently, it was not long before multiple base hospitals situated in Europe, formally organized and staffed by medical school faculty and physicians and surgeons from civilian hospitals in the United States, became a standing feature of the "new" army medical department. Originally, the American Red Cross had proposed the organization of such structures, but Crile took the concept one step further when he suggested, at a symposium on military surgery at the 1915 Clinical Congress, the "unit idea" for management of American military base hospitals. Communities from all over America took great pride in their overseas hospital units, and this public support aided in the collection of relatively large funds to equip the new facilities. As Crile told surgeons, "mediocrity well organized is more efficient than brilliancy combined with strife and discord."

Six base hospital units reached Europe prior to the American military build-up. Sent abroad at an early date to take over facilities for the British, each hospital consisted of twenty-three doctors, two dentists, sixty-five nurses, and one hundred and fifty enlisted men from the army's medical department. Each unit was equipped to care for five hundred wounded men. Unit No. 4, under the leadership of George Crile and organized at Lakeside Hospital, Cleveland, was the first unit to reach Europe in May 1917. It remained with the British Expeditionary Force in France during its entire overseas existence, operating as No. 9 General Hospital. It was soon followed by Unit No. 5, commanded by Harvey Cushing (1869–1939) of Harvard University; Unit No. 2, led by George Brewer (1861–1939) of the Presbyterian Hospital in New York City; Unit No. 22 directed by Frederic Belsey of Northwestern University; Unit No. 10 headed by Richard Harte (1855–1925) of Pennsylvania Hospital; and Unit No. 21 of Washington University with Fred Murphy (1872–1948) in charge. By the end of the war, some fifty base units had been established, the vast majority under the leadership of well-known specialists in surgery from virtually every major city in the United States.

Base Hospital Unit No. 18 was organized by The Johns Hopkins Hospital and Medical School to serve as a five-hundred-bed facility. Its evolution and activities serve as an apt example of how most of these units were arranged and utilized. Shortly before the United States entered the war, a group of prominent Baltimore businessmen put together a luncheon and raised over $30,000 to equip the unit. The purchase of beds and specified equipment, particularly for operating rooms, was supervised by the administrative office of The Johns Hopkins Hospital. All the surgical dressings, operating gowns, sheets, pillow cases, and towels were hand-made by Baltimore women volunteers working under the auspices of the local Red Cross chapter. Most of these preparations proceeded at a rather leisurely pace. However, a sudden decision in late May by the War Department called for Unit No. 18 to be dispatched immediately to France to support the First Division of the Army. John Finney was named director, and with essentially no training and little warning, the medical personnel boarded the troop ship *Finland* on June 9th and set sail for France escorted by the cruiser *Charleston*. On board were twenty-four medical officers, including surgeons William Baer, Bertram Bernheim, Harvey Stone, and George Heuer, some sixty Hopkins-trained nurses, and 148 enlisted men, among whom were thirty-two third-year medical students.

By July 1917, the Hopkins unit had been transported across France to occupy a French barracks-type hospital of 1,000 beds at Bazoilles-sur-Meuse in the Vosges ("Bacillus-on-the-Mess"), at the headwaters of the River Meuse. In fulfilment of the time-honored motto "hurry up and wait," coupled with the fact that the great American offensives had not yet begun, the members of the unit had little to do surgically until mid-1918. Not until the fighting in June and July at Château-Thierry, where American and French troops defeated German fighting forces, did freshly wounded soldiers begin to be seen. In September, the Allies swept toward the Meuse-Argonne region. American soldiers took over a large portion of the combat activities and helped break through the fortified Hindenburg line. Almost 1,200,000 Americans fought in the Battle of the Meuse-Argonne, and one in ten was killed or wounded.

For the Hopkins' surgeons, a period of intense day-and-night activity occurred throughout September and October 1918. The facility was so close to the front lines that No. 18 served as an immediate evacuation hospital giving primary surgical care to many of the wounded, who had received little more than perfunctory first aid on the battlefield. All personnel worked around-the-clock shifts, and for weeks on end the operating room was in virtually continual use. There is little doubt that the surgeons were both exhausted and exhilarated in performing their duties. Writing in his wartime diaries, *From A Surgeon's Journal* (1936), Cushing described what the surgical personnel were up against:

[The Passchendaele Battles] August, 1917
Pouring cats and dogs all day - also pouring cold and shivering wounded, covered with mud and blood.... The preoperation room is still crowded - one can't possibly keep up with them; and the unsystematic way things are run drives one frantic. The news, too, is very bad. The greatest battle of history is floundering up to its middle in a morass...Gott mit uns was certainly true for the enemy this time. Operating from 8.30 a.m. one day till 2.00 a.m. the next; standing in a pair of rubber boots, and periodically full of tea as a stimulant, is not healthy. It's an awful business, probably the worst possible training in surgery for a young man, and ruinous for the carefully acquired technique of an oldster.... A lot of wounded must have drowned in the mud...a large batch of wounded were unexpectedly brought in...men who have been lying out for four days in craters in the rain, without food. It is amazing what the human animal can endure. Some of them had maggots in their wounds.... One English officer who had been six days thus in transport, with a musket for a splint tied to a compound fracture of the femus, no dressing whatsoever, almost no food or drink; he was in delirium when he arrived.

The neurological nature of many of the wounds was simply devastating. There seemed to be so many, perhaps related to the soldiers' habit of peering imprudently over the tops of the unprotected trenches only to be shot in the head. Not only were there protean injuries from shell blasts, but other conditions common to this type of warfare were seen all too often. Trench foot was ubiquitous, or as Cushing described it, "erythromelalgia-like feet - painful, blue, cold, macerated-looking extremities:

5. Because the fields of France and Belgium had been cultivated for centuries with animal manure used as fertilizer, the ground was laden with *Bacillus welchii* and other gas–producing pathogens. When trench warfare made its debut in World War I, it was therefore inevitable that gas gangrene would soon complicate battlefield wounds. The disease process became a major problem, necessitating extensive wound debridement with an often fatal outcome. (*Courtesy of Stanley B. Burns, M.D., and The Burns Collection and Archive*)

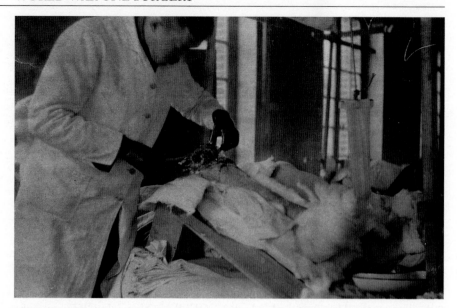

from continuous standing without change of boots in the muddy trenches in the almost unceasing rain." As a result, extremity amputation became one of the more common operations. Tetanus was rife early in the war until an antitetanus serum became available. Enormous numbers of men were incapacitated by "shell-shock": pure psychological breakdown secondary to the tremendous strain of trench warfare and incessant shelling.

As satisfying from a professional standpoint as surgical service might have been, the surgery of war is a sorry spectacle. To look at the mangled bodies of young men, with life so needlessly stripped away, does little to bolster one's faith in humankind. Many surgical stories came out of World War I, but that involving Harvey Cushing, William Osler (1849–1919), and the latter's son Revere Osler (1896–1917) is one of the saddest. The elder Osler was professor of medicine at The Johns Hopkins Hospital (1889–1904) when Cushing was serving his surgical residency under William Halsted. Cushing always regarded Osler as his intellectual mentor and had a much closer relationship with the professor of medicine than with the professor of surgery. Cushing had watched Revere grow up, and for William Osler, his only child was the source of greatest happiness and soon-to-be overwhelming sorrow. William Osler left Baltimore to become Regius Professor of Medicine at the University of Oxford (1904), where he would remain until his death. Revere Osler, having spent his adolescence in England and in the patriotic fervor of the times, joined the British military service's Royal Artillery Force. Assigned to an area in Flanders, Lieutenant Osler was serving on the front lines when, in the late afternoon of August 29th, he was wounded in the chest and abdomen by a German shell. It took almost four hours to get Osler to a casualty clearing station, where Revere's first words to the medical officer were "This will take me home." As fate would have it, many of William Osler's surgical friends were on duty in that immediate vicinity. Crile came from Rémy and joined George Brewer and William Darrach (1876–1948). Cushing, who was nearby consulting, arrived within thirty minutes of being summoned. Osler's field ambulance card read "G.S.W. multiple - chest, abdomen, thigh." In Cushing's words, "It could not have been much worse...one traversing through the upper abdomen, another penetrating the chest just above the heart, two others in the thigh." With nighttime at its peak, nearly eight hours following the injury, a surgical operation was begun. Crile began transfusing blood obtained from one of Osler's own less seriously wounded men brought in at the same time. Darrach, assisted by Brewer, opened the abdomen and found "bleeding from two holes - in the upper colon and the mesenteric vessels." Osler's condition never stabilized, and just before sunrise, as Cushing wrote in his wartime diaries, "this world lost this fine boy, as it does many others every day." Cushing, in a poignant *arrière-pensée*, described the burial of the young man he had known so well:

> A soggy Flanders field beside a little oak grove to the rear of the Dosinghem group - an overcast, windy, autumnal day - the long rows of simple wooden crosses - the new ditches half full of water being dug by Chinese coolies wearing tin helmets - the boy wrapped in an army blanket and covered by a weather-worn Union Jack, carried on their shoulders by four slipping stretcher-bearers. A strange scene - the great-great grandson of Paul Revere under a British flag, and awaiting him a group of some six or eight American Army medical officers - saddened with the thoughts of his father. Happily it was fairly dry at this end of the trench, and some green branches were thrown in for him to lie on. The Padre recited the usual service - the bugler gave the "Last Post" - and we went about our duties. Plot 4, Row F.

For the men and women of Unit No. 18, the inflow of casualties, even during the few weeks following the November armistice, continued unabated. Then, just as abruptly as it had started, there was no longer a need for their services. On January 31, 1919, No. 18's officers and men boarded the *Finland* for friendlier shores, followed by the nurses a month later. So the war ended, with the results of the conflict proving disastrous to the central powers (Austria-Hungary, Bulgaria, Germany, and the Ottoman Empire) and especially to German-speaking surgeons. Europe took on a new look after the signing of the Peace of Paris. Three independent countries, Austria, Czechoslovakia, and Hungary, emerged from the defeated Austro-Hungarian empire. Allied diplomats created a new Poland out of old Austrian, German, and Russian territories. Yugoslavia was formed, and the area of Romania was doubled. The Ottoman Empire lost most of its land in the Middle East, and its territorial claims in Africa were dismissed. Estonia, Finland, Latvia, and Lithuania declared their independence from Russia.

The demise of Germany's status as the world leader in surgery occurred after the war. Economic ruin and deprivation were evident throughout the land. Erwin Payr, professor of surgery and director of the university clinic in Leipzig, wrote in a letter to Halsted in 1919:

> There are only sad things to report. The saddest is that in each nation a few hotblooded politicians and radical nationalists exert more influence on the masses than 99% of the rational thinking intellectuals.... This stupidity destroyed a nation which was capable to excel intellectually in any area for 50 years or more.... Our science is heavily threatened by poverty. Perhaps people will start writing poetry and philosophize again, at least they don't cost anything. Undoubtedly, technology, the natural sciences and medicine are finished.

The conclusion of World War I signaled the true beginnings of the ascent of American surgery to its current position of international leadership. Initially, however, the country's surgical supremacy was more a matter of default than of actual deserving. War had destroyed much of Europe—if not its physical features, then a large measure of its scientific and intellectual fervor. As a result, a vacuum existed internationally in both surgical research and clinical therapeutics. It was only natural and inevitable that surgeons from the United States, the industrialized country least affected emotionally and physically by the war's aftermath, would so easily fill this void.

There is a certain irony in the fact that one of the most important surgical triumphs to be associated with a war that involved Americans fighting on European soil concerned a European surgeon, who felt he had to emigrate to North American shores in order to seek his surgical greatness. Alexis Carrel (1873–1944) was born near Lyon, France, and obtained his medical degree from that city's university in 1900. He served as a surgical house officer for four years while training with several excellent French surgeons, including Antonin Poncet (1849–1913) and Mathieu Jaboulay (1860–1913). Having already authored some widely read papers, and upset by the apparently minimal interest expressed by both peers and professors for his

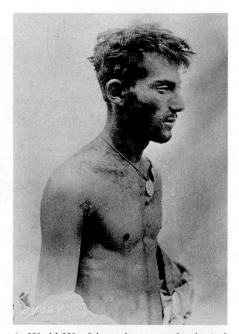

6. World War I brought new technological weapons, such as flame throwers and liquid fire devices. Along with these new devices came surgical problems previously unseen. When the injury was unusual, photographic documentation was employed so that other practitioners could learn about the problem. (*Courtesy of Stanley B. Burns, M.D., and The Burns Collection and Archive*)

proposed further studies in vascular and transplantation surgery, Carrel left France in May 1904. He traveled to Montreal, where he remained until August. The results of his prior experimental studies and recently completed research efforts attracted the attention of American surgeons, and Carrel was offered and accepted an assistantship in the Hull Physiology Laboratory at the University of Chicago. Over the next two years, he collaborated with Charles Guthrie (1880–1963) on their now famous series of experiments that perfected a technique for suturing severed blood vessels. Carrel's growing reputation for technical surgical skills was met by increasingly receptive surgical audiences. The fifth annual meeting of the Society of Clinical Surgery was held in Chicago in October 1905. George Crile, Harvey Cushing, Rudolph Matas, and other members went to inspect Carrel's laboratory facilities. There, the technique of vascular anastomosis was demonstrated on the carotid artery of a dog. This meeting was a major turning point in Carrel's scientific life. It resulted in what was to become a lifelong friendship with Cushing and his surgical coterie.

By late 1905, Carrel had proved himself to his American colleagues. At that time, finding a laboratory, with a suitable work environment and facilities for conducting experimental surgical research, was difficult. The lack of financial support for the continuation of his work was becoming a major frustration. He was offered a clinical professorship in Chicago but did not accept. He thought he would have to support his experimental work by developing a busy private practice, something he did not wish to pursue. In the United States, the only full-fledged surgical research laboratory was the Hunterian Laboratory of The Johns Hopkins Hospital, of which

7. "First Aid Station, Argonne" (circa 1918) as depicted by George Harding, official artist to the American Expeditionary Forces. (*Historical Collections, College of Physicians of Philadelphia*)

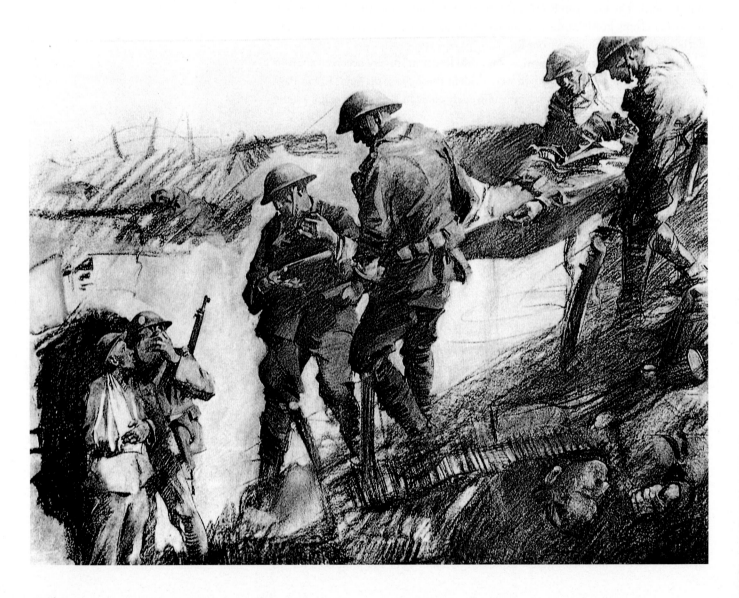

Cushing was director. Additional funding was difficult to obtain at the Baltimore facility, and as a result, Cushing was unable to offer Carrel a position on the Hunterian staff. However, a serendipitous event was about to change Carrel's professional life. Simon Flexner (1863–1946), brother of Abraham Flexner and director of the newly founded Rockefeller Institute in New York City, had read a recent surgical publication of Carrel's describing the functions of a transplanted kidney. Flexner asked Cushing to arrange a meeting with the Frenchman. Flexner quickly offered Carrel a Rockefeller Scholarship, and the French surgeon moved East in September 1906. His association with the Institute was to last until his retirement in June 1939.

Carrel would soon go on to perfect his technique of end-to-end anastomosis of blood vessels; the application of this skill to the transplantation of organs; the use of hypothermia to maintain blood vessels, skin grafts, and other tissues in storage before using them for transplantation; and the development of techniques in the field of tissue cultivation. For his work on vascular surgery and organ transplantation, Carrel was awarded the Nobel Prize for 1912 in Physiology and Medicine. Carrel never sought citizenship in the United States, and as a French citizen he received mobilization orders from France in the fall of 1914. It is difficult to comprehend the politics involved, but this Nobel Prize-winning surgeon was originally stationed in a railroad yard in Lyon performing little more than routine administrative medical tasks. Dissatisfied with his circumstances, and noting the growing number of battlefield casualties who were dying from the ravages of wound infection, Carrel asked for and received a transfer to the Hôtel Dieu in Lyon. There he began the systematic study of infected war wounds.

As the number of wounded increased, Carrel realized that the current methods of wound treatment were completely inadequate to deal with the problems of gas gangrene. Consequently, his interests soon focused on the development of an antiseptic agent with which to irrigate the fresh injury. Although he tried to persuade French authorities to appropriate funds to aid in the establishment of a laboratory and to assist in the hiring of a chemist, his efforts remained unsuccessful. In November 1914, through the influence of James Hyde (1876–1959), a wealthy American industrialist, Carrel's plans were finally directed to the proper governmental agencies. Carrel received permission to establish a hospital and research facilities at Compiègne in the old Rond Royal Hotel; thus, Hôpital Complémentaire 21 came to be, situated some eight miles from the front.

Unfortunately, the provision of hospital facilities was the extent to which the French government was willing to commit funds to Carrel's endeavors. Through the sustained efforts of Hyde, additional support was obtained from the Rockefeller Institute and other interested organizations in the United States. In addition, Flexner was able to find the ideal chemist in Henry Dakin (1880–1952), an English citizen, who was interested in the optical activity of organic compounds, its influence on their biological activity, and their acceptability as nutrients. Under Carrel's directions, the tedious process of testing solutions for the needed properties of maximal bacterial antisepsis with minimal wound irritation was begun. After several months of preliminary trials, they settled on a solution of sodium hypochlorite buffered with sodium bicarbonate (Dakin's solution). Later, an antiseptic paste, Dichloramin-T, was also produced. Carrel concurrently set forth his system of wound management, which included mechanical cleansing, surgical debridement of injured and necrotic tissue, and adequate chemical sterilization through copius irrigation with the new antiseptic solution. In addition, Carrel recommended that a bacteriological smear be taken daily of the wound and that secondary closure not be performed until the cultures demonstrated complete absence of bacterial growth.

Dakin's solution was suspended over an injured patient in a bottle and allowed to flow down through glass distributing tubes with many branches, each leading to a separate portion of the wound. The skin around the injury was protected by compresses of Vaseline gauze. A pinchcock on the distributing tube allowed precise adjustment of the speed of irrigation. There was one decided disadvantage with the overall method: it demanded greater care, precision, personnel, and equipment than were usually available in a wartime setting. Military surgeons found it too elaborate for use near the front. Only in a well-protected and less busy atmosphere could the proper pH of the solution be maintained, irrigations continuously applied, and frequent bacterial counts accurately completed.

The acceptance of the Carrel–Dakin method of wound management was rather slow. Many prominent American, English, and French surgeons doubted its genuine efficacy. Not until the end of 1916, at an interallied surgical conference, was the method finally adopted as the approved treatment for war injuries. Despite all the controversy surrounding the general effectiveness of the treatment and its eventual approval, it remains a little-appreciated surgical discovery from World War I. Nevertheless, Dakin's solution continues currently to be used as a disinfectant agent for minor wounds.

As Carrel's method was grudgingly accepted into civilian practice, numerous papers on the progress and validity of his work began to appear in the surgical literature. Two such reports were read before the June 1917 meeting of the American Surgical Association. In addition, Carrel wrote a surgical textbook, *The Treatment of Infected War Wounds* (1917), and his wife authored a companion manual for nurses, *Technic of the Irrigation Treatment of Wounds by the Carrel Method* (1917). Simultaneously, William Keen brought out his 169-page *Treatment of War Wounds* (1917), which included an approving prefatory note, "I am gratified to be able to add…two most important contributions to our knowledge…the new antiseptic, Dichloramin-T, and the simplified technic of Dakin for the treatment of infection in wounds." Crile, too, was compiling his *Notes on Military Surgery* (1924) in the autumn of 1917 at the request of the medical section of the Council of National Defense. Although it was intended for immediate publication "as one of the stop-gap war series," Crile noted that in the confusion of government activities at the time of the Armistice, its publication was delayed. During the same years, the Philadelphia publishing firm of Lea & Febiger brought out a series of medical war manuals authorized by the Secretary of War. Included among the eight titles was *Military Ophthalmic Surgery*, *Military Orthopedic Surgery*, *Military Surgery of the Zone of the Advance*, and *Military Surgery of the Ear, Nose, and Throat*, all in 1918. From 1921 to 1929, the Surgeon-General's Office authorized publication of a fifteen-volume set,

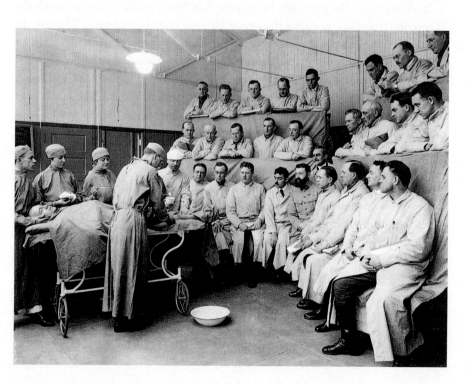

8. Alexis Carrel *(white cap)* lecturing to a surgical class at Rockefeller Institute's War Demonstration College. *(Courtesy of the Rockefeller University Archives)*

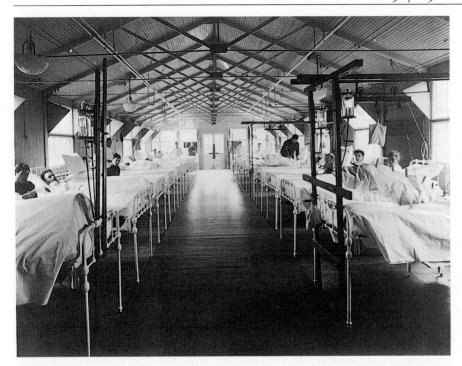

9. The Rockefeller Institute's War Demonstration College also had its own hospital ward. This scene is particularly revealing for the bottles of Dakin's solution hanging at the foot of each patient's bed. (*Courtesy of the Rockefeller University Archives*)

The Medical Department of the United States Army in the First World War, which summarized the war's medical and surgical developments.

As the United States was drawn into the European conflict, the governing board of the Rockefeller Institute began to discuss its responsibility to the country and the future crisis. The board members settled on a plan to teach the Carrel-Dakin method to American physicians and surgeons. Flexner agreed to set up a center for this purpose, and he asked Carrel to return to New York City and assume command of the War Demonstration Hospital to be located adjacent to the Institute. The sixty-six-bed facility, housed in sixteen portable buildings, occupied the whole southwest corner of the Institute's grounds. The expressed purpose of this "self-sufficient" facility was to train American military surgeons in the treatment of infected wounds and to offer courses to civilian surgeons on the care of trauma patients.

The first class reported in August 1917, and the last group departed in March 1919. The initial patients were civilians suffering from a variety of infected wounds; they were slowly replaced, after American forces entered combat, by wounded soldiers sent home from France. Twice monthly a new class of medical officers settled in to learn the Carrel-Dakin method. In addition, laboratory specialists were given short courses in the preparation of Dakin's antiseptic solution and in the bacteriological testing and control of the surgical treatment.

The War Demonstration Hospital attracted much attention in professional, military, and governmental circles. Even Winston Churchill (1874–1965), serving as England's Secretary for War and Air, visited the hospital and Carrel's laboratory in April 1918. Despite the well-recognized success of Carrel's method of wound treatment, the usual professional jealousies crept into the picture when Arthur Dean Bevan, a professor of surgery from Chicago, wrote a highly critical letter of the facility to the *Journal of the American Medical Association* (November 1917). Pettiness aside, it seemed that much of the adverse criticism came from those who had not visited the War Demonstration Hospital for any considerable length of time. In the end, Carrel's work at the hospital, and the very fact that a private organization like the Rockefeller Institute was able to fund such an undertaking, pointed to the growing maturity of American medicine.

The war was coming to an end, albeit with a lingering bitterness on the part of some American surgeons. At the 1918 meeting of the American Surgical Association, its governing council suggested that any "fellow, active or honorary, aiding the enemy in the war...be struck from the list of the Association." William Mayo, in discussing the resolution, noted that one of the active fellows, Otto Kiliani, a New York City surgeon who had been on staff at that city's German Hospital, was now serving in the German Army and had even received the Iron Cross. Kilani was summarily expelled from the membership, never to be reinstated. What was never introduced into the official records of the Association was that Kilani seemed to have partially redeemed himself in November 1923, when he took an active part in suppressing Adolf Hitler's (1889–1945) attempt to seize the Bavarian government in Munich in what became known as the Beer Hall *Putsch*.

With the conclusion of hostilities, American surgery emerged stronger than ever. Many authorities believed that the greatest boon from the war effort was the return to civilian practice of good surgeons practicing good surgery. Surgeons did return and go about their work much as before in their communities and universities, but whether there was a truly perceptible change in the conduct of American surgical practice is difficult to ascertain. The population of the country was approximately 100 million, and over half the physicians in the United States still listed themselves as general practitioner-surgeons, only some fifteen to twenty-five hundred confining their practices entirely to what would be termed general surgery. Lewis Pilcher summed up the world's calamity from a surgical standpoint in his presidential address before the 1919 meeting of the American Surgical Association: "The traumatic surgery of this war has constituted a tremendous vivisection experimental laboratory in which not mice, nor rabbits, nor guinea-pigs, nor dogs have been the subjects of experiments, but humans being, the choicest young men of the civilized world."

1920	1925	1930	1935	1940	1945	1950	1955	1960

DAILY LIFE

Jack Dempsey becomes world heavyweight boxing champion (1919)

Nineteenth amendment (women's suffrage) passed (1920)

Sacco and Vanzetti convicted of murder (1921)

First commercially sponsored radio broadcast (1922)

Cecil B. DeMille directs and produces *The Ten Commandments* (1923)

Leopold and Loeb sentenced to life imprisonment for kidnapping (1924)

Scopes "monkey trial" (1925)

Book-of-the-Month Club (1926)

Charles Lindbergh flies the Atlantic Ocean solo (1927)

Walt Disney releases first Mickey Mouse cartoon (1928)

St. Valentine's Day Massacre in Chicago (1929)

318 prisoners at the Ohio State Penitentiary at Columbus burn to death (1930)

George Washington Bridge between New York City and New Jersey is completed (1931)

Depression reaches lowest point with average monthly unemployment of 12 million (1932)

President Franklin Roosevelt begins "fireside chats" (1933)

Shirley Temple sings "On the Good Ship Lollipop" (1934)

Social Security Act (1935)

Baseball Hall of Fame is established at Cooperstown, New York (1936)

Amelia Earhart disappears on a flight across the Pacific Ocean (1937)

Orson Welles' "Invasion from Mars" causes widespread panic when aired on radio (1938)

Pan American World Airways begins regular transatlantic passenger service (1939)

Ernest Hemingway writes *For Whom the Bell Tolls* (1940)

Mount Rushmore National Monument (1941)

France's greatest ocean liner, *S.S. Normandie,* burns and capsizes at a New York City pier (1942)

Pentagon completed (1943)

Meat rationing ends, except for steak and choice cuts of beef (1944)

B-52 bomber flies into the 78th and 79th floors of the Empire State Building (1945)

U.S.A. POPULATION

1920	=	110 million
1930	=	123 million
1940	=	132 million

HISTORY AND POLITICS

Paris Peace Conference, Treaty of Versailles, and League of Nations (1919)

Warren Harding and Calvin Coolidge elected president and vice president, respectively (1920)

Bureau of the Budget created (1921)

Fordney-McCumber Tariff raises duties on manufactured goods (1922)

Teapot Dome scandal (1923)

Immigration Act of 1924 (1924)

U.S. agrees to drastic reduction of war debts owed by European countries (1925)

Congress creates the Army Air Corps (1926)

U.S. Marines land in Nicaragua (1927)

Herbert Hoover and Charles Curtis are elected president and vice president, respectively (1928)

Standard Oil Company found guilty of violating the Sherman Antitrust Act (1929)

Hawley-Smoot Tariff (1930)

Congress passes Veterans Compensation Act over President Hoover's veto (1931)

Reconstruction Finance Corporation established (1932)

President Roosevelt declares national bank holiday, suspending activity of Federal Reserve System (1933)

Securities and Exchange Commission (SEC) authorized (1934)

Works Progress Administration (WPA) (1935)

Soil Conservation and Domestic Allotment Act (1936)

Congress resists President Roosevelt's scheme to increase the number of Supreme Court justices (1937)

Congress establishes the House Committee on Un-American Activities (1938)

Hatch Act prohibits political campaign activities by most federal employees (1939)

Selective Service System, the first U.S. peacetime program of compulsory military service (1940)

Japan attacks U.S. naval base at Pearl Harbor, Hawaii (1941)

U.S. warplanes defeat Japanese fleet at the Battles of the Coral Sea and Midway (1942)

U.S. Marines win decisive victory against Japanese forces at Guadalcanal (1943)

D-Day invasion of France (1944)

President Roosevelt, Prime Minister Churchill, and Premier Stalin meet at Yalta in the Crimea (1945)

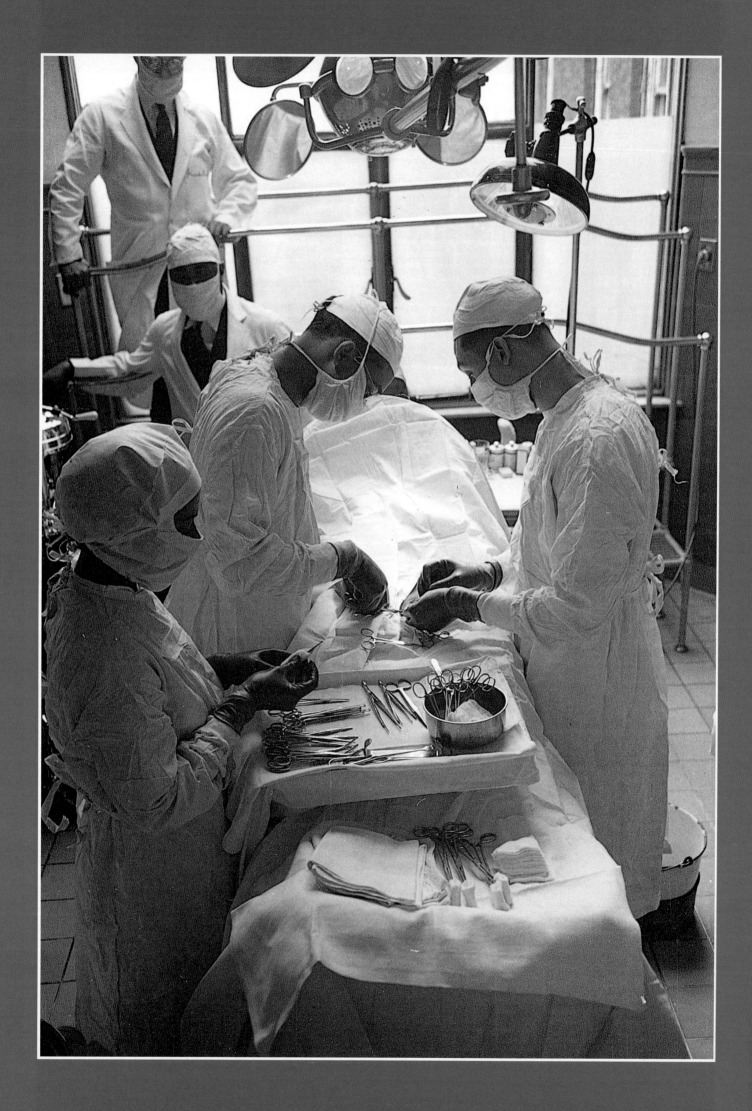

CHAPTER 9

CONSOLIDATION AND SPECIALIZATION
1919–1940

he 1920s proved a prosperous time for American society and its surgeons. During that decade, described as an era of "wonderful nonsense," there was a palpable revolt against the standards of the prewar years. In the wake of Henry Ford's (1863–1947) "putting America on wheels" and the flourishing of oil companies, a web of macadamized highways began to spread across the nation. Charles Lindbergh's (1902–1974) thrilling flight across the Atlantic Ocean from New York to Paris in 1927 roused the nation to a fever pitch of excitement and helped stimulate the new aviation industry. Responding to these events, citizens began spending ever greater amounts of money on such recreational activities as travel and sports. Flappers, speak-easies, and bootlegging, despite a 1919 Constitutional ban on the manufacture and sale of intoxicating liquor, flourished everywhere. Canned foods, ready-made clothing, and household appliances began to free women from much of the centuries-old tedium of household chores. Based on what was believed to be a solid foundation of industrial, scientific, and technologic development, the "new" American way of life seemed fundamentally secure.

The future looked bright when Herbert Hoover (1874–1964) was inaugurated as President in March 1929. Unfortunately, the prosperity of the era had brought about an inordinate speculation in stocks, creating the allure of paper wealth. At the same time, Congress, yielding to lobbying interests, passed the Hawley-Smoot Tariff Act. The law raised tariffs to extremely high levels, and despite protests by every important industrialized foreign nation against the bill's *raison d'état*, and a petition by more than a thousand American economists who urged Hoover to veto the act, the president went ahead and signed it. The effect on foreign trade was disastrous, and that, combined with a decline in industrial growth, made the stock market crash of October 1929 an unfathomable inevitability. The country was plunged into the most acute financial depression in its history, one that lasted through the beginnings of World War II.

By the early 1930s, millions of Americans had lost every dollar they owned. Banks failed, factories shut down, small businesses closed, all levels of government could not collect taxes, and foreign trade came to a virtual halt. The urgent demand for change was met by the election of Franklin Roosevelt as president in 1932. Roosevelt promised a "New Deal," and in the first one hundred days of his administration, the Democratic Congress passed an onslaught of important bills. One act created a Federal Emergency Relief Administration (FERA) and another established the Civilian Conservation Corps (CCC). From these two agencies came the Works Progress Administration (WPA). The National Recovery Administration (NRA), although later ruled unconstitutional by the Supreme Court, attempted to restrengthen industry by shortening work hours, raising wages, and stopping cut-

1. *(facing page)* An operative scene from the Provident Hospital in Chicago (circa 1930s). *(Collection of the Library of Congress)*

2. "Trapper 'Peg Leg Smith' Amputating His Own Leg." A vignette from Bernard Zakheim's frescoe (circa 1935–1938) on early California medicine. Thomas "Peg Leg" Smith was a well-known western pioneer prospector and trapper, who, according to legend, was wounded in a skirmish with Native Americans. Forced into amputating his own leg (presumably gangrenous changes had occurred) Smith placed a self-made tourniquet around the extremity and proceeded with the operation. He sits on a rock in which is carved an old Spanish proverb, "Of medicine, poetry, and insanity, we all have a little." *(Courtesy of Masha Zakheim and the University of California Medical Center, San Francisco)*

throat competition. The establishment of a Labor Relations Board (LRB) added to the luster of the American Federation of Labor (AFL) and led to the organization of a new labor movement, the Congress of Industrial Organizations (CIO). A Securities and Exchange Commission (SEC) was organized, and the Federal Securities Act was passed, requiring sworn statements about all securities for sale to be filed with the Federal Trade Commission (FTC). Roosevelt was of the opinion that the federal government should act in the broadest possible way to assure the long-term welfare of all American citizens. As a result of these beliefs, Congress framed the Social Security Act of 1935, which set the stage for the providing of pensions to the aged, insurance to the unemployed, and benefit payments to the blind, crippled children, and dependent mothers.

Despite the depression, it continued to be a heady time for American surgeons. A therapeutic positivism, spurred on by scientific advancements, was felt throughout the growing profession of surgery. There was an underlying faith that the matura-

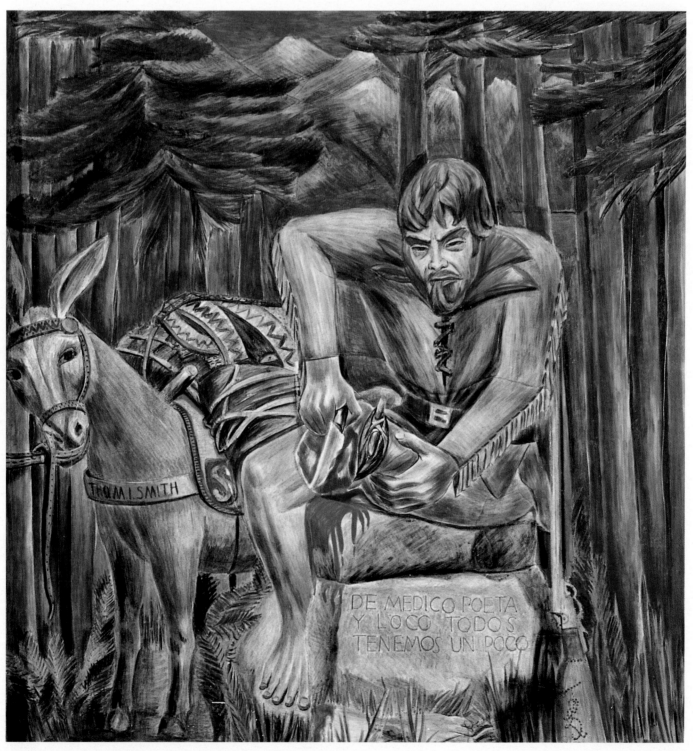

tion of clinical surgery would permanently bring together humane considerations and scientific and technical acumen in ways never before thought imaginable. Passionate debates within the medical and lay communities were beginning to take shape with regard to the future structure of the nation's system of health care delivery. On a national level, questions about the socialization of American medicine and the growing influence of medical insurance companies became paramount. Specialization in surgery, while still under attack, was becoming increasingly common, especially as powerful educational, institutional, and social forces fostered this trend. So too, the overwhelming role of economics acting to hasten the acceptance of specialization by the medical profession was quite evident. In other words, it did not take long for the physician-surgeon to realize that the specialist in surgery could command larger fees even though both might perform the same technical service.

THE CONSOLIDATION OF PROFESSIONAL POWER

During the decade of the twenties a consolidation of professional power was finally achieved. Physicians' incomes dramatically increased; and surgeons' prestige, aided by the ever-mounting successes of medical science, became securely established in American culture. In 1932, the *Report of the Committee on the Costs of Medical Care* confirmed this growing influence of the medical professional in daily American life. Out of concern about nationwide costs and distribution of medical care, a privately funded body, the Committee on the Costs of Medical Care, was established by economists, physicians, and public health specialists in 1926. Among the areas under investigation was a determination of the effect of specialization on physicians' earnings.

It had long been believed that the popularity of certain specialties, although somewhat linked to the prestige enjoyed by specialists among lay and professional groups, was more closely related to financial concerns. Not unexpectedly, the Committee's findings showed that the full-time specialist had an average annual net income of $10,000, compared with $6,100 for partial specialists and $3,900 for general practitioners. As the authors of the *Report* stated: "from the point of view of financial returns...surgery, whether practiced as a partial or a complete specialty, is one of the most remunerative fields of medicine." These observations were corroborated in a second survey conducted by the editors of the journal *Medical Economics* in 1939. They found that the average annual gross income for full-time specialists ranged from a high of $13,354 for radiologists to a low of $6,933 for proctologists. Other income levels included "surgery - $12,161," "eye, ear, nose and throat - $11,310," "ophthalmology - $11,089," "orthopedics - $10,000," "ear, nose and throat - $9,879," "urology - $9,299," and "obstetrics/gynecology - $9,273."

Also evident in the 1932 *Report* was that the distribution of physicians among the various specialties was apportioned almost entirely according to economic factors. Of the approximately 150,000 total American physicians, almost 48,000 considered themselves either full- or part-time specialty practitioners. And, of the specialists, almost two-thirds were distributed solely among the surgical specialties: surgery, 13,700; obstetrics/gynecology, 6,410; eye, ear, nose, and throat, 4,994; urology, 2,360; ear, nose, and throat, 1,920; and, orthopedics, 891. Six years later, the United States Public Health Service published the results of a National Health Survey, which provided further evidence that surgical science had become integral to modern medical therapeutics. In this, the first report of its kind, the number of surgical procedures performed on a random population of 8,758 Caucasian families in eighteen states was ascertained. The authors found that over 6,500 procedures per 100,000 population per year were being conducted; tonsillectomies accounted for almost one-third of all operations, setting a fractured bone second, and appendectomies third.

It was believed that one of the many reasons for the performance of so many surgical operations was a continued lack of regulation within American medicine of who could or should be allowed the right to practice surgery. There remained virtually no limits on the manner in which general practitioners entered specialty practice.

Therefore, it only made sense, as the socioeconomics of medical practice evolved, that if fees for surgical operations were going to be high, the absolute number of completed operative procedures would likewise increase. Such a basic capitalistic tenet as the increase of one's personal wealth held as much appeal for physicians and surgeons as for any citizen, and it probably accounted significantly for the desire of so many medical practitioners to proclaim themselves part-time and eventually full-time surgical specialists. In fact, by 1940, out of 157,000 total physicians in the United States, almost 37,000 individuals were now describing themselves as strictly full-time specialists. Among their declared specialties were ophthalmology and otorhinolaryngology (7,608), surgery (6,645), obstetrics and gynecology (2,551), urology (1,723), and orthopedics (1,078). For a financially struggling physician, especially during the 1930s, what easier way was there to increase personal income then to also perform surgical procedures?

Unfortunately, there was no one educational pathway that provided entrée into the surgical specialty field. Bona fide general surgical residency programs, patterned after Halstedian precepts, remained scarce. As late as 1922, there were fewer than a dozen such approved programs scattered throughout the country. Not until three years later did the American Medical Association's Council on Medical Education publish its first list of hospitals having residencies, then only twenty-nine. Of these, seventeen were in surgery, but the duration of training was not indicated. Besides the lack of formal educational opportunities in specialty training, there was no legal way to distinguish the well-trained surgeon, who limited his work to general surgery or one of the subspecialties, from the vast majority of physicians, inadequately trained in surgery and simultaneously practicing general medicine.

This noticeable lack of standards and regulations in specialty practice became a serious concern to leaders in the profession. In 1913, the Council on Medical Education recommended that the Association should become more involved in the establishment of standards for postgraduate education and training. Among the Council's unstated aims was a perceived opportunity to destroy the taint of commercialism that persisted in graduate education, as had been accomplished via the Flexner report on undergraduate medical schooling. Recommendations for a two-year standard of specialty graduate training, in addition to a one-year internship, were proposed. Not unexpectedly, it proved difficult to realize such standards because of a noticeable lack of legal and voluntary coordination on a national level. The difficulties of World War I further accentuated the realistic need for specialty standards when many of the physicians who were self-proclaimed surgical specialists were found to be unqualified by military examining boards. In ophthalmology, for example, over 50 percent of tested individuals were deemed unfit to treat diseases of the eye.

By the mid-1920s, virtually every surgical specialty had already established numerous nationally recognized fraternal educational organizations; they included the American Otological Society, the American Association of Genito-Urinary Surgeons, the American Association of Obstetricians and Gynecologists, and the Clinical Orthopaedic Society. As these professional associations evolved socially and politically, there was a growing clamor for a clearer definition of specialty work. Full-time specialists attempted to raise the standards for admission to specialty practice by making the completion of an approved residency as accepted minimum requirement. A further question also arose: should not the public be protected from unqualified specialty practitioners by some type of legal structure beyond that of a residency? Not unexpectedly, state medical licensing boards were loath to get involved in the question of specialty identification.

The result, from a governmental and legal standpoint, was that the general medical license, obtained by a physician from the state in which he or she practiced, would continue to entitle the holder to the unrestricted pursuit of virtually any type of allopathic therapeutic activity deemed not physically harmful. As in the nineteenth century, the lack of governmental response seemed to have consigned the problem of licensure, in this case involving specialty work, to voluntary professional organizations. There was little doubt that the medical profession and its rapidly evolving hierarchy of specialties were given a strong message by American society and its elected officials that any attempts at specialty regulation would have to emanate from the profession itself. Although this was not a new precedent, it provided further impetus for physicians and surgeons to remain sheltered from outside monitoring activities. A pattern was thus established that led over the next six decades to much of the currently perceived inability of American physicians and surgeons to police their own profession.

It has long been recognized that the integrity of any profession is guaranteed largely by the control it exercises over the professional competence of its members. Therefore, the question of licensing, whether mandated by the government by voluntary submission, and how it is controlled becomes one of crucial importance. In a certain abstract sense, the granting of a medical/surgical license forms the nexus between professional education and training and private practice, and it serves as an all-important interphase with the public that the profession needed to preserve. Accordingly, the first surgical specialty to attempt to rein in practitioners by licensure was ophthalmology. Unlike most of their fellow surgeons, ophthalmologists had long been established on the American medical scene. Despite their organized presence for well over half a century, they remained beset with significant political problems. Following the turn of the century, non-medically schooled optometrists began to make claims, through extensive advertising campaigns, of greater competency in correcting refractive errors than allopathic practitioners. Both full-time and part-time ophthalmologists were restrained from advertising their services by the ethical code of the medical profession. As a result, they could do little to effectively counter the boasts of their optometric competitors. Even more problematic to full-time ophthalmologists was the simple fact that growing numbers of general practitioners, after attending a postgraduate course lasting only for several weeks, were beginning to trumpet their investiture as "ophthalmologists" under the pretext that they were now trained refractionists and could even capably treat eye diseases.

Leaders in ophthalmology were outraged at what they perceived as the usurping of hard-earned professional skills. Most worrisome of all was the unmistakeable reality that there were no established criteria with which to distinguish the well-qualified ophthalmologist from the "upstart" optometrist or to clarify the differences in clinical expertise between the well-trained, full-time specialist and the inadequately trained, part-time general practitioner. In recognition of the gravity of the situation, the self-patrolling concept of a professional examining board, sponsored by leading

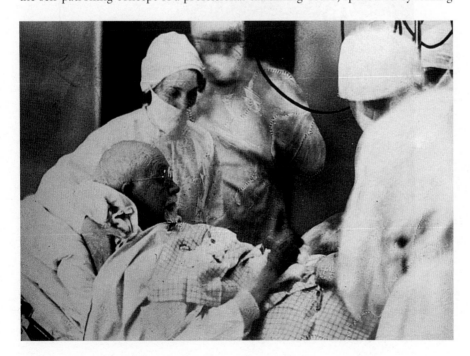

3. Nowhere can the advances in modern surgery (i.e., anesthesia and antisepsis) be more aptly summarized than in this photograph of Evan O'Neill Kane, a Pennsylvania surgeon, performing his own inguinal hernia repair (circa 1925). Whether he was fool or phenom, Kane's skill and self-confidence are clearly present. He appears to be calm and without pain. The operation proved a success, but by this time Kane had already become renowned for self-surgery, since he had previously astounded the medical world in 1921 when he removed his own appendix. *(Courtesy of Stanley B. Burns, M.D., and The Burns Collection and Archive)*

voluntary ophthalmological organizations (e.g., the American Ophthalmological Society and various regional societies), was proposed as a mechanism for certifying competency. In 1916, uniform standards and regulations were set forth in the form of minimal educational requirements and written and oral examinations, and the American Board for Ophthalmic Examinations (later changed to the American Board of Ophthalmology) was formally incorporated.

During the 1920s, two other surgical specialty groups followed the ophthalmologists in creating boards to examine and certify those who wished to be recognized as qualified specialists. A National Board of Examiners in Otolaryngology was formalized in 1924 (its name was later changed to the American Board of Otolaryngology), representing the joint interests of several nationally recognized organizations in this field. Four years later, a committee meant to organize the country's obstetricians and gynecologists began to consider a similar course of action. Composed of representatives from the American Association of Obstetricians, Gynecologists and Abdominal Surgeons; the American Gynecological Society; and the Section on Obstetrics, Gynecology and Abdominal Surgery of the American Medical Association, the American Board of Obstetrics and Gynecology was incorporated in 1930. The new Board required its applicants to undergo a minimum of three years of residency training in obstetrics and gynecology subsequent to a year of internship, and to provide proper assurance of their wholehearted intention to limit their practice to the specialty. The first written examination of candidates for certification by the American Board of Obstetrics and Gynecology took place in March 1931, followed by oral, clinical, and pathological examinations two months later.

In the early 1920s, recognizing the importance of specialty licensure, the American Medical Association's Council on Medical Education began to again consider the question of specialties. Its members recommended that a defined period of postgraduate training be established by national voluntary specialty organizations, followed by

4. Cover to a dinner program (April 1922) during which a gold medal was presented to William Halsted by the National Dental Association honoring his "discovery of conduction anesthesia." For this joyous occassion, less than six months prior to Halsted's death, the well-known medical illustrator Max Brödel created an eloquent emblematic drawing symbolizing Halsted's scientific achievements as an instrumental building block in the evolution of surgery. In the lower left corner, a figure symbolizing a historical scribe of surgery is dressed in the style of ancient Greece. Behind him, two muscular men erect a wall of surgical history, guided by what appear to be godlike hands. In the distance is a Greek healing temple of Aesculapius. The building blocks bear various surnames; those of Theodor Billroth, John Hunter, Theodor Kocher, Bernhard von Lagenbeck, Joseph Lister and, now, William Halsted can be deduced. (Author's Collection)

DINNER
IN HONOR
OF
DR.W.S.HALSTED

some form of certifying examination. However, by its very nature, the American Medical Association has no true legal authority over any facet of the country's health care delivery system. As a result of these legal "handcuffs," as well as the overt influence of concerned general practitioners within its rank and file, the American Medical Association was forced to proceed cautiously toward any embrace of specialty work.

Quite appropriately, general practitioners feared that surgeons and other medical specialists would block access to hospital staff privileges and similarly deny them opportunities to obtain specialty training, formal or otherwise. They reasoned that their economic livelihood would be destroyed, especially for physicians in the more rural areas of the country, who out of sheer geographic necessity performed surgical work. In many instances, these part-time surgical operators were a lingering after-effect of the massive numbers of physicians who obtained rudimentary surgical skills at the time of the Civil War. In no uncertain terms, many of the inadequately trained, mid-nineteenth century "surgeon-fathers" begot poorly trained "surgeon-sons," who by the 1930s begot ill-prepared "surgeon-grandsons." The result of all this political jockeying by members of the American Medical Association meant that the system of standards and regulations governing medical and surgical specialty work in the United States was ultimately forced to evolve outside the Association's organizational framework.

It was fast becoming apparent to America's specialist physicians that a means of efficiently and intelligently coordinating all the various specialities' certifying activities needed to be developed. Maladroit attempts at the creation of further specialty boards, in the absence of a central controlling body, threatened to undermine one of the very reasons why boards were contemplated in the first place: an orderly restructuring of the country's health care delivery system. To remedy this perceived lack of leadership, an Advisory Board for Medical Specialties, representing an independent coalition of the three existing surgical specialty boards, some seventy medical schools, state licensing committees, and various hospitals—all tied together with extremely weak links to the American Medical Association's Council on Medical Education—was formed in 1933. One year later, it issued a written statement, "Essentials for an Approved Special Examining Board," which declared that future boards should be organized under the joint auspices of the American Medical Association, the various national specialty societies, and would have to meet final approval by the Advisory Board. Among the proposed generic requirements for candidates applying for specialty certification were at least three years of training after an internship of at least one year, an unrestricted license to practice medicine and surgery, and membership in the American Medical Association or an acceptably equivalent specialty organization. Following the adoption of these standards and the promise of appropriate implementation, specialty boards were organized in rapid succession. By the end of 1940, twelve more specialty boards were established, including six within surgery: orthopedic (1934), colon and rectal (1934), urology (1935), plastic (1937), surgery (1937), and neurologic (1940).

As the desire for specialty training grew, there was a concomitant need to increase the number of "approved" hospital residency positions. As had happened following the founding of the American College of Surgeons, when growing numbers of candidates for fellowship directly caused their hospitals to take corrective actions relative to standards of patient care, many hospitals seeking approval for residency training positions were forced to upgrade their educational and training facilities. The net result was that from 338 hospitals having 2,028 approved residency positions in 1930, there came to be 610 approved hospitals listing 5,256 residency positions by 1941.

Despite the best of intentions, the truth was that without federal or state government involvement, specialty boards never had legal or any other type of power to prevent uncertified doctors from practicing as specialists. Nor, for that matter, could boards compel hospitals to employ the boards' certification as a requirement for admitting privileges relative to patient care. This became unmistakeably evident in the case of the American College of Surgeons and its more academic members. For ten years, the College had attempted to upgrade the standards of American surgical practice by opening its doors to large numbers of individuals who practiced surgery (trained or untrained, full-time or part-time) and exposing them to "wet" clinics, dry demonstrations, and clinical lectures by leading surgeons of the day. In accomplishing this task, it was necessary to set what some surgeons considered as rather low standards for membership despite the intended goals set forth in the organization's by-laws.

By 1924, College membership had reached nearly 7,000 "surgeons" and, in the opinion of certain members of the academic segment of the profession, was continuing to increase at too alarming a rate. That year, the American College of Surgeons received petitions from members of both the Society of Clinical Surgery and the Eclat Club, two exclusive and elitist surgical societies. The petitions expressed concern over the growing number of fellows admitted over the past few year and what was assessed as their poor quality. The petitioners demanded more "rigid tests of character, training, and intelligence." In essence, surgical academicians flung down a gauntlet to self-taught and part-time surgeons. The result was the surfacing in surgical politics of the entire split between academicians and private practitioners over what the nation's largest surgical organization should truly represent.

Initially, little action came about, possibly because of a lack of unanimity of opinion but more likely because, as William Mayo wrote to Franklin Martin: "A group of men who thought they had this College killed years ago, suddenly found it had become a great institution and they would like to take over the running of it.... Personally I think the treatment they have had for all these years, letting them holler, has been successful and should be continued." Still, the lingering questions over competency levels could not be easily quelled, and the "town-gown" argument spilled onto the national arena. Samuel Harvey (1886–1953), professor of surgery at Yale University, stated that "compared with the analagous organization in Great Britain, the American College of Surgeons has about the relative standards of a 5 and 10 cent store as compared with any first class department store." This was countered by the assertion of George Muller (1877–1947), a Philadelphia surgeon, that "the American College of Surgeons has done a splendid thing for surgery. The title of F.R.C.S. usually comes as a reward for work done, but the title of F.A.C.S. signifies an inducement to do good work. I have an idea that things surgical would have been very chaotic in this country had it not been for the College." In a disparaging afterthought aimed at the academic community, Muller added, "the majority of surgeons are a bit impatient with the group that belongs to the American Surgical Association...except for a wearisome grind with papers read at the annual meeting the...Association is a club, a mutual admiration society, and has done nothing of a constructive nature."

In the midst of all these arguments, a decided trend was developing in American medical education. As a consequence of World War I and the subsequent imposition of quotas, immigration had come to a crashing halt. Demographers and leaders of American medicine were coming to the opinion that with a stabilized population, any increase in the number of medical practitioners would be undesirable. The result of extensive bickering was a reduction in the size of entering medical school classes from 7,578 acceptances out of 12,128 applicants in 1933, to 6,211 acceptances out of 11,800 applicants in 1940. Whether this political maneuvering provided a logical consistency in helping streamline the country's health care delivery network remains conjectural. What cannot be denied, however, is that this decrease in the number of medical and surgical practitioners in the United States assured the economic viability of private solo practice.

Some advocates of a reduced number of medical school matriculants believed that more specific measures needed to be taken, in particular against certain immigrant groups. Arthur Dean Bevan (1861–1943), professor of surgery at Rush Medical College and an important voice in American surgery, urged that special action be

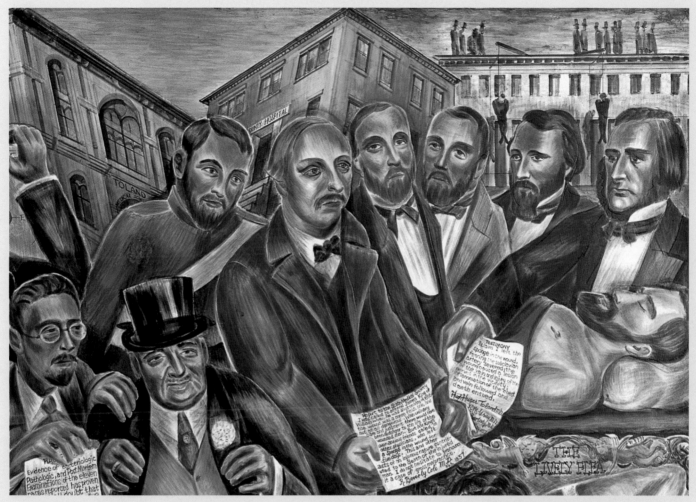

5. Completed during the New Deal (circa 1935–1938), Bernard Zakheim's twelve-panel fresco on early San Francisco medicine included a vignette on the infamous "retained surgical sponge" malpractice case of 1856. Although there are no reliable statistics regarding the total number of medical malpractice actions initiated before the Civil War, numerous suits were known to have been filed involving questions of forensic medicine. The disputed death of James King of William (he adopted the strange name from his father's given name, William, to distinguish him from all the other James Kings residing in California), a crusading journalist, is one such example. King of William was shot by James Casey, a corrupt politician, in the left side of the chest. He was immediately taken to his office at the *Pacific*

Express, which ultimately became his death chamber, as tens of physicians manually explored the wound and in a cacophony of divided opinion decided to have a sponge inserted in the bullet entrance site to tamponade further bleeding. Five days later King of William expired, following the onset of purulent drainage from the wound. Almost immediately, cries of surgical malpractice were initiated by R. Beverly Cole (1829–1901), a physician who had been a close friend of King of William, against the many other doctors involved in the management of the case, particularly Hugh H. Toland (1806–1880), the state's best-known surgeon. Cole, who felt he had been personally humiliated by Toland during the discussions at King of William's bedside, argued that the retained sponge had directly

contributed to King of William's demise by creating putrefaction in addition to the general confusion caused by so many consulting physicians. In May 1857, the well-publicized legal battle to affix the guilt of King of William's death began. Toland argued that death resulted from a subclavian vein phlebitis and "shock" in a man with poor resistance. The jury returned a verdict of no medical malpractice, stating that regardless of the sponge, King of William would have died of the bullet wound. In modern parlance, he probably died of an overwhelming bacterial infection, secondary to a gunshot injury, causing septic shock. *(Courtesy of Masha Zakheim and the University of California Medical Center, San Francisco)*

taken against Jewish applicants from New York City. Bevan noted that Jewish-sounding surnames had increased steadily from 10 percent of all applicants in 1926 to almost 20 percent by 1936. In a speech to the American Medical Association, Bevan, as long-standing chairman of its Council on Medical Education, enunciated his opinion that in the "present over-crowded condition, no group should be permitted to enter medicine in such numbers as to crowd out of medicine the members of other groups who desire to enter." Bevan proposed that zero growth of the profession be achieved by setting a ceiling on admission to medical schools and creating designated quotas for certain groups of applicants, particularly Jews. Bevan even went so far as to assure his audience that influential "leaders of Jewish thought and

6. George Heuer, surgeon-in-chief at New York Hospital, conducts a surgical lecture at Cornell University Medical College, addressing the students on the subject of skull fracture (circa 1930s). *(Courtesy of the Medical Archives, New York Hospital–Cornell Medical Center)*

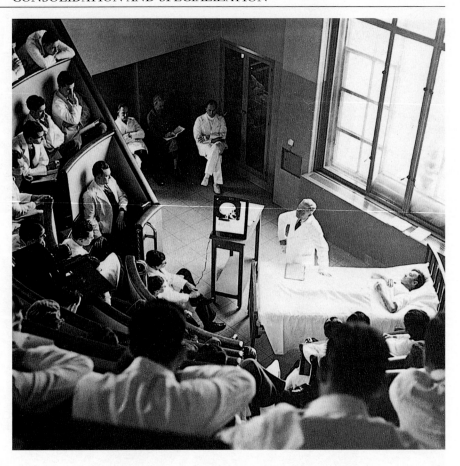

culture…are making a determined effort through Jewish publications and societies to lower the great number of Jewish students who are overcrowding into medicine." However, Bevan's attempt to depict such an "effort" as being representative of mainstream Jewish organizations was speculative at best.

Bevan's "zero-growth" suggestions were never explicitly adopted, but little doubt exists that elements of his attitude insinuated themselves into the whole of 1920s and 1930s American medicine and extended into American surgery. There might have been an objectionable number of individuals practicing medicine, but just as serious was the reverse indictment that many worthwhile persons were being excluded. So strong were ethnic and religious prejudices, especially against African Americans but also Jews and Roman Catholics, that in 1936, alone, almost two thousand individuals went abroad to attend European medical schools—a number that must have far exceeded any record established during the earlier trek to German universities.

Bevan was a remarkable personality, who served during World War I as director of general surgery in the surgical division of the Surgeon General's office. An individual of great authority, with a noticeable disdain for personal criticism, Bevan held many important positions throughout organized surgery. From 1892 till his death, he was on the surgical staff of Chicago's Presbyterian Hospital, serving as chief of surgery during most of that time. In 1906 he was named chairman of the American Medical Association's Section on Surgery and Anatomy, and twelve years later he was elected president of the Association. Furthermore, Bevan was a member of the first Board of Governors of the American College of Surgeons, president of the Inter-State Post-Graduate Medical Assembly in 1931, and president of the American Surgical Association in 1932. As a surgeon, Bevan developed several operative procedures, and his name was long associated with an operation for cryptorchidism. He also developed the "hockey-stick" incision for cholecystectomy and performed the first operation in which ethylene oxide was used as an anesthetic.

It is self-evident that the religious attitudes and elements of racial prejudice held by Bevan and others constituted more than a minor role in the overall evolution of American medicine. Similarly, it would be historically wrong to deny the long-whispered belief held by various members of the Jewish medical community that prior to the 1950s, anti-Semitism was particularly rife in general surgery, contrasted to the rest of medicine. This is evidenced in the fact that by the end of World War II, although Jews had held responsible political positions in virtually all surgical subspecialties, no general surgeon of acknowledged Jewish heritage would assume the presidency of the American College of Surgeons nor the American Surgical Association until the late 1950s and early 1960s, when Isidor Ravdin (1894–1972), professor of surgery at the University of Pennsylvania, held both. Unfortunately, this lack of Jewish representation in the political power structure of general surgery would repeat itself into the 1990s.

By the mid-1930s, the entrenched control of the American College of Surgeons by the likes of Franklin Martin, the Mayo brothers and George Crile, was coming to an end. At the 1935 meeting of the American Surgical Association, president Edward Archibald (1872–1945) of Montreal, Canada, appointed a committee to investigate the "elevation of surgical standards." Thomas Orr (1884–1955), a surgeon from Kansas City, Missouri, remarked that in the private practice of surgery there existed "only a sprinkling of surgeons" but a "deluge of operators." Spurred on by that remark, the Association's committee, headed by Evarts Graham (1883–1957) of St. Louis, decided that a more representative national body should be invested with the authority to organize a qualifying board of surgery. There were acrimonious discussions between officials of the American Surgical Association and the American College of Surgeons, but by early 1936, a National Committee for the Elevation of the Standards of Surgery was formally established. The Committee consisted of three men each from national organizations (American College of Surgeons, American Medical Association, and American Surgical Association) and one man each from certain regional surgical societies (Southern, Western, Pacific Coast, and New England).

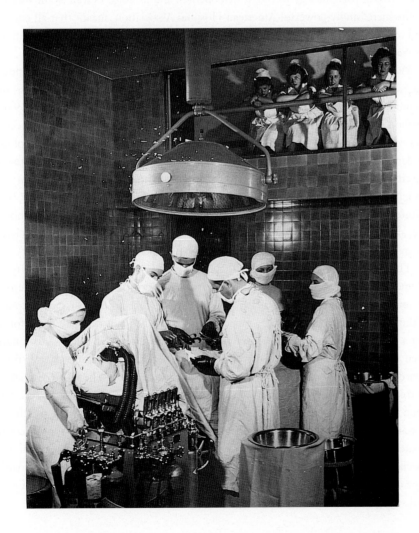

7. During this era of consolidation and specialization, dramatic changes were occurring in the physical makeup of an operating room. As demonstrated in this scene (circa 1935) the viewing audience (in this case nurses rather than physicians) was now clearly distanced from the patient as sterilization and aseptic techniques were expanded to include both surgeon and spectator. In only a few more years, visitors' galleries would be completely enclosed by glass. *(Courtesy of Stanley B. Burns, M.D., and The Burns Collection and Archive)*

8. By the 1920s, decoratively framed operative scenes were an important part of hospital halls and surgical offices. Such "artwork" imbued a psychological confidence in the accomplishments of the institution and its practitioners. The physical act of surgery was no longer a public event, and modern medicine was rapidly turning into a profession separated from the general population by education and scientific convention. Consequently, the only views of surgical operations for mass consumption were framed icons and/or the pictures found in weekly magazines. *(Courtesy of Stanley B. Burns, M.D., and The Burns Collection and Archive)*

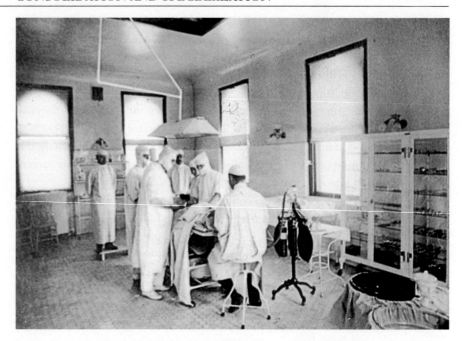

THE AMERICAN BOARD OF SURGERY AND THE EVOLUTION OF SPECIALTIES

As Graham would find out, the political complexities involved in the evolution of the American Board of Surgery proved especially difficult. Unlike the surgical subspecialty boards, which affected small numbers of practitioners, the American Board of Surgery would have an important and forceful impact in upgrading the quality of all surgical training throughout the United States. However, the often disparate objectives of the three national organizations and of previously founded surgical specialty boards, in particular gynecology, orthopedics, and urology, as well as the interest of the increasingly powerful American Hospital Association, meant that all entities had to mesh their vested interests in order to accomplish this difficult and politically charged feat.

Well before the American Board of Surgery was formalized, the organizational fragmentation of American surgical specialization was occurring. In particular, the founding of the American Boards of Obstetrics and Gynecology (1930), Orthopaedic Surgery (1934), and Urology (1935) dashed any hopes that all specialties could be grouped under one familial surgical umbrella. Unlike ophthalmology, otolaryngology, and obstetrics, which were considered topical specialties related to specific regions of the human body, gynecologic, orthopedic, and urologic surgery all fell under the rubric of general surgery. Thus, the question remained: what constituted general surgery? The answer in negative came from gynecologic, orthopedic, and urologic surgeons, who by establishing their own certifying boards, declared themselves fundamentally different from general surgeons.

The emergence of these subspecialty boards raised political questions: what types of operations would general surgeons be certified to perform? The entire concept of generalism in American medicine was assuming increasingly negative tones. Although a surgeon of the 1920s and 1930s might feel equally competent performing a bowel resection, a hysterectomy, and a prostatectomy, and setting a comminuted fracture of the lower extremity, in the public's opinion a full-time, board-certified orthopedic surgeon was increasingly assumed to be more competent in treating the comminuted fracture than the general surgeon. Conversely, the surgeon who restricted his practice to urologic and gynecologic procedures, which was not an uncommon choice, was not eligible for certification by either the American Board of Obstetrics and Gynecology or the American Board of Urology, as each subspecialty board required its members to restrict their clinical affairs to that board's type of surgery. He was ipso facto a general surgeon, but truly did not perform general surgical operations!

It was a politically difficult time in the evolution of American surgery. With eye, ear, nose, throat, bone, female pelvic, male and female urologic, and, shortly, plastic and reconstructive surgery removed from their primary jurisdiction, the general surgeon was pushed into defending his monopoly of what remained in the abdomen, breasts, neck, and thorax. The American College of Surgeons, the American Surgical Association, and the fledgling American Board of Surgery were faced with a great politico-socio-economic dilemma of sense of purpose. As Evarts Graham, and the other young turks who wished to bring vigorous new academic blood into these organizations, were confronted with the growing power of the surgical subspecialty boards, they would find that it was too late to totally control their overall development.

The American Board of Surgery held its formal organizational meeting in January 1937. Though born in conflict and soon to be under attack by varied forces, who considered that such an all-encompassing board would lead to overstandardization and regimentation and would also limit the number of general surgical specialists for socioeconomic reasons, the American Board of Surgery soon became a powerful force on the surgical stage. In only a short while, the value of surgical certification—a sort of unofficial license—became recognized by the better-educated public and by more reform-minded physicians. Still, there was no legal requirement for certification, and well into the 1960s it was commonly known that many less sophisticated families continued to be surgically served almost entirely by general practitioner-surgeons. As the boards evolved in stature, it also became obvious that their diplomates were beginning to receive preferential treatment. In World War II, board-certified surgeons obtained generally higher military rank and were given more responsible managerial and clinical positions than surgeons without board certification. Following the war, some hospitals even began to limit surgical privileges to only board-certified individuals.

As order was introduced into specialty training and the process of certification, it was apparent that the continued growth of residency programs carried important implications for the future structure of American medical practice and the social relations of medicine to overall society. Professional power had been consolidated, and specialization, which had been evolving since the time of the Civil War, was now recognized as an essential if not integral part of modern medicine. Although the creation of surgical specialty boards was justified under the broad imprimatur of raising the educational status and evaluating the clinical competency of specialists, undeniably board certification began to restrict entry into the specialties. Perhaps their critics secretly wished that one long-term direct effect of the boards would be to decrease the number of specialists to relatively small cadres of individuals with insurmountable professional competence, and thus strengthen the "threatened position" of general practitioners. But such hypothetically reasonable results never materialized. Instead, the more persuasive roles played by economics and sociology in the acceptance of specialization by the medical profession and the lay public meant that patients began to consult the specialist directly and avoid the general practitioner "middleman."

This uncoordinated drift toward increasing dependence on specialism, enhanced by ever more amazing technologic feats, foreshadowed the complete breakdown of old-fashioned general practice. For various reasons, from the very outset of formalized medical and surgical specialization in the 1920s and 1930s, American medicine never developed the kind of two-tiered health care delivery system found in England and several other European countries. General practitioners in the United States remained politically unable to secure for themselves the sinecure of the expansive role of their counterparts in England, where patients could consult a specialist only by direct referral from a general practitioner. By the late 1960s, the result of this failure to obtain a mediating role in the delivery of American health care would bring about a socioeconomic collapse of the American family doctor.

As the specialties evolved, the political influence and cultural authority enjoyed by the profession of surgery was growing. This socioeconomic strength was most prominently expressed in reform efforts directed toward the modernization and standardization of America's hospital system. With the ascent of scientific surgery and the maze of available new technologies, the country's surgeons were performing ever more intricate surgical operations. Any vestiges of "kitchen surgery" had essentially disappeared, and other than for numerous small private hospitals predominantly constructed by surgeons for their personal use, the only facilities where major surgery could be adequately conducted and postoperative patients appropriately cared for were the well-equipped and physically impressive modern hospitals. For this reason, the American College of Surgeons and its growing list of fellows had a strong motive to ensure that the country's hospital system was as up-to-date and efficient as possible.

The organization and function of a hospital's surgical clinic was increasingly defined by the adjunctive ability to conduct bacteriological, pathological, chemical, and other special examinations. In addition to performing surgical procedures, the surgeon was being asked to act as diagnostician, pathologist, and bacteriologist. To ensure such capabilities, there was need for better regulation of hospital practices and procedures, particularly professional accountability vis-à-vis quality assurance, or, in the parlance of the times, "standardization." In 1912, Edward Martin, clinical professor of surgery at the University of Pennsylvania, in his role as president of the Clinical Congress of Surgeons of North America, appointed a Committee on the Standardization of Hospitals. Martin named Ernest Codman (1869–1940), a Boston surgeon, as chairman and included Allen Kanavel (1874–1938) and William J. Mayo as staff members. Codman, the son of a Boston Brahmin family, had attended Harvard College (1891) and Harvard Medical School (1895). Following his graduation from medical school, he served a surgical internship at Massachusetts General Hospital, remained on the surgical staff, and rose to the position of assistant surgeon in the outpatient department. Almost from the outset of his remarkable career, Codman demonstrated an interest in evaluating the efficacies of surgical practice contrasted with pure laboratory research or clinical scientific investigations. This was first evidenced during his internship when he, with Harvey Cushing, jointly devised the first system of ether charts (i.e., anesthetic records) to monitor a patient's vital signs during the conduct of an operation. Codman had a pragmatic nature, and his concern with surgical outcomes led to his decade-long (1900–1910) development of the "end-result plan" of tracking hospital surgical patients long enough to determine the effectiveness of treatments so that the competence of hospital surgeons and staff could be evaluated. Prior to Codman's interest in determining whether or not surgical treatment had been successful, no such structured system had been in place in any American hospital. In virtually all instances, surgeons remained ignorant of how their patients, as a statistical group, were doing both on a short-term and a long-term basis.

As chairman of the Committee on Hospital Standardization, Codman began a personal crusade to improve and standardize hospital treatment nationwide. His system was essentially an in-house audit with standardized measures, which allowed for intra- and inter-institutional and personnel comparisons. The phrase "therapeutic efficiency" became Codman's rallying cry, punctuated by his warnings that without such a selfless goal, the profession of surgery and the American College of Surgeons in particular could offer little to differentiate themselves from a trade union. Utilizing the results of standardization, surgeons could begin to concentrate on the procedures at which they were best, rather than be beholden to external socioeconomic considerations. The heretical aspect of Codman's beliefs was that surgical seniority in hospitals should henceforth be based on patient outcomes rather than long-established nepotistic policies and politics. Even more radical was Codman's assertion that hospitals needed to publish their end-result data so that concerned citizens could choose their hospitals intelligently. In the spring of 1913, Codman gave an important speech to the Philadelphia County Medical Society in which he spoke for the first time of the "products of a hospital." The talk was so

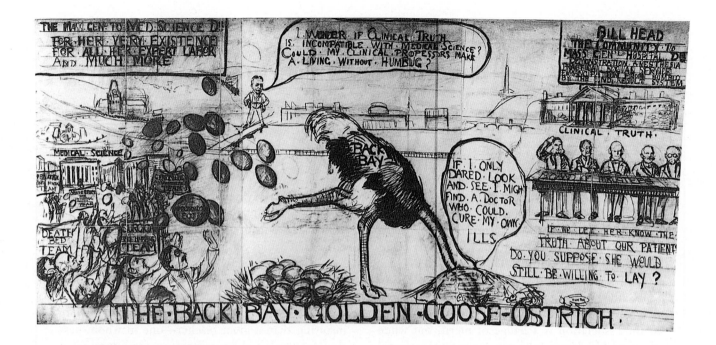

well received that within a year it had been published in *Surgery, Gynecology & Obstetrics* and widely distributed as a reprint. Codman's underlying theme was that results in American industry were being measured by quality of products, and that various "commodities" of the medical profession, including patient care, student education, house staff, nursing care, ancillary services, and residency programs, had to be similarly "qualified" by some type of end-results system.

Codman was viewed as part of a larger group of avant-garde physicians, surgeons, and hospital administrators who were trying to bring together scientific management or industrial efficiency techniques to medicine and surgery. If American factories were assuring that their products were demonstrably good, then hospitals needed to do the same. Codman remained distrustful of surgeons' abilities to police themselves and to be held accountable for their operative blunders. As this great skeptic of all things surgical wrote in the dedication to his book *A Study in Hospital Efficiency* (1917), others "want to reform the bottom of the profession, while I think the blame belongs at the top."

HOSPITAL REFORM AND POLITICAL DIFFICULTIES

Throughout 1913 and 1914, both the American Medical Association and the fledgling American College of Surgeons were evaluating their role in the movement to reform American hospitals. Codman's committee had correctly surmised that the Clinical Congress was not well enough structured to pursue the matter of hospital standardization. Consequently, the committee recommended either the American Hospital Association or the American Medical Association as possible organizations to complete such a vast project. The latter group had hoped to receive a grant from the Carnegie Foundation, which had similarly funded the Flexner report, to support intensive studies of hospitals in the thirty or forty largest population centers of the country. But no monies were forthcoming.

During these back-and-forth discussions, the American College of Surgeons hired its first full-time director. John Bowman (1877–1952) held a doctorate of philosophy, not a doctorate of medicine, and was more administrator than scientist. He had been president of the University of Iowa, and his managerial style easily complemented Franklin Martin's mania for College growth. Traveling throughout the country to discuss College affairs with fellows, Bowman became convinced of the need for adequate hospital records and regulation in order to bring about the proper evaluation of applicants for fellowship.

9. In January 1915, Ernest Codman was serving as chairman of the Surgical Section of the Suffolk District Medical Society in Boston. At the conclusion of the meeting, having anticipated that there would not be enough candidness in discussing the members' surgical results, he displayed this eight-foot-long cartoon, which he had previously drawn. Depicting the Boston Brahmin Back Bay populace as little more than an ostrich with its head in a hill of "humbugs," Codman showed the animal kicking golden eggs of appendectomies and other surgical operations into the waiting hands of the Harvard Medical School faculty, who ignored any pretense of medical science while vainly enriching their wallets. Harvard's President Abbott Lowell (1856–1943) questions "if clinical truth is incompatible with medical science?" while wondering if his "clinical professors [could] make a living without humbug?" Not unexpectedly, Codman's attempt at satire caused a huge brouhaha. He was forced to resign from his medical society position and lost his instructorship in surgery at Harvard. (*The Francis A. Countway Library of Medicine*)

THE CAREER OF A SURGEON

Each surgeon has, to a large extent, the power to fashion his career after his own liking.... Which of the numerous ways does the surgeon elect to follow? His choice with persistence of effort very definitely fixes his career. Down in the bottom of his heart does he desire the limelight more than anything else? Is it his wish to have the conspicuousness and power that accrue to the holders of offices in medical societies? Is he attracted by the exclusiveness of membership in certain surgical associations? Does he mistake the chaff for the wheat? An office filled because of good professional or scientific work or because of faithful and worthy service to the association is a badge of merit, but when obtained like kisses by favor, because of political pull or friendship and influence with the powers that be, the office becomes only a token of political efficiency and ceases to be desirable.

A surgical career can only be truly satisfactory to one who is interested in the science as well as in the art of surgery. The acquiring of the technic of an operation and the possesion of manual dexterity, necessary to its performance, are essential; but an intimate acquaintance with the anatomy, physiology and pathology of the tissues involved in the operation are just as important as the carrying out of a mechanical technic. A knowledge of physiology and of the biologic processes that go with tissue repair is peculiarly important in operations on the gastrointestinal tract, the brain, the lungs, and the urinary system. A practical acquaintance with pathology is a great aid in the treatment of tumors, inflammatory and bacterial affections, and proves a scientific stimulus throughout the surgeon's career.... With an interest in pathology goes the desire for post mortem examinations in all patients that die.... This is not merely scientific curosity, but have a great practical bearing.... Surgeons who do not have necropsies of at least most of their operative deaths are greatly to be pitied.

The career of a surgeon who is merely an operator—a "cutter"—is of very doubtful benefit to himself or to humanity. A certain degree of manual skill is essential to good results, though a surgeon who is not imbued with a knowledge of biologic principles, who is not particularly interested in pathology, but becomes intoxicated with his own dexterity, may be a source of very real danger...

Nothing is more helpful and stimulating to a surgeon than to have some research problem in mind. It may be a simple problem.... But if the surgeon acquires the habit of looking for such problems they are more readily seen.... Who shall deny the possibility of discoveries by the isolated surgeon in these modern days as long as an active scientific curiosity is encouraged and the will to get at the bottom of things exists? The word "research" often has too formidable a sound and discourages a humble undertaking that might be of distinct value.

Universities and great clinics are extremely valuable for the training of a surgeon. Nothing is more inspiring than a great teacher—one in whom passion for truth and an enthusiasm for imparting it burn fiercely. But after learning laboratory and clinical methods, the surgeon must deal directly with the diagnosis of cases and the treatment of patients.... The method of dealing with each case should be mentally reviewed when the case has been completed and an honest conclusion reached whether the best thing was done in this particular instance...

And such experiences, when courageously faced and honestly pondered, do more than merely add to the efficiency of the surgeon's work. They make character. No one should be permitted to embark on a surgical career unless he is first of all a good citizen, unless he stands for what is best in his community, unless he has a keen sense of right and wrong, and the courage of his convictions to do what is right, unless he has a human touch.... Can any one doubt that these things make character and so increase the value of the individual to his community and to his country?

The necessity for intelligence, for preliminary education, and for adequate training of a surgeon are constantly emphasized. The foundation upon which his career should firmly rest is intelligence, training and character—these three, and the greatest of these is character.

J. Shelton Horsley (1870–1946): The chairman's address to the section on surgery of the Southern Medical Association. *The Southern Medical Journal*, vol. 18, pages 1–5, 1925.

The College's Board of Regents appealed to Arthur Dean Bevan, chairman of the American Medical Association's Council on Medical Education, that any activity relative to hospital standardization should come under the auspices of his committee. In reply, Bevan spoke of the tremendous expense involved in such an undertaking and unambiguously stated that the Association's Board of Trustees had flat-out decided not to accept responsibility for the task. When asked if there would then be any objections to the American College of Surgeons undertaking the task of hospital regulation, Bevan expressed no disapproval. Indeed, the relative poverty and uncertain future of the College probably suggested to the leaders of the American Medical Association that no great competition to its own further limited activities in hospital standardization could be envisioned. However, the persuasive powers of Bowman, who had recently served as executive secretary of the Carnegie Foundation and remained quite friendly with its president, Henry Pritchett, were not appreciated.

In January 1916, the College received $30,000 from the Foundation for the expressed purposes of studying hospital standardization. Later that year, the College received formal written notice that the American Hospital Association and the Catholic Hospital Association (at that time, approximately one-half of hospital beds in the country were in Catholic-run institutions) would cooperate fully in the proposed project. Within eighteen months, the first nationwide conference on hospital standarization was organized. Thus, the American Medical Association, despite its interlocking of leadership with the College (indeed, the guidance of the medical profession at that time was largely dominated by surgeons) lost the initiative in the hospital standardization movement. The American College of Surgeons became the dominant force behind hospital reform, not merely from the standpoint of its fellows, around whom standards had largely developed, but in terms of all other medical and surgical specialties. If the College could not control the soon-to-come fragmentation of American surgery, as embodied in the founding of numerous specialty certifying boards, it at least enjoyed the possibility of partially directing subspecialty growth within the institutional setting.

At that first hospital standardization conference called by the College in October 1917, the attendees (some three hundred surgeon and physician members of state Committees on Standards and sixty hospital superintendents) clearly articulated support for turning hospitals into "workshops to serve professional needs." It was becoming evident through public opinion that unless change was forthcoming, both hospitals and surgeons would lose credibility regarding their questionable dedication to science and public service. Not unexpectedly, surgeons remained reluctant to concede control over the introduction of change in institutions, nor could they allow themselves to be viewed as mere technicians in an industrialized hospital. That would have meant that they were once again being regarded as little more than unthinking practitioners of a manual or trade craft—the very two-thousand-year-old opinion that the ascent of scientific surgery had recently put to rest. The motive for these new ideals was reflected in Alan Kanavel's remarks that "dividends must be sought in scientific knowledge…rather than in dollars and cents…. The trustees and superintendents must cease to feel that their duty ends when they have provided food and beds…. Carpentry in surgery must end. Laxness or laziness in diagnosis should be branded a crime. The hospital must become a diagnostic and teaching center if it is to realize its highest ideals of service to physicians, the patients, and the community."

For two years, a preliminary analysis of hospitals was quietly pursued. During the first half of 1919 alone, College staff and members of state standardization committees conducted twenty hospital conferences in the western half of the United States and Canada. Physicians, surgeons, hospital administrators and trustees, county medical societies, chambers of commerce, service organizations, and the general public were issued invitations. The College's program of hospital evaluation was explained,

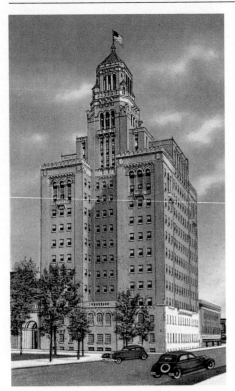

10. The growth and sophistication of the country's hospital system was epitomized by the Mayo Clinic (circa 1928). *(Copyright Curt Teich Postcard Archives, Lake County (IL) Museum)*

pros and cons discussed, and questions answered. In October 1919, John Bowman enunciated the concept of the minimum standard, stating that it would now be possible to know "if any unnecessary surgical operations are performed in the hospital; or if incompetent surgical operations are performed; or if lax, lazy, or incomplete diagnoses are made." Five years after the Board of Regents formally adopted Bowman's ideas, Franklin Martin extolled, "This document has now achieved international fame, and has become to hospital betterment what the Sermon on the Mount is to a great religion."

Minimum standards called for the keeping of case records, the establishment of a clinical laboratory, prohibition against fee splitting, and requirements for a staff organization. During the years 1918 and 1919, field representatives visited 671 hospitals of one hundred beds or more in North America. So poor was the initial performance of most hospitals that only eight or nine institutions surveyed were able to pass muster. Still, the program won public notice primarily when the editors of a general periodical, *World's Work*, assigned a writer to report on it. Appearing in the June 1920 issue, the article proclaimed that the minimum standard brought about "conscientious care that every patient in every hospital has a right to expect. From coast to coast the idea is changing the conditions in hospitals. Everywhere there is the ferment of development, the activity of improvement…The world of the hospital is changing." Other articles in the general literature were also being published, and before long the success of the hospital standardization program became hemispheric in scope. In 1924, at the Third Pan–American Scientific Congress held in Lima, Peru, official endorsement of minimum standards was approved. Shortly thereafter, forty hospitals in South America were surveyed and several were placed on the College's approved list.

The first printed enumeration of approved hospitals appeared in the January 1921 *Bulletin of the American College of Surgeons*. Only 198 institutions came close to satisfying the criteria for minimum standards, but the program proved an important start in the modernization of America's hospital system. Each year, the list of approved hospitals appeared in community newspapers throughout the country. This enabled local townspeople to see how their hospital stood in comparison to others. By 1922, 677 out of 812 hospitals (83 percent) of one hundred or more beds were approved, and 342 out of 811 institutions (42 percent) of fifty to ninety-nine beds met standards. Two decades later, of 4,045 hospitals surveyed, almost 81 percent were on the approved list. However, the fewer beds the hospital had, the more difficult it was to satisfy all the requirements; whereas 93 percent of facilities having more than one hundred beds were approved, only 40 percent of those maintaining between twenty-five and forty-nine beds were placed on the College's list.

As the evaluation process evolved, commencing in 1926, a yearly *Manual of Hospital Standardization* was published. Regarded as the "bible" for every hospital administrator who sought approval for his institution, the detailed text was closely followed by College surveyors in the field. Starting out only eighteen pages in length, the hospital standardization manuals were printed and distributed in the tens of thousands. Revised every two to three years, the manual contained not only instructions on how to apply the principles of minimum standard but a statement concerning the "By-Products of Standardization," based on 13,360 surveys over the years 1918 to 1926. In this self-congratulatory message, the College assured its critics that the first nine years of institutional evaluations had brought about greater attention to patients' concerns; better organization of persons, facilities, and procedures; and enhanced inter-institutional cooperation and coordination— all resulting in improved end results relative to patient care. By 1946, the *Manual* had grown to 118 pages in length, including a stern proscription against fee-splitting by members of a hospital staff, "Principles of Financial Relations in the Professional Care of the Patient," and a thoroughly revised "Rules and Regulations for the Staff."

Throughout its eighty-plus years, one of the cardinal principles on which the American College of Surgeons was founded—the deceptive division of professional fees—has been consistently upheld. Fee-splitting was considered among the most egregious of vices that permeated the American health care delivery system. In this form of economic blackmail, the general practitioner, upon referring his patient, was given, through a prearranged scheme, a portion of the fee paid the surgeon. The family doctor in return might possibly assist at the operation or provide postoperative care, but it was all a premeditated sham. The impropriety of the system was its obvious dishonesty: the patient paid a fee to one person, part of which surreptitiously ended up in the wallet of another. Of even greater threat to the patient's welfare was the simple reality that fee-splitting produced a biased referral system based entirely on socioeconomics rather than quality of care. A technically incompetent surgeon who was willing to participate in this devious division of professional fees could create large-scale physical mayhem. Not only were inadequate medical and surgical services rendered, along with the inevitable performance of unnecessary surgical operations, but there was a deadening of scientific and research incentives in the profession. Consequently, for many of the founders of the College, the question of how to combat division of fees became a professional obsession.

To do away with this pernicious practice, the College early on mounted a major crusade against any form of fee-splitting. In fact, no one ethical qualification of a candidate for fellowship received so much intense scrutiny as that concerning the division of fees. In a final act of prohibition, a ban on division of fees was incorporated into one part of the Fellowship Oath: "I pledge myself, so far as I am able, to avoid the sins of selfishness; to shun unwarranted publicity, dishonest money-seeking, and commercialism as disgraceful to our profession; to refuse utterly all money

---

THE MINIMUM STANDARD

1. That physicians and surgeons privileged to practice in the hospital be organized as a definite group or staff. Such organization has nothing to do with the question as to whether the hospital is "open" or "closed," nor need it affect the various existing types of staff organization. The word STAFF is here defined as the group of doctors who practice in this hospital inclusive of all groups such as the "regular staff," "the visiting staff," and the "associate staff."

2. That membership upon the staff be restricted to physicians and surgeons who are (a) full graduates of medicine in good standing and legally licensed to practice in their respective states or provinces; (b) competent in their respective fields and (c) worthy in character and in matters of professional ethics; that in this latter connection the practice of the division of fees, under any guise whatever, be prohibited.

3. That the staff initiate and, with the approval of the governing board of the hospital, adopt rules, regulations, and policies governing the professional work of the hospital; that these rules, regulations, and policies specifically provide:

   (a) That staff meetings be held at least once each month. (In large hospitals the departments may choose to meet separately.)

   (b) That the staff review and analyze at regular intervals their clinical experience in the various departments of the hospital, such as medicine, surgery, obstetrics, and other specialties; the clinical records of patients, free and pay to be the basis for such review and analyses.

4. That accurate and complete records be written for all patients and filed in an accessible manner in the hospital - a complete case record being one which includes identification data; complaint; personal and family history; history of present illness; physical examination; special examinations; such as consultations, clinical laboratory, X-ray and other examinations; provisional or working diagnosis; medical or surgical treatment; gross and microscopical pathological findings; progress notes; final diagnosis; condition on discharge; follow-up and, in case of death, autopsy findings.

5. That diagnostic and therapeutic facilities under competent supervision be available for the study, diagnosis, and treatment of patients, these to include, at least (a) a clinical laboratory providing chemical, bacteriological, serological, and pathological services; (b) an X-ray department providing radiographic and fluoroscopic services.

Bulletin of the American College of Surgeons (January 1924)

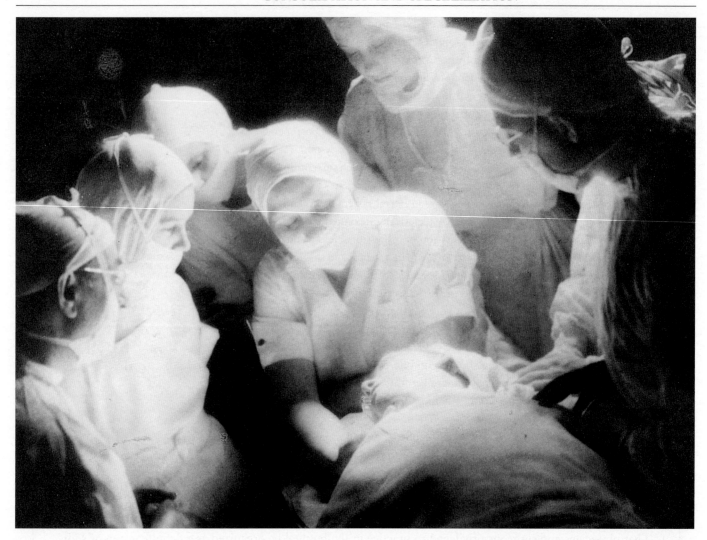

11. Max Thorek was not only renowned as a surgeon but widely respected for his skills as an amateur photographer. Founder of the Photographic Society of America, Thorek also authored the little-known text *Creative Camera Art*. In this gelatin silver print titled "Suspense," Thorek, the photographer, depicts tension in the operating room through artistic utilization of lights and shadows on an already dramatic subject. *(Courtesy of the George Eastman House, Rochester, New York)*

trades with consultants, practitioners or others…to expect the practitioner to obtain his compensation directly from the patient…and to avoid discrediting my associates by taking unwarranted compensation." Though governmental action outlawed the practice of fee-splitting by physicians in many states, the current fellowship pledge of the American College of Surgeons, several revisions later, still requires its candidates to "take no part in any arrangement, such as fee splitting or itinerant surgery, which induces referral or treatment for reason other than the patient's best welfare."

INTERNATIONAL COLLEGE OF SURGEONS

Unfortunately, questionable accusations of fee-splitting, along with unbridled contempt of certain surgeons' business practices, were occasionally used as a method to deny fellowship. As a result, some prominent American surgeons were permanently blackballed and were never permitted the privilege of membership. Among those individuals was Max Thorek (1880–1960), a well-known Chicago surgeon, co-translator of the renowned German surgeon Fedor Krause's (1856–1937) monumental three-volume *Surgery of the Brain and Spinal Cord* (1909–1912), and author of several important and controversial textbooks, *The Human Testis* (1924), *Surgical Errors and Safeguards* (1932), *Plastic Surgery of the Breast and Abdominal Wall* (1942), and *The Face in Health and Disease* (1946). Born in the old Austro-Hungarian empire, Thorek graduated from Rush Medical College but was long perceived by the leaders of Chicago surgery, most of whom were influential in the American College of Surgeons, as an immigrant "outsider." Known for his uncompromising ways (in his autobiography, *A Surgeon's World*, he admits to being "stubborn at times" and "turning a deaf ear to…admonitions"), Thorek was bit of a grandstander and economically entrepreneurial in his attitude toward surgical practice. Three times he applied for fellowship in the American College of Surgeons, and on each occasion he was denied membership by the local credentials committee. Thorek felt that the injustice of exclusion needed to be rectified and ostensibly organized an American chapter of the International College of Surgeons. Members, many of whom had similarly been refused membership in the American College of Surgeons, quickly began to designate themselves fellows of the International College of Surgeons and to use the inititals F.I.C.S., so that the perceived discrimination of the American College with its F.A.C.S. could be partially alleviated.

The true origins of the International College of Surgeons remain cloaked in mystery, although it was known to have been nominally organized in Geneva, Switzerland, in 1935, and headed by Albert Jentzer, chairman of the department of surgery at the University of Geneva. From its inception, the International College was intended to serve as a liaison between existing colleges and surgical societies in the various countries of the world. However, it was long suspected by the likes of Arthur Dean Bevan, Evarts Graham, and Rudolph Matas that Thorek was solely responsible in founding the rival college, and through his Old World political connections manipulated its incorporation papers in Switzerland. As other prominent individuals who had been denied membership in the American College of Surgeons joined the fray (for example, André Crotti of Columbus, Ohio, and Richard Leonardo (1895–1950) of Rochester, New York) unflattering accusations flew across international boundaries, and European surgeons were dragged into the American surgical political scene.

Bitter recriminations between both Colleges continued off and on over the next two to three decades. For instance, in 1946, the American chapter of the International College of Surgeons organized an International Board of Surgery. Diplomas similar in form to those issued by the established American boards in surgery and the surgical specialties were to be awarded. Political passions were aroused by this impudent action, and five years later the Board of Regents of the American College of Surgeons passed a resolution deploring the establishment of certifying boards "other than those approved by the Advisory Board for Medical Specialties." It was further stated that the "application of standards fixed by the boards of the International College of Surgeons...constitute a menace to present standards in the practice of surgery and to their further elevation." Late in 1951, the general counsel for the International College of Surgeons supposedly threatened legal action against the American College of Surgeons for this "violation of antitrust laws." The leadership of the American College was thrown into a tizzy, although little in the way of formal retribution occurred and the matter lay largely unresolved. Charges were traded back and forth, but finally in 1958, Isidor Ravdin, chairman of the Board of Regents of the American College of Surgeons, was informed that the Executive Council of the American Chapter of the International College had voted, back in January 1952, not to proceed with any type of legal action against the American College. Furthermore, the American College was assured by the International College that its International Board of Surgery was also abolished at that time.

During all this bickering, many physicians were puzzled about why the American College of Surgeons would even bother to take up the cause of the various American boards of surgery and surgical specialties when the boards themselves had initially showed little concern with the actions of the International College and its upstart International Board of Surgery. Although maintaining standards of surgical care was given as the primary explanation, an element of self-protection probably played some role.

As time passed and individuals died the American chapter of the International College of Surgeons has faded into relative obscurity. Conversely, by the mid-1960s, the American College of Surgeons was a decidedly more egalitarian organization and, despite the fact that certain remnants of the "blackball" system remained, had grown considerably in size. In the end, the International College of Surgeons' stated goals of elevating the art and science of surgery, creating greater understanding among the surgeons of the world, and affording a means of international postgraduate study never came to full fruition, in part because the American College of Surgeons vehemently opposed the establishment of the International College's American chapter. For the modern surgeon, the internecine surgical "wars" between the American and International Colleges of Surgeons are largely forgotten and remain little more than a curious chapter in the history of American surgery.

As in other eras, many of the issues that shaped the practice of surgery mirrored events that transpired in American life. Beginning at the turn of the century, there was a growing grass-roots movement to politically mandate compulsory health insurance. For the majority of physicians, this was regarded as the initial step towards the socialization of medicine. Consequently, it was not long before the American Medical Association began to lead the visible opposition. By the end of the Hoover administration in 1933, the severe economic depression was making it difficult for many citizens to continue receiving fee-for-service medical and surgical care. At the same time, advances in surgery along with many technical improvements were making the increasingly costly modern hospital the center of a surgeon's practice. The coming of President Roosevelt's New Deal made it seem that federally mandated health insurance was a *fait accompli*.

To help reduce medical costs, group and contract practices began to be established, as well as innovative insurance plans. As with other developments that perturbed the traditional socioeconomics of medical practice, the American Medical Association continued to voice its disagreement with the spread of any compulsory insurance plans, especially the concept of providing health care via prepayment schemes. This latter concept was becoming more common in areas of the country where massive public works projects ensued. It was typified by Sidney Garfield, a young surgeon, and several of his associates who, beginning in 1933, provided medical care on a prepaid basis for approximately 5,000 workers involved in the building of an aqueduct across the California desert to the burgeoning city of Los Angeles. In this particular insurance strategy, workmen's compensation insurance companies paid the Garfield group a pre-established percentage of their premium income to take care of accident cases. In addition, workmen contributed another five cents out of their wages for other medical services. By 1938, Garfield had begun a similar service for men building the Grand Coulee Dam in eastern Washington for industrialist Henry J. Kaiser. In this case, because workers had brought their families with them and established their own community, Garfield decided to expand his prepaid coverage to all dependents. In the early years of World War II, Kaiser asked Garfield to organize medical care for the thousands of individuals and their families who went West to be employed at Kaiser's shipyards and steel mill. Experience with these three special population groups amply demonstrated that the organization of prepaid medical and surgical care could be economically viable. Following the war, Kaiser's physicians were asked to not only continue the program but expand it to the general public. Thus was born the Kaiser-Permanente Medical Care Program.

In 1934, the American College of Surgeons, through the forceful intent of Franklin Martin, who used his prestige on behalf of the concept, endorsed compulsory health insurance. Quite naturally, newspapers seized on the controversy over which organization had the right to speak publicly for the medical profession. The *New York Times* announced, on June 11, 1934, **Surgeons Back Health Insurance Vote to Lead National Movement - Regents Adopt Program for System of Voluntary Prepayments for Hospitalization and Medical Care to Aid Persons of Moderate Means** and on June 12, **Doctors Resent Health Insurance - Resolution Opposing Stand of Surgeons Offered...- American Medical Association Rebukes Surgeons for Advocating Socialized Medicine.** Such headlines served as a noticeable source of confusion to the lay public.

Following Martin's death in 1935, the College quickly rescinded its somewhat lukewarm endorsement. However, the furors attendant on the natural evolution of changes in the social and economic fabric of the United States, as they affected medicine and surgery, continued unabated. Uncomfortable with its confrontation with the College and disturbed by several other socioeconomic developments that raised doubts over its leadership of the medical profession, the American Medical Association went all out to convince the public and any skeptical physicians of the dangers of compulsory health insurance. The crusade proved successful when Congress found itself at an impasse over the passage of any laws on the subject. The defeat of national health insurance meant that payments for medical services in the United States would remain predominantly private, although the specific organizational structure of these evolving free enterprise insurance plans remained unclear. Despite past difficulties, it was also evident by the time of World War II that in waging so successful and expansive a campaign against mandatory health insurance, the Association had wrested titular leadership of American medicine out of the grasp of the College and its many member surgeons.

SURGICAL RESEARCH AND THE
ESTABLISHMENT OF CANCER CLINICS

Between the two world wars, basic surgical research became an established reality in most medical schools in the United States. This ability to conduct research depended entirely on financial support for surgical laboratories and equipment, but most especially for the surgeon-researcher. However, as in earlier surgical eras, the government at first was minimally involved in providing funds. Instead, the majority of monies came from private sources such as university endowments and several

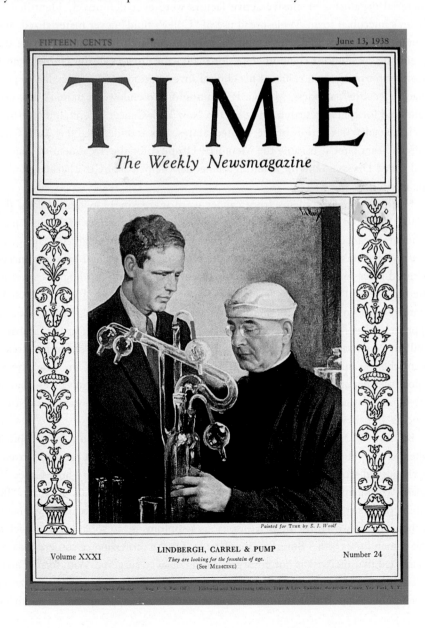

FIFTEEN CENTS • June 13, 1938

TIME
The Weekly Newsmagazine

Painted for TIME by S. J. Woolf

Volume XXXI

LINDBERGH, CARREL & PUMP
They are looking for the fountain of age.
(See MEDICINE)

Number 24

12. Famed aviator Charles Lindbergh pictured on the cover of *Time* (June 1938) with Alexis Carrel. In 1931, the year before his son's sensational kidnapping, Lindbergh began working with Carrel at the Rockefeller Institute on a perfusion pump that would allow the cultivation of whole organs *in vitro*. (*Copyright 1938 Time Inc., reprinted by permission*)

325

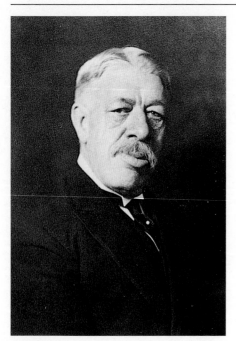

13. William Bradley Coley. *(Courtesy of The New York Academy of Medicine)*

generously financed foundations. Such a combination of private philanthropy and empirical clinical research was especially evident in the study and treatment of cancer, for which surgical intervention seemed most helpful. This was epitomized in the clinical work of William Coley (1862–1936), a New York City surgeon. Coley graduated from Harvard Medical School in 1888 and served a two-year internship at New York Hospital. He was soon appointed to the surgical staff of New York's Hospital for the Ruptured and Crippled, for over forty years was surgeon to the Memorial Hospital, and from 1909 until his death was chairman of the faculty research fund at Cornell University Medical college. Considered an authority on abdominal surgery, Coley was among the first in America to adopt the Bassini method of inguinal herniorrhaphy. He was best known for his research interest in malignant tumors, and his development of Coley's toxin, a chilled preparation consisting of killed cultures of *Streptococcus erysipelatis* (*S. pyogenes*) combined with toxins of *Bacillus prodigiosus*. Coley's interest in a causative link between bacteria and cancer grew out of his observations concerning the supposed regression of an untreatable lymphosarcoma in a surgical patient, who had recently suffered through a severe infection of erysipelas. Coley empirically reasoned that there must be some type of relationship between sarcoma and bacteria, and he launched a lifelong study of the effects of bacterial products on cancer. For years, "Coley's fluid" was given to patients, usually those with inoperable sarcoma or as a prophylactic measure after surgery for bone sarcoma, although not for malignant tumors in general. Cures were claimed, but despite any number of major investigative searches, no causative bacterial organisms or elusive active factors were ever definitively identified in Coley's microbial toxin. Widespread use of "Coley's fluid" never materialized, and therapeutic failures aside, his empirical surgical research is considered to be the beginning of adjuvant chemotherapy for malignant diseases in the United States. More importantly, as a result of his clinical investigations, Coley was able to persuade a wealthy patroness, Mrs. C. P. Huntington, to endow the nation's first private fund for cancer research. In 1884, the New York Cancer Hospital, the earliest such specialty institution in the United States, was founded in New York City. Fifteen years later it became the Memorial Hospital for the Treatment of Cancer and Allied Diseases, and the Huntington bequest helped assure the permanency of the institution.

Health-related problems from cancer were increasingly evident during the 1930s, when the population grew 7 percent and the total number of deaths 2 percent, while cancer-related mortalities increased 35 percent. So marked a change in just one decade's time suggested some measure of environmental or other unrecognized forces as the etiologic agents. But without an understanding of cancer at the biochemical and cellular levels, surgery, with its advocacy of early and complete removal of malignant tumors, remained the most promising therapeutic approach. Illustrious American surgeons, such as Harvey Cushing, Evarts Graham, William Mayo, and Hugh Young (1870–1945) provided the only "definitive" treatment then available for the salvage of patients with cancers of the head, neck, colon, rectum, and uterus. Still, surgical intervention, despite its advances, shared the limitations of all cancer therapies. They might cure or ameliorate the disease process, but they could not prevent its formation.

By May 1913, public concern about cancer deaths had reached a fevered pitch when Samuel Hopkins Adams (1871–1958), a prominent journalist, wrote an extensively quoted article in the *Ladies Home Journal*, "What Can We do About Cancer?" Adams' comments contained many of today's familiar admonitions about cancer, "Be careful of persistent sores or irritations, external or internal. Be watchful of yourself, without undue worry. At the first suspicious symptoms go to some good physician and demand the truth." But, most importantly for the profession of surgery, Adams concluded that the "risk is not in surgery but in delayed surgery." With further articles appearing in *Collier's* and *McClure's* magazines, Adams was able to galvanize so much public support that an organization to combat cancer, composed of volunteer professionals and nonprofessionals, including the surgeons Thomas Cullen (1868–1953) and Joseph Bloodgood (1867–1935), was founded in New York City: the American Society for the Control of Cancer.

It seemed only normal, considering that the then "definitive" treatment of cancer remained firmly in the hands of surgeons, that from the outset there would be close cooperation between the American College of Surgeons and the American Society for the Control of Cancer. The Society grew steadily, and many fellows of the College were also members of Society chapters. Newspaper articles about the recognition and curability of cancer, placards displayed in public places, and special meetings of medical societies devoted to the subject of the prevention and treatment of cancer were the results of joint College and Society efforts. The slogan "fight cancer with knowledge" became a readily recognized symbol of the desire of both organizations to educate the public about the danger signals of cancer. In 1926, the first international symposium on cancer was held under the auspices of the American Society, and its proceedings were published in the College's journal *Surgery, Gynecology and Obstetrics*.

A decision was now made that would have an enormous impact on the future treatment of cancer in the United States. While public education remained the main theme for the Society and the College, the participation of various clinicians in educational programs revealed that such efforts would also have to be directed at the general physician. If the surgeon was going to successfully extirpate a malignant growth, then it was essential for the family practitioner to recognize the disease process at a relatively early stage so that treatment could be instituted without delay. To do otherwise would undermine two decades' worth of public education efforts.

One strong impetus for the College's activities in this education of the professional occurred as early as 1921, when, at the instigation of Ernest Codman, a Registry of Bone Sarcoma was established. The Registry was organized around the nomenclature of bone tumors first suggested in 1921 by Bloodgood, Codman, and James Ewing (1866–1943), a New York pathologist. A uniform classification of bone tumors was officially adopted in 1923 and revised in 1928 and again in 1939. It was soon utilized by surgeons, pathologists, and radiologists throughout America, introducing order into a previously chaotic field. In 1922, a Committee on the Treatment of Malignant Diseases by Surgery, Radium, and X-ray, under the chairmanship of Robert Greenough (1871–1937) from the Massachusetts General Hospital, was also formalized by the Board of Regents of the College. This committee established local committees to investigate the care of cancer patients within hospitals in eleven American cities. After a five-year effort, statistical studies of cancer of the cervix, breast, and mouth nationwide were available. In this way, both general practitioners and specialists could be more aware of the extent of the cancer problem.

The Board of Regents of the College remained in a quandary on how to best continue the programs of public and professional education. Could it be accomplished by assisting in the organization of a moderate number of specialty cancer hospitals, staffed with all manner of physicians and surgeons, or was it more expedient to encourage the establishment of cancer clinics in general hospitals located throughout the country? After thorough discussion, it was decided that the latter concept would bring a larger number of family doctors into cancer educational projects and lend itself to more streamlined diagnostic and treatment possibilities. During the same time, the American Society had begun to decentralize its efforts as a response to the mounting problem of coordinating the work of various local organizations and health care delivery institutions. In 1929, a committee appointed by the Society and chaired by the celebrated James Ewing, the country's first full-time practitioner of medical oncology, called for a more widespread organization of cancer clinics in acute-care hospitals. Since the College was already deeply involved in the evaluation of America's hospitals, it only seemed natural that it should further develop the cancer clinic concept. The following year, the College formulated a minimum standard for cancer clinics in general hospitals, and shortly thereafter, it began to survey exist-

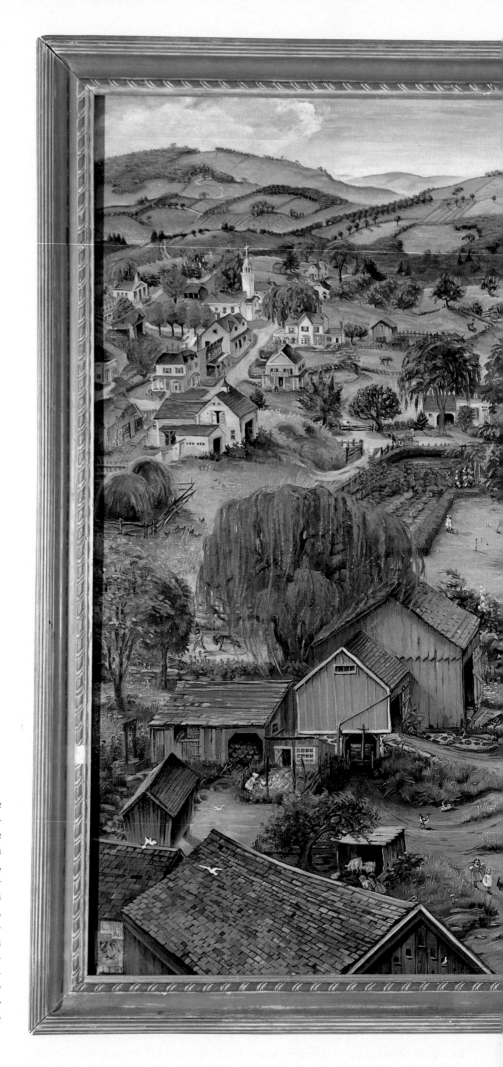

14. Through the end of World War II, the general practitioner, represented by the country doctor, remained representative of the American health care system. Specialization might have been making its presence known, but in pictorial arts the kindly general practitioner-surgeon remained dominant. Lauren Ford's panoramic scene of small town life, "Country Doctor" (circa 1930–1940), embodies the importance of the rural practitioner to a tranquil and content United States. The physician-surgeon is at the heart of the scene, having arrived in his horse-drawn carriage, ready to dispense whatever type of medical and/or surgical expertise is necessary. *(Canajoharie Library and Art Gallery, Canajoharie, New York)*

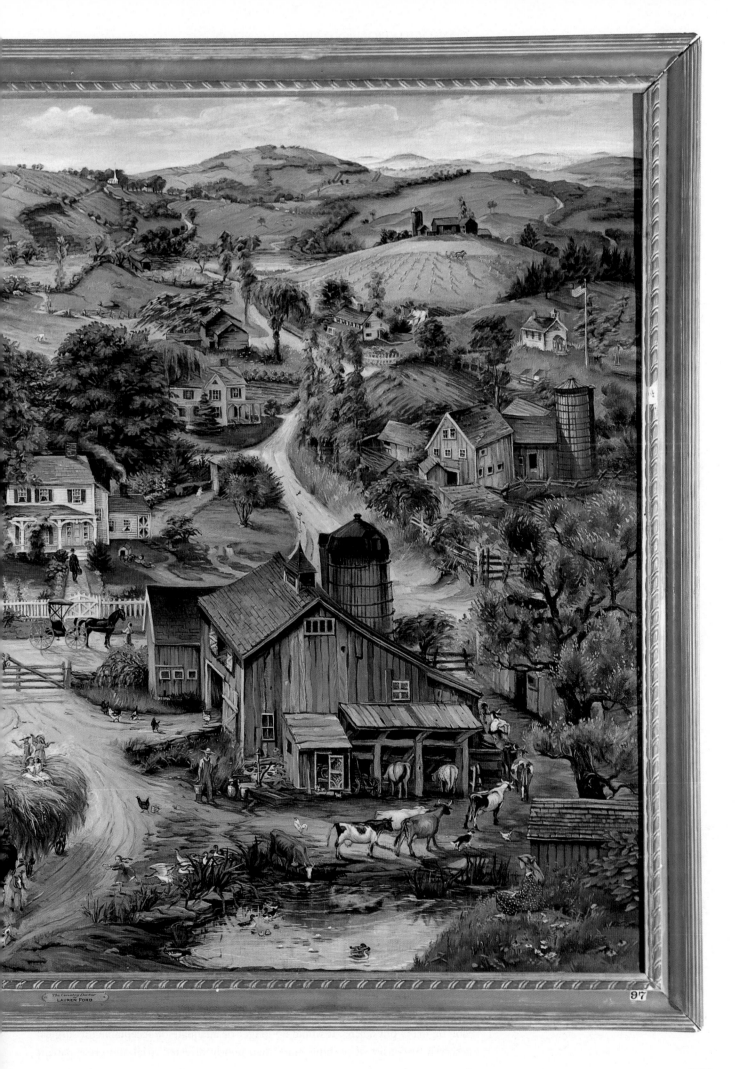

The Country Doctor
by LAUREN FORD

97

329

ing facilities. In 1932, the first list of one hundred approved cancer clinics was published. Eight years later, there were 345 approved clinics, constituting 23 percent of the general hospitals having one hundred or more beds. This effort, alone among the many projects undertaken by the health care industry in pre–World War II America, had the greatest effect on bringing uniformity to the treatment of cancer and established the organizational model for cancer care for decades to come.

By 1937, it was estimated that some $700,000 was the total amount available annually in the United States for cancer research. In that year, Yale Medical School received a $3.5 million grant from the Jane Coffin Childs Fund, which immediately became the largest private endowment for cancer research in the nation. Through such continued funding efforts, numerous surgeons were beginning to make a name for themselves solely in the field of cancer surgery and clinical research. In 1944, the M. D. Anderson Hospital for Cancer Research in Houston, Texas, was founded, and a surgeon, Randolph Clark, became director. Other surgeons, typified by Alexander Brunschwig (1901–1969) and Alan Oldfather Whipple (1881–1963) of New York City, achieved notable prominence for their technical skills in performing complex oncologic surgery.

During World War II, directors of the American Society for the Control of Cancer decided to expand the organization on a greater national basis. Part of this broadening of its base was predicated on the fact that fundamental research into the causes and prevention of cancer was becoming of prime concern. It would no longer be adequate for cancer research to be conducted solely in the clinical setting. The basic science of cancer needed investigation if scientists were to have a detailed understanding of the disease process at the cellular and molecular levels. The Society decided that from then on, approximately one-third of the funds derived from its annual fund raising campaigns would be allocated to basic research. In 1944, only $780,000 had been raised. The following year, Albert and Mary Lasker, prominent and wealthy citizens, joined the efforts, and through their social and political connections were able to raise $4 million for the Society. In 1946, the Lasker-led philanthropy group brought in almost $10 million. With a new board of directors and with its financial security intact, the name of the organization was formally changed to the American Cancer Society. Although surgeons were direct beneficiaries of this massive infusion of research funds, the postwar period represented the beginnings of a fundamental shift away from the concept that the "definitive" treatment of cancer could be found only in surgery. For the first time, surgeons were not to be the sole arbiters of cancer care in the United States. They would now serve as part of a multidisciplinary approach to this most perplexing of modern health care dilemmas.

Although it might seem that this era's surgical evolution was closely focused on socioeconomic and political issues, a wide variety of clinical and research activities also occurred. Most prominent was the ascendancy of the laboratory-based, research-oriented surgeon, who had knowledge not only of the scalpel but also of experimental science. Since time immemorial, surgeons had been categorized by their technical expertise. This was easily understandable, since the more adept the surgeon was with the knife, the less pain a patient was forced to endure while undergoing a surgical operation. The technically renowned surgeon of the past was always considered the innovator and naturally bore the designation of "surgical researcher." However, it was evident that such larger-than-life personalities as John Deaver, John Murphy, and even William Mayo were more skillful surgical technicians than able surgeon-scientists. Accordingly, if surgery were going to be considered a mainstay of the scientific community, then a cadre of research surgeons would have to be developed. In this way, the phrase "surgical research" would not be denigrated as a modern oxymoron.

By the 1920s, a growing reliance on the research facility to furnish answers to the most fundamental surgical problems was creating an indelibly positive impression on many physicians. It would no longer be adequate or acceptable for surgical research to consist of nothing more than poorly directed, trial-and-error patient studies. The new surgeon-scientist looked to the experimental laboratory for answers to complex problems involving the basic functioning of the human organism. After all, to make a meaningful contribution to the art and science of surgery, was it absolutely essential that an individual be first and foremost a superb clinical surgeon or was it equally important that research surgeons, with perhaps only a passing interest in the clinical practice of surgery (e.g., Alexis Carrel and Charles Huggins), be encouraged in their laboratory activities and considered just as integral to the growth of the profession?

Several earlier events helped implement this conjunction of clinical and research methods. In 1901, a group of enterprising physicians in Buffalo, led by surgeon Roswell Park (1852–1914), successfully petitioned the New York State legislature for an appropriation for the study of cancer, which helped establish the New York State Institute for the Study of Malignant Diseases. The Institute, a direct descendent of Park's Gratwick Laboratory, represented the first important American governmental contribution to cancer research and brought sophisticated clinical and laboratory surgical research under the same roof. Two years later, Harvey Cushing organized the country's first university-sponsored experimental surgical laboratory at The Johns Hopkins Hospital. Stimulated by his mentor, William Halsted, Cushing recognized the importance of teaching experimental surgical techniques to third-year medical students. Thus, the laboratory was initially used for a course in practical animal surgery for junior-year students in which they performed on animals many of the more important procedures used in surgical operations. As a result, numerous

15. The Hunterian Laboratory at The Johns Hopkins Hospital contained its own paddock for animals outside the rear of the building, a well-lighted room for student operating teams and extensive research facilities for faculty of the departments of medicine, pathology, and surgery. Built at the behest of Harvey Cushing in 1905, the two-story brick structure utilized the innovative concept of skylights to provide greater illumination when animal experiments were being conducted. (*The Alan Mason Chesney Medical Archives of The Johns Hopkins Medical Institutions*)

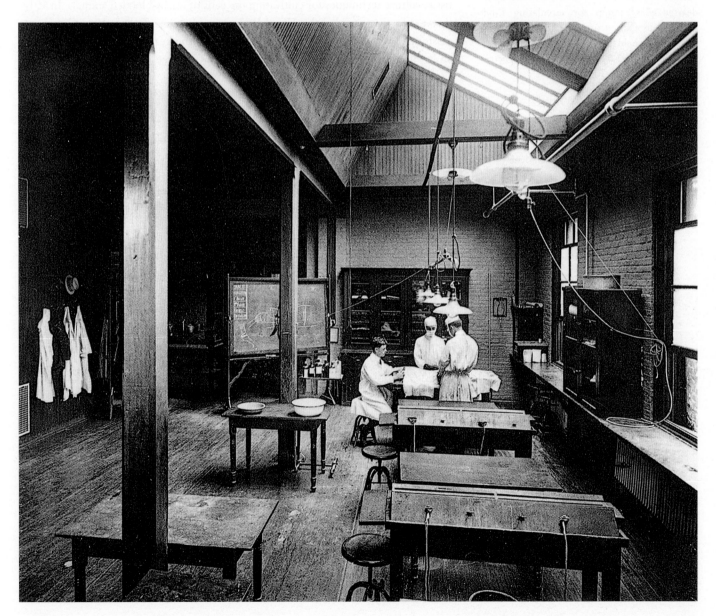

students were led into various phases of physiological and surgical research. Both faculty and students were enthralled with the new classes. In the summer of 1905, a separate building was erected on the hospital's campus; half of its space was alloted to pathological research and the other half to surgery. The structure became known as the Hunterian Laboratory for Experimental Medicine, in honor of the great English surgeon John Hunter (1728–1793). Its nickname, "old Hunterian," mystified many Baltimoreans who believed it referred to pointers, retrievers, and setters.

The experimental surgical laboratory at Hopkins had several distinctive features. First, the excellence and meticulousness of performance demanded in the operating rooms of The Johns Hopkins Hospital were required of all workers in the laboratory. Second, virtually all of the problems studied were basic problems; clinical patient investigations were not part of the laboratory's goals. Finally, a spirit of creative scholarship pervaded the atmosphere of the "old Hunterian," which proved an immeasurable influence on students, faculty, and, most importantly, visitors from America and abroad. It was these foreign guests, who, when they visited the United States always included Baltimore on their itinerary, established growing links between surgical research communities on both sides of the Atlantic. By observing what was accomplished at Halsted's and Cushing's laboratory, European surgeons provided the facility with the international imprimatur that was necessary for American surgery to become a leader in world surgery.

Other examples of basic surgical research could be found scattered throughout the country. At the Rockefeller Institute in New York City, Alexis Carrel developed tissue culture techniques for cultivating the cells of warm-blooded animals. In 1912, the year he was awarded the Nobel Prize in medicine and physiology, Carrel successfully transplanted connective tissue cells from the heart of an embryo chick into an in vitro culture, which was maintained for over three more decades. This spec-

16. Alexis Carrel, working in conjunction with Charles Lindbergh, developed a method to culture organs. They exhibited their newly devised glass pump for circulating fluid through an excised organ at the 1939–1940 World's Fair held in New York City. *(Historical Collections, College of Physicians of Philadelphia)*

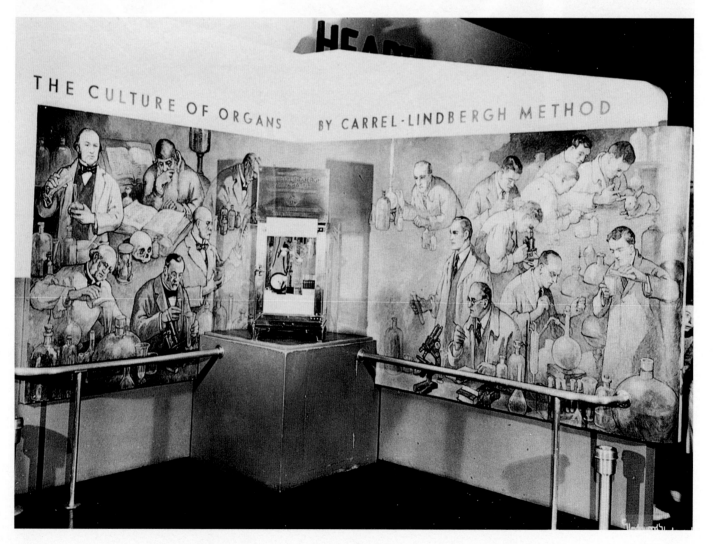

tacular laboratory feat attracted much public attention to the seemingly incredulous fact that cells, and maybe even organs, could be grown in "bottles" far removed from a living body. A measure of immortality was achieved through the hands of a surgeon. The press, for whom the "chicken heart culture" seemed to have a romantic and perhaps even morbid appeal, followed Carrel's reports with unabashed interest. The surgeon-scientist had finally begun to receive a measure of the respect that had previously been afforded only the clinical surgeon. During the 1930s, Carrel in collaboration with Charles Lindbergh (1902–1974), of transatlantic fame, developed a sterilizable glass pump for circulating a culture fluid through an excised organ, by means of which the organ could be kept alive for a short time. This joint effort so intrigued the public that a picture of Carrel and Lindbergh graced the cover of *Time Magazine* in 1938.

Such spectacular surgical research feats were not necessarily isolated to well-endowed institutions. George Crile (1864–1943) is important to American surgical history as a mover of clinicians to the laboratory for the purpose of studying the systemic effects of the diseases they were called upon to treat. He was an extremely bright, enthusiastic, and industrious individual, who finished medical school in 1887 at Wooster College (later Western Reserve Medical School) in Cleveland. Demonstrating an interest in surgical research from the earliest days of his professional life, Crile obtained desultory instruction in investigative laboratory techniques from mentors scattered throughout Europe and the United States. Having first joined the histology faculty (1889–1890) and then the physiology faculty (1890–1893) at his poorly equipped and financially strapped alma mater, Crile persevered through monetary difficulties in setting up his own experimental laboratory in order to study the treatment of traumatic shock. Through laboratory experimentation with various classes of drugs, Crile noted that stimulation of the vasomotor center as a method of treating shock was not only ineffective but potentially dangerous. He concluded that adrenalin raised blood pressure by causing intense and occasionally harmful peripheral arteriolar vasoconstriction. Conversely, the administration of saline would sustain pressure but without many of the negative side effects. The actions of saline were only fleeting, and Crile experimented with other replacement fluids, finally settling on whole blood. In an audacious act, he began to administer whole blood to surgical patients in shock. This intrepid step was completed without benefit of donor-recipient cross-matching and soon led to further studies and the first large-scale use of blood to treat shock during World War I. Crile's contributions to the safer handling of surgical patients extended far beyond his investigations into shock. He popularized the monitoring of blood pressure in surgical procedures and was responsible for many advances in surgical technique, especially in thyroid surgery. Crile called attention to the effect of emotions on the thyroid and adrenal glands and the importance of the patient's mental state in preparation for surgery. He advanced the concept of "anoci-association" in which local and general anesthesia are combined in sequence to eliminate preoperative fear and tension. Crile's reliance on the laboratory to provide answers to many of these problems made an indelibly positive impression on his surgical peers, nearly all of whom had relied on empirical treatment, especially clinical signs and symptoms. Increasing numbers of younger surgeons were now looking to the surgical research laboratory for answers to complex clinical problems, particularly as the scope of operative intervention widened. Crile was a bold proselytizer of physiological principles and their relationship to the practice of surgery. He thoroughly enjoyed the public spotlight as much as the research laboratory or the surgical amphitheater, and his unique combination of talents was crucially important to the promotion of scientific surgery in America. Crile would go on to become a founder of the Cleveland Clinic, and he served as president of both the American College of Surgeons (1917) and the American Surgical Association (1924). A measure of his amazing creativity can be noted in his prolific literary output, including such prominent textbooks as *An Experimental Research into Surgical Shock* (1899), *Experimental Research into the Surgery of the Respiratory System* (1899), *An Experimental and Clinical Research into Certain Problems Relating to Surgical Operations* (1901), *Blood-Pressure in Surgery* (1903), *Hemorrhage and Transfusion* (1909), *Anemia and Resuscitation* (1914), *Anoci-Association* (1914), *The Origin and Nature of the Emotions* (1915), *Surgical Shock and the Shockless Operation* (1920), *Notes on Military Surgery* (1924), *The Bipolar Theory of Living Processes* (1926), *Diseases Peculiar to Civilized Man* (1934), *The Phemonena of Life, a Radio-Electric Interpretation* (1936), and *Intelligence, Power and Personality* (1941).

A small nucleus of research-oriented surgeons had been formed, many of whom would assume increasingly important positions within organized medicine and surgery. Alfred Blalock (1899–1964), a second-generation successor to William Halsted as professor of surgery at The Johns Hopkins Hospital, worked in the "old Hunterian" in 1920 while a medical student. Blalock would go on to achieve his greatest fame as co-developer, with Helen Taussig (1898–1896), of the "blue-baby" operation for the relief of congenital defects of the pulmonary artery. What is frequently overlooked in the career of Blalock is that among his most valuable contributions was his fundamental laboratory research, confirming Crile's observations, that surgical shock is not due to the elaboration of toxins or to reflex neurologic mechanisms but to decreases in the circulating blood volume. Following his surgical training, Blalock took a faculty position at Vanderbilt University in Nashville, Tennessee. He devoted himself to laboratory work, moving from the general study of cardiorespiratory function to the problem of shock and eventually into the etiology of hypertension. In a sign of the times, Vivien Thomas (1910–1985), an African American forced for lack of funds to leave his first year of college, was hired by Blalock in 1930 as a laboratory assistant. In short order, Thomas learned to operate on animals and to perform chemical analyses crucial for further experimental studies, and he was instrumental in maintaining the surgical protocols necessary to keep the laboratory functioning efficiently. When Blalock assumed the surgical professorship at his alma mater in 1941, Thomas moved with him and eventually became director of personnel at the Hunterian Laboratory. Thomas's manual skill at involved operative techniques was legendary, and it was he who developed, in animal models, the techniques needed to perform the celebrated subclavian pulmonary artery anastomosis. Years later, Blalock reflected to an associate that he should have encouraged Thomas to complete his college education. As an ingenious and technically gifted individual, Thomas helped train a generation of Hopkins-educated surgeons, accomplishing this task within the confines of the surgical research laboratory. Although Thomas was rightfully bitter about the racial prejudice he experienced throughout his entire career, his stature in the field of experimental surgery was officially recognized when he was awarded an Honorary Doctor of Laws degree from The Johns Hopkins University in 1976 and simultaneously received a formal appointment to the faculty of The Johns Hopkins School of Medicine as instructor in surgery.

Other surgical scientists were also at work in the research laboratory. Dallas Phemister (1882–1951) served as Arthur Dean Bevan's first assistant early in his career, and later became professor of surgery at the University of Chicago. He established a department characterized by its production of academic surgeons, distinguished for their contributions to basic experimental research and clinical applications. Phemister worked on the problem of shock contemporaneously with Blalock and arrived at many of the same conclusions concerning the role of hypovolemia. His research interests extended to orthopedic surgery: he employed epiphysiodesis in an animal model to inhibit bone growth in the treatment of bony deformities. In clinical surgery, he demonstrated that for some sarcomas, a length of bone and muscle could be resected, and the function of the limb restored by grafting.

Charles Huggins (1901–1997) was the first native-born American surgeon to win the Nobel Prize in Physiology and Medicine. He obtained his medical degree from Harvard University in 1924 and received his surgical training under Frederick Coller (1887–1964) at the University of Michigan. In 1927, Huggins joined the

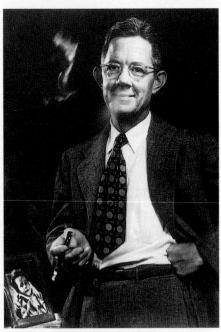

17. Alfred Blalock as photographed by Yousuf Kharsh. The Kharsh studies emerged from two days of photographing Blalock around The Johns Hopkins Hospital at the time the official "1,000th blue baby" photograph was taken in 1950. What makes this particular image unique is the child pictured in the lower left. The youngster's likeness was sent to Blalock by her parents, as he had completed his operation for tetralogy of Fallot upon her in 1947, at the time of his triumphal reception in London and Paris. *(The Alan Mason Chesney Medical Archives of The Johns Hopkins Medical Institutions)*

surgical faculty of Phemister's department, where he was encouraged to pursue laboratory-based investigative work in the field of urology. Huggins traveled abroad to further his knowledge of organic chemistry and its relation to cell multiplication at the Lister Institute in London, under the direction of Robert Robinson (1883–1941). Robinson himself would be awarded the Nobel Prize in Chemistry in 1947. Upon his return to the United States, Huggins was appointed by Phemister to be chief of urology at the University of Chicago's newly built Billings Hospital. Despite appearances, patient care in the newly created urology ward was scant, and Huggins had more than ample time to pursue his interests in the experimental surgical laboratory. He and his co-workers devised a simple surgical technique for collecting prostatic secretions from dogs. In the early 1940s, he demonstrated androgenic regulation of prostatic function and its inhibition by estrogens. This observation ultimately resulted in the ability to clinically retard the growth of prostatic carcinoma through hormonal manipulation. Huggins further observed that following orchiectomy for advanced prostatic carcinoma, the prostate shrinks in size and its secretion ceases. Suspecting a correlation between adrenocortical function and the progression of advanced prostatic carcinoma, Huggins performed the first bilateral adrenalectomy for advanced prostatic carcinoma in 1944. His observations were soon applied to additional organs and led to widespread use of endocrine-ablative or "physiological-surgery" procedures (the removal of a normal structure in order to heal a disease in some other region of the body), particularly for cancers of the breast and prostate. Huggins's accomplishments in the surgical research laboratory and application of his findings to the clinical setting were reason enough for him to receive the Nobel Prize in 1966.

Much as the ascendancy of the surgeon-scientist brought about changes in the way in which the public and the profession viewed surgical research, the introduction of increasingly sophisticated technologies had an enormous impact on the practice of surgery. Throughout the history of American surgery, the practice of surgery—the art, the craft, and finally the science of working with one's hands—had been largely defined by its tools. From the crude flint instruments of Native Americans, through the simple tonsillotomes and lithotrites of the early nineteenth century, up to the increasingly complex surgical instruments developed at the turn of the twentieth century, new and improved instruments usually led to a better surgical result. Progress in surgical instrumentation and surgical technique went hand in hand. Beginning in the 1920s, however, advances in scientific technologies introduced new possibilities into surgical practice that were not necessarily related to

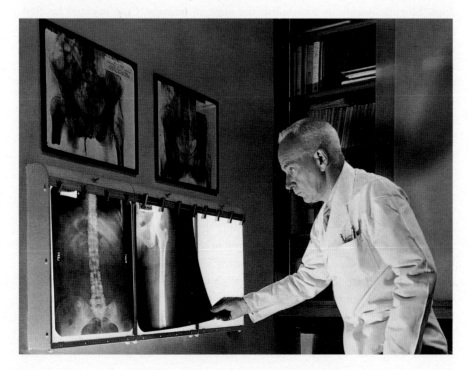

18. Charles Huggins (circa 1959), the William B. Ogden Distinguished Service Professor and Director of the Ben May Laboratory for Cancer Research at the University of Chicago. (*University of Chicago Medical Center*)

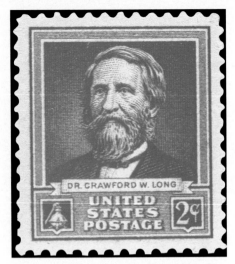

19. Seven surgeons have been honored by having their likenesses placed on United States postage stamps. The first such issue was a depiction of Crawford Long as part of the "Famous American" series (1940). (*Author's Collection*)

improvements in technique. The domain of surgery was so well established that the foundation of basic operative procedures to be performed was already completed. Surgical techniques would, of course, become more sophisticated with the passage of time, but by the conclusion of this surgical era, all organs and areas of the body had been fully explored. In consequence, there were few technical surgical mysteries left. What the profession needed to sustain its continued growth was the ability to diagnose surgical diseases at earlier stages, to locate malignant growths while they remained small, and to have more effective postoperative treatment so that patients could survive ever more technically complex operations.

An apt example of the blending of new technologies to aid the growth of surgery was the introduction in 1924 of cholecystography by Evarts Graham (1883–1957) and Warren Cole (1898–1990). From 1919 to 1951, Graham served as Bixby professor of surgery at Washington University in St. Louis and during that time dominated much of organized American surgery. A graduate of Rush Medical College (1907), he was widely recognized for his work with the U.S. Army's Empyema Commission during World War I. Experiences during the hostilities showed that a significant improvement in mortality rates from thoracic injuries and diseases could be achieved by delaying operation until the acute phase of a pulmonary infection had subsided. Like other experimental surgeons of the period, Graham had spent a considerable amount of time in the intensive study of a nonsurgical science. In his case, he spent three years as a university fellow in chemistry at the University of Chicago. Warren Cole was a surgical resident in Graham's program when he was approached by his chief to undertake an assignment in the experimental laboratory. It had recently been shown that when sodium iodide was injected into a vein and x-rays were taken of the region of the kidney, the chemical was concentrated and then excreted by the kidneys in such a way that an x-ray image of the kidneys, ureters, and urinary bladder could be obtained. Graham's knowledge of chemistry led him to believe that a similar substance could be found to enable visualization of the gallbladder by x-rays. Graham wanted Cole to chemically devise such a substance so that physicians could diagnose human gallbladder disease earlier and more accurately. Graham suggested that if a heavier halogen such as iodine could be chemically attached to a phenolphthalein radical, the bile that is concentrated and stored in the gallbladder, and which would also incorporate the phenolphthalein, might then become impervious to x-rays. Obtaining suitable halogenated compounds from the Mallinckrodt Chemical Works in St. Louis, and after five months of disappointing results, Cole finally obtained a faint gallbladder shadow on the x-ray of one of the dogs. Moving quickly to accomplish the same in humans, Cole injected his first patient with the chemical mixture on Feburary 21, 1924. Despite numerous initial problems of drug toxicity, the surgeons soon learned how to minimize these adverse reactions. Graham and Moore went on to understand that if the patient's gallbladder was healthy, a shadow would begin to appear on x-ray films about four hours after intravenous administration and reach maximum density in another eight hours. If the drug was taken orally, the shadow appeared in ten hours and reached maximum density in twenty hours. They also surmised that if a shadow did not appear on the x-ray, then the gallbladder was diseased because it was unable to store the dye. The Graham-Cole test was originally described in the *Journal of the American Medical Association*, whose large and influential readership brought the two surgeons much national attention. Like many great medical discoveries, cholecystography quickly spread throughout the country and abroad. For seventeen years, Cole's tetraiodophenolphthalein remained the drug of choice for physicians to visualize the human gallbladder on x-ray films. By the early 1940s, a less toxic contrast agent was found, and more modern methods of oral cholecystography evolved. Even today, when ultrasound and other noninvasive imaging methods are available, oral cholecystography remains quite popular. To the profession of surgery, the discovery of cholecystography proved most important not only because it brought about more accurate diagnoses of cholecystitis but because it created an influx of surgical patients where few had previously existed. If the profession were to grow, then large numbers of individuals with surgical diseases were needed. The influence of Graham and Cole's discovery was so great that within a few years time, cholecystectomy, the surgical removal of a diseased gallbladder, had become, and remains today, the most commonly performed abdominal operation, with over 650,000 completed annually in the United States.

As in other surgical eras, clinical advances were also being made in the operating room. Among the highlights were the introduction in 1935 of pancreaticoduodenectomy for cancer of the pancreas by Allen Whipple, a report in 1943 on vagotomy for operative therapy for peptic ulcer by Lester Dragstedt (1893–1976), and the publication of numerous papers in the 1930s about the importance of identifying the recurrent laryngeal nerve during the course of thyroid surgery by Frank Lahey (1880–1953). Owen Wangensteen (1898–1981) successfully decompressed mechanical bowel obstructions using a newly devised suction apparatus in 1932; George Vaughan (1859–1948) completed a successful ligation of the abdominal aorta for aneurysmal disease in 1921; Max Peet (1885–1949) presented his splanchnic resection for hypertension in 1935; Walter Dandy (1886–1946) performed intracranial sections of various cranial nerves, including the trigeminal and glossopharyngeal nerves in the 1920s; Walter Freeman (1895–1972) described prefrontal lobotomy as a means of treatment for various mental illnesses in 1936; Harvey Cushing, assisted by W. T. Bovie, a physicist, introduced electrocoagulation in neurosurgery in 1928; Marius Smith-Petersen (1886–1953) described a flanged nail used for pinning a fracture of the neck of the femur in 1931 and introduced vitallium cup arthroplasty in 1939; Samuel Kopetzky (1876–1950) improved the technique for the fenestration operation to restore hearing loss in otosclerosis in 1941; Vilray Blair (1871–1955) and James Brown (1899–1971) popularized the use of split-skin grafts to cover large areas of granulating wounds; Earl Padgett (1893–1946) devised an operative dermatome, which allowed calibration of the thickness of skin grafts, in 1939; Elliott Cutler performed a successful section of the mitral valve for relief of mitral stenosis in heart disease in 1923; Evarts Graham completed the first successful removal of an entire lung for cancer in 1933; Claude Beck (1894–1971) implanted pectoral muscle into the pericardium and attached a pedicled omental graft to the surface of the heart, thus providing collateral circulation to that organ, in 1935; Robert Gross (1905–1988) reported the first successful ligation of a patent arterial duct in 1939 and a resection for coarctation of the aorta with direct anastomosis of the remaining ends in 1945; and John Alexander (1891–1954) resected a saccular aneurysm of the thoracic aorta in 1944.

From 1919 to 1945, the evolutionary process of American surgery gathered tremendous momentum. A consolidation of professional power, inherent in the movement toward specialization, predominated most events of this era. Ironically, the United States, which had been much slower than European countries to recognize surgeons as a distinct group of clinicians separate from physicians, would now spearhead the move toward surgical specialization with great alacrity. Clearly, the course of surgical fragmentation into specialties and subspecialties was gathering tremendous speed as the dark clouds of World War II settled over the globe. The era coming to an end helped propel American surgery onto the world stage and, in so doing, brought about a fundamental change in the way surgeons viewed themselves and their interactions with the society in which they lived and worked.

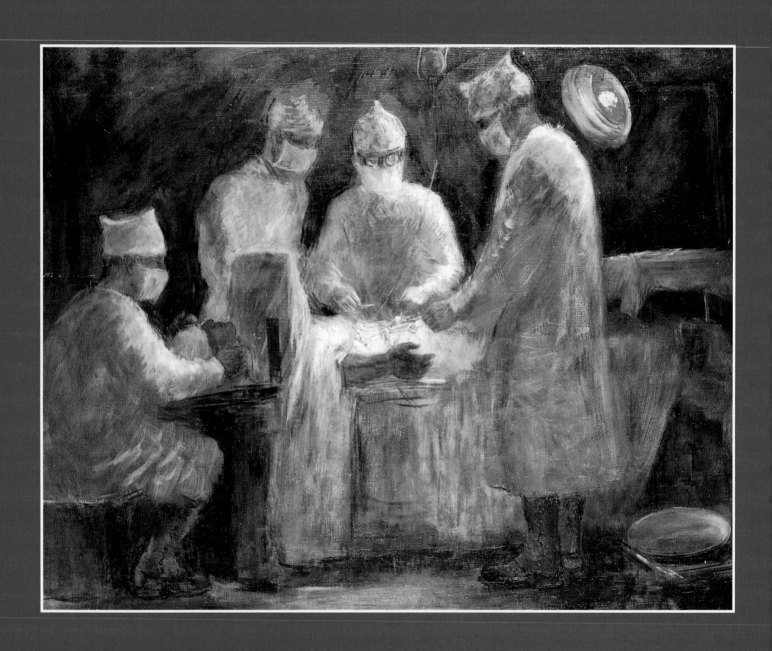

CHAPTER 10

WORLD WAR TWO SURGERY
1941–1945

The impact of World War II on the American profession of surgery was profound and long-lasting. For the first time in the history of the country, deaths from military action (291,577) exceeded those from diseases and causes not primarily related to hostilities (113,842). Despite some 670,000 soldiers being wounded, the mortality rate from wounds (4.5 percent) was almost half that of what it had been in World War I. Accordingly, from a surgical viewpoint, World War II was the most successful military campaign in which American armed forces had ever been engaged. Various factors contributed to this accomplishment, including better organization of the U.S. Army Medical Department and its personnel; recognition that early surgery was paramount in the resuscitation effort; improvements in the management of surgical shock, including the mass availability of blood and plasma; the use of sulfa drugs and penicillin for the treatment and prevention of wound infections, especially cellulitic sequelae; a directive making it mandatory to leave all amputation wounds open, followed by delayed closure; more rapid evacuation of the wounded by hand-held litter, motorized ambulances, and airplanes; the establishment of specialized treatment centers for seriously wounded casualties; and the effective use of mobile surgical teams on all fronts plus well-staffed hospital ships in the island-hopping campaigns of the Pacific combat theater.

From the surgeon's perspective, what set the two world wars apart was an ability by the 1940s to pursue more aggressive surgical management of battle-incurred abdominal and thoracic injuries. This change in attitude, from what had previously been a form of military surgical "abstention" when surgical expertise was still evolving, resulted not only from the medical and surgical experience gained in World War I but, more importantly, from the intervening accomplishments in civilian surgery. There was little denying the fact that American surgery had evolved to the point where operating on the abdomen, chest, or head was a readily accepted part of American culture and medical therapeutics. Surgeons had clearly attained a scientific and technical maturity that brought about new confidence in their ability to treat traumatic and other pathological processes that in the past would have caused the demise of a patient. Accordingly, in World War II an easily promulgated official policy was to operate, as promptly as possible, on all wounded personnel in whom the mere act of surgical intervention would not prove fatal. The maturing of surgery as an accepted therapeutic modality is evidenced by the fact that only a small number of injured (less than 1 percent) constituted this latter category of non-operable and mortally wounded. This was vastly different from what had transpired during previous conflicts, when young Americans were left to die without benefit of medical or surgical assistance.

1. *(facing page)* "Front Line Surgery" (circa 1943) by John Steuart Curry (1897–1946). Curry became most famous for his dramatic scenes of Midwestern rural life, having belonged to the movement among artists of the 1930s known as Regionalism. *(Courtesy of the U.S. Army Center of Military History)*

The policy of prompt surgical intervention was made possible by tremendous strides in surgical research on preoperative resuscitation and its clinical application. In World War I, it was not uncommon for a soldier to expire because he could not be revived to a level where a surgical operation might be safely performed. In World War II, a small number of patients died while resuscitation was in progress, but at least the attempt had been made to bring them to a status in which surgical intervention could be physiologically tolerated. The military surgeon had at his disposal new techniques for whole blood and/or plasma transfusion, including the innovative concept of blood banking, which became a central feature of preoperative resuscitation. When transfusion was combined with competently administered anesthesia, surgical operations of great magnitude could be completed on injured individuals whose initial conditions were such that in a prior era they would have been left to die. In addition, the performance of "negative exploratory laparotomies" was widely accepted. This meant that the prompt surgical exploration in every case when there was any suspicion of foreign body penetration of the abdominal or thoracic cavities was regarded as entirely justified. In view of the almost zero percent mortality associated with such an exploration, contrasted with the morbidity and mortality risks involved in the nonsurgical management of penetrating abdominal and thoracic wounds, the concept of negative exploration became part of standard military trauma care. Although they may have been regarded as unnecessary emergencies, the ability to safely complete negative explorations illustrates the changing surgical philosophy that directed the management of most injuries in World War II.

The long-term status of any wounded soldier was most notably influenced by the methods employed and the elapsed time needed to transport him from the site where injury occurred to a field facility for treatment. Initial care occurred on the battlefield, where medical corpsmen rendered first aid: control of hemorrhage, dressing of wounds, initiation of sulfonamide therapy, control of pain with morphine, splinting of fractures, and evacuating the wounded to the battalion aid post. That the army medical corpsmen, or medics, had a difficult and dangerous responsibility is attested to by the fact that more than 2,000 of them were killed in the European theater of action.

Definitive resuscitation began at the battalion aid post, where a junior medical officer was usually in attendance. Ordinarily located some five hundred yards behind the line of combat, it was reached either by foot or by hand-held litter. There, the main objective was to ensure that the wounded soldier remained transportable and to refrain from any medical or surgical action that would make him unfit for further evacuation. Therapies were accordingly limited to such simple but stabilizing measures as further control of gross hemorrhage, including placement of tourniquets and administration of plasma as needed; application of more elaborate splints and bandages; closure of sucking chest wounds; and giving of tetanus toxoid and further doses of morphine. At this location, also, a field medical record was initiated to accompany each casualty.

From the battalion aid post, evacuation to a collecting post, positioned about a mile farther to the rear, was completed by foot, hand litter, jeeps with improvised litter racks, or even an occasional ambulance. As in the battalion aid post, treatment was limited to what was absolutely essential and consisted at times of nothing more than simple inspection. Dressings could be reinforced if necessary but were never taken down, since each change added further contamination. Hot drinks were available, and the field medical record was further filled out.

From a multitude of collecting stations, the injured were brought approximately five miles by ambulance to the rearmost point in the combat zone of the division, the clearing station, which housed a hundred to a hundred and fifty patients at a time. There the formal triage of patients began. The soldier's health status was carefully reappraised. Lightly injured soldiers and those who were not seriously ill could be held for as long as necessary and returned to duty without leaving the organizational limits of their division. Adjacent tented units were available for special functions, including the care of venereal disease, neuropsychiatric problems, and trench foot. Battle casualties were divided into two groups: those who were seriously injured and in need of immediate surgical care and those who could withstand an additional journey of tens of miles to an evacuation hospital. This sorting was of such importance that only experienced medical officers were given the responsibility. Whole blood was available at the clearing station, as was penicillin. In the early years of the war, sulfonamide therapy started on the battlefield was continued to the level of the evacuation hospital, and many wounded soldiers received simultaneous treatment with both sulfonamide and penicillin. By the middle of the war, as supplies of penicillin increased, the continued use of sulfonamides gradually diminished until it became practically reserved, other than the initial doses on the battlefield, for areas where penicillin was in short supply.

Prompt and definitive surgical care was available at all field hospitals. These facilities were established in juxtaposition to the clearing station, so that wounded soldiers whose injury precluded any further evacuation could be expediently carried from one to the other by hand litter. The field hospital was a tented surgical complex capable of handling three platoons, with a capacity of one hundred beds for each platoon. It was equipped to support all manner of emergency surgery and had the theoretical capability of being able to maintain patients for up to twelve postoperative days, although such lengthy respites rarely took place. Soldiers needing care at the field hospital level usually had sustained life-threatening injuries to the abdomen, chest, and head and neck; had such obstructed respiration that they required immediate tracheotomy, or were in so poor a condition that further evacuation jeopardized any chance of survival. Not unexpectedly, surgical conditions in a field hospital were far from ideal. The medical staff was small, surgeons were not the most experienced, and overall resuscitation capabilities were less than those found in an evacuation hospital. The field hospital was always far forward, usually near or sometimes just in front of heavy artillery positions. Incessant bombarding made it difficult for the recently operated-on soldier to obtain necessary rest, and during periods of intense military action, adequate postoperative care might not be available. It is not surprising that many of these independently functioning field hospitals existed in a state of chronic confusion of structure and function. The 1943

2. An outdoor operating room at an evacuation field hospital in DeCambre, France, June 11, 1944. This operative unit occupies an impromptu site necessitated by the overwhelming events of the D-Day invasion. The stark white operating gowns against the dark background of military canvas emphasizes the concern for sterility even in the face of less than ideal operating conditions. (*Courtesy of Stanley B. Burns, M.D., and The Burns Collection and Archive*)

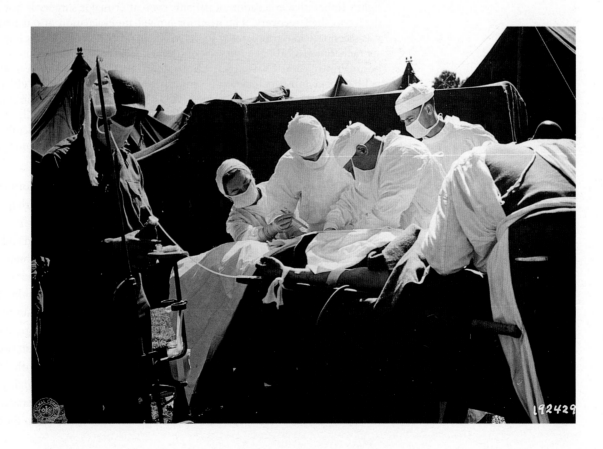

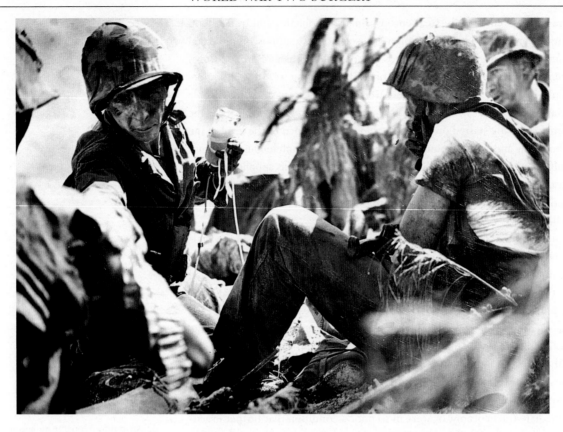

3. Of all the surgical advances in World War II, the giving of blood plasma had the most far-reaching effect in saving the lives of countless numbers of wounded soldiers. In this dramatic photograph from the battle of Saipan (June 1944) a wounded marine receives an intravenous injection of the life-saving humor. (*Courtesy of Stanley B. Burns, M.D., and The Burns Collection and Archive*)

annual surgical report to the Surgeon-General's Office said this about clearing stations and field hospitals in the North African theater of operations:

> Most of the work is done under quite adverse circumstances without the essentials, to say nothing of the niceties and decorum of a well-regulated operating room. Clearing Stations...are not adequately equipped for the performance of major surgery.... The lack of any suction apparatus, particularly in abdominal surgery, was keenly felt. Lighting facilities were...inadequate and uncertain. One abdominal operation, with multiple small and large bowel perforations, was performed with the only source of illumination being furnished by flashlights. Imperative evacuation of patients soon after major surgery is not conducive to their recovery. The need for immediate evacuation of our patients was secondary to our proximity to the front, a poorly defended front line with sporadic fluctuations, and our lack of hospital facilities and trained nurses for postoperative care. That surgery can be done in a Clearing Platoon is admitted but in so doing its function is seriously impaired and maximum efficiency of the surgical teams is not obtained. We, who were elected to fill in the gap between the front line and the Evacuation Hospitals 100 to 150 miles to the rear...in an installation not designed for major surgery, will welcome the opportunity of doing our work in the future under circumstances more conducive to the recovery of our patients.

Evacuation hospitals handled the great bulk of the wounded in the forward combat area. They received over 90 percent of total cases, with the small group of first-priority cases diverted to the field hospitals constituting less than 10 percent of the injured. The evacuation hospitals were fully equipped with well-trained and experienced surgeons who were fully proficient in initial wound management. By all accounts, these facilities served as the backbone of the Army medical service.

One indication of the complete acceptance of surgical specialization by the profession concerned the next level of evacuation/convalescence in the European theater of operations. General hospitals had one thousand beds and more, and were designed for injured soldiers who could not return to combat duty within two weeks following medical or surgical therapy. These facilities were frequently grouped together in what were termed hospital centers so as to increase the flexibility of care and decrease the number of highly trained personnel required. On average, it took from three to five days for a wounded or postoperative patient to reach the general hospital. The grouping of general hospitals together as a hospital center made it possible to provide specialty care for various types of injuries. Such specialization usually included centers for hand surgery, maxillofacial surgery, neurosurgery, plastic and reconstructive surgery, and thoracic surgery. In the early part of the war effort, hospital centers were mainly situated in Great Britain and Ireland, but their locations changed as military successes were achieved. The grouping of casualties under highly trained surgical specialists provided these specialists the opportunity to improve on technically complex procedures that would have taken years to evaluate in civilian life. The final portion of the evacuation scheme concerned air and sea transportation back to the United States for those patients deemed unable to return to active duty.

What made this casualty management plan so unique, at least for the European, North African, and Mediterranean theaters of combat, was their inherent organizational flexibility regarding surgical personnel and patients. When casualties were reaching 40,000 to 50,000 per month, the ability to expeditiously shift patients between field, evacuation, and general hospitals and/or return to America was an absolute necessity if the wounded were to receive maximum levels of surgical care. In addition, the availability of rapidly deployable auxiliary surgical teams, usually headed by a board-certified general surgeon and sent to field and evacuation hospitals to bolster the staff where there were insufficient numbers of experienced surgeons for the load imposed, was instrumental in decreasing surgical mortality rates and increasing daily morale.

THE OVERALL ORGANIZATION OF SURGICAL CARE

Professional aspects of the care of the wounded were carefully prescribed in various clinical directives from the Office of the Chief Surgeon. The willingness to abide by a form of standardization of clinical surgical methods was crucial in maintaining an acceptable level of overall medical care. This was especially important because large numbers of young and inexperienced physicians and surgeons, due to the exigencies of the time, were pressed into military service having received a bare minimum of medical and postgraduate education. In many instances, medical students matriculated in three years and completed their formal surgical training in about the same time.

From an education and training standpoint, the experiences of World War II provided evidence that the seven- to ten-year residency made famous by William

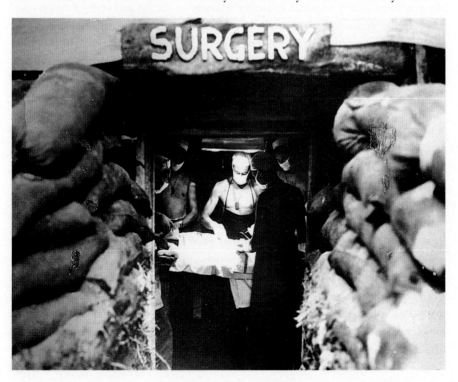

4. Bougainville, the largest of the Solomon Islands, became part of the Territory of New Guinea in 1920. Japan captured the island in 1942, and United States Marines landed there in November, 1943. This cramped operating room in the jungle, quite typical of the working conditions that surgeons found themselves in, was protected by sandbags against enemy shelling. *(Courtesy of Stanley B. Burns, M.D., and The Burns Collection and Archive)*

343

5. In the evacuation field hospital, 3rd Marine Division, Bougainville, Territory of New Guinea, a surgical team prepares to operate on the leg of a wounded marine (November 1943). *(Courtesy of Stanley B. Burns, M.D., and The Burns Collection and Archive)*

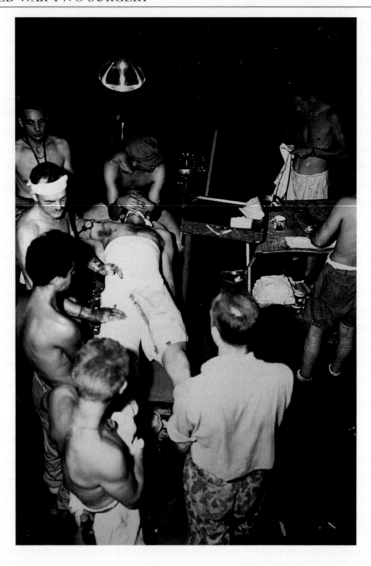

Halsted's program at The Johns Hopkins Hospital and those established since then were not essential to learning the technical aspects of surgery. Necessary dexterity could be learned more quickly than had previously been thought. However, the lessons of military surgery clearly showed that the passage of four to six postgraduate years was ideally required to enable mastery of the art and craft of surgery and the restraint engendered by sound clinical judgment. The insatiable demands of the Air Force, Army, and Navy for surgeons created a vast proliferation of surgical training programs and forced those already in existence to speed up their residency process. The result was that by the war's conclusion, a veritable flood of active and mostly capable young surgeons returned home eager to begin their civilian practices.

Over 97 percent of the almost 20,000 Medical Corps officers who served in the African, European, and Mediterranean combat theaters were recently commissioned civilian physicians. Most of them had been in private practice, and their willingness to conform to standardized methods of therapy, with which they might not agree, showed remarkable solidarity towards the war effort. The Chief Surgeon of the European Theater of Operations, U.S. Army, was Paul Hawley (1891–1965), a native of Indiana. Hawley was a career military medical officer and, following his graduation from medical school, received what little surgical training he had by working with his father, a rural family physician-surgeon. Hawley was more administrator than clinician, and under his command the treatment of the wounded, the administration of the Medical Corps in the European combat zone, and his office's cooperation with the high command and the Allies was considered unsurpassed in efficiency. Although officially designated surgeon, Hawley was commander of all American medical forces serving in Europe. In mid-1942, he established the Division of Professional Services, which coordinated the activities of physicians and surgeons through a surgical consultant system. James Kimbrough (1887–1956), a well-known urologist and, following the war, chief of the genitourinary service at Walter Reed Army Hospital, was named Director of Professional Services. The consultant organization was set up according to the Regular Army surgical service in large Army hospitals. In such a hierarchy, a general surgeon was chief of the overall surgical service, and specialist surgeons headed the various surgical sections. Since all surgical consultants in the European theater held prestigious positions in university hospitals and medical schools in the United States, this subordination to a general surgeon caused some dissatisfaction among the specialists. The specialist surgeons objected to the designation "senior consultant," as contrasted to the title "chief consultant," who had to be a general surgeon. By early 1945, in an attempt to mollify political squabbles, surgical specialties in army hospitals were given the higher status of a service, or department, similar to the organizational scheme in most large civilian hospitals.

Surgical consultants in the European theater were arranged in five hierarchal groups. Those of highest rank were assigned to Hawley's Chief Surgeon's Office. It was Hawley and Kimbrough who jointly selected Elliot Cutler (1888–1947), Moseley Professor of Surgery at Harvard Medical School, to be chief consultant in surgery. Cutler received both his undergraduate and medical degrees from Harvard University, interned (1913–1915) with Harvey Cushing, studied immunology with Simon Flexner (1863–1946) at the Rockefeller Institute for Medical Research, and following service in World War I, completed his surgical training (1919–1921) at the Peter Bent Brigham Hospital. For three years, Cutler remained on the surgical faculty of his alma mater, until he was appointed professor of surgery and chairman of the surgical department at Western Reserve University Medical School and Lakeside Hospital in Cleveland, Ohio. In 1932, he was asked to succeed his mentor, Cushing, as surgeon-in-chief at the Brigham. Cutler, who had a magnetic personality and was considered an outstanding teacher, pioneered thoracic and cardiac surgery, being the first American surgeon to operate successfully on a heart valve in a patient in 1923. He was elected president of the American Surgical Association in 1947 but died of metastatic prostate cancer prior to his formal induction at the 1948 meeting. Among Cutler's other numerous accomplishments was coauthoring with Robert Zollinger (1903–1992), who served his surgical residency under Cutler at the Peter Bent Brigham, the renowned *Atlas of Surgical Operations* (1939), which is still perennially re-edited.

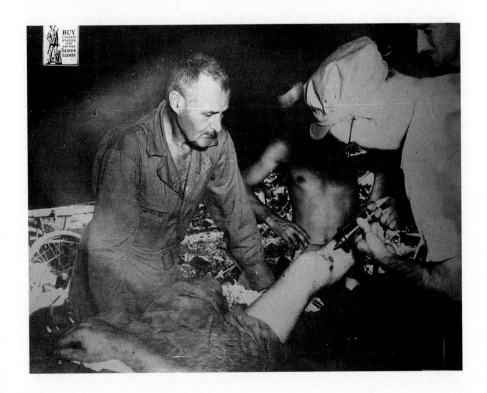

6. In a tent dressing station on New Georgia, part of the Solomon Islands, surgeons remove bomb fragments from a soldier's wounded knee. (*Courtesy of Stanley B. Burns, M.D., and The Burns Collection and Archive*)

345

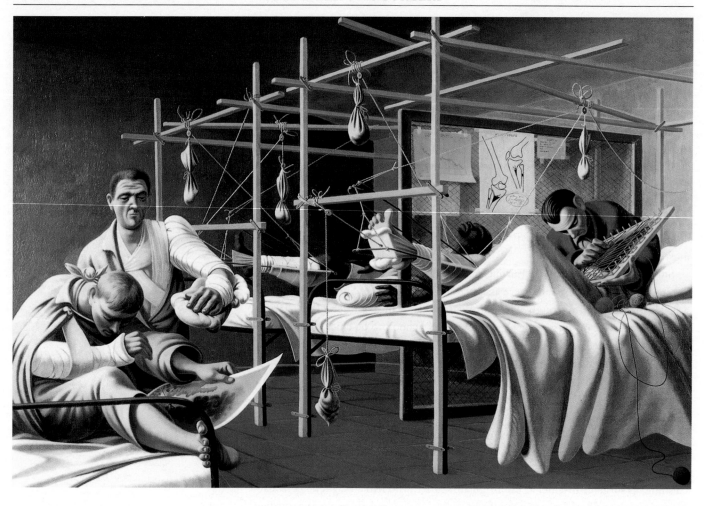

7. "Fracture Ward" by Peter Blume (circa 1943) is a scene of geometric intricacies. The Rube Goldberg-like Balkan frames, in addition to the angular likenesses of wounded soldiers, provide a complex compositional design. *(Courtesy of the U.S. Army Center of Military History)*

The reasons why Cutler was chosen to be chief consultant in surgery in the European Theater of Operations, a position similar to that held by John M. T. Finney (1863–1942), the Johns Hopkins-based surgeon with the American Expeditionary Forces in World War I, were inextricably rooted in that "war to end all wars." Cutler had served as a civilian in 1915 on the Harvard Unit of the American Ambulance Hospital in Paris. Following this three-month tour, he returned to the United States and soon received a commission in the Medical Corps Reserve as a first lieutenant. During this period (1915–1916), Cutler also served as a resident surgeon at the Massachusetts General Hospital. In May 1917, Cutler sailed for France with Base Hospital No. 5, a unit affiliated with the Harvard Medical School, under the command of Cushing. Cutler worked closely with Cushing on various surgical teams, particularly in neurosurgery, and later served as an adjutant of an evacuation hospital. Cutler was discharged as a major in April 1919 and returned to Boston to complete his surgical residency under Cushing at the Brigham. Following completion of his formal postgraduate training in 1921, Cutler reactivated his commission in the Medical Corps Reserve and from then on kept in constant contact with personnel in the Army Medical Department. Throughout the 1920s and 1930s, Cutler was well known to various Surgeon-Generals of the time, and he was a logical candidate for the chief consultancy in surgery in World War II. Much to the dismay and objections of the president of Harvard University and the trustees of Peter Bent Brigham Hospital, Cutler eagerly accepted the military position in July 1942.

Cutler's appointment and promotion to colonel were soon approved, and he was joined by various senior surgical consultants, including: James Brown (1900–1974), professor of clinical and oral surgery at Washington University in St. Louis, accompanied by Eugene Bricker (born 1908), who succeeded Brown within six months, in plastic surgery; Loyal Davis (1896–1982), professor of surgery at Northwestern

University, in neurosurgery; Derrick Vail (1898–1973), professor of ophthalmology at the University of Cincinnati, in ophthalmology; Rex Dively of Kansas City, in orthopedics; Norton Canfield, professor of otolaryngology at Yale University, in otolaryngology; and Ambrose Storck (1903–1975), of the Charity Hospital in New Orleans, in general surgery. During the course of the war effort, John Scarff (1898–1978), assistant professor of neurosurgery at Columbia University, and later Glenn Spurling, clinical professor of neurosurgery at the University of Louisville, succeeded Davis in neurosurgery; Mather Cleveland (1889–1979), assistant professor of anatomy and instructor of orthopedic surgery at Columbia University, was placed in charge of orthopedic surgery after Dively became head of a separate rehabilitation division; Robert Zollinger replaced Storck in general surgery; and John Robinson (1903–1967), a urologist at Columbia University, replaced Kimbrough, who had been serving in the dual capacity of Director of Professional Services and senior consultant in urology.

There was a huge hierarchy of command within the medical division of the armed forces, and it inevitably grew as the hostilities expanded. The second-ranking level of surgical consultants in the European theater were the base section surgical consultants, who changed command frequently. Regional consultants and coordinators in the hospital centers constituted the third group of surgical consultants. These individuals were usually the senior outstanding surgeons of one of the general hospitals of the center and served as consultants in addition to their duties as chiefs of the surgical services or sections of the hospitals to which they were assigned. The fourth level were Army surgical consultants. Each field army had an assigned surgical consultant who functioned under the direction of the army surgeon. Finally, the Army Air Force developed a limited system of consultation as necessary within its own command structure.

The rapidity of the mobilization effort, from a consultants' standpoint, meant that they initially had little concept of the duties or responsibilities in an overseas combat theater. However, each consultant would, in turn, build his own staff by arranging the appointments of consultants from other specialites. For instance, Edward Churchill of the Massachusetts General Hospital was named chief surgical consultant to the North African and Mediterranean theater of operations and soon brought in, among others, John Stewart (1892–1983) (shock and fluid management), Oscar Hampton (1905–1977) (extremity wounds), and Eldridge Campbell (1901–1956) (neurosurgery) as his senior surgical consultants. As a chief consultant, Churchill relates in his fascinating book *Surgeons to Soldiers, Diary and Records of the Surgical Consultant Allied Force Headquarters, World War II* (1972), what the concept of "undefined duties" implied:

> I started with a complete lack of definition and understanding of what the post of Surgical Consultant to a Theater Surgeon really meant. However...it proved to be a great advantage...to take up a position for which the duties were not defined.... [No one] had definite ideas about the scope of an overseas consultant's job. They did know that somebody was needed...with sufficient professional prestige to speak for and represent American surgery. With few exceptions, the names of the high ranking officers of the regular Medical Corps were unknown outside Army circles, and the Army had to cloak itself with civilian professional prestige.... When I finally left Washington for North Africa, my ignorance of the Army was still so great that I would not have been surprised to have found General Eisenhower meeting me...I was that impressed by the importance of my mission as I saw it...I received no briefing in military etiquette. Being commissioned as a colonel...I escaped what my confreres in the 6th General Hospital had been getting for months - namely, drill, etiquette and unit organization regulations.

The politics were maddening, aggravated by strong surgical personalities who were forced to be at each other's bidding in the coordination of far-flung activities. As in World War I, various civilian hospitals and medical schools organized and staffed general hospitals, which were called into service soon after the United States

347

entered the war. These affiliated units, usually assuming the roles of evacuation and general hospitals, were mobilized to every battlefront. The facilities were sometimes located physically near an actual combat zone, but they were more likely farther back in the chain of evacuation. For instance, the 5th and 105th General Hospitals were situated in Europe and represented Harvard University and the Peter Bent Brigham Hospital. Within their command structure were such well-known surgeons as J. Engleburt Dunphy (1908–1981) and Robert Zollinger. This was prior to the latter's July 1944 promotion to senior surgical consultancy status. The Massachusetts General Hospital controlled the 6th General Hospital, which was initially based in Northern Ireland and later moved to Salisbury, England, while the Roosevelt Hospital in New York City organized the 9th Evacuation Hospital. The 9th was a "heavy" (750-bed) mobile facility often expanded to house over 1,000 patients under canvas and served in both the North African and European campaigns. The 2nd General Hospital, staffed by medical officers from Columbia University College of Physicians and Surgeons and Presbyterian Hospital, was established in southern England at Oxford, while the 30th General Hospital was initially located in the English Midlands at Mansfield and comprised physicians and surgeons from the University of California School of Medicine in San Francisco. Ashley Oughterson (1895–1956) commanded the 39th General Hospital, which was affiliated with Yale. Located to Nouméa, New Caledonia, in what was claimed to have been a house of ill repute, the 39th served all of its time in the Pacific theater.

The surgical consultant command structure in the Pacific Ocean areas was not as easily coordinated as in Europe. Liaison between the Army, Navy, and Air Force left much to be desired and caused difficulties in the efficient evacuation of casualties. Oughterson was eventually promoted by General Douglas MacArthur (1880–1964) to be chief surgical consultant in the Pacific combat zone, but he faced a more diffi-

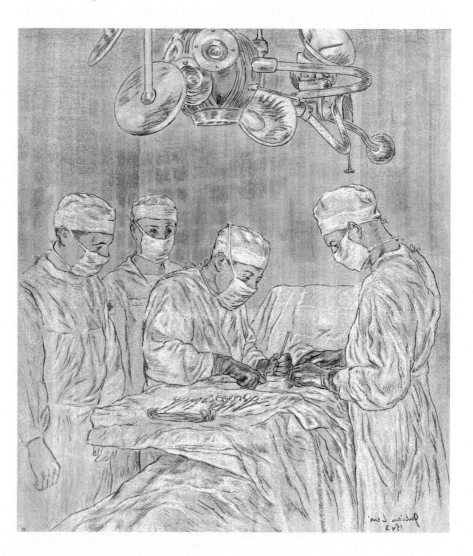

8. "Operation" by Julian Levi (circa 1943). *(Courtesy of the U.S. Naval Historical Center)*

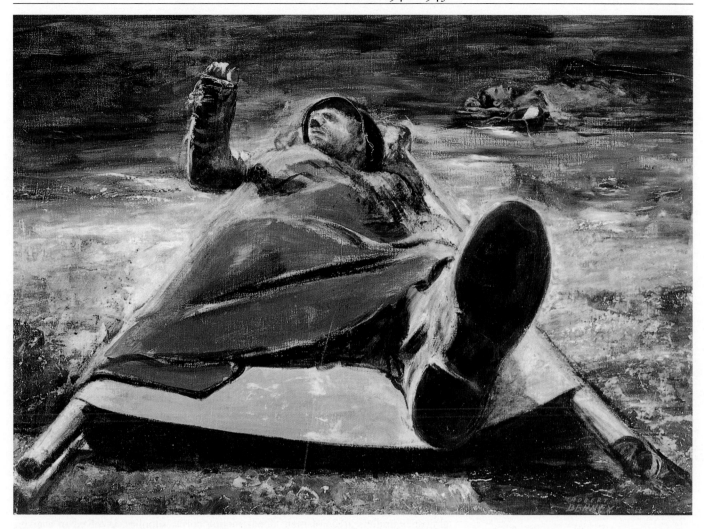

9. "Just Off The Line-Amputation" by Robert Benney (circa 1944). (*Courtesy of the U.S. Army Center of Military History*)

cult command task than Cutler and Churchill. Unlike some of his associates, Oughterson criticized the policy of sending younger, less experienced surgeons to the far front, rather than senior medical officers and surgical specialists. His European-based colleague, Cutler, agreed somewhat and organized the placing of surgical teams in the clearing station area. Yet, Cutler was adamant that the "team personnel should be general surgeons, not specialists." Churchill believed that auxiliary surgical groups represented the best method by which specialized and more senior surgical skill and talent could be selectively deployed as needed. Oughterson pointed out that hospital units affiliated with medical schools or well-known stateside institutions, by remaining intact with all of their clinical specialists, created an uneven distribution of surgical talent. Portable surgical hospitals were not able to properly function because they lacked qualified surgical personnel. While Cutler and Churchill covered hundreds of miles around Europe and North Africa as chief surgical consultants, Oughterson traveled thousands of miles, usually by air, throughout the western and south Pacific. Oughterson even went so far as to follow the troops up the small island chains from Guadalcanal, Bougainville, Tarawa, Makin, and Peleliu on to the Philippines, where he was present for the landings at Leyte and Luzon. Perhaps it was the difference in sheer size of the European and Pacific combat theaters that accounted for the variation in chief surgical consultants' opinions regarding how to best deploy medical and surgical personnel. With European combat being mostly land based, and Pacific action combining both land and sea operations, differing war strategies could easily cause disagreements over questions of surgical administration.

For instance, Cutler had long been convinced of the necessity for land-based mobile surgical units, as opposed to only mobile surgical teams, and asked Zollinger to coordinate such a project. Mainly through the latter's efforts, and in time for the

Normandy invasion in June 1944, a scheme was devised to have mobile units ready for deployment by limiting supplies to those that could be transported in a single two-and-a-half ton United States 4 x 4 Army truck. All personnel were similarly transported in a single weapons carrier. In addition to tentage, eighteen standard-issue Army metal trunks were filled and labeled. One trunk might contain plaster of Paris, cast cutter, plastic knives, and padding. Another would hold the anesthetist's tray, while a suction apparatus was separately packaged. Portable lighting equipment with electricity was supplied by a small 2.5-KV gasoline-operated generator. Several collapsible operating tables were added, which could support stretchers if need be. Three sterilizing metal drums holding two thousand 4 x 4 and sixty 4 x 8 gauze sponges were placed in another trunk. It was believed by Zollinger and his staff that such a mobile surgical unit had the capacity to complete fifty to one hundred major surgical operations or two hundred minor procedures before having to restock. Such mobile surgical units helped support the rapidly advancing 3rd Army commanded by General George Patton (1885–1945), and they earned his continuing gratitude. Although Zollinger's mobile surgical units never played a predominant role in the European Medical Department's evacuation scheme for casualties, they became the acknowledged forerunner of the MASH units (mobile army surgical hospitals) that were popularized and used so extensively during the Korean War.

To provide efficient and effective military surgical care, it was paramount that clinical standardization be accepted. However, since the psychological profile of most surgeons includes a relatively strong ego, efforts at directing surgical care from afar were a concept alien to the recently inducted, civilian-oriented "cutter." As Loyal Davis noted in *From One Surgeon's Notebook* (1967), "Undoubtedly, it requires a suitable temperament for a practicing doctor to be inducted suddenly into the Armed Forces without having had previous military experience. Many of the difficulties which were encountered were due to an ignorance of the reasons upon which a given method or procedure was based, and a failure to grasp the enormity of the almost boundless areas of men, departments, corps, supplies, involved in a given decision." Despite the problems of professional individuality, virtually all aspects of the care of the sick and wounded were carefully enunciated in various clinical manuals and "circular letters." Clinical directives from the Office of the Surgeon-General of the Army were usually established by surgical consultants after careful study of patient data, which were being constantly updated and compiled. These advisories instructed medical officers in what should be done to the wounded soldier, all the way from the battlefront to the rearmost hospital. Details were given about the use of blood and plasma for resuscitation, proper dosage of the sulfonamides and penicillin, débridement of a wound, and methods of caring for fractures, both during transportation and the period of healing in a General Hospital. Much like the surgical manuals utilized during the Civil War, the World War II works included drawings to illustrate appropriate methods of débridement, decompression of tension pneumothorax, and so on. Several circular letters became particularly well known because they enunciated surgical principles that subsequently became fundamental in the care of civilian trauma patients:

Circular Letter No. 91 - April 26, 1943
The guillotine or open circular method of amputation is the procedure of choice in traumatic surgery under war conditions and is especially indicated in gunshot wounds and in controlling infection. Primary suture of all wounds of extremities under war conditions is never to be done.

Circular Letter No. 178 - October 23, 1943
In large bowel injuries, the damaged segment will be exteriorized by drawing it out through a separate incision, preferably in the flank. In order to facilitate subsequent closure the two limbs of the loop should be approximated by suture for a distance of about 2 1/2 inches and then returned to the abdomen, leaving the apex exteriorized with a short length of rubber tubing or other suitable material beneath it. If the segment cannot be mobilized, the injury should be repaired and a proximal colostomy done.

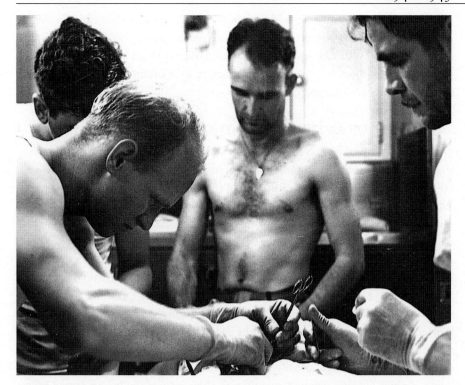

10. An emergency appendectomy on board the submerged submarine U.S.S. *Silversides* (December 23, 1942) performed by pharmacy mate first class Thomas A. Moore on George M. Platter. The *Silversides* was then in enemy waters in the Solomon Islands, and despite Moore's not being a trained surgeon, Platter returned to duty within a few days of the operation. (*National Archives*)

Strict adherence to these standardized policies was essential if the results of surgical operations were to be maximized. For instance, the policy of exteriorization of the bowel and colostomy shortened the time necessary to care for wounds of the colon and saved additional lives by making earlier treatment possible for other wounded men. A directive by Surgeon-General of the Army Norman Kirk (1888–1960) concerning open wound management was far-reaching in allowing amputated limbs to heal faster, reducing the threat of secondary infection and gangrene, and permitting soldiers to commence rehabilitation in a more expedient fashion.

The one item in surgical care that distinguished this war from all those before it, as well as the single reason most directly responsible for the improvement in morbidity and mortality statistics, was the resuscitation of the wounded soldier. It came to be believed that proper preoperative resuscitation transcended in importance any other single method of therapy employed during the hostilities. In World War I, the pulse rate and the presence of nausea, sweating, and vomiting were utilized as valuable signs and symptoms in delineating shock. However, surgical research conducted by Blalock, Crile, Phemister, and others during the period between the wars showed these indicators were not necessarily accurate. During World War II, such signs and symptoms were thought to be related more to the character of the wound or to psychological factors, or even physiological responses to the administration of morphine, which was claimed to be routinely given in too large doses. Blood pressure, degree of thirst and the patient's mental status, none of which received much attention in World War I, were now noted to be extremely useful in evaluating the degree of shock. Still, the diagnosis of surgical shock all too often remained confusing and needed to be clarified.

In response to this problem, preoperative shock wards and shock teams were organized. By the last year of combat in the European zone, all casualties thought to be in shock were admitted to shock wards or tents, regardless of whether or not it was believed that they would require a surgical operation. In a field hospital, the officer in charge of the shock ward was usually chosen from among the internists or junior surgeons on the staff. It was too important a position for a totally inexperienced officer to be in charge, but the prolonged assignment (quick rotation of personnel merely promoted inefficiency) of experienced surgeons was not considered appropriate because their technical skills were better used in the operating room.

Yet, by the end of hostilities, the importance of the function of the officer in charge of the shock ward was so evident that many senior surgeons were forced to assume this supervisory role. The legacy of the World War II shock ward is noted in the modern surgical intensive care unit with its cadre of specialized intensive care specialists and trauma care experts.

THE USE OF ANTIBIOTICS AND ADVANCES IN BURN CARE

Of the many medical lessons learned in World War II, the importance of antibiotics to surgical therapeutics was among the most important. In 1928, Alexander Fleming (1881–1955), of London, discovered a mold (*Penicillium notatum*), which produced a substance that strongly inhibited the growth of common infectious disease causing microorganisms. By the early 1940s, the clinical importance of penicillin had been demonstrated, but efforts to produce the antibiotic in large quantities had not been realized. Several United States pharmaceutical manufacturers began to apply to the penicillin production problem the experience gained in other industries using yeasts and molds, most notably beer brewing. By mid-1943, larger quantities of penicillin were being produced, but because of the war effort and the surgeons' need for unrestricted availability of the antibiotic, the federal government took control of the entire penicillin output. Prior to May 1944, injured soldiers were treated with one of the sulfonamide drugs, usually parenterally. At that time, penicillin was finally being produced in large enough quantities to allow routine use by our armed forces and those of our allies. Virtually every injured soldier began receiving an intramuscular injection of penicillin in the division clearing stations. By war's conclusion, it was believed that penicillin had proved to be more efficacious than the sulfonamides in the prevention and treatment of peritonitis secondary to war wounds of the abdomen and had helped save numerous lives.

Advances in surgical care during the war years were not associated solely with military events. In Boston, the Coconut Grove was a large and popular nightclub situated near the Commons, just off Charles Street. In November 1942, the newly refurbished club, sporting groves of imitation palm trees, overhead hangings, and draperies was packed with almost one thousand patrons. At about 10:15 in the evening, some of the draperies and other flammable decorations caught fire, followed by a horrendous deflagrating situation. Within five minutes, the entire nightclub was filled with smoke and flames. Although the Boston fire department extinguished the blaze within thirty minutes, the structure was a smoldering ruin, and hundreds of victims lay inside and overflowed onto the sidewalk. Trapped inside because of locked exits or doors that opened only inward, 490 individuals died. It was later estimated that there were 440 immediate survivors. The largest number of dead and injured, approximately 300, were taken to Boston City Hospital. Of these, 132 were alive when they got there, 36 of whom soon died. The Massachusetts General Hospital received 114 casualties; 39 of those patients were still alive after the first few hours. Ten had severe burns, while 29 had mostly pulmonary injuries. Two months later, there were still 9 severely burned individuals in the Massachusetts General facility receiving surgical care and undergoing skin grafting.

The treatment of burns has long been the purview of the surgeon. Consequently, surgical methods, including gentleness in handling burned tissue, frequent dressing changes, and performance of skin grafting at the appropriate time, had steadily evolved since the last decades of the nineteenth century. What remained a puzzle though, were the subsequent pulmonary problems suffered at the time of thermal injury. Many victims with seemingly innocuous physical burns succumbed to lung damage, which was difficult to detect and virtually impossible to treat. As a direct result of the Coconut Grove fire, a series of surgical investigations was begun at the Massachusetts General Hospital under the leadership of Oliver Cope (1904–1994), a senior member of the surgical staff with an ongoing interest in burn therapeutics.

Cope had primary responsibility for care of the Coconut Grove patients. He used a newly devised type of wound dressing, boric-petrolatum gauze, and began to investigate pulmonary injury in burns. The care of such patients was of obvious importance to military surgeons, and the results of Cope's efforts had an immediate impact on official channels in Washington. This was aided by the fact that Edward Churchill, in his position as Cope's mentor and professor of surgery at the Massachusetts General Hospital, was about to leave for military service and assume the chief surgical consultancy for the Mediterranean theater. Churchill immediately promulgated disaster management measures, which were relevant not only to national defense but also to American industry. Older chemical dressings were eliminated and the introduction of simple local applications, à la Cope's gauze, was begun. Most importantly, the Coconut Grove conflagration proved a crucial turning point in the scientific assessment and treatment of direct lung injuries in burns. As a result, the surgical investigations instigated by the Boston disaster helped clarify the treatment of burns in the military setting.

The explosion of atomic devices over Hiroshima and Nagasaki signaled more than the end of World War II. The detonations demonstrated how a concatenation of basic and applied sciences could yield technological breakthroughs never before thought possible. For the surgeon, new paths were to be opened that brought surgical therapeutics beyond the simple manual craft of just a few decades before. From a technical and logistical standpoint, American surgeons were about to inherit the mantle of world surgical leadership. The demand for surgery would soon be so great as to force the profession to undergo a socioeconomic revolution that in the end would provide direction for its forseeable future.

1945	1950	1955	1960	1965	1970	1975	1980	1985

Mother Frances X. Cabrini canonized as first American to be made a Roman Catholic saint *(1946)*

Jackie Robinson becomes first African-American major-league baseball player *(1947)*

Idlewild International Airport (renamed Kennedy Airport in 1963) *(1948)*

Rodgers and Hammerstein produce *South Pacific,* starring Mary Martin *(1949)*

Brinks armored car robbery in Boston nets $1 million in cash *(1950)*

First transcontinental television broadcast *(1951)*

Panty raids carried out on college campuses *(1952)*

Playboy founded by Hugh Hefner *(1953)*

Salk vaccinations for poliomyelitis *(1954)*

African Americans boycott segregated city bus lines in Montgomery, Alabama *(1955)*

Elvis Presley achieves national fame with his song "Heartbreak Hotel" *(1956)*

Hurricane Audrey and a tidal wave strike Louisiana and Texas coastlines, leaving 531 dead *(1957)*

Transatlantic jet service begun by Pan-American World Airways *(1958)*

Alaska and Hawaii become the 49th and 50th states, respectively *(1959)*

Alfred Hitchcock releases the suspense thriller *Psycho (1960)*

First intercontinental ballistic missle (ICBM) fired *(1961)*

John *Steinbeck* awarded the Nobel Prize in literature *(1962)*

U.S.S. Thresher, a nuclear-powered submarine, is lost in the Atlantic Ocean with 129 men on board *(1963)*

Beatlemania sweeps the United States *(1964)*

On November 9th, a massive power failure blacks out New England, New York, and parts of New Jersey and Pennsylvania *(1965)*

Uniform Time Act establishes daylight saving time throughout the country, from the last Sunday in April until the last Sunday in October *(1966)*

Trapped in the Apollo capsule of a Saturn 1-B rocket on the ground, astronauts Roger Chaffee, Ed White, and Gus Grissom are killed when fire erupts *(1967)*

Stanley Kubrick's *2001: A Space Odyssey (1968)*

Neil Armstrong and Edwin Aldrin land on the moon *(1969)*

Environmental Protection Agency (EPA) *(1970)*

Charles Manson and his followers are convicted of mass murder *(1971)*

First woman rabbi in the United States, Sally J. Priesand, ordained in Cincinnati *(1972)*

Secretariat wins horse racing's triple crown *(1973)*

Gasoline shortage inconveniences Americans through winter months *(1974)*

U.S.A. POPULATION

1950	=	151 million
1960	=	179 million
1970	=	205 million

DAILY LIFE

HISTORY AND POLITICS

Government lifts most wage and price controls *(1946)*

Secretary of State George Marshall proposes the European Recovery Program (the Marshall Plan) *(1947)*

United States recognizes the new state of Israel *(1948)*

Senate ratifies agreement establishing the North Atlantic Treaty Organization (NATO) *(1949)*

President Harry Truman authorizes the use of United States forces in Korea *(1950)*

General Douglas MacArthur relieved of his Far Eastern command by President Harry Truman *(1951)*

Dwight Eisenhower and Richard Nixon elected president and vice president, respectively *(1952)*

Department of Health, Education, and Welfare *(1953)*

Supreme Court in *Brown v. Board of Education of Topeka* rules that segregation in public schools violates the Fourteenth Amendment of the Constitution *(1954)*

American Federation of Labor (AFL) and the Congress of Industrial Organizations (CIO) merge *(1955)*

Federal Aid Highway Act authorizes a thirteen-year intra- and interstate highway building program *(1956)*

United States occupation forces leave Japan *(1957)*

U.S. Marines sent to Lebanon to restore order after uprising by Arab nationalists *(1958)*

Supreme Court upholds injunction under the Taft-Hartley Act, ending 116-day steel strike in Pittsburgh *(1959)*

U-2 photographic reconnaissance plane shot down over Soviet territory, and pilot Francis Gary Powers is captured *(1960)*

United States breaks diplomatic relations with Cuba *(1961)*

Cuban missle crisis brings the United States and the Soviet Union to the brink of nuclear war *(1962)*

President John F. Kennedy is assassinated in Dallas *(1963)*

Congress passes Tonkin Gulf Resolution, which gives President Lyndon Johnson power to use any action necessary to repel armed attack on United States forces, particularly in North and South Vietnam *(1964)*

Martin Luther King, Jr., leads civil rights march from Selma to Montgomery, Alabama *(1965)*

United States increases its military strength in South Vietnam and its bombing of North Vietnam *(1966)*

Selective Service System cancels draft deferments for college students who interfere with military recruiting *(1967)*

Martin Luther King, Jr., assassinated in Memphis *(1968)*

United States–North Vietnamese peace talks in Paris are expanded to include Viet Cong and South Vietnamese government *(1969)*

National Guard Troops kill four student Vietnam War protesters at Kent State University, *(1970)*

New York Times publishes classified Pentagon papers obtained by Daniel Ellsberg about United States involvement in Vietnam *(1971)*

President Richard Nixon visits China and the Soviet Union *(1972)*

United States and South Vietnam sign cease-fire with North Vietnam and Viet Cong, ending Vietnam War *(1973)*

Congress recommends three articles of impeachment against President Richard Nixon, and he resigns *(1974)*

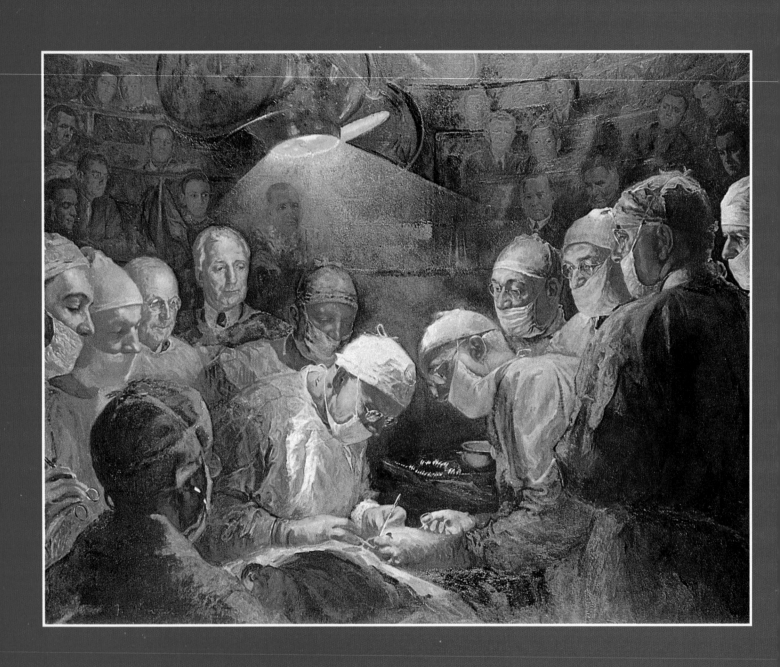

CHAPTER 11

AMERICAN SURGICAL SUPREMACY *1946–1974*

The decades of economic expansion after World War II had a dramatic impact on the scale of American medicine and surgery. Between 1950 and 1970, the number of individuals in the health care work force increased from 1.2 to 3.9 million. Total expenditures on the nation's health care delivery system grew from $12.7 billion to $71.6 billion, an increase from 4.5 to 7.3 percent of the gross national product. Spending on health, adjusted to 1995 dollars, was approximately $1,125 per capita in 1965. Ten years later, the figure had increased to $1,750, a 55 percent jump in a decade's time. It was as if medicine had become big business overnight, with the singleminded pursuit of health care rapidly becoming society's largest growth industry. Spacious hospital complexes were built, which not only represented the scientific advancement of the healing arts but vividly demonstrated the strength of America's postwar socioeconomic boom.

Society was willing to give medical science unprecedented recognition as a prized national asset. This was especially evidenced in 1963, when Congress passed the Health Education Assistance Act, which for the first time provided unrestricted federal funds for the construction, renovation, and/or equipping of medical schools. Whereas only eleven American medical colleges had been founded between 1940 and 1965, twenty-six new institutions opened and admitted students during the eight-year period 1966 to 1973, bringing the total number of accredited schools to 112. In 1950, 7,042 individuals were matriculating in the first-year classes of American medical schools. Ten years later the number increased to 8,103, and in the year ending this surgical era (1975), a total of 14,763 first-year medical students were beginning their medical education. With graduation rates approaching 100 percent, it was evident that American citizens were anticipating a rapid rise in the aggregate of their physicians and surgeons.

The overwhelming impact of World War II on surgery was the sudden expansion of the profession and the extensive distribution of surgeons throughout the country. Many of these individuals, newly baptized to the rigors of technically complex trauma operations, became leaders in the construction and improvement of hospitals, multispecialty clinics, and surgical facilities in their hometowns. Large urban and community hospitals established surgical education and training programs, finding it relatively easy matter to attract interns and residents. For the first time, residency programs in general surgery were rivaled in growth and educational sophistication by those in all the special fields of surgery. The rapid and ongoing expansion of postgraduate internship and residency programs, initially a result of the exigencies of World War II, soon became the reason for further increases in the number of students entering surgery. Before the war, the great majority of physicians in active clinical practice (77 percent in 1940) classified themselves as either general practitioners

1. *(facing page)* "The Babcock Surgical Clinic," Painted by Furman J. Finck (born 1900) in 1944–1945, this is a commemorative group portrait rather than a tribute to one great surgeon. W. Wayne Babcock was a legendary surgical figure who, in 1904, was named the first professor and head of the department of surgery at Temple University School of Medicine. In honor of Babcock's retirement, Finck invoked the memory of Philadelphian Thomas Eakins' portrayal of Samuel Gross and D. Hayes Agnew by incorporating numerous onlookers (most of whom were surgical residents but also including Babcock's wife and Finck himself) into the subdued background. Grouped around Babcock, shown holding a scalpel, are ten of his former students and/or associates, all surgeons: *(left to right)* George Rosemond, W. Emory Burnett, William A. Steele, William N. Parkinson, Daniel J. Preston, James N. Coombs, John Leedom, George M. Astley, Valentine Ness, and Harry E. Bacon. In the institutional custom of the day, the surgeon's mask was situated beneath the nose, and Finck makes certain that this quirk of surgical individualism was obvious to all. In the immediate foreground is Helen Krause, a nurse anesthetist, who often administered anesthesia to Babcock's patients. The actual surgical operation being conducted remains both an artistic and a medical mystery. *(Temple University School of Medicine)*

2. In a rear-line hospital operating room in Pusan, Korea (July 26, 1950), a surgeon debrides a soldier's thigh wound. While members of mobile army surgical hospitals in the Korean War received notoriety for their supposed casualness under fire, this surgeon in a non-M.A.S.H. unit demonstrates a similar demeanor, operating in street clothes, with a South Korean map or guidebook in his back pocket. *(Courtesy of Stanley B. Burns, M.D., and The Burns Collection and Archive)*

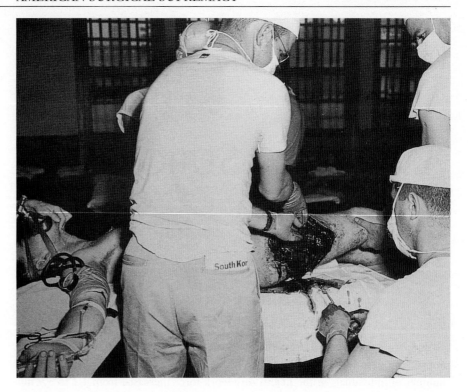

or part-time specialists. By the end of that decade, the 23 percent of doctors reporting themselves as full-time specialists had increased to 37 percent. Ten years later, the number of full-time specialists had grown to 55 percent; by 1975, it was nearly 80 percent of all American physicians. So profound was this trend toward specialization that a threatened extinction of the old-fashioned general practitioner seemed inevitable. By 1970, of the 302,966 physicians in active practice (clinical and non-clinical), only 58,919 were considered family physicians.

This change in practice demographics of the American doctor was most dramatic for the surgical specialties. In 1930, 10 percent of the medical profession considered themselves surgeons. Thirty years later, the proportion had risen to 26 percent, and by the conclusion of this era of American surgical supremacy, over one third of all physicians were full-time practitioners of either general surgery or one of the surgical specialties. According to the American Medical Association's *Directory of Approved Internships and Residencies*, in 1970, of 46,785 total residency positions offered, 17,385 (37 percent) were in the surgical sciences. The emergence of surgical programs as the most sought-after residencies reflected the growing economic strength of America's surgeons. Not only did surgeons command the highest salaries (the average cardiac surgeon by the mid-1970s was earning $200 to $300 thousand per year), but the public was enamored with the drama of the operating room. Television series, movies, novels, and the more than occasional live performance of a heart operation on network broadcast beckoned the lay individual.

As the population of surgeons increased, telltale signs of overcrowding and the inevitable after-effect of loosened indications for surgical operations (i.e., unnecessary surgery) became evident. In 1970, John Bunker, an anesthesiologist and epidemiologist from Stanford University, authored in the *New England Journal of Medicine* a widely quoted and somewhat disturbing study showing that not only were there twice as many surgeons in an average American city as in an English city, but twice as many surgical procedures were performed per capita. It was earlier suggested, in a 1969 study on variations in the incidence of elective surgery in Kansas, that a surgical form of Parkinson's law existed in the United States: patient admissions for surgery naturally expanded to fill beds, operating suites, and total surgical manpower. Yet, despite such a large volume of surgical practice in America, no appreciable direct short-term or long-term health related benefits were noted. Death rates from surgical diseases in England and the United States were essentially the same, even though the people of the latter country were spending more monies on health systems and consequently receiving higher levels of patient care.

This change was occurring at a time when surgeons and physicians were about to be overwhelmingly affected by federal and state fiscal policies. Since the founding of the country, the practice and governance of "physick" and "chirurgery" had been a more or less *laissez faire* proposition. Yes, the government had become increasingly involved in maintaining licensure and discipline, but no attempt to mandate change in the actual delivery of health care (i.e., implementation of health insurance) proved successful. From 1904, when the Socialists became the first political party to endorse national health insurance, through President Theodore Roosevelt's 1912 championing of such a measure on behalf of the Progressive Party, through the American Medical Association's call for national insurance (1916), to the Association's flip-flop to a hard-line denunciation of compulsory insurance (1932), all proposals were defeated by special interest groups.

Three months after the end of World War II, President Harry Truman called on Congress to create a single insurance system for all citizens and to expand budget money for hospital construction, medical research, and education. Although Truman acknowledged that it would be a costly proposition, he justified the action by stating that health care accounted for just 4 percent of the gross national product. The American Medical Association opposed the "enslavement of the medical profession," and along with Congressional Republicans termed compulsory health insurance "socialized medicine." Once again, basic socioeconomic reform of the country's health care delivery system was defeated.

For the American College of Surgeons, the postwar years presented a precarious financial situation. Poor management, including the inefficient arrangement of having two associate directors of the College instead of a single chief executive officer, created financial havoc. In 1950, with the College administration advised of the likely need for deficit spending, its surgeon trustees made a decision that would have an important impact on the future of American health care. Paul Hawley, who assumed the newly created office of Director of the College in March 1950, was authorized to discuss with George Bugbee, executive director of the American Hospital Association, the possibility that the Association might share the financial burden of the College's Hospital Standardization Program. The College took great pride in the fact that almost 3,300 hospitals were on the approved list. However, the increasing economic hardship in managing the expanding Standardization Program threatened the financial stability of many of the College's other educational programs. Over the years, the American Hospital Association had become a financially sound organization and was more than willing to participate and even assume the cost of evaluating its member institutions. Negotiations were begun between the two organizations, despite the accusation by certain segments of College membership that their trustees were "selling out to laymen."

In the midst of this complicated political maneuvering, members of the Board of Trustees of the American Medical Association became aware of the approaching imbroglio. Sensing an opportunity to undo their previous exclusion from the hospital reform movement, the Association asked to be included in the bargaining process. Committees were appointed, and in December 1951, the Joint Commission on Accreditation of Hospitals was formally organized. The new Board of Commissioners had nineteen voting members, including three each from the American College of Surgeons and American College of Physicians, with the remainder apportioned between the American Hospital Association and the American Medical Association. When a ceremony formally conveying the American College of Surgeons' Hospital Standardization Program to the Joint Commission was held in late 1952, it marked the end of a remarkably successful three and a half decades of voluntary effort by the College to improve the country's patient care.

Over the next fifteen years, the Joint Commission carried on its regulatory work, receiving scant notice from the public or from most medical professionals. As it

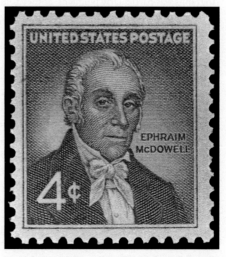

3. Ephraim McDowell (1959). (*Author's Collection*)

existed without true legal power, its member institutions participated in the regulatory programs on a strictly voluntary basis. Business practices dramatically changed in 1965 when Congress passed Public Law 89-97, the Medicare Act. This legislation decreed that any hospital would have to meet requirements established by the Joint Commission in order to qualify for medical payments from the federal government. The Commission was immediately catapulted onto the national health care scene and cast into the new role of a "quasi-public-legal" licensing authority.

Despite the increasing powers of the Joint Commission, there continued to be no stronger delineation of clinical privileges, particularly with regard to physicians performing surgical operations. Attempts were made by members of the American College of Surgeons and the American Board of Surgery to have the Joint Commission adopt rules stating that surgery could be performed in its member hospitals only by qualified surgeons (i.e., board-certified individuals), but these attempts failed for sundry political reasons on many occasions. This inability to introduce board certification as a national standard for clinical practice continued a policy reflective of an era when less than fully trained surgeons were conducting the majority of surgical procedures in the United States. Accordingly, it was suggested throughout the 1950s, 1960s, and early 1970s that the only thing that prevented the Joint Commission from adopting a regulation requiring surgery to be practiced by qualified surgeons was an anticipated roar of protest from the many non-board-certified and ill-prepared individuals who would have to give up their lucrative surgical practices at fully accredited member hospitals,

To offset this problem of partially and poorly trained surgeons, a review system was developed to better assure the integrity and desirability of the surgical residency system. As early as 1938, the American College of Surgeons established the Committee on Graduate Training in Surgery to investigate, analyze, and evaluate the opportunities for the training of surgeons. One year later, the College began to publish an annual list of approved residencies in surgery. The College also distributed a *Manual of Graduate Training in Surgery*, which was similar to the American Medical Association's *Essentials of Approved Residencies and Fellowships*. As obvious rivals in attempting to direct graduate education and training programs in the United States, the American College of Surgeons and the American Medical Association continued the duality of evaluating the same surgical programs through the late 1940s. At that time, an agreement was reached by representatives of the American Board of Surgery, the American College of Surgeons, and the Council on Medical Education of the American Medical Association about the establishment of a unified accrediting program for surgical residencies.

The resulting Conference Committee on Graduate Training in Surgery became effective in 1950. This development of a multibased committee for surgical residency review was a watershed in cooperative arrangements and obviated the need for labor-intensive multiple inspections of the same hospitals. In its first year of activity, the Conference Committee approved 224 four-year and 258 three-year residency programs in general surgery. Its members also began to lobby for the introduction of mandatory four-year residency programs, progressively graded in work responsibility. The working theory behind the tripartite organization approach was that the Conference Committee could focus on enforcing standards in training, while the specialty board could concentrate on establishing educational standards and developing appropriate written and oral surgical examinations.

Over the next decade, the American College of Surgeons and the Council on Medical Education established similar joint relations with the American Board of Otolaryngology, the American Board of Plastic Surgery, and the American Board of Obstetrics and Gynecology. These early relationships led to the concept of formal residency review committees for each separate surgical specialty and remains in effect today. Residency review committees have had a significant impact on upgrading the quality of residency training in all medical and surgical specialties by providing a level of specialty regulation not previously available. Empowered to act in

4. *(facing page)* In 1948, *Life* Magazine sent W. Eugene Smith to photograph Ernest Ceriani, a Colorado-based rural physician-surgeon at work. Smith spent four weeks living with the doctor and snapped pictures of all his various medical activities. One series of photographs was particularly poignant, as they told the story of two-and-a-half-year-old Lee Marie Wheatly. Ceriani was called to perform emergency surgery *(top)* after the youngster was kicked in the face by a horse. While the anxious parents looked on, Ceriani closed a severe laceration of the left side of the forehead *(bottom left)*. Concerned that the little girl would lose vision in her eye, the family doctor had to tell the parents the sad news. Ceriani was typical of that era's rural physicians who provided general medical care but also performed major surgical operations. At the end of another long day, a haggered but still gowned Ceriani relaxes over a cup of coffee in a hospital kitchen following completion of an operation that lasted until 2 in the morning *(bottom right)*. *(W. Eugene Smith, Life Magazine, Copyright Time)*

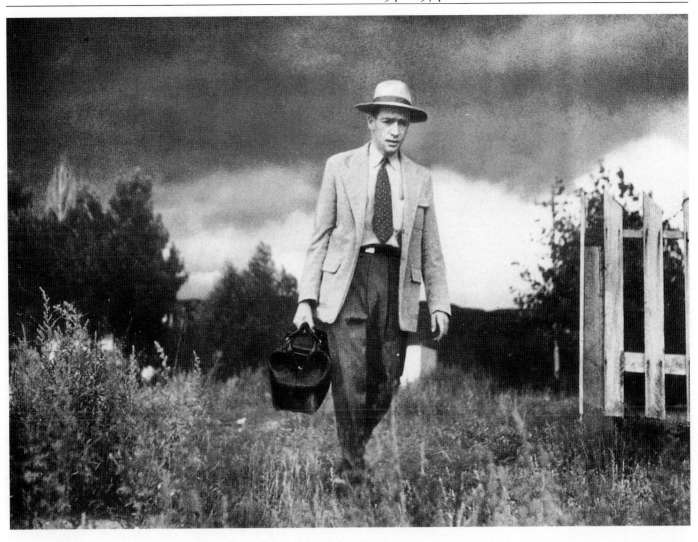

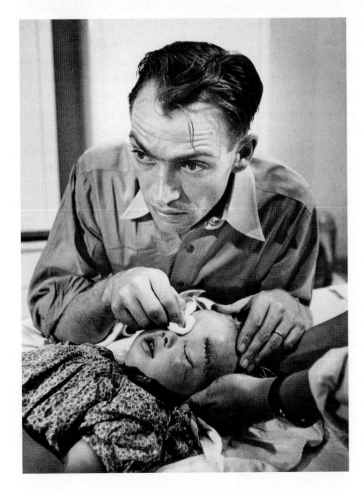

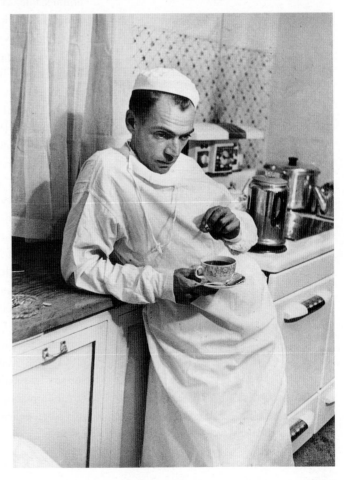

approving residency programs on behalf of their constitutient organizations, residency review committees make recommendations about the requirements for education and training programs in the specialty, although the specifications of such requirements remain the responsibility of the specialty board and, in some instances, a specialty society.

Following three and a half centuries of growth, the American profession of surgery seemed finally ready to assume its role as leader of world surgery. After all, the physical destruction of World War II had brought an end to any semblance of European surgical superiority. But in America everything seemed in place, from the acceptance of surgery as a medical science, through the blossoming of specialization, to the establishment of parameters regarding surgical education and training. The 1946–1974 surgical era would showcase American surgical greatness while setting the stage for an inevitable but unwelcome socioeconomic transformation of medicine and surgery.

CARDIAC SURGERY AND ORGAN TRANPLANTATION

Two developments epitomized the magnificence of post-World War II American surgery and concurrently fascinated the public: the maturation of cardiac surgery as a new surgical specialty and the emergence of organ transplantation, which together stand as signposts along this well-traveled scientific highway. In addition, when Dwight Eisenhower (1890–1969) became the first president of the United States to undergo major abdominal surgery (ileotransverse colostomy for intestinal obstruction secondary to regional ileitis) during his term in office and experienced a relatively uneventful postoperative course, the life-saving value of modern surgical therapeutics was clearly demonstrated to all.

Fascination with the heart goes far beyond that of clinical medicine. From the historical perspective of art, customs, literature, philosophy, religion, and science, the heart has represented the seat of the soul and the wellspring of life itself. Such reverence has also meant that this noble organ was long considered surgically untouchable. While the late nineteenth and twentieth centuries witnessed a steady march of surgical triumphs for opening successive cavities of the body, the final achievement awaited the perfection of methods for surgical operations in the thoracic space, especially the human heart. Such a scientific and technological accomplishment can be traced back to the repair of cardiac stab wounds by direct suture and the earliest attempts at fixing faulty heart valves. Although the world's first successful surgical repair of a pericardial wound was completed in 1891 by Henry Dalton (1847–1916), professor of abdominal and clinical surgery at the Marion Sims College of Medicine in St. Louis, it was Luther Hill (1862–1946) who performed in 1902 the country's first known successful suture of a wound that penetrated a cardiac chamber. Hill, a physician-surgeon from Mobile, Alabama, and recipient of postgraduate surgical training at John Wyeth's New York Polyclinic Medical School and Hospital and Joseph Lister's King's College Hospital Clinic, had to sew up a left ventricular wound in a heart beating over one hundred times a minute. This technically demanding feat was accomplished on an old kitchen table in a slum district shack, utilizing only the light from two kerosene lamps.

As triumphant as these successes were, not until the 1930s could the development of safe intrapleural surgery be counted on as something other than an occasional event. Edward Churchill of Boston completed the first successful pericardial resection in the United States in 1929. Almost a full decade later, Robert Gross (1905–1988) at the Boston Children's Hospital ushered in the modern era of cardiac surgery by repairing a cogenital cardiac anomaly known as patent ductus arteriosus (an abnormal opening between the left pulmonary artery and the descending aorta) in a seven-year-old girl. Gross's technical tour de force presupposed profound precision and a personal boldness dictated by the inescapable fact that loss of control of

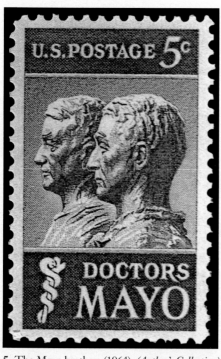

5. The Mayo brothers (1964). (*Author's Collection*)

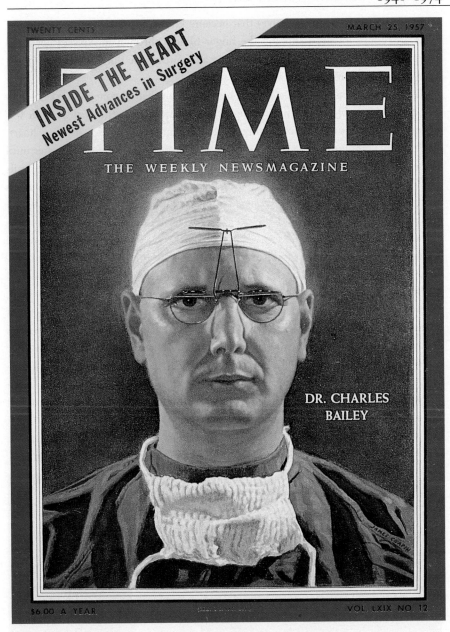

6. With Charles Bailey's appearance on the cover of *Time* (March 25, 1957), the supremacy of American surgery was becoming evident. *(Copyright 1957 Time Inc., reprinted by permission)*

these blood vessels, for even a few minutes, would result in the immediate death of the patient.

Notwithstanding Gross's achievement, the clinical reality was that most fields of surgery had been largely based on extirpation until this time. If an organ failed or an extremity was injured beyond salvage, then it was unceremoniously removed. However, the future of cardiac surgery demanded that reparative surgery be performed. Since the heart was nothing more than a sophisticated mechanical device with a muscle power source and uniflow valves, its more than occasional breakdowns needed to be fixed. Such structural failures necessitated repair, as opposed to removal, and efforts to provide the necessary clinical acumen set the stage for direct cardiac surgery.

During World War II, Dwight Harken (1910–1993), a Boston-based surgeon, gained extensive experience by removing 142 bullets and shrapnel in or in relation to the heart and great vessels, without a single fatality. In so doing, he shattered the long-held medical myth of the heart as an organ so complex and vital that it was sacrosanct from surgical intervention and that surgeons should be reluctant to even touch it. Building on his battlefield experiences in 1948, Harken, and also Charles Bailey (1910–1993) of Jefferson Medical College, proceeded to expand intracardiac surgery by independently developing an operation for mitral valve stenosis (scarring and narrowing of the mitral valve) that became known as mitral commissurotomy. This procedure involved slipping the finger blindly through the heart's left atrial chamber, pushing a scalpel along the finger, and cutting the fibrous lateral commissure of the faulty mitral valve.

Despite mounting clinical successes, heart surgeons had to contend not only with the quagmire of blood flowing through the area where a difficult dissection was occurring but with the unrelenting to-and-fro movement of a beating heart. Technically complex cardiac repair procedures could not be developed further until these problems were solved. Therefore, if open-heart surgery was to be made available to the mass of patients, cardiac contractions had to be stopped while circulation to the remainder of the body was maintained. Fortunately, one American surgeon had perceived this requirement back in the early 1930s and had been quietly working on its implementation. John Gibbon, Jr. (1903–1973), son of the renowned Philadelphia surgeon John Heysham Gibbon (1871–1956), received his undergraduate education at Princeton University (1923) and attended Jefferson Medical College (1927). Following a two-year internship at the Pennsylvania Hospital, Gibbon served as a research fellow in surgery at the Massachusetts General Hospital. In 1931, while under the direction of Edward Churchill, Gibbon was involved in the care of a female patient who, fifteen days following removal of her gallbladder, developed severe substernal chest pain, accompanied by marked elevation of pulse and respiratory rates and a decrease in blood pressure. With death imminent, a diagnosis of massive pulmonary embolus was made, and Churchill attempted a technically challenging pulmonary embolectomy, knowing that no such surgical operation had been successfully performed in the United States. Despite the

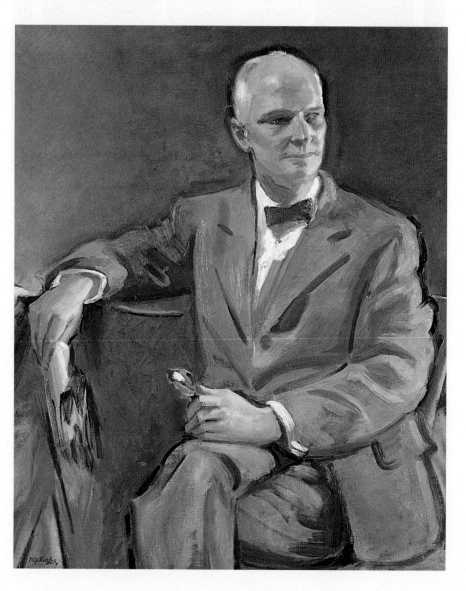

7. John Heysham Gibbon, Jr. as painted in 1953 by Charles Hopkinson (1869–1962). (*Courtesy of the College of Physicians of Philadelphia*)

364

rapidity of the procedure, the patient's condition soon deteriorated to the point where she could not be revived. During the night-long ordeal, the twenty-eight-year-old Gibbon reasoned that if a pulmonary embolus obstructed blood flow through the lungs, it might be possible to save a patient's life if a machine could be developed that would draw off the patient's oxygen-poor blood, reoxygenate it, and return it to the body's circulation.

This might have seemed a far-fetched fantasy at the time, but Gibbon's tenacity in the research laboratory was to become legendary. Working with Churchill's chief technician, Mary Hopkinson, who later became his wife, Gibbon soon devised an apparatus by means of which an obstructed pulmonary artery could be successfully bypassed in an experimental animal. By 1935, the Gibbons had demonstrated that life could be maintained by an extracorporeal blood circuit containing a pump serving as an artificial heart and a device for oxygenating the blood. More importantly, it was shown that even after the blood had been excluded from the animal's own heart and lungs for almost forty minutes, these organs were able to resume their normal activity when the artificial circuit was closed and circulation reestablished. From 1936 until 1941, the next phase of Gibbon's research was carried out at the Harrison Department of Surgical Research at the University of Pennsylvania School of Medicine. During these years, his research team showed that no permanent physiological or pathological damage had occurred to any animal that had had its cardiorespiratory functions maintained for lengthy periods of time on the artificial heart and lung. Following World War II, Gibbon continued his laboratory work as professor of surgery and director of surgical research at Jefferson Medical College. From 1956 to 1967 he served as Samuel D. Gross Professor of Surgery and chairman of the department of surgery. Because the extracorporeal project demanded ever-increasing amounts of engineering know-how, Gibbon sought out Thomas Watson (1874–1956), chairman of the board of International Business Machines Corporation, to make use of the company's engineering expertise. The mechanical question was how to construct an artificial lung with an oxygenating capacity great enough to sustain human patients as opposed to smaller laboratory animals. Working with a team of engineers, and paid for entirely by International Business Machines Corporation, Gibbon's six-year venture reached fruition when it was discovered that the creation of turbulence in the blood passing through the oxygenator increased the oxygenation level approximately eight times. Having tested the device thoroughly on experimental animals, Gibbon used it in May 1953 on an eighteen-year-old girl with a large opening in her atrial septum. All of Cecelia Bavolek's cardiopulmonary functions were maintained by the heart–lung machine for twenty-six minutes, while Gibbon and his assistant, Frank Allbritten, Jr. (born 1914), completely repaired the defect by direct suture-closure.

This first successful open heart operation in the world, using a heart-lung machine, was a momentous surgical contribution and stands as one of the landmarks of American surgical achievements. Gibbon, a self-effacing and intensely private individual, insisted that his success receive no undue publicity. Consequently, few individuals in the profession of surgery were aware that an extracorporeal device had been used successfully in a clinical cardiac operation. At first, Gibbon was reluctant to even report his accomplishment in the medical literature. However, in the fall of 1953, Gibbon was asked to present a paper about the heart-lung machine at a symposium on advances in cardiovascular surgery at the University of Minnesota. It was suggested to Gibbon that if he would submit the paper he was about to present, the report would be expeditiously published in *Minnesota Medicine*. Thus, this most astounding and momentous of surgical events was first described in a regional, not a national, periodical. More to the point, the only working prototype was Gibbon's machine, and it would be several years before the apparatus became readily available and surgeons familiar with its use. Through single-mindedness of purpose, Gibbon's research paved the way for open-heart surgery, including procedures for correction of congenital heart defects, repair of heart valves, and heart transplant. Most importantly, his work allowed the physician and the surgeon direct entrée to the disease process that is the most common cause of death in modern America-myocardial ischemia-and its surgical treatment, coronary artery bypass. In the final analysis, the development of the heart–lung machine must be considered a high point in the surgical family of remarkable achievements in this century, as it allowed heart surgery, a vision in 1950, to become practical by 1955 and routine by the 1960s.

The public's fascination with heart surgery was piqued by the newest communications tool, live television broadcasts. In June 1952, the first surgical operation televised coast-to-coast was transmitted through the auspices of the National Broadcasting Company, originating from Chicago's Wesley Memorial Hospital. Samuel Fogelson completed a three-and-a-half-hour procedure for duodenal ulcer, during which an eight-minute segment was shown live. The broadcast was soon followed by other performances and, for cardiac surgery, culminated in the on-air correction of a congenital anomaly in three-year-old Mabel Chin in May 1958. As the viewing public looked on with fear and fascination, the child's operation was completed without complication, and she was discharged from New York's University Hospital twelve days later, able to ride her "velocipede without difficulty."

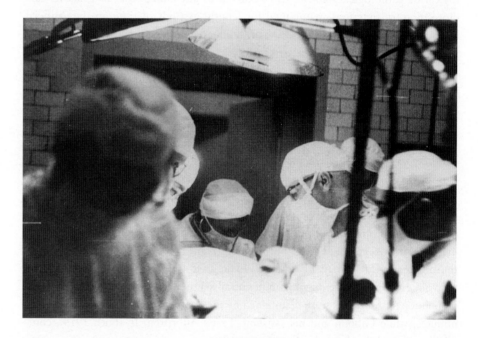

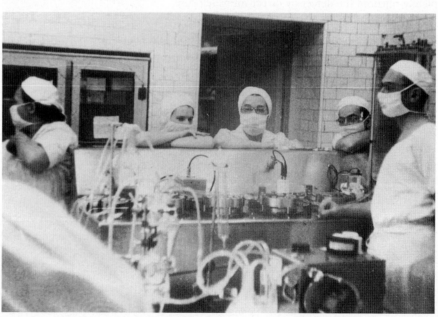

8. John Heysham Gibbon, Jr. *(right center in the full white mask)* and Frank Allbritten, Jr. *(left center, partially obscured in a white mask) (top)* and their operating room team *(surrounding the heart-lung apparatus) (bottom)* during the first successful cardiac bypass surgery using a pump oxygenator, May 6, 1953. *(Thomas Jefferson University Archives, Philadelphia, PA)*

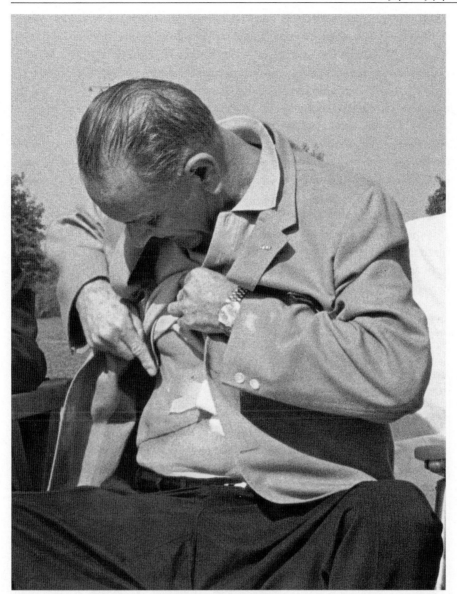

Increasing press coverage of developments in American surgery was particularly evident following President Dwight Eisenhower's surgical procedure for intestinal obstruction secondary to regional enteritis. It was an altogether risky situation, involving a surgical controversy over bypass versus excision of the involved ileal segment, and was made more difficult by the fact that the president had suffered a severe myocardial infarction just nine months previously. After the president had endured crampy lower abdominal pains for over twenty-four hours, a series of x-rays demonstrated an unrelenting small bowel obstruction. At 2:20 in the morning on June 9, 1956, an exploratory laparotomy revealed "30-40 cm. of the terminal ileum involved by a chronic, dry type of regional enteritis." The surgical team at Walter Reed General Hospital, which included Isidor Ravdin, completed an ileotransverse colostomy performed in continuity approximately 12 to 15 cm. proximal to the diseased small intestine. The president's course was generally uneventful, except for a prolonged ileus necessitating use of a nasogastric tube until the fifth postsurgical day, at which time he was also allowed to begin transacting official state business. Eisenhower was discharged on the twenty-first day after his operation.

What made this event so unique was that a sitting President had undergone an abdominal operation for the first time in the annals of American surgery. Significantly, not only were the intra- and perioperative periods free of untoward difficulties, but the entire saga and safe outcome of Eisenhower's surgery was dramatically reported by the press corps. Banner headlines in the *New York Times* of June 10th read: **Doctors Say President Can Run; Condition "Most**

Satisfactory;" Hospital Stay Is Put At 15 Days. The following day, Eisenhower's surgical condition remained page one news: **President Walks 30 Feet With Aid And Sits In Chair**. In the midst of all this hullabaloo, it was the surgeon who reigned supreme. One reporter ascribed to Leonard Heaton (1902–1983), leader of the surgical team, a savoir-faire complimentary to the world of surgery at large: "At the end, as at the start, he appeared to be the coolest and perhaps the calmest person in the room, which had been heated to oven-like temperatures by klieg lights and the presence of about seventy reporters and photographers." There was little doubting that the Eisenhower episode helped allay society's fear of the surgical unknown and put surgical science in a positive light as an accepted part of established medical treatment.

Less than a decade later, in October 1965, President Lyndon Johnson (1908–1973) underwent an elective cholecystectomy that was regarded as so routine the surgical event barely caused a ripple in the daily life of the nation. A few days later, in an act of surgical machismo, Johnson proudly displayed his six-inch incision to a news photographer. With a picture of the president of the United States showing off

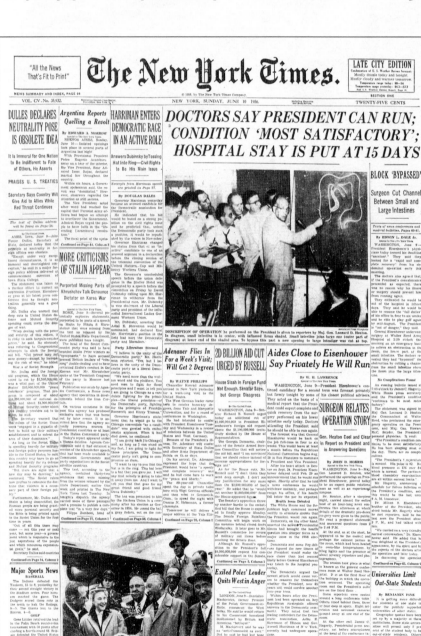

10. *(left)* June 10, 1956, *The New York Times;* *(right)* October 9–10, 1965, *The New York Times. (Courtesy of the New York Times)*

his newly acquired "trophy" splashed across virtually every newspaper and magazine in the country, could there be any lingering question about the social acceptability of surgery?

Although success and approbation in the biomedical sciences are difficult to achieve, one measure of both in the twentieth century has been the awarding of the Nobel Prize in Medicine and Physiology. In 1990, Joseph Murray (born 1919) won the coveted honor and became the second native-born American surgeon to be so recognized. Murray was cited for his discovery of "organ and cell transplantation in the treatment of human disease," specifically the first successful transplants of vascularized human organs. A graduate of Harvard Medical School (1943), Murray served as a major at the Valley Forge General Hospital from 1944 to 1947. Returning to his alma mater, where he received his surgical training, Murray was board certified in general surgery in 1952 and plastic and reconstructive surgery in 1954. By 1970 he had risen to the rank of full professor of surgery at Harvard Medical School and chaired the plastic and reconstructive surgery department at the Harvard-affiliated Peter Bent Brigham and Boston Children's Hospitals. Murray

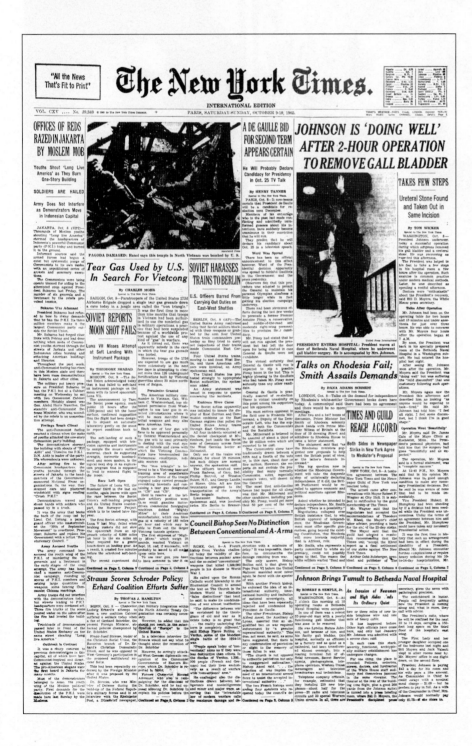

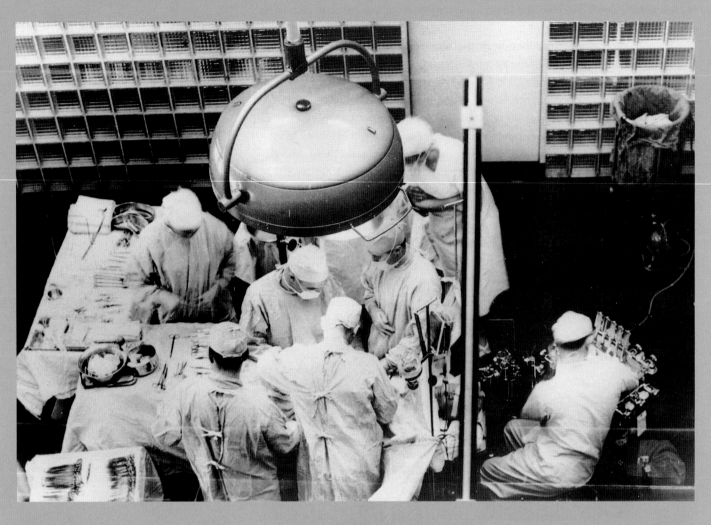

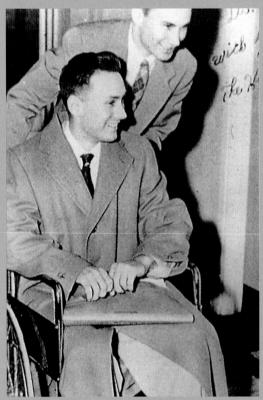

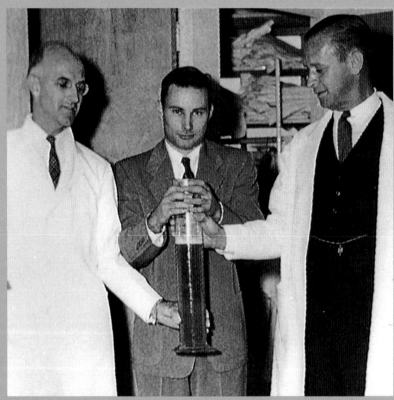

retired from the active clinical faculty in 1989 and has since served in an emeritus status. His numerous other honors include serving as president of the American Association of Plastic Surgeons in 1964 and chairing the American Board of Plastic and Reconstructive Surgery in 1969.

The efforts of both Gibbon and Murray were aided by two unique features of American surgical research after World War II: large-scale federal government funding of basic science and clinical investigative projects and the widespread availability of dogs and other animals (e.g., primates) as ideal laboratory models. Not surprisingly, during this era of American surgical supremacy, funding by the National Institutes of Health, via its Surgical Study Section for such projects as extracorporeal circulation and transplantation of organs, was at its peak. The latter undertaking, however, would come to represent the epitome of modern-day surgical élan. After all, in the late 1940s and early 1950s, the very thought of surgically replacing diseased or worn-out body parts with healthy organs verged on scientific fantasy.

For Murray, the three renal transplant operations lauded by the Nobel committee had been preceded by vast amounts of experimental and clinical work conducted by both himself and others. For instance, several unsuccessful attempts at kidney transplantation in humans, using organs obtained from fresh cadavers, were carried out between 1936 and 1951. In each case, the implanted kidney was summarily rejected by its host through a series of intervening immunological events. The result was always the same: blood appeared in the urine, production of urine decreased, and the kidney shut down. Before Murray began his particular research efforts at the Peter Bent Brigham Hospital, David Hume (1917–1973) and John Merrill (1917–1986), working in the same surgical department and under the admirable direction of Francis Moore (born 1913), the newest in a line of distinguished Moseley Professors of Surgery, had transplanted cadaver kidneys by inserting them into a pocket fashioned in the thigh skin of patients. These surgical pioneers, laboring without an understanding of tissue matching or an availability of biochemical immunosuppressants, in addition to the fact that the anastomosis of renal vessels to femoral artery and vein as well as the ureter's drainage of urine onto the skin were anatomically unsatisfactory, miraculously managed to achieve a six-month success in one patient.

Shortly after completing his residency, Murray began to focus his formidable technical skills on the problem of improving kidney transplant outcomes by situating the new organ within the abdomen. This would become an essential step in the research process, since the orthotopic location (the normal or usual position) is virtually impossible to recreate for kidney transplantation. Utilizing the method of autotransplantation in dogs with contralateral nephrectomy (removing both kidneys, but then reanastomosing one in a different position while the other is destroyed), Murray showed that such an implanted kidney would function perfectly well for a prolonged time. Having secured this technical insight, Murray was still confronted with the staggering problem of tissue immunology. He was forced to become familiar with the implications of rejected human-to-human skin grafts, incompatible blood transfusions, and the freemartin phenomenon. The last is an immunological rule stating that when two persons who as fetuses shared blood in the placental mix, even though they are neither genetically identical nor monozygotic, they can accept each other's tissue for transplantation. Still, from a genetic point of view, the ideal situation for any organ transplant would be identical twins, in whom blood and tissue types were compatible.

In the fall of 1954, a twenty-four-year-old man dying of renal failure was admitted to the Peter Bent Brigham Hospital. The individual had a healthy twin brother, and tests were conducted to verify whether the two brothers were indeed identical twins. The results, most notably a successful skin graft from the healthy to the sick twin, confirmed the immunological suspicion of identicality. Although the patient had been initially maintained by an artificial kidney, his condition eventually deteriorated to the point where it was decided to proceed with the procedure of last resort:

11. *(facing page)* The first successful kidney transplantation in a human being, December 23, 1954. Joseph Murray stands on the patient's right. Opposite Murray is his first assistant, John Rowbotham; to his left is Edward Gray; and to Murray's left is Dan Pugh. Leroy Vandam *(back turned)* is the anesthetist. In the upper right is Edith Comiskey, the circulating nurse, and upper left, Miss Rhodes, the scrub nurse *(top)*. A few weeks later the joyous Herrick twins *(donor Ronald pushing his recipient brother Richard)* leave the Peter Bent Brigham Hospital *(bottom left)*. Celebrating the successful outcome and making claims about the new kidney's urinary output are Murray *(left)*, Ronald Herrick *(middle)*, and J. Hartwell Harrison *(right)* *(bottom right)*. *(Collection of Joseph P. Murray, M.D.)*

renal transplantation. Accordingly, on a cold December day, the healthy twin's normal kidney was removed by J. Hartwell Harrison (1909–1984), and ninety minutes later Murray had transplanted the donor organ into the dying twin's body. In this instance, the kidney, instead of being placed into the thigh, was positioned in the surgically accessible hollow of the pelvis, while the ureter was directly implanted into the bladder so that the urine would follow a natural course rather than being drained to the outside. Although seemingly simple in hindsight, these were all innovative technical surgical details that Murray had previously perfected on canine models in the research laboratory. As for Murray's patient, his uremia, secondary to the buildup of poisonous waste from the previous lack of adequate kidney function, cleared up rapidly. Six weeks after this momentous surgical feat, the patient was well enough to undergo removal of his own diseased kidneys, which helped bring his blood pressure within an acceptable range. The transplanted kidney continued to function well, and over the course of the next several months, the patient gained weight and returned to normal health.

In December 1959, Murray performed the second in his triad of notable renal transplant operations. This was a procedure carried out between two fraternal, rather than identical, twins, with whole-body irradiation used to obtain immuno-suppression. Two and a half years later, the final transplant listed in the Nobel committee's citation was completed between unrelated individuals. This 1962 operation was particularly significant because azathioprine was employed as immunosuppressive chemotherapy for the kidney from a cadaver donor. It became the first prolonged successful organ transplant from a non-twin donor based on drug immunosuppression and has served as the model for essentially all organ transplants since that time.

Murray's Nobel Prize-winning efforts led to a world-wide blossoming of transplant surgery. By the end of this surgical era, a total of almost 18,000 kidney transplants had been completed, the vast number having taken place in the United States. Just fifteen years later, over 10,000 renal transplants were occurring annually in America, about 80 percent of which involved unrelated donors, all using various immunosuppressive chemotherapeutic agents. That same year (1990), there were 2,700 liver transplants, 2,100 heart transplants, 202 lung transplants, 50 heart-lung transplants, and 549 pancreas transplants. Thus, by the beginning of the last decade of the twentieth century, more than 15,000 organ transplants were being completed in this country annually with the overall number steadily increasing each year.

As enthusiastically as the American public received each new surgical triumph, there were also several unseemly developments. Such difficulties usually arose as a result of the commercial exploitation of surgical procedures by persons who lack an adequate scientific or ethical background. This occurs because surgery sometimes lends itself to hasty endorsements and initial overapplications. As a result, many surgical operations have been performed for years based on minimal scientific rationale or a lack of empirical efficaciousness. The phenomenon of therapeutic abuse usually comes to a halt following harsh criticism or abandonment of the procedure from within the profession. However, this remains an unwieldy and generally ineffective manner with which to police the profession. One little discussed example of such a surgical circumstance concerns Owen Wangensteen (1898–1981) and his trumpeting, in the late 1950s and early 1960s, of the concept of "gastric freezing" as a cure for peptic ulcer disease. Wangensteen, a graduate of the University of Minnesota School of Medicine (1922), spent virtually his entire career at his alma mater. Recognized as one of America's true surgical geniuses, he assumed the chairmanship of the university's department of surgery at the age of thirty-one and held the post for thirty-seven years. He made many investigative and clinical contributions; among his most important written works is *The Therapeutic Problem in Bowel Obstruction: A Physiological and Clinical Consideration* (1935). Wangensteen, much like William Halsted before him, brought his department to a position of world renown as a center for innovative research and a veritable training ground for a generation

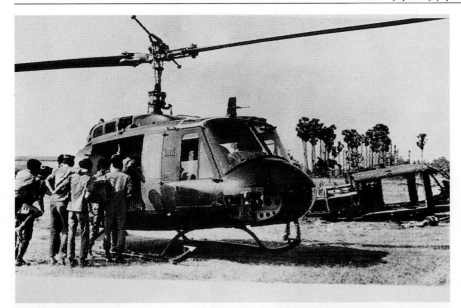

12. The ability to expeditiously evacuate wounded soldiers has always been a key component of any successful military campaign. In the Vietnam War, the routine use of helicopters enabled a traumatized individual to be on an operating room table within minutes of the injury. This was a far cry from the hand-held litter and horse-drawn cart evacuations of the Civil War or the motorized ambulances of World Wars I and II. *(Courtesy of Stanley B. Burns, M.D., and The Burns Collection and Archive)*

of surgical leaders, particularly in abdominal, cardiac, and transplant surgery. Following his retirement in 1967, Wangensteen concentrated his efforts in the field of surgical history and, together with his wife, wrote the classic text *The Rise of Surgery, From Empiric Craft to Scientific Discipline* (1978). Wangensteen was intimately involved with the surgical power structure in America, having served as president of the American College of Surgeons (1959) and the American Surgical Association (1969). In addition, he was chairman of the Surgical Study Section of the National Institutes of Health (1953) and consultant to the Surgeon General of the United States (1956–1967).

Beginning in 1958, Wangensteen was tantalized by the belief that "peptic ulcer diathesis could be favorably influenced through the use of cold." It was his contention that by freezing the inside mucosal lining of the stomach, bleeding from "duodenal ulcer, gastric erosion, and gastric varices…with lesser levels of sustained effectiveness in gastric ulcer, steroid ulcer, and hemorrhagic gastritis" could be controlled. Marshalling the vast resources of his department and laboratories, Wangensteen attempted to determine the effect of gastric freezing on acid secretion, the most effective methods of producing gastric freezing, and the indications for such a "surgical" procedure. By the mid-1960s, Wangensteen and his collaborators had published almost fifty papers on the subject in the most prestigious of American surgical journals. To achieve gastric freezing, Wangensteen inserted a crescent-shaped rubber balloon through the mouth and then had it swallowed into the stomach. The device was connected to an elaborately designed mechanical apparatus that delivered coolant at an inflow temperature of -17° to -20°C.

Wangensteen, a forceful and persuasive surgical personality, was invited to give numerous guest lectures on his new "cure" for peptic ulcer. In the process, with his surgical colleagues clamoring to climb on board the gastric freezing craze, Wangensteen's balloons and freezing machines were sold to virtually every mid-size to large hospital in the country. Although monies had been spent on buying the devices and tens of thousands of patients were undergoing the newest in surgical fads, gastric freezing never gained widespread acceptance as a therapeutic procedure because, when empirically tested throughout the surgical community, it was found to be generally ineffective. There is little doubt that Wangensteen was a true believer in his gastric freezing methodology, but some critics contend that his scientific reasoning was partially clouded with his personal reputation at stake and the indirect financial interest he held in the development and selling of the vast army of deployed gastric freezing machines. Clearly, Wangensteen had conceived a technique in search of a disease. As gastric freezing faded from the picture, Wangensteen's apparati were consigned to the back storage rooms of hospitals or the harsh spotlights of

13. By the mid-1970s, modern aspects of surgery had allowed patients to become more blasé in their attitude toward surgical operations. This is evidenced by medical personnel performing minor surgery on a crewman while he reads a book in sick bay on board the amphibious assault ship U.S.S. *Guadalcanal*. *(U.S. Naval Historical Center)*

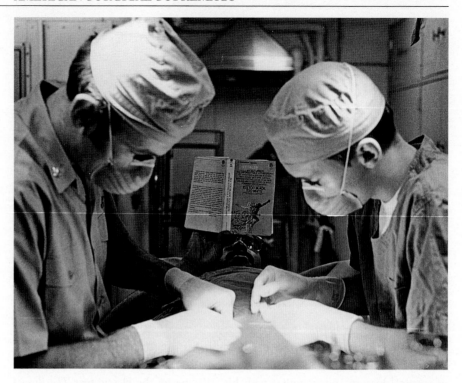

medical museums, where they joined a long list of dubious surgical inventions. What this entire expensive episode points out is how readily a surgical operation can be embraced by the profession, strictly on the strength of a master surgeon's proselytizing, even when the scientific and empirical evidence supporting its purported intent are problematic.

SOCIOECONOMIC INFLUENCES

The 1950s and 1960s witnessed some of the most magnificent advances in the history of American surgery, but by the 1970s, socioeconomic changes were starting to overshadow many of the clinical triumphs. It was the beginning of a schizophrenic existence for surgeons: complex and dramatic life-saving operations were performed by surgeons who received innumerable accolades, while concurrently, public criticism of the economics of medicine, in particular surgical practice, portrayed the scalpel bearer as an acquisitive, financially-driven, selfish individual. This was in sharp contrast to the relatively selfless and sanctified image of the American doctor prior to the growth of specialty work and the introduction of government involvement in health care delivery. Although they are philosophically inconsistent, the dramatic and theatrical features of surgery that make surgeons heroes from one perspective, and symbols of corruption, mendacity, and greed from the opposite point of view, are the very reasons why society demands so much of its surgeons. There is the precise and definitive nature of surgical intervention, the expectation of success that surrounds an operation, the short time frame in which outcomes are realized, the high income levels of most surgeons, and the almost insatiable inquisitiveness by lay individuals concerning all aspects of the act of consensually cutting into another human being's flesh. These phenomena, ever more sensitized in an age of mass media and instantaneous telecommunication, make the surgeon seem more accountable than his medical colleague and, simultaneously, symbolic of the best and the worst in American medicine.

What became clear by the mid-1970s was that lay institutions (i.e., business, government, and industry), prodded by unassailable socioeconomic market forces, would from then on determine how health services were to be financed and ultimately provided, rather than medical professionals. Ominously, American surgeons, long accustomed to a cottage industry mentality of small-scale private practices with fee-for-service payment schemes, were stagnating in a political thought process at least two to three decades behind the social and economic implications of increasing specialization and rapidly rising health care costs. Organized surgery had long viewed itself as the proper interpreter of the nation's surgical health. However, public interest was rapidly emerging as the dominant decision maker, and surgical leaders appeared unattuned to the changes about to engulf their profession.

The establishment of the Medicare and Medicaid health care insurance plans in 1965 signaled a watershed in the long history of medical and surgical professionalism in the United States. Created by President Lyndon Johnson's administration as part of his Great Society social reforms, the programs were bitterly opposed by the American Medical Association and the American College of Surgeons, with physicians in every specialty threatening to go on strike when the plans were to be implemented in 1966. The vociferousness of their arguments reflected more than a rationalization of pecuniary shortsightedness or vested interests. Instead, it was a knee-jerk reaction to the long-standing tradition that organized medicine was the sole arbiter of the country's medical well being. For two centuries, the federal government had essentially abdicated any direct responsibility for the daily management of the health care delivery system. Suddenly, things were about to change, and the sinecure-like appeal of medicine no longer seemed apparent. More to the point, the cohesiveness of the profession, which had been so vital to its past political successes, was beginning to noticeably unravel.

Initially, what surgeons could not first perceive about Medicare soon became a welcome reality. The new system was going to make them wealthier than they had ever been in the past. As the government's insurance plan expanded, income levels never before deemed possible were being attained by surgeons in every specialty area. However, with health care costs rising out of control, economic dilemmas soon displaced scientific progress as the focus of public attention. Distorted fee structures, which grossly favored the performance of manually performed procedures over cognitive services (i.e., talking to patients), heightened the already existing economic biases in the health care system. Consequently, simple economic facts of life encouraged young doctors to enter surgical specialties and procedure-oriented medical fields such as radiology, gastroenterology, and cardiology in greater numbers than society truly needed. There was a skewing of resources with surgeons and medical procedurists claiming an ever larger percentage of both government and commercial insurance dollars.

Within a few years, the cost of both Medicare and Medicaid exceeded all original calculations. Figures for 1970 placed the expenditure level of Medicare at $5.5 billion (original estimate, $2.9 billion) and the price tag for Medicaid similarly at $5.5 billion (original estimate, $3.5 billion). The escalation continued. Within five years, the rapidly increasing costs under Medicare and Medicaid brought the entire health care industry under greater critical financial scrutiny than ever before. With the federal government fast becoming the single major procurer of health services, it was inevitable that elected officials would have to intervene in unprecedented ways. By 1971, President Richard Nixon (1913–1994) was already calling for Medicare cutbacks as part of his economic stabilization program, including a 2.5 percent annual increase cap on physicians' fees and the establishment of health maintenance organizations as a new method to control health costs.

Despite its clinical supremacy, the American profession of surgery was on the verge of losing its hard-earned mandate. No longer the master of its own fate, surgery was becoming divided, not just between academic medicine and private practice but, more significantly, from an inter-subspecialty perspective. No longer did a single unifying voice speak for the American surgeon. The blossoming of specialization had eroded the support base of the American College of Surgeons. Since its founding, the College had promoted itself as representing all surgical specialties, particularly when its membership roles encompassed a large number of surgeons in the subspecialties.

By the 1970s, specialty societies such as the American College of Obstetricians and Gynecologists, the American Orthopedic Association, and the American Urological Association had usurped this role, being perceived by their constituents as better able to articulate the clinical and socioeconomic difficulties that confronted the specific specialties. With subspecialists providing larger amounts of financial support to their own societies, the American College of Surgeons became increasingly unable to galvanize the whole of surgery relative to major issues of the day.

It is ironic that in the United States, a country much slower than its European counterparts to recognize surgeons as a distinct group of clinicians separate from physicians, the move toward surgical specialization and subspecialization was ultimately pursued with alacrity and forcefulness. Yet, it is this unimpeded fragmentation into increasingly focused surgical specialty societies (e.g., Society for Pediatric

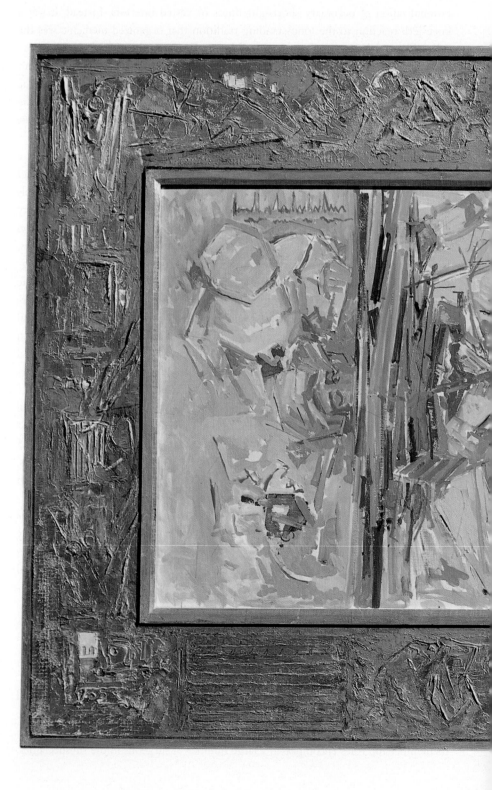

14. "Open heart surgery." This oil, gold leaf, and silver leaf on canvas by Lamar Dodd incorporates implements of heart surgery into the surrounding gilded "border." *(Collection of the artist and permission of W. Robert Nix, photographer)*

Urology, American Society of Ophthalmic Plastic & Reconstructive Surgery, American Society for Surgery of the Hand) that contributes to the present lack of political unison within the profession. Accordingly, unless a clear and demonstrable intercommunication is established between all the disparate specialties and subspecialties, the survival of surgery as a unified discipline remains in jeopardy.

Surgeons circumvented Nixon's wage and price controls by raising fees and, some critics would argue, by performing additional and perhaps unnecessary operations. This occurred because the structure of the surgical market place before the 1970s was such that surgeons were not bound by normal supply-and-demand curve economics. In the business world, the price of a product results from an interplay of supply and demand in a free market setting. Prices should be high when the demand is comparatively great and low when the supply is relatively large. As the absolute

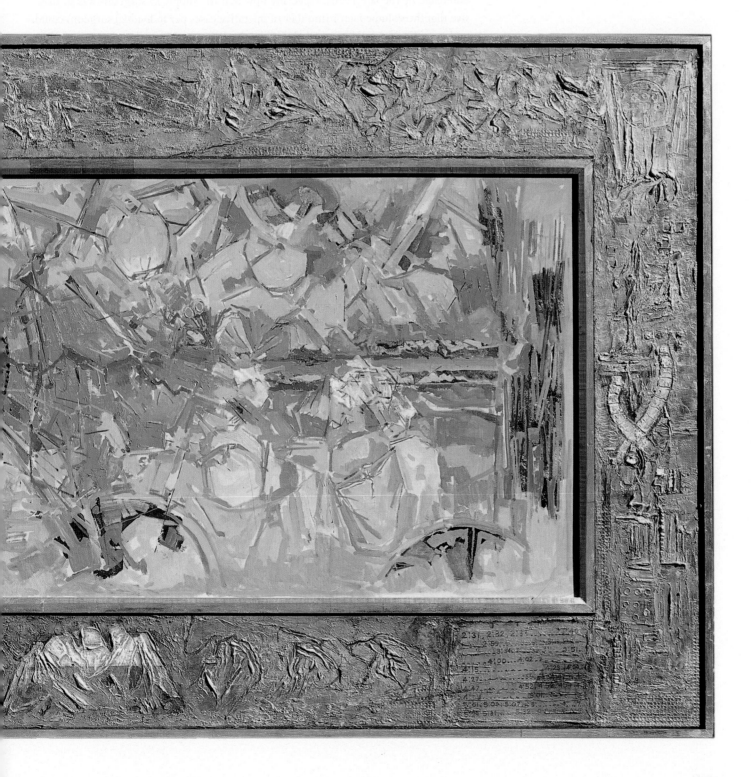

number of surgeons began to increase in the post- World War II era, surgical fees should theoretically have decreased. The reality was that the exact opposite happened. Not only did surgeons manage to increase their operative fees in response to normal inflation, but with the growing social acceptance of surgical intervention, ever-greater numbers of operations were being performed. From 1970 to 1974, the total supply of general surgeons increased 5 percent while the absolute number of general surgical operations increased 16 percent. Similar sequelae were noted in every surgical subspecialty, ranging from a 7 percent increase in obstetrician-gynecologists accompanied by a 40 percent increase in obstetric-gynecologic operations to a 15 percent gain in orthopedic surgeons while numbers of orthopedic cases rose 28 percent. Not unexpectedly, surgeons prospered in this type of environment and enjoyed spectacular income levels throughout most of the era of surgical supremacy.

The economic scenario of the 1960s and early to mid-1970s was becoming untenable by the late 1970s, especially now that the supply of surgeons was so massive that the volume factor (number of operative cases per individual surgeon) could no longer be positively controlled. Unlike the 1970 to 1974 period, a converse situation (fewer procedures per individual surgeon) was present. From 1979 to 1985, the total number of general surgical operations increased just 1 percent while the absolute number of general surgeons increased 19 percent. The same effect was noted in every surgical subspecialty, including a 2 percent decrease in the number of urologic operations in face of a 22 percent increase in urologists, as well as a 26 percent decrease in otolaryngologic cases with a 19 percent rise in otolaryngologists. If American surgeons were to maintain high income levels and prosper financially in this new era of social and economic transformation, then they were left with only one viable option: an escalation of fees far beyond that of any reasonable inflation factor. This distorted pricing system, without evidence of effective restraint, left surgeons in a particularly vulnerable position, especially when general dissatisfaction with excessive medical costs beckoned strong societal and political corrective action.

With surgeons forced to practice in this increasingly controlled environment, it was only natural that queries about the overall efficacy and efficiency of surgical health care delivery were being raised. Concerns were directed to three areas: (1) increasing doubts over the necessity and appropriateness of many surgically related services, (2) recognition that surgical care may contain important differentials in the quality of service and results achieved, and (3) questions about how to deliver appropriate surgical services in the most cost-efficient manner consistent with high-quality results. By 1975, political decision makers made it clear the delivery of surgical health care was about to become a priority in federal policy and research. The future evolution of surgery would become more affected by socioeconomic and governmental factors, in contrast to the past's unique clinical accomplishments. More pointedly, the vast socioeconomic and political transformation that engulfed all of American medicine, now appears to control the fate of the individual surgeon to a greater degree than surgeons, as a collective force, are able to direct their own profession.

With socioeconomic concerns assuming greater relevance in the delivery of surgical health care, it was not long before surgically oriented studies were being completed on various administrative and management-related topics. A 1973 report by Jack Wennberg and Alan Gittelsohn, two nonsurgeons, demonstrated extreme geographic variations, up to 1,000 percent, in the patterns of use of nine common surgical procedures in the states of Vermont and Maine. These authors even proposed the concept of "population at risk of organ loss" as a major component in determining realistic age- and sex-standardized surgical rates. Their principle reflects the fact that once a person has undergone an operation for removal of an organ, he or she can no longer be considered at risk for a similar procedure. So high was the risk of organ loss that the estimated percentage of women in certain states with an intact uterus by age sixty years was only 64 percent.

Much of the surgical health services research of the early 1970s pointed to a growing concern about the rapid and continuous rise in rates of elective surgical operations. Studies of the problem had proved contradictory relative to the exact amount of change, but nonetheless there was a sense that rates of surgical procedures and subsequent health care expenditures needed to be controlled. It is rare that publication of a single article in a medical journal can stimulate fundamental changes in the health care delivery system. But in December 1974, such an article appeared in *The New England Journal of Medicine*, detailing the results of an investigation concerning pre-surgical screening consultations, commonly termed second opinion programs. By having a patient, previously recommended for elective surgery, undergo a second surgical opinion, it was found that almost one-quarter of all surgical procedures cleared by one surgeon were not confirmed by the second surgeon. The reaction to the paper was immediate and centered on purported cost savings that could be realized by decreasing elective surgical rates through second opinion programs. Within a few years, most state Medicaid systems had recruited surgeons to provide second opinions. Over 50 percent of the nation's Blue Cross-Blue Shield plans instituted mandatory second opinion consultations for their insured population. Nationally, the federal government established a 24-hour toll-free telephone service to answer any questions and direct a patient to a second surgical opinion. For certain operations such as coronary artery bypass, hemorrhoidectomy, hernia repair, hysterectomy, and varicose vein procedures, Medicare mandated that second opinions be obtained before any patient could be finally certified for surgery.

Second opinion programs rapidly invaded the daily routines of most surgeons and thus exemplified how modern-day economic pressures can readily impact on the practice of surgery. In many aspects, second opinion programs proved helpful to the surgeon. They made patients more cognizant of the surgical credentialing process, including board certification. Programs were instrumental in reinforcing the many positive aspects of patient autonomy that have affected surgery throughout the United States. Whether these undertakings increased the overall quality of surgical health care has yet to be resolved. Second opinion programs were originally intended to curb health care costs, but there has been no confirmatory evidence that this occurred. For many elective operations, it was clearly redundant to require second opinions. Consultations for obvious groin hernias, stones in the gallbladder, or cancer of the uterus represented duplication of individual effort and caused dollars to be expended in needless and often pointless second opinions. However, what second opinion programs lacked in economic effect they made up in a practical sense by measurably affecting the surgeon's daily work routine. Surgeons were forced to deliver health care in a more fiscally prudent but patient-friendlier environment. Most importantly, second opinion programs proved a harbinger of the socioeconomic and political transformation that would overwhelm all of American surgery in the 1980s and 1990s.

1975	1980	1985	1990	1995	2000

Apollo 18 docks with *Soyuz 19,*
first joint United States and Russian
manned space endeavor *(1975)*

Women win 13 of 32 Rhodes scholarships
given to Americans; first time the award
is available to women *(1976)*

Legionnaires' disease kills 29 persons
in Philadelphia *(1977)*

Mass murder-suicide of 911 individuals
at Peoples Temple, Jonestown, Guyana *(1978)*

Three Mile Island nuclear power plant
disaster near Middletown, Pennsylvania *(1979)*

Winter Olympics held in Lake Placid,
New York *(1980)*

12,000 air traffic controllers go on strike
and are dismissed *(1981)*

Disney World, Florida, opens EPCOT
(Experimental Community of Tomorrow) *(1982)*

United States loses yachting's America's Cup
Race after 132 years of unbroken victories:
Australia II beats *Liberty,* 4 races to 3 *(1983)*

Standard Oil of California acquires Gulf for
$13.2 billion; world's largest corporate merger
(1984)

Pete Rose makes the 4,192nd hit of his
baseball career, breaking Ty Cobb's record
set in 1928 *(1985)*

Space shuttle *Challenger* explodes on
takeoff *(1986)*

Black Monday: Wall Street's Dow Jones Index
falls by 508 points, a 23 percent decline *(1987)*

Fires burn 88,000 acres of Yellowstone National
Park *(1988)*

Exxon Valdez disaster in Alaska causes
the world's largest oil spill (11 million gallons)
(1989)

Vincent Van Gogh's *Portrait of Dr. Gachet*
is sold in New York City for a world record
amount of $82.5 million *(1990)*

Carl Lewis leads United States athletes
at Tokyo Olympics *(1991)*

Supreme court reaffirms a woman's
right to abortion *(1992)*

World Trade Center is bombed by
Islamic terrorist group *(1993)*

Major earthquake hits Los Angeles
region, causing widespread destruction
(1994)

Federal office building in Oklahoma
City is destroyed by terrorist bomb,
causing 168 deaths *(1995)*

Historic blizzard of '96 buries
the American Northeast in
thirty-plus inches of snow *(1996)*

Hale-Bopp comet inspires group
suicide of 39 Heaven's Gate
members who hope to catch
spaceship travelling in its wake
(1997)

DAILY LIFE

U.S.A. POPULATION

1980 = 227 million

1990 = 249 million

2000 = estimated to reach
275 million

HISTORY AND POLITICS

Attorney General John Mitchell and presidential aides John Ehrlichman and H. R. Haldeman are found guilty of perjury, conspiracy, and obstruction of justice in the Watergate coverup and receive jail sentences *(1975)*

Jimmy Carter and Walter Mondale are elected president and vice president, respectively *(1976)*

Presidential pardon given to most draft evaders of the Vietnam War period *(1977)*

Senate ratifies new Panama Canal treaty, giving full control of the Canal to Panama in 1999 *(1978)*

50 hostages taken by Islamic fundamentalists at United State embassy in Teheran, Iran *(1979)*

Chrysler Corporation receives government-guaranteed $400 million loan *(1980)*

John Hinckley attempts to assassinate President Ronald Reagan *(1981)*

Dedication of the Vietnam Veterans' War Memorial in Washington, D.C., with the names of more than 58,000 dead inscribed on the black monument *(1982)*

President Reagan dubs the Soviet Union the "Evil Empire" and proposes a new antimissile defense system, the Strategic Defense Initiative (nicknamed "Star Wars") *(1983)*

Ronald Reagan resoundingly defeats Walter Mondale in the presidential election *(1984)*

A Trans World Airline jet is hijacked by Arab terrorists, who hold 39 American passengers hostage for 17 days *(1985)*

President Reagan admits secret arms deals with Iran in breach of the U. S. embargo (the "Irangate" scandal) *(1986)*

For the first time in history, the proposed budget of the United States is over one trillion dollars *(1987)*

The U.S.S. *Vincennes* mistakenly shoots down an Iranian airliner over the Persian Gulf, resulting in 290 fatalities *(1988)*

President George Bush and Premier Mikhail Gorbachev hold a two-day summit in Malta *(1989)*

Panamanian General Manuel Noriega surrenders to United States troops and is extradited on drug-trafficking charges *(1990)*

United States and Allied soldiers destroy Iraqi Army in the Persian Gulf War *(1991)*

Bill Clinton defeats incumbent George Bush in the presidential election *(1992)*

President Clinton hosts Yitzhak Rabin, Prime Minister of Israel, and Yasir Arafat, Chairman of the Palestine Liberation Organization at the White House in signing of Middle East peace accord *(1993)*

United States troops land in Haiti and restore Jean-Bertrand Aristide as president *(1994)*

Bosnia peace treaty requires sending of U. S. troops to enforce agreement *(1995)*

U.S. Congress passes bill to severely restrict welfare benefits *(1996)*

Supreme Court rules that a sitting President can be sued for actions outside the scope of his official duties *(1997)*

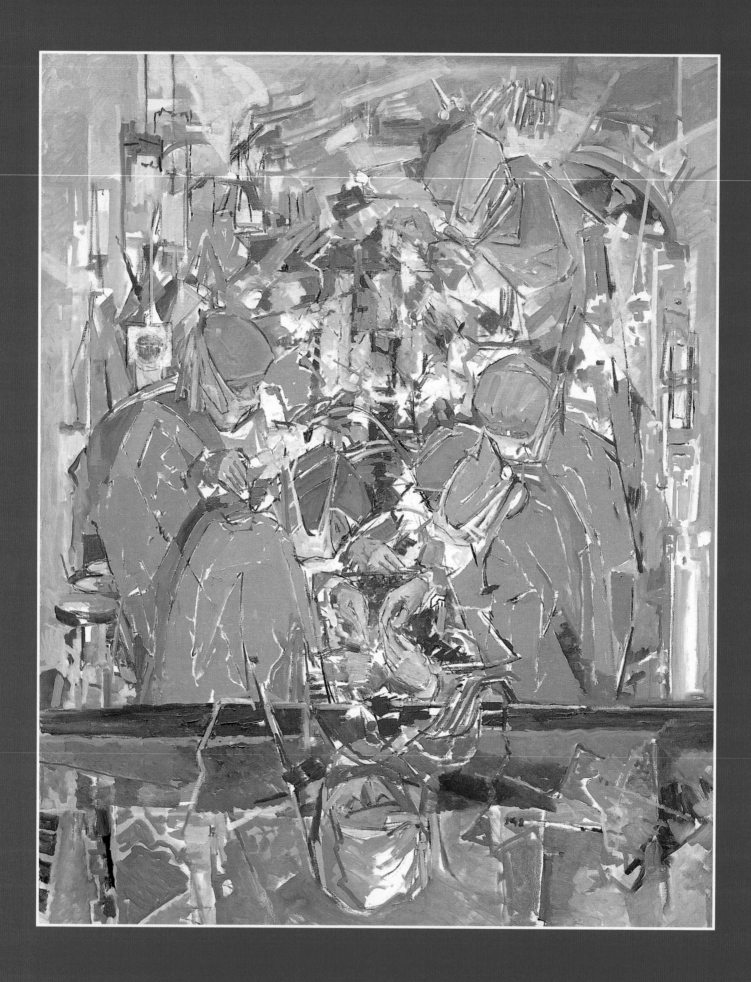

CHAPTER 12

SOCIOECONOMIC AND POLITICAL TRANSFORMATION
1975–1997

The socioeconomic and political transformation of American medicine in the 1980s and 1990s brought harsh financial times to its surgeons. Highlighted by economic concerns that had not previously affected the profession, the relationships between surgeons and their patients also changed from fairly simple to numbingly complex. Many of these fundamental restructurings were stimulated by the advent of a strong consumers' movement, which contributed to articles appearing in the lay press, government publications, and scientific journals alluding to the performance of certain common surgical procedures without proper clinical and pathological justification. In January 1976, a Congressional study, *Cost and Quality of Health Care: Unnecessary Surgery*, provoked a huge storm of criticism regarding surgical health care in the United States. The report concluded that "second opinion consultations before surgery can cut down on unnecessary surgical procedures...surgical payments by the fee-for-service mechanism encourages surgery in questionable situations...there were approximately 2.4 million unnecessary surgeries performed in 1974 at a cost to the American public of almost $4 billion, and...these unnecessary surgeries led to 11,900 deaths." In the same month, a five-part series of front page articles in the *New York Times* featured sensational accusations of both unnecessary and incompetent surgery, with the reporter writing that "at least some surgeons 'make work' for themselves by doing operations that are unnecessary."

One of the great illusions of surgeons in the mid-1970s was that federal government policies were the cause of these problems. From 1975 to 1977, a series of Medicare amendments seemed to justify this position: Section 222 supported mandatory rate-setting programs, Section 223 disallowed any costs unnecessary to efficient delivery of health care, and the Professional Standards Review Organizations monitored quality of federally funded care. However, this was an overly simplistic reaction to an ever-expanding loss of professional autonomy brought about by a scrambled series of socioeconomic events. Even though this era of surgical transformation lacks the benefit of a mature historical perspective, it seems evident that leaders of the profession were generally unwilling to acknowledge that the looming surplus of surgeons could contribute to their loss of traditional patient control. Nothing points to this lack of understanding better than the profession's own self-analysis, the massive *Study on Surgical Services for the United States (SOSSUS)*.

The roots of *SOSSUS* go back to January 1969, when Owen Wangensteen, as president of the American Surgical Association, appointed a committee chaired by Jonathan Rhoads (born 1907), John Rhea Barton professor of surgery at the

1. *(facing page)* "Operation Proceeding Number 2" (circa, 1978–1979). The style of Lamar Dodd (1909–1996), chairman emeritus of the Department of Art at the University of Georgia, ranged from near-abstraction to moody realism. *(Collection of the artist and permission of W. Robert Nix, photographer)*

University of Pennsylvania, to study the future course of that organization. Rhoads's report in April 1970 recommended a broad approach to the major issues facing surgery in the United States. This led to the formation of a committee on issues under the chairmanship of George Zuidema (born 1928), successor to Alfred Blalock at The Johns Hopkins Hospital. At the same time, the American College of Surgeons' Board of Regents appointed a steering committee on distribution and adequacy of surgical health care delivery under the chairmanship of Francis Moore. As these two parallel studies began, it became obvious to members of both organizations that the duplicative efforts could be pursued more effectively by combining the resources of the two associations. In July 1970, a somewhat uneasy alliance was formalized, and *SOSSUS* came into existence with Zuidema as chairman and Moore as vice-chairman.

The five-year effort should have represented one of American surgery's finest hours. With the stated aim of gathering data on all aspects of surgical manpower; organization, delivery, and financing of surgical services; legal and ethical issues in surgery; community-physician relations; interprofessional relations; surgical research; quality of surgical care; and government relations, *SOSSUS* was meant to be the most introspective analysis in which any segment of American medicine had ever engaged. It was massive in scope and intent. Over 10,000 surgeons were questioned concerning their practice habits and daily work schedules. In addition, an in-depth analysis of surgery in four diverse geographic areas of the country was completed on another 2,700 physicians. The results of *SOSSUS* were presented in a three-volume, hardbound, 2782-page report in the spring of 1976.

The findings were startling, particularly the data on workloads and manpower. Surgeons were found to be vastly underemployed and their services underutilized. Approximately 15 percent of the nation's active board-certified surgical specialists carried out fewer than fifty operations a year, and 31 percent between 100 to 199, or fewer than four per week. Just slightly more than 33 percent performed two hundred or more procedures. Even more worrisome was that 25 percent of physicians who perform surgery in the United States did not have the established credentials of the specialty boards. The study's authors concluded that far too many physicians perform surgical operations and that the workloads of surgical specialists were much more modest than originally expected. Further, it was suggested that the total volume of operations performed in the country could be handled by a substantially smaller cadre of busier board-certified surgeons. In order to accomplish this goal, two straightforward recommendations were made: the number of training programs should be reduced and identified more closely with university centers as affiliated hospitals, and the total number of persons entering practice who have surgical board certificates should be decreased over the next ten year with many of the tasks completed by residents to be assumed by allied health personnel.

The wholly unanticipated *SOSSUS* findings were soon corroborated by other independent studies. These in turn prompted several further recommendations, closely paralleling those of the *SOSSUS*, all based on the obvious underutilization of costly and highly specialized surgical skills in the United States. As proposals to place constraints on surgical manpower became more vociferous, the *SOSSUS* recommendations were soon questioned by—of all authorities—the American College of Surgeons. In a bizarre twist of self-denial and internal surgical Machiavellianism, the College directly challenged the accuracy of certain findings by disclaiming in its September 1976 *Bulletin*: "Unreliable data such as those cited in *SOSSUS* provide a poor basis for manpower estimates or for advanced planning." Despite the fanfare associated with its publication and the quality and quantity of its data, within less than half a year of its release the *SOSSUS* had become an orphan in the world of surgical politics, permanently disowned by its creator and likely never to achieve its hoped-for impact on American surgery.

Why the American College of Surgeons refused to endorse the major findings of a study it itself had financed and organized has never been fully explained. Clearly, issues of surgical manpower have affected the College's course since its founding, and for decades its succession of leaders have espoused the easily proselytized concept that there are not too many surgeons but too many "other" individuals, that is, non-board-certified and nonsurgically trained physicians, performing surgical operations. From historical hindsight, this position in the 1970s and 1980s seems tenuous and shortsighted at best. Amid professional bitterness, Francis Moore, organizer of the *SOSSUS* section on manpower, writing in 1984 in the journal *Surgery*, viewed the surgical surplus as a realistic problem that needed to be faced squarely "rather than adopting the juvenile view that surgeons are such wonderful people that one can never imagine a situation in which there are actually too many of them."

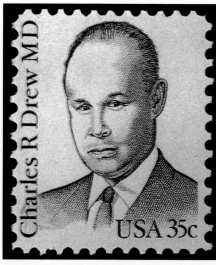

2. Charles Drew (early 1980s). *(Author's Collection)*

The generally expansionist policies for physician manpower, recommended by medical and governmental commissions and implemented by medical schools and state and federal governments during the 1960s and 1970s, had finally begun to have a noticeable effect on the delivery of United States surgical health care. By 1985, over 16,000 physicians were graduating from the country's schools of medicine each year, a figure that has since stabilized. Between 1960 and 1986, the absolute number of total physicians grew 119 percent (260,000 to 569,000) while the country's population increased just 35 percent. In 1986, there were 60 percent more physicians per 100,000 population than there had been a quarter of a century earlier. That same year, of the 569,000 physicans in the United States, 129,000 (23 percent) designated themselves as surgeons. Clearly, government and society had managed to increase the total population of physicians, but real-life economic imbalances between surgeons' and physicians' incomes skewed the number of residents entering surgical specialties. This overabundance of surgeons and undersupply of primary care physicians was partially responsible for the passage of the Health Professional Educational Assistance Act of 1976, which required medical schools to reserve training positions in internal medicine, family practice, and pediatrics in order to receive federal capitation grants.

Because of continuing concerns about the supply of physicians and the adverse effect that a surplus might have on health care expenditures, the *Graduate Medical Education National Advisory Committee (GMENAC)* was chartered in April 1976 by the federal government's Secretary of Health, Education, and Welfare. Published in 1980, *GMENAC* concurred with the *SOSSUS* findings and even provided a numerical estimate for the anticipated surplus of surgeons by specialty in 1990: general surgeons, 11,800; obstetrician-gynecologic surgeons, 1,450; orthopedic surgeons, 5,000; ophthalmologic surgeons, 4,700; neurosurgeons, 2,450; urologic surgeons, 1,650; plastic surgeons, 1,200; thoracic and cardiovascular surgeons, 850; and otolaryngologic surgeons, 500. Much criticism was directed at *GMENAC* and its methodology. However, the major findings in support of the *SOSSUS* results could not be easily discounted.

As with *SOSSUS*, no major surgical organizations came forward to lend support to the *GMENAC* findings. And, five years later (June 1985), the *Bulletin of the American College of Surgeons* carried a scathing denunciation of the *GMENAC* manpower projections. Although the College has never formally acknowledged the existence of a surplus of surgeons, their further analysis of surgeons' caseloads in 1987 showed that the average number of operative procedures completed by a general surgeon decreased 25 percent from 1982 to 1985. During the same time period, there was a decrease from 60 percent to 48 percent of general surgeons who felt that their practice workload was satisfactory. Conversely, there was an increase from 17 percent to 29 percent of general surgeons who considered their workload too light. By the late 1980s, the delivery of surgical health care was undergoing such profound changes that styles of practice could now dramatically change from one three-year period to the next.

In view of diminishing operative case loads, surgeons were forced to continually increase their fees in order to maintain income levels. This occurred at a time in the nation's economic history when health care expenditures were deemed out of con-

3. "Surgeons as Heroes." Painted by Joseph Wilder (born 1920) in 1995. This powerful portrait transforms the sometimes humdrum operative work of a surgeon into a more valorous setting. Wilder, formerly director of surgery at the Hospital for Joint Diseases and Medical Center, New York, and professor emeritus of surgery at Mount Sinai School of Medicine, has distinguished himself as an athlete, surgeon, and, most recently, painter. *(Collection of the artist)*

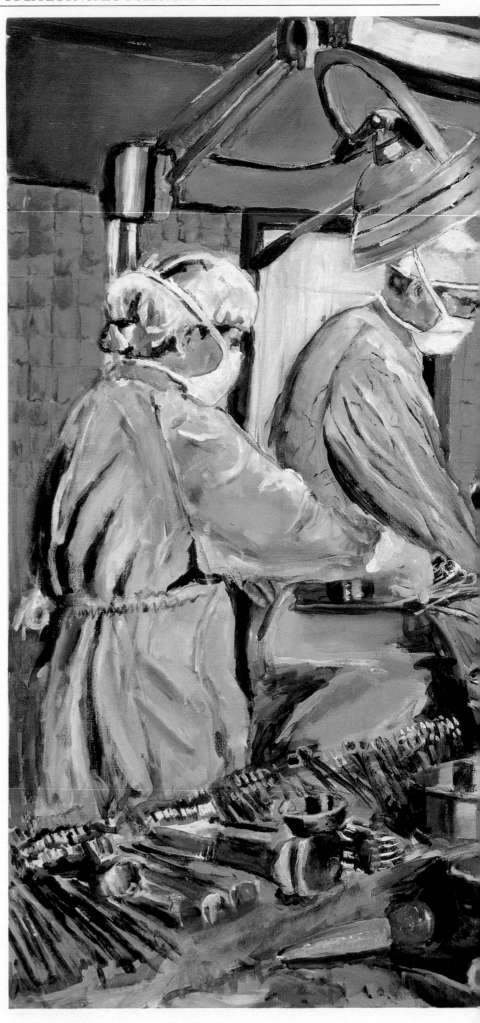

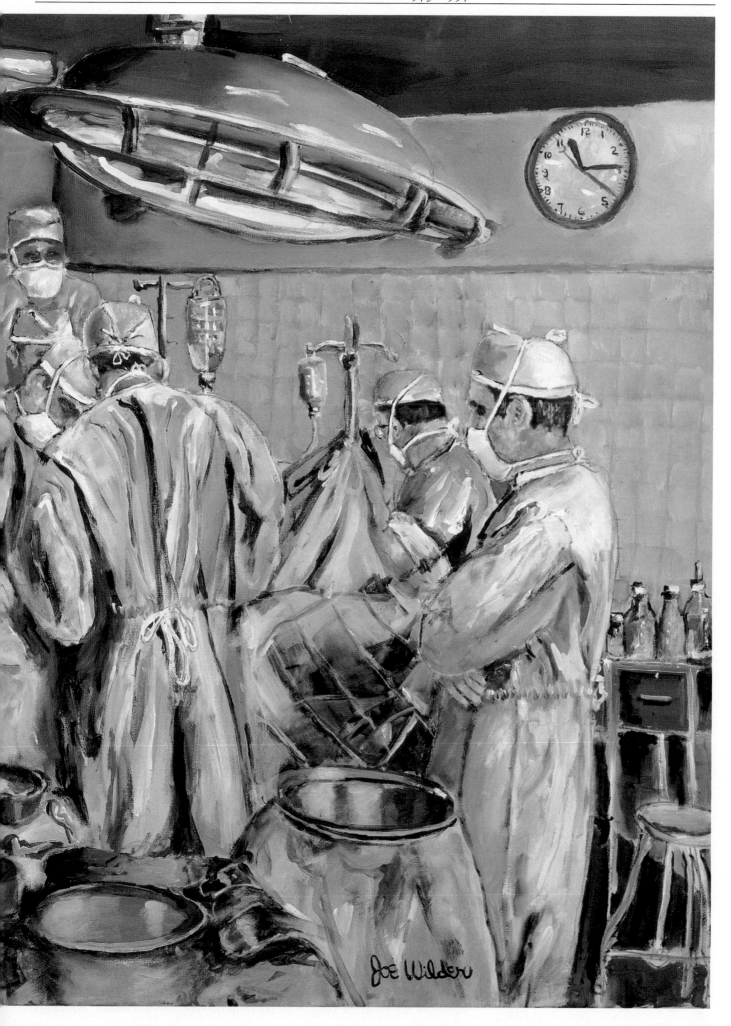

Joe Wilder

trol. In 1980, society was spending almost $300 billion annually on health care (approximately 9 percent of gross domestic product), but by the end of the decade, costs had risen to approximately $600 billion, or 12 percent of gross domestic product. In 1995, the country's health care costs broke the $1 trillion mark, or almost $3 billion daily. Few would deny that the country had overdeveloped its medical capacity and led the world in performing expensive diagnostic and therapeutic procedures. Still, there seemed no guarantee that such monumental spending assured better surgical health care for Americans. The surgeons' worst fears were slowly being realized. They were no longer able to garner increasingly larger shares of the health care dollar, and their ever-rising number was beginning to contribute to conflict and fragmentation within the profession.

CHANGES IN MEDICAL ECONOMICS

By the mid-1980s, with health expenditures rising out of control, serious attempts to ratchet down costs became especially evident. In 1984, a fifteen-month freeze on physicians' fee increases in Medicare's customary and prevailing charges was signed into law. This legislation altered the terms of physicians' participation in Medicare by requiring that they accept Medicare's reimbursement as payment in full for their services. Eight years later, Medicare started reimbursing physicians and surgeons using a relative value scale, which takes into account physician practice behavior, including price and volume of services, in an effort to establish greater control over physician payments. The results of such a system drastically restructured medical reimbursements, so that physicians receive a greater portion of the total dollar than they did in the past. Correspondingly, surgeons' incomes proportionately decreased.

To make matters even more difficult for the surgeon, in the 1990s, the reality of managed care, as typified by health maintenance organizations and other centralized insurance networks, became a growing socioeconomic force. Studies have begun to show that such entities will inevitably drive down the utilization of surgical services further by moving from a fee-for-service to a pre-paid structure. Managed care networks optimally operate with significantly lower ratios of surgeons to patients than does the country as a whole. Accordingly, when surgery is potentially avoidable, it is less likely to occur under the auspices of a managed care contract than in a less regulated system. Furthermore, the rising supply of surgeons will aggravate the already existing price advantages of managed care networks over conventional insurance, since prepayment plans will be able to hire surgeons on more favorable financial terms. As these scenarios come to fruition, the growing surplus of surgeons will be magnified even further than the *SOSSUS*, *GMENAC*, or other studies predicted.

Perhaps it is not surprising that the journal *Medical Economics* headlined, in October 1993, **Surgeons' Earnings: Are the Clouds Rolling In**? One year later, and for the first time in the post–World War II history of American surgery, the lead caption expressed a more troublesome message: **Surgeons' Earnings Take a Plunge.** According to the journal's annual wage survey, "physicians' income hasn't declined so steeply since the Great Depression" with surgical specialists netting 12 percent less than the year before. Not surprisingly, surgeons' median net earnings rose cumulatively at only half the rate of inflation. Despite it all, the average net income in 1994 still averaged $187,000 for surgical specialists, ranging from the survey's high of $244,000 for orthopedic surgeons to a low of $152,000 for general surgeons.

This era has become a confusing and distressing time for surgeons, as they can no longer anticipate steadfast increases in numbers of procedures, and they have little ability to increase their fees per case. The surplus of surgeons leaves the profession and society with seemingly unsolvable social and economic predicaments from which there is little evident escape. The oversupply of surgeons will have a potentially far-reaching impact not only on surgeons' livelihoods but, significantly, on society's ability to obtain efficient and affordable surgical health care. The simple reason for this economic conundrum concerns the time-honored maxim "experience is the best teacher." Technical surgical proficiency cannot be taught or learned through textbooks and/or passive observation at the operating room table. It can be mastered only with repetitive hands-on performance. The completion of a surgical operation can be a technically demanding feat, and studies have begun to document the relationship between a surgeon's operative volume and his or her surgical morbidity and mortality rates. For this reason, if the large number of young surgeons in today's residency system and during the formative years of practice do not have large enough patient bases to allow them to procure these skills, their technical proficiency must become suspect. It is axiomatic that surgeons, like all individuals, do best what they do most often. It becomes difficult to forsee how, in the future, a surgeon who performs just two or three major operations a week will maintain technical competency. This is perhaps one of the reasons why regionalization of surgical health care and super-specialization—that is, a surgeon's performing only one type of operation in a high-volume practice—have begun to appear on the American health care scene.

How will the problem of surgical manpower affect patients' rights? If future caseloads are decreased to the level where clinical competence can be questioned, are surgeons ethically and morally bound to inform the public of their overall experience, including complications, with particular operations? Or is it more likely that the health insurance industry will begin to employ (i.e., reimburse) only surgeons with proven clinical records, suggesting that patients will no longer have to fend for themselves in researching a surgeon's credentials? Trends do not necessarily represent fate, and images of the future sometimes reflect little more than caricatures of present-day situations. However, what clinical situations may emerge from the current perplexities involving surgical health care? As surgeons perform fewer operations, their technical skills might decline most notably for more complex but less frequently completed procedures. This could lead to increased postoperative morbidity and mortality. In any attempt to increase volume, the indications for surgical operations may become less stringent, leading to unnecessary surgery. Because of shrinking operative caseloads, surgeons may be forced to practice nonsurgical—that is, primary care—medicine to maintain their livelihoods. This will further erode their technical skills and shift them into clinical areas for which they have received little formal postgraduate training. Ultimately, society might invest more in the cost of training a surgeon than the surgeon returns to it in the way of surgical skills. Yet, if past performance is any indicator of present possibilities, it appears unlikely that the surgical supply-and-demand marketplace will respond to these concerns in the immediate future.

Instead, it is more conceivable that the current direction will inevitably produce two classes of surgeons: those who are splendid technicians and perform large numbers of surgical operations, and a larger dispirited and deprived group who complete little in the way of operative surgery. This polarization will be further aggravated, because the introduction of expenditure caps by Medicare in the 1990s and the increasing use of capitation fee structures by managed care networks implies that the financial gains of one surgeon or group of surgeons will have to come at the expense of other of their colleagues. The practice of surgery, like much of American medicine, will be more of a zero-sum financial reimbursement game, wherein every surgeon can no longer be a livelihood "winner." All this points to a potentially crippling and tragic effect on the future quality of the country's surgical health care. Solutions are difficult at best, but a proper balance of surgeons and surgical operations will have to be achieved. One fact remains certain: unless the profession and the nation are willing to confront these important questions in an expeditious manner, it is likely that further unwanted restrictions on the practice of surgery will occur, causing possible dire consequences on the overall delivery of health care.

In this era of economic, political, and social transformation, developments outside the surgeon's world jeopardize the profession's control of its own organizations and standards of clinical judgment. Ironically, this comes at a time when American

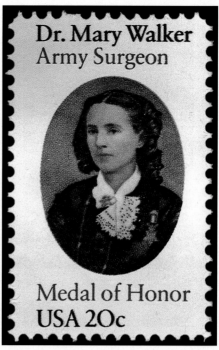

4. Mary Walker (1982). (*Author's Collection*)

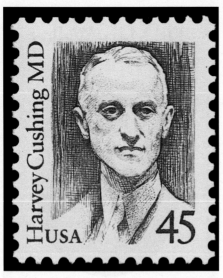

5. Harvey Cushing (circa 1990). (*Author's Collection*)

surgeons continue to produce a steady stream of superlative clinical accomplishments. Although most surgeons conceptualize surgical advances as new operative techniques or technologic breakthroughs, the landmark innovation in American surgical care during the 1980s and 1990s has been the shift from inpatient to outpatient surgery. Admittedly a prosaic and sometimes overlooked phenomenon, ambulatory surgery currently accounts for more than 50 percent of all surgical operations performed in the United States.

Sustained by patient and societal preference, so-called day surgery is primarily a reflection of rapidly changing socioeconomic and technologic realities. This occurs at a time when the delivery of American surgical health care is so decentralized that it has become increasingly difficult to provide exact figures on how many total surgical operations are performed and by whom. For instance, in 1993, the American Hospital Association's annual survey of its 5,261 acute-care hospitals showed that an estimated 22.8 million surgical procedures were completed in these institutions. However, many of these "surgical procedures" consisted of little more than removing a mole or completing a vasectomy. The American Hospital Association's data did, however, demonstrate that 55 percent of these total operations were completed on an outpatient basis, compared with just 27 percent in 1984. Paralleling these statistics is the fact that freestanding outpatient surgical facilities have become one of American health care's fastest growing market segments, with almost 2,000 units now open. Since the majority of these ventures are privately owned, surgical operations performed in them are not included in the American Hospital Association's figures. The result is that at present, in consideration of the dramatic shift from inpatient to outpatient venues, the total number and types of operations completed annually in the United States remain somewhat conjectural.

The steady growth of ambulatory surgery has dramatically changed the manner in which American surgeons engage in their professional activities. Common elective procedures, such as hernia repair, mastectomy, cataract removal, and knee surgery, now require little more than a few hours' stay in a health care facility. The full extent of this transformation is difficult to ascertain, but it seems unmistakable that outpatient surgery has become a totally accepted and expected component of the health care delivery system. This occurred because outpatient surgery represents one of those rare socioeconomic and political phenomena in which all participants benefit. The public is interested in it and demands it, the surgeons are satisfied, increasing numbers of patients are participating, and, most importantly, third-party payers encourage and mandate it.

The shift to ambulatory surgery has been primarily fostered by three independent variables: an economic realization that patients can no longer be kept in hospitals for lengthy postoperative courses; increasing sophistication in surgical therapeutics, mainly the introduction of safer though expensive technologies; and clinical confidence regarding anesthesia and the ability to have patients safely up and about shortly after a procedure has been completed. These three factors have conspicuously converged in relation to this era's other important surgical advance: endoscopic and laparoscopic surgery. Based on the concept of surgical minimalism relative to incisions and tissue dissection, these technology-dependent techniques revolutionized the manner in which surgeons approach numerous disease processes. For instance, a traditional cholecystectomy (removal of the gallbladder) required a lengthy abdominal incision, which once resulted in a postoperative hospital stay of several days. As inpatient settings became increasingly expensive, it was financially necessary to decrease post-cholecystectomy hospitalization time to a bare minimum. Laparoscopic cholecystectomy gave the profession the wherewithal to accomplish this task via the development of radically innovative surgical instrumentation. With a "viewing" laparoscope and accompanying miniature scissors and other surgical implements easily introduced into the abdominal cavity through a series of half-inch puncture wounds, the gallbladder is readily dissected free from its attachments and brought out through the laparoscope. Such a technological feat caused an immediate revolution in the management of this most common surgical disease (over 650,000 cholecystectomies are performed annually in the United States). Laparoscopic cholecystectomy was indisputably safe and efficacious, and it afforded greater patient comfort. With a resultant shorter hospital stay, health care economists eagerly looked forward to a pronounced reduction in the total monies spent on gall bladder disease.

What was not taken into account was that as the operation became easier to perform, the relative indications for cholecystectomy also changed. These "loosened" indications precipitated increased demand, which led to a rise in the total number of cholecystectomies. As a consequence, the aggregate (i.e., social) expenditure on gall-bladder surgery increased despite an appreciable reduction in the unit (i.e., patient) cost for cholecystectomies. Similarly, although the unit operative mortality associated with laparoscopic cholecystectomy was less than that after traditional or open cholecystectomy, there was no change in the aggregate number of cholecystectomy-related complications and deaths because of the increase in the operative rate. For the surgeons of the 1980s and earlier, the assessment of outcome of cholecystectomy was restricted to feasibility, complications, and mortality, all at the level of the individual patient. In the 1990s, the issue of relevance had to be expanded to include additional social costs and benefits. Accordingly, there is little denying that indications for laparoscopic cholecystectomy need to reflect a better balance between patient and societal expectations.

The saga of laparoscopic cholecystectomy demonstrates how surgeons, who have always prided themselves on self-reliance, individual achievements, and independence of thought and action, can fall victim to an emerging socioeconomic tyranny of surgical technology. Simultaneously, advances in many worthwhile surgical devices and the procedures that require their use have tended to raise aggregate spending, while unwarranted emphasis on certain high-cost, low-benefit therapies has pushed the surgical system well beyond the point at which marginal costs exceed marginal benefits. The latter situation is evidenced by the controversies surrounding laparoscopic hernia repair. Since over 80 percent of the almost 750,000 groin hernia operations performed annually in the United States are already completed on an ambulatory or same-day basis, the idea that a laparoscopic approach will decrease facility or hospital costs by shortening an impending inpatient stay appears spurious. In fact, the laparoscopic approach for groin hernia surgery ultimately costs more because a considerable amount of expensive equipment must be purchased in order for the laparoscopic operation to be performed. This is in obvious contradistinction to other types of laparoscopic and endoscopic surgery (e.g., cholecystectomy, knee repair, hiatal herniorrhaphy, pulmonary resection), where the lengthy and expensive hospitalizations necessitated by open surgical techniques, have truly been shortened. Not only do modern open methods of groin hernia repair obviate the need for expensive instrumentation, but these nonlaparoscopic techniques permit the patient to be discharged one to two hours after surgery and to resume full normal daily activities the following day.

The case of laparoscopic groin hernia repair is a striking example of socioeconomic tyranny caused by surgical technology. Through public relations and massive advertising campaigns, corporate manufacturers of laparoscopic hernia equipment attempt to convince surgeons and the public of the necessity to perform hernia repairs via the gimmickry of laparoscopy. The financial stakes are enormous for the equipment makers, since groin hernias represent one of the most common procedures performed by the general surgeon. However, patients cannot engage in normal activities any more rapidly after a laparoscopic groin hernia repair than they can following several commonly employed existing nonlaparoscopic techniques. What equipment manufacturers never acknowledge is that by encouraging the mass utilization of their laparoscopic hernia products, they are able to greatly increase their company's profits, but at the expense of patient and societal economic well-being. The overwhelming clinical success of laparoscopic cholecystectomy and its acceptance by the public and profession clearly epitomizes the increasing dependence on technology. Conversely, though, the clinical and financial dubiousness of laparoscopic groin hernia repair makes the nation and its surgeons victims of a technology-driven socioeconomic tyranny and helps underscore the socioeconomic and political transformation that characterizes this era of American surgery.

THE OUTLOOK FOR THE FUTURE

The years since 1975 have witnessed some of the most far-reaching changes ever to affect the scientific discipline of surgery. With success rates of over 90 percent at one year and 70 percent at ten years for live donor kidney transplants, and 80 percent at one year and almost 50 percent at ten years with cadaveric kidneys, any past surgical impossibilities seem ready to be conquered. Yet, surgeons have essentially explored all the cavities of the body. Nor are there are new organs left to discover or legions of radically bold operating techniques waiting to be improvised. What will more likely transpire within the profession is an increasing sophistication in the methods of performing time-honored surgical procedures. The clinical need to remove a diseased gallbladder will not change, at least not in the forseeable future. What will evolve is the manner in which excision is performed (e.g., open versus laparoscopic cholecystectomy). This increasing sophistication in surgical techniques should lead to less invasive technical methodologies, further shortened convalescence times, and diminished postoperative discomfort.

In 1874, London's John Erichsen wrote that "the abdomen, chest, and brain will forever be closed to operations by a wise and humane surgeon." A decade or so later, Vienna's Theodor Billroth (1829–1894) supposedly remarked, "A surgeon who tries to suture a heart wound deserves to lose the esteem of his colleagues." Both Erichsen and Billroth were incorrect in their assessments of surgery's future. Surgery, which began as a manual and much feared therapy within the whole of medicine, has gloriously evolved into an integral aspect of modern science and technology. What the future will hold for American surgeons remains unknown. Writing in 1876, a prophetic Samuel Gross told of the "cultured and refined American physician" who is a "prince among men." Gross felt the future to be "full of bright promises" and "the dignity, and the glory of American surgery" to be safe in the keeping of his "younger brethren." Looking one hundred years ahead, he rhapsodized that "the century closing with the year 1976 will open for medicine one of the brightest pages in the history of human progress."

Gross was correct in his scientific surmises, although the magnificent technical achievements that he so greatly appreciated, pursued by a few dominant individual personalities, are no longer part of the modern surgical scene. What Gross could not have envisioned are the numerous concerns that must now be addressed relative to socioeconomic and political pressures and technological breakthroughs. The obvious transformation of American surgery from "cottage industry" to mammoth governmental-industrial-medical complex is undeniable. The central question for the profession then becomes: how does it view itself in relation to social and cultural change and where does surgery fit into a rapidly altered health care delivery environment? Private insurers, employers, government officials, and the public want surgical expenditures controlled, with medicine placed under some form of financial constraints. For the surgeon, this presents previously unimagined socioeconomic and political perplexities.

The technological advances of the half century since World War II clearly reveal the continuing importance of basic science research to surgical evolution. For centuries, surgeons depended heavily on discoveries and important advances in other medical disciplines for its own progress. Following the advent of anesthesia and antisepsis, surgical researchers came into their own while garnering respect within the world's scientific community. Feeling the impact of allied technologies, surgeons must currently seek interdependence with their basic science colleagues. It is no

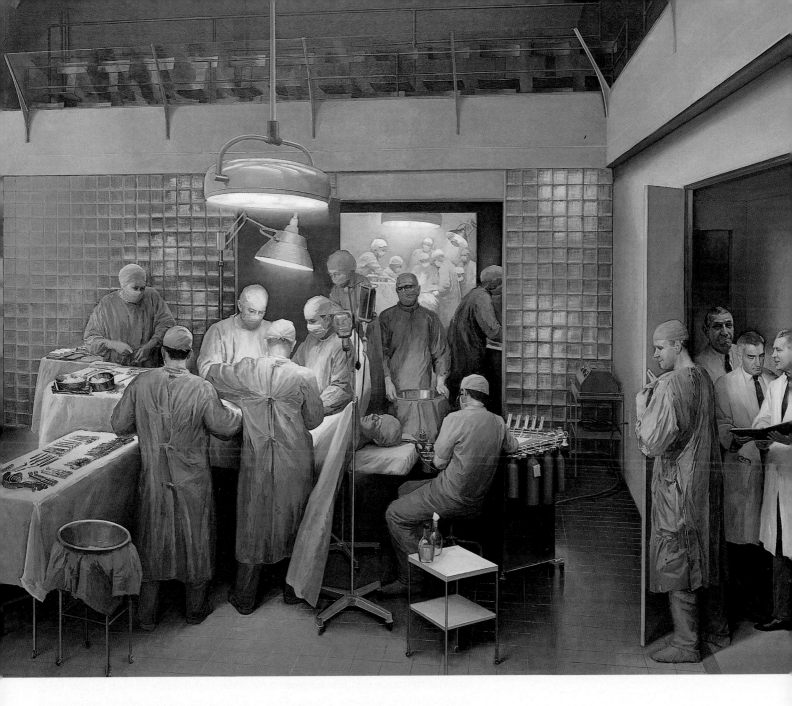

6. "The First Successful Kidney Transplantation—December 23, 1954." Completed by Joel Babb in 1995–1996, this painting of a monumental event in the history of American surgery and Harvard Medical School hangs directly opposite Robert Hinckley's "The First Operation Under Ether" in The Francis A. Countway Library of Medicine. In Babb's recreation of a composite scene, Joseph E. Murray, the Nobel Prize-winning surgeon, is standing at the patient's right side. Opposite him is John Rowbotham, the assistant surgeon. Aiding them are Edward Gray and Daniel Pugh. The scrub nurse is Miss Rhodes, while the circulating nurse, Edith Comiskey, peers over the surgeons' shoulders. The patient, Richard Herrick, is under spinal anesthesia administered by Leroy Vandam. Hartwell Harrison has just completed the donor nephrectomy, entered the operating room on the right-hand side, and pulled down his mask to converse. Francis Moore, surgeon-in-chief at the Peter Bent Brigham Hospital, is seen bringing the donor kidney in a surgical basin. Looking in on the progress of the transplantation procedure are pathologist Gustave Dammin, dialysis physician John Merrill, and physician-in-chief George Thorn. *(The Harvard Medical Library in The Francis A. Countway Library of Medicine)*

longer realistic to define surgical research as experimental investigations completed strictly by surgeons in a surgical research facility. The interdisciplinary facets of biochemistry, biophysics, bioradiology, and biomechanical engineering need to be incorporated into the world of the surgeon.

Throughout the narrative of this illustrated history of American surgery, the practice of surgery has been largely defined by its tools and the manual aspects of the craft. The last decades of the twentieth century have seen unprecedented progress in the development of new instrumentation and imaging techniques. These refinements have not come without noticeable social and economic cost. Advancement will assuredly continue, for if the study of surgical history offers any lesson, it is that progress can always be expected, at least relative to technology. There will be more sophisticated surgical operations with better results. Eventually, automation may even robotize the surgeon's hand for certain operations. Still, the surgical sciences will always retain their historical roots as, fundamentally, a manual-based art and craft.

Although it may be easier to relate to modern surgery of the last few decades than to the seemingly primitive practices of prior eras, writing the history of modern surgery and predicting its future is in most respects more difficult than describing distant developments. One reason for this abstruseness is the ever quickening pace of scientific development. The art and science of surgery remains in constant flux, and the more rapid the change, the more difficult it is to obtain satisfactory historical perspective. Only the adequate passage of time permits a truly valid historical analysis. However, in the future, one thing that can be anticipated is that any surgeon who wishes to positively affect the health care delivery system will also need additional education in the social sciences. The future leaders of American surgery must be more than excellent clinicians who also investigate the basic surgical sciences. They will be increasingly asked to make critical public policy decisions, and without proper education and experience, they will be more likely to make ill-informed and potentially damaging ones.

Most important to the future conduct of surgery will be the participation of surgeons in the planning of health services research. Although surgeons who participate in basic biomedical research will always be an integral part of the profession, a similar need now exists for surgeons who can conceive and conduct original investigations into the socioeconomics of the country's health care delivery system. It is unfortunately true that few surgeons have additional training in such diverse fields as biostatistics, business administration, economics, epidemiology, government affairs, health services administration, public health, policy formation, and sociology. Until a critical mass of surgeons adopts an interdisciplinary approach to understanding the many nuances of modern surgical health care delivery, the crucial and often difficult process of making appropriate surgical policy decisions will be largely left to those outside the profession.

It is imperative that departments of surgery in major teaching medical centers establish formalized groups that have as their principal function the study and conduct of research into the organization and delivery of surgical care. The leadership of organized surgery must begin to understand the importance of this message and correct the current inbalance in surgical research priorities. Surgical chairmen should not only encourage their residents to enter the basic science laboratory but also direct them into formal degree programs in areas such as business administration, health care economics, and public policy. It is a sad truth that the most important issue now faced by surgeons is not how to perform a better pancreaticoduodenectomy (excision of the pancreas and duodenum), for example, but how best to determine the financial ramifications of performing such an operation when the patient's life expectancy is known to be less than a year.

Professional autonomy has long been protected by the institutional autonomy of hospitals. This is coming to an end, with multihospital chains and managed care networks depriving surgeons of much of the power they are accustomed to wielding over institutional policies. To partially offset this loss of influence, surgeons should once more reevaluate themselves with a *SOSSUS*-like study. National databases need to be established to allow proper analyses of numbers of operations that are performed and to evaluate who is completing them and where. Without such basic background data, much of surgical health care delivery research will prove ineffective, and surgeons will lose even more control of their profession.

The surgical community must learn to accept with equanimity the changes that are taking place in the overall health care system. Power has shifted: the once dominant role of the surgeon has declined. Surgeons are the heroes of yesteryear, and the many dramatic alterations in the conduct of surgical practice will have to be acknowledged with a sanguine outlook. Surgeons need to clarify their newfound role in the coming transformation of American medicine. The practice of surgery can be conducted in a businesslike manner. This does not imply that the humanitarian aspects of medicine should be forsaken. The commitment to act on behalf of a sick patient and to be compassionate to those less fortunate should always be preserved. Surgical health care must remain a right, not a privilege, of American society. What remains to be answered is: to what dollar amount does that right extend? Should all individuals be guaranteed a liver transplant if they have alcoholic cirrhosis, or a heart and lung transplant if they continue to smoke cigarettes? Should surgical care be rationed? From the perspective of the mid-1990s, it appears that some rationing will be inevitable. If so, upon whom will the responsibility for making this surgical judgment fall?

Surgeons must provide effective leadership in determining the economic constraints that need be imposed to control expenditures and make services available to the poor and the uninsured. The highest priority that the United States, the most affluent society on this planet, can ensure is that the surgical interests of the economically and socially disadvantaged and those who have limited access to health care will be guaranteed. Surgeons cannot consider themselves among the true heirs of Hippocrates if they are interested solely in patients who can pay for their care.

To study the history of American surgery is a wonderful adventure. With its many magnificent personalities and outstanding scientific and social achievements, it mirrors the growth of America itself. To a certain extent, if surgeons in the future wish to be regarded as more than mere technicians, the profession needs to appreciate again the value of its past experiences. American surgery has a distinguished heritage that is in danger of being forgotten. The present rests on the past, but it is the past that leads us into the future.

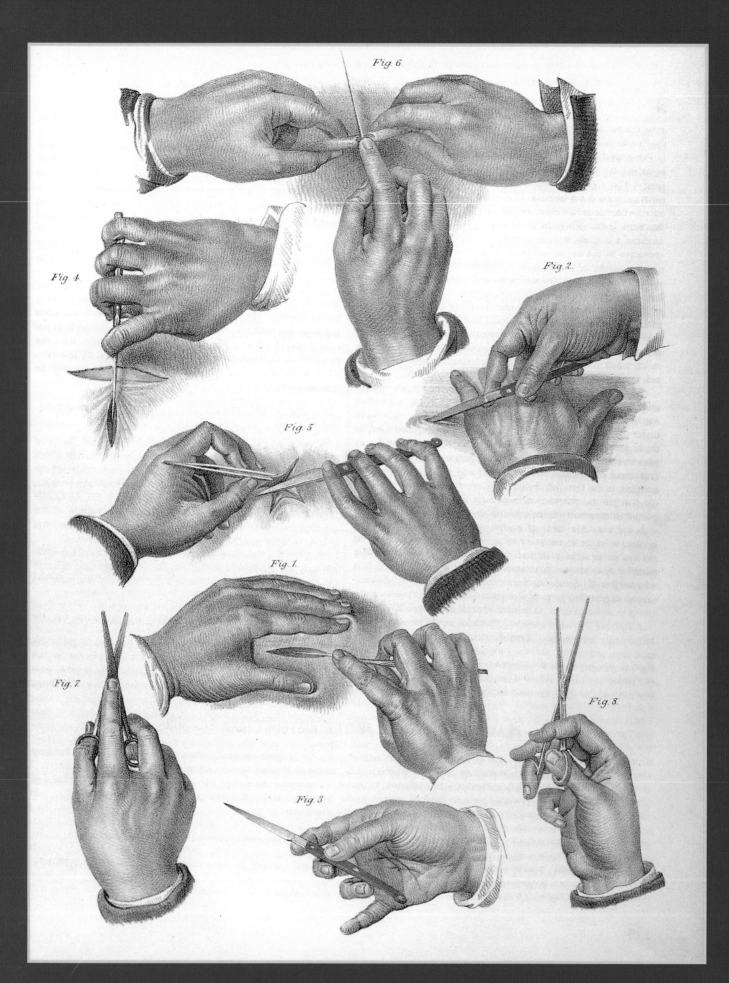

Fig. 6.

Fig. 4.

Fig. 2.

Fig. 5.

Fig. 1.

Fig. 7.

Fig. 8.

Fig. 3.

CHAPTER 13

GENERAL SURGERY

eneral surgery was the substrate from which the surgical sciences flourished. Consequently, the attendant development of surgical specialization and subspecialization brought about an encroachment upon the broad clinical territories presided over by so-called general surgeons. In effect, the general surgeon represents a leftover by-product of this ongoing evolutionary drive toward surgical specialism. Before surgical specialization was widely accepted in the United States, a surgeon was expected to perform all classes of surgical operations. Thus, the average late-nineteenth-century American surgeon could perform a gynecologic procedure with as much technical expertise as an orthopedic operation. Through the first decade of the twentieth century, a single surgeon could still author an all-encompassing surgical text, such as Nicholas Senn's *Practical Surgery for the General Practitioner* (1901) or Albert Ochsner's *Clinical Surgery for the Instruction of Practitioners* (1902).

Like its many specialty offshoots, general surgery is also considered a bona fide surgical specialty, and in the United States it is so recognized by the country's official arbiter of such decisions, the American Board of Medical Specialties. Yet, there remains a semantic difficulty in that the misnomer "general" is applied to this mother of all surgical specialties. General surgeons no longer practice general surgery; instead, they have been unceremoniously left with whatever the other surgical specialties have not been able to, or do not choose to, treat. Therefore, the technical scope of general surgery remains constantly contracting and in need of continous redefinition. Paradoxically, general surgery and its practitioners continue to assume dominant roles on medical faculties and in the design of medical school curricula.

Only since the spread of surgical specialization has the American public's perception of the role of general surgery within the whole of surgery become less distinct. Part of this problem stemmed from the simple reality that through the mid-1970s, many physician-surgeons continued to perform simple "general" surgical operations such as appendectomy, cholecystectomy, and herniorrhaphy. These family practitioner-surgeons, mostly in rural locations, represented the multigenerational vestiges of individuals who received surgical experience during the Civil War. With the evolution of modern clinical practice, however, family practice and general internal medicine have become recognized medical specialties with their own examining boards. As these medical and primary care specialties have been redefined, and in consideration of the ethical and moral ramifications of surgical operations performed by inadequately trained individuals in today's legal climate, present-day family practitioners and internists neither learn nor perform surgical operations. Instead, essentially all surgery in the United States is now conducted by individuals trained in either general surgery or one of the other surgical specialties.

1. *(facing page)* Exacting surgical technique must be learned by every surgeon-to-be, and Joseph Pancoast stressed this point by including an illustration on "positions of the bistoury and scissors" in his 1844 atlas. *(Author's Collection)*

2. Peter Parker (1804–1888) was a Presbyterian minister and physician (Yale Divinity School and Yale Medical College, class of 1834), who traveled to China as a medical missionary. Combining the message of Christian scriptures with the mercies of the surgeon's scalpel, Parker was the first Western physician to perform surgery on a woman in China and the first health care worker in that country to employ sulfuric ether and chloroform as surgical anesthetics. During his extended sojourn in the Far East, a well-known Chinese artist, Lam Qua, painted almost eighty of Parker's most interesting surgical cases. These two oil paintings on canvas (1836–1837) record the before-and-after views of the first voluntary amputation of a limb in China. Po Ashing, a 23-year-old man, had twice fractured his left humerus. Because of an unhealed fracture, the extremity became useless, and in November 1836 Parker performed an amputation, which according to his notations "did not exceed a minute from the application of the scalpel till the arm was laid upon the floor....it weighed 21¼ pounds." *(Yale University, Harvey Cushing/John Hay Whitney Medical Library)*

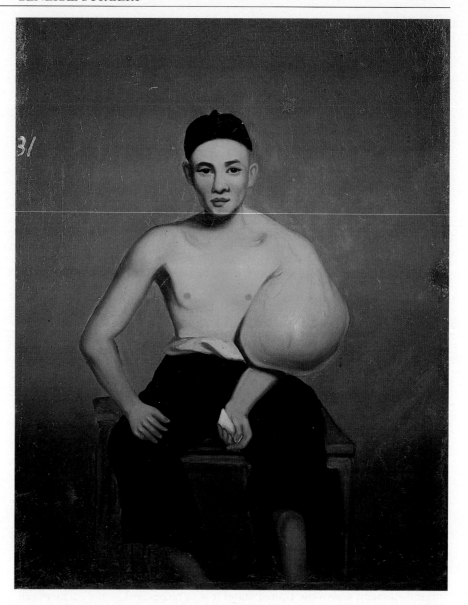

In 1937, general surgery in the United States began to garner the imprimatur of a duly recognized surgical specialty when the American Board of Surgery was incorporated as an examining body for all individuals interested in performing "general" surgical operations. Since then, the definition of "general surgery" has been periodically updated, so that by the mid-1990s, the general surgeon is delineated by the Board as having specialized knowledge and skill relating to nine areas of primary responsibility: alimentary tract; abdomen and its contents; breast, skin, and soft tissue; head and neck; vascular system; endocrine system; surgical oncology, including coordinated multimodality management of the cancer patient by screening, surveillance, surgical adjunctive therapy, rehabilitation, and follow-up; comprehensive management of trauma; and complete care of critically ill patients with underlying surgical conditions. As a reminder of its historical roots, the American Board of Surgery also expects its diplomates to have an "understanding of the management of the more common problems in cardiac, gynecologic, neurologic, orthopedic, and urologic surgery." Applicants for certification must have completed a minimum of five years of "progressive education following graduation from medical school" including "twelve months in the capacity of chief resident in general surgery."

In addition to awarding general certificates in the overall specialty of surgery, the American Board of Surgery recently began to offer examinations leading to certificates of special or added qualifications in the disciplines of pediatric surgery (1975), general vascular surgery (1982), surgical critical care (1986), and surgery of the hand (1989). Prior to 1980, 25,442 general certificates had been awarded by the American

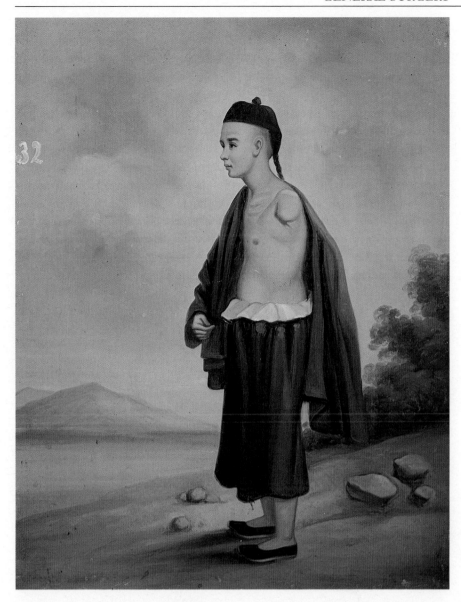

Board of Surgery. During the fifteen-year period 1980 through 1994, an additional 14,479 general certificates in surgery were issued, or an average of 965 per year. As of mid-1995, a total of 40,377 general surgeons had been certified since the Board's founding. In addition, there were 644 diplomates in pediatric surgery, 1,527 diplomates in general vascular surgery, 1,413 diplomates in surgical critical care, and 172 diplomates in surgery of the hand.

The American Medical Association, through its annual survey of physicians' characteristics and distribution, provides historical and current data on American physicians. As of January 1995, there were approximately 621,000 physicians in active practice in the United States. Among this total, some 145,000 (23 percent) designate themselves as surgical specialists, and almost 38,000 (6.1 percent) are considered general surgeons. Of the general surgeons, 22,700 (60 percent) are board certified. The majority of the non–board-certified group fall into two categories: older surgeons who began practice when board certification was not as important as it is now, and younger surgeons who are in the middle of postgraduate training or have just completed it and have not yet taken the board examination. However, it can be expected in the future that it will be the rare practicing surgeon who does not have the full credentials of his or her specialty board.

Of the almost 38,000 physicians who consider themselves general surgeons, approximately 3,000 (8 percent) are women and some 8,000 (21 percent) are international medical graduates. Among the total pool of general surgeons, approximately 10,200 (27 percent) are under 35; 9,300 (24 percent) are 35 to 44 years old; 8,100

(21 percent) are 45 to 54 years old; 6,200 (16 percent) are 55 to 64 years old; and 4,100 (11 percent) are 65 years old and older. Of the 3,000 or so female general surgeons, almost 2,700 (90 percent) are under 44 years of age. This is contrasted with the approximately 35,300 male general surgeons, of whom 18,400 (53 percent) are under 44 years of age.

Unlike other surgical specialists, general surgeons do not have a long-standing professional organization incorporating the words "general surgeon" within its appellation. This unwieldy circumstance has come about because many of the major extant American surgical societies, initially organized during the last thirty years of the nineteenth century and the first quarter of the twentieth, were originally intended to encompass all surgeons. However, since surgical specialization brought about a spate of specialty societies, some of the older surgical organizations have assumed the role of primarily serving the general surgeon by default Among the most well known are the American Surgical Association (1880) and five regional surgical societies: the Southern Surgical Association (1886), the Western Surgical Association

3. Although intestinal surgery was rarely performed before the 1880s, Pancoast's *Treatise on Operative Surgery* (1844) did demonstrate the repair of wounded small intestine secondary to an abdominal wall injury and subsequent eventration. This colored plate shows how to enlarge the abdominal wall injury in order to permit reduction of the herniated small bowel, as well as intestinal suturing techniques. (*Author's Collection*)

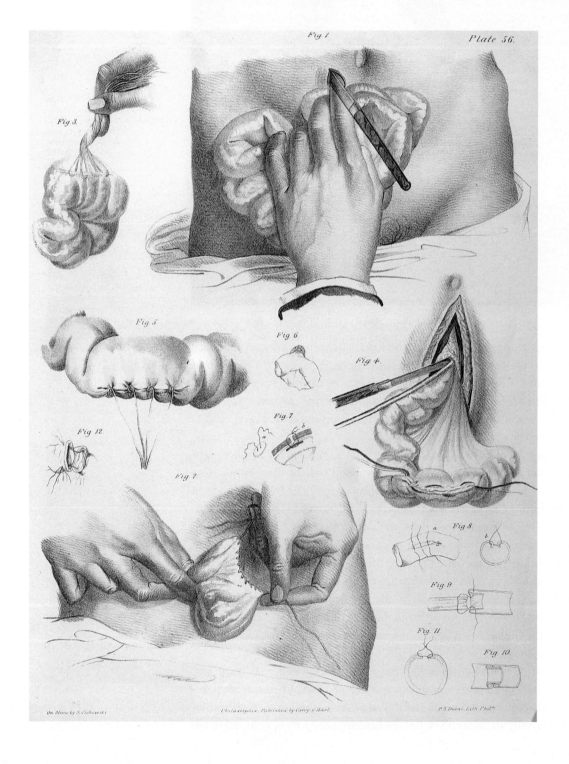

(1890), the New England Surgical Society (1916), the Pacific Coast Surgical Association (1926), and the Central Surgical Association (1940). Other national organizations also represent the collective interests of general surgeons, including the Society of University Surgeons, the Association for Academic Surgery, the Society for Surgery of the Alimentary Tract, the American Association for the Surgery of Trauma, the Joint Council of the Vascular Societies, and the Society of Surgical Oncology. Although the American College of Surgeons regards itself as a society for the whole of American surgery, the majority of its fellows are general surgeons. Throughout its history, leaders of the College have steadfastly assumed the doctrinaire position that all branches of surgery must be served via the College's various functions. However, present-day pragmatism and political realities suggest that the College is increasingly oriented toward the socioeconomic and educational goals of the country's general surgeons.

Although the general surgeon has a vast number of peer-reviewed surgical journals to peruse, the five most influential and their past editors-in-chief are *Annals of Surgery* (Lewis S. Pilcher, 1885–1935; Walter E. Lee, 1936–1946; John H. Gibbon, Jr., 1947–1956; John H. Mulholland, 1957–1970; Jonathan E. Rhoads, 1971–1973; David C. Sabiston, Jr., 1974–1997; and Layton F. Rikkers, 1997–??); *American Journal of Surgery* (Walter M. Brickner, 1905–1927; Thurston S. Welton, 1928–1957; Robert M. Zollinger, 1958–1985; and Hiram C. Polk, Jr., 1986–??); *Surgery, Gynecology and Obstetrics* (whose name was changed in 1994 to *Journal of the American College of Surgeons*) (Franklin H. Martin, 1905–1935; Alan B. Kanavel, 1935–1938; Loyal Davis, 1939–1981; G. Tom Shires, 1982–1993; Samuel A. Wells, Jr., 1994–1996; and Seymour Schwartz, 1997–??); *Archives of Surgery* (Dean Lewis, 1920–1940; Waltman Walters, 1941–1942 & 1946–1961; Lester Dragstedt, 1943–1945; J. Garrett Allen, 1962–1969; Richard Warren, 1970–1976; Arthur Baue, 1977–1988; and Claude H. Organ, Jr., 1989–present); and *Surgery* (Alton Ochsner and Owen Wangensteen, 1937–1970; Theodore Drapanas, 1971–1975; Walter F. Ballinger, 1971–1997; and George D. Zuidema, 1976–1997; and Andrew L. Warshaw, 1997–??, and Michael G. Sarr, 1997–??).

TWO CENTURIES OF SURGICAL PROGRESS

Systematic review of the highlights of the surgical specialties has been facilitated by consultation of a wise and worldly compilation of texts and periodical articles illustrating the history of medicine. *Morton's Medical Bibliography* (affectionately known as "Garrison-Morton" or "G-M") is an authoritative and thoroughly annotated work that provides a chronological bibliography of the most important contributions to the history and development of the medical sciences. Almost 9,000 individually numbered entries encompass virtually every area of medical knowledge from the time of the ancient Egyptians through the modern era. During the last two centuries, numerous advances have been made by American general surgeons in the operative treatment of esophageal, gastric, and intestinal diseases. The first serious attempt at research into repairing intestinal injuries in the United States, and the earliest reported use of dogs for experimental surgery, was authored by Thomas Smith (1785–1831) in his *Essay on Wounds of the Intestines* (1805). About the same time, Philip Syng Physick reported the first use of a stomach tube for gastric lavage in 1812 and described his operation for "artificial anus" (colocutaneous fistula formed as a result of mortification from a strangulated inguinal hernia) in 1826. John Davidge authored the country's first description of a parotid extirpation in 1823. Two decades later, Samuel Gross reported in the *Western Journal of Medicine and Surgery* a series of experiments on dogs to determine the most efficacious way to treat intestinal wounds. In 1844, John Watson (1807–1863) described an esophagotomy for relief of stricture of the esophagus; that was followed by Frank Maury's (1840–1879) use of gastrostomy for esophageal obstruction in 1870. William Halsted commenced his momentous surgical advances in 1887 when he proposed fundamental rules regarding intestinal anastomosis. The following year, Nicholas Senn suggested a method of detecting intestinal perforation by insufflation with hydrogen. Robert Abbe, a New York City-based surgeon, introduced catgut rings for intestinal suturing in the late 1880s. Shortly thereafter, John Benjamin Murphy described the now classic "Murphy's button" for cholecystointestinal, gastrointestinal, and enterointestinal anastomosis without sutures. Much of the extensive experimentation in gastrointestinal anatomosis was summed up by Senn in his 1893 report "Enterorrhaphy: its history, technique and present status" in the *Journal of the American Medical Association*. John Baldy (1860–1934) claimed credit in 1898 for having performed America's first gastric excision five years previously. However, that claim was vehemently contested by Augustus Bernays (1854–1907), and while Baldy probably deserves priority, the point is moot, since neither Baldy's nor Bernay's operation was successful. At the beginning of the twentieth century, William Mayo described his procedure of partial gastrectomy for malignant diseases of the stomach and pylorus. In 1902, Robert Weir proposed a method of appendicostomy in the surgical management of "obstinate colitis." John Finney assisted Halsted in the management of the residency program at The Johns Hopkins Hospital and authored a paper on a new method of gastroduodenostomy, or widened pyloroplasty, in 1903. A decade later, Henry Janeway (1873–1921) of New York City developed a technique for gastrostomy in which he wrapped the anterior wall of the stomach around a rubber catheter and sutured it in place, establishing a permanent fistula. In 1932, Burrill Crohn (1884–1983), along with the surgeon Leon Ginzburg, authored a report on regional ileitis and its operative treatment. Owen Wangensteen first reported on an apparatus for the relief of acute intestinal obstruction in 1932 and followed that work with his classic monograph *The Therapeutic Problem in Bowel Obstruction* in 1937. N. Logan Leven described repair of congenital esophageal atresia through an extrapleural ligation of the fistulous communication and cervical esophagostomy in 1941. In 1943, Lester Dragstedt reported on his results of vagotomy for cure of peptic ulcer disease. Twelve years later, Robert Zollinger and Edwin Ellison first described Zollinger-Ellison syndrome (familial polyendocrine adenomastosis).

American surgical highlights in treating liver, gallbladder, and pancreatic diseases began in 1868, when John Bobbs, of rural Indiana, reported the world's first known account of a cholecystotomy for the removal of gallstones. Five years later, J. Marion Sims, while residing in London, duplicated Bobb's success. Senn reviewed the world literature regarding surgery of the pancreas in a 134-page report presented to the American Surgical Association in 1886. He concluded that complete extirpation of the pancreas was invariably followed by death but that partial excision was feasible and justifiable. In 1899, Halsted reported the first successful operation for a primary cancer of the ampulla of Vater. Evarts Graham and Warren Cole introduced cholecystography in 1924. Allen Whipple was serving as professor of surgery at Columbia University in New York City when he devised pancreaticoduodenectomy for cancer of the pancreas in 1935. Two years later, Alexander Brunschwig, also of New York City, further modified the operation.

The first important early report on the surgical treatment of appendicitis in the United States appeared in 1867 when Willard Parker advocated the opening of appendicular abscesses at an early stage. Until then, such abscesses had been incised and drained only when they "pointed" on the skin's surface. By 1880, Henry Sands had collected a series of twenty-six patients on whom he had operated for "perityphlitis"; the surgery was successful in all but two patients. The conclusive demonstration of the pathology and symptoms of disease of the vermiform appendix was accomplished by Reginald Fitz, a pathologist at the Massachusetts General Hospital, in 1886. He coined the term "appendicitis" and convinced physicians and surgeons of the need to remove the appendix immediately if threatening symptoms did not subside within twenty-four hours of presentation. That same year, Richard Hall

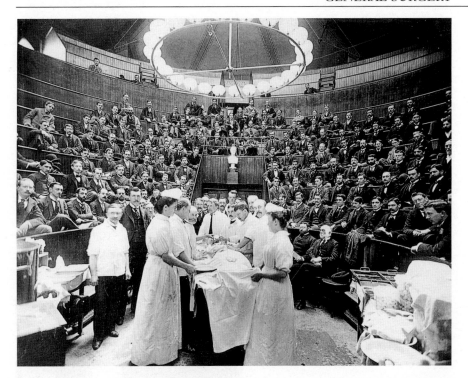

4. William Williams Keen operating in the surgical amphitheater at Jefferson Medical College in Philadelphia, November 1904. Born in 1837, Keen lived until 1932, witnessing and contributing to the evolution of American surgery from its beginning as a trade to its becoming a profession based on scientific principles. At the time of his death he was one of the last surviving surgeons to have served in the Civil War. Keen *(third from the left)* is the slight bearded figure in the operating team. *(Historical Collections, College of Physicians of Philadelphia)*

(1856–1897) reported the first case of survival after removal of a perforated appendix. Thomas Morton (1835–1903), of the Pennsylvania Hospital, was one of the first to deliberately operate for and remove an inflamed appendix after correct preoperative diagnosis (1887). In 1889, Charles McBurney described McBurney's point, the "seat of greatest pain" in early appendicitis. Albert Ochsner was professor of clinical surgery at the University of Illinois when he clarified diffuse peritonitis as a sequela complicating appendicitis in 1901. Howard Kelly and Elizabeth Hurdon (1869–1941) published their classic and massive *The Vermiform Appendix and its Diseases* in 1905.

Although groin hernias have long given difficulty to *Homo sapiens*, advances by American surgeons greatly added to the understanding of this anatomical defect. In the 1870s, Henry Marcy stressed the importance of reconstruction of the internal ring following reduction of the hernia sac and the utilization of antiseptic ligatures (carbolized catgut) in the radical cure of hernia. In 1892, he authored one of the country's most visually spectacular surgical monographs, *The Anatomy and Surgical Treatment of Hernia*. Joseph Warren (1831–1891) of Boston introduced the injection method of treating hernia in his 1880 textbook, *Hernia, Strangulated and Reducible, with Cure by Subcutaneous Injections*. For the next half century, the injection method, although it was minimally effective, remained a mainstay of hernia therapy. William Halsted devised one of the modern operations for the radical cure of inguinal hernia in 1889. Working with Halsted, Joseph Bloodgood described a method of transplantation of the rectus muscle in certain cases of inguinal hernia in 1898. At the same time, Edward Andrews (1856–1927) of Chicago began to imbricate aponeurotic flaps in hernia repairs (1895). Alexander Ferguson (1853–1912), also of Chicago, described his methods of herniorrhaphy in *The Technic of Modern Operations for Hernia* (1907). Paul LaRoque (1876–1934) of Richmond, Virginia, combined a superior transperitoneal gridiron incision with a repair based on the method of Bassini (1919). During the 1940s, Chester McVay began to popularize a method of hernia repair based on the pectineal, or Cooper's, ligament.

The treatment of breast cancer was radically altered in the 1890s when Halsted began to publish numerous reports on its surgical therapy. Bloodgood of Baltimore authored his theory on the causation of chronic mastitis in 1906 and followed it with a description of blue dome cysts in 1921. In 1931 Max Cutler (1899–1984), of New

York City, in collaboration with George Cheatle (1865–1951), of London, published the important monograph *Tumours of the Breast*. In that same year, Cutler detailed his systemic use of ovarian hormone in the treatment of chronic mastitis. Two years later, Frank Adair (1887–1982) provided the first description of plasma-cell mastitis.

The treatment of vascular diseases has become a mainstay of the twentieth-century general surgeon's practice. In 1909 Halsted introduced a metal band in place of a ligature for the progressive occlusion of arterial aneurysms. Four years later Bertram Bernheim (1880–1957), a surgeon from Baltimore, authored America's first textbook on the subject, *Surgery of the Vascular System*. George Vaughan of Georgetown University completed a successful ligation of the abdominal aorta for aneurysmal disease in 1921. In 1924, Barney Brooks (1884–1952), professor of surgery at Vanderbilt University in Nashville, Tennessee, introduced clinical angiography and femoral arteriography. Half a decade later, William Babcock (1872–1963), chief of surgery at Temple University in Philadelphia, proposed his

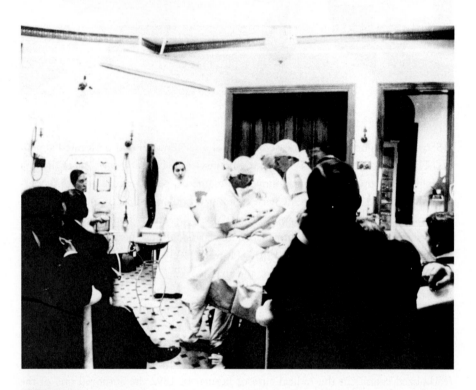

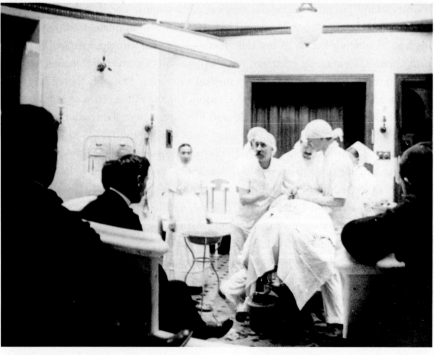

5. Henry Orlando Marcy was a formidable presence on the American surgical scene. In the 1880s he established a private hospital in Cambridge, Massachusetts, where he devoted his efforts exclusively to surgery. His womens' clinic became the focal point of numerous activities, especially the education and entertainment of visiting surgeons. Demonstrated in these previously unpublished and candid photographs (circa late 1880s), is Marcy the consummate surgical showman. *(Courtesy of Stanley B. Burns, M.D., and The Burns Collection and Archive)*

operative decompression of aortic aneurysm by carotid–jugular anastomosis. Max Peet (1885–1949), of Ann Arbor, Michigan, described splanchnic resection for hypertension in 1935.

The identification of more recent contributions to general surgical therapy is difficult. Few histories of surgical specialties cover the period after World War II, and establishing the important clinical and research advances can involve undeniable subjectivity. When the *Study on Surgical Services for the United States* was undertaken in the 1970s, a surgical research subcommittee was established to identify important contributions to surgical health care in the post–World War II era. On the basis of responses to a questionnaire survey of over 250 surgical specialists (general and thoracic surgery, neurosurgery, ophthalmology, orthopedics, otolaryngology, pediatric surgery, plastic surgery, and urology) the advances were placed in one of three ordered categories. These rankings are the only known instance in which a group of American surgeons, in both academic and private practice, attempted to

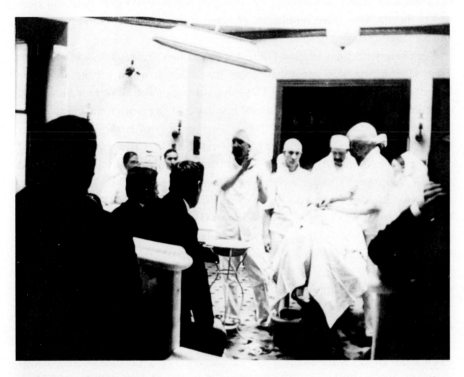

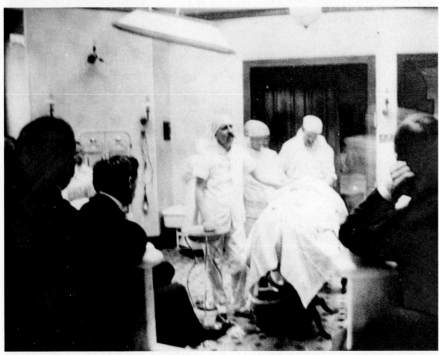

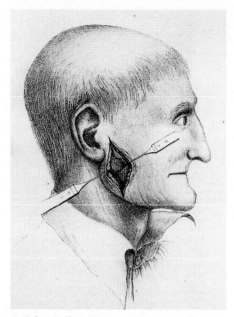

6. John Collins Warren was among the most experienced American surgeons of his era in the treatment of neuralgia by division of nerves. This engraving (*Boston Medical and Surgical Journal*, vol. 1, pages 1–6, 1828) shows how he divided and excised a portion of the submaxillary nerve, providing complete relief of the patient's pain. (*Historical Collections, College of Physicians of Philadelphia*)

quantitatively appraise the relative importance of scientific advances in their respective specialties.

General surgeons considered kidney transplantation, the replacement of arteries by grafts, vagotomy and antrectomy for peptic ulcer, intravenous hyperalimentation, hemodialysis, the effect of hormones on cancer, and resuscitation and topical chemotherapy of burns to be of first-order importance. Of second-order importance were chemotherapy for cancer, Zollinger-Ellison syndrome, endocrine surgery, metabolic response to trauma, and portacaval shunt. Colectomy for ulcerative colitis, endarterectomy, the Fogarty balloon catheter, continuous suction drainage of wounds, and indwelling intravenous catheters were of third-order importance. Among the infrequent selections were ileal conduit, operations for hypertension, fiberoptic endoscopes, cancer immunotherapy, the no-touch technique for colon cancer, pathophysiology of reflux esophagitis, surgical staging of Hodgkins disease, and prospective randomized clinical studies. Excluded by definition (i.e., not developed solely or mainly by surgeons, or conceived before 1945) were fluid and electrolyte therapy, controlled ventilation, physiological monitoring, blood transfusion and banking, treatment of shock, and antibiotics.

Beginning with John Watson (1807–1863) and his *Medical Profession in Ancient Times* (1856), American general surgeons have been active in writing about the history of their profession. Samuel D. Gross, although more known for his clinical achievements, was an important surgical historian, having written the classic paper "A century of American surgery" in the *American Journal of the Medical Sciences* (1876) and the almost eight-hundred page *Lives of Eminent American Physicians and Surgeons on the Nineteenth Century* (1861). At the turn of this century James Mumford wrote *A Narrative of Medicine in America* (1903) and *Surgical Memoirs* (1908). During the 1940s, Richard Leonardo was writing *History of Surgery* (1943), *History of Gynecology* (1944), and *Lives of Master Surgeons* (1948). More recent surgical historical texts include Richard Meade's (born 1897) *An Introduction to the History of General Surgery* (1968) and *A History of Thoracic Surgery* (1961); Loyal Davis's *J. B. Murphy, Stormy Petrel of Surgery* (1938) and *Fellowship of Surgeons; A History of the American College of Surgeons* (1960); Allen O. Whipples' *The Evolution of Surgery in the United States* (1963), *The Story of Wound Healing and Wound Repair* (1963), and *The Role of the Nestorians and Muslims in the History of Medicine* (1967); Owen Wangensteen's *The Rise of Surgery from Empiric Craft to Scientific Discipline* (1978); Harris Shumacker's (born 1908) *History of the Society of Clinical Surgery* (1977), *Leo Eloesser, MD, Eulogy for a Free Spirit* (1982), and *The Evolution of Cardiac Surgery* (1992); and Mark Ravitch's (1911–1989) *A Century of Surgery, the History of the American Surgical Association* (1981).

Although biographies alone do not constitute an adequate basis for understanding surgical history, there is an understandable thrill in reading about the life exploits of renowned surgeons of the past. Biographies, as the essence of hagiographic glorification, provide a different but necessary perspective on the evolution of surgery as a profession. The following vignettes afford a sampling of the accomplishments of individual general surgeons, apart from developments within the whole of surgery. However, in no way should the listing be regarded as an inclusive group of prominent twentieth-century American general surgeons.

BIOGRAPHIES OF GENERAL SURGEONS

George Tully Vaughan (1859–1948) received his medical education at the Bellevue Hospital Medical College (1880) and pursued postgraduate work at the New York Polyclinic Medical School and Hospital. He began private practice in Virginia and then, in 1888, entered the U.S. Marine Hospital Service, where he rose in rank, eventually serving as assistant surgeon-general (1902). During his years of public service, he also studied at the University of Berlin (1894) and Jefferson Medical College (1905). Resigning his commission in 1906, Vaughan continued his career at

Georgetown University Medical School, where he became professor and chairman of the department of surgery. Among his pioneering clinical efforts was the first successful ligation of the abdominal aorta in 1921. A founding member of the American College of Surgeons, Vaughan authored the 569-page *Principles and Practice of Surgery* (1902) and a collected work, *Papers on Surgery and Other Subjects* (1932). He served as an operating surgeon for the U.S. Navy at Vera Cruz in 1914 and as chief surgeon on board the U.S. Transport *Leviathan* during World War I. Vaughan was buried with full military honors at Arlington National Cemetery.

Rudolph Matas (1860–1957) received his medical education at the University of Louisiana (later Tulane University) and graduated in 1880. He had such a long and distinguished career that his many accomplishments and honors are astounding. From 1885 to 1895, Matas served on the anatomy faculty of his alma mater, and from 1894 to 1927 on the surgical faculty of the same institution. At Tulane, he held the chair of surgery while also working at Charity Hospital and the Touro Infirmary. During World War I, Matas organized Base Hospital 24 (Tulane Unit) and directed the New Orleans School for Intensive Surgery War Training, Medical Reserve Corps. Although Matas never authored a textbook of surgery, he did make numerous contributions to the periodical literature. In 1888 he reported the world's first known aneurysmorrhaphy, which garnered the eponym Matas' operation. During the 1890s Matas performed some of the earliest successful preplanned attempts at intraspinal cocainization. At the turn of the century he developed a test to determine the adequacy of the collateral circulation before performing surgery on the great vessels. Among Matas' many honors were presidencies of the American Surgical Association (1909), the Southern Surgical Association (1911), the American Association for Thoracic Surgery (1920), and the American College of Surgeons (1924). His lifetime habit of exhaustive reading combined with a remarkable memory and a rich vocabulary made Matas one of the country's most sought-after surgical lecturers. He remained intellectually vigorous throughout most of his ninety-seven years and was the subject of Isidore Cohn's exhaustive *Rudolph Matas: A Biography of One of the Great Pioneers in Surgery* (1960).

William James Mayo (1861–1939) is one of the most famous figures in American surgery. He was born in Rochester, Minnesota, and attended the University of Michigan School of Medicine (1883). Mayo immediately left for New York City to receive further training at the New York Post-Graduate Medical School (1884) and the New York Polyclinic Medical School (1885). Although his formal training was modest, beginning in 1889, Mayo took annual study leaves, both in the United States and abroad. His entire professional life was spent in practice with his father, William Worrall Mayo, and his brother Charles. The three men made the Mayo Clinic one of the world's foremost centers for surgical care, training, and research, and they demonstrated the advantages of group practice in a private setting. William Mayo's professional career included the presidencies of the American Medical Association (1906), the Society of Clinical Surgery (1911), the American Surgical Association (1913), the American College of Surgeons (1919), and the Congress of American Physicians and Surgeons (1925). His name is linked with several surgical operations, including an excision of the pylorus and exclusion of the duodenum with posterior gastrojejunostomy, the cure of umbilical hernia, and the excision of the rectum with removal of the neighboring lymph glands for cancer. Mayo is eponymically associated with the prepyloric vein. He never wrote a textbook of surgery but contributed more than six hundred papers to the periodical literature. Many of these reports were brought together in the two-volume *William J. Mayo and Charles H. Mayo, A Collection of Papers Published Previous to 1909* (1912).

Malcolm LaSalle Harris (1862–1936) was born in Rock Island, Illinois, and received his medical education at Rush Medical College (1882). His entire professional career was spent in Chicago, where he was professor of surgery in the Chicago Polyclinic Medical School and Hospital. Harris also served continuously as secretary

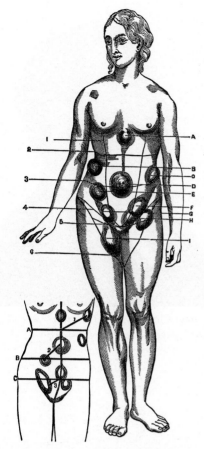

7. Greensville Dowell (1822–1881) was professor of surgery at Texas Medical College in Galveston. In his *Treatise on Hernia* (1876), the country's first monograph concerning the operative treatment of abdominal wall hernias, Dowell utilized this plate to demonstrate the locations of various hernias. *(Author's Collection)*

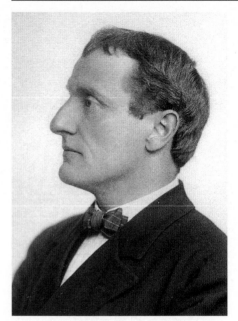

8. John Chalmers DaCosta. *(Historical Collections, College of Physicians of Philadelphia)*

of the board of trustees of Henrotin Hospital from 1889 until he retired as president emeritus in 1935. Among his honors were the chairmanship of the American Medical Association's Section on Surgery (1899) and the presidencies of the Western Surgical Association (1907) and the American Medical Association (1929). His name is eponymically associated with the Harris segregator or separator: a double catheter, the beaks of which are separated when in the bladder, a ridge being formed between the two by a sound in the rectum making upward pressure; the urine from each kidney thus collects in its own pouch and is aspirated out through the catheter on that side.

John Chalmers DaCosta (1863–1933) was born in Washington, D.C. An unfortunate childhood injury caused loss of vision in his right eye. After the accident he became interested in medicine and ultimately in surgery. DaCosta graduated from Jefferson Medical College in 1885 and served an internship at the Philadelphia General Hospital, then known as the Old Blockley Asylum. He was soon appointed demonstrator in anatomy at his alma mater (1887), and at about the same time became office assistant to William W. Keen, professor of surgery, while also serving as an associate in the surgical outpatient department at the Jefferson Hospital. DaCosta advanced through various academic ranks and became clinical professor of surgery in 1896. As his reputation grew he was offered several alluring positions in rival medical schools, but Jefferson kept him by promoting him to full professor of the principles and practice of surgery at the age of 37. On Keen's retirement in 1907, DaCosta was appointed his successor and became the first incumbent of the Samuel D. Gross Chair of Surgery. DaCosta remains best known for his textbook *A Manual of Modern Surgery* (1894), which went through ten editions, the last appearing in 1931. Encyclopedic in scope, it was for almost forty years among the most used surgical texts in the country. In 1905 DaCosta edited the American edition of Henry Gray's *Anatomy, Descriptive and Surgical.* Following his early retirement due to rapidly progressing arthritis deformans, a collective work, *The Papers and Speeches of John Chalmers DaCosta* (1931) was published. A posthumous printing of some of his written papers, *The Trials and Triumphs of the Surgeon*, appeared in 1944. DaCosta was also a poet, and a book of his written verse was published in 1942.

John Miller Turpin Finney (1863–1942) was born in Natchez, Mississippi, the son of a Presbyterian minister. Finney received his undergraduate education at Princeton University (1884) and his medical degree from Harvard (1887). Following eighteen months of training at the Massachusetts General Hospital (and six months before that as a substitute intern at Boston's Lying-in Hospital), he joined William Halsted's original staff and faculty at The Johns Hopkins Hospital in 1889, a few months after the hospital opened. An individual of enormous charm, Finney remained on the Hopkins' faculty until 1933, despite offers of numerous professorships of surgery and even the presidency of Princeton University. Well known for his advocacy of private practice, Finney joined the staff of Baltimore's Union Protestant Infirmary (later Union Memorial Hospital) and helped transform it into a modern urban hospital that included the country's first surgical residency outside a formal academic setting. During World War I he served as a brigadier general and chief surgical consultant of the American Expeditionary Forces. Particularly renowned for his contributions to gastric surgery, Finney developed that era's standard operating procedures for the relief of duodenal ulcer (Finney's pyloroplasty and gastroduodenostomy). He served as first president of the American College of Surgeons (1913–1916) and president of the American Surgical Association (1921). Among his publications were his autobiography, *A Surgeon's Life* (1940), and a collection of written essays, *The Physician* (1923).

George Cleveland Hall (1864–1930) was educated at Lincoln University (1886) and received his medical degree from Bennett Medical College (1888), a proprietary institution. His entire professional life was spent in Chicago on the staff of Provident Hospital. He was considered the leading African-American surgeon of that city and

9. John Miller Turpin Finney. *(Historical Collections, College of Physicians of Philadelphia)*

a strong rival to Daniel Hale Williams. Because Hall was a left-handed surgeon and had graduated from a nonaccredited medical school, and for various personal reasons, Williams willfully attempted to destroy Hall's professional reputation. These public slights proved little more than soon-to-be-forgotten embarrassments, and Hall continued giving surgical clinics throughout the country in order to teach other African-American surgeons his ideas and operative techniques. As a member of the board of trustees and chief of staff of Provident Hospital, Hall played a major role in the institution's development and daily management. He organized and directed the hospital's first postgraduate course for African-American physicians, which led to a program that became, by the 1930s, a national center for postgraduate education and training. Deeply involved in humanitarian and fund-raising activities, Hall was a founder of the Cook County Physician's Association of Chicago.

10. "Extirpation of the mammary gland," drawn on stone by S. Cichowski for Pancoast's *Treatise on Operative Surgery. (Author's Collection)*

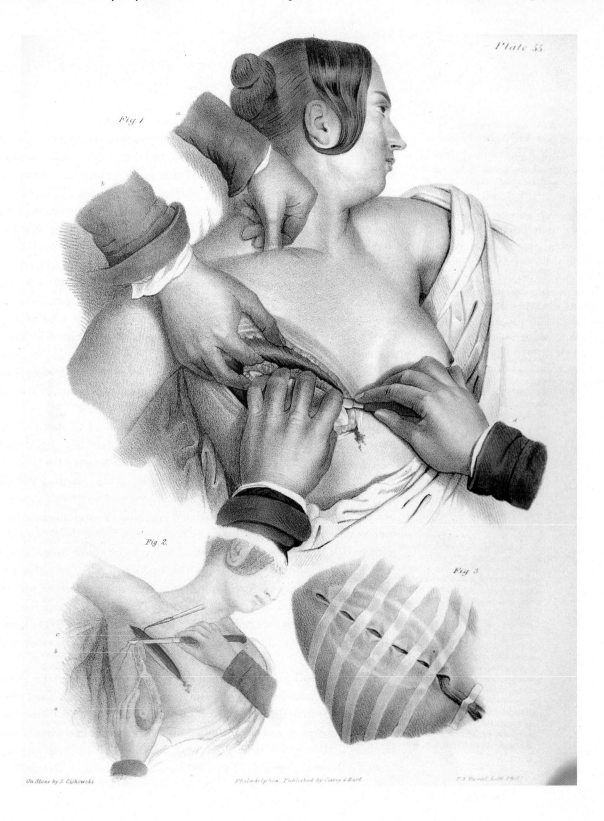

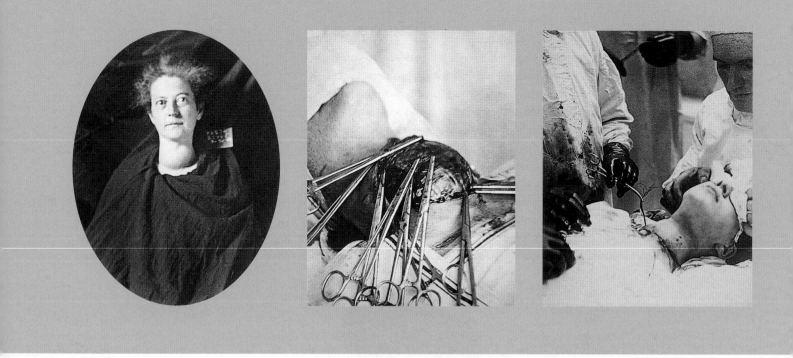

11. Stringent hemostasis by use of multiple blood vessel clamps and attention to technical details allowed surgical operations to be completed on previously inaccessible internal organs. The highly vascularized thyroid gland is one such example. It was rarely extirpated in the nineteenth century, but the work of such pioneer American surgeons as William Halsted, George Crile, and the Mayo brothers brought about a revolution in endocrine surgery. In this series of photographs (September 1909) Charles Mayo completes a thyroidectomy on a female patient with Graves' disease, or hyperthroidism, and obvious exophthalmos, or protrusion of the eyeballs. *(Courtesy of Stanley B. Burns, M.D., and The Burns Collection and Archive)*

Adolf Gundersen (1865–1938) was born in Norway, received his medical degree from the University of Christiania in 1890, and served as a resident surgeon at the Rigshospitalet in Christiania. To gain further surgical experience and repay educational debts to a maternal uncle, he emigrated to La Crosse, Wisconsin, in 1891. There he joined Christian Christensen as an assistant and remained in practice with him until 1918, when the partnership dissolved. During these years Gundersen also took additional surgical study in Austria, Germany, and Switzerland. In 1924 Gundersen founded, with his three sons, the Gundersen Clinic, which became one of Wisconsin's largest and most successful group practices. Gundersen wrote little, but he reputedly performed the first appendectomy in the state in 1894, and he set standards for surgical practice throughout western Wisconsin. One of the original clinical preceptors for the University of Wisconsin Medical School, he delivered the opening address before the Scandinavian Surgical Society meeting in Copenhagen in 1905. He was knighted by the king of Norway for his service to Norwegian physicians in 1925, and he served as a member of the Board of Regents for the University of Wisconsin.

Charles Horace Mayo (1865–1939) was the brother of William and one of the Mayo family members who established the Mayo Clinic. He received his medical education at the Chicago Medical College (later Northwestern University), graduating in 1888. After a period of postgraduate study at the New York Polyclinic and the New York Post-Graduate Medical School, he joined his brother in private practice in Rochester, Minnesota. Although not as prolific or surgically innovative as his brother, Mayo was well regarded and served as president of the Society of Clinical Surgery (1912), the Clinical Congress of Surgeons of North America (1914), the American Medical Association (1916), the American College of Surgeons (1924), and the American Surgical Association (1932). His name is associated with the operative treatment of tic douloureux, in which the affected nerve branch is exsected and the foramen of exit in the skull is plugged by a silver screw to prevent reunion, and with a bunionectomy, the principal feature of which is the resection of the first metatarsal head.

Arthur Carroll Scott (1865–1940) was born in Gainsville, Texas, where he served an apprenticeship to a local family practitioner. In 1886, Scott received his medical degree from Bellevue Hospital Medical College, and for the next two years he served as an intern and resident surgeon at the Western Pennsylvania Hospital in Pittsburgh. Moving back to his home town, Scott became a railway surgeon for the Santa Fe Railroad. From 1892 to 1940 he was in practice in Temple, Texas, and founded, with Raleigh White, the Scott and White Clinic. As senior surgeon and long-time president of the institution, Scott became an authority on the diagnosis and surgical treatment of cancer. Scott was a member of the Board of Governors of the American College of Surgeons (1927–1933) and chairman of the Texas Committee of the American Society for the Control of Cancer (1913–1925).

Joseph Colt Bloodgood (1867–1935) received his undergraduate education at the University of Wisconsin in 1888 and his medical degree from the University of Pennsylvania School of Medicine in 1891. The following year he served as an assistant resident surgeon at The Johns Hopkins Hospital, and in 1893 he attended various European clinics and hospitals. Upon Bloodgood's return to Baltimore, he became Halsted's resident surgeon and remained in this position until 1897. As a surgeon, Bloodgood practiced at St. Agnes Hospital in Baltimore while also serving on the surgical faculty at The Johns Hopkins University. For many years he directed the laboratory of surgical pathology at the Hopkins and made basic contributions to the pathology of bone tumors and their diagnosis and treatment by x-ray and radium. Bloodgood impressed on both physicians and the lay public the importance of early detection and treatment of cancer, especially so-called precancerous lesions such as "black moles" and "ulcers." He is particularly remembered for Bloodgood's hernia operation, which involved a transplantation of the rectus muscle when the conjoined tendon has been obliterated, and his theory of the causation of chronic mastitis. Bloodgood's interest in the latter led to his describing the "blue-domed" breast cyst.

Austin Maurice Curtis (1868–1939) graduated from Lincoln University in 1888 and the Northwestern University School of Medicine in 1891. He became the first intern at the newly established Provident Hospital in Chicago where he worked closely with Daniel Hale Williams. From 1892 to 1898 Curtis engaged in the private practice of surgery, during which time he became the first African-American physician to receive a regular staff appointment at a "white" Chicago hospital (Cook County Hospital, 1896), when the County Commissioners agreed to open a staff position for one African-American doctor. Considered among the most prominent African-American surgeons of his era, Curtis was recruited to be surgeon-in-chief of the Freedmen's Hospital in Washington, D.C. in 1898. He soon joined the surgical faculty at Howard University and in 1928 was appointed professor of surgery. Curtis was the first African American to hold Howard University's surgical chair and was highly regarded for his bedside teaching skills and operative expertise. He gave numerous surgical demonstration clinics at African-American hospitals throughout the South and headed the National Medical Association in 1911. With one of his three physician sons, Curtis established a surgical hospital for African-American private patients (1925–1933) in Washington, D.C.

Jabez North Jackson (1868–1935), born in Labadie, Missouri, received his medical degree from the University Medical College of Kansas City. This was followed by graduate work at the New York Polyclinic Hospital. From 1891 to 1896 Jackson was demonstrator of anatomy at his alma mater, then professor of surgical anatomy and adjunct professor of surgery until 1900, when he became professor of the principles and practice of surgery (1900–1911). During the Spanish-American War he served as a brigade surgeon in charge of the Second Division Hospital of the Second Army Corps. Among his numerous honors were presidencies of the Western Surgical Association (1913) and the American Medical Association (1927). His name is eponymically linked with Jackson's membrane or veil, a thin vascular membrane or veil-like adhesion, covering the anterior surface of the ascending colon from the cecum to the hepatic flexure, that can cause obstruction by kinking of the bowel.

Ernest Amory Codman (1869–1940) was a leading crusader for the reform of hospital standards. He was born in Boston and attended Harvard College (1891) and Harvard Medical School (1895). After completing a surgical house-officership at the

Massachusetts General Hospital, he joined that institution's surgical staff and became a member of the Harvard faculty. He lost his staff privileges at the Massachusetts General Hospital in 1914 in a dispute over evaluating the competence of surgeons (eventually the seniority system was abolished), which resulted from his zealous efforts to improve and promote the standardization of hospital treatment nationally. Thus, to test his management concepts, Codman was forced to establish his own private hospital in Boston. His ideas and results were enumerated in a privately printed pamphlet, *A Study in Hospital Efficiency, As Demonstrated by the Case Report* (1915 and 1920). In the early 1920s Codman established the first bone tumor registry in the United States, which set the precedent for a national exchange of information on bone tumor cases. This effort culminated in his authoring *Bone Sarcoma, An Interpretation of the Nomenclature* (1925). He described subdeltoid bursitis, was also among the country's earliest experts on diseases and injuries of the shoulder, and wrote the now classic textbook *The Shoulder: Rupture of the Supraspinatus Tendon and Other Lesions in or about the Subacromial Bursa* (1934). Codman's name is linked with a clinical sign of hunching of the shoulder that occurs when the deltoid muscle contracts in the absence of rotator cuff function, and with a chondroblastoma.

Arthur Emanuel Hertzler (1870–1946) was born in West Point, Iowa, and received his medical education at Northwestern University (1894). His postgraduate education included stints with Wilhelm Waldeyer and Hans Virchow in Berlin and the obtaining of a master of arts degree from Illinois Wesleyan in 1897. Most of Hertzler's career was divided between teaching in Kansas City and developing a multispecialty clinic in Halstead, Kansas. The latter institution was formally established in 1902 and was repeatedly expanded along the model of the Mayo Clinic. In 1933 it was formally transferred to the Sisters of Saint Joseph. For five years (1902–1907), Hertzler was professor of histology and pathology at the University Medical College of Kansas City. For the last forty years of his life, he was on the surgical faculty of the University of Kansas School of Medicine, becoming full professor in 1919. Hertzler always considered himself a family physician first and a surgeon second. However, he ranks among the most accomplished surgical pathologists of his era. From the outset of his career, he saved virtually every surgical specimen he excised and amassed a collection of 150,000 slides. This remarkable assemblage allowed Hertzler to author ten lengthy monographs on surgical pathology (1930–1938) under the direction of the J. B. Lippincott Company. Hertzler was one of the most prolific surgeon-authors of the twentieth century and counted among his other works *Laboratory Guide in Bacteriology* (1903), *A Treatise on Tumors* (1912), *Surgical Operations with Local Anesthesia* (1912), the two-volume *The Peritoneum* (1919), the two-volume *Clinical Surgery by Case Histories* (1921), *Diseases of the Thyroid Gland* (1922), *Minor Surgery* (1930), and *Surgery of General Practice* (1934). He achieved worldwide popular acclaim with the 1938 publication of his autobiography, *The Horse and Buggy Doctor*, which sold more than 200,000 copies the first year (it was a Book-of-the-Month Club choice) and eventually was translated into almost twenty languages. Hertzler soon followed his autobiography with *The Doctor and His Patients, The American Domestic Scene as Viewed by the Family Doctor* (1940), *The Grounds of an Old Surgeon's Faith* (1944), and *Ventures in Sciences of a Country Surgeon* (1944). Irascible in his professional views, Hertzler was no different in his private life, having been married and divorced three times.

William Wayne Babcock (1872–1963) was born in East Worcester, New York, and attended the College of Physicians and Surgeons in Baltimore (1893). He became a resident physician at St. Mark's Hospital in Salt Lake City but considered his medical education to have been inadequate and matriculated at the University of Pennsylvania Department of Medicine, where he received his medical degree in 1895. After several years of house officership at various Philadelphia hospitals, Babcock was appointed demonstrator and lecturer in pathology and bacteriology at the Medico-Chirurgical College of Philadelphia. In 1903 he was named as professor

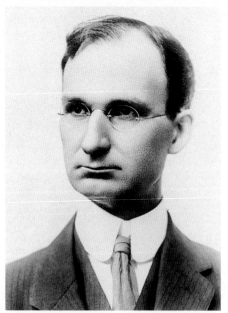

12. Arthur Emanuel Hertzler. *(Historical Collections, College of Physicians of Philadelphia)*

of gynecology at Temple University School of Medicine, and the following year he became professor and head of the department of surgery, a position he held until 1943. Babcock was best known for his originality in devising several surgical procedures, including an extirpation of the varicosed saphenous vein by introducing an olive-tipped sound, fastening the vein to it, and then drawing the latter out (1907), and the operative decompression of an aortic aneurysm by carotid–jugular anastomosis (1929). His major textbook was the *Principles and Practice of Surgery* (1928). Less than 5'3" in height, Babcock was considered an authoritative individual with a sometimes abrupt personality.

William David Haggard, Jr. (1872–1940), the son of a surgeon, was born in Nashville and received his medical degree from the University of Tennessee Medical Department in 1893. Three years later, Haggard was appointed assistant professor of gynecology at his alma mater and, in 1900, professor of gynecology and abdominal surgery. He served in the latter capacity until 1912, when he became professor of surgery and clinical surgery at the Vanderbilt University Medical School. He remained in this position until his death. Among his many honors was serving as chairman of the American Medical Association's Surgical Section (1916) and president of the American College of Surgeons (1925), the American Medical Association (1925), and the Southern Surgical Association (1933). During World War I, Haggard was named to the national Advisory Board of the Division of Surgery and acted as surgeon to Evacuation Hospital No.1 in Toul, France. Renowned as an investigator of clinical subjects, especially the abdominal and pelvic region of the body, he originated the concept of the periodic health examination. In his presidential inaugural speech to the American Medical Association, Haggard stated that "prevention runs a thread of gold through the fabric of medicine." Respected for his skills in undergraduate medical teaching, he authored *The Romance of Medicine and Other Addresses* (1927) and *Surgery, Queen of the Arts and Other Papers and Addresses* (1935).

Allen Buckner Kanavel (1874–1938) was born in Sedgwick, Kansas. The son of a Methodist minister, Kanavel received both his undergraduate education (1896) and his medical degree (1899) from Northwestern University. Following graduation from medical school, Kanavel went abroad, studying in Vienna for six months. On

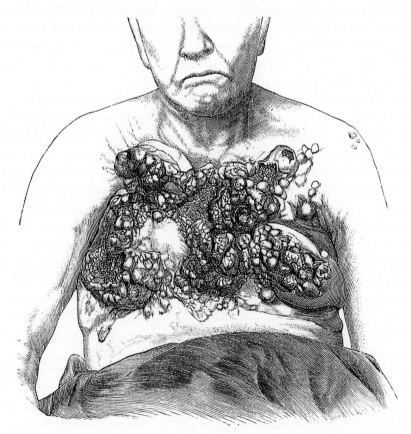

13. Samuel Weissell Gross authored an early text (1880) on tumors of the mammary glands. Most of the illustrations were elementary wood engravings, including this "disseminated simple carcinoma of the breast." Gross's work was preceded by Homer Ostrom's *Treatise on the Breast and its Surgical Diseases* (1877), the first surgical text written in the United States dedicated solely to breast disease. *(Author's Collection)*

413

returning to the United States, he undertook an internship at Cook County Hospital. In 1901 Kanavel opened offices on the south side of Chicago for general practice. Within one year's time he was dissatisfied with private practice and accepted a position as instructor of clinical surgery at his alma mater. From 1908–1917 he was assistant professor of surgery, and two years later was appointed professor of surgery. In 1920 Kanavel was named chairman of the division of surgery at Northwestern. Early in his surgical career, Kanavel became interested in severe infections of the hand that did not respond well to the era's standard treatment. Believing that much crippling of hands and fingers might be prevented with improved surgical technique, he developed a wholly original method of studying the tendon sheaths and fascial spaces of the hand. In so doing, he produced an efficient system of drainage for every anatomical compartment. His research resulted in a monograph, *Infections of the Hand* (1912), that is the first comprehensive treatise on the subject and the classic work on tendon and bursal hand spaces relevant to the management of hand infections. Kanavel was a founding member of the American College of Surgeons and served as its president in 1931. In addition, he was an associate editor of *Surgery, Gynecology & Obstetrics* at its inception and became editor-in-chief in 1935. Kanavel was killed in a car accident near Mojave, California.

Dean DeWitt Lewis (1874–1941) was born in Kewanee, Illinois, and received his bachelor of arts degree from Lake Forest University (1895) and his doctor of medicine degree from Rush Medical College (1899). He served an internship at Cook County Hospital and, upon completion of this service, accepted a position as instructor of anatomy at the University of Chicago. From 1903 to 1924, Lewis taught surgery at his alma mater, being named professor of surgery in 1920. Beginning in the mid-1920s, he received offers from several medical schools to head their departments of surgery, and in January 1925 he assumed the professorship of surgery at the University of Illinois. Lewis remained for just six months and was then named professor of surgery at The Johns Hopkins Hospital as successor to William Halsted. During World War I, Lewis was actively involved in the management of numerous base hospitals, and after the armistice he was promoted to lieutenant colonel and placed in command of General Hospital No. 28 at Fort Sheridan, Illinois. Lewis remains best known for editing the widely used twelve-volume *Loose-Leaf Practice of Surgery* as well as for his lengthy chief editorship of the *Archives of Surgery* (1920-1940). Among his honors was serving as chairman of the American Medical Association's Section on Surgery (1919) and as president of the Association in 1933. The last few years of his life were marked by increasing senility, necessitating his removal from clinical activities.

Irvin Abell (1876–1949) was born in Lebanon, Kentucky, and received his medical education at the Louisville Medical College (1897). He continued his postgraduate studies at the Universities of Berlin and Marburg and, in 1900, began practice in Louisville. From 1900 to 1908, Abell served as assistant in surgery at his alma mater. In 1908, he was appointed professor of surgery in the University of Louisville, where he remained until his death. Actively involved in all aspects of organized medicine and surgery, Abell was president of the Southern Surgical Association (1925), the Kentucky Medical Association (1926), the American Medical Association (1938), and the American College of Surgeons (1946). During World War I he was a lieutenant colonel commanding Base Hospital No. 59, and later he was president of the Association of Military Surgeons of the United States. From 1943 to 1946, Abell was a member of the surgical committe of the National Research Council. Relative to his interest in surgical history, he served as chairman of the Ephraim McDowell Committe in 1936, whose members were instrumental in purchasing the McDowell ancestral home in Danville, Kentucky, and aided in its restoration.

John Homans (1877–1954), a native Bostonian, graduated from Harvard College in 1897 and Harvard Medical School in 1901. He interned at the Massachusetts General Hospital, under Maurice Richardson, and remained on its surgical staff. In 1908, Richardson arranged for Homans to work in the Old

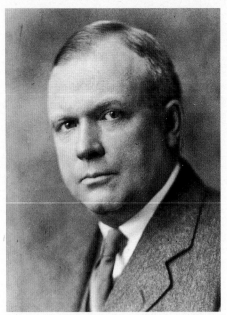

14. Dean DeWitt Lewis. *(Historical Collections, College of Physicians of Philadelphia)*

Hunterian Laboratory at The Johns Hopkins Hospital under the direction of Harvey Cushing. The research efforts of Homans and another laboratory assistant, Samuel Crowe, resulted in the first experimental evidence of the relationship between the pituitary body and the reproductive system (1910). Homans also spent time in London working with the English physiologist Ernest Starling (1866–1927). In 1912, Homans and David Cheever (1876–1955) were selected by Cushing to form the nucleus of the new department of surgery at the soon-to-open Peter Bent Brigham Hospital. Except for the period of World War I and a year-long research sabbatical spent at the Yale School of Medicine, Homans remained on the surgical faculty at the Brigham for the remainder of his life. Among his writings were two important book-length works, *A Textbook of Surgery* (1931) and the influential *Circulatory Diseases of the Extremities* (1939). Undoubtedly, Homans is best remembered eponymically for Homan's sign, a slight pain at the back of the knee or calf when the ankle is forcibly dorsiflexed, indicative of incipient or established thrombosis in the veins of the leg.

Edward Starr Judd (1878–1935) was born in Rochester, Minnesota, and matriculated at the University of Minnesota School of Medicine, where he received his doctor of medicine degree in 1902. He was an intern at St. Mary's Hospital in Rochester for a year and then was named Charles Mayo's first assistant. In 1904, Judd became the first surgeon invited to join the Mayo brothers' practice when they were no longer able to deal with their ever-increasing volume of surgical cases. Later, Judd was appointed chief of the surgical staff at the Mayo Clinic as well as professor of surgery in the Graduate School of the University of Minnesota. Recognized for his technical abilities, Judd had exceptional surgical judgement, which was displayed in 339 separate contributions to the periodical literature. Among his many honors were the presidencies of the Western Surgical Association (1912), the American Medical Association (1931), and the Society of Clinical Surgery (1932). Judd also served as a long-time member of the editorial board of the *Archives of Surgery*. He had a fanatical surgical work schedule, which began promptly at 7:00 am, with two operating rooms and two scrub teams required to deal with the large number of procedures he performed each day. While visiting Chicago, Judd contracted pneumonia and, in that preantibiotic era, succumbed to the ravages of the disease.

Donald Guthrie (1880–1958) was born in Wilkes-Barre, Pennsylvania, and received his undergraduate education at Yale University (1901) and medical degree

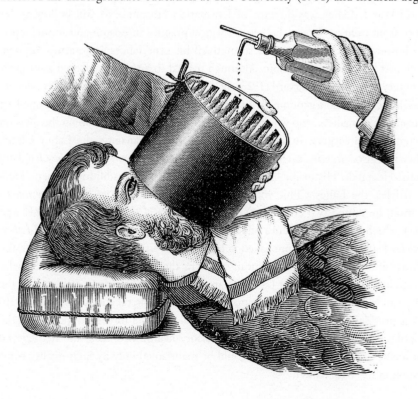

15. An ether inhaler designed by Oscar Allis (1836–1921), as shown in Laurence Turnbull's (1821–1900) *Advantages and Accidents of Artificial Anaesthesia* (1878). The mode of using the apparatus, its application to the patient's mouth, and use of a protective towel placed across the chest in case of nausea and vomiting are demonstrated. (*Author's Collection*)

415

from the University of Pennsylvania (1905). Following an internship at the Wilkes-Barre General Hospital, he entered the Mayo Clinic as a surgical assistant. After three and a half years on staff in Minnesota, Guthrie was appointed surgeon-in-chief of the Robert Packer Hospital in Sayre, Pennsylvania (1901), and remained in this position until his death. Like many of the young surgeons who trained under the Mayo brothers, Guthrie tried to emulate their clinical and managerial successes by developing his own multispecialty institution, the Guthrie Clinic. In connection with the Packer Hospital, Guthrie's facility became one of the first successful clinics in the East with a full-time staff. Although not recognized in the academic arena for most of his life, Guthrie did make numerous contributions to the periodical literature and was ultimately appointed, at the age of seventy, professor of clinical surgery of the Graduate School of Medicine of the University of Pennsylvania.

William Edwards Ladd (1880–1967) was born in Milton, Massachusetts, and received his undergraduate (1902) and medical (1906) education at Harvard University. He trained at Boston City Hospital (1906–1910) and became an office assistant to Edward Reynolds, a gynecologist and surgeon. In 1909 Ladd joined the surgical staff of that city's Children's Hospital, eventually being named chief of surgery in 1927. He was also on the Harvard faculty, being named clinical professor of surgery in 1935, and after 1940 he served as the Ladd Professor of Child Surgery. Considered the father of American pediatric surgery, Ladd devised the standard operation for malrotation of the intestines (Ladd's bands). An authority on anomalies of the esophagus, he performed the earliest successful operation for esophageal atresia in 1939 and also improved the management of diaphragmatic hernia. Along with Robert Gross, who served as his chief resident, Ladd authored the classic pediatric surgical textbook, *Abdominal Surgery of Infancy and Childhood* (1941). Among his honors was the presidency of the American Association of Plastic Surgeons (1937) and being a member of the founders' group of the American Board of Surgery and the American Board of Plastic Surgery.

Frank Howard Lahey (1880–1953) was born in Haverhill, Massachusetts, son of a wealthy bridge contractor, and received his medical degree from Harvard University in 1904. After serving as intern and house surgeon in the Long Island Hospital (1904–1905) and as surgeon in the Boston City Hospital (1905–1907), Lahey became resident surgeon of the Haymarket Square Relief Station in 1908. He was intermittently on the surgical faculty of his alma mater from 1908 to 1924 while also working as an assistant professor of surgery at the Tufts Medical School. During World War I, Lahey was director of Evacuation Hospital No. 30. Following his return from military service, he began surgical practice in Boston and started a private hospital, which, through the strength of his experiences as an army surgeon, developed into the Lahey Clinic. Although named to an unprecedented joint chair in surgery at Tufts and Harvard (1923–1924), Lahey resigned within a year to devote himself fully to his burgeoning facility. He believed that surgery could be done best by teams of specialists, who would share advanced techniques, including the division of complicated surgery. In addition to his efforts in managing the Lahey Clinic, Lahey was also surgeon-in-chief of the New England Deaconess and New England Baptist Hospitals. His major literary contributions were, in addition to many journal articles, the Lahey Clinic volumes of the *Surgical Clinics of North America*. In addition, he edited two editions of *Surgical Practice of the Lahey Clinic* (1941 and 1951), which were the resident's bible of surgery in their day. *Frank Howard Lahey: Birthday Volume* (1940) was published in honor of his sixtieth birthday. However, the writings are not those of Lahey but of surgeons throughout the United States who had studied with him. Among Lahey's many honors were serving as chairman of the American Medical Association's Section on Surgery, General and Abdominal (1930) and as president of the Association in 1941. Lahey was a forceful opponent of the adoption of group health plans and compulsory health insurance, and he believed that medical and surgical standards could be maintained only by high-quality competition in the free market.

Allen Oldfather Whipple (1881–1963) was born in Urmia, Persia (later Risaiyeh, Iran), where his father was performing missionary work as a Presbyterian clergyman. Whipple graduated from Princeton University (1904) and then matriculated at the Columbia University's College of Physicians and Surgeons (1908). From 1908 to 1910 he completed postgraduate work at Roosevelt Hospital in New York City. Whipple began the practice of medicine by joining the surgical staff at the Sloane Hospital and at his alma mater, and he spent the remainder of his professional career on the school's faculty. In 1921 he was named the Valentine Mott professor and director of surgical services at Presbyterian Hospital. During World War II, Whipple was a member of the National Research Council's Committee on Surgery. Among his numerous honors were serving as president of the New York Surgical Society (1934), the Society of Clinical Surgery (1936), and the American Surgical Association (1940). In addition, he was a trustee of the American University of Beirut (1941–1957) and Princeton University (1951–1963). Eponymously known for his triad of criteria of hyperinsulism with islet tumors, Whipple is best remembered by the surgeon for Whipple's operation (pancreaticoduodenectomy or radical excision of the head of the pancreas for carcinoma, 1935). However, his most important and long-lasting contribution was the creation of the spleen clinic in the surgery department at Columbia University, which led to many important advances, including prosthetic materials for aortic grafting and the measurement and treatment of portal hypertension. Following his retirement from Columbia, Whipple revised the medical training program at Memorial Hospital in New York City (1946–1951). He was editor-in-chief of *Nelson's Loose-Leaf Surgery* for almost twenty years and a member of the editorial board of the *Annals of Surgery* (1932–1946). Among his writings were three monographs relating to medical and surgical history, *The Story of Wound Healing and Wound Repair* (1963), *The Evolution of Surgery in the United States* (1963), and *The Role of the Nestorians and Muslims in the History of Medicine* (1967).

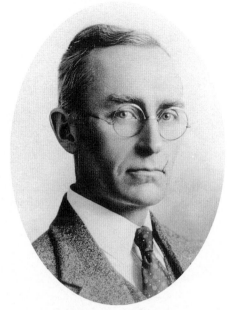

16. Allen Oldfather Whipple. *(Historical Collections, College of Physicians of Philadelphia)*

George Julius Heuer (1882–1950), born in Madison, Wisconsin, graduated from the University of Wisconsin in 1903 and obtained his medical degree with honors from The Johns Hopkins School of Medicine in 1907. He completed his surgical training under William Halsted, serving as the latter's thirteenth resident surgeon (1911–1914). In June 1914, Heuer participated in the first international exchange of surgical residents when he traveled to Hermann Küttner's clinic in Breslau, Germany (now known as Wroclaw and located in southwestern Poland), and Felix Landois (1879–1945) from Breslau assumed a position in Baltimore. Because of the onset of World War I, Heuer's stay in Breslau lasted only six weeks, but this experiment in surgical education set the stage for all future exchanges of residents. Following his return, Heuer was immediately made a captain in the medical corps of the American Expeditionary Forces and placed in charge of Evacuation Hospital No. 10 in France. From 1919 to 1922, Heuer remained at The Johns Hopkins Hospital until his appointment as the first Christian R. Holmes professor of surgery at the University of Cincinnati. He introduced the same Halstedian type of postgraduate training, including the use of full-time clinical teachers, that he had himself experienced, and the Cincinnati program became an early model for surgical residencies throughout the United States. After nine years in Cincinnati, Heuer assumed the chairmanship of the department of surgery at Cornell University and became chief surgeon at the New York Hospital, positions he held until his retirement in 1947. Heuer was a member of the founders' group of the American Board of Surgery and served as president of the American Association for Thoracic Surgery. Of the seventeen resident surgeons appointed by William Halsted, it was Heuer who made the greatest contributions to perpetuating the Halsted school of surgery, as a forceful advocate for the meticulous surgical technique first introduced into American surgery by his mentor. Accordingly, it was not surprising that immediately after his retirement, Heuer began work on a biography of his former chief. Owing to Heuer's untimely death, the work was never brought to fruition, although completed portions of the manuscript were published as a special 105-page supplement to the February 1952 *Bulletin of the Johns Hopkins Hospital.*

James Tate Mason (1882–1936), a native of Lahore, Orange County, Virginia, received his medical degree from the University of Virginia in 1905. After two years of postgraduate study at the Philadelphia Polyclinic and Municipal Contagious Hospital, he was appointed a ship's surgeon and left on a voyage around Cape Horn to Seattle. Arriving in the Northwest, Mason practiced for two years for the Pacific Coast Coal Company in Black Diamond and Franklin, Washington, after which he moved to Seattle, where he remained until his death. Mason soon developed an extensive surgical practice and from 1914–1922 was superintendent and surgeon of the King's County Hospital. In 1917, he organized the Mason Clinic and two years later, he and seven associates established the Virginia Mason Hospital, where he served as surgeon-in-chief. A leading specialist in goiter surgery, Mason was chairman of the American Medical Association's Section on Surgery, General and Abdominal (1927) as well as president of the American Medical Association (1936) and the Pacific Coast Surgical Association (1933). Mason wrote little and suffered an untimely death from a circulatory disturbance resulting in multiple emboli, which occluded blood vessels in his lower extremities and disturbed his cerebral circulation.

Dallas B. Phemister (1882–1951) attended Valparaiso University as an undergraduate and received his medical education at Rush Medical College (1904). He interned at Cook County Hospital and subsequently spent two years in private general practice. Unsatisfied with the extent of his postgraduate training, Phemister traveled to Europe and pursued two years of further study in Berlin, Paris, and Vienna. In 1911, he was appointed the Senn Fellow and surgical assistant to Arthur Dean Bevan at Rush Medical College and the Presbyterian Hospital. During the World War I Phemister headed an operating team behind enemy lines at the battles of Château Thierry and the Argonne. Returning to his alma mater, Phemister conducted surgical research into bone pathology and physiology that culminated in his use of epiphysiodesis to inhibit bone growth of a longer leg (1933). In 1925 he was named the first professor and chairman of the University of Chicago Department of Surgery, a position he held until retiring in 1947. During his chairmanship, the surgical department was widely recognized for producing a large number of academic surgeons distinguished for their contributions to basic science research and its application to clinical surgery. Among Phemister's numerous honors were the chairmanship of the American Medical Association's Section on Surgery, General and Abdominal (1925) and the presidencies of the Society of Clinical Surgery (1934), the American Surgical Association (1938), and the American College of Surgeons (1948). In a touch of surgical irony, Phemister died of a pulmonary embolism following an emergency appendectomy.

Evarts Ambrose Graham (1883–1957), born in Chicago, graduated from Princeton University in 1904 and from Rush Medical College in 1907. He interned at Presbyterian Hospital in Chicago and became a university fellow in chemistry at the University of Chicago (1907–1909). For five years, Graham served as an assistant surgeon at his alma mater, but then decided to enter private practice in Mason City, Iowa (1915–1918). With the beginnings of World War I, he joined the Army Medical Corps with the rank of captain and was later promoted to major. Through Graham's work with the Army's Empyema Commission, a significant improvement in mortality rates was achieved by delaying operation until the acute phase of the pulmonary infection had passed, and the danger of open drainage with an unfixed mediastinum was established. In 1919 Graham was named chairman of surgery at Washington University in St. Louis. As Bixby professor of surgery, he remained there until his retirement from active clinical practice in 1951. By the late 1920s he had developed an outstanding training program in chest diseases and thoracic surgery. With Warren Cole, Graham introduced cholecystography in the mid 1920s, and he reported the world's first successful one-stage pneumonectomy in 1933.

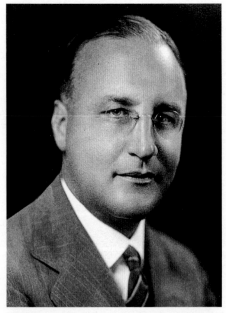

17. Evarts Ambrose Graham. *(Historical Collections, College of Physicians of Philadelphia)*

Throughout the remainder of his career, he concentrated his research efforts on the problem of bronchogenic carcinoma, culminating in a series of articles during the 1950s on the carcinogenicity of cigarette tar and the links between smoking and cancer. Graham dominated the politics of American surgery from the mid-1930s until his death, including the revitalization of the American College of Surgeons and the creation and organization of the American Board of Surgery, of which he was the first chairman. Among his many honors were the presidency of the American Surgical Association (1937) and the American College of Surgeons (1941).

William Randolph Lovelace (1883–1968) was born in a rural area near Dry Fork, Missouri, and received his medical education at St. Louis University School of Medicine (1905). His internship at St. Mary's Hospital in St. Louis was interrupted by the onset of tuberculosis, and Lovelace moved to the New Mexico Territory to regain his health. He became a surgeon to the Lantry Sharp Construction Company and the Santa Fe Railroad in Sunnyside. Performing much in the way of "kitchen surgery," Lovelace eventually relocated to Albuquerque, where he remained a railroad surgeon and joined the staff of various area hospitals. In 1922 he combined his medical practice with that of his brother-in-law, Edgar T. Lassetter, and the following year they founded the Lovelace Clinic. The institution was patterned after the Mayo Clinic, and this model was further strengthened in 1946, when Lovelace's nephew, **William R. Lovelace, II,** (1907–1965), a Mayo-trained surgeon, moved to Albuquerque to head a section of surgery at his uncle's facility. In 1947 the assets of the Lovelace Clinic were donated to establish the Lovelace Foundation for Medical Education and Research. The elder Lovelace was a founding member of the International College of Surgeons and a long-standing member of the University of New Mexico Board of Regents, serving in 1936 as its president. The younger Lovelace had completed important research in aviation physiology during his postgraduate years at the Mayo Clinic. In 1938, William R. Lovelace, II, reported the first acute case of recognized decompression sickness and also authored an article in the *Proceedings of the Mayo Clinic* describing an apparatus for the administration of oxygen, or oxygen and helium, by inhalation at high altitudes. The younger Lovelace would go on to become distinguished in the field of space medicine and was responsible for selecting and training the seven astronauts for Project Mercury. In 1964, President Lyndon Johnson appointed him director of space medicine in the manned flight space division of the National Aeronautics and Space Administration.

Thomas Grover Orr (1884–1955) was born in Carrol County, Missouri, and attended the University of Missouri (1907) and The Johns Hopkins School of Medicine (1910). He received postgraduate training in New York City (1911–1913) at the New York Hospital, the Hudson Street Hospital, and St. Mary's Free Hospital for Children. In 1915 Orr was named professor of bacteriology at the University of Kansas School of Medicine and soon was appointed instructor in the department of surgery. From 1924 to 1949 he was professor of surgery and chairman of the department, remaining clinically active until 1954. Surgery was Orr's sole vocation and avocation; he authored or shared in writing 231 scientific articles. In addition, he wrote two textbooks, *Modern Methods of Amputation* (1926) and *Operations of General Surgery* (1944). Among his other responsibilities were serving as editor-in-chief of *The American Surgeon*, and varied activities on the editorial boards of *General Practice Clinics, International Record of Medicine, Quarterly Review of Surgery,* and *Surgery.* Orr was a founding member of the American Board of Surgery and president of the Western Surgical Association and the American Surgical Association in 1950.

Ulysses Grant Dailey (1885–1961) was born in Donaldsonville, Louisiana, attended Straight College (now Dillard University), and received his medical education at Northwestern University (1906). For the next two years, Dailey interned at Provident Hospital, and in 1908 he became an assistant to Daniel Hale Williams while also serving in a civil service position as an ambulance surgeon for the city of Chicago. In 1910 Daily was promoted to associate professor at Provident Hospital, and from 1912 to 1926 he was a full attending surgeon. To further his surgical skills,

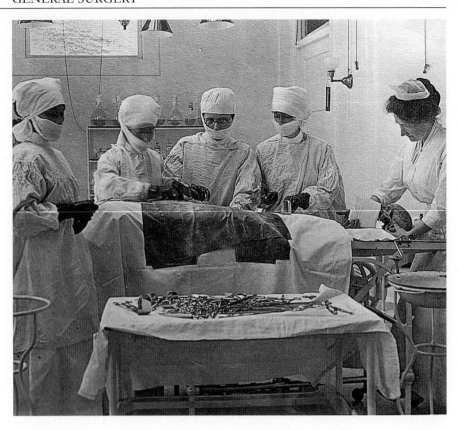

18. Although this looks like an ordinary operating room scene of the mid-1920s, a closer glance shows a skull being given anesthesia. The photograph was a satirical attempt by female surgeons and nurses to poke fun at male domination of the profession. *(Courtesy of Stanley B. Burns, M.D., and The Burns Collection and Archive)*

Dailey studied in Europe (1925), visiting medical centers in Leeds, London, Manchester, Paris, and Rome. After seven months he returned to Chicago, but he remained frustrated by the racial barriers and political problems that beset Provident Hospital and the Chicago African-American medical community. To assume more personal control over his surgical practice, Dailey purchased two large houses at the corner of 37th Street and Michigan Boulevard and opened the Dailey Hospital and Sanitarium. It is estimated that almost 1,600 surgical procedures were completed by Dailey and his co-workers at his new facility during its six years of existence. Following the death of Williams, Dailey recommitted his efforts to fostering surgical education for African-American physicians and returned to Provident Hospital, where he was appointed director of the surgical residency program. He remained at this institution through 1961, when he retired from active clinical practice. Dailey proved to be an important and long-time leader in African-American organized medicine, particularly in his relationship with the National Medical Association. He served as its president (1915) and participated in numerous editorial capacities for its *Journal*. A founding member of the John A. Andrew Clinical Society in Tuskegee, Alabama, Dailey was increasingly in demand for named lectureships and clinical demonstrations, especially in the rural South. During the 1950s he did health organizational work in Pakistan and Haiti. A well-recognized author with over sixty publications to his credit, Dailey was one of the earliest African-American surgeons to become a diplomate of the American Board of Surgery (1942) and was a fellow of the American College of Surgeons (1945). He was a founding member of the International College of Surgeons and, through his association with Max Thorek, became the first African-American physician to participate on an international surgical panel.

Fred Wharton Rankin (1886–1954) was born in Mooresville, North Carolina, and received his bachelor of arts degree from Davidson College in 1905 and his doctor of medicine degree from the University of Maryland in 1909. Following graduation, he became a resident surgeon at University Hospital in Baltimore (1909–1912) and was assistant demonstrator of anatomy and associate in surgery at his alma mater from 1913 to 1916. During these years, Rankin also received a master's degree in English (1913) at St. John's College in Annapolis. In an effort to strengthen his surgical skills, Rankin joined the Mayo Clinic as a fellow in surgery (1916) and other than a stint as a major in the medical corps during World War I, remained in Minnesota through the beginning of 1923. At that time, he moved to Kentucky to become professor of surgery at the University of Louisville and chief of the surgical staff of the City Hospital. Within one year, political difficulties arose, and Rankin left Louisville to join the Lexington Clinic. He returned to the Mayo Clinic in 1926 as head of a surgical section and remained for seven years. In January 1933, Rankin left the Mayo Clinic for the last time and returned to the private practice of surgery in Lexington, Kentucky, where he joined the staffs of St. Joseph's and Good Samaritan Hospitals. Rankin was brusque, impatient, and intolerant to those he believed did not measure up to his standards of decisiveness and incisiveness. Married to Edith Mayo, daughter of Charles Mayo, Rankin had a difficult relationship with William Mayo, which contributed to his ultimate ouster from the Mayo Clinic. So strained were the personal animosities that Rankin returned to the Mayo Clinic only once after he last left the institution in 1933, and that was to attend the funeral of his father-in-law. Rankin never appeared to be truly interested in teaching and was regarded as being almost antagonistic to academia. During World War II he was a chief consultant in surgery to the armed forces of the United States, with particular responsibility for the assignment of surgical personnel. He was an expert clinical surgeon, and his bibliography consists of almost three hundred articles, the majority of which deal with gastrointestinal surgery. He also authored two surgical texts, *The Colon, Rectum and Anus* (1932) and *Cancer of the Colon and Rectum* (1939). Rankin was a natural leader and accordingly became an important figure in the politics of American surgery. He had the distinction of being one of only three surgeons in the history of American surgery (the Mayo brothers were the others) to be president of the American Medical Association (1942), the American Surgical Association (1949), and the American College of Surgeons (1953). A measure of Rankin's stature is indicated by the fact that six universities (Davidson, Kentucky, Louisville, Maryland, Northwestern, and Temple) awarded him honorary degrees.

Harrison Shoulders (1886–1963), born in Whitleyville, Jackson County, Tennessee, received his undergraduate education at Potter Bible College in Bowling Green, Kentucky, and his medical degree from Nashville Medical College (later Vanderbilt University) in 1909. He served an internship at St. Thomas Hospital in Nashville (1909–1910) and was house surgeon of Fonts Infirmary from 1910 to 1912. Shoulders then became assistant director of the Tennessee State Department of Health until 1917. After being commissioned a captain in the United States Army Medical Corps (1917–1919), he sought further surgical training in New York City as house surgeon on William Coley's service at the Hospital for the Ruptured and Crippled. From 1922 to 1955, Shoulders was in the private practice of surgery in Nashville while serving on the clinical faculty of his alma mater as associate professor of surgery. He was the organizer and first president of the Nashville Surgical Society and a member of the founders' group of the American Board of Surgery. Shoulders aided the advancement of American surgery through his impressive leadership skills, which culminated in his serving as the one hundredth president of the American Medical Association in 1946.

Arthur Wilburn Allen (1887–1958), born in McKinney, Kentucky, graduated from The Johns Hopkins School of Medicine in 1913. He immediately went on to spend his entire surgical career at the Massachusetts General Hospital, starting as an intern and eventually becoming chief of that institution's East Surgical Service (1936–1948) and lecturer in surgery at Harvard Medical School (1936–1948). In World War I he was a captain in the medical corps, serving in France and Germany with the Fourth Division. His major contribution to surgery was as a superb clinician and as a demanding and much beloved postgraduate teacher who trained hundreds of surgeons. Although he was not recognized as a writer, Allen's stature is indicated by the numerous offices he held in organized surgery, including chairman of the Surgery Section of the American Medical Association (1942), and president of the Boston Surgical Society (1942), the American College of Surgeons (1947), the Society of Vascular Surgery (1948), the Massachusetts Medical Society (1949), and the Pan-Pacific Surgical Society (1955–1958). In addition, Allen was chairman of the Board of Regents of the American College of Surgeons from 1948 to 1951.

Frederick Amasa Coller (1887–1964) was born in Brookings, South Dakota, and received bachelor's (1906) and master of science (1908) degrees from South Dakota State College. He attended Harvard Medical School (1912) and pursued surgical training at the Massachusetts General Hospital (1912–1915). Coller's studies were interrupted by the outbreak of World War I, when he was asked to join the surgical staff of the American Ambulance Hospital based at Neuilly-sur-Seine, France. He later joined a Harvard unit that arrived in Flanders to work with the Royal Army Medical Corps of the British Expeditionary Force. After six months in France, he went to England, where he was named assistant director of the American Woman's War Hospital in Paighton, Devonshire (1916). Returning to America, Coller joined his father in private surgical practice in Los Angeles (1916–1917). In a bizarre turn of events for the young surgeon, when the United States formally entered the war, Coller was drafted despite his prior voluntary service. He was once again sent abroad with a field hospital unit attached to the 91st Division. Coller accompanied the troops through northern France and Belgium in the final battles of the war, and on demobilization (1919) he reentered private practice in California. In mid-1920, Coller was invited by Hugh Cabot (1872–1945) to join the surgical faculty at the University of Michigan. Coller remained in Ann Arbor until his retirement in 1957, having been promoted to professor of surgery (1925) and head of the department (1930). During World War II he was a member of the surgical committee of the National Research Council and special consultant to the Surgeon General of the United States Army. Coller was internationally respected as a clinical surgeon, medical investigator, and outstanding teacher. Working with Eugene Potter, he conducted extensive studies of water and electrolyte metabolism in surgical patients (1930s). Their research demonstrated that the insensible fluid loss of the sick surgical patient averaged two liters per day and that such abnormal water and electrolyte depletion could lead to severe cardiovascular collapse. Coller developed a course of therapy aimed at replacement of urinary losses of sodium, potassium, and water that was utilized by surgeons throughout the world. Among his honors was serving as president of the American Surgical Association (1943) and the American College of Surgeons (1949). In 1947 Coller's many surgical protégés established the Frederick A. Coller Surgical Society, and four decades later he was the subject of a full-length biography written by James Robinson.

Mont Rogers Reid (1889–1943) was born near Oriskany, Virginia, attended Roanoke College (1908), and received his medical degree from The Johns Hopkins Medical School in 1912. He was appointed an intern under William Halsted and the following year (1913–1914) was named an assistant resident in pathology. Subsequently, Reid returned to surgery and held the position of assistant resident surgeon (1914–1918). In 1918 Halsted appointed Reid to be his resident surgeon, a position he occupied for three years. When George Heuer was nominated for the chair of surgery at the University of Cincinnati in 1922, he invited Reid to join him. A decade later, when Heuer departed for New York Hospital, Reid was chosen to be his successor. In 1925 Reid was visiting professor of surgery to the Union Medical College of Peking, China. He returned to Cincinnati a victim of malaria, which for a time considerably impaired his health. Under the leadership of Heuer and Reid, the University of Cincinnati became one of the nation's outstanding training centers for surgeons. Reid's principal scientific contributions were experimental and clinical studies of surgery of the thyroid gland and of the large blood vessels. In 1939 he was offered the professorship of surgery at The Johns Hopkins Hospital, but he declined the appointment. Reid's premature death was met by an outpouring of public sympathy in Cincinnati, where the city hall flag was flown at half mast.

Roscoe Conkling Giles (1890–1970), born in Albany, New York, received his undergraduate education at Cornell University (1911), and was the first African American admitted to that institution's school of medicine (1915). Because of the racial attitudes of that time, Giles could consider only African-American hospitals for his postgraduate training, and so began his life-long relationship with Provident Hospital in Chicago. In 1917 he passed a Civil Service examination to be a junior physician at the Municipal Tuberculosis Sanitarium and Oak Park Infirmary, but he was denied appointment on racial grounds. Through the intervention of a Chicago alderman, Giles was eventually appointed a supervisor in the Chicago Health Department. From 1917 to 1970 Giles was an attending surgeon at Provident Hospital, and during the last twenty-five years of his life he was an assistant professor of surgery at Chicago Medical School. Seeking to expand his surgical skills, Giles took postgraduate surgical work in Vienna (1931) and, in 1933, studied bone pathology and anatomy at the University of Chicago. Five years later he became the first African-American surgeon to be certified by the American Board of Surgery. Giles was actively involved in many aspects of the National Medical Association; he was on its executive committee for ten years (1926–1935) and served as its president in 1937. He also chaired the National Medical Association's committee that succeeded in having the abbreviation "col." (colored) removed from the names of all African-American physicians listed in the American Medical Association's Directory (1938–1940). Giles was an important figure in the NAACP campaign to open Bellevue Hospital in New York City to African-American interns (1915), and following World War II he worked to secure the inclusion of African-American physicians on the local and appeals boards of the Selective Service System and to open military hospitals to African-American officers. In 1945 Giles was made a fellow of the American College of Surgeons and was invited to become a founding fellow of the International College of Surgeons.

Louis Tompkins Wright (1891–1952) of LaGrange, Georgia, attended Clark University in Atlanta (1911) and received his medical education at Harvard Medical School (1915). Unable to secure an internship at either Boston City, Peter Bent

19. Some of the most unheralded works of nineteenth-century American surgeons are their personal surgical journals. In many instances, these mostly unpublished private diaries provide unique insights into the professional doings of well-known medical personalities. Lewis Sayre's casebook of the late 1860s *(left)* contains his own drawings of various patients, including this six-year-old girl with deformities of the spine and hip. She underwent a surgical operation to remove necrotic bone from her left acetabulum but succumbed to miliary tuberculosis two years later. John Syng Dorsey's notebook from about 1811 *(right)* shows his rendering of an iliac artery aneurysm. In treating this patient, Dorsey became the first surgeon in America to successfully ligate the external iliac artery. *(left: Courtesy of The New York Academy of Medicine) (right: Historical Collections, College of Physicians of Philadelphia)*

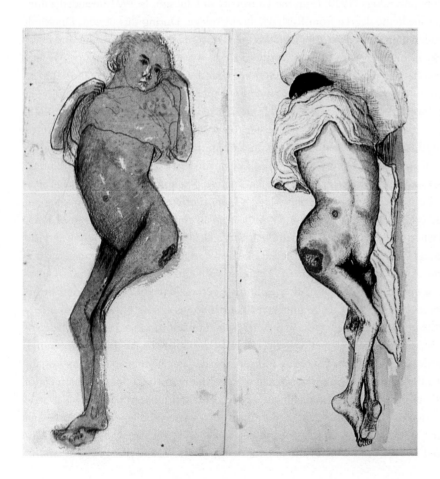

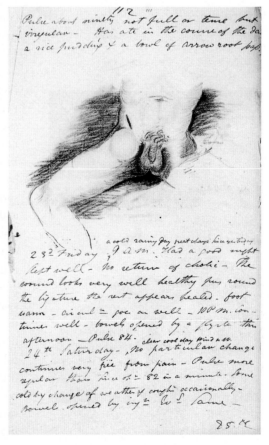

Brigham, or Massachusetts General hospitals, Wright interned at Freedmen's Hospital in Washington, D.C. (1915–1916) and soon began general practice in Atlanta. During his internship Wright demonstrated the validity of the Schick test in African Americans, a fact that Bela Schick (1877–1967) himself had previously denied. In 1918 Wright introduced a new method of intradermal vaccination against smallpox. During World War I he was commissioned a first lieutenant in the Medical Corps and assigned to the 92nd Division stationed in France. At Field Hospital No. 366, the triage facility of the division, Wright was head of the surgical wards. Having been gassed with phosgene and suffering permanent pulmonary damage, Wright was awarded the Purple Heart. Returning to the United States, he opened his office in Harlem and was appointed clinical assistant visiting attending at Harlem Hospital Center, the lowest rank in the outpatient clinic. Yet, with this seemingly minor position, Wright became the first African-American physician to be appointed to the staff of a New York City Hospital. A decade later he became the the first African-American physician to hold the position of police surgeon in a major United States city. From 1943 until his death, Wright was surgical director of Harlem Hospital. During the later years of his life, he was mainly involved in administrative duties, including the directorship of the Harlem Hospital Cancer Research Foundation, the founding of the *Harlem Hospital Bulletin*, and membership on the Advisory Council and Executive Committee of the New York City Department of Hospitals. Wright also served as chairman of the Board of Directors of the National Association for the Advancement of Colored People (1932–1952) and was a cofounder and influential member of the strongly antisegregationist Manhattan Central Medical Society. Among his other clinical achievements was pioneering the use of aureomycin (1948), inventing a brace for cervical vertebrae fractures (1936), and devising a blade-plate for operative treatment of knee-joint fractures. Wright was a diplomate of the American Board of Surgery (1938) and the second African-American surgeon to become a fellow of the American College of Surgeons (1934).

Lester Reynold Dragstedt (1893–1975) was born in Anaconda, Montana, and received his bachelor of science (1915), master of science (1916), and doctor of science in physiology (1920) from the University of Chicago. In 1921 he added a doctor of medicine degree from Rush Medical College. During this period, Dragstedt considered himself primarily a basic scientist and joined the pharmacology and physiology faculties at the State University of Iowa. After serving in the Army Medical Corps he was appointed to the physiology staff at his alma mater, and later he became chairman of the department of pharmacology and physiology at Northwestern University (1923–1925). Dragstedt's second career began in 1925, when he was invited by Dallas Phemister to become a member of the newly formed surgical faculty at the University of Chicago. In designing research facilities for his new department, Phemister employed Dragstedt as a consultant to the architect. Impressed with Dragstedt's scientific knowledge, Phemister is alleged to have stated, "I can teach surgery to a physiologist; I am interested in teaching physiology to surgeons." Dragstedt studied surgery in European clinics throughout most of 1925, and when he returned, he rejoined Phemister's faculty, receiving on-the-job surgical training. In 1947 Dragstedt succeeded Phemister as chairman and continued the tradition of an academic department of surgery with a heavy orientation toward laboratory investigation. One of the leading surgeons of the alimentary tract of his generation, Dragstedt made important contributions to the physiological understanding of pancreatic function and gastric secretion and advanced the knowledge of the cause of gastric and duodenal ulcer. In 1936 he isolated a fat-utilizing hormone, lipocaic, secreted by the pancreas, and seven years later he reintroduced and established the value of vagotomy combined with gastroenterostomy for the treatment of peptic ulcers. This surgical technique replaced the more hazardous and older style operation of total gastric resection. Minimally involved with the politics of American surgery, Dragstedt was more a creative researcher and clinician, who wrote or coauthored 364 scientific articles and one full-length work, *The Physiology and Treatment*

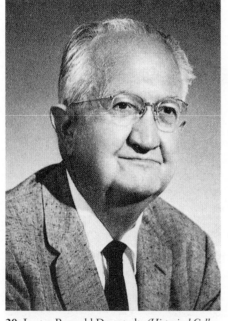

20. Lester Reynold Dragstedt. *(Historical Collections, College of Physicians of Philadelphia)*

of Peptic Ulcer (1959). When he retired from his surgical chairmanship (1959), Dragstedt moved to Gainesville and joined the surgical research faculty at the University of Florida, then under the direction of his former resident and collaborator, Edward R. Woodward.

Daniel Collier Elkin (1893–1958) was born in Louisville, attended boarding school at the Phillips Andover Academy in Massachusetts, and graduated from Yale University in 1914. Following military service, Elkin matriculated at Emory University School of Medicine, where his uncle was dean, and graduated with honors (1920). Serving as an assistant resident surgeon at New York City's Lying-In Hospital until mid-1921, Elkin moved to Boston and completed an additional two years of postgraduate training at the Peter Bent Brigham Hospital under Harvey Cushing. Returning to Atlanta in the fall of 1923, Elkin entered surgical practice with his uncle, William S. Elkin. Primarily interested in vascular surgery, he began to pursue clinical research into aneurysms and arteriovenous fistulae. In 1930 Elkin was appointed professor of surgery and chairman of the department of surgery and surgeon-in-chief to the Grady Hospital. Nine years later he was named the Joseph B. Whitehead professor of surgery and head of the surgical department at the Emory University Hospital. During World War II, Elkin's expertise in vascular surgery led to his assignment as chief of the surgical service at the U.S. Army's Ashford General Hospital, a referral center for vascular problems. Few surgeons have received as many honors as were bestowed on Elkin, including the presidencies of the Southern Surgical Association (1946), the Society of Clinical Surgery (1947), the American College of Surgeons (1956), and the American Surgical Association (1952). In addition, he served as chairman of the surgical section of the American Medical Association.

Isidor S. Ravdin (1894–1972), born in Evansville, Indiana, received his undergraduate degree from the University of Indiana (1916) and his medical education at the University of Pennsylvania (1918). He undertook most of his surgical training at his alma mater with John Deaver and George Muller. In 1927–1928, Ravdin spent a year in Edinburgh working with David Wilkie and Sharpey Shafer. Returning to Philadelphia, he was appointed professor of surgical research, and seven years later he became the Harrison professor of surgery (1935). He was among the first American surgical scientists to emphasize the importance of physiologic and biochemical approaches to surgical diseases, contrasted solely with anatomic and pathologic considerations. During World War II, Ravdin headed the surgical unit for the 20th General Hospital in India and subsequently was promoted to the rank of brigadier general. In 1945 he was appointed the John Rhea Barton professor and chairman of the department of surgery at the University of Pennsylvania. A major force in American surgery for almost three decades, Ravdin's research emphasis on the nutrition of the surgical patient helped his successor, Jonathan Rhoads and Stanley Dudrick, develop total parenteral nutrition. Retiring from his surgical chair in 1959, Ravdin became vice president for medical affairs of his alma mater and continued his prodigious fund-raising activities for the Hospital of the University of Pennsylvania and its sister institution, the School of Medicine. Among Ravdin's many honors were the presidencies of the American Surgical Association (1959) and the American College of Surgeons (1960). In 1956, he assisted Leonard Heaton in the emergency operation for ileitis that was performed on President Dwight Eisenhower.

Loyal Davis (1896–1982), born in Galesburg, Illinois, attended Knox College (1914) and the Northwestern University School of Medicine (1918). He interned at the Cook County Hospital and soon came under the influence of Allen Kanavel, who helped Davis pursue his interest in neurosurgery. The latter's surgical residency set the initital pattern at Northwestern University of a combination of basic science, surgical research laboratory work, and clinical experience as a model for future postgraduate training. Davis pursued master of science (1921) and doctor of philosophy (1923) degrees in the neurologic sciences, aided by a National Research Council Fellowship. He then spent a year with Harvey Cushing (1923–1924) in Boston, completing basic research while studying numerous neurosurgical patients.

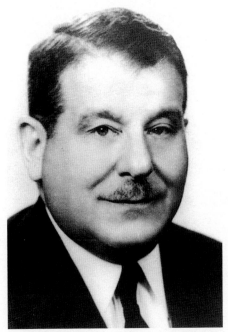

21. Isidor S. Ravdin. *(Historical Collections, College of Physicians of Philadelphia)*

Davis returned to Chicago as the first neurosurgical specialist in the Midwest and was soon appointed director of the laboratory of surgical research at his alma mater. At the age of thirty-six, Davis was named chairman of the department of surgery at Northwestern University (1932). During World War II he was the chief consultant in neurosurgery of the European Theater of Operations. An indefatigable personality, he played an important role in establishing policies in surgical education and training for several generations of surgical residents. Davis was one of the country's most prolific surgical writers. Among his full length works were *Neurologic Diagnosis* (1923), *Intracranial Tumors of Childhood, Roentgenologically Considered* (1933), *Peripheral Nerve Injuries* (1933), *Neurological Surgery* (1936), *J. B. Murphy, Stormy Petrel of Surgery* (1938), *Go In Peace* (1954), *Fellowship of Surgeons, A History of the American College of Surgeons* (1960), *From One Surgeon's Notebook* (1967), and *A Surgeon's Odyssey* (1973). In addition, Davis served as the main editor for Christopher's *Textbook of Surgery*, beginning with the 6th edition in 1956 and ending with the 9th edition in 1968, and was editor-in-chief of *Surgery, Gynecology and Obstetrics* from 1939 to 1981. A powerful influence in American surgery, Davis served as president of the American Surgical Association (1957) and the American College of Surgeons (1962). In addition, he was chairman of the American Board of Surgery and the Board of Regents of the American College of Surgeons. In later years, Davis gained further recognition from the fact that his stepdaughter, Nancy Davis Reagan, was married to President Ronald Reagan.

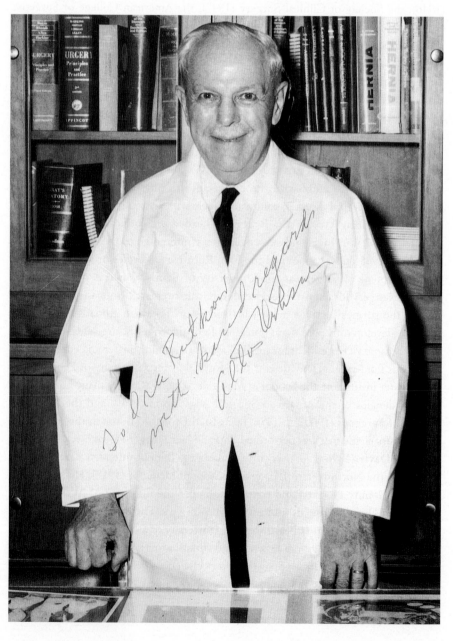

22. E. W. Alton Ochsner. *(Author's Collection)*

Edward William Alton Ochsner (1896–1981), born in Kimball, South Dakota, received a bachelor of arts degree from the University of South Dakota in 1918 and a doctor of medicine degree from Washington University in 1920. Following graduation, he served a year as an assistant resident in medicine at Barnes Hospital under internist George Dock (1860–1951). Ochsner then moved to Chicago for a surgical residency (1921–1922) supervised by his uncle, Albert J. Ochsner, who was professor of clinical surgery at the University of Illinois. Through his uncle's support and counsel, Ochsner continued his surgical training in Europe, where he studied with Paul Clairmont in Zurich and Viktor Schmieden (1874–1945) in Frankfurt. Returning to the United States, Ochsner was appointed instructor in surgery at Northwestern and subsequently assistant professor at the University of Wisconsin. After only one year in Madison, the 31-year-old Ochsner was named chairman of the department of surgery at Tulane University in New Orleans, thus becoming the successor to Rudolph Matas. Actively involved in academic research, Ochsner was also convinced that participation in private practice was a necessary component of any surgeon's professional life. Accordingly, he and other colleagues founded the Ochsner Clinic in 1942, despite much professional opposition from various elements of the medical community. Regarded as a superior clinician, Ochsner completed over 20,000 surgical operations during his lifetime, while his research activities led to over 500 contributions to the surgical literature. He was one of the first physicians to recognize the relationship between cigarette smoking and lung cancer, and this prompted his crusading effort from lecture platforms and in books and magazine articles. Among his numerous honors was serving as president of the Southern Surgical Association (1944), the Southeastern Surgical Association (1945), the Society for Vascular Surgery (1947), the American Cancer Society (1949), the American College of Surgeons (1952), the International Society of Angiography (later the International Cardiovascular Society) (1955), the International Society of Surgery (1962), and the Pan-Pacific Surgical Association (1962). Ochsner was also one of the founders and first co-editor-in-chief of the journal *Surgery*, planned in cooperation with Owen Wangensteen (1937). Ochsner was the subject of a full-length biography written by John Wilds and Ira Harkey in 1990.

Arthur Hendley Blakemore (1897–1970) was born in Senora, Virginia, and attended the College of William and Mary (1918) and The Johns Hopkins School of Medicine (1922). He received his formal surgical training at his alma mater (1922–1923), Henry Ford Hospital in Detroit (1923–1924), and the Roosevelt Hospital in New York City (1924–1926). In 1927 Blakemore was a United States Marine surgeon at Cordova General Hospital and Territorial Commissioner of Health, Cordova, Alaska Territory. He returned to New York City in 1928 and joined the surgical staff at Columbia-Presbyterian Medical Center, where he spent the remainder of his professional career working with his long-time friend and mentor, Allen O. Whipple. Widely respected for his clinical research capabilities, Blakemore was director, during World War II, of the National Research Council project in anastomosis of blood vessels for the wounded. Considered one of the country's pioneer vascular surgeons, he developed, in conjunction with Jere W. Lord (born 1910), the vitallium tube nonsuture blood vessel anastomosis technique for bridging arterial defects (1945). Working with Arthur B. Vorhees, Jr. (1921–1992), he introduced prosthetic materials (Vinyon "N" cloth) for aortic grafting (1952). Well known for perfecting balloon tamponade of the esophogeal varix (1950), Blakemore earlier proposed the application of porto-systemic anastomoses to the problem of portal hypertension, and later he directed the development of the Sengstaken-Blakemore esophageal balloon device (1954). Not one to be overly involved in surgical administration and national medical politics, Blakemore quietly retired in 1962.

Warren Henry Cole (1898–1990) was born in Clay Center, Kansas, attended the University of Kansas (1916), and received his medical education at Washington University (1920). A seminal event that influenced Cole to study surgery was the death of his mother in 1904 after a botched kitchen-table hysterectomy in the family's farmhouse. So bitter was Cole's father against the medical profession that he almost prevented the young Cole from later attending medical school. In 1920 and 1921, Cole was an intern in medicine at City Hospital in Baltimore under Thomas Boggs (1875–1938). Returning to St. Louis, Cole began a surgical residency at his alma mater under the newly named professor of surgery, Evarts Graham, and completed his postgraduate training in 1926. During this period, Cole and Graham introduced cholecystography to the profession (1924). By the mid-1930s several medical schools, most prominently Vanderbilt University and the University of Louisville, had begun attempting to woo Cole away from Barnes Hospital. Finally, in 1936, Cole succumbed to an offer from the University of Illinois and was appointed chairman of its department of surgery. Unlike his immediate predecessor, Carl A. Hedbloom (1879–1934), Cole established a full-time faculty system that brought about much in the way of research activities and expansive growth. Among Cole's many contributions to the surgical literature were the full-length works *Textbook of General Surgery* (1936), *The Breast* (1944), *Operative Technic* (1949), and *Chemotherapy of Cancer* (1970). In 1959 the Warren H. Cole Society was established by his hundreds of surgical protégés. In recognition of his scientific and administrative contributions to American surgery, Cole served as president of the American College of Surgeons (1955) and the American Surgical Association (1959). Having never had children, Cole and his wife established the Warren H. and Clara Cole Foundation (1957) to assist the activities of the University of Illinois department of surgery, the Cole Society, and selected individuals in the early stages of their careers in surgical research. A biography entitled *Warren Cole, MD, and the Ascent of Scientific Surgery* by Dennis Connaughton was published in 1991.

John Hugh Mulholland (1900–1974), a New York City native, attended New York University as an undergraduate (1921) and medical student (1925). His surgical training began with his internship (1925) at Bellevue Hospital (New York University), where he later became chief resident on the Third Surgical Division. Accepting an appointment to his alma mater's surgical faculty, Mulholland began research into such diverse fields as protein metabolism, fracture healing, and the effects of denervation on the autonomic nervous system. During World War II he entered the Army Medical Corps as a lieutenant colonel and was surgical chief of the Bellevue Unit, which became the First General Hospital located in France. In 1946 he was discharged, having received a Bronze Star and a promotion to colonel. Returning to New York City, Mulholland was named George David Stewart Professor and chairman of New York University's department of surgery, a position he held until his retirement in 1965. Mulholland served on numerous national panels, most notably the Committee on Surgery of the National Research Council and the Surgical Study Section of the United States Public Health Service, and was a member of the American Board of Surgery 1949–1953. In addition, he was president of the American Surgical Association in 1957. Mulholland's greatest impact on American surgery came through his lengthy association with the *Annals of Surgery* and his chairmanship of its editorial board from 1957 to 1970.

Frank Glenn (1901–1982) was born in Marissa, Illinois, and attended Washington University for both his undergraduate (1923) and medical (1927) degrees. He completed a medical internship at Strong Memorial Hospital in Rochester, New York (1927–1928), and then commenced surgical training at the Peter Bent Brigham Hospital under Harvey Cushing. In 1931–1932, Glenn was named Gorham Peters Traveling Fellow and worked in the surgical research laboratories at the University of Edinburgh, Scotland. Following Cushing's forced retirement from Harvard in 1932, Glenn transferred to the New York Hospital-Cornell Medical Center, where he completed his surgical residency under George Heuer (1935). Subsequently appointed an assistant to William Andrus, Glenn began work in the Laboratories of Surgical Research at Cornell. During World War II he joined the Army Medical Corps and served as surgical consultant to the Sixth Army in the Southwest Pacific. While in military service he was awarded a Bronze Star, and he

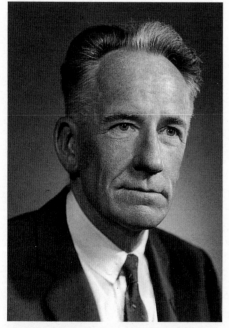

23. Frank Glenn. *(Author's Collection)*

was discharged in 1946 with the rank of lieutenant colonel. In 1947 Glenn was named first Lewis Atterbury Stimson Professor of Surgery at Cornell University Medical College and surgeon-in-chief of the New York Hospital, positions he held until he retired in 1967. In addition to his 28 chapters for surgical textbooks and 407 original articles to the periodical literature, he authored five major textbooks, *Mitral Valvulotomy* (1959), *Surgery in the Aged* (1960), *Atlas of Biliary Tract Surgery* (1963), *Surgery of the Adrenal Gland* (1968), and *Common Duct Stones* (1975). Considered among the world's leading authorities on gallbladder disease and a pioneer in cardiac surgery, Glenn developed one of the most highly respected surgical training programs in the United States. He was president of the American College of Surgeons (1954, succeeding to the post when Fred Rankin died unexpectedly) and chairman of the American Board of Surgery and the Executive Committee of Cardiovascular Surgery of the American Heart Association.

James Taggart Priestley (1903–1979) was born in Des Moines, Iowa, and received his bachelor of arts (1923) and doctor of medicine (1926) degrees from the University of Pennsylvania. He served a two-year internship at his alma mater and then went to Rochester, Minnesota, as a fellow in surgery at the Mayo Graduate School of Medicine. During his surgical residency, Priestley earned a master of science degree in experimental surgery (1931) and a doctor of philosophy degree in surgery (1932) from the University of Minnesota. In 1934 he was appointed head of a section of surgery at the Mayo Clinic, and the following year he was awarded the J. William White Scholarship for Foreign Travel. Priestley received certification from the American Board of Surgery in 1940, and three years later he was commissioned in the Army Medical Corps, eventually commanding the 237th Station Hospital in the Pacific theater. Returning to Minnesota, he advanced steadily in academic rank, becoming professor of surgery in the Mayo Graduate School of Medicine in 1948 and senior surgeon of the Mayo Clinic in 1963. Priestley is best remembered for his tireless activities on behalf of organized surgery, including the presidencies of the Central Surgical Association (1953), the Society of Clinical Surgery (1957), the Western Surgical Association (1959), and the American College of Surgeons (1964). In addition, he was chairman of the Board of Regents of the American College of Surgeons (1962) and served an eight-year stint as chairman of the Mayo Clinic's Board of Governors (1956–1964). In 1965, his former first assistants established the James Priestley Surgical Society, a select group of nationally renowned surgeons.

Robert Milton Zollinger (1903–1994) was born in Millersport, Ohio, and attended Ohio State University as an undergraduate (1923) and medical student (1927). Appointed to begin a surgical internship at the Peter Bent Brigham Hospital under Harvey Cushing, Zollinger spent a six-month interim period working with Elliot C. Cutler at Western Reserve University in Cleveland. On the completion of his surgical internship, Zollinger returned to Cleveland and became one of Cutler's surgical residents and the Crile Fellow in charge of the university's surgical research laboratory. When Cutler succeeded Cushing in 1932, he named Zollinger as his accompanying chief resident. From 1933 through 1946, Zollinger rose in academic rank from instructor to assistant professor of surgery at Harvard University. During the war years he was recruited by Cutler to join the surgical staff at the 5th General Hospital, Harvard Unit, and eventually became its commanding officer. Returning from the army, Zollinger was recruited to Ohio State University and was appointed professor and chairman of its department of surgery in 1947. His research contributions were legendary, including the eponymically recognizable Zollinger-Ellison syndrome. Among his many written works are the *Atlas of Surgical Operations* (1939), *The Influence of Pancreatic Tumors on the Stomach* (1974), *General Surgery, Principles in Practice* (1981), and *Elliott Carr Cutler and the Cloning of Surgeons* (1988). Actively involved with all aspects of organized American surgery, Zollinger served as president of the American College of Surgeons in 1962 and the American Surgical Association in 1965. In addition, he was a founder of the Society of University

Surgeons (1938) and chairman of the American Board of Surgery. As a long time editor-in-chief of the *American Journal of Surgery* (1958–1985), Zollinger left an indelible mark on the surgical literature of the mid-twentieth century.

Charles Richard Drew (1904–1950) was born in Washington, D.C., attended Amherst College (1926), and received his medical degree and master of surgery degree from McGill University (1933). From 1933 to 1935 he was an intern and resident at the Montreal General Hospital. As an African American he initially pursued surgical training at the Freedmen's Hospital in Washington, D.C. (1936–1937), but from 1938 to 1940 he was a surgical resident at Presbyterian Hospital in New York City. Working additionally as a graduate student at Columbia University, Drew earned a doctor of science degree in 1940, authoring a thesis entitled "Banked Blood, A Study in Blood Preservation." Drew's mentors in New York City included Allen Whipple and John Scudder, who aided him as he completed research on problems of fluid balance, blood chemistry, and blood transfusion and established the Presbyterian Hospital's first blood bank in 1939. Upon completing his course work, Drew returned to Howard University as an assistant professor of surgery and as an attending surgeon at Freedmen's Hospital. When World War II began, Drew was chosen by the board of the Blood Transfusion Association in New York to be the medical supervisor of the Plasma for Britain Project. Moving back to New York City, he and other colleagues established uniform procedures for procuring and processing blood and for shipping the plasma. Soon thereafter he was appointed medical director of the American Red Cross blood bank program and assistant director of blood procurement for the National Research Council in charge of blood for use by the United States armed forces (February 1941). But a few weeks later, an official directive from the armed forces to segregate Caucasian blood from other blood, and the acceptance of that directive by the Red Cross over the strenuous objections of Drew and other scientists, led to his resignation in protest. In April 1941 Drew received certification by the American Board of Surgery, and soon he was made an examiner for the Board itself. At the same time he was named professor and chairman of the department of surgery at Howard University and chief surgeon at Freedmen's Hospital, where he remained until he was killed in a car accident in rural North Carolina. Drew was a remarkable individual who accomplished much in a short lifetime, particularly in the face of unrelenting bigotry. In 1944, he received the Spingarn Medal from the National Association for the Advancement of Colored People for his seminal work on blood banks. Drew accepted fellowship in the International College of Surgeons (1946) but refused membership in the American College of Surgeons because of what he perceived as its racist attitude in not accepting other capable and well-qualified African-American surgeons. He has been the subject of several full-length biographies, including Richard Hardwick's *Charles Richard Drew: Pioneer in Blood Research* (1967), Charles Wynes' *Charles Richard Drew: The Man and the Myth* (1988), and Spencie Love's *One Blood, the Death and Resurrection of Charles R. Drew* (1996).

Henry Nelson Harkins (1905–1967) was born in Missoula, Montana, and received his bachelor's (1925), master's (1926), and doctor of philosophy (1928) degrees from the University of Chicago and his medical education at Rush Medical College (1930). He interned at Presbyterian Hospital in Chicago and in 1931 did postgraduate work at the University of Edinburgh, Scotland, and the National Hospital, London. Returning to his medical school alma mater, Harkins finished his surgical residency in 1938. During the following year he received a Guggenheim Memorial Fellowship in surgery and enjoyed a *wanderjahr* at universities in Edinburgh, Ghent, Belgium, Frankfurt, and Uppsala, Sweden. In 1939 he joined the surgical staff at Henry Ford Hospital, Detroit, and he was also associated with the surgical faculty at Wayne University College of Medicine (1943). Harkins was rejected for military service for physical reasons, and Alfred Blalock invited him to join the faculty at The Johns Hopkins Hospital as associate professor of surgery (1943–1947). During his Baltimore years he also served as secretary of the subcommittee on shock in the Office of Science, Research and Development of the National Research Council (1943–1945). In 1947 Harkins began a new career path when he was named professor of surgery and first chairman of the department of surgery at the University of Washington School of Medicine in Seattle. Aside from the dean, Harkins was the first full-time clinical appointee at the new institution. He remained as departmental chairman until his retirement from active clinical service in 1964. Harkins aided the development of American surgery through his research, teaching, and editing. He made numerous experimental studies of gastric physiology and related subjects and developed new methods for the surgical treatment of peptic ulcer (by selective and highly selective gastric vagotomy) and hernia. A prolific writer, Harkins authored or helped coauthor numerous textbooks, including *The Treatment of Burns* (1942), *The Billroth I Gastric Resection* (1954), *Surgery: Principles and Practice* (1957), *Surgery of the Stomach and Duodenum* (1962), and *Hernia* (1964). In addition, he served as editor-in-chief of the *Quarterly Review of Surgery* (later *Review of Surgery*) from 1943 to 1967, and was on the editorial boards of the *Annals of Surgery* and *the Western Journal of Surgery*. He died of a coronary occlusion while attending a surgical department picnic.

Claude E. Welch (1906–1996) was born in Stanton, Nebraska, and attended Doane College, Crete, Nebraska as an undergraduate (1928) and Harvard Medical School (1932). He pursued surgical residency training at the Massachusetts General Hospital from 1932 to 1937 and was certified by the American Board of Surgery in 1939. From 1937 to 1942, Welch worked as a first assistant with Arthur W. Allen and also served as a surgeon for the Harvard University Health Service. During World War II, Welch laid important groundwork for much of his later career by serving in North Africa and Italy with the Sixth General Hospital, a sort of Massachusetts General expeditionary force, the members of whose surgical staff, having bonded with one another in wartime, returned home after the war to become leaders of the medical profession. Welch resumed his affiliation with the Massachusetts General Hospital, rising in rank to become clinical professor of surgery. Recognized as a specialist in abdominal surgery, Welch authored nearly 300 scientific publications and delivered so many important lectures that he earned an international reputation. He was one of six physicians summoned to Rome in 1981 to consult about the surgical treatment of Pope John Paul II after the Pontiff was wounded in the abdomen by an assassin's bullet. Welch's bibliography includes four textbooks: *Surgery of the Stomach and Duodenum* (1951), *Intestinal Obstruction* (1959), *Polypoid Lesions of the Gastrointestinal Tract* (1964), and *Manual of Lower Gastrointestinal Surgery* (1980). He also served as editor-in-chief of *Advances in Surgery* and was on the editorial boards of *Surgery* and the *American Journal of Surgery*. Among his numerous honors were the presidencies of the American College of Surgeons (1973), the American Surgical Association (1976), and the American Chapter of the International Society of Surgeons (1979). In spite of Welch's many accomplishments, he failed in his 1975 bid to become president of the American Medical Association. In 1992 he authored an autobiography, *A Twentieth-Century Surgeon, My Life in the Massachusetts General Hospital.*

George Washington Crile, Jr. (1907–1992), son of George Crile, Sr., was born in Cleveland and graduated from Yale University (1929) and Harvard Medical School (1933). He completed a one-year internship at Barnes Hospital, St. Louis, and then completed a three-year surgical residency at the Cleveland Clinic. Subsequently, Crile joined his father in practice in 1937, and they remained partners until World War II intervened. Crile joined the United States Navy and served in the South Pacific with a team of enlistees from the Cleveland Clinic. Returning to Cleveland, Crile began the private practice of surgery, but his wartime experiences had convinced him of the necessity to take up the cudgels against surgical orthodoxy. As was noted in his three-columns obituary in the *New York Times*, Crile was soon branded a "foe of unneeded surgery." He angered the medical establishment by insisting that many radical procedures for breast cancer and other disease processes,

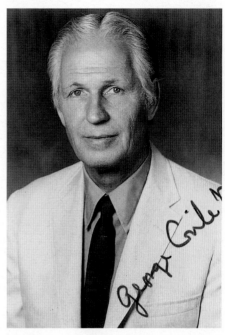

24. George Washington Crile, Jr. *(Author's Collection)*

in particular thyroid surgery, met only the surgeon's needs as contrasted with the patient's. Crile waged an endless battle against unnecessary surgery, and two decades of controversy swirled around his vigorous campaign opposing radical mastectomy. Like his father, Crile was a prolific author and wrote on a variety of topics, both surgical and nonsurgical. Among his full-length works are *Hospital Care of the Surgical Patient* (1943), *Practical Aspects of Thyroid Disease* (1949), *Treasure Diving Holidays* (1954), *Cancer and Common Sense* (1955), *More Than Booty* (1965), *A Biological Consideration of the Treatment of Breast Cancer* (1967), *A Naturalistic View of Man* (1969), *Above and Below: A Journey Through our National Underwater Parks* (1969), *To Act as a Unit: The Story of the Cleveland Clinic* (1971), *What Women Should Know About the Breast Cancer Controversy* (1973), *Surgery: Your Choices, Your Alternatives* (1978), and an autobiography, *The Way It Was, Sex, Surgery, Treasure, and Travel, 1907–1987* (1992). Crile was never part of the American surgical mainstream, but his crusades affected the lives of countless people, many of whom never heard his name. Crile's first wife, the former Jane Halle, succumbed to cancer in 1963. His second marriage was to Helga Sandburg, the daughter of the poet Carl Sandburg (1878–1967).

John Englebert Dunphy (1908–1981), born in Northampton, Massachusetts, attended Holy Cross College (1929) and received his medical degree from Harvard University (1933). He entered surgical training at Peter Bent Brigham Hospital and served as resident surgeon in 1940. During his residency, he broadened his clinical background by spending one year on the hospital's pathology service, several months as a fellow at the Lahey Clinic, a period of time as the George Gorham Peters Traveling Fellow, and twelve months as the Arthur Tracy Cabot Research Fellow at Harvard. During World War II Dunphy served on the surgical service of the Fifth General Hospital, the Peter Bent Brigham's overseas health care unit. In 1943 Dunphy succeeded Robert Zollinger as chief of the Fifth, and with the end of hostilities, Dunphy was discharged as a lieutenant colonel. On returning to the United States, Dunphy rejoined the Brigham's surgical faculty, and in 1955 he was named director of the Fifth Surgical Service (Harvard) and Sears Surgical Laboratory at the Boston City Hospital. Four years later, he was appointed Kenneth A. J. MacKenzie professor of surgery and chairman of the department of surgery at the University of Oregon Medical School. In 1964, Dunphy accepted the chairmanship of the department of surgery of the University of California School of Medicine, San Francisco. He remained in this position until his retirement in 1975. Broadly interested in general surgery, particularly abdominal surgery, Dunphy played a major role in American surgery and in national and international surgical societies. He served as president of both the American Surgical Association (1962) and the American College of Surgeons (1964). His written works number over 300 journal articles and six textbooks, including *Physical Examination of the Surgical Patient* (1953), *Repair and Regeneration, The Scientific Basis for Surgical Practice* (1969), *Current Surgical Diagnosis and Treatment* (1973), and *Fundamentals of Wound Management* (1979).

David Milford Hume (1917–1973) was born in Muskegon, Michigan, and attended Harvard University (1940) and the University of Chicago School of Medicine (1943). He completed his internship and surgical residency at the Peter Bent Brigham Hospital (1943–1951). As senior resident under Elliott Cutler and chief resident under Francis Moore, Hume helped pioneer kidney transplantation and the modern evolution of pituitary endocrinology. Starting in 1949, he began to carry out experimental animal work on kidney transplantation that culminated in a series of cadaver kidney transplants (1950–1951) in human subjects dying of renal failure. There were no survivors, but this experience led directly to the first successful twin transplantation performed by his colleagues David Murray and John Merrill. Hume also studied the suprapituitary control of the secretion of adrenocorticotrophic hormone and developed the first quantitative bioassay for serum adrenocorticotrophic hormone. This latter work was completed while Hume was on his second tour of duty in the United States Navy (his first had been wartime service in 1945–1946) assigned to the National Naval Medical Research Institute in Bethesda,

Maryland (1953–1954). In 1955 Hume was appointed professor of surgery at the Medical College of Virginia in Richmond. He went on to play a leading role in the development of Virginia Commonwealth University and helped establish a large surgical research laboratory renowned for its research in kidney transplantation. Among his many written contributions was the textbook *Principles of Surgery* (1969). Hume was killed while flying a small plane near Chatsworth, California.

W. Dean Warren (1924–1989), born in Miami, Florida, graduated from Dartmouth College in (1946) and its two-year preclinical medical school curriculum (1948) and completed his medical education at The Johns Hopkins School of Medicine (1950). Warren interned at The Johns Hopkins Hospital. He began his surgical residency at the University of Michigan under Fred Coller and finished as chief resident with Carl Moyer (1910–1970) at Barnes Hospital in St. Louis. Warren received his first academic appointment as assistant professor of surgery at the University of Virginia (1960–1963) under William Müller (born 1919). Having received a Markle Scholarship, Warren began studies in pancreatic physiology and portal circulation. In 1963 he was appointed chairman of the department of surgery at the University of Miami. There his work on the pathophysiology of portal hypertension came to fruition with the close collaboration of Robert Zeppa (1924–1993). They devised the eponymic selective distal-splenorenal shunt as a logical method of ameliorating portal hypertension and the subsequent devastating encephalopathy that so often follows a portosystemic shunt. In 1967 Warren assumed a new position as dean of the University of Miami School of Medicine, and the following year he became vice president of medical affairs. Three years later (1971) Warren became professor and chairman of surgery at Emory University in Atlanta. He remained there until his death from a recurrent squamous cell carcinoma of the left zygoma and orbit. Warren was closely involved with organized American surgery, having served as vice chairman of the American Board of Surgery (1973–1975) and chairman of the Residency Review Committee for Surgery (1976–1978). Among his many honors were the presidencies of the American Surgical Association (1987) and the American College of Surgeons (1986). Warren served on the editorial boards of the *American Journal of Surgery*, *Surgery*, and *Surgery, Gynecology and Obstetrics*.

Samuel Lee Kountz (1930–1981) was born in Lexa, Arkansas, and graduated from that state's Agricultural, Mechanical and Normal College in 1952. He then earned a master's degree in chemistry (1954) and a doctor of medicine degree (1958) from the University of Arkansas. Kountz completed seven years of postgraduate surgical training on the Stanford Service at San Francisco General Hospital (1958–1965) and was named assistant professor of surgery in 1966. During his residency years Kountz was awarded a Bank of America Giannini Fellowship, which allowed him to spend time at the Postgraduate Medical School, Hammersmith Hospital, London, with additional work at that city's St. Bartholomew Hospital (1962). In 1965 he was awarded a Visiting Fulbright Professorship to the United Arab Republic, where he spent almost four months performing surgical operations and working on research projects. By 1967, Kountz had been elevated to associate professor of surgery, and five years later (1972) he was appointed professor of surgery at the University of California, San Francisco, where he was director of the transplant service. He and Folkert O. Belzer (1931–1995), working in collaboration, established a spectacularly successful program in clinical kidney transplantation (introducing the perfusion and preservation system), which served as an international model for such centers. In 1972 Kountz was named professor and chief of the department of surgery at the State University of New York Downstate Medical Center, Brooklyn, New York. He remained there until his untimely death after a four-year lingering illness with severe neurologic deficits, presumably due to encephalitis. Kountz, one of American surgery's pioneers in renal transplantation, served on the editorial boards of *The Journal of Hypertension and Renal Disease*, *The Kidney*, and *Surgery* and was president of the Society of University Surgeons in 1975.

433

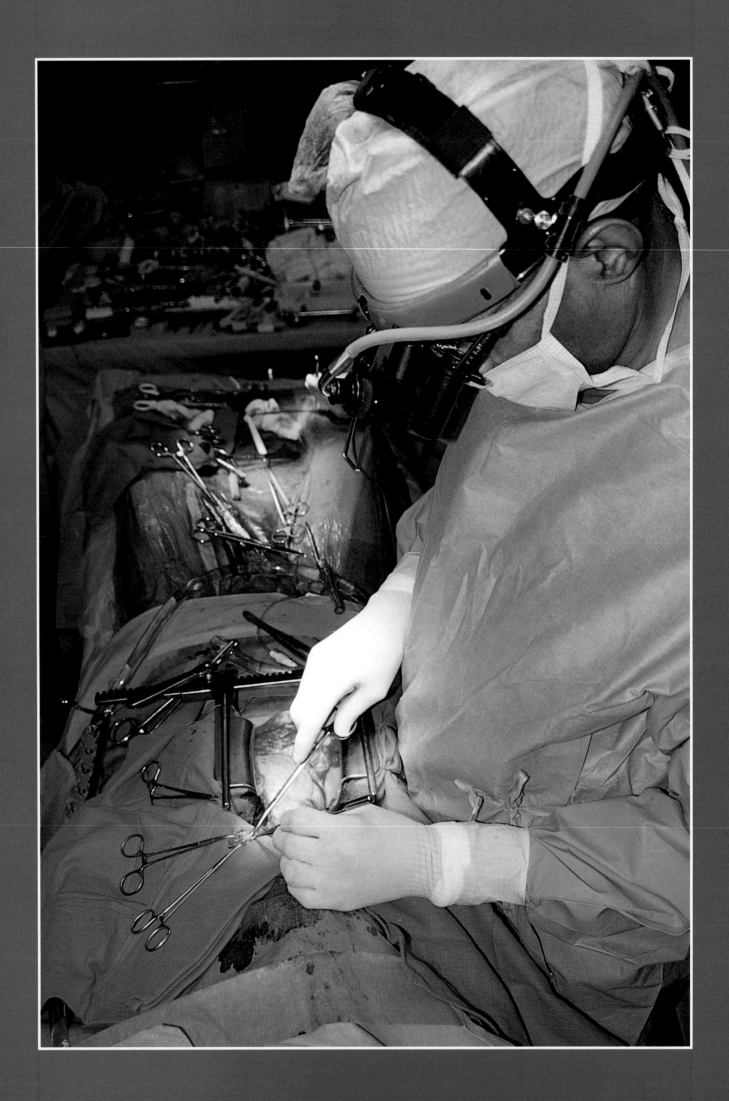

CHAPTER 14

CARDIOTHORACIC SURGERY

The opening of the thoracic cavity for both cardiac and pulmonary surgical operations involved physiological problems far more complicated than those involving the abdomen. Through the last decades of the nineteenth century, such operative intervention usually resulted in a fatal outcome. Accordingly, little practical interest was expressed in the establishment of cardiothoracic surgery as a specialty. However, as greater numbers of papers on pulmonary surgery were presented during the first years of the twentieth century this attitude changed.

In 1898, John Murphy gave a lengthy oration on thoracic surgery at the annual meeting of the American Medical Association. This lecture, later published as a four-part article more than sixty pages long in the *Journal of the American Medical Association*, was one of the more important contributions to surgery of the lungs in nineteenth-century United States. Murphy proposed that tuberculosis be treated by artificial pneumothorax, and he would later utilize thoracoplasty for the collapse treatment of the disease. Oddly, in spite of his masterful oration, Murphy never demonstrated any further sustained interest in this branch of surgery. Yet, his lecture, combined with concurrent scientific developments, provided the impetus for the eventual establishment of various thoracic surgical societies and for the acceptance of thoracic surgery as a bona fide surgical specialty.

In 1917, the New York Society for Thoracic Surgery, the first such organization worldwide, was founded. It was followed in the same year by the formation of the American Association for Thoracic Surgery. An immediate problem of the fledgling organizations was the publication of papers read at their annual meetings. Initially, New York's *Medical Record* was designated the periodical of choice, but after a few years the journal could not bear the extra cost of reproducing numerous x-rays. When the American Medical Association's *Archives of Surgery* was established in 1920, its editors took over responsibility for publishing the thoracic society's articles, which appeared in every January issue along with a special supplement. A decade later (1931), the American Association for Thoracic Surgery arranged with the C. V. Mosby Company in St. Louis to publish the *Journal of Thoracic Surgery*. Evarts Graham was appointed editor-in-chief and remained in this position until his death in 1957. A few years later, the name was changed to *The Journal of Thoracic and Cardiovascular Surgery* to reflect the growth of cardiac surgery and the significant role it would assume in the evolution of the specialty. Following Graham, the other editorial chairmen have been Emile Holman, 1957–1962; Brian Blades, 1962–1977; Dwight C. McGoon, 1977–1987; John W. Kirklin, 1988–1994; and John A. Waldhausen, 1995–??. The other influential and widely read peer-reviewed cardiothoracic journal is the *Annals of Thoracic Surgery*. Its editors-in-chief have included

1. *(facing page)* Coronary artery bypass has become one of the most common surgical operatios in the United States. With the patient's chest opened and his heart exposed, the cardiac surgeon prepares a venous graft to be used to bypass the obstructed coronary artery. In the background of this photograph, the operative area on the patient's leg where the vein graft was obtained is visible. *(Courtesy of Stanley B. Burns, M.D., and The Burns Collection and Archive and the permission of Valavanur A. Subramanian, M.D.)*

John D. Steele, 1965–1969; Herbert Sloan, 1969–1984; and Thomas B. Ferguson, 1984–??.

The possibility of certifying thoracic surgeons via written and oral examinations was first discussed by members of the American Association for Thoracic Surgery in 1936. At that time, the consensus was that no need for certification existed, since so few individuals were primarily interested in thoracic surgery. However, ten years later, as a direct result of the advances made in treating chest injuries during World War II, the need for a specialty board in thoracic surgery became apparent. Carl Eggers (1892–1956) and Alton Ochsner were appointed to form a committee to meet with members of the American Board of Surgery in order to consider establishing a subsidiary board of thoracic surgery. This committee reported to the Association at the 1947 meeting, and the executive board of the Association voted to establish a board of thoracic surgery. Ochsner, as incoming President of the American Association, appointed a larger committee to organize the new board, establish a founders' group, appoint an examining committee, and establish requirements for the education, training, and certification of thoracic surgeons. Through lengthy negotiations, a plan of organization was approved by the American Board of Surgery and the American Association for Thoracic Surgery at their respective meetings in Quebec in 1948. The first organizational meeting of the Board of Thoracic Surgery was held in Detroit in October of that year. In 1971, the Board of Thoracic Surgery changed its name to the American Board of Thoracic Surgery and was made a member of the American Board of Medical Specialties, an organization that encompasses the twenty-four primary specialty boards.

Currently, the American Board of Thoracic Surgery defines the specialty as encompassing the operative, perioperative, and surgical critical care of patients with acquired and congenital pathologic conditions within the chest, including heart lesions and congenital and acquired conditions of the coronary arteries, valves, and myocardium. Also included are pathologic conditions of the lung, esophagus, and chest wall; abnormalities of the great vessels; tumors of the mediastinum; and diseases of the diaphragm and pericardium. The management of airway difficulties and injuries to the chest are also considered within the domain of the thoracic surgeon. Applicants for certification must be already certified by the American Board of Surgery after five years of postgraduate training and then undergo an additional two years of residency in thoracic and cardiovascular surgery.

By 1995, of the approximately 621,000 total physicians in active practice in the United States, 2,300 (less than 1 percent) designated themselves as cardiothoracic surgeons. Within this cadre of cardiothoracic surgeons, 2,000 (87 percent) are board certified. (During the fifteen-year period 1980 through 1994, 2,057 certificates in cardiothoracic surgery were issued, or an average of 137 per year.) Forty (1.7%) are women and 365 (16 percent) are international medical graduates. Among the total pool of cardiothoracic surgeons, approximately 275 (12 percent) are younger than 35; 635 (28 percent) are 35 to 44 years of age; 555 (24 percent) are 45 to 54; 535 (23 percent) are 55 to 64; and 310 (13 percent) are 65 and older. Of the 40 female cardiothoracic surgeons, 32 (80 percent) are under 44 years of age, in contrast with the approximately 2,260 male cardiothoracic surgeons, of whom 880 (39 percent) are under 44 years of age.

The clinical advances in thoracic surgery made during the twentieth century have been legendary, starting with the avoidance of lethal hypoventilation during open thoracotomy, a conundrum that occupied the attention of surgeons for many years. Although the advantages of positive pressure endotracheal anesthesia had already been demonstrated in surgical research laboratories by 1905, it was not routinely adopted for clinical use until many years later. Instead, surgeons such as Willy Meyer constructed large pressure chambers in operating suites and were forced to complete their procedures in an all-too-clumsy manner. In 1909, Samuel Meltzer (1851–1920) and John Auer (1875–1948) experimented with the new method of intratracheal insufflation. The following year, Charles Elsberg (1871–1948) of New York City described for the first time the successful performance of open chest surgery, using positive pressure endotracheal anesthesia. During this first decade of the twentieth century Chevalier Jackson (1865–1958) of Philadelphia developed direct vision laryngoscopy, making it possible to introduce the endotracheal tube more easily. Jackson became a pioneer in the art of endoscopy and demonstrated it in his textbook *Tracheo-Bronchoscopy, Esophagoscopy and Gastroscopy* (1907), the world's first on the subject. Three decades later, he wrote one of the most comprehensive treatises on a closely related topic, *Diseases of the Air and Food Passages of Foreign Body Origin* (1937).

Although pulmonary tuberculosis was the foremost problem for early thoracic surgeons, other infections of the chest cavity and lungs proved equally difficult to treat. The first case of thoracoplasty for the sequalae of empyema was completed by George Fowler in 1893. Chronic inflammation with bronchial dilation, known as bronchiectasis, was long regarded as a surgeon's nightmare because of the inflammation around the hilum of the lung. However, by 1929 Harold Brunn (1874–1950) had clearly established the principles for a one-stage pulmonary lobectomy. Four years later, Evarts Graham and Jacob Singer (1882–1954) reported the first successful removal of an entire lung for carcinoma of the bronchus. That same year, Howard Lilienthal (1861–1946) authored an article in the *Journal of Thoracic Surgery* on total pneumonectomy. In 1935, Samuel Freedlander (1893–1969) began the modern era in lung resection for tuberculosis when he performed the first planned lobectomy for the disease. The pre-World War II successes in thoracic surgery concluded with Edward Churchill's (1895–1972) article in 1939 on segmental pneumonectomy in bronchiectasis. Following the war, several changes occurred that altered the dimensions of thoracic surgery as suddenly as endotracheal anesthesia had done two decades earlier. First was the development of antibiotics, which virtually eliminated the need for pulmonary surgery for bronchiectasis and tuberculosis; second was the overshadowing development of cardiac surgery; and third was an explosive rise in the incidence of carcinoma of the lung.

2. Frederick Parham (1858–1927), a New Orleans surgeon, authored the first important report on tumors of the chest wall to appear in the American surgical literature (*Transactions of the Southern Surgical and Gynecological Association*, vol. 1, pages 223–369, 1899). His paper included a remarkable photograph showing one of his patients following an operation for a massive tumor of the left thoracic cage. Parham's article was also notable because it decribed the earliest use of artificial respiration via an endotracheal tube during a surgical procedure. (*Historical Collections, College of Physicians of Philadelphia*)

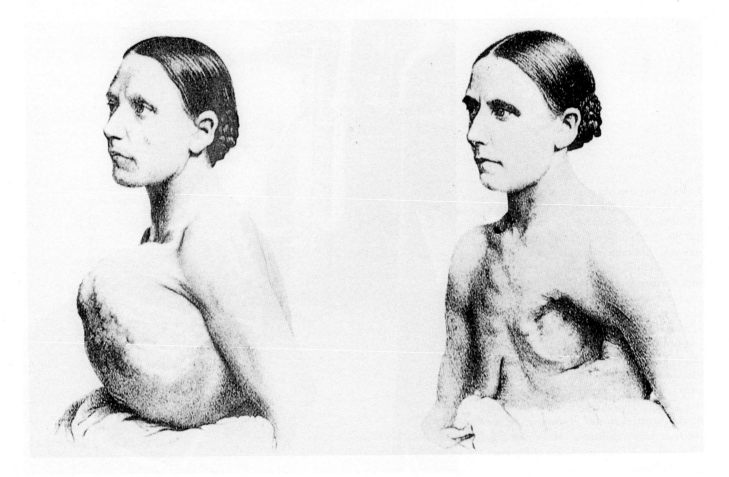

Following the development of safe intrapleural surgery, cardiac operations were beginning to be undertaken with great verve. However, rudimentary surgery on the heart and its surrounding structures had been taking place since the last quarter of the nineteenth century. John B. Roberts (1852–1924) was still a house officer at Pennsylvania Hospital when he authored his first report on cardiac surgery in 1876. As his experience with paracentesis of the pericardium increased, Roberts became interested in the act of operating on the actual myocardium. In the early 1880s, he wrote a number of reports on heart suture, although none included clinical examples. In an 1897 report to the American Surgical Association, Roberts concluded that open drainage of the pericardium using a chondroplastic method of pericardotomy with a trap-door excision of costal cartilage was indicated as soon as a diagnosis of "suppurative pericarditis" was established.

Solon Marks (1827–1914) was professor of military surgery, fractures, and dislocations at the Wisconsin College of Physicians and Surgeons when he presented this country's first published report on true mediastinal surgery. In remarks to members of the American Surgical Association in 1883, Marks described how he dissected a V-shaped flap from the sternum and removed a Minie ball that had been lodged in a patient's mediastinum since the Civil War. Two years later, Joseph Bryant became the first American to report on a surgical approach to the posterior mediastinum.

During the early 1890s, the surgical treatment of stab wounds to the heart began to garner much attention. In 1893, Heine Marks (born 1853), superintendent of the City Hospital in St. Louis, authored a little-known report in an obscure periodical, the *Medical Fortnightly*, describing a successful operation for a stab wound of the myocardium. The following year, Henry Dalton (born 1847), professor of abdominal and clinical surgery at Marion-Sims College of Medicine in St. Louis, reported

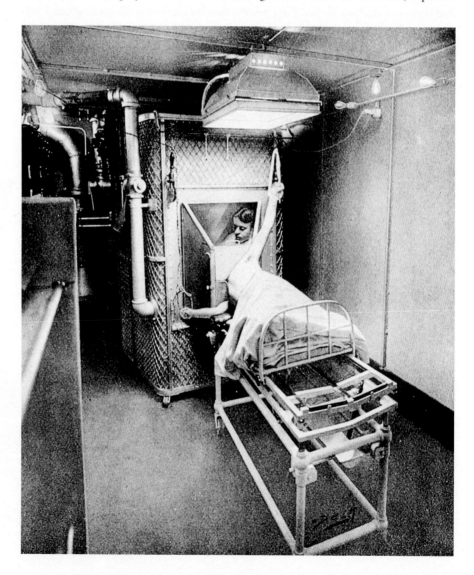

3. Willy Meyer used a positive pressure chamber at the Lenox Hill Hospital in New York City. During the operation, the patient's head and the anesthetist were on the positive pressure side. After the procedure was complete, the nurse remained within the device, along with the patient from his shoulder up, and an attendant was outside. Pneumothorax was prevented by the positive pressure and by a sheet of rubber dam applied over the drained thoracotomy wounds, with zinc oxide ointment, acting as a flutter valve. The operating room itself, with appropriate supportive equipment, was the negative pressure chamber portion of the system. This photograph comes from Meyer's article in the *Transactions of the American Surgical Association*, vol. 36, page 296, 1918. *(Historical Collections, College of Physicians of Philadelphia)*

to the Medical Association of the State of Missouri what was probably the first successful evacuation of a traumatic hemopericardium and placement of a suture in the pericardium. Dalton's surgical triumph occurred in September 1891, and his patient made an uninterrupted, rapid recovery. Daniel Hale Williams authored his famous account of the 1893 stabbing of James Cornish and the successful suturing of his pericardium in the *Medical Record* in 1897. His claim that this case was "the first successful or unsuccessful case of suture of the pericardium that has ever been recorded" was incorrect. He had been preceded by Marks and Dalton. However, Williams' paper provided a more substantive effect on American surgery because of the greater prestige of the journal in which it was published. In 1902, Luther Hill performed the country's first successful operation for a stab wound of the actual myocardium (left ventricle) in a thirteen-year-old boy. Much of this early work in cardiac surgery was given credence by Charles Elsberg's (1871–1948) important paper in the *Journal of Experimental Medicine* (1899) reviewing the entire literature on penetrating cardiac trauma, and his conduct of numerous experiments on rabbits, demonstrating that the mammalian heart could withstand much greater manipulation than had previously been believed. By 1907, Carl Beck (1856–1911), professor of surgery at the New York Post-Graduate School of Medicine, had written the country's first textbook on thoracic surgery, *Surgical Diseases of the Chest*.

Although John Munro (1858–1910) of Boston first suggested the feasibility of ligating a patent ductus arteriosus in 1907, not until the mid-1920s did cardiac surgery become a reasonable reality. From that time on, three major areas of heart surgery evolved: operations for congenital cardiovascular defects, operations on heart valves, and surgical treatment of coronary artery disease. The important landmarks in modern American cardiac surgery began in 1923, when Elliott Cutler completed a successful section of the mitral valve for relief of mitral stenosis. Wayne Babcock proposed an operation for thoracic aneurysm in 1926. By the end of that decade, Edward Churchill was able to report a successful pericardiectomy for constrictive pericarditis (1929). Claude Beck (1894–1971) implanted pectoral muscle into the pericardium and attached a pedicled omental graft to the surface of the heart in 1935, thus providing collateral circulation to that organ for relief of myocardial ischemia. Three years later, Robert Gross completed the first successful ligation of a patent ductus arteriosus. The 1930s concluded with John Gibbon constructing a prototypical heart–lung machine that was used in laboratory animals.

A congenital anomaly that attracted the attention of surgeons relatively early in the evolution of cardiac surgery was coarctation of the aorta. This narrowing of the aorta causes the heart to work against increased pressure and eventually results in cardiac failure. In the mid-1940s, Gross reported a resection of coarctation and direct anastomosis of the aortic ends. John Alexander (1891–1954), of the University of Michigan, resected a saccular aneurysm of the thoracic aorta in 1944. That same year, Alfred Blalock, working with Helen Taussig (1898–1986), a pediatrician, devised an operation for the relief of congenital defects of the pulmonary artery. The Blalock-Taussig subclavian–pulmonary artery shunt for increasing blood flow to the lungs of the "blue baby" proved an important event in the history of American surgery. From 1945 to 1950, more than 1,000 cyanotic children were subjected to operation by Blalock's surgical team. Not only was it a pioneering technical accomplishment, but it managed to give many very ill children a relatively normal existence. The salutary effect of such a surgical feat on the explosive growth of American cardiothoracic surgery, and its public relations value, cannot be overstated. Willis Potts (1895–1968) of Chicago soon improved on the Blalock-Taussig operation when he devised a small surgical clamp that allowed the surgeon to anastomose the aorta to the pulmonary artery more easily, thus obviating the need to sever the subclavian artery (1946).

Also during the late 1940s, Charles Bailey of Jefferson Medical College developed an operation that became known as mitral commissurotomy. This surgical technique involved slipping the finger through the heart's left atrium, pushing a specially constructed knife along the finger, and cutting the lateral commissure of the diseased mitral valve. Bailey completed his first successful commissurotomy in June 1948. A few days later, Dwight Harken of Boston performed an essentially similar procedure (valvuloplasty) for mitral stenosis. During that same year, Edward Bland and Richard Sweet (1901–1962) took the indirect route to correct mitral stenosis by performing the world's first pulmonary–azygos shunt operation in Boston.

When John Gibbon successfully used a pump oxygenator in May 1953 to complete an intracardiac operation in a patient on total heart–lung bypass, open cardiac surgery truly came of age. A little earlier, in 1951, Charles Hufnagel (1916–1989) had designed and inserted the first workable prosthetic heart valve in a human being. The following year, 1952, John Lewis closed an atrial septal defect using immersion hypothermia. In 1953, Michael DeBakey (born 1908) and Denton Cooley (born 1920) reported in the *Journal of the American Medical Association* their successful repair of a thoracic aorta aneurysm and its replacement with a synthetic vascular graft. C. Walton Lillehei (born 1918) closed a ventricular septal defect with controlled cross circulation (human heart–lung "machine") in March 1954. He went on to utilize this technique to repair various other congenital defects, including atrioventricularis communis and tetralogy of Fallot. Cooley resected a ventricular aneurysm with the patient on cardiopulmonary bypass in 1959. By the end of the decade, the experimental use of intracardiac pacemakers, with external power sources, for the correction of total heart block had been presented at the Surgical Forum of the Clinical Congress of the American College of Surgeons.

Beginning in 1960, Norman Shumway (born 1923) reported on the orthotopic homotransplantation of the canine heart, and four years later, James Hardy (born 1918) of the University of Mississippi performed an unsuccessful heart transplant from a chimpanzee into a man. Shumway was the leader in human heart transplantation throughout the late 1960s and 1970s. In 1981, Bruce Reitz, working in Shumway's surgical department at Stanford University, completed the world's first successful heart–lung transplant. The first fully implantable pacemaker was described by William Chardack in 1960. The following year, Albert Starr (born 1926) authored an important paper in the *Journal of Thoracic and Cardiovascular Surgery* on the first replacement of the mitral valve in a human, using shielded ball valve prostheses.

Surgical treatment of coronary artery disease gained momentum during the 1970s, and by the end of the decade, more cardiac operations were being completed for coronary artery insufficiency than for all other types of cardiac disease together. Although René Favaloro's (born 1923) coronary artery bypass procedure at the Cleveland Clinic in 1967 has been regarded as the first truly successful surgical approach to coronary artery disease, Edward Garrett (born 1926) and Michael DeBakey had completed a similar procedure three years earlier. However, they did not report their case until 1973 in the *Journal of the American Medical Association*.

It is also important to note that thoracic surgeons, queried about developments in their specialty, reported in the *Study on Surgical Services for the United States* that from 1945 to 1970, cardiopulmonary bypass, open and closed correction of congenital cardiovascular disease, prosthetic heart valves, closed chest resuscitation for cardiac arrest, and cardiac pacemarkers should be considered of the first-order importance. Of second-order importance was coronary bypass for coronary artery disease. Excluded by definition, having been developed before 1945, was pulmonary resection. Many individuals were instrumental in making these landmark advances. The following biographical listing provides an all-too-brief overview of the life accomplishments of some of these pioneer cardiothoracic surgeons.

BIOGRAPHIES OF CARDIOTHORACIC SURGEONS

Willy Meyer (1858–1932) was born in Minden, Germany, and studied at the universities of Bonn and Erlangen, receiving a medical degree from the former institution in 1880. After a year as an army surgeon, Meyer returned to Bonn and served

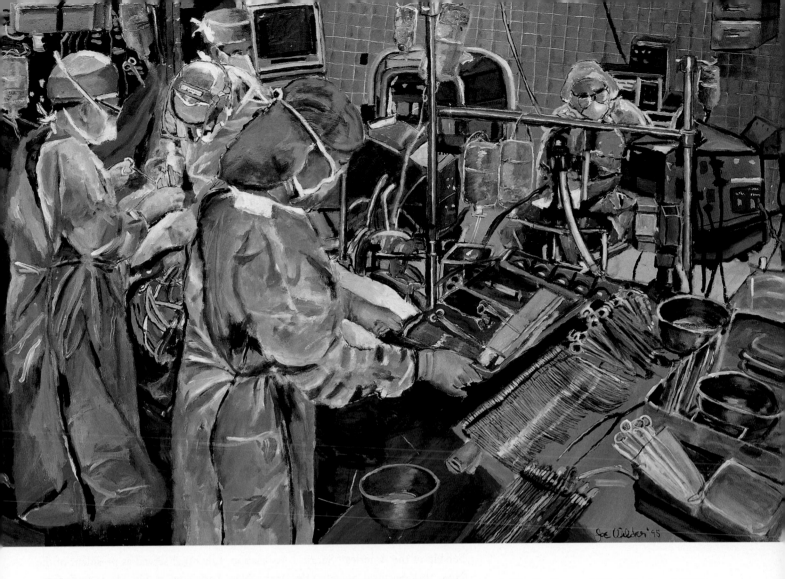

4. "Cardiac Surgery." Painted by Joseph Wilder in 1994. *(Collection of the artist)*

(1880–1883) as a clinical assistant to Friedrich Trendelenburg (1844–1924). In 1884, prompted by his family's close friendship with Abraham Jacobi (1830–1919), considered the "father of American pediatrics" and founder of New York City's German Hospital (now the Lenox Hill), Meyer emigrated to North America and promptly developed a successful general practice in Manhattan. Within two years, Meyer was able to limit his clinical activities to surgery and obtained appointments to the surgical staffs of that city's Woman's Medical College, Skin and Cancer Hospital, German Hospital, and Post-Graduate Hospital. The scope of Meyer's clinical activites was extensive and included the introduction to American physicians of many advances made by European surgeons. Among them were cystoscopy (1897), catheterization of the ureters in the male with the aid of the electric cystoscope (1896), staged prostatectomy (1897), and newer methods of gastrostomy. In 1894, and independently of William Halsted, Meyer described a radical operation for cancer of the breast. Of all his contributions, there is little question that his work in thoracic surgery remains best known. An early advocate of the controlled pressure chamber for thoracotomy, especially the negative-pressure cabinet developed by Ernst Sauerbruch (1875–1951) in Johann von Mikulicz-Radecki's (1850–1905) surgical department in Breslau, Meyer went so far as to have a double chamber built at the German Hospital. Convinced of the need to form a specialty society devoted to thoracic surgery, in February 1917 Meyer invited twenty of his friends to his office, where they agreed to form the New York Society for Thoracic Surgery with Meyer serving as chairman. The following month, a national list of prospective members was asked to attend an organizational meeting of a national society. The first scientific meeting of the newly formed American Association for Thoracic Surgery was held in Chicago in June 1918; Meyer was elected president. At that initial meeting, Meyer provided a *raison d'être* for the new society by giving a wide- ranging review of the state of thoracic surgery. He died suddenly while at a session of the New York Academy of Medicine, defending his surgical approach to breast cancer. Meyer is eponymically remembered for a reagent solution of phenolphthalein and sodium hydroxide, which in the presence of minute traces of blood turns purple or blue-red.

Howard Lilienthal (1861–1946), born in Albany, New York, received his undergraduate degree (1883) and medical diploma (1887) from Harvard University. He completed a year of house officership at Mt. Sinai Hospital in New York City and immediately commenced his surgical training as an assistant (1889–1897) to Arpad Gerster. Lilienthal soon joined the surgical faculty at New York's Polyclinic Medical School and Hospital and was also appointed a member of the surgical staff at Mt. Sinai. He remained at the latter institution for his entire professional career while also serving on the clinical surgery faculty at Cornell University Medical College. During World War I, Lilienthal was in the Medical Corps, U.S. Army Reserve, and was also appointed surgical director of the Mount Sinai Hospital Unit (Base Hospital No. 3) located in Vauclaire, Dordogne, France. Lilienthal made important contributions to the surgical literature and to operative and diagnostic techniques. He invented a portable operating table and a rib retractor, and he is eponymically known for Lilienthal's electric probe used to search for metal objects. His broad interest in all fields of surgery, particularly urologic and abdominal operations, was quite typical of his times. Early on, Lilienthal espoused open reduction and fixation of fractures, and he was one of the first American surgeons to adopt emergency cholecystectomy as the treatment for acute cholecystitis. Following the war, he concentrated most of his clinical efforts on the emerging specialty of thoracic surgery. He became one of the great pioneers in the field, completing pulmonary resections for suppurative disease, draining lung abscesses, and treating cancer of the lungs and esophagus. In 1925, Lilienthal authored the now classic two-volume *Thoracic Surgery*, which became the standard textbook on the subject in pre-World War II America. His motion picture of "major intercostal thoracotomy with lung mobilization" for empyema (1917) was the first such production presented before the membership of the American Surgical Association. Lilienthal served as president of the New York Surgical Society (1903), the New York Society for Thoracic Surgery (1921), and the American Association for Thoracic Surgery (1923). In addition, he helped establish the American Cancer Society.

Ralph Charles Matson (1880–1945) was born in Brookville, Pennsylvania, and received his medical education at the University of Oregon Medical School (1902). He served three years (1902–1905) as an intern and resident at the Good Samaritan Hospital in Portland, Oregon, and received postgraduate training at Cambridge Hospital and St. Mary's Hospital in London (1906–1907). Other than for periods of foreign study, Matson's entire professional career was spent in Portland, where he was on the medical faculty of his alma mater. He spent 1911 and 1912 at universities in Berlin, Dusseldorf, and Vienna, and from 1923 to 1925 he received additional postgraduate training at Victoria Park and St. Mary's Hospitals (London) and the University of Vienna. During World War I, Matson served with the Harvard University surgical unit that supported the British Expeditionary Forces (1916) and was also in the Royal Army Medical Corps (1917). An international authority on tuberculosis and chest surgery, Matson originated an electrosurgical method of cutting adhesions in artificial pneumothorax, and during World War II he devised a new method of irrigating thoracic wounds. Considered a pioneer in the emerging specialty of thoracic surgery, he was president of the American College of Chest Physicians (1939) and editor-in-chief of the journal *Diseases of the Chest* (1941–1945). His twin brother, **Ray William Matson** (1880–1934), had a remarkably similar medical career, including a five-year stint as surgical consultant to the U.S. Veterans Administration Hospital in Portland. Ray Matson was also interested in the early diagnosis and collapse therapy of tuberculosis, and he championed oleothorax and phrenic neurectomy.

Leo Eloesser (1881–1976), a native of San Francisco, received his undergraduate education at the University of California at Berkeley (1900) and a medical diploma from the University of Heidelberg (1907), following studies at Kiel and Breslau.

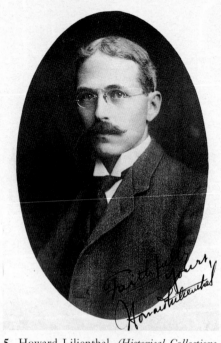

5. Howard Lilienthal. *(Historical Collections, College of Physicians of Philadelphia)*

An inveterate traveler, he undoubtedly led one of the most peripatetic and extraordinary lives of any American surgeon. Eloesser's surgical training was obtained principally at the clinics of Heidelberg under Vincenz Czerny (1842–1916) and Albert Narath (1864–1924), in Kiel with Anschutz, and in Berlin with Fedor Krause. He also spent a few months in the research laboratories of Almroth Wright (1861–1947) at St. Mary's Hospital in London. Returning to the United States in 1909, Eloesser interned at the San Francisco City and County Hospitals, and he eventually became professor of surgery at Stanford and chief of that university's surgical services in those hospitals. His humanistic qualities (he was fluent in almost ten languages) and remarkably independent thinking notwithstanding, Eloesser took part in more than his share of warfare. With the onset of World War I, he volunteered to help German war wounded and headed a base hospital in Karlsruhe. The sinking of the Lusitania in 1915 convinced him to leave Germany, and he returned to America, where he was commissioned a major in the medical corps. Denied his request for duty at the French front, he was assigned to Letterman Hospital, where he worked as chief of the orthopedic service until his discharge in 1919. He organized and headed a field service unit supporting the Republican Army in the Spanish Civil War (1938) and, after a grueling and disheartening period of service, escaped across the Pyrennes to France when the Republican government fell. Too old for active duty in World War II,

---

The New England
Journal of Medicine

Volume 310   FEBRUARY 2, 1984   Number 5

CLINICAL USE OF THE TOTAL ARTIFICIAL HEART

William C. DeVries, M.D., Jeffrey L. Anderson, M.D., Lyle D. Joyce, M.D., Fred L. Anderson, M.D., Elizabeth H. Hammond, M.D., Robert K. Jarvik, M.D., and Willem J. Kolff, M.D., Ph.D.

Abstract We report here our first experience with the use of a total artificial heart in a human being. The heart was developed at the University of Utah, and the patient was a 61-year-old man with chronic congestive heart failure due to primary cardiomyopathy, who also had chronic obstructive pulmonary disease.

Except for dysfunction of the prosthetic mitral valve, which required replacement of the left-heart prosthesis on the 13th postoperative day, the artificial heart functioned well for the entire postoperative course of 112 days. The mean blood pressure was 84±8 mm Hg, and cardiac output was generally maintained at 6.7±0.8 liters per minute for the right heart and 7.5±0.8 for the left, resulting in postoperative diuresis and relief of congestive failure.

The postoperative course was complicated by recurrent pulmonary insufficiency, several episodes of acute renal failure, episodes of fever of unidentified cause (necessitating multiple courses of antibiotics), hemorrhagic complica-tions of anticoagulation, and one generalized seizure of uncertain cause.

On the 92nd postoperative day, the patient had diarrhea and vomiting, leading to aspiration pneumonia and sepsis. Death occurred on the 112th day, preceded by progressive renal failure and refractory hypotension, despite maintenance of cardiac output. Autopsy revealed extensive pseudomembranous colitis, acute tubular necrosis, peritoneal and pleural effusion, centrilobular emphysema, and chronic bronchitis with fibrosis and bronchiectasis. The artificial heart system was intact and uninvolved by thrombosis or infectious processes.

This experience should encourage further clinical trials with the artificial heart, but we emphasize that the procedure is still highly experimental. Further experience, development, and discussion will be required before more general application of the device can be recommended. (N Engl J Med 1984; 310:273-8.)

HEART disease continues to exact the greatest toll of human life, causing approximately 1 million deaths each year in the United States. The idea of replacing the function of the heart with mechanical devices has stimulated conjecture and experimentation for well over a century.[1] These efforts eventually led to the heart–lung machine, which allows temporary circulatory support during open-heart surgery. Cardiac-assistance devices to provide support for intermediate periods have also been developed; an example is the intraaortic balloon pump for clinical use. Progress has also occurred in recent years toward the ultimate goal of an implantable device to provide long-term replacement of all cardiac function. Since the mid-1960s, approximately $160 million in federal funds have been used for research in the development of an artificial heart. Important advances in biomaterials and pump and energy systems, as well as experiments in animals, have now led to the clinical possibility of implantation of a total artificial heart in human beings.[1,2] We report here the initial clinical applica-tion of the total artificial heart developed at the University of Utah.

Methods

The current clinical model of the Utah total artificial heart (model Jarvik-7) is the culmination of 20 years of developmental research (Fig. 1). The heart consists of two approximately spherical ventricles with anatomic transitions to the great vessels and atria. Each ventricle is pneumatically powered. Air is intermittently pulsed through the ventricular air chambers at adjustable rates of 40 to 120 beats per minute. The ventricles are constructed of a smooth blood surface made of segmented polyurethane. Each ventricle has a stroke volume of 100 ml. The cardiac valves consist of clinical-grade pyrolytic-carbon tilting-disk prostheses (currently Bjork–Shiley devices). Connections to the natural atria are achieved by cuffs made of Dacron felt. These are connected to the total artificial heart by a system consisting of rigid polycarbonate segments. Connections to the great vessels are made by means of Dacron vascular prosthetic grafts.

The drive lines out of the ventricular air chambers consist of reinforced polyurethane tubing (thickness, 0.64 cm; internal diameter, 1.6 cm). These lines are covered at the skin level with customized Velour skin buttons, which are designed to enhance tissue ingrowth around the skin despite external movement by the patient. These internal tubes connect with two 2-m external drive-system tubes, which lead to the heart-drive system. The drive tubes are further secured to the patient's body by an abdominal belt.

The Utah pneumatic heart driver is connected to sources of compressed air, vacuum, and electricity. The electrical system is backed up by rechargeable batteries in order to compensate immediately for any interruption of electricity. Drive frequency and pressure are selected and regulated independently to the right and left ventricles.

From the Departments of Surgery, Medicine, and Artificial Organs, University of Utah College of Medicine, Salt Lake City, Utah. Address reprint requests to Dr. DeVries at the Department of Cardiovascular Surgery, University of Utah Medical Center, 50 N. Medical Dr., Salt Lake City, UT 84132.

6. The first published report on the use of a total artificial heart. (*Historical Collections, College of Physicians of Philadelphia*)

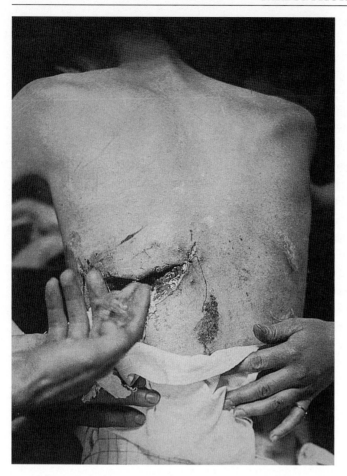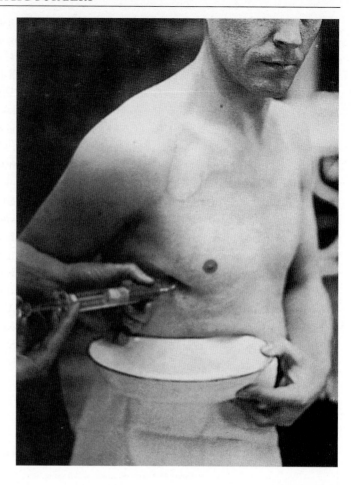

7. Late-nineteenth and early-twentieth-century thoracic surgery grew largely out of the medical necessity to treat tuberculosis. The primary affected organs were the lungs, where pockets of tuberculous pus would form, occasionally breaking through the skin to drain spontaneously. Surgical treatment, when possible, consisted of debridement and washing of detritus from the cavities as well as the manual breaking up of loculations. In this preantibiotic era, bismuth nitrate was then injected into the wound in an attempt to treat the resulting empyema. *(Courtesy of Stanley B. Burns, M.D., and The Burns Collection and Archive)*

Eloesser went to China with the United Nations Relief and Rehabilitation Administration in 1945 as a specialist in thoracic surgery. Following two years of practice in Nationalist China, he gained entry into the communist North, where he organized courses for training rural medical personnel, sanitarians, and midwives. In 1949, he moved to New York City and served with the United Nations International Children's Emergency Fund. Three years later, Eloesser retired to Mexico, returning to the United States annually for the meetings of the American Surgical Association and the American Association of Thoracic Surgery. Although his surgical interests were varied, it was in thoracic surgery that his major contributions are found. He developed the skin flap procedure for empyema and was the first to utilize suction drainage for tuberculous cavitation. In 1934 he set up a thoracic surgical ward in the First University Surgical Clinic in Moscow. Eloesser served on a committee of the American Association for Thoracic Surgery to consider establishing a specialty examining board and was president of the Association in 1937. In 1982, Harris Shumacker (born 1908) authored a full-length biography titled Leo Eloesser, M.D., Eulogy for a Free Spirit.

Elliott Carr Cutler (1888–1947) was born in Bangor, Maine, and received both his undergraduate (1909) and his medical education (1913) at Harvard University. Graduating first in his medical school class, he immediately undertook a five-month grand tour of Europe that included studying pathology at the university clinic in Heidelberg. Cutler returned to the newly built Peter Bent Brigham Hospital, where he served a surgical houseofficership (1913–1915) under Harvey Cushing. After spending a few months overseas with the Harvard Unit American Ambulance Hospital in Paris, he traveled back to Boston and was appointed a resident surgeon (1915–1916) at the Massachusetts General Hospital. During the winter of 1916–1917, Cutler was a voluntary assistant at The Rockefeller Institute in New York City, working in the laboratory of Simon Flexner (1863–1946). When the United States formally entered World War I, Cutler joined Base Hospital No. 5, the Harvard Unit, and was shipped overseas in May 1917. He was eventually assigned to

U.S. Evacuation Hospital No. 1 as chief of the surgical service and participated in offensive actions at Argonne-Meuse, Champagne, and San Mihiel. Awarded the Distinguished Service Medal, our country's highest noncombat award, Cutler returned to Boston and completed his surgical training at the Peter Bent Brigham (1919–1921). He was appointed to the faculty as an associate in surgery and director of the laboratory of surgical research at Harvard. In 1924, Cutler was appointed professor of surgery at the Western Reserve University Medical School and surgical director of Lakeside Hospital in Cleveland. Eight years later, he returned to the Peter Bent Brigham Hospital and succeeded Cushing as Moseley Professor of Surgery, remaining in this position until his early death of metastatic prostate cancer. During World War II, he served as the chief surgical consultant in the European Theater of Operations and was responsible for many organizational improvements in military surgery. Following the war, he effected a nationwide improvement in Veterans Administration hospitals by arranging for affiliations with nearby university teaching hospitals and by better integrating the house and senior staffs. Cutler was a master surgeon, especially remembered as a pioneer in cardiac and thoracic surgery. He was the first American to operate successfully on a heart valve (1923) and one of the earliest to resect the pericardium for constrictive pericarditis. In 1934 he announced that he had achieved permanent relief from angina pectoris through excision of normal thyroid glands, but the operation was soon abandoned because of the resulting athyroidism. Cutler served on the editorial boards of several periodicals, including *American Heart Journal, American Journal of Surgery, British Journal of Surgery, Journal of Clinical Investigation,* and *Surgery.* In addition to over two hundred contributions to the surgical literature, Cutler, along with Robert Zollinger, wrote the acclaimed *Atlas of Surgical Operations* (1939). Among Cutler's many professional honors was serving as president of the Society of Clinical Surgery (1941–1946) and the American Surgical Association (1947). In 1988, a biography by Robert Zollinger was published: *Elliott Carr Cutler and the Cloning of Surgeons.*

Emile Holman (1890–1977), born in Moberly, Missouri, received his undergraduate degree from Stanford University (1911). For three years following graduation, Holman served as personal secretary to David Starr Jordan (1851–1931), president of the university. At Jordan's suggestion, Holman successfully applied for a Rhodes scholarship and began his medical studies at St. John's College, Oxford. The third year of his scholarship was spent as a casualty house surgeon at the Radcliffe Infirmary. This advanced clinical work enabled Holman to enter the fourth year at The Johns Hopkins University School of Medicine, from which he received his medical degree in 1918. Holman's first postgraduate year was spent in the Hunterian Laboratory for Surgical Research as part of William Halsted's surgical residency staff. After serving as an assistant resident surgeon for two years, Holman was appointed resident surgeon (1921–1922) remaining until Halsted's death in September 1922. In 1923, Holman took a position with Harvey Cushing at the Peter Bent Brigham Hospital and gained further surgical experience under the tutelage of David Cheever, Elliott Cutler, and John Homans. Cutler left to become chief surgeon at the Lakeside Hospital in Cleveland, and Holman joined him there in 1924. While there, Holman worked in the laboratory with Claude Beck (1894–1971), as Cutler gave him few clinical responsibilities. In 1926 Holman was offered the professorship of surgery at Stanford, and he remained there until his retirement. He immediately set out to establish a true academic department of surgery, the first such endeavor in the American far West. Although his surgical interests were broad, Holman was increasingly interested in matters of cardiothoracic surgery and introduced cardiac surgery to California, performing the first operations there for patent ductus arteriosus, coarctation of the aorta, tetralogy of Fallot, and mitral stenosis. In so doing, he provided the impetus for the internationally recognized program in cardiac surgery that later developed at Stanford.

John Alexander (1891–1954), born in Philadelphia, received both his bachelor's (1912) and medical degrees (1916) from the University of Pennsylvania. Shortly

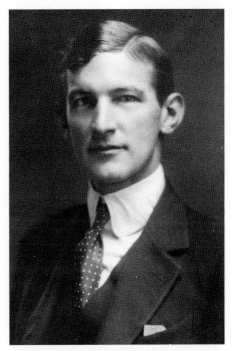

8. Elliott Carr Cutler. *(Historical Collections, College of Physicians of Philadelphia)*

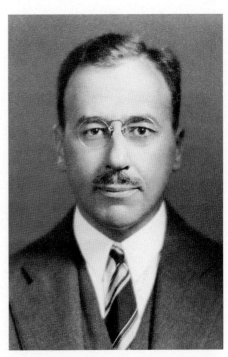

9. John Alexander. *(Historical Collections, College of Physicians of Philadelphia)*

thereafter, he enlisted in an American unit attached to the French Army but transferred to the U.S. Army Medical Corps in 1919 when the United States entered the war. In 1919 Alexander worked briefly at Leon Bérard's clinic in Lyon, France, learning the technique of paravertebral thoracoplasty as a treatment of tuberculosis. Returning to the United States, Alexander served on Charles Frazier's surgical staff at the University of Pennsylvania. In the fall of 1920, Alexander was recruited by Hugh Cabot to join the surgical faculty at the University of Michigan. Alexander's work in Ann Arbor was soon interrupted by his own tuberculosis and its sequelae of pleural effusion, kidney infection, and Pott's disease of the spine. Forced to undergo protracted bed rest, Alexander went to the Trudeau Sanatorium at Saranac Lake in upper New York State, where he was alternately put into a full body cast and placed in a Bradford frame. While there, he wrote his book, *The Surgery of Pulmonary Tuberculosis* (1925), for which he was awarded the Samuel D. Gross prize of the Philadelphia Academy of Surgery. Alexander returned to the University of Michigan in 1926 and, within two years, devoted himself exclusively to thoracic surgery. In the late 1920s, Alexander began a formal program to train thoracic surgeons, which had increased by 1932 to a formal two-year committment, similar in requirements to that later adopted by the Board of Thoracic Surgery. He was renowned for his writings in the field of surgical therapy for pulmonary tuberculosis, and his recommendations for staging of thoracoplasty operations did much to improve the mortality of the procedure. His comprehensive classic, *The Collapse Therapy of Pulmonary Tuberculosis*, was published in 1937. In the field of cardiac surgery, Alexander was the first surgeon to resect a saccular aneurysm of the thoracic aorta that had developed secondary to a coarctation (1944). In recognition of his many accomplishments, he was elected president of the American Association for Thoracic Surgery in 1935. Alexander eventually succumbed to the ravages of tuberculosis.

Samuel Oscar Freedlander (1893–1971) was born in Wooster, Ohio, and attended Adelbert College, Western Reserve University (1915) and Western Reserve University School of Medicine (1918). From 1918 to 1921 he served an internship and residency at Cleveland City Hospital and then traveled to Vienna and took training in pathology (1922). Following his return to the United States, Freedlander joined the surgical faculty at his alma mater and was resident surgeon-in-charge at Cleveland City Hospital (1924–1929). From 1932 to 1953, he was chief of the institution's surgical division and head of thoracic surgery. In addition, Freedlander was director of surgery at Cleveland's Mt. Sinai Hospital (1945–1959) and surgeon-in-charge at the Sunny Acres Sanitarium (1932–1959). While at Mt. Sinai, he also directed the Katz-Sanders Laboratory for Surgical Research. A founding member of Forest City Hospital, Freedlander helped draft legislation for organizing the Community Health Foundation (forerunner of the Kaiser Foundation) and also served as a member of the National Advisory Council for the Health Professions (1964–1966). Although not viewed as an academic surgeon, Freedlander did author thirty-five articles for the surgical literature, and he began the modern era in lung resection for tuberculosis when he completed the first planned lobectomy for the disease (1935).

Claude Schaeffer Beck (1894–1971) was born in Shamokin, Pennsylvania, and attended Franklin and Marshall College (1916) and The Johns Hopkins University School of Medicine (1921). He interned at The Johns Hopkins Hospital (1922–1923), but because of the administrative disarray that followed William Halsted's death, he transferred for a short time to the Yale-New Haven Hospital as an assistant resident surgeon. Through the influence of Harvey Cushing, Beck soon received the Arthur Tracy Cabot Fellowship in Surgical Research at Harvard's Peter Bent Brigham Hospital (1923–1924). In 1924, the Brigham's Elliott Cutler left Boston to be professor of surgery at Western Reserve University, and he invited Beck to join him as the Crile Fellow in Surgery. Following that time, Beck became resident surgeon in the University Hospital of Cleveland (1926–1927). This was to be Beck's final career move, as he remained in Ohio for the rest of his professional life. His academic appointments included instructor in surgery (1925–1928), assistant professor (1928–1933), associate professor (1933–1940), and professor of neurosurgery (1940–1952). Despite professorial titles, Beck was mainly engaged in cardiothoracic surgical research throughout most of his career, and he was eventually named professor of cardiovascular surgery (1952–1965), the first such academic appointment in the United States. During World War II, he was surgical consultant, 5th Service Command, with a rank of colonel in the U.S. Army Medical Corps. Among his many contributions to cardiothoracic surgery are the first mitral valve operation (1924), the first successful removal of a cardiac tumor (1942), the first successful defribrillation of a surgical patient, with the chest opened and the paddles applied directly to the myocardium (1947), and the earliest successful reversal of a near-fatal heart attack (1955). He is eponymically remembered for the Beck I operation (1941), a procedure designed to increase the blood supply to the myocardium, consisting in abrasion of the epicardium and lining of the parietal pericardium, application of an irritant to these surfaces, partial occlusion of the coronary sinus at its opening into the right atrium, and grafting of omental and mediastinal fat and the parietal pericardium to the surface of the heart; and for the Beck II procedure, a two-stage surgical operation to increase blood flow to the myocardium by placement of a vein graft between the aorta and the coronary sinus; later the coronary sinus is partially occluded to increase the pressure therein and thereby induce retrograde flow of arterial blood into the coronary capillaries. Beck's name is also linked with a test for acute cardiac compression (rising venous pressure, falling arterial pressure, and the small quiet heart of cardiac tamponade). In 1949, as professor of neurosurgery, Beck attempted to revascularize the brain in children with mental retardation and convulsive disorders by creating a cervical arteriovenous fistula. This attempt at reversing circulation in the veins through a carotid–jugular anastomosis resulted in an

10. "Triptych: Dr. Carver and Team." Painted by Lamar Dodd in 1982–1983, in oil, gold leaf, silver leaf, and palladium leaf on canvas plus Masonite panels. *(Collection of the artist and permission of W. Robert Nix, photographer)*

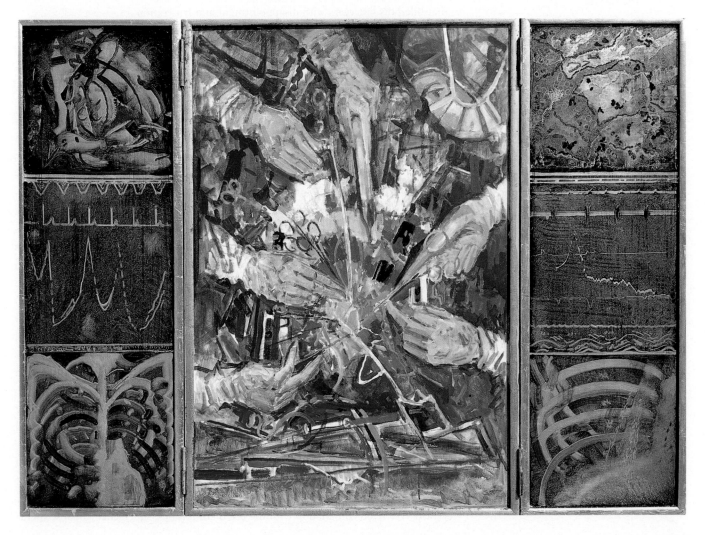

11. In 1984, William Shroeder had a mechanical heart, powered from outside the body, inserted into his thoracic cavity. As he is about to take his first step following the surgical operation, William De Vries, the cardiac surgeon, assists him. The death of all of De Vries' "mechanical heart patients" proved a disappointing episode in modern surgical history. *(Courtesy of William Strode Associates)*

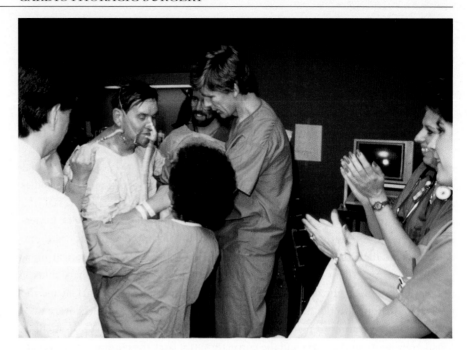

academic imbroglio, which plagued his later career. Beck established the first teaching course in cardiac resuscitation in the United States and was a forceful advocate for the installation of defibrillators in emergency rooms and elsewhere. His proselytizing efforts led to the wide acceptance of cardiopulmonary resuscitation when the closed chest method of cardiac massage was developed. Despite a lifetime of superb clinical accomplishments, Beck held few honorary positions in organized American surgery. His recognition was far greater abroad than in the United States, a situation that filled his last years with disappointment and frustration.

Edward Delos Churchill (1895–1972) was born in Chenoa, Illinois, and graduated from Northwestern University with bachelor's (1916) and master's (1917) degrees and from Harvard Medical School (1920). He took his internship and residency at the Massachusetts General Hospital (1920–1924) and also received further postgraduate training in Europe as a Moseley Traveling Fellow (1926–1927). Essentially all of Churchill's professional career was spent on the surgical faculty of his alma mater and the surgical staff of the Massachusetts General Hospital. From 1928 to 1930, he also served as an associate surgeon and director of Harvard's Surgical Research Laboratory at the Boston City Hospital. Churchill was eventually named John Homans Professor of Surgery and chief of the general surgical services at the Massachusetts General Hospital. His career was particularly distinguished by his military service during World War II, when he was chief surgical consultant to the North African–Mediterranean theater of operation. From his vast military experiences, Churchill authored *Surgeon to Soldiers* (1972), a detailed account of combat surgery and progress in military medicine. Following the war, he was named chairman of a medical advisory board to the secretary of war (1946–1948) and served on the surgical committee of the National Research Council (1946–1949). From 1948 to 1951, Churchill was an influential member of the Armed Forces Medical Advisory Committee to the Secretary of Defense. For over twenty years (1953–1972), he acted as senior civilian consultant in thoracic surgery to the Surgeon-General. While acting as a Rockefeller Foundation consultant (1958), Churchill visited medical centers throughout India and was instrumental in helping to establish a residency program at Lucknow University's King George Medical College. The following year, Churchill spent several months on the surgical faculty of the American University in Beirut, Lebanon. Churchill advanced the frontiers of cardiothoracic surgery through numerous technical breakthroughs, including one of the earliest segmental pneumonectomies for bronchiectasis (1939), which, after World War II, in conjunction with the use of antibiotics, superseded collapse therapy in the treatment of pulmonary tuberculosis. He also completed the first successful operation in the United States to relieve constrictive pericarditis, and established the role of parathyroidectomy in the treatment of hyperparathyroidism. A scholarly individual, Churchill developed an outstanding academic department of surgery at the Massachusetts General Hospital, and many of his residents became renowned surgeons in their own right. Among his many honors were serving as president of the American Surgical Association (1946), American Association for Thoracic Surgery (1948), and the Society of Clinical Surgery (1949). Churchill was a prolific contributor to the surgical literature and edited the autobiographical memoirs of John Collins Warren, *To Work in the Vineyard of Surgery* (1958). In 1990, J. Gordon Scannell (born 1914) edited Churchill's unpublished memoirs of his year as a Moseley Traveling Fellow, *Wanderjahr, the Education of a Surgeon, Edward D. Churchill.*

Willis J. Potts (1895–1968) was born in Sheboygan, Wisconsin, and received his undergraduate education at Hope College (1918). He also studied for a Bachelor of Science degree from the University of Chicago (1920) and took his medical education at Rush Medical College (1924). Potts served an internship and residency at the Presbyterian Hospital in Chicago (1923–1925) and then spent two years as the Logan Fellow in Surgery at Rush Medical College. Following completion of his postgraduate studies, Potts joined the surgical staff of the Presbyterian Hospital (1928–1942) while also being appointed to the faculty at his alma mater. He held the position of clinical assistant professor of surgery from 1936 to 1939 and was clinical associate professor from 1939 to 1946. Potts had a distinguished record in the Armed Forces, having served as a sergeant in the Chemical Warfare Service during World War I. During the World War II, he organized and became unit director of the 25th Evacuation Hospital, which was stationed in the New Hebrides Islands, South Pacific. Upon his return to Chicago, Potts was named surgeon-in-chief at the Children's Memorial Hospital and professor of surgery at Northwestern University, positions he held until his retirement in 1960. He became internationally known for his work in pediatric cardiac surgery, and his name is eponymically linked with Pott's operation or anastomosis, a direct side-to-side anastomosis between the aorta and pulmonary artery as a palliative procedure in Fallot's tetralogy (1946). Towards the end of his career, Potts devoted ever greater amounts of time to the general care of children and authored two books indicative of his abiding interest in their welfare, *The Surgeon and the Child* (1959) and *Your Wonderful Baby* (1963).

Alfred Blalock (1899–1964), born in Culloden, Georgia, graduated from the University of Georgia in 1918 and The Johns Hopkins University School of Medicine in 1922. He served two years as a surgical resident at his alma mater, primarily on Hugh H. Young's (1870–1945) urology service but, having been refused a reappointment to the surgical house staff, was forced to accept an externship in otolaryngology under Samuel Crowe (1883–1955), chief of the institution's otolaryngology service for one year, 1924–1925. In July 1925, Blalock moved from Baltimore to Nashville and became resident surgeon for a year under Barney Brooks (1894–1952), newly appointed professor of surgery at Vanderbilt University. After completing his postgraduate studies in 1926, Blalock joined the surgical faculty at Vanderbilt and remained there until 1941. During his Nashville years he demonstrated that surgical shock resulted from the loss of blood and popularized the use of plasma or whole-blood transfusions to treat the condition. Blalock was an outstanding surgical researcher and combined clinical talents with a knowledge of basic surgical science. He was already well established as a thoracic surgeon with an important series of pericardiectomies and the first deliberate treatment of myasthenia gravis by thymectomy (1939) when he was appointed chairman of the department of surgery at The Johns Hopkins Hospital. Blalock remained in Baltimore until his death of metastatic retroperitoneal carcinoma. At Hopkins, Blalock met Helen Taussig, head of pediatric cardiology, who theorized that the poor circulation of "blue babies" was due to a lack of oxygenated blood caused by a narrowness, or obstruction, of passages from the heart to the pulmonary arteries. After numerous animal experiments, Blalock, with the assistance of Vivien Thomas his laboratory technologist, developed an operation to bypass the congenital deformity by surgically joining the subclavian artery to the pulmonary artery (1945). Hence was born the Blalock-Taussig shunt, an operation that saved the lives of thousands of babies born with congenital cyanotic heart disease. This surgical success had been preceded by his development of a bypass operation for coarctation of the aorta (1944) and would lead to the Blalock-Hanlon operation, which entailed the creation of a large atrial septal defect as a palliative procedure for the treatment of complete transposition of the great blood vessels leading to and from the heart (1948). Perhaps Blalock's greatest contribution to modern surgery was the establishment of a school of surgery in which a generation of influential American surgical leaders were trained. Highly involved in the world of surgical politics, Blalock served as president of the American College of Surgeons (1954) and the American Surgical Association (1956). In 1991, William P. Longmire, Jr. (born 1913), one of Blalock's most distinguished surgical residents, privately published a full-length biography entitled *Alfred Blalock, His Life and Times*. A two-volume set of Blalock's collected papers was edited (1966) by Mark M. Ravitch (1912–1989), another of Blalock's renowned trainees.

Cameron Haight (1901–1970) was born in San Francisco and received his undergraduate degree from the University of California (1923) and medical diploma from Harvard University (1926). He began surgical training on Harvey Cushing's service at the Peter Bent Brigham Hospital (1926–1928). In his second year, Haight missed the diagnosis of a subdural hematoma and was summarily dismissed by the imperious Cushing. He then completed his surgical residency at New Haven Hospital (1928–1931). In 1931, he moved to the University of Michigan and pursued further study in thoracic surgery with John Alexander. Remaining in Ann Arbor, Haight joined the surgical faculty and advanced through the academic ranks, becoming professor of surgery in 1950. Four years later, following Alexander's death, Haight was named chief of the university's section of thoracic surgery, a position he held for the next sixteen years. In 1932 Haight received international recognition for being the first American, and second surgeon in the world, to remove an entire lung successfully. Eight years later, he pioneered transnasal tracheo-bronchial aspiration. Haight's greatest clinical achievement was the surgical correction of esophageal atresia and tracheoesophageal fistula in the newborn. His ablation of an tracheoesophageal fistula with primary end-to-end esophageal anatomosis was first achieved in 1941. A founding member of the Board of Thoracic Surgery (1949), Haight served as chairman of the American Board of Thoracic Surgeons (1952–1954). In 1957 he was given the distinction of being elected president of the American Association of Thoracic Surgeons. Although not known as a prolific writer, Haight served on the editorial board of the *Journal of Thoracic and Cardiovascular Surgery* from 1954 until the time of his death.

Richard H. Overholt (1902–1990) was born in Ashland, Nebraska, and received his medical degree from the University of Nebraska. He received surgical training at the University of Pennsylvania and then joined the surgical staff of the Lahey Clinic in Boston in 1930. Overholt remained at the Lahey Clinic until 1937, when he entered full-time private practice and founded his own Overholt Thoracic Clinic in Boston. Although Overholt held a teaching position at Tufts Medical School and taught surgical residents at both the New England Baptist and Quincy City Hospitals, he never had a true academic title. While at the Lahey Clinic, he performed the first successful removal of a right lung on a cancer patient, and he went on to make important technical contributions to pulmonary segmentectomy. His book *The Technique of Pulmonary Resection* (1949) contributed to the worldwide diffusion of modern pulmonary surgery. Overholt was also among the first to recommend a simultaneous thoracoplasty with resection for tuberculosis (1950) and to perform simultaneous bilateral pulmonary resections (1952). He remains best known for his lifelong crusade against cigarette smoking. In the early 1930s, while operating on tuberculosis patients, Overholt observed that the lungs of nonsmokers recovered faster than those of smokers. By the mid-1930s he was addressing doctors and urging them to support measures to curb smoking, and he adopted a personal policy of refusing to treat patients unless they gave up cigarettes. Not unexpectedly, the medical establishment initially viewed Overholt as little more than a gadfly, but by the mid-1960s, he had the satisfaction of seeing smoking condemned by the profession. Overholt held few honorary positions in organized surgery, but he did serve as president of the American College of Chest Surgeons. The Overholt Foundation, established in the late 1930's, financed research and patient care for many years.

Robert E. Gross (1905–1988) graduated with honors from Carleton College (1927) and Harvard Medical School (1931). He spent two years as a pathology resident and then entered surgical residency at the Peter Bent Brigham Hospital. After three years of general surgical training, Gross decided to devote his talents to pediatric surgery. He was appointed chief resident in surgery at the Boston Children's Hospital, where he worked with William E. Ladd, who was then occupying the first chair of pediatric surgery in the country. In 1939, having devised in the research laboratory a surgical approach to the closure of patent ductus arteriosus, Gross went on to successfully complete the procedure in a human patient. Six years later, Gross performed a resection of a coarctation of the aorta with direct anastomosis of the remaining ends. In 1947 Gross was named professor of children's surgery at Harvard Medical School and surgeon-in-chief of the Children's Hospital. Gross became cardiovascular surgeon-in-chief in 1964, retiring eight years later. His contributions to the literature included the classic textbooks *Abdominal Surgery of Infancy and Childhood* (1941) and *The Surgery of Infancy and Childhood* (1953). The latter work was the first modern comprehensive text on the specialty of pediatric surgery and brought Gross much respect and prominence. In 1970 he authored his third and final book, *An Atlas of Children's Surgery*, which included a wide range of pediatric cardiac surgical procedures. Gross was elected president of the American Association for Thoracic Surgery in 1964 and served as the first president of the American Pediatric Surgical Association (1970).

Brian Brewer Blades (1906–1977) was born in Scottsville, Kansas, and graduated from the University of Kansas in 1928 and Washington University School of Medicine in 1932. He interned at Henry Ford Hospital in Detroit and completed a surgical residency at New York City's Bellevue Hospital. Blades returned to St. Louis for further training in thoracic surgery under Evarts Graham, and he remained on staff as an assistant professor of surgery. During World War II he served as chief of thoracic surgery at Walter Reed Hospital in Washington. In 1946, Blades was appointed professor and chairman of the department of surgery at The George Washington University School of Medicine. This chair was subsequently endowed as the Lewis Saltz Chair of Surgery, and Blades remained in this capacity until 1970. He was president of the American Association for Thoracic Surgery in 1958 and authored a well-received textbook, *Surgical Diseases of the Chest*, but his longest-lasting influence on American thoracic surgery was achieved through his long-time editorship of the *Journal of Thoracic and Cardiovascular Surgery* (1962–1977).

Frederick Douglass Stubbs (1906–1947), born in Wilmington, Delaware, graduated magna cum laude from Dartmouth College (1927) and received his medical education at Harvard Medical School (1931). He interned at Cleveland City Hospital, being the first African American to do so, and then took a thoracic fellowship at the same institution (1932–1933), serving under Samuel Freedlander. Stubbs soon moved to Philadelphia, where he was a resident in surgery at the Douglass Memorial Hospital (1933–1934). For three years he was engaged in private medical and surgical practice with his father-in-law. Not satisfied with his prior training or his experiences in practice, Stubbs took another year of thoracic training with P. N. Coryllos at Sea View Hospital in New York City (1937–1938). Returning to Philadelphia, Stubbs, the only trained African-American thoracic surgeon in the United States, became an associate in general surgery at the Douglass Memorial

Hospital and was soon appointed its chief of thoracic surgery. At the same time, he was organizing a department of thoracic surgery at Mercy Hospital. In 1941, Stubbs was named medical director of Douglass Memorial Hospital, which would soon merge with Mercy, and also joined the visiting surgical staff at Atkinson Memorial Hospital in Coatesville, Pennsylvania. Stubbs was the first African-American board-certified surgeon (1943) in Philadelphia, and although he applied for fellowship in the American College of Surgeons in 1942, his application was not approved until 1946. In 1947, Stubbs was named chief of the Tuberculosis Division of Jefferson Medical School, but he died of an apparent myocardial infarction before assuming his duties. As the leading African-American medical figure in Philadelphia, Stubbs served as president of the Pennsylvania Medical, Dental, and Pharmaceutical Association. Although not a prolific author, Stubbs was a contributing editor to the *Journal of the National Medical Association* and served as the Association's vice-president.

James Richard Laurey (1907–1964), was born in East St. Louis, Illinois, attended the College of the City of Detroit (now Wayne State University), graduating in 1925, and received his medical degree from the same institution in 1933. He interned at Provident Hospital in Chicago and remained for an additional year as senior assistant in surgery (1933–1934). In 1934–1935, Laurey was resident surgeon at the Parkside Hospital in Detroit. Most of his career was spent at Howard University, where he started as an assistant in physiology (1935–1936) and was soon promoted to assistant in surgery. The years 1939–1941 involved postgraduate training as a General Education Board Fellow in thoracic surgery at the University of Michigan. Returning to Howard University in 1941, Laurey was appointed associate professor of thoracic surgery, and six years later he became a full professor. In 1950 he was named chief of thoracic surgery and, following the death of Charles Drew, was elected to the chairmanship of the department of surgery. He remained in this capacity until 1955, when he resumed his former position as professor and chief of thoracic surgery. In 1947 Laurey became a consulting thoracic surgeon to the Glenn Dale Tuberculosis Sanitorium in Washington, and from 1950 to 1955 he served as a consultant thoracic surgeon to the Denmar Sanitorium in West Virginia, a United Mine Workers' tuberculosis hospital. He was a diplomate of the American Board of Surgery (1942) and a member of the founders' group of the Board of Thoracic Surgery (1949). Among his many contributions, Laurey was instrumental in opening the doors of District of Columbia hospitals to African-American physicians by demonstrating his and his surgical staff's clinical competence when asked to fill in for Caucasian physicians regularly drawn from George Washington and Georgetown Medical Schools (1947). This action paved the way for an agreement, reached in 1948, allowing Howard University physicians to join the staff at Gallinger (now D.C. General) Hospital.

Charles Philamore Bailey (1910–1993) of Wanamassa, New Jersey, attended Rutgers University (1928) and Hahnemann Medical College (1932). He also earned master of science and doctor of science degrees at the University of Pennsylvania. Bailey was chief of thoracic surgery at Hahnemann University Hospital in the 1940s and 1950s and director of cardiovascular surgery at the Deborah Heart and Lung Center in Browns Mills, New Jersey from 1956 to 1961. In addition, he was professor and director of general surgery at the New York Medical College and Flower-Fifth Avenue Hospitals (1959–1962). Long considered a maverick personality, Bailey began studying evenings at Fordham Law School in the late 1960's, eventually became a consultant to law firms and insurance companies, and by the mid-1970s had retired from all active clinical responsibilities. His professional career was somewhat uneven because of his aggressive and volatile nature. Never one to shun controversy, Bailey was an intrepid pioneer in cardiac surgery and performed the first successful operation for mitral stenosis (1948). This mitral commissurotomy represented a significant landmark in modern heart surgery and demonstrated that the human heart could withstand manipulations previously considered impossible. Bailey was a prolific author; his surgical texts included *Diagnosis and Management of*

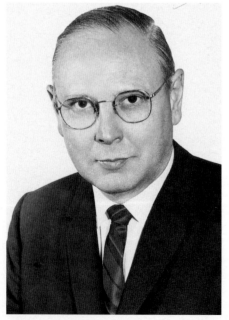

12. Charles Philamore Bailey. (*Author's Collection*)

the Thoracic Patient (1945), *Surgery of the Heart* (1955), and *Cardiac Surgery* (1960). He continued his legal work up to the time of his death, having three years before written a legal monograph, *Liability in Medical Practice* (1990).

Dwight E. Harken (1910–1993) was born in Osceola, Iowa, and earned his bachelor's and medical degrees from Harvard University. Following surgical training at Bellevue Hospital in New York City, he was awarded a New York Academy of Medicine Fellowship in London. There, Harken focused his attentions on diseases of the chest and began devising surgical approaches to treat cardiac infections. During World War II he served with the U.S. Army Medical Corps in England. Assigned to the 106th General Hospital, Harken was sent to Cirencester as director of the 15th Thoracic Center, a facility to which thousands of D-Day and post-invasion casualties would soon be evacuated. It was at Cirencester that Harken achieved his initial renown when he removed bullets and shrapnel from the hearts of 134 wounded soldiers without a single fatality. In so doing, Harken and his surgical team shattered the long-held myth that the heart was so complex and vital that it should be viewed as sacrosanct from any type of surgical intervention. Returning to the United States, Harken joined the surgical faculty at Tufts Medical School for two years and then transferred to Harvard Medical School and its Peter Bent Brigham Hospital, where he was chief of cardiothoracic surgery from 1948 to 1970. He also held a similar position at Mount Auburn Hospital in Cambridge, Massachusetts. In 1948, Harken completed a successful valvuloplasty for mitral stenosis, a landmark procedure in the evolutionary pathway of modern cardiac surgery. Three years later, Harken established the world's first intensive surgical care unit at the Peter Bent Brigham Hospital. He was a tireless critic of tobacco smoking and a cofounder of Action on Smoking and Health. Harken was a member of the founders' group of the Board of Thoracic Surgery and served as president of the American College of Cardiology and the Association for the Advancement of Medical Instrumentation. The author of more than two hundred journal articles, he served on the editorial board of eight different periodicals.

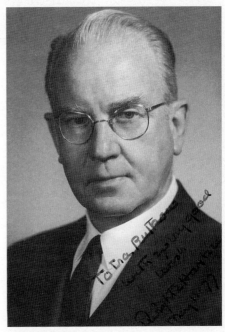

13. Dwight E. Harken. (*Author's Collection*)

Charles Anthony Hufnagel (1915–1989) was born in Louisville, Kentucky, and graduated from the University of Notre Dame in 1937 and Harvard Medical School in 1941. His surgical training was at the Peter Bent Brigham Hospital, interspersed with one year at Boston Children's Hospital working with Robert Gross. From 1947 to 1950, Hufnagel served as director of the Surgical Research Laboratory at Harvard, where he began research into the feasibility of engineering cardiac and vascular replacement parts. In 1950 he joined the faculty at Georgetown University School of Medicine as professor of experimental surgery. Two years later, he inserted an artificial heart valve into a thirty-year-old woman. This first workable prosthetic ball-valve device was one of the most important milestones in the development of cardiac surgery in the period before the advent of the heart–lung machine. In 1953 Hufnagel was named associate professor of surgery, and sixteen years later he was appointed professor and chairman of the Georgetown University's Department of Surgery. He remained in this capacity for ten years. On his retirement he continued a private surgical practice and also joined the faculty at the Uniformed Services University of the Health Sciences in Bethesda, Maryland. In 1974, Hufnagel was appointed chairman of a three-man medical team by Judge John Sirica, of Watergate fame, to examine former President Richard Nixon (1913–1994) at his home in San Clemente, California, to determine whether the president was medically fit to testify at the Watergate trial. Nixon was recovering from a venous ligation for a chronic phlebitis condition, and Hufnagel's panel concluded that he was unfit to appear. The physicians made a point of protecting the medical confidentiality of the former president and refused to cite a reason for recommending against his testimony. A prolific contributor to the surgical literature, with over four hundred papers, Hufnagel served on the editorial boards of numerous journals.

Fig. 1.

Plate 2.

Fig. 2.

Fig. 3.

Fig. 6.

Fig. 4.

Fig. 5.

Fig. 7.

CHAPTER 15

COLORECTAL SURGERY

*I*n few countries of the world is colorectal surgery recognized as a surgical specialty distinct from general surgery. However, in the United States, the vagaries of surgical politics in the 1930s and 1940s conjured a certifying board for colon and rectal surgery. Loosely organized as the American Board of Proctology in 1934, it was the sixth Board to be so recognized and represented efforts of the membership of the American Proctologic Society (now the American Society of Colon and Rectal Surgeons) to seek specialty status. The political maneuvering around the new board was intense, and colorectal surgeons were markedly disappointed not to receive "primary board" status as previously deemed by the Council on Medical Education of the American Medical Association and the Advisory Board for Medical Specialties for other specialty boards. Three years later, with the founding of the American Board of Surgery, it was considered more politically expedient for the certifying of colon and rectal surgeons to be included under the purview of a subsidiary board of the new American Board. Accordingly, in 1940, provisions were made for the certification of proctologists by the American Board of Surgery and for a committee of proctologists known as the Central Certifying Committee in Proctology of the American Board of Surgery. The arrangement was highly unsatisfactory to general surgeons, proctologists, and candidates for examination. Hence, nine years later, the Advisory Board for Medical Specialties and the Council on Medical Education and Hospitals granted the status as a primary board to the American Board of Proctology. It thus became the eighteenth specialty board approved by these organizations. In 1961, the board formally changed its name to the American Board of Colon and Rectal Surgery.

To be eligible for board certification in colon and rectal surgery, an applicant must have completed at least a five-year training program in general surgery and one additional year in an approved colon and rectal residency. Furthermore, the candidate must have had previous certification by the American Board of Surgery. A colon and rectal surgeon is expected to deal with conditions such as colon and rectal cancer, diverticulitis, inflammatory bowel disease, polyps, and anal pathology, including abscesses, fissures, fistulas, and hemorrhoids. In addition, colon and rectal specialists must have the in-depth knowledge of intestinal and anorectal physiology required for the treatment of constipation, diarrhea, and incontinence.

As of 1995, of the approximately 621,000 total physicians in active practice, 965 (less than 1 percent) designate themselves as colorectal surgeons. Within this cadre of colorectal surgeons, 850 (88 percent) are board certified (from 1980 through 1994, 588 certificates in colorectal surgery were issued, or an average of 39 per year); 45 (1 percent) are women; and 220 (23 percent) are international medical graduates. Among the total pool of colorectal surgeons, approximately 80 (8 percent) are under

1. *(facing page)* George Bushe's *A Treatise on the Malformations, Injuries, and Diseases of the Rectum and Anus* (1837) was the first text on colon and rectal surgery to be published in the United States. The work is unique in the annals of American medicine, since it is the only nineteenth-century surgical monograph with a separate atlas of plates, a practice already established in Europe. This illustration shows two views of internal hemorrhoids from a patient whom Bushe had operated on two years earlier. *(Author's Collection)*

35 years old; 355 (37 percent) are 35 to 44; 275 (28 percent) are 45 to 54; 140 (15 percent) are 55 to 64; and 115 (12 percent) are 65 years old and older. Of the 45 female colorectal surgeons, 40 (89 percent) are under 44, in contrast to the 920 male colorectal surgeons, of whom 395 (41 percent) are under 44 years of age.

The roots of this specialty in the United States can be traced back to the itinerant rectal surgeons of medieval Europe. In the nineteenth century in this country, the itinerant role was most prominently assumed by Milton Mitchell (1834–1887), a native Kentuckian. He attended the proprietary Kentucky School of Medicine for less than a year in the late 1860s and shortly began to limit his practice to the injection treatment of hemorrhoids. Like all itinerants, Mitchell was essentially self-taught and unpublished, and he led a peripatetic existence (Jacksonville, Illinois; Carrollton, Missouri; Wichita, Kansas). Territory rights were sold relative to his treatment, and there are numerous accounts of questionable activities regarding his overall venture. Still, in the strictest sense of the definition, he was the country's first rectal specialist, and he inspired several well-intentioned followers, including Jacob Albright, Charles Blanchard, Alexander Brinkerhoff, and Eugene Hoyt.

From about the late 1870s on, the Midwest was overrun with itinerant "pile doctors." The most well known was Brinkerhoff (died 1887), who was considered by the allopathic medical community to be both a nuisance and a quack. He made monthly tours of such towns as Chillicothe, Lima, Portsmouth, and Springfield, Ohio, and Fort Wayne, Winchester, and other places in Indiana. Plying his trade of curing piles, Brinkerhoff was even so bold as to privately publish a lengthy monograph, *Diseases of the Rectum and New Method of Rectal Treatment* (1881). The 266-page volume was little more than a massive advertisement for the Brinkerhoff treatment of piles and other rectal and anal problems.

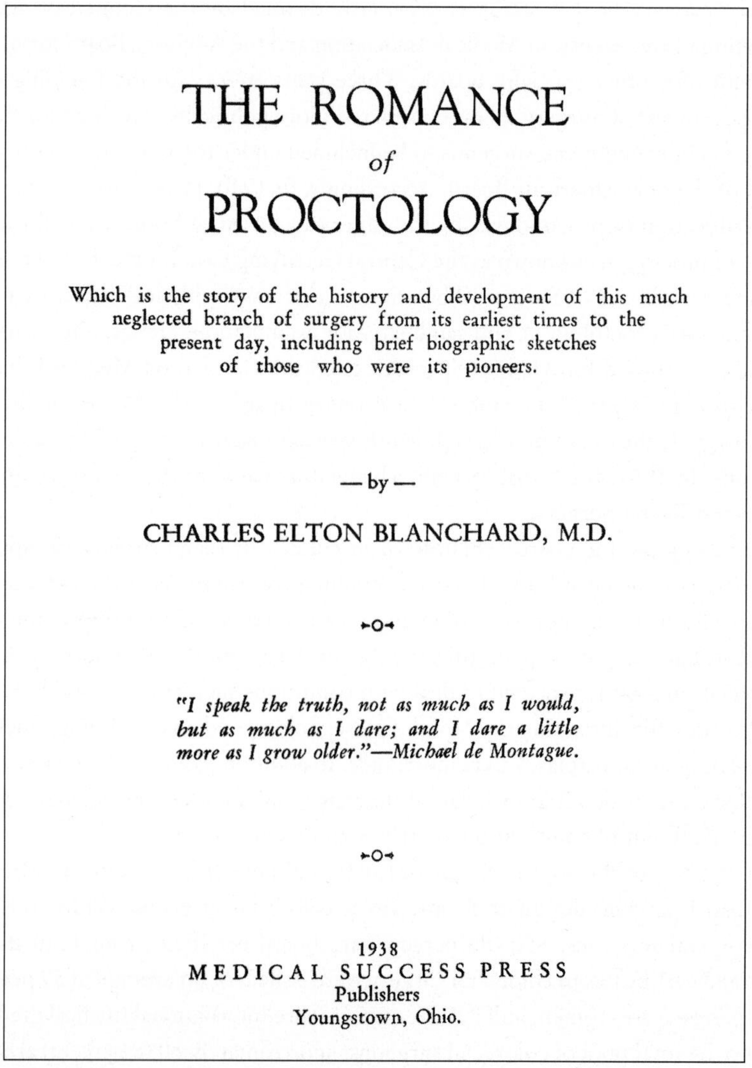

THE ROMANCE
of
PROCTOLOGY

Which is the story of the history and development of this much neglected branch of surgery from its earliest times to the present day, including brief biographic sketches of those who were its pioneers.

— by —

CHARLES ELTON BLANCHARD, M.D.

"I speak the truth, not as much as I would, but as much as I dare; and I dare a little more as I grow older."—Michael de Montague.

1938
MEDICAL SUCCESS PRESS
Publishers
Youngstown, Ohio.

2. Although the title of this historical monograph might be considered an oxymoron, proctology has long been considered an area for specialty work. Including the quacks of last century and their fanciful hemorrhoidal treatments, the history of colon and rectal surgery has been among the most colorful of all surgical specialties. (*Author's Collection*)

In 1888, Edmund Andrews and his son Edward exposed the spurious methods of the "pile doctors" when they authored a monograph entitled *Rectal and Anal Surgery, with a Description of the Secret Methods of the Itinerants*. The Andrews were quick to point out that these quacks "divided up the United States into districts, and sold local 'rights' to practice the plan, after the manner of patent rights, each purchaser being solemnly sworn, or pledged, to confine his practice to his own district, and to keep the secret of the methods." The itinerant rectal specialist faded rapidly from the health care delivery scene, but their questionable brand of medical therapeutics did manage to compel allopathic physicians to pay more attention to the neglected subject of rectal diseases.

Although modern American colon and rectal surgery is usually stated to have begun with the work of Joseph Mathews (1847–1928), some earlier nineteenth-century surgeons took an interest in studying anal and rectal pathology. George M. Bushe (1793–1836) authored the country's first colorectal text with a separate atlas of plates, *A Treatise on the Malformations, Injuries, and Diseases of the Rectum and Anus* (1837), but succumbed to tuberculosis shortly before the work was published. Ten years later, William Bodenhamer (1808–1905), an 1839 graduate of Worthington Medical College of Ohio University, began to write on anal and rectal diseases. Much like the Midwestern itinerants, Bodenhamer also led a disquieting existence. In his privately printed first monograph, *Practical Observations on Some of the Diseases of the Rectum, Anus, and Contiguous Textures* (1847), Bodenhamer wrote in the addenda that any patients who wish to visit him should know that he divides his time between Louisville and New Orleans in order to bring his medical advice to as many people as possible. In 1859, Bodenhamer settled in New York City and began to produce an impressive body of full-length written texts on colorectal diseases: *A Practical Treatise on the Etiology, Pathology, and Treatment of the Congenital Malformations of the Rectum and Anus* (1860); *Practical Observations on the Etiology, Pathology, Diagnosis, and Treatment of Anal Fissure* (1868), and *A Theoretical and Practical Treatise on the Hemorrhoidal Diseases* (1884). Whether Bodenhamer was the country's earliest specialist in rectal diseases, as opposed to the Midwest's Mitchell, is open to historical inquiry. In the 1870s, Bodenhamer listed himself as "professor of the diseases, injuries, and malformations of the rectum, anus, and genitourinary organs." He never named the medical institution at which he held professorial rank, and he clearly did not limit himself to rectal difficulties.

As interest in rectal surgery grew, various physicians began to clamor for a society dedicated to proctologic diseases. In 1895, Samuel T. Earle of Baltimore, during the annual meeting of the American Medical Association, invited a group of men to his home to discuss organizing the physicians interested in this special field. Nothing came of this effort until four years later when, in response to a call issued by Thomas C. Martin (1864–1926) a group of those interested met at the Chittenden Hotel in Columbus, Ohio. Thus, the American Proctologic Society was begun with Martin, Lewis Adler, William Beach (died 1930), George Cook (1844–1920), A. Bennett Cooke (1853–1946), Samuel T. Earle, George B. Evans (1834–1930), Samuel Gant, Joseph M. Mathews, John Pennington (1856–1927), B. Merrill Rickets (died 1910), Leon Straus (1861–1913), and James P. Tuttle (1857–1913) serving as charter members.

During the 1890s, three important proctologic textbooks were published that established treatment guidelines for the growing specialty: Joseph Mathew's *A Treatise on Disease of the Rectum, Anus, and Sigmoid Flexure* (1892), Samuel Gant's *Diagnosis and Treatment of Diseases of the Rectum, Anus, and Contiguous Textures* (1896), and Charles Kelsey's *Surgery of the Rectum and Pelvis* (1897). The Society had not been organized very long before other books of proctology began to appear regularly. Jacob Albright's (1870–1926) *A Practical Treatise on Rectal Diseases, Their Diagnosis and Treatment by Ambulant Methods* (1909) and A. B. Cooke's *Treatise on Diseases of the Rectum and Anus* (1916) were particularly influential. In 1913, a movement was started to form a Section of Proctology within the American Medical Association. Members of the American Gastroenterological Association were likewise seeking a similar goal. The Committee on Sections decided that the limited attendance at such sections, one medical, the other surgical, would not justify their separate creation. As a matter of compromise, the proctologists joined with the gastroenterologists, and in 1917 the first meeting of the Section of Proctology and Gastroenterology of the American Medical Association was held in New York City.

Important clinical contributions were also being made. In 1910, Donald Balfour (1882–1963) at the Mayo Clinic described his method of anastomosis for resection of the sigmoid colon. That same year, William Mayo presented a series of 120 cases concerning a radical operation for carcinoma of the rectum. Numerous textbooks were published during the 1920s, including Martin Bodkin's *Diseases of the Rectum and Pelvic Colon* (1925), Joseph Montague's *The Modern Treatment of Hemorrhoids* (1926), and William Minor's *Clinical Proctology* (1929). In 1933, Lawrence Goldbacher of Philadelphia authored his important *Rectal Diseases in Office Practice*, an attempt to demonstrate to the profession that the majority of proctologic work could be carried out successfully in the office instead of the hospital. Five years later, Louis Buie of the Mayo Clinic wrote *Practical Proctology*, a now classic text. In the *Study for Surgical Services for the United States*, the Committee on Surgical Research felt that no clinical colorectal contributions between 1945 and 1970 could be rated as being of first- or second-order importance. However, colectomy for ulcerative colitis was named of third-order importance, while the no-touch technique for colon cancer was cited as an infrequent selection.

Throughout the years, the most influential periodical for the colorectal specialist has been *Diseases of the Colon and Rectum*. Published monthly, its editors-in-chief included Louis A Buie, 1958–1966, John R Hill, 1966–1986, and Robert W Beart, Jr., 1987-??. Many individuals have made major contributions to the development of American colon-rectal surgery through both their writings and their clinical successes. The following is but a sampling of what should be a longer list of biographies.

BIOGRAPHIES OF COLORECTAL SURGEONS

Joseph McDowell Mathews (1847–1928) was born in New Castle, Kentucky, and received his medical education at the University of Louisville (1867). Returning to his birthplace, Mathews entered a general medical practice and remained there until 1872. He then moved to Louisville, where he continued general practice but became increasingly interested in the diagnosis and treatment of rectal diseases. In an unusual career move, Mathews went to London (1877) and studied colon and rectal surgery with William Allingham (1829–1908), senior surgeon at St. Mark's Hospital. Imbued with a new sense of purpose, Mathews entered the full-time practice of proctology in Louisville and practiced that specialty exclusively from 1878–1912. In 1880 he was appointed professor of surgery in the Kentucky School of Medicine, and three years later, when a department of proctology was established, he was named its head. Mathews is often called America's first true proctologist and the first allopathic physician anywhere in the world to limit his practice to rectal diseases. He took proctology out of the hands of charlatans and itinerants and placed it on a true scientific basis. Interestingly, Mathews exerted a conservative influence in rectal surgery by introducing British surgical methods for the treatment of diseases of the colon and rectum, thereby opposing most radical operations because of their demonstrated failure to save or prolong life. Lacking modern diagnostic and laboratory tools, he was able to develop the art of manual diagnosis of rectal diseases to a high level of sophistication. A well-respected author, Mathews wrote his *Treatise on Diseases of the Rectum, Anus, and Sigmoid Flexure* in 1892, the first proctology textbook by an American orthodox physician. Two years later, he started *Mathews' Medical Quarterly*, the first journal on proctology in the United States. Mathews' other medical book was the popular *How To Succeed in the Practice of Medicine* (1902). In 1899, he helped organize the American Proctologic Society and served as its first president. At the same time, he was appointed president of the Kentucky State Board of Health and, during a service of ten years, initiated many important reforms.

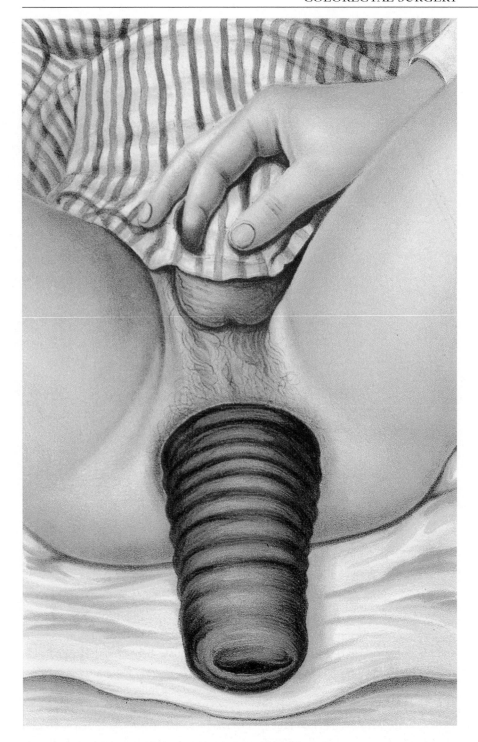

3. Samuel Gant's *Diagnosis and Treatment of Diseases of the Rectum, Anus, and Contiguous Textures* (1896) was an amazing written effort in that Gant was only twenty-seven years old when the work was completed. The chromolithographic plates were quite graphic yet strikingly artistic in their renderings, as typified by this figure showing a case of procidentia recti, or rectal prolapse. *(Author's Collection)*

Mathews also served as president of the Kentucky State Medical Society (1898–1899). He is also remembered for having been the fifty-first president of the American Medical Association (1899), the youngest physician up to that time to hold the office. Mathews retired from active practice in 1913 and moved to Seattle for four years, after which he resettled in Los Angeles, where he died.

Charles Boyd Kelsey (1850–1917) was born at Farmington, Connecticut, and received his undergraduate education at the College of the City of New York (1870) and a medical degree from that city's College of Physicians and Surgeons (1873). For three years, he served as house surgeon at St. Luke's Hospital (1873–1876), and subsequently he was appointed assistant demonstrator of anatomy at his alma mater (1876–1879). For ten years he was in private practice in New York City, where he was staff surgeon at St. Paul's Infirmary for Diseases of the Rectum and consulting surgeon for diseases of the rectum at Harlem Hospital. In 1889, Kelsey was named professor of diseases of the rectum at the University of Vermont. He remained for

4. Samuel T. Earle (1849–1931), professor of proctology at the University of Maryland and author of *Diseases of the Anus, Rectum and Pelvic Colon* (1911), about to perform a hemorrhoidectomy (circa 1910). *(Courtesy of Stanley B. Burns, M.D., and The Burns Collection and Archive)*

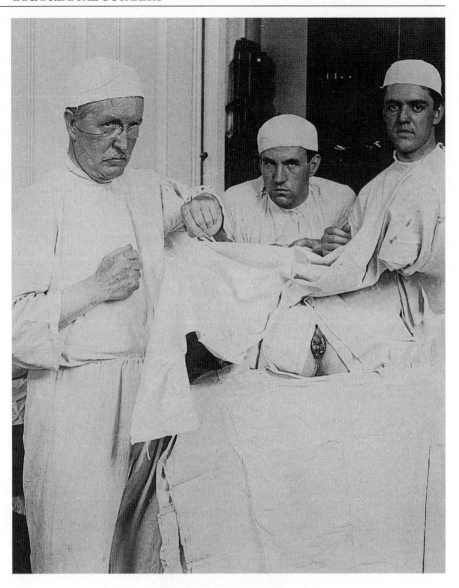

only one year, returning to New York City to occupy the chair of professor of pelvic and abdominal surgery in the New York Post-Graduate School and Hospital. He resigned in 1898 and remained in private practice. Kelsey was among the most prolific of early American proctologists, having authored the following full-length texts: *Diseases of the Rectum and Anus* (1882), *The Pathology, Diagnosis, and Treatment of Diseases of the Rectum and Anus* (1884), *The Diagnosis and Treatment of Haemorrhoids; With General Rules as to the Examination of Rectal Diseases* (1887), *Surgery of the Rectum and Pelvis* (1897), and *The Office Treatment of Hemorrhoids, Fistula, Etc. Without Operation* (1898).

John Rawson Pennington (1856–1927), born in Indiana, graduated from the University of Maryland School of Medicine in 1887. Following his graduation, he entered practice in Kentucky and there came under the direct influence of Joseph Mathews, who persuaded him to study in London at St. Mark's Hospital (1893). Returning to the United States, Pennington decided to limit his clinical activities to proctology and settled in Chicago. He had numerous hospital affiliations and was professor of rectal surgery at the Chicago Polyclinic Hospital and later professor in the Illinois Post-Graduate School of Medicine. Pennington was a charter member of the American Proctologic Society and served as its president in 1904. In 1922 he was elected chairman of the Section on Gastroenterology and Proctology of the American Medical Association. Regarded as a mechanical genius, Pennington devised numerous instruments for the diagnosis and treatment of diseases of the rectum and colon. He authored a wide variety of papers for the surgical literature, but his most influential work is the encyclopedic *Treatise on the Diseases and Injuries of the Anus, Rectum, and Pelvic Colon* (1923). A man of strong beliefs, Pennington was quick-tempered and infamous for an incident in which he punched out Leon Straus (1861–1913), a fellow charter member of the American Proctologic Society, at the 1907 annual meeting, when the latter made a critical remark about a clamp Pennington had developed.

James Percival Tuttle (1857–1913) was born in Fulton, Missouri, and graduated from Westminster College in 1877 and the University of Pennsylvania School of Medicine in 1881. Having served an internship at Blockley Hospital in Philadelphia, Tuttle eventually settled in New York City and joined the staff at that city's Polyclinic Hospital. In 1893 he was instrumental in establishing a department of rectal and intestinal surgery, and subsequently he was named professor. Because the Polyclinic served as a fertile training ground for so many of that era's physicians, Tuttle's influence on prostelytizing the advantages of specialization in colorectal diseases was undeniable. He was a charter member of the American Proctologic Society, serving as temporary chairman at its organizational meeting and becoming president in 1900. Tuttle's lone textbook, the 961-page *A Treatise on Diseases of the Anus, Rectum, and Pelvic Colon* (1902), was so well received that within five years it had gone through three editions. The final years of his life were ravaged by the complications of adult-onset diabetes.

Samuel Goodwin Gant (1869–1944) was born in Knoxville, Missouri, and received his medical degree from Missouri Medical College in 1889. After obtaining surgical training, he initially practiced proctology in Wichita and in Kansas City, Kansas, where he served as professor of diseases of the rectum and anus at the University of Missouri and Woman's Medical College and lecturer on intestinal diseases at the Scarritt Training School for Nurses. Gant later moved to New York City, where he was appointed professor of diseases of the colon, rectum and anus at the New York Post-Graduate Medical School and Hospital and attending surgeon for rectal diseases at St. Mary's Hospital and the German Polyclinic Dispensary. A charter member of the American Proctologic Society, Gant's earliest textbook, *Diagnosis and Treatment of Diseases of the Rectum, Anus, and Contiguous Textures* (1896), is an amazing effort, since he wrote it when only twenty-seven years old. Among his other books were *Constipation and Intestinal Obstruction (Obstipation)* (1909), *Diarrheal, Inflammatory, Obstructive, and Parasitic Diseases of the Gastro-Intestinal Tract* (1915), and the massive three-volume *Diseases of the Rectum, Anus, and Colon* (1923).

Louis Jacob Hirschman (1878–1956) was born in Republic, Michigan, and received his medical education at the Detroit College of Medicine (1899). He served as a house physician at Harper Hospital in Detroit (1899–1900) and in 1904 was appointed proctologist and chairman of the department of proctology at that institution. Five years later, Hirschman was named professor of proctology at his alma mater (now known as Wayne State University), and he remained in this position until 1946. He also was proctologist to Detroit Women's Hospital, Charles Jennings Hospital, Detroit Receiving Hospital, and the Deaconess Hospital. Active in many areas of organized medicine, Hirschman was a member of the Michigan State Board of Health (1927–1938), spending the last year as president. During World War I he was a major in the U.S. Medical Corps and was stationed in Dijon, France as a surgeon at Base Hospital No. 17, the Harper Hospital Unit. A member of the founders' group of the American College of Surgeons, Hirschman was a president of the Michigan State Medical Society (1928) and vice-president of the American Medical Association (1930). An early president of the American Proctologic Society, he was chairman of the Central Certifying Committee of the American Board of Surgery (1940–1945) and, through his experience in this position, served in a similar role with the Certifying Committee in Proctology. Hirschman was an original member of the American Board of Proctology (1948–1953). A prolific author, he served on the editorial boards of the *American Journal of Surgery* and the *American Journal of Digestive Diseases* while also editing the *American Year Book of Anesthesia* (1915). His

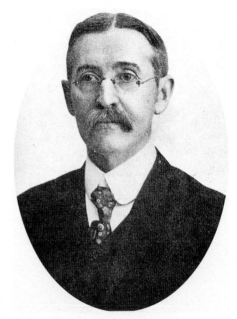

5. James Percival Tuttle. *(Historical Collections, College of Physicians of Philadelphia)*

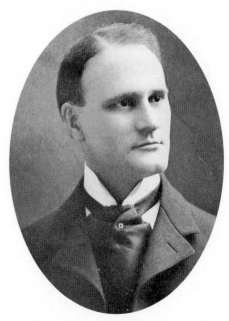

6. Samual Gant. *(Historical Collections, College of Physicians of Philadelphia)*

461

textbooks were *Handbook of Diseases of the Rectum* (1909) and *Synopsis of Ano-Rectal Diseases* (1937).

Louis Arthur Buie (1890–1975), born in Kingstree, South Carolina, did his undergraduate work at the University of South Carolina (1911) and his medical training at the University of Maryland (1915). He completed an internship at his alma mater and then entered the Mayo Graduate School as a fellow in surgery. Following two years of service in the Army Medical Corps in Italy during World War I, Buie returned to the Mayo Clinic in 1919 and was asked by William Mayo to establish a section of proctology. He was head of the section until two years before his retirement in 1955, when he became a senior consultant. Buie was a founder of the American Board of Proctology and played a leading role in the development of proctology and subsequently colon and rectal surgery as a specialty. Among his many honors were serving as president of the American Proctologic Society and the Minnesota State Medical Association, and as chairman of the Section of Gastroenterology and Proctology of the American Medical Association. The author of *Proctoscopic Examination and the Treatment of Hemorrhoids and Anal Pruritus* (1931) and *Practical Proctology* (1938), Buie was the founding editor of *Diseases of the Colon & Rectum* and served as its editor-in-chief from 1957 to 1967. Buie is best remembered for introducing the concept of marsupialization as a treatment for pilonidal sinus.

Anthony Wayne Martin Marino, Sr. (1894–1980) was born in New York City and graduated from the Long Island College of Medicine in 1916. He interned at St. Mary's Hospital in Rochester, Minnesota, and pursued postgraduate training in surgery at the Mayo Clinic (1917–1918), where he then served as a clinical assistant in gastroenterology (1919–1921) and was also chief of the rectal clinic (1922–1924). Marino remained at the Mayo Clinic until 1933, when he moved to New York City and was appointed attending surgeon at the Brooklyn Hospital and proctologist at the Kingston Hospital. He worked mostly at the Brooklyn Hospital until his retirement in 1963. Marino also served as a consulting proctologist to the Wyckoff Heights Hospital (1934–1956) and St. Mary's Hospital (1951–1970). In addition, he was instructor in surgery (1933) and later assistant (1943), associate (1948), and clinical professor of surgery (1954) at the State University of New York College of Medicine (Downstate) in Brooklyn. A member of the founders' group of the American Board of Proctology, Marino was twice president of the American Board of Colon and Rectal Surgery (1958, 1963). He represented colon and rectal surgery in the American Medical Association's House of Delegates for many years and was instrumental in establishing a separate section of Colon and Rectal Surgery in the American Medical Association. Among his honors were serving as president of the American Society of Colon and Rectal Surgeons in 1954 and being on the editorial board of *Diseases of the Colon and Rectum*.

Harry Ellicott Bacon (1900–1981), born in Philadelphia, received his medical degree from Temple University Medical School in 1925. After an internship at Philadelphia General Hospital, he became a fellow in proctologic surgery at the Graduate School of Medicine of the University of Pennyslvania (1926–1927). Bacon pursued further training at St. Mark's Hospital in London, Hospital Saint Antoine in Paris, and Allgemeine Krankenhaus in Vienna. He returned to his alma mater as lecturer in anatomy (1932–1934) and later was named associate professor of proctologic surgery at the University of Pennsylvania (1938–1942). From 1942 to 1971 he served as professor and head of the department of colon and rectal surgery at Temple University. Between 1971 and 1976 Bacon was chief of the department of colon and rectal surgery at St. Luke's and Children's Medical Center in Philadelphia. Actively involved in the politics of American proctology, he was a member of the Council of the American Proctologic Society (1942–1950), serving as president in 1949. A founder of the American Board of Proctology, Bacon was president in 1955, and that year he also served as chairman of the American Medical Association's Section on Gastroenterology and Proctology. He was president of the American Society of

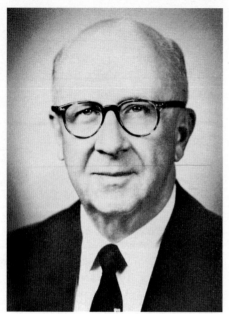

7. Louis Arthur Buie. *(Historical Collections, College of Physicians of Philadelphia)*

Colon and Rectal Surgeons in 1948. He was elected president of the International College of Surgery in 1958 and was later president of the International Society for the Study of Diseases of the Colon and Rectum (1961–1964). A principal organizer of the journal *Diseases of the Colon and Rectum*, Bacon was a prolific author, contributing over four hundred articles to the scientific literature. Among his textbooks are *Anus, Rectum, Sigmoid Colon: Diagnosis and Treatment* (1938), *Essentials of Proctology* (1943), *Atlas of Operative Technique: Anus, Rectum and Colon* (1954), *Proctology* (1956), *Ulcerative Colitis* (1958), *Surgical Anatomy of the Colon, Rectum and Anal Canal* (1962), and *Cancer of the Colon, Rectum and Anal Canal* (1964). A man not limited to science, Bacon had considerable literary and musical talents, which included the publication of three volumes of poetry. In 1979 he earned a Ph.D. in literature from Villanova University.

Robert Turell (1902–1990) graduated from the University of Wisconsin School of Medicine in 1927. After pursuing several years of peripatetic postgraduate education and training, he joined the Mount Sinai Hospital in New York City as a resident in gynecology. He soon switched his specialty work to proctology and remained at Mount Sinai for the next half century as a well-known proctologist and surgical educator. Turell authored hundreds of articles for professional journals and wrote two important textbooks, *Treatment in Proctology* (1949) and the two-volume *Diseases of the Colon and Anorectum* (1959). In addition, he edited two editions of the *Surgical Clinics of North America* devoted to colon and rectal surgery (1965, 1972).

Rupert Beach Turnbull, Jr. (1913–1981) was born in Pasadena, California, and attended Pomona College (1936) and McGill University School of Medicine (1940). After an internship at South Pacific Hospital in San Francisco, he spent a few months in the Panama Canal Zone at Gorgas Memorial Hospital (1941). During World War II, Turnbull served in the South Pacific as a field surgeon and later in Tientsin, China, as director of a general hospital. Following the war, Turnbull completed his surgical training at the Cleveland Clinic, where he ultimately joined its staff. From 1949 to 1979 he was chief of that institution's department of colon and rectal surgery. Much of Turnbull's interest in colon and rectal surgery was directed at stomal problems and their management. He codesigned the first postoperative pouch for ostomy patients, and through his encouragement the nursing specialty of enterostomal therapy was developed. Turnbull was on the editorial board of many scientific journals, including *Diseases of the Colon and Rectum*, and authored the definitive *Atlas of Intestinal Stomas* (1967). He was president of the American Society of Colon and Rectal Surgeons in 1974.

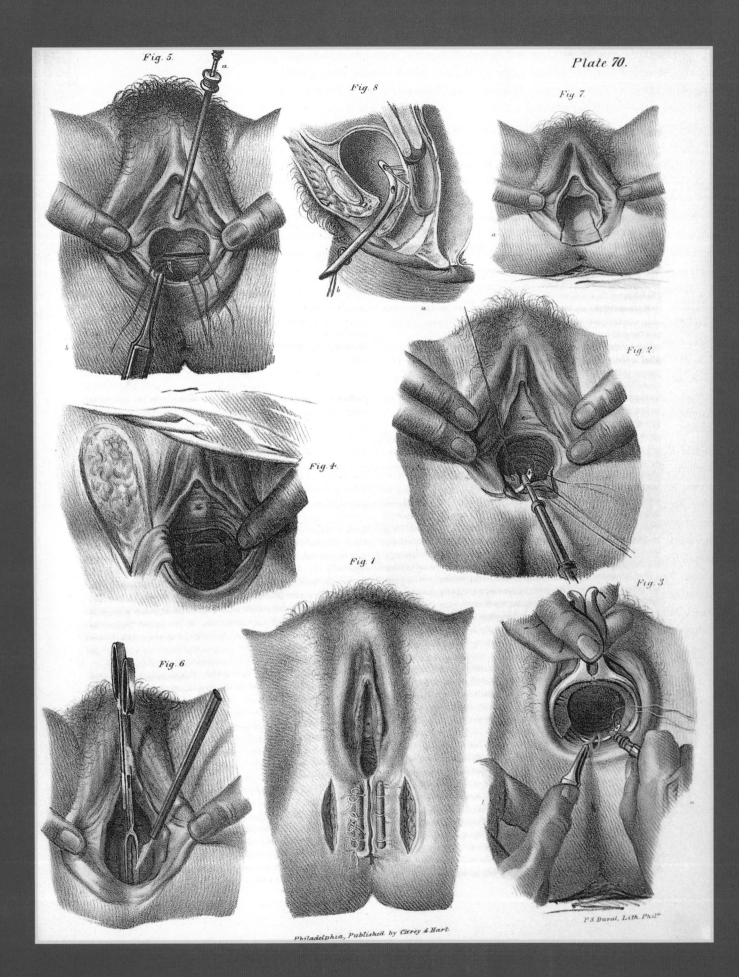

Fig. 5.

Plate 70.

Fig. 8.

Fig 7.

Fig. 2.

Fig. 4.

Fig. 1.

Fig. 3.

Fig. 6.

Philadelphia, Published by Carey & Hart.

CHAPTER 16

GYNECOLOGIC SURGERY

t the end of the nineteenth century, a looming clinical and socio-economic question for American gynecologists, obstetricians, and surgeons was whether or not gynecology should be independent of obstetrics and considered a subspecialty within the whole of operative surgery. It was a complicated relationship, made more difficult by the pragmatic fact that most surgeons included gynecologic cases within their purview but blithely dismissed routine obstetrical care as belonging to midwives. Although gynecologic surgery as an organized specialty would never exist, many well-intentioned hospital administrators and influential surgeons managed to continue the controversy well past the midpoint of the present century.

For instance, at Harvard, formal instruction in obstetrics began in 1815 when Walter Channing (1786–1876) was designated lecturer on obstetrics and medical jurisprudence. Six decades later, a separate chair of obstetrics was finally established. Instruction in gynecology was first offered in 1871, but not until seventeen years later was a chair of gynecology organized, with William H. Baker (1845–1914) serving as professor of gynecology. Following Baker's resignation in 1895, the Harvard faculty voted to merge the department of gynecology with William L. Richardson's (1842–1932) department of obstetrics. Separatism arose again in the pre-World War I era, when a distinct department of gynecology was reestablished under the direction of William P. Graves (1870–1933). Gynecology and obstetrics at Harvard were taught separately until 1959, when they were again united, apparently for the final time, under Duncan E. Reid (1905–1973).

Such organizational confusion was also apparent at The Johns Hopkins Hospital where, in 1889, Howard Kelly was initially appointed "gynecologist and obstetrician." Four years later, the trustees of The Johns Hopkins University School of Medicine named him professor of obstetrics and gynecology. Yet, within a few short years (1896), Kelly expressed his desire that a separate department of obstetrics be created and J. Whitridge Williams (1866–1931) be named professor of obstetrics. At first the trustees of the hospital were reluctant to acquiesce to Kelly's recommendations, but in 1899 the chair of obstetrics and gynecology was formally divided, and Williams became professor of obstetrics and obstetrician-in-chief to The Johns Hopkins Hospital. Both departments remained fully autonomous until Kelly resigned his position at the hospital in 1919, when the board of trustees voted to appoint Thomas S. Cullen (1868–1953) as professor of clinical gynecology but stated that "hereafter gynecology be regarded as a sub-department of Surgery." Complicating the new administrative arrangements of the department of gynecology was its continuing ambiguous relationship to the department of obstetrics. Cullen was among the more vocal, on both local and national levels, who continued to resist

1. *(facing page)* The plates in Joseph Pancoast's *Treatise* were exceedingly lifelike. These figures shows a vaginal fistula and suture of the lacerated female perineum. Religious purists were offended by the realistic drawings, and this plate and one on "lithotomy in the female" were frequently removed from the book in order not to offend a reader's modesty. *(Author's Collection)*

the union of obstetrics and gynecology. He stated his opposition whenever possible, most notably in his chairman's address before the American Medical Association's Section on Obstetrics, Gynecology, and Abdominal Surgery (1915). In 1939, Richard W. TeLinde (1894–1989) succeeded Cullen. His appointment reflected a victory for the separatists, who continued to favor independent departments of obstetrics and gynecology. TeLinde also suggested that gynecology be given an independent status, separate from the department of surgery, and his proposal was accepted. Despite it all, TeLinde foresaw the increasing role of gynecology as a close clinical partner of obstetrics and later named Georgeanna Seegar Jones (born 1912) to head a gynecology subsection of reproductive endocrinology. This appointment was, in fact, a joint project of the departments of gynecology and obstetrics. When Williams died, he was succeeded by Nicholson J. Eastman (1895–1973), who strongly advocated a joint department. Coincidentally, TeLinde and Eastman retired in the same year, and such propitious political timing finally brought about a unification of the two specialties under one leader, Allan C. Barnes (1911–1982), appointed in 1964 as director of the combined department of obstetrics and gynecology.

More numerous than the separatists or "resisters" were the proponents of a unified specialty. Thaddeus Reamy (1829–1909) founded the first hospital for women west of the Allegheny Mountains. Based in Cincinnati, he persistently argued in vain during the last decades of the nineteenth century for a combining of gynecology with obstetrics. Matthew Mann (1845–1921), professor of obstetrics and gynecology at the University of Buffalo, stated in his 1895 presidential address to the American Gynecological Society that obstetrics and gynecology "can never be sep-

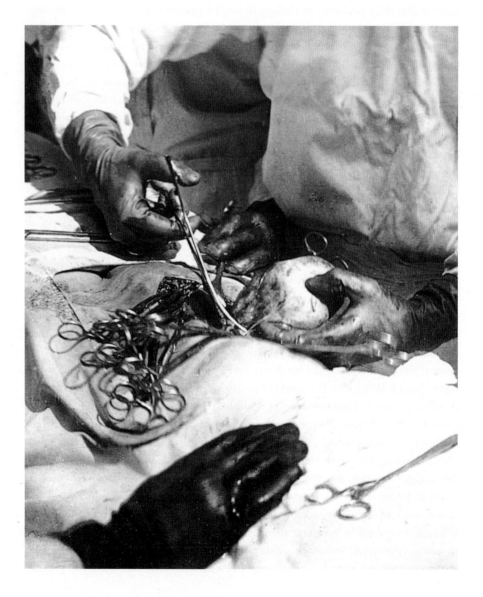

2. The hands of master surgeon Howard Kelly, in the process of clamping the vascular pedicle to an ovarian dermoid cyst (circa 1908). This photograph is from Kelly's *Stereo Clinics*, an interesting departure in the illustration of operations. First appearing in 1908, and issued in eighty-four sections over ten years, the *Clinics* was an attempt to teach practitioners the specific principles of modern surgery through stereophotographs. Kelly and his assistants and photographers spared no expense in making these stereograms as perfect as possible. The photographers traveled to many hospitals and clinics to secure representations of operations by surgeons renowned in their field. In 1909 and 1910, Kelly himself visited clinics abroad and arranged to photograph the work of prominent European surgeons. Each series of the *Clinics* was accompanied by a text descriptive of every important operative step and a clear analysis such as the surgeon would present to students during an actual operation. Using a viewing stereoscope, the reading physician was made to feel as if he were actually present in the master surgeon's operating room. *(Courtesy of Stanley B. Burns, M.D., and The Burns Collection and Archive)*

arated." Rhetoric aside, there did not exist a politically powerful society to bring about the hoped-for amalgamation. Although the American Medical Association's Section on Obstetrics and Gynecology was established in 1860, it was more of an educational and scientific forum than an effective lobbying tool. Many local societies also emerged, including the New York Obstetrical Society (1863), the Obstetrical Society of Philadelphia (1868), the Cincinnati Obstetrical Society (1876), the Chicago Gynecological Society (1878), the Obstetrical Society of Boston (1881), and the Brooklyn Gynecological Society (1890), but they rarely brought gynecologist and obstetrician together.

The first nationwide organization for gynecologists was the American Gynecological Society (1876), and the founding of the American Association of Obstetricians and Gynecologists (1888) soon followed. The memberships of both these groups were deliberately limited by the founding members. Consequently, a rapidly growing corps of obstetrical and gynecological specialists in the United States could not exist. As late as 1912, Williams showed, in a questionnaire survey of the teaching of obstetrics and gynecology in American medical schools, that only one fifth of the respondents noted a unified department. In 1927, a joint committee on the standardization of requirements for obstetric and gynecologic specialists was established by the American Association of Obstetricians, Gynecologists and Abdominal Surgeons and the American Gynecological Society. The members of this committee, in turn, recommended that they be joined in their efforts by three members of the Section on Obstetrics, Gynecology and Abdominal Surgery of the American Medical Association. Within one year, an agreement had been reached to incorporate a formal certifying body, the American Board of Obstetrics and Gynecology. The board's first written examination of candidates for certification was held in March 1931, followed by oral, clinical, and pathological examinations in May.

By 1934, combined departments of obstetrics and gynecology were found in 60 percent of America's medical schools. Yet, as late as 1952, this figure had increased to only 78 percent. A nationwide attempt had been made to correct the situation in 1944, when the National Federation of Obstetric-Gynecologic Societies was formed. To make their institution more egalitarian, the federation members decided in 1951 that the organization should be reconstituted into an inclusive national body based on individual membership and known as the American Academy of Obstetrics and Gynecology. Five years later the Academy changed its name to the American College of Obstetricians and Gynecologists.

Despite the presence of the combined certifying board, the American Academy of Obstetrics and Gynecology, and the growing number of departments of obstetrics and gynecology, a cadre of diehards still persisted in their efforts to maintain a separate identity for gynecologic surgeons. In 1950, Joe V. Meigs (1892–1963), in a presentation to the American Surgical Association, succeeded in having its Executive Committee pass a motion calling for the American Board of Obstetrics and Gynecology to provide "separate certification of obstetricians and gynecologists...and should this fail...have a Board of Gynecologic Surgery established as a subsidiary to the American Board of Surgery." In a bizarre move, the leadership of The American Board of Obstetrics and Gynecology assented to the proposition, and such separate certification was authorized for candidates who had graduated from medical school before 1939 and who had been in practice for at least five years after their training. Not surprisingly, only a few single certificates in either obstetrics or gynecology were ever issued, and the disintegrative policy was silently discontinued in 1965.

Attempts to recognize gynecologic surgery as an independent surgical specialty are no longer heard, and presently, when combined with obstetrics, it becomes the only specialty in the United States that enjoys both surgical and primary care status. At present, candidates for certification are required to complete four years of graduate medical education with no less than thirty-six months of clinical obstetrics and gynecology. As defined by the American Board, obstetrician-gynecologists are physicians who possess "special knowledge, skills and professional capability in the medical and surgical care of the female reproductive system and associated disorders." Because it is recognized that obstetrician-gynecologists may develop more focused types of clinical practices, the Board also began to award, in 1974, certificates of special qualifications in gynecological oncology, maternal-fetal medicine, and reproductive endocrinology.

In 1995, approximately 621,000 total physicians were in active practice in the United States, 36,650 (5.9 percent) of whom designated themselves as obstetric and gynecologic surgeons. Within this cadre of obstetric and gynecologic surgeons, 24,480 (67 percent) were board certified. (By contrast, during the fifteen years from 1980 through 1994, 15,633 certificates in obstetric and gynecologic surgery were issued, or an average of 1,042 per year; and of the special certificates, 1,007 were awarded during the 1980s.) Of the total number in 1995, 10,000 (27 percent) were women and 7,140 (19 percent) were international medical graduates. Among the total pool of obstetric and gynecologic surgeons, approximately 7,690 (21 percent) were younger than 35 years old; 11,225 (31 percent) were 35 to 44 years old; 8,595 (23 percent) were 45 to 54 years old; 5,990 16 percent) were 55 to 64 years old; and 3,150 (9 percent) were 65 years old and older. Of the 10,000 female obstetric and gynecologic surgeons, 7,970 (80 percent) were under 44 years of age, in contrast to the 26,650 male obstetric and gynecologic surgeons, of whom 10,940 (41 percent) were under 44 years of age.

As with most surgical specialties, until the last half of the nineteenth century, few works on gynecologic surgery were published. Although William Dewees (1768–1841) authored the country's first "gynecologic" text in 1826, *A Treatise on the Diseases of Females*, it was mostly concerned with medical gynecology. Immediately following the Civil War, William Byford (1817–1890), professor of obstetrics and diseases of women and children at Chicago Medical College, authored the first gynecologic treatise to mention surgery in the title, *The Practice of Medicine and Surgery, Applied to the Diseases and Accidents Incident to Women*. By the end of the 1860s, two important monographs on gynecologic surgery were published: J. Marion Sims' (1813–1883) *Clinical Notes on Uterine Surgery* (1866) and Thomas A Emmet's (1828–1919) *Vesico-Vaginal Fistula from Parturition and Other Causes* (1868). Emmet dedicated his effort to his mentor, Sims, and said that "the work established my reputation as a surgeon." During that same era, Thomas G. Thomas (1831–1903) authored *A Practical Treatise on the Diseases of Women* (1868). This massive textbook was the most complete and systematic treatise on all aspects of gynecology by an American surgeon up to that time. It surpassed all other gynecologic texts of the era in popularity; was translated into Chinese, French, German, Italian, and Spanish; went into six editions, the last being edited by Paul F. Mundé (1846–1902) in 1891; and sold over sixty thousand copies. The 1870s were notable for the appearance of Emmet's *The Principles and Practice of Gynaecology* (1879). Heavily oriented toward gynecologic surgery, the book was the first thoroughly scientific and comprehensive tome on the subject. Also published during this decade was Edmund Peaslee's (1814–1878) *Ovarian Tumors; Their Pathology, Diagnosis, and Treatment, Especially by Ovariotomy* (1872). In 1887 and 1888, Matthew Mann edited the first American gynecologic textbook to be written by more than one author, the two-volume *A System of Gynecology*. Two years later, Andrew Howe (1825–1892), professor of surgery at the Eclectic Medical Institute in Cincinnati, authored the country's first textbook dedicated strictly to operative gynecology. During the first half of the 1890s, John Baldy's (1860–1934) *An American Textbook of Gynecology, Medical and Surgical* (1894) appeared. Part of *The American Text-Book Series* brought out by W. B. Saunders, Baldy's text became one of the company's most successful nineteenth-century publishing ventures. The turn of the century was largely domi-

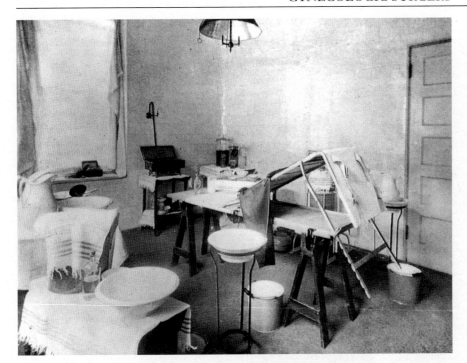

3. A gynecologic operating room in the Gynecean Hospital in Philadelphia, as shown in John Baldy's (1860–1934) *An American Text-Book of Gynecology* (1894). *(Author's Collection)*

nated by the prolific writings of Howard Kelly. Within a ten-year span he managed to write the two-volume *Operative Gynecology* (1898), the two-volume *Gynecology and Abdominal Surgery* (1907) coauthored with Charles Noble (1863–1935), and the single-volume *Medical Gynecology* (1908). This series of textbooks was important for several reasons. Not only did it proclaim to the world Kelly's leadership in all aspects of clinical gynecology, but the works introduced a new standard of excellence to medical illustration in America by showcasing the artistic talents of Max Brödel (1870–1941). At about the same time, William Ashton's (1859–1933) *A Text-book on the Practice of Gynecology* (1905) appeared and managed to obtain some prominence. Eleven years later it was superseded by William Graves' *Gynecology*.

Much as textbooks have played an integral part in the development of surgical specialties, so too has been the impact of the periodicals. In 1881, James Chadwick (1844–1905), one of the founders of the American Gynecological Society, published an article on the world's obstetric and gynecological literature in the *Boston Medical and Surgical Journal*. Chadwick noted that in the United States four separate journals and two annual volumes of society transactions were being printed, compared with a total of sixteen such publications from all the countries of Western Europe. Such excesses were not about to end, and by the turn of the century, almost a dozen obstetric and/or gynecologic journals had been or were still being published. Of these, the *American Journal of Obstetrics and Diseases of Women and Children* was the most influential. Originally edited by Emil Noeggerath (1827–1895), after fifty years of publication it was discontinued in 1919, when the journal was no longer economically viable. Two years later the periodical was revived as the *American Journal of Obstetrics and Gynecology* under the leadership of George Kosmak (1873–1954). It now ranks as one of the most important journals in the specialty. Its editors-in-chief and the years of their stewardship have included Kosmak, 1921–1942; Hugo Ehrenfest, 1935–1942; William J. Dieckmann, 1952–1957; Howard C. Taylor, Jr., 1952–1969; Alan C. Barnes, 1969–1971; John I. Brewer, 1969–1990; Frederick P. Zuspan, 1991–??; and E. J. Quilligan, 1991–??. The other influential peer-reviewed journal is *Obstetrics and Gynecology*, popularly known as the "Green Journal." It was founded in 1953 as the official publication of the newly organized American Academy of Obstetrics and Gynecology. Ralph A. Reis (1895–1978) served as its first editor-in-chief through 1965. Since then, the editorial mantle has been assumed by S. Leon Israel, 1966–1971; Richard F. Mattingly, 1971–1986; and Roy M. Pitkin, 1986–??.

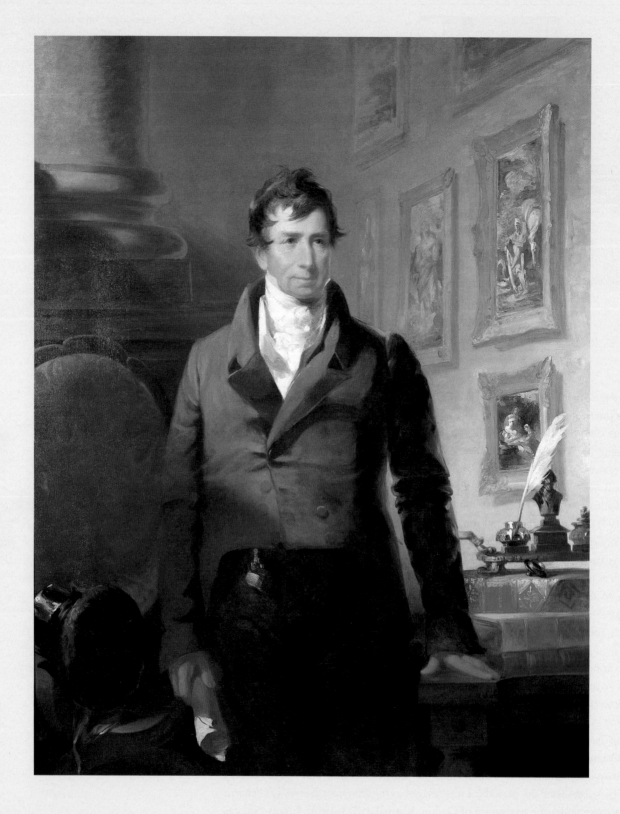

4. One of the finest portraits of an early nineteenth-century American physician-surgeon (circa 1833), William Dewees, author of the country's first textbook on gynecology, is impressively rendered by John Neagle (1796–1865). The renowned obstetrician is brightly illuminated, and his vigor is suggested by a penetrating stare, romantically tousled hair, and a sturdy pose. The oil painting emphasizes Dewees' intellectual attainments, metaphorically noted by enormous literary volumes on the table as well as the elegant inkstand and quill pen. Only in the elaborately framed lowest painting on the wall is there an oblique hint of Dewees' professional occupation: the discovery of baby Moses in the bulrushes. Dewees was such an outstanding figure in his field that no less an authority than Samuel Gross wrote, "No woman of any social position in Philadelphia considered herself safe if she could not have Dewees in her confinement." *(Courtesy of the University of Pennsylvania School of Medicine)*

Many magnificent clinical advances have been made in American gynecologic surgery during the twentieth century. In 1900 Cullen authored his monumental *Cancer of the Uterus*, which included the first detailed clinical and pathologic study of hyperplasia of the endometrium. That same year, George Noble (1860–1932) described, to members of the Southern Surgical and Gynecological Association, a flap operation for atresia of the vagina. In 1901 George Edebohls (1853–1908), of New York City, successfully completed a panhysterocolpectomy, a new method of treatment for uterine prolapse. John C. Webster (1863–1950) described his operation for certain cases of retroversion of the uterus in the *Journal of the American Medical Association* in 1901. Within one year's time, John Baldy had devised a modification of Wester's procedure. James Baldwin (1850–1936) proposed the formation of an artificial vagina by means of intestinal transplantation in 1904. A decade later, William Cary (1883–1969) became the first individual to perform salpingography. At about the same time, Isador Rubin was conducting his own experimentation on uterotubal insufflation (1915). Rubin expanded on his original research five years later (1920), when tubal insufflation was used for the diagnosis and treatment of sterility caused by occlusion of the fallopian tubes. Cullen wrote *Embryology, Anatomy, and Diseases of the Umbilicus Together with Diseases of the Urachus* in 1916. This magnificent volume, with extraordinary illustrations, contained the first reference to a clinical sign of periumbilical darkening of the skin caused by the presence of free blood in the abdomen, usually associated with ruptured ectopic gestation. John Sampson (1873–1946), of Albany, New York, first accurately described ovarian endometriosis and its pathognomonic hallmark, the chocolate cyst, in the *Archives of Surgery* (1921). In 1934, Meigs authored his classic monograph, *Tumors of the Female Pelvic Organs*. Meigs' syndrome, or fibroma of the ovary with pleural effusions, was fully described on pages 262–263 of that work. Irving Stein (1887–1976) and Michael Leventhal (1901–1971) reported a syndrome of amenorrhea associated with bilateral polycystic ovaries in 1935. In 1941 George Papanicolaou (1883–1962) observed, while working in New York City, that he could recognize cancer cells in a microscopic examination of vaginal smears.

Obstetrical highlights included the publication of Williams' *Obstetrics*, among the most famous of American textbooks of obstetrics (1903). In 1915 Frank Lynch (1871–1945) described the use of nitrous oxide gas analgesia as a method of achieving easy childbirth. Six years later, Irving Potter (1868–1956), writing in the *American Journal of Obstetrics and Gynecology*, detailed his operation of podalic version. Spalding's sign of intrauterine death was presented by Alfred Spalding (1874–1942) in 1922. A decade later (1931), Maurice Friedman devised a simple laboratory test for the diagnosis of early pregnancy. Maternal pulmonary embolism by amniotic fluid as a cause of "obstetric shock and unexpected deaths in obstetrics" was reported by Paul Steiner (born 1902) in the *Journal of the American Medical Association* 1941. A quarter of a century later, Cecil Jacobson (born 1936) used amniocentesis to diagnose genetic disorders in utero.

Of all the surgical specialties in the United States, obstetrics and gynecology has been admirably served by the medical historian. Herbert Thoms (1885–1972) wrote *Chapters in American Obstetrics* in 1933, and Harold Speert (born 1915) authored his wonderfully detailed *Obstetrics and Gynecology in America: A History* (1980) in addition to *Obstetric and Gynecologic Milestones, Essays in Eponymy* (1958). The most notable of recent gynecological historians was James Ricci, clinical professor of gynecology and obstetrics at New York Medical College, whose masterful works include the trilogy *The Genealogy of Gynaecology, History of the Development of Gynaecology Throughout the Ages, 2000 BC–1800 AD* (1943), *One Hundred Years of Gynaecology, 1800–1900* (1945), and *The Development of Gynaecological Surgery and Instruments* (1949). Notwithstanding attempts to understand the specialty from the broad perspective of clinical, economic, and sociologic changes, individual achievements are sometimes best described through biographical vignettes. The following are more reflective of gynecologic surgeons than of obstetricians, and represent but a small fraction of the many men and women who have so wonderfully contributed to the development of American obstetrics and gynecology.

BIOGRAPHIES OF GYNECOLOGIC SURGEONS

William Heath Byford (1817–1890) was born in Eaton, Ohio, and received his initial medical education as an apprentice to Joseph Maddox, a general physician-surgeon living in Vincennes, Indiana. Considered capable in less than two years' time, Byford successfully passed an examination before an Indiana State Board of Commissioners and was granted a license to practice medicine. He began practice in the town of Owensville in 1838 and resettled in Mt. Vernon two years later as an associate of Hezekiah Holland. Having married Holland's daughter, Mary Ann, in 1840, Byford remained in Mt. Vernon for ten years. During this time he attended a course of lectures at the Ohio Medical College, and he graduated from that institution in 1845. Five years later Byford was appointed to the chair of anatomy in the Evansville Medical College, and in 1852 he was elected to the chair of the theory and practice of medicine. The Evansville Medical College, a proprietary facility, ceased to exist in 1854, but Byford remained in Evansville as a private practitioner while assisting in the editing of the *Indiana Medical Journal*. In 1857 he accepted the professorship of obstetrics and diseases of women and children at Rush Medical College in Chicago. Two years later he helped found the Chicago Medical College, where he was nominated to a professorship similar to that at Rush. Byford remained at this school for almost twenty years, but in 1879 he was recalled to Rush to assume the professorship of gynecology, which had been especially created for him. Byford was active in Chicago medical politics and helped organize the Women's Medical College (1870), serving as president of the faculty as well as on the board of trustees. In addition, he was one of the founding members of the American Gynecological Society and later a president. A respected writer, Byford edited the *Chicago Medical Journal and Examiner* and the *Northwestern Medical and Surgical Journal*. Most of his later career was spent in the full-time practice of gynecology. He is remembered for his two gynecologic textbooks, *A Treatise on the Chronic Inflammation and Displacement of the Unimpregnated Uterus* (1864) and *The Practice of Medicine and Surgery, Applied to the Diseases and Accidents Incident to Women* (1865). In addition, he authored *The Philosophy of Domestic Life* (1869) and *A Treatise on the Theory and Practice of Obstetrics* (1870).

Nathan Bozeman (1825–1905), born in Greenville, Alabama, initially studied medicine in the office of James A. Kelly in Coosa County and later received a medical degree from the University of Louisville (1848). For a few months, Bozeman had the good fortune to be a private assistant to Samuel Gross (1805–1884) when the latter taught in Louisville. Following his graduation, Bozeman was a demonstrator of anatomy at his alma mater under Thomas G. Robinson while also serving as an assistant in the Louisville Marine Hospital. In 1849 Bozeman began medical practice in Montgomery, Alabama, and for a time was associated with the soon-to-be famous J. Marion Sims (1813–1883). Four years later, Bozeman developed his "button suture," whose virtues he promoted for the rest of his professional career. Two years before, Sims had shown that vesicovaginal fistulae could be repaired by freshening the wound edges and bringing them together with silver wire sutures. Bozeman modified Sims' concept by inserting a lead plate over the line of closure of the fistula and fastening the silver sutures, through holes in the plate, to buttons on the device. Although this type of repair was more tedious, Bozeman claimed that the results were far superior to those of Sims. Bozeman's relationship with Sims deteriorated into one of the most bitter feuds in nineteenth-century American surgery: Sims claimed that Bozeman had stolen his concepts for repair of vesicovaginal fistula, and Bozeman retaliated that his "button-suture" had nothing to do with Sims' work. In 1858, Bozeman visited Europe and made a triumphal tour, repairing vesicovaginal

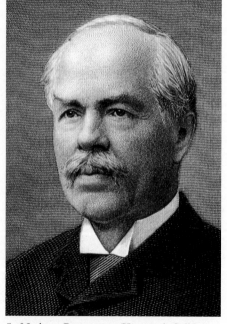

5. Nathan Bozeman. *(Historical Collections, College of Physicians of Philadelphia)*

fistulae in Edinburgh, Glasgow, London, and Paris. After returning to the United States he opened a private hospital in New Orleans for the treatment of women and was appointed attending surgeon to the Charity Hospital (1861). During the Civil War Bozeman was a surgeon in the Confederate States Army, but most of his efforts were spent on a medical board for the examination of surgeons. In 1866 Bozeman moved to New York City, where he practiced for eight years, specializing in gynecologic conditions. For two years (1874–1876) he lived in Europe and demonstrated the practicability of his "button-suture" repair throughout Austria, France, and Germany. Resettling in New York City in 1877, Bozeman was appointed to the attending staff of the New York Woman's Hospital (1878–1889), and in 1889 he opened a private hospital for women. While at the Woman's Hospital, Bozeman specialized in bladder, kidney, and ureteral surgery. Among the most difficult clinical conditions to treat at that time was chronic pyelitis secondary to vesical and fecal fistulae. Bozeman dealt with this complication by catheterization of the ureter through a vesicovaginal opening. His name remains eponymically linked with the Bozeman-Fritsch catheter, a slightly curved double-current uterine catheter with several openings at the tip; the Bozeman operation, hysterocystocleisis for uterovaginal fistula; the Bozeman or knee-elbow position; and the Bozeman speculum, a bivalve vaginal speculum, the long blades of which remain parallel when separated.

Emil Oscar Noeggerath (1827–1895) was born in Bonn, Germany, received his medical degree from his native city's university in 1852, and studied with several influential European gynecologic surgeons over the next five years. In 1857 he decided to emigrate to the United States, intending to accept a professorship in St. Louis, but when he arrived he was not satisfied with the offered position and, instead, was forced to relocate to New York City. Appointed to the staff of the female department of the German Hospital, Noeggerath was eventually named professor of obstetrics and diseases of women at New York College of Medicine. In addition, he was surgeon to the Woman's Hospital and consulting surgeon to St. Mary's Hospital for Women. Noeggerath was a founding member of the American Gynecological Society and presented his important paper on "latent gonorrhea" at its first annual meeting. In 1858, he authored an influential article that reintroduced epicystotomy, or suprapubic cystotomy, to the American surgeon. Along with Abraham Jacobi (1830–1919), Noeggerath founded the *American Journal of Obstetrics* in 1868 and edited it for five years. He was vice-president of the American Gynecological Society in 1882. Three years later Noeggerath retired from active clinical practice because of poor health. He returned to Germany, where he lived the remaining ten years of his life.

Robert Battey (1828–1895) was born in Augusta, Georgia, attended preparatory school at the Phillips Academy in Andover, Massachusetts, and took medical apprenticeships with his brother George M. Battey in Rome, Georgia (1856), and with Ellwood Wilson (1822–1889) of Philadelphia (1857). In addition, Battey received a medical degree from Jefferson Medical College in 1857. His entire professional career was spent in Rome, Georgia, except for the years 1859–1860, when he studied in Paris, and 1872–1875, when he was professor of obstetrics at Atlanta Medical College. During the Civil War Battey was surgeon of the Nineteenth Regiment of Georgia Volunteers and Hampton's Brigade. While residing in Atlanta, Battey edited the *Atlanta Medical and Surgical Journal*. Battey is eponymically linked with Battey's operation, in which normal ovaries were removed to induce artificial menopause for the cure of uterine fibroids and other conditions. Battey was convinced that removing the ovaries, whether they were diseased or not, would do away with disturbances of menstruation accompanied by various nervous manifestations, including severe headaches, pelvic pain, and hystero-epileptic attacks. He first broached the subject of "normal ovariotomy" in 1872 and presented his findings on ten such operations to the American Gynecological Society four years later. Despite his erroneous beliefs, which for a time were widely accepted, Battey contributed to

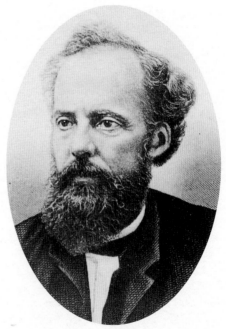

6. Robert Battey. *(Historical Collections, College of Physicians of Philadelphia)*

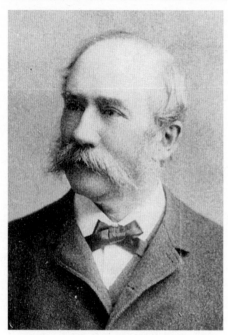

7. Thomas Addis Emmet. *(Historical Collections, College of Physicians of Philadelphia)*

the development of pelvic and abdominal surgery and helped establish the functional relationship between ovaries and menstruation, thus stimulating the beginnings of endocrinology as a science. He served as president of the American Gynecologic Society in 1888 and of the Medical Association of the State of Georgia in 1876.

Thomas Addis Emmet (1828–1919) was born on the campus of the University of Virginia, where his father, John Patten Emmet (1797–1842), was professor of natural history and later of chemistry and materia medica. The younger Emmet studied at the University of Virginia but was a poor student and never graduated. At the coaxing of his mother, he attended lectures given by John K. Mitchell (1793–1858), a friend of the family, at Jefferson Medical College. Emmet found medicine to his liking and graduated from Jefferson in 1850. Moving to New York City, where he had previously lived for a time with his uncle's family, Emmet was named resident physician at the Emigrant Refuge Hospital on Ward's Island. At the same time he commenced general practice, but in 1855 Emmet lost his position at the Emigrant because of New York City politics. Fortuitously, he met J. Marion Sims at the same time, and Emmet became Sims' assistant surgeon at the Woman's Hospital (1855–1861). When Sims left for an extended sojourn to Europe, Emmet found himself, at the age of 33, surgeon in chief to the institution (1861). Seven years later, Emmet's classic text *Vesico-Vaginal Fistula from Parturition and Other Cases; with Cases of Recto-Vaginal Fistula* was published, providing minutely detailed accounts of 273 patients. Emmet remained surgeon in chief at the Woman's Hospital until 1872, when an irked Board of Governors put an end to his one-man autocratic rule. Although he remained on staff until 1900, it was only in the capacity of visiting surgeon. In 1879 he authored his most important and influential work, *The Principles and Practice of Gynaecology*. Emmet made numerous contributions to medical literature, including work on the treatment of dysmenorrhea and sterility resulting from anteflexion of the uterus (1865), surgical repair of lacerations of the cervix, or Emmet's operation of trachelorrhaphy (1869), vaginal cystotomy for chronic cystitis (1872), and a technique for perineorrhaphy, known as Emmet's method (1883). He is eponymically remembered for a surgical needle with the eye in the point, having a wide curve and set in a handle. Among Emmet's many honors was serving as president of the American Gynecological Society in 1882. Emmet, a prolific writer, authored a lengthy autobiography, *Incidents of my Life, Professional-Literary-Social with Services in the Cause of Ireland* (1911). As a renowned genealogist and Irish patriot, he also wrote *The Emmet Family with Some Incidents Relating to Irish History* (1898); *Ireland Under English Rule, or a Plea for the Plaintiff* (1903), and *Memoir of Thomas Addis and Robert Emmet with their Ancestors and Immediate Family* (1915). Toward the end of his career, Emmet sold a valuable piece of property at 94 Madison Avenue. He stipulated in the sale that when a proposed skyscraper was built it must contain a suite reserved for him on the top floor. Emmet spent the last years of his life as a virtual recluse in this apartment, cut off from visitors by deafness and age.

Theodore Gaillard Thomas (1831–1903) was born on Edisto Island near Charleston, South Carolina, and received his medical education at the Medical College of the State of South Carolina (1852). He completed a year-long internship at Bellevue Hospital and the Emigrant Refuge Hospital in New York City. From 1853 to 1855 Thomas studied medicine in Europe, paying special attention to obstetrics and gynecology in the Rotunda Hospital in Dublin. Returning to New York City, he joined John T. Metcalfe (1818–1883) in practice while also establishing a "quiz class" for medical students in connection with the University of New York. Thomas remained a partner with Metcalfe for fifteen years, during which time he devoted himself to obstetrics and was named replacement for Gunning Bedford (1806–1870) as professor of obstetrics at Bellevue Hospital and the University Medical College (1855–1863). In 1863 Thomas resigned to become adjunct professor of obstetrics and the diseases of women and children at the College of Physicians and Surgeons, a position he held until 1879, when he was appointed professor of gynecology at the same institution. From 1872 to 1887, Thomas also served as an attending surgeon at the Woman's Hospital. His most important written work was the massive *A Practical Treatise on the Diseases of Women* (1868). Having purposefully and methodically narrowed the field of his professional work in order to devote his entire time to gynecology, Thomas was convinced of the necessity for a textbook that would suit students but would also serve as a reference book for the busy practitioner. The *Treatise* was translated into five other languages, and over 60,000 copies were eventually sold. Thomas is also remembered for his contributions to the periodical literature, including a report on the first vaginal ovariotomy (1870) and the use of gastro-elytrotomy as a substitute for cesarean section (1871). His other full-length text is *Abortion and its Treatment, from the Stand-Point of Practical Experience* (1890). A founding member of the American Gynecological Society, Thomas was its president in 1879. Long associated with the social life in Southampton, Long Island, Thomas was an active member of the Shinnecock Golf Club from its founding in 1896. He died while on vacation in Thomasville, Georgia, of a ruptured aortic aneurysm.

Alexander Johnston Chalmers Skene (1837–1900) was born in Fyvie, Scotland, briefly studied medicine in King's College, Scotland, and emigrated to the United States at the age of nineteen (1857). Three years later he began to again study medicine, this time in Toronto, Canada. He soon relocated to the University of Michigan (1861–1862) and finally graduated from the Long Island College Hospital Medical School in 1863. He entered military service as an assistant surgeon in the United States Volunteers and served at Port Royal, Charleston Harbor, and David's Island. In 1865 Skene commenced medical practice in Brooklyn, and three years later he was named professor of gynecology at Long Island College Hospital. He served this institution in several capacities, including dean and president (1886–1893). Skene was also professor of gynecology in the New York Post-Graduate Medical School (1883–1886), and during those years he opened up a private sanitarium in Brooklyn. Shortly before his death he established Skene's Hospital for Self-Supporting Women. A pioneering gynecologist, Skene is best remembered eponymically for describing the paraurethral glands in females (1880). He authored several important clinical textbooks, including *Diseases of the Bladder and Urethra in Women* (1878), *Treatise on the Diseases of Women* (1888), *Medical Gynecology* (1895), and *Electro-Haemostasis in Operative Surgery* (1899). In addition, he wrote *Education and Culture as Related to the Health and Diseases of Women* (1889). Skene was an associate editor of the *Archives of Medicine*, the *American Medical Digest*, and the *New York Gynecological and Obstetrical Journal*. He was one of the founders of the American Gynecological Society and its tenth president (1886). In a little appreciated historic fact, Skene served as mayor of the city of Brooklyn before it became a borough of New York City, and his statue stands in the entrance of Prospect Park.

James Read Chadwick (1844–1905) was born in Boston, attended that city's public schools, and graduated from Harvard College in 1865. After an extended trip abroad, he matriculated at Harvard Medical School and received his degree in 1871. That year, Chadwick married Katherine Lyman, daughter of George Lyman (1819–1891), one of Boston's most renowned gynecologists. The married couple moved to Europe, where Chadwick pursued further medical studies for two years in Berlin, London, Paris, and Vienna. Returning to his native city in 1873, he built a house at 270 Clarendon Street and lived there for the remainder of his life. Appointed gynecologist to the outpatient department of the Boston City Hospital, Chadwick later opened a private gynecologic dispensary, where he also instructed Harvard medical students following his appointment to Harvard's surgical faculty as clinical instructor in gynecology (1881–1887). With his father-in-law, Chadwick became a guiding force in the founding of the American Gynecological Society, serving as its first secretary and eventually as its president (1897). In 1890 he organized the Harvard Medical Alumni Association, which he served as president for its first four years. A well-respected bibliophile, Chadwick was instrumental in founding the Boston Medical Library, which has since been amalgamated with the Harvard Medical Library and currently constitutes The Francis A. Countway Library of Medicine. Chadwick is best remembered for his description of a dark bluish or purplish discoloration of the vulvovaginal mucous membrane, which is considered a presumptive sign of pregnancy (1887). A firm believer in cremation, Chadwick reorganized the New England Cremation Society and was long called the father of cremation in New England. He died at his summer home in Chocorua, New Hampshire, as the result of a fall from a porch roof.

Matthew Derbyshire Mann (1845–1921), born in Utica, New York, received his undergraduate education at Yale (1867) and his medical degree from New York City's College of Physicians and Surgeons (1871). Coming from a well-to-do family, Mann spent the two years following medical school graduation in Europe, where he pursued postgraduate studies in Heidelberg, London, Paris, and Vienna. Returning to the United States, he began practice in New York City (1873–1879) but later relocated to Hartford, Connecticut (1879–1882), where he was regarded as a specialist in the diseases of women. He was appointed clinical lecturer in gynecology at Yale in 1880 and 1881, and from 1882 to 1910 he served as professor of

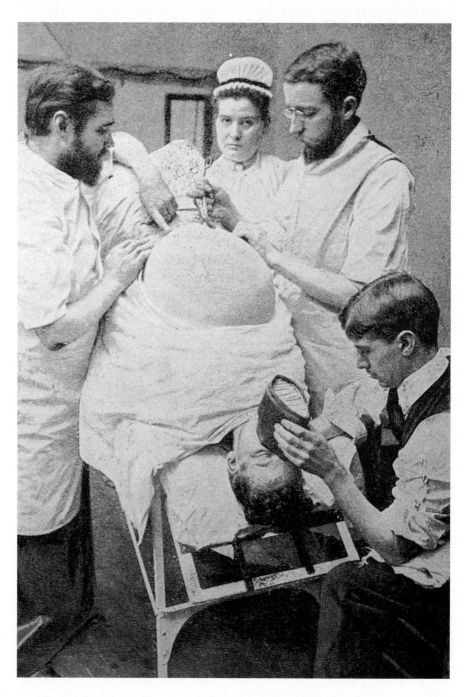

8. As late as the early 1880s, the performance of a cesarean section in the United States was fraught with danger for both mother and child. A decade later there was a spectacular decline in the previously prohibitive cesarean section mortality rates when more modern anesthetic methods and uterine sutures came into use. In this photograph (mid-1890s), the attending surgeons appear to be utilizing a low transverse incision with the patient in a steep head-down position. *(Courtesy of Stanley B. Burns, M.D., and The Burns Collection and Archive)*

obstetrics and gynecology at the University of Buffalo. He also held the position of dean of the faculty at Buffalo and was instrumental in securing the establishment of departments of pharmacy and dentistry there. Long considered a pioneering gynecologic surgeon, Mann brought the newer methods of gynecology, as practiced by J. Marion Sims and Thomas A. Emmet, to western New York. He served as president of the American Gynecological Society in 1895 and was a founding member of the International Congress of Obstetricians and Gynecologists, as well as its vice president in 1901. Because of his esteem in Buffalo medical circles, Mann served as chief surgeon in charge of President William McKinley (1843–1901) following the assassination attempt in 1901, and remained with him until his death. Mann is best remembered for editing the first American gynecologic textbook written by more than one author, the massive two-volume *A System of Gynecology by American Authors* (1887–1888), which crystallized and successfully promulgated many newer surgical techniques. The author of over eighty papers in the periodical literature, Mann also wrote *A Manual of Prescription Writing with a Full Explanation of the Methods of Correctly Writing Prescriptions* (1878).

Fernand Henrotin (1847–1906) was born in Brussels, Belgium, and brought to the United States in 1857, where he attended public high school in Chicago. He graduated from Rush Medical College in 1868 and soon joined his father in a lucrative private practice. Although he was on staff at Cook County Hospital, it was at the Alexian Brothers Hospital that Henrotin did most of his gynecological operating. He was also consulting gynecologist to St. Joseph's and the German Hospitals. As professor of gynecology at the Chicago Polyclinic, his memory was perpetuated in a building erected at the turn of the century called the Henrotin Hospital. The facility survived for nine decades but was finally forced to close in the early 1990s as the result of economic misfortunes and changing neighborhood socioeconomic conditions. Henrotin regarded his specialty as operative gynecology, and although not known for his writings, he did make several worthwhile contributions to various books of that era in the form of lengthy chapters. A long-standing member of the American Gynecological Society, Henrotin also helped found the International Congress of Obstetrics and Gynecology.

Joseph Price (1853–1911) was born in Rockingham County, Virgina, and attended Union College in Schenectady, New York, for one year (1871–1872). He left college to join the engineering department of the New York Central Railroad but eventually returned to his schooling and received his medical degree from the University of Pennsylvania in 1877. Over the course of the next year, Price served as surgeon on a transatlantic passenger steamer between Antwerp, Liverpool, and Philadelphia, making three voyages in all. Settling in Philadelphia, he became head of the obstetrical department of the Philadelphia Dispensary and soon created its gynecological department. From 1887 to 1894, Price was the resident physician at the Preston Retreat, a philanthropic maternity hospital. During those years he also helped found the Gynecean Hospital with Charles Penrose (1862–1925) and established his own private facility, the Joseph Price Hospital. The latter became the largest private institution in the country for abdominal surgery. A devoted admirer of J. Marion Sims and Thomas A. Emmet, Price was instrumental in bringing gynecological surgery into the modern era. As a leading obstetrician and gynecologist in late-nineteenth-century Philadelphia, he was a pioneer in attempting to evaluate surgical outcomes statistically. Price was a leading proponent of the use of abdominal drainage and concomitant irrigation of the peritoneal cavity, and he authored an important paper on "pus in the pelvis," which was presented to the Southern Surgical and Gynecological Association (1890). He was a founder and president (1896) of the American Association of Obstetricians and Gynecologists.

Howard Atwood Kelly (1858–1943) was born in Camden, New Jersey, and educated at the University of Pennsylvania, as both an undergraduate (1877) and a medical student (1882). He interned for a year at Episcopal Hospital in the Kensington area of Philadelphia, Pennsylvania, and shortly thereafter helped found the

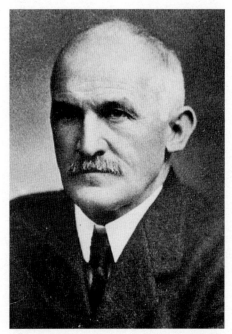

9. Joseph Price. *(Historical Collections, College of Physicians of Philadelphia)*

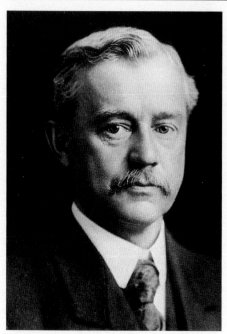

10. Howard Kelly. *(Historical Collections, College of Physicians of Philadelphia)*

Kensington Hospital for Women, one of the country's earliest institutions devoted exclusively to the surgical treatment of women's diseases. Kelly remained in private practice while associated with this specialty facility from 1883 to 1888. During those years he dealt with both obstetric and gynecologic problems. In 1888 he was named associate professor and, within a few months, professor of obstetrics at his alma mater. In 1889 Kelly moved to Baltimore, where he began his lengthy association with The Johns Hopkins Hospital and School of Medicine as professor of gynecology. Kelly soon developed a long-term residency program in gynecology that proved a fundamental contribution to the future evolution of gynecology in the United States. In 1892, when Hunter Robb (1863–1940), who had been Kelly's first resident, was offered the chair of gynecology and obstetrics at Western Reserve University in Cleveland, Kelly facilitated his move by taking over his small private sanatorium on Eutaw Place. Eventually renamed the Howard A. Kelly Hospital, it was the site of Kelly's pioneering use of radium for treating cancer of the female reproductive tract. In 1917 his institution had 5 1/2 grams of radium, said to be the largest amount then in any clinic in the world. After serving for a full three decades as chief gynecologist to The Johns Hopkins Hospital and professor of gynecology at its affiliated medical school, Kelly voluntarily retired in 1919 because of his disapproval of the full-time system which the faculty was being forced to accept. With a very successful private hospital, Kelly was placed in an economically difficult position of having to relinquish his teaching responsibilities in order to maintain his lucrative private practice. Kelly was a major figure in the development of gynecological and abdominal surgery and was vociferous in establishing gynecology as a field distinct from that of obstetrics. He made many fundamental contributions, but his most important clinical legacy was his teaching of the technique of bimanual pelvic examination. Before Kelly's unrelenting advocacy of bimanual pelvic examination while the patient was in the lithotomy position, gynecologic physical examination consisted mostly of inspection and palpation of the cervix. Kelly was the author of over five hundred articles to the periodical literature. Among his most important contributions were papers on hysterorrhaphy (1887), the introduction of aeroscopic examination of the bladder in women and catheterization of the ureters (1893), a method of ureteroureteral anastomosis that included the use of the catheter as a temporary ureteral splint (1894), the removal of pelvic inflammatory masses via the abdomen after bisection of the uterus (1900), the use of wax on a bladder catheter tip so that it registers any pressure resulting from sharp stones, thus providing an important means of diagnosing calculi (1901), and the design of various rectal and vesical speculums (1903). Most impressively, Kelly authored or coauthored a wide array of textbooks, including *Operative Gynecology* (1898), *The Vermiform Appendix and its Diseases* (1905), *Gynecology and Abdominal Surgery* (1907), *Medical Gynecology* (1908), *Myomata of the Uterus* (1909), *Diseases of the Kidney, Ureters, and Bladder* (1914), and *Electrosurgery* (1932). Another interesting work was *The Stereo Clinics* (1908–1915), comprising eighty-four sections of stereograms depicting gynecological operations photographed throughout the United States and Europe. Kelly was also a medical historian of major repute and wrote *Walter Reed and Yellow Fever* (1906), *Some American Medical Botanists* (1914), the two-volume *Cyclopedia of American Medical Biography, Comprising the Lives of Eminent Deceased Physicians and Surgeons from 1610–1910* (1912), *American Medical Biographies* (1920), and a *Dictionary of American Medical Biography* (1928). An individual of many talents and varied tastes, Kelly devoted himself to manifold moral, public, religious, and social interests and during his lifetime contributed nearly $1 million to philanthropic projects. Strongly committed to the tenets of the Roman Catholic Church, Kelly wrote *A Scientific Man and the Bible* in 1925. His religious-oriented civic efforts, including renting a large house at his own expense so that prostitutes could have refuge and care until they were able to find suitable employment and housing, brought him into frequent philosophical conflict with another distinguished

Baltimorean, Henry L. Mencken (1880–1956), writer, editor, and social critic. Kelly also gathered the most extensive private collection of books on mycology in the country and later donated it to the University of Michigan. An authority on snakes, Kelly allowed several to run free in his house and even authored a well-respected monograph, *Snakes of Maryland* (1936). Kelly and his wife of fifty-four years had nine children. The Kellys died less than twelve hours apart. A biography, *Dr. Kelly of Hopkins, Surgeon, Scientist, Christian* was written by Audrey Davis (1959).

Bertha Van Hoosen (1863–1952) was born in Stony Creek, Michigan, and graduated from the University of Michigan with bachelor's (1884) and medical (1888) degrees. She took four years of postgraduate training at the Woman's Hospital in Detroit, the Kalamazoo State Hospital for the Insane, and the New England Hospital for Women and Children in Boston (1888–1892). In 1892 she relocated to Chicago and opened a private obstetrical practice. The following year, Van Hoosen was appointed to the anatomy and embryology faculty of the Northwestern University Woman's Medical School. After holding this position for ten years, she joined the clinical gynecology faculty of Illinois University Medical School (1902–1912). In 1913 Van Hoosen became chief of the gynecological staff at Cook County Hospital, the first time a woman had received this appointment, which was granted on the basis of a competitive civil service exam. Seven years later, she was also named chief of obstetrics. From 1918 to 1937, Van Hoosen was professor and head of obstetrics at the Loyola University Medical School. An outstanding surgeon, Van Hoosen was the first woman to head a medical division at a coeducational university. She traveled extensively and performed surgery in several countries. In 1915 she organized the first national medical women's association. Van Hoosen trained scores of female surgeons, whom she referred to as her "surgical daughters" in lieu of the fact that she was never married. In 1948 she authored an autobiography, *Petticoat Surgeon*.

Thomas James Watkins (1863–1925) was born on a farm near Utica, New York, and attended the University of Michigan School of Medicine from 1880 to 1883 but never finished his degree requirements. He eventually transferred to New York City's Bellevue Hospital Medical College, from which he graduated in 1886. He pursued postgraduate training at the Utica City Hospital, St. Peter's Hospital in Brooklyn, and the Woman's Hospital in New York. At the last institution, Watkins worked with Thomas Emmet and developed an interest in vaginal reconstructive surgery. In 1889, Watkins moved to Chicago and for the next thirty-four years served on the surgical faculty of Northwestern University, where he was subsequently promoted to professor of gynecology (1916). He also held attending gyne-

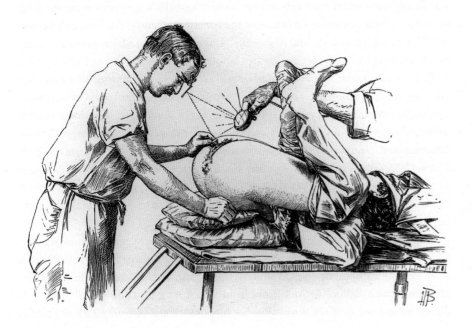

11. When Howard Kelly wrote his two-volume *Operative Gynecology* (1898), his leadership in American gynecology was firmly established. With over 550 original illustrations, including numerous images by Max Brödel, it also helped revolutionize medical illustration. In this drawing, an "examination of the bladder in the dorsal position, with elevated pelvis" is demonstrated. The electric light held close to the symphysis pubis is reflected by the head mirror into the bladder. (*Author's Collection*)

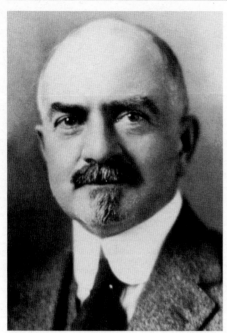

12. Thomas Stephen Cullen. *(Historical Collections, College of Physicians of Philadelphia)*

cologist status at Mercy, St. Luke's, and Wesley Hospitals in Chicago. Watkins is best remembered for his interposition operation, in which he used the uterine fundus as an obturator for the defective anterior pelvic diaphragm and a buttress for the base of the bladder (1899). A founding member of the American College of Surgeons, he was elected president of the American Gynecological Society in 1915. In addition, Watkins was chairman of the American Medical Association's Section on Obstetrics, Gynecology and Abdominal Surgery in 1919.

Thomas Stephen Cullen (1868–1953) was born in Bridgewater, Ontario, Canada, and received his medical degree from the University of Toronto in 1890. He interned for a year at the Toronto General Hospital, during which he had a chance meeting with Howard Kelly. Impressed with Kelly's operative techniques, Cullen relocated to Baltimore and worked for a year in The Johns Hopkins' pathology laboratories of William Welch (1850–1934) and William Councilman (1854–1933). Cullen eventually succeeded in obtaining an appointment as intern at The Johns Hopkins Hospital (1892–1893). Imbued with the enthusiasm of Kelly and other faculty members, Cullen decided to pursue his further training in Baltimore. In the latter part of 1893, Cullen was granted a six-month leave of absence to conduct research at the pathology laboratory of Johannes Orth (1847–1923) in Göttingen, Germany. Upon his return to Maryland, Cullen was placed in charge of gynecologic pathology at The Johns Hopkins Hospital (1893–1896) and was soon appointed instructor in gynecology (1895). In 1896 Cullen finally attained the coveted resident surgeon position under Kelly and was able to complete his residency training. The following year, Cullen entered the private practice of surgery while also being named an associate in Kelly's department. Although he maintained close relations with The Hopkins, Cullen performed most of his early surgical and gynecological work at the Cambridge-Maryland Hospital. In 1908, he became chairman of the Church Home and Infirmary and Episcopal Hospital and was also named gynecologist-in-chief. He established a highly regarded surgical clinic, which became an important teaching center for gynecologic surgery. Upon Kelly's retirement in 1919, Cullen was named professor of clinical gynecology, with the title changed to professor of gynecology in 1932. He remained professor through 1939, when he retired from clinical activites. Cullen was the first to publish on the use of formalin in preparing frozen sections for pathologic evaluation (1895). Two and a half decades later, he described the "blue navel," or Cullen's sign for diagnosis of ruptured ectopic (extrauterine) pregnancy. An irrepressible evangelist when committed to a cause, Cullen stimulated the first public campaign in the United States for the control of cancer, acting as chairman of the American Medical Association's Cancer Campaign committee in 1914. He was firmly convinced that gynecology should remain a specialty separate from obstetrics. Cullen served as chairman of the American Medical Association's Section of Obstetrics, Gynecology, and Abdominal Surgery in 1915 and was president of the Southern Surgical and Gynecological Association in 1916. From 1929 to 1953 Cullen served on the Maryland State Board of Health and, during this time, was also appointed chairman of the Chesapeake Bay Authority Conservation Committee concerning the area's dwindling oyster population. He was a prolific writer, whose textbooks included *Cancer of the Uterus: its Pathology, Symptomatology, Diagnosis and Treatment* (1900), *Adenomyoma of the Uterus* (1908), *Myomata of the Uterus* (1909), and *Embryology, Anatomy, and Diseases of the Umbilicus* (1916). He also authored a biography, *Henry Mills Hurd, the First Superintendent of The Johns Hopkins Hospital* (1920). A full-length biography, *Tom Cullen of Baltimore*, was written by Judith Robinson in 1949.

Eugene Theodore Hinson (1873–1960) was born in Philadelphia and graduated from the Institute for Colored Youth in 1892. He worked as a school teacher from 1892 to 1894 but soon decided to study medicine and matriculated at the University of Pennsylvania School of Medicine, from which he graduated in 1898. He was denied an internship at his alma mater because of race and instead joined the staff at

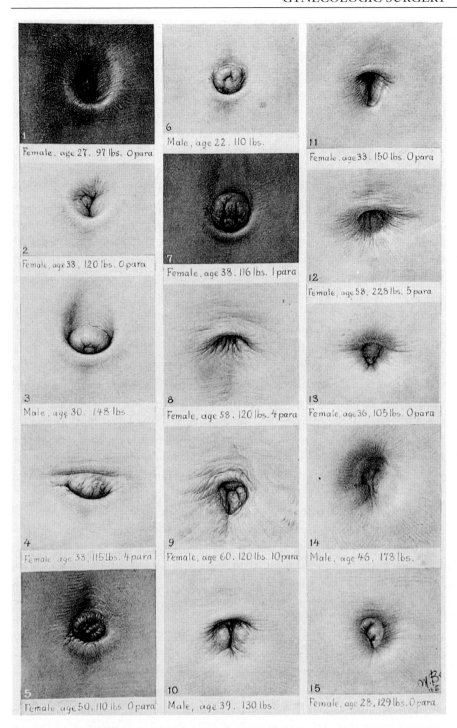

1
Female, age 27. 97 lbs. O para

6
Male, age 22. 110 lbs.

11
Female, age 33. 150 lbs. O para

2
Female, age 33, 120 lbs. O para

7
Female, age 38. 116 lbs. 1 para

12
Female, age 58, 228 lbs. 5 para

3
Male, age 30. 148 lbs

8
Female, age 58. 120 lbs. 4 para

13
Female, age 36, 105 lbs. O para

4
Female, age 33, 115 lbs. 4 para

9
Female, age 60. 120 lbs. 10 para

14
Male, age 46, 178 lbs.

5
Female, age 50, 110 lbs. O para

10
Male, age 39. 130 lbs.

15
Female, age 28, 129 lbs. O para

13. Many textbooks on seemingly obscure and sometimes mundane topics have been authored by American surgeons. Thomas Cullen's massive treatise on "belly buttons" (*Embryology, Anatomy, and Diseases of the Umbilicus*, 1916) must be considered in this grouping. Despite its quirky subject, the work contains extraordinary illustrations by Max Brödel, including a series of truly remarkable variations in belly buttons. (*Historical Collections, College of Physicians of Philadelphia*)

the Frederick Douglass Memorial Hospital in Philadelphia. He remained there until 1905, when he transferred to the newly established Mercy Hospital and served as its chief of gynecology until his retirement in 1955. Hinson was instrumental in founding Mercy, the second oldest institution for African-American physicians in Philadelphia, because he felt that opportunities for personal development should be greater than those offered at Douglass Hospital. Hinson was a highly respected gynecologist and was actively involved in African-American community improvement through his relationships with the National Association for the Advancement of Colored People and other similar organizations. He was also a cofounder, with Henry M. Minton (1870–1946), of Sigma Pi Phi, the first African-American Greek letter fraternity.

Emily Dunning Barringer (1876–1961) was born in Scarsdale, New York, took medical preparatory courses at Cornell University (1894–1897), attended the Medical College of the New York Infirmary (1897–1898), and received her medical

481

degree from Cornell Medical School (1901) after it absorbed students from the New York Infirmary. She completed some postgraduate work in Vienna and, from 1902 to 1904, served as a house officer at Gouverneur Hospital, which was part of New York City's municipal hospital system. Barringer was briefly associated with Mary Putnam Jacobi (1842–1906) but later commenced the private practice of gynecology, with the majority of her clinical activities centered at the New York Infirmary and the Kingston Avenue Hospital. In 1940 she retired from the Kingston facility, having completed twenty-one years of service, much of it as director of gynecology. Barringer remains most remembered for becoming the first woman to win a coveted residency position at Gouverneur, then considered a "feeder" hospital for further postgraduate training at Bellevue. In 1904 she became chief resident at Bellevue, thereby winning recognition as the "first woman ambulance surgeon" in New York City." During World War I she was appointed by New York City's Board of Health to take charge of a large venereal disease service for women in "an effort to safeguard the health of troops embarking overseas." A tireless social reformer, Barringer was active in the National Prison Association and served on the General Medical Advisory Board of the American Social Hygiene Association. During World War II she campaigned tirelessly for the commission of women physicians in the armed services, and she was president of the American Woman's Medical Association in 1941. For several sessions, Barringer was a delegate from the Medical Society of the State of New York to the American Medical Association's House of Delegates. Although never a member of the American Gynecological Society, Barringer was a fellow of the American College of Surgeons. Barringer married Benjamin Barringer, also a physician, in 1905, and raised two children. In 1950 she authored an autobiography, *Bowery to Bellevue, the Story of New York's First Woman Ambulance Surgeon.* Twelve years later, Iris Noble wrote a full-length biography, *First Woman Ambulance Surgeon—Emily Barringer.*

Catharine MacFarlane (1877–1969) was born in Philadelphia and received a "certificate in biology" from the University of Pennsylvania (1895) and a medical diploma from Woman's Medical College of Pennsylvania (1899). She interned at her alma mater and then pursued rather peripatetic residency training at The Johns Hopkins Hospital (gynecological urology), Royal Charité in Berlin (obstetrics), University of Vienna's Frauenklinik (gynecology), and Radium Hemmet in Stockholm (radiology). Once MacFarlane established a practice, all of her career was spent in Philadelphia, where, at her alma mater, she advanced from instructor in obstetrics (1898) to professor of gynecology (1922). In 1940, she was named interim dean of the institution; two years later, appointed research professor of gynecology; and in 1946, became vice president of its Board of Corporators. She also held several staff positions at various hospitals throughout Philadelphia, where she was simultaneously engaged in the private practice of gynecology. MacFarlane was best known for her Cancer Control Research Project, which was a specific cancer-screening effort within the department of gynecology at Woman's Medical College. This project, the first of its kind in Pennsylvania, was designed to detect early signs of uterine cancer. Although it was originally conceived as a five-year study, the screening continued for fifteen years with a permanent facility and detection program being established at the medical school in the mid-1950s. During the study, pelvic examinations were conducted every six months on 1,319 presumably well women who volunteered to participate. In addition to her cancer research, MacFarlane was an active proponent of birth control, appearing on the speaker's platform with Margaret Sanger (1879–1966) at the first Pennsylvania State Conference on Birth Control in 1922. MacFarlane authored numerous articles in the field of obstetrics and gynecology, but her only full-length work was *A Reference Hand-Book of Gynecology for Nurses* (1908). Active in supporting the role of women in the medical profession, she was president of the American Medical Women's Association (1936) and vice-president of the Medical Women's International Association (1937–1947). MacFarlane was the

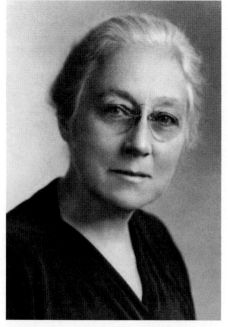

14. Catharine MacFarlane. *(Historical Collections, College of Physicians of Philadelphia)*

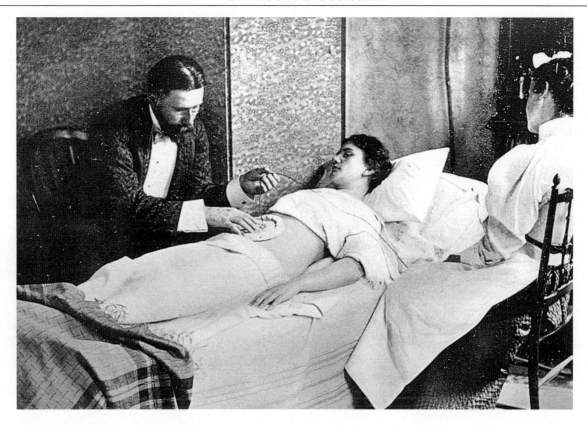

first female member of the College of Physicians of Philadelphia (1932) and the first woman president of the Obstetrical Society of Philadelphia (1943).

William Clarence McNeill (1878–1964), born in Lake Waccamow, North Carolina, graduated from Howard Academy in 1900 and from the Howard University School of Medicine in 1904. For some months following his medical school graduation, he served as an assistant to the secretary-treasurer of his alma mater. From 1905 to 1907, McNeill was an assistant surgeon at Freedmen's Hospital in Washington, D.C. On completing this training, he joined the surgical staff at his alma mater, where he was professor of gynecology from 1910–1943. Following his retirement from Howard's faculty, McNeill pursued private practice in the Washington area through the late 1950s. A respected teacher at Howard for four decades, McNeill developed a reputation for noticing and financially helping many needy Howard medical students. He was an influential figure in the administration of Howard University School of Medicine and served as secretary-treasurer of the institution from 1907 to 1920. He was instrumental in raising money from private sources so that the school could improve its facilities in order to meet the accreditation standards of the American Association of Medical Colleges (1911) and to match General Education Board endowments in the post-World War I period.

Isador Clinton Rubin (1883–1958) was born in Vienna, Austria, and brought to the United States at an early age. He was educated at the College of the City of New York and received a medical diploma from that city's College of Physicians and Surgeons (Columbia) in 1905. Rubin took postgraduate training at Mount Sinai Hospital (1905–1908) and then spent 1909 at the gynecologic pathology laboratory in the University of Vienna. Upon his return to New York City, Rubin was made associate pathologist and adjunct gynecologist at the Beth Israel Hospital, and from 1934 to 1937 he served as director of its gynecologic service. In 1916 he was concurrently appointed to the visiting staff of the Mount Sinai Hospital, where he eventually rose to the rank of attending gynecologist (1937–1945). From 1937 to 1947, Rubin was on the obstetrics and gynecology faculty of his medical alma mater, and he later held similar positions at New York University and New York Medical College. He was elected president of the New York Obstetrical Society in 1928, and

15. Throughout the latter half of the nineteenth century, American physicians sought applications of electricity to their practice. In gynecologic surgery, electrotherapy was used for conditions such as ectopic pregnancy, uterine displacements and fibroids, and even ovarian tumors. Numerous textbooks were written, including John Byrne's (1825–1902) *Clinical Notes on the Electric Cautery in Uterine Surgery* (1873) and Franklin Martin's *Lectures on the Treatment of Fibroid Tumors of the Uterus, Medical, Electrical and Surgical* (1897). Despite its great promise, electrotherapy was never found to have any positive effects, and by the end of the century it had reached its zenith. In this scene Issac Massey (1838–1898) of Philadelphia applies electric stimulators to a patient's abdomen (circa, 1889). *(Courtesy of Stanley B. Burns, M.D., and The Burns Collection and Archive)*

16. Several important statues of American surgeons can be found. Among the most prominent are those of Crawford Long by J. Massey Rhind, in Statuary Hall of the United States Congress, and of Samuel Gross by Alexander Stirling Calder, originally located (1897) on the grounds of the Smithsonian Museum but moved to make way for the Hirshhorn Art Museum and rededicated (1970) at the rear of the Scott Memorial Library at Jefferson Medical College. In New York City, a prominent monument was erected in honor of James Marion Sims and placed in Bryant Park in 1894. Four decades later, the city fathers of Manhattan decided that the statue was not sufficiently important to remain a city landmark. It was consigned to a storage bin, from which influential physicians had to rescue it and have the bronze piece placed in a niche in the Central Park wall on Fifth Avenue at 103rd Street, opposite the New York Academy of Medicine. *(Courtesy of The New York Academy of Medicine)*

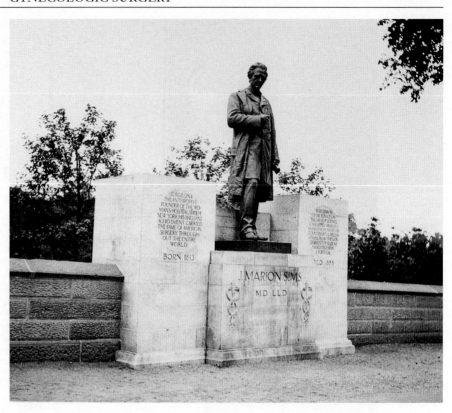

almost three decades later served the American Gynecological Society in a similar capacity (1955). Rubin was also president of the American Association of Obstetricians, Gynecologists and Abdominal Surgeons. One of the first to use x-rays in gynecology, Rubin is eponymically remembered for the introduction of tubal insufflation with a gaseous medium for the diagnosis and treatment of sterility due to occlusion of the fallopian tubes (1920). A founding fellow of the American Board of Obstetrics and Gynecology and the American Academy of Obstetrics, Rubin helped edit numerous journals, including the *International Journal of Fertility*, *Gynécologie Pratique, Excerpta Medica, Fertility and Sterility*, and the *American Journal of Obstetrics and Gynecology*. Among his written efforts are *Symptoms in Gynecology* (1923), *Uterotubal Insufflation* (1947), and the three-volume *Integrated Gynecology* (1956). He died of a myocardial infarction while attending the International Cancer Congress in London.

Peter Marshall Murray (1888–1969), born in Houma, Louisiana, was educated at New Orleans University, now Dillard University (1910), and the Howard University School of Medicine (1914). He served an internship at Freedmen's Hospital in Washington, D.C., and the following year was assistant to the dean and to the professor of surgery at Howard University. Murray took postgraduate study in surgery and gynecology at both the New York Post-Graduate School and Bellevue Hospital. During 1917 and 1918 he was a medical inspector in the public schools of Washington, and from 1918 to 1920 he was appointed surgeon in chief of Freedmen's Hospital. Murray entered the private practice of gynecology in New York City in 1921, but owing to the segregated and racist policies then in existence, he found most hospital staffs closed to him. Sharing office space with Wiley M. Wilson, a Harlem physician, Murray completed the majority of his gynecologic surgery, for about fifteen years, at Wilson's private sanitarium. Murray joined the Harlem Hospital in 1928 as a "provisional assistant adjunct visiting physician in gynecology" and eventually became its director of gynecological services. During these years, Murray was also consulting gynecologist to the Sydenham Hospital, becoming director of the department of obstetrics and gynecology in 1954. In addition, he was on the surgical staffs of St. Clare's Hospital in New York City and the Beth Israel Hospital in Newark, New Jersey. Murray was the first African-American member of the American Medical Association's House of Delegates (1949–1961), and the first African-American president of the Medical Society of the County of New York (1955), a constituent society of the American Medical Association. A long-standing member of the Howard University Board of Trustees (1924–1958), Murray was also president of the National Medical Association (1932) and chairman of its publication committee (1942–1957). Murray was a fellow of the American College of Surgeons and the International College of Surgeons, and the first member of his race to become a certified diplomate of the American Board of Obstetrics and Gynecology (1931). He was a leader in numerous national causes to further African-American improvement, especially health concerns and the relationship of African-American physicians to the profession. In 1958, Murray was appointed to the Board of Hospitals of the City of New York, a nine-member board that directed the city's twenty-nine municipal hospitals.

Joe Vincent Meigs (1892–1963) was born in Lowell, Massachusetts, and graduated from Princeton in 1915 and Harvard Medical School in 1919. He received postgraduate training at the Massachusetts General Hospital while also serving as a full-time assistant to William Graves, professor of gynecology at the Free Hospital for Women in Brookline, Massachusetts. In 1927 Meigs was appointed gynecologist to the Pondville State Cancer Hospital of the Massachusetts Department of Public Health. He subsequently became director of gynecology at the Vincent Memorial Hospital, Massachusetts General Hospital, and Palmer Memorial Hospital. In 1942 he was promoted to clinical professor of gynecology at Harvard Medical School. Meigs served as president of the Society of Pelvic Surgeons, the Boston Surgical Society, and the Boston Obstetrical Society. He authored *Tumors of the Female Pelvic Organs* (1934), edited a volume entitled *Surgical Treatment of Carcinoma of the Cervix* (1954), and coedited *Progress in Gynecology* (1946). He is eponymically remembered for a syndrome involving fibromyoma of the ovary and hydroperitoneum and hydrothorax.

Richard Wesley TeLinde (1894–1989) was born in Waupun, Wisconsin, and educated at the University of Wisconsin (1917) and The Johns Hopkins University School of Medicine (1920). He completed an internship and residency at The Johns Hopkins Hospital (1920–1925) and soon entered the private practice of gynecology. He was named an associate gynecologist at The Hopkins in 1936, and three years later was appointed professor of gynecology and successor to Thomas Cullen. TeLinde remains best known for his classic textbook, *Operative Gynecology* (1946), which was written to fill a void that he perceived in the area of gynecological surgery. So influential was TeLinde's work that it has gone through a total of eight editions, incorporating the further editorial guidance of Richard Mattingly (born 1925), John Rock (born 1927), and John Thompson (born 1927). Considered a pivotal figure in the field of gynecologic education and training, TeLinde received many honors, including the presidency of the American Gynecological Society in 1953.

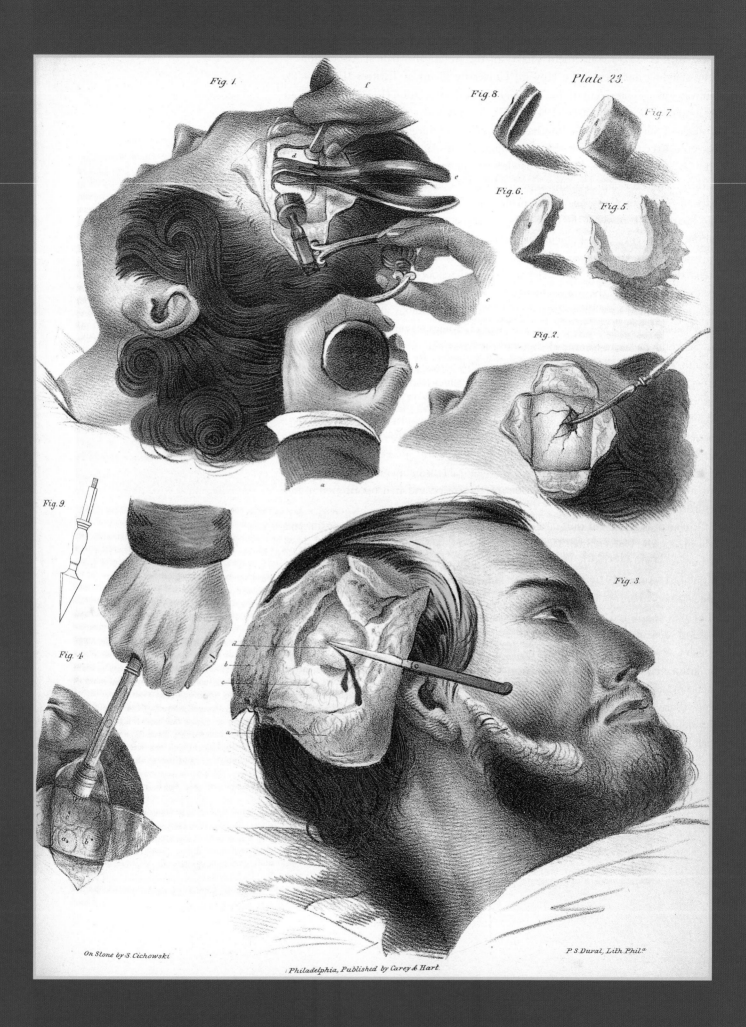

Fig. 1.

Fig. 8.

Plate 23.

Fig. 7.

Fig. 6.

Fig. 5.

Fig. 2.

Fig. 9.

Fig. 3.

Fig. 4.

On Stone by S. Cichowski

P S Duval, Lith. Phila.

Philadelphia, Published by Carey & Hart.

CHAPTER 17

NEUROLOGIC SURGERY

*A*t the end of the nineteenth century, neurologic surgery was primarily performed by a few surgeons who had acquired a special interest in the central nervous system. Among these American pioneers, William W. Keen was the most clinically bold and surgically prominent. Beginning in the late 1880s, he reported numerous cases of cerebral surgery in the *American Journal of the Medical Sciences*. The journal's prestige, combined with Keen's successful removal of various types of brain tumors, helped bring about a burgeoning of more effective neurosurgical care. During these years, Keen also completed studies on tapping the cerebral ventricles (1890) and performed widely hailed neurosurgical operations for torticollis (1891) and tic douloureux (1894).

In 1893, Moses Allen Starr (1854–1932), professor of diseases of the mind and nervous system at New York City's College of Physicians and Surgeons, authored the country's first true neurosurgical textbook, *Brain Surgery*. Starr was not a surgeon, and as was common at the time, the neurologist usually diagnosed the tumor and then directed a surgeon, in Starr's case Charles McBurney, in the conduct of the operation. Other surgeons were also becoming renowned in the field, including James Mears, who first suggested Gasserian ganglionectomy for trigeminal neuralgia in 1884; Robert Weir (1838–1927) for the second (1887) and third (1888) published reports of removal of a brain tumor in the American periodical literature, and Frank Hartley (1856–1913) for his intracranial neurectomy for facial neuralgia (1892).

More than any other single surgical specialty, surgery of the central nervous system in the twentieth century owes its development to the scientific genius of one man, Harvey W. Cushing (1869–1939). He realized the need to develop related sciences such as neuroophthalmology, neuropathology, and neuroradiology while also organizing an extensive training program in neurologic surgery for surgeons who had already acquired basic training in general surgery. With such luminaries as Cushing, Charles Frazier (1870–1936), and Walter Dandy (1886–1946) leading the way, the years 1905–1945 mark the growth of the neurosurgical specialist and neurosurgery as a surgical specialty. Three distinct phases of maturation are recognizable: first, the development of operative and diagnostic skills permitting the neurosurgeon to locate the lesion, reach it, and deal effectively with it without prohibitive mortality; second, the establishment of a classification of tumors excised at operation and the correlation of pathologic specimens with various clinical syndromes; and third, the application of research methods in the basic science laboratory to the study of the human living brain in the operating room.

As the number of neurological surgeons increased, individuals began meeting to discuss their mutual interests. In 1920, Cushing conceived the idea of a society

1. *(facing page)* Joseph Pancoast's 1844 volume *A Treatise on Operative Surgery* contained some of the most outstanding mid-nineteenth-century American surgical illustrations. This patient, without any evidence of pain on his face, undergoes a trepanning, or trephining, of the cranium. *(Author's Collection)*

487

devoted exclusively to the study and improvement of neurologic surgery. The Society of Neurological Surgeons became so successful in helping to advance the subject in the United States that similar groups were formed in other countries. Eleven years later, the Harvey Cushing Society (now the American Association of Neurological Surgeons) was founded, and it soon became the most influential of all national organizations.

With the specialty growing in popularity, and recognizing the need for detailed training and special qualifications for the practice of neurologic surgery, representatives of the Society of Neurological Surgeons and the Harvey Cushing Society held an informal meeting in March 1939. This group was later expanded to include representatives from the Section on Nervous and Mental Diseases of the American Medical Association, the Section on Surgery of the American Medical Association, the American Neurological Association, and the American College of Surgeons. This group decided that a separate board would be formed for certification in neurosurgery. In 1940 the American Board of Neurological Surgery was formally created, following approval by the Advisory Board of Medical Specialties of the American Medical Association. Four years later the *Journal of Neurosurgery* was organized, and it became the specialty's most influential peer-reviewed journal. Its first editor-in-chief was Gilbert Horrax. Recent editors and their years of stewardship are Henry L. Heyl (1965–1974), Henry G. Schwartz (1975–1984), William F. Collins (1985–1989), Thoralf M. Sundt, Jr. (1990–1992), and John A. Jane (1993–??).

The current eligibility requirements for board certification, after a medical degree has been received, include at least one year of clinical skills training (internship) and an additional five years of neurosurgical residency in an approved program. In 1995, of the approximately 621,000 total physicians in active practice, 4,710 (less than 1 percent) designated themselves as neurologic surgeons. Within this cadre of neurologic surgeons, 2,935 (62 percent) were board certified. (By contrast, during the fifteen years between 1980 and 1994, 1,643 certificates in neurologic surgery were issued, or an average of 110 per year.) Of the 1995 total, 175 (4 percent) were women, and 730 (15 percent) were international medical graduates. Among the total pool of neurologic surgeons, approximately 905 (19 percent) were younger than the age of 35; 1,340 (28 percent) were 35 to 44 years old; 1,135 (24 percent) were 45 to 54 years old; 920 (20 percent) were 55 to 64 years old; and 410 (9 percent) were 65 years old and older. Of the 175 female neurologic surgeons, 150 (85 percent) were younger than 44, in contrast to the approximately 4,535 male neurologic surgeons, of whom 2,095 (46 percent) were under 44.

In 1900, Harvey Cushing had just completed his surgical training under William Halsted at The Johns Hopkins Hospital. Cushing, who was born in Cleveland, Ohio, was an 1891 graduate of Yale University and the recipient of a Harvard medical education (1895). After a year as a house officer (1895–1896) at the Massachusetts General Hospital, he decided to relocate to Baltimore. Four stressful years as one of Halsted's residents culminated in a twelve-month study period in Bern, Switzerland, under the auspices of Theodor Kocher (1841–1917). At about this time, Cushing authored his first important clinical paper in the field of neurosurgery. In developing a new method of total extirpation of the Gasserian ganglion for trigeminal neuralgia, Cushing began to advance the development of modern neurosurgical operative techniques. One year later, Charles Frazier, at the suggestion of William Spiller (1863–1940), successfully relieved trigeminal neuralgia by simply dividing the sensory root behind the ganglion (i.e., intracranial trigeminal neurotomy). This procedure eliminated the inherent operative risks of earlier procedures, and Gasserian ganglionectomy was eliminated from the neurosurgeon's repertoire.

As the furor over the surgical treatment of trigeminal neuralgia gradually subsided, a new neurosurgical interest was becoming evident: the development of palliative decompressive procedures for the relief of intracranial pressure. In 1905 Cushing described, in the inaugural volume of *Surgery, Gynecology and Obstetrics*, his

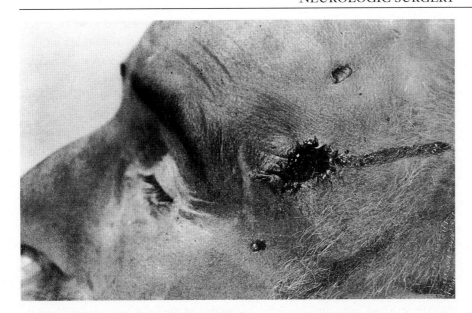

2. Charles Phelps's (1834–1913) *Traumatic Injuries of the Brain and its Membranes, with a Special Study of Pistol-Shot Wounds of the Head in Their Medico-Legal and Surgical Relations* (1897) was one of the country's earliest monographs on a neurosurgical topic. The vast majority of the forty-nine illustrations are clinical photographs of cadavers taken in the coroner's office in New York City. *(Author's Collection)*

technique of subtemporal decompression. By maintaining decompression under the supporting temporal or occipital muscles, Cushing relieved the intracranial tension enough to stop headaches and preserve vision without incurring the unsightly herniation of the brain. One year later, Frazier and Spiller detailed their experience with decompressive procedures in fourteen patients.

After developing satisfactory temporary decompressive procedures, the early neurosurgeons were better able to focus their attention on the problem of directly exposing and resecting brain tumors. Neurosurgery as a specialty would now be able to expand rapidly. Cushing, newly appointed associate professor of surgery at The Johns Hopkins Hospital, addressed this point in a November 1904 speech before the Academy of Medicine at Cleveland. He was adamant that "those whose inclinations follow the branch of neurology must do their own surgery…and not depend on the help supplied by the lukewarm assistance of other departments." The time constraints of a single lecture gave Cushing little opportunity to discuss the many new technical procedures available to the neurosurgeon, including his own innovative use of pneumatic tourniquets to measure blood pressure during the conduct of a craniotomy, and his successful operative interventions in intracranial hemorrhage of the newborn. However, Cushing's next major publication on neurological surgery sounded the keynote to the specialty's development over the following half century.

When William Keen invited Cushing to contribute a section on "surgery of the head" for his multivolume *Surgery: Its Principles and Practice*, he limited him to eighty printed pages. Work on the manuscript occupied the greater part of Cushing's leisure time during the years 1906 and 1907, but in his usual brash and authoritative manner, he delivered a manuscript of almost eight hundred typed pages plus 154 illustrations. Realizing the significance of Cushing's work, Keen agreed to publish essentially all of the content, compressing it into a printed monograph of 273 pages. With its publication in 1908, neurological surgery became recognized almost immediately as a special field of surgical endeavor.

Not only had "Surgery of the Head" succeeded in making brain surgery a recognized specialty, it also brought increased attention to the clinical activities of Cushing, especially his attempts to treat brain tumors. During 1902 and 1903 he had completed a total of just seven operations for intracranial tumors. Five years later, the number had increased to only ten a year, still with a continued prohibitive mortality. Frazier had a similar, albeit larger, experience, but his principal interests in neurosurgery lay elsewhere than with brain tumors. In fact, from 1908 to 1920 Frazier authored no statistical reviews of tumor removal.

For Cushing, the year 1909 proved a renaissance in his clinical approach to cerebral tumors. In January 1910, he published in *Lancet* a report of sixty-four cases of brain tumor seen personally by him during the preceding ten months, in which eighty-four operations had been performed by either George Heuer, his surgical assistant, or himself. Amazingly, one-quarter of the patients had their lesions removed "with restoration of function," while only 10 percent died. In 1911 Cushing authored a paper of great historical significance on technical advances in operative surgery, specifically the use of silver clips in neurosurgery. Four years later he established his preeminence in the surgery of brain tumors by detailing results far superior to those of any of his European contemporaries. Cushing's 1915 paper was a major milestone and signaled a victory in the fierce struggle to overcome the forbidding mortality that had generally attended operations on brain tumors before 1909. Even a decade and a half later, remarkably, Cushing's mortality figures remained exactly the same as those he had reported in 1915: an admirable 8.7 percent.

Concurrently with his study of brain tumors, Cushing began devoting special attention to the pathophysiology of the pituitary gland and the possibilities of surgical treatment for its various disorders. The subject was to absorb a large share of his research activities and culminate in his description of the basophilic adenoma and its pathological correlation with the clinical syndrome with which he is eponymically linked (1932). As early as 1906, Cushing demonstrated interest in the subject by

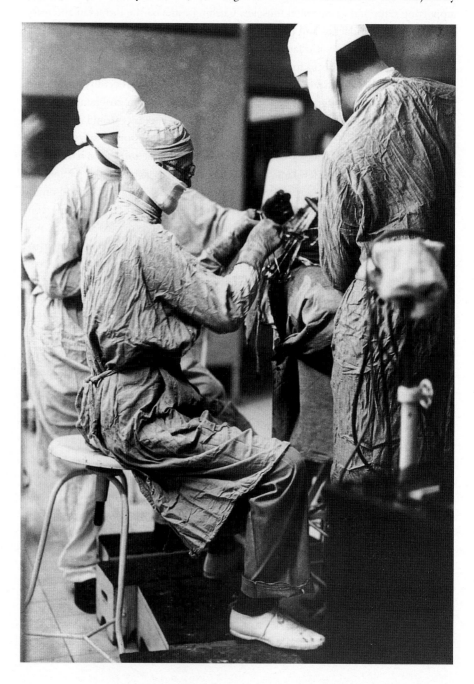

3. Harvey Cushing operating on the 2,000th verified brain tumor in his series, on April 15, 1931. In honor of the occasion, his staff made elaborate preparations for photographs and a movie to be taken. The distinguished photographer Walter W. Boyd took dozens of pictures while Cushing excised a growth of the pituitary body from a woman suffering from "a mild grade of acromegaly associated with bad headaches." *(Yale University, Harvey Cushing/John Hay Whitney Medical Library)*

publishing a paper on "sexual infantilism with optic atrophy in cases of tumor affecting the hypophysis cerebri." In 1910 he authored papers on "the functions of the pituitary body" and "experimental hypophysectomy," and less than twenty-four months after his first operation upon a hypophyseal tumor, Cushing managed to author his now landmark monograph in endocrinology, *The Pituitary Body and its Disorders* (1912). He described his use of a transsphenoidal operation, a surgical approach that led to an operative mortality of less than 10 percent. In what appeared to be an ongoing rivalry concerning all things neurosurgical, Frazier trumpeted an intracranial (transfrontal) technique. Frazier's procedure did not prove successful in the hands of surgeons without special expertise in neurosurgery, and mainly for this reason, Cushing's transsphenoidal procedure became the operation of choice for hypophyseal tumors, evolving into the sophisticated inferior nasal, sublabial operation of Cushing. For approximately two decades (1912–1931), the transsphenoidal approach was the universal method of choice. However, by the time Cushing issued his important monograph *Papers Relating to the Pituitary Body, Hypothalamus, and Para-Sympathetic Nervous System* (1932), he had begun to exclusively use the transfrontal operation.

In the years leading up to World War I, Cushing also developed methods for operating on intracranial tumors of the acoustic nerve. By 1915 he had concentrated on cerebellar pontine angle tumors (tumors of the nervus acusticus), as distinguished from other tumors in the posterior fossa, and two years later he wrote another landmark monograph, *Tumors of the Nervus Acusticus and the Syndrome of the Cerebello-Pontile Angle* (1917). He reported in great detail his results in twenty-nine verified acoustic neurinomas, and once again his demonstrated low operative mortality (11 percent) stood in sharp contrast to that found elsewhere (75 percent) in the world.

In a short two decades, Cushing had single-handedly changed the face of neurosurgery. Although mortality figures for surgical excision of brain tumors, including difficult hypophyseal and cerebellar pontine angle tumors, were stabilized in the area of 10 percent, it would take one more creative Cushing spark to bring neurosurgical techniques into the modern era. In 1928, he and an engineer colleague, William Bovie, introduced electrocoagulation in neurosurgery via the development of "a new surgical-current generator." Affectionately called the "Bovie" by subsequent generations of neurosurgeons and other surgeons alike, electrocoagulation proved a great boon. It speeded the control of bleeding vessels and proved particularly important in the piecemeal removal of meningiomas. As a result of this final technical contribution, the first and basic phase in the evolution of neurosurgical techniques was concluded, earmarked by two of Cushing's textbooks, *Intracranial Tumours* (1932) and *Meningiomas, Their Classification, Regional Behavior, Life History, and Surgical End Results* (1938).

Harvey Cushing was one of the most eclectic personalities in American surgery. His clinical accomplishments are legendary, but just as impressive are his achievements outside the world of medical science. He found time to write the two-volume *Life of Sir William Osler* (1925), for which he was awarded a Pulitzer Prize in 1926. In addition, he authored *Consecratio Medici and Other Papers* (1928), *From a Surgeon's Journal, 1915–1918* (1936), and *The Medical Career and Other Papers* (1940). Cushing was a renowned medical and surgical historian and bibliophile. His extensive collection was bequeathed to Yale University and summarized in *The Harvey Cushing Collection of Books and Manuscripts* (1943). Cushing himself has been the subject of two full-length biographies, *Harvey Cushing, a Biography* written by John Fulton (1983) and *Harvey Cushing, Surgeon, Author, Artist* authored by Elizabeth Thomason (1950). And, in a little-known fact of American surgical arcanum, Cushing's daughter Betsey married James Roosevelt, son of Franklin D. Roosevelt, in June 1930. This union produced two grandchildren before ending in a bitter divorce.

Cushing's overall leadership in the field of American neurosurgery was never seriously challenged, although several individuals proved similarly brilliant in their clin-

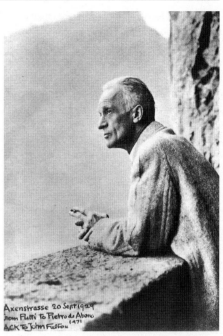

Axenstrasse 20 Sept 1929
from Flüti To Pietro de Abano
ACK To John Fulton (471)

4. While on an extended visit to Europe in September 1929, Cushing was traveling from Italy to Switzerland via the St. Gotthard route and its famed Axenstrasse. There his companion, Arnold Klebs (1870–1943), took this well-known photograph, which was later used as the frontispiece for John Fulton's (1899–1960) masterful *Harvey Cushing, A Biography* (1946). (*Yale University, Harvey Cushing/John Hay Whitney Medical Library*)

5. Among Harvey Cushing's many talents was his artistic ability. This drawing, completed by him in 1906 and first issued in William Keen's multivolume *Surgery, Its Principles and Practice* (1908), demonstrates the exposed motor area of the brain from a patient having focal epilepsy secondary to a bullet wound. In a bit of surgical reverence, the face is that of Cushing's hero, William Osler. *(Yale University, Harvey Cushing/John Hay Whitney Medical Library)*

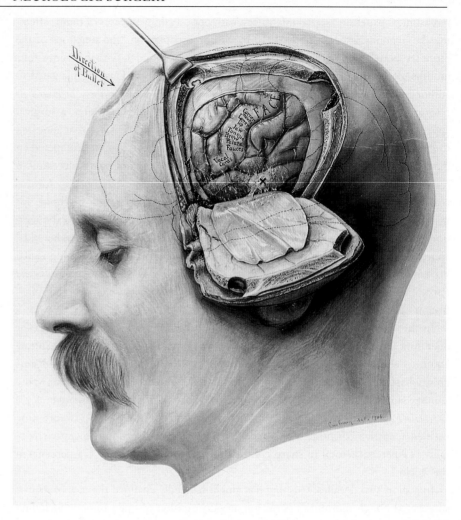

ical contributions. In 1914 Walter Dandy (1886–1946), then on the surgical residency staff at The Johns Hopkins Hospital, experimentally produced hydrocephalus. Four years later Dandy described a method for visualizing the cerebral ventricles by replacing the intraventricular fluid with gas. Thus ventriculography was introduced–a diagnostic process that would have an incalculable effect on the further development of neurosurgery. Writing in the *Annals of Surgery* in 1919, Dandy also detailed how visualization of the ventricles of the brain followed the injection of air into the lumbar subarachnoid sac (i.e., pneumoencephalography). Much of Dandy's inspiration had been based on William Luckett's prior observation of finding air in the ventricles following a fracture of the skull (1913). Dandy's championing of pneumoroentgenology made possible direct surgical attack on a large variety of intracranial tumors that had previously been unlocalizable by any clinical method of examination. Most importantly, it provided a technique for investigating various intracranial conditions other than brain tumors, such as hydrocephalus. Dandy went on to clarify the pathologic difference between obstructive (noncommunicating) and nonobstructive (communicating) hydrocephalus by devising a simple test for differentiating clinically between the two types. In 1918 he described the extirpation of the choroid plexus of the lateral ventricles in communicating hydrocephalus and also developed ventriculostomy for the obstructive type (1922). Additional innovative surgical procedures to treat hydrocephalus were further described by other neurosurgeons throughout the 1930s. However, by the end of the 1940s, the development of plastic tubing, which was less irritating to tissues than ordinary rubber tubing, provided a new class of surgical operations (cerebrospinal fluid shunts) relative to draining obstructed cerebrospinal fluid out of the ventricles or subarachnoid spaces into organ systems or body cavities other than the natural cerebrospinal fluid channels.

From World War I through the end of World War II, enormous accomplishments were made in virtually all fields of neurosurgery. In 1916 Harris Mosher (1867–1942) initiated the modern method of trephining and draining inflammatory processes of the brain. Max Peet (1885–1949), at the University of Michigan, devised a method of resecting the trigeminal nerve, while conserving its motor root, for treatment of trigeminal neuralgia in 1918. James Ayer (1882–1963) introduced cisternal puncture in 1920, and John Hunter (1898–1924) demonstrated the sympathetic innervation of skeletal muscle and, proceeding on this finding, devised the technique of sympathetic ramisection in 1924. The following year, Dandy completed an intracranial section of the sensory root of the trigeminal nerve at the level of the pons for glossopharyngeal neuralgia. Leo Davidoff (1898–1975) described lumbar encephalography in 1932. Two years later, Tracy Putnam reported, in the *New England Journal of Medicine*, a method of treatment of hydrocephalus by endoscopic coagulation of the choroid plexus. Walter Freeman (1895–1972) and James Watts (1904–1990) reported a case of prefrontal lobotomy in agitated depression in 1936, the first such operation in North America. Six years later, the two surgeons authored their classic textbook *Psychosurgery: Intelligence, Emotion, and Social Behavior Following Prefrontal Lobotomy for Mental Disorders* (1942).

As diagnostic capabilities and clinical techniques became more sophisticated, surgery of the spine became an area of heightened interest. Charles Elsberg (1871–1948) was the country's earliest authority on the subject; he wrote *Diagnosis and Treatment of Surgical Diseases of the Spinal Cord and its Membranes* (1916) and followed it a decade later with *Tumors of the Spinal Cord and the Symptoms of Irritation and Compression of the Spinal Cord and Nerve Roots* (1925). A greater awareness of the clinical significance of ruptured intervertebral discs in the lumbar region was provided by William Mixter's 1934 report establishing the clinicopathologic syndrome of the small laterally extruded nucleus pulposus causing typical symptoms of low backache and sciatic pain. Elsberg summed up clinical developments in surgery of the spinal cord when he authored *Surgical Diseases of the Spinal Cord, Membranes, and Nerve Roots* (1941).

When neurosurgeons were queried by members of the research subcommittee of the *Study on Surgical Services for the United States* regarding important surgical contributions from 1945 to 1970, four areas were deemed of first-order importance: corticosteroids and osmotic diuretics for cerebral edema, shunts for hydrocephalus, stereotaxic neurosurgery, and microneurosurgery. Percutaneous cordotomy and dorsal column stimulation for pain were considered of second-order importance, and surgery for aneurysms of the brain of third-order importance.

The history of neurosurgery has been particularly well served by American neurosurgeons. A. Earl Walker (1907–1995) authored his monumental *A History of Neurological Surgery* in 1951. Ernest Sachs (1879–1958) soon followed with *The History and Development of Neurological Surgery* in 1952. That same year, Gilbert Horrax (1887–1957) wrote *Neurosurgery, An Historical Sketch*. Louis Bakay, professor of neurosurgery at the State University of New York at Buffalo, has written *An Early History of Craniotomy: From Antiquity to the Napoleonic Era* (1985) and *Neurosurgeons of the Past* (1987). In 1965, Robert Wilkins edited *Neurosurgical Classics*. The authoritative *A History of Neurosurgery, in its Scientific and Professional Contexts*, under the editorship of Samuel H. Greenblatt, was published by the American Association of Neurological Surgeons in 1997. The following biographical samplings provide a historical glimpse into the lives of several individuals who have contributed to the development of American neurosurgery.

BIOGRAPHIES OF NEUROLOGIC SURGEONS

Charles Harrison Frazier (1870–1936) was born in Philadelphia, graduated from the "college department" of the University of Pennsylvania in 1889 and from its medical school in 1892. Following time as a surgical house officer at his alma mater, Frazier studied for a year in Berlin, Germany. After an early probationary period of

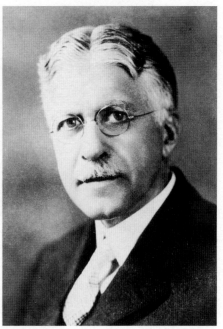

6. Charles Harrison Frazier. *(Historical Collections, College of Physicians of Philadelphia)*

493

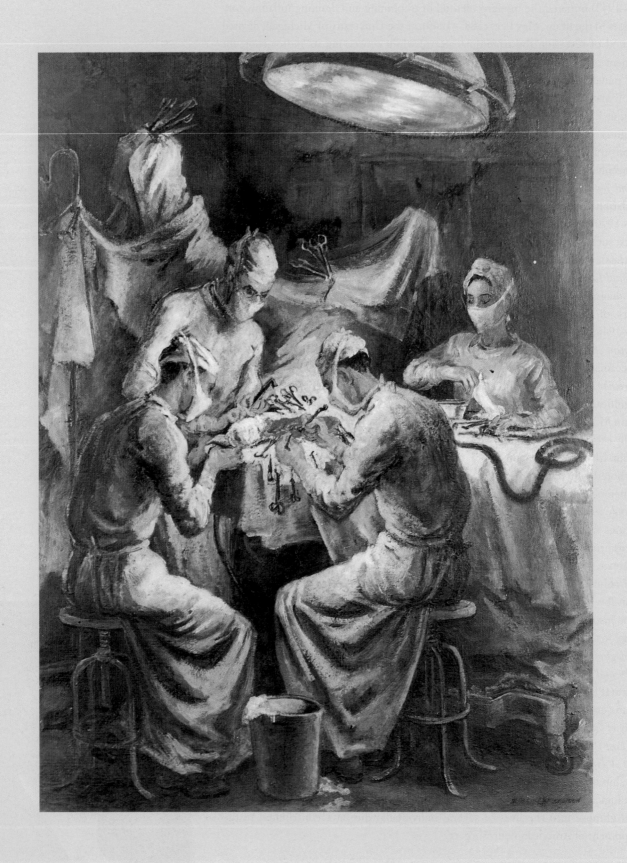

7. "Neurosurgery" by Marion Greenwood
(circa 1944). *(Courtesy of the U.S. Army Center of
Military History)*

service in subordinate positions in surgery at the University, Episcopal, and Philadelphia General Hospitals (1896–1901), he was elected professor of clinical surgery at his alma mater and devoted himself to general surgery during the next decade and a half. Frazier's subsequent professional activities were confined to the University of Pennsylvania, where he also served a ten-year tenure as dean of the medical school. During World War I he was consultant in neurosurgery to the Surgeon-General of the Army and directed a government hospital for the care of neurosurgical patients sent back from France. From about 1918 throughout the remainder of his active clinical work, Frazier devoted himself almost exclusively to the development of neurosurgical techniques and the rise of neurosurgery as a bona fide surgical specialty. As early as 1901, while working with the Philadelphian neurologist William Spiller (1863–1940), Frazier introduced intracranial trigeminal neurotomy for the relief of tic douloureux, using a modification of the techniques of Victor Horsley (1857–1916). As an early pioneer in American neurosurgery, Frazier also accomplished the transfrontal approach to the pituitary region, the development of cordotomy, and extensive experience with peripheral nerve surgery. He was also engaged in many clinical studies that are less widely appreciated: palliative decompressive operations for the treatment of brain tumors, the localization and organization of the human motor cortex, the treatment of spasticity and athetosis by posterior rhizotomy, intracranial division of the auditory nerve for persistent aural vertigo, intradural nerve anastomoses, and observations on the surgical treatment of epilepsy. Frazier is eponymically linked with a metal needle for draining lateral ventricles of the brain, and with subtemporal trigeminal rhizotomy.

Charles Albert Elsberg (1871–1948) graduated from New York City's College of Physicians and Surgeons in 1893. He interned at the Mount Sinai Hospital and then traveled to Germany, where he studied with Johannes von Mikulicz-Radecki (1850–1905). Returning to Mount Sinai, Elsberg was appointed assistant pathologist and later adjunct surgeon. His first paper on neurological surgery concerned two cases of cerebellopontine tumor (1904). Over the next five years he devoted greater amounts of his time to neurological surgery, and by 1910 he had essentially stopped performing general surgical cases. Elsberg introduced Samuel Meltzer's (1851–1920) and John Auer's (1875–1948) method of intratracheal insufflation in the *Annals of Surgery* (1910), thus beginning modern endotracheal anesthesia. In 1913 he authored his first report on laminectomies, and three years later he wrote *Diagnosis and Treatment of Surgical Diseases of the Spinal Cord and its Membranes*. In 1925 he completed *Tumors of the Spinal Cord and the Symptoms of Irritation and Compression of the Spinal Cord and Nerve Roots: Pathology, Symptomatology, Diagnosis, and Treatment*. Elsberg's most influential monograph was *Surgical Diseases of the Spinal Cord, Membranes, and Nerve Roots* (1941). When the Neurological Institute of New York was established in 1909, Elsberg was one of its founding members. He remained clinically active in that institution until his retirement in 1937.

Ernest Sachs (1879–1958) was born in New York City and attended Harvard University (1900) and The Johns Hopkins School of Medicine (1904). He pursued postgraduate education and training at Mount Sinai Hospital in New York City, where he came under the guidance of Arpad Gerster. Sachs remained at Mount Sinai for less than two years, at which time his uncle, the renowned neurologist Bernard Sachs (1858–1944), persuaded him to undertake further specialty training in neurosurgery. Sachs moved to Europe, where he spent three years, most of the time working with Victor Horsley at the National Hospital at Queen Square. Returning to New York City, Sachs was soon asked by Fred Murphy to become a member of the newly organized surgical faculty at Washington University in St. Louis. Shortly after World War I, Sachs was named the institution's first professor of neurological surgery, and he immediately gave up the clinical practice of general surgery entirely. By 1921, Sachs was training "fellows" in neurological surgery, and although he was considered a formidable taskmaster, his neurosurgical residency produced some of the most famous names in American surgery. Upon his retirement from

Washington University in 1945, he was invited to become a member of the surgical faculty at Yale University School of Medicine, where he continued his interest in teaching but did little clinical work. The honors bestowed upon Sachs were numerous. He was a founding member and first secretary of the Society of Neurological Surgeons. Later he became the president of this society, and in 1943 he served as president of the American Neurological Association. When the American Board of Neurological Surgery was established in 1940, Sachs was one of its first members and examiners. A prolific writer, Sachs produced the clinical texts *The Diagnosis and Treatment of Brain Tumors* (1931) and *The Care of the Neurosurgical Patient, Before, During and After Operation* (1945). In addition, he authored *The History and Development of Neurological Surgery* (1952), *Prerequisites of Good Teaching and Other Essays* (1954), and *Fifty Years of Neurosurgery, A Personal Story* (1958).

Howard Christian Naffziger (1884–1961) was born in Nevada City, Nevada, and received his undergraduate and medical education at the University of California. He was a resident in neurosurgery at The Johns Hopkins Hospital, and although he was invited by Cushing to join the staff of the Peter Bent Brigham Hospital, he decided to return to the Far West. There he served as professor of surgery and chief surgeon at the University of California Medical Center from 1929 to 1947, and he was named professor of neurological surgery and head of a separate department of neurological surgery in 1947. Naffziger trained relatively few neurosurgical specialists in the early years of his chairmanship, but he had a profound influence on surgical education in the West and helped increase standards of excellence in the general field of surgery nationally. Among his many honors was being a founding member of the American Board of Surgery and serving as president of the American College of Surgeons (1939), the American Surgical Association (1954), and The Society of Neurological Surgeons. In addition, Naffziger was chairman of the American Board of Neurological Surgery for several terms. He was a major force in the great expansion of the medical schools of the University of California and was an influential regent of the university from the time of his retirement from active clinical practice (1952) until his death.

Max Minor Peet (1885–1949) was born in Detroit and graduated from the University of Michigan in 1908 and its medical school two years later. After a two-year internship in the Rhode Island General Hospital, Peet obtained the Porter Fellowship in Research Medicine at the University of Pennsylvania. From 1913 to 1915 he was assistant instructor in surgery, and from 1914 to 1916, assistant chief surgeon at the Philadelphia General Hospital. While in Philadelphia, Peet spent considerable time working with Charles Frazier, and it was there that his interest in neurosurgery first began. Peet returned to the University of Michigan in 1916 as an instructor in surgery, but within a few years his clinical activities were confined to neurological surgery. In 1918 he reported to the Michigan State Medical Association on resection of the trigeminal nerve with conservation of the motor root for treatment of trigeminal neuralgia. Peet remains best known for his vast operative experience with splanchnicectomy for arterial hypertension. He carried out the initial research during the mid-1930s and went on to complete over two thousand surgical operations for hypertension.

Walter Edward Dandy (1886–1946) was born in Sedalia, Missouri, and received his undergraduate education at the University of Missouri (1907). In 1910 he graduated from The Johns Hopkins School of Medicine and immediately began working in the Hunterian Laboratory under the direction of Harvey Cushing. Dandy became Cushing's clinical assistant in The Johns Hopkins Hospital during 1911–1912, the year preceding Cushing's departure to assume the professorship of surgery at Harvard. Both Cushing and Dandy were high-strung, temperamental individuals, and their personalities clashed on several occasions. Such difficulties would last for the remainder of their professional association and resulted in Cushing's not tendering Dandy an "expected" offer to assume a surgical residency position at the Peter Bent Brigham Hospital. After a year of personal confusion, including work with

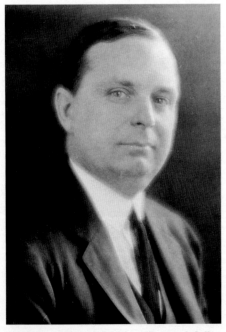

8. Walter Edward Dandy. *(Historical Collections, College of Physicians of Philadelphia)*

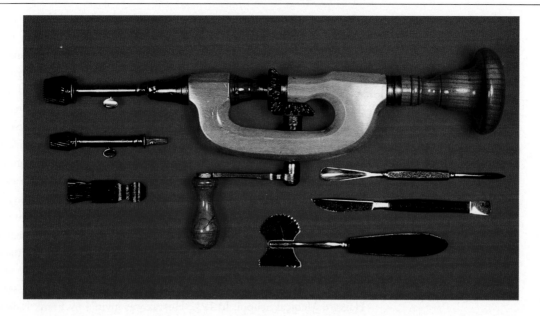

Kenneth Blackfan (1883–1941) in the Hunterian, where the two elucidated the pathophysiology of hydrocephalus and its diagnosis and treatment by surgery, Dandy was finally asked to remain in William Halsted's training program. In 1917–1919, Dandy served as resident surgeon, and during these years he introduced air contrast ventriculography for the diagnosis and localization of brain tumors, often termed the single greatest advance in brain surgery. Dandy also developed pneumoencephalography for using x-rays to visualize the subarachnoid space (1918). In 1922 he devised a procedure for the total removal of tumors of the acoustic nerve, and three years later he introduced surgical procedures for the treatment of painful facial neuralgias. For glossopharyngeal neuralgia, Dandy divided the ninth cranial nerve intracranially in 1928, and at the same time he developed an operation that was highly successful in the treatment of Ménière's disease, an affliction that causes extreme dizziness, nausea, and deafness in one ear. Considered by many authorities to have been the greatest neurosurgeon of his time, Dandy found surgical cures for intracranial aneurysms. He also demonstrated that a ruptured vertebral disc is often the cause of low backache and sciatica, and he devised tests and operations for this ailment. In 1941 he even designed a protective helmet for professional baseball players. Dandy was a stern taskmaster to all who worked with him, including his own resident staff at The Hopkins, where he remained on the surgical staff for his entire professional career, eventually serving as professor of neurosurgery. He was an aloof and moody individual, intensely preoccupied with his clinical and research work, who held few national offices in the growing specialty of neurosurgery. Dandy is eponymically linked with third ventriculostomy, suboccipital trigeminal rhizotomy, and hydrocephalus in infants associated with atresia of the foramen of Magendie. In 1984, William L. Fox authored a biography, *Dandy of Johns Hopkins*.

Alfred Washington Adson (1887–1951) was born in Terril, Iowa, and graduated from the University of Pennsylvania School of Medicine in 1914. Following medical school, he began a three-year surgical fellowship at the Mayo Clinic, where he came under the guidance of not only the Mayo brothers but E. Starr Judd, Walter Sistrunk (1880–1933), and Emil Beckman (1872–1916). After Beckman's untimely death from a cavernous sinus thrombosis secondary to a nasal furuncle, Adson was asked to join the Mayo surgical staff as junior surgeon in January 1917. As part of his responsibilities, Adson was responsible for the care of the few neurosurgical patients who came to the clinic. Like many of the early neurosurgeons, Adson was essentially a self-taught neurosurgical technician. He traveled extensively to visit and observe leading neurosurgeons such as Cushing, Elsberg, and Frazier. From 1917 to 1919 Adson became engrossed in the details of the needs of his patients with neurologic problems. The Section on Neurologic Surgery was established at the Mayo Clinic in 1919, and

9. A surgeon has long been defined by his surgical tools, and the nineteenth-century American physician-surgeon needed to be prepared for any clinical calamity. Particularly difficult to manage were skull fractures and the need for trephination. Consequently, without satisfactory trephining tools, the doctor was essentially helpless. This trepan set (circa 1860s) was hand-manufactured by the firm of Horatio B. Kern in Philadelphia and would have been an integral part of any surgeon's personal equipment. *(Collection of Alex Peck, Antique Scientifica)*

Adson was appointed head of the section. He remained in this position until 1946, when he became senior consultant. Adson was a founding member of the Society of Neurological Surgeons, the American Board of Surgery and the American Board of Psychiatry and Neurology. In addition, he was an influential sponsor of the formation of the American Board of Neurological Surgery and later served as its chairman. Adson was president of the American Society of Neurological Surgeons in 1932.

Gilbert Horrax (1887–1957) was born in Glen Ridge, New Jersey, and graduated from Williams College in 1909 and The Johns Hopkins University School of Medicine in 1913. He served as intern and assistant resident surgeon at the Peter Bent Brigham Hospital under Harvey Cushing. Horrax was named an Arthur Tracey Cabot Fellow at Harvard University and completed his surgical residency at Massachusetts General Hospital. During World War I he joined the staff of Harvard's 5th Base Hospital unit in France. He was chiefly interested in brain and spinal injuries. At the time of discharge he had been promoted to major in the U.S. Army Medical Corps. From 1919 to 1932 Horrax was closely associated with Cushing at the Brigham, where he was appointed assistant professor of surgery at Harvard Medical School. In 1932 Horrax was invited by Frank Lahey to develop a

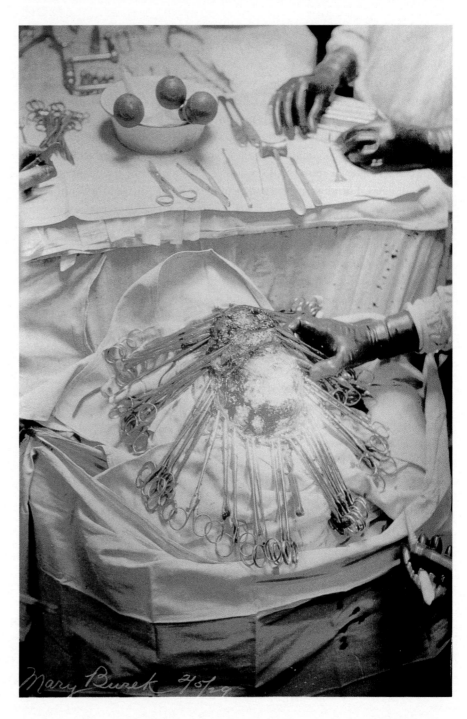

10. There can be no more dramatic example of how vascular the brain is then this operation on a cerebral tumor. Taken at The Johns Hopkins Hospital (circa 1929), this illustration shows the more than fifty blood vessel clamps used to control bleeding. It was about this time that Harvey Cushing and William Bovie first began to utilize electrocoagulation in neurosurgery, a technologic breakthrough that would reduce the number of needed vascular clamps. *(Courtesy of Stanley B. Burns, M.D., and The Burns Collection and Archive)*

498

department of neurosurgery at the Lahey Clinic while he was also serving on the neurosurgical staffs of the New England Baptist and New England Deaconess hospitals. Horrax remained chief of the neurosurgical service at the Lahey Clinic for the remainder of his professional life. Among his many honors were serving as president of the Society of Neurological Surgeons and the Boston Society of Psychiatry and Neurology. Among his written efforts was *Neurosurgery: An Historical Sketch* (1952). Horrax died of cancer of the lung.

Winchell McKendree Craig (1892–1960) was born in Washington Court House, Ohio, and received his undergraduate degree from Ohio Wesleyan University (1915) and his medical education at The Johns Hopkins School of Medicine (1919). He completed internships at the New Haven Hospital in New Haven, Connecticut, and Roosevelt Hospital in New York City, and an abbreviated residency in surgery at Saint Agnes Hospital in Baltimore (1919–1921). From 1921 to 1924 Craig was a fellow in surgery at the Mayo Foundation Graduate School, University of Minnesota. In 1930 he received a master of science degree in surgery. He was formally appointed to the attending surgical staff at the Mayo Clinic in 1926 and eventually transferred to its neurologic surgery faculty, where he remained until retiring in 1957. During World War II Craig was on the surgical staff of the U.S. Naval Hospital in Corona, California (1941–1942), and he later joined the faculty at the National Naval Medical Center in Bethesda, Maryland (1942–1945). In 1946 he was appointed director of the Graduate Training Program of the Bureau of Medicine and Surgery in Washington, D.C., and is believed to be the first civilian physician to attain the rank of rear admiral. Active in all areas of organized medicine, Craig was a field representative to the Council on Medical Education and Hospitals of the American Medical Association (1959) and also served as special assistant for health and medical affairs to Arthur S. Flemming, U.S. Secretary of Health, Education and Welfare (1960). A pioneer in the development of modern neurosurgery, Craig was distinguished for his clinical work on the sympathetic nervous system, the surgical treatment of hypertension, and the classification of tumors of the brain and spinal cord. He greatly improved surgical techniques and apparatus in his field, and introduced the Craig headrest (1953), which was used for many years in ventriculography and other neurosurgical procedures. Among his many honors were serving as president of the Society of Neurological Surgeons (1946), the Harvey Cushing Society (1948), and the Association of Military Surgeons of the United States (1953). Craig was a long-time member of the editorial board of the *Journal of Neurosurgery* (1944–1957).

Eldridge Houston Campbell, Jr. (1901–1956) was born in Alderson, West Virginia, and elected to Phi Beta Kappa at the University of Virginia, where he earned his bachelor of science degree in 1922. After one year of study at the University of Virginia Medical School, Campbell was awarded a Rhodes scholarship, and he attended Balliol College of Oxford University from 1923 to 1925. Returning to the United States, Campbell matriculated at The Johns Hopkins School of Medicine (1927). Following his graduation, he entered the surgical residency program at The Johns Hopkins Hospital, where he spent one year working with Walter Dandy. Completing his surgical training, and in anticipation of assuming a faculty appointment at Albany Hospital in Albany, New York, with responsiblity for neurosurgical cases, Campbell spent an additional three months under Dandy's tutelage. By the end of the 1930s, Campbell's clinical activities were focused almost entirely on neurosurgical diseases. He steadily advanced through the academic ranks, becoming professor of surgery at Albany Medical College (1937) and ultimately head of neurosurgery and chairman of the department of surgery (1946). During World War II, Campbell directed the 33rd General Hospital, which was activated for service in North Africa and Italy. He was discharged in September 1945 with the rank of colonel, having been awarded the Legion of Merit. Campbell was a scholar of history and translated from Latin into English the two-volume *Surgery of Theodoric* (1955–1960).

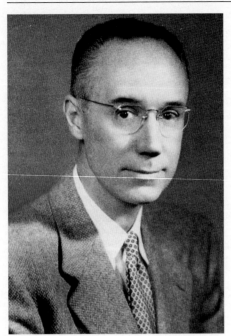

11. James Winston Watts. *(Historical Collections, College of Physicians of Philadelphia)*

Clarence Sumner Greene (1901–1957) was born in Washington, D.C., and attended the University of Pennsylvania for two years (1920–1922), eventually graduating from its school of dentistry in 1926. He completed a year of dental practice in Long Island, New York, but was unsatisfied with his career choice. Greene then matriculated at Harvard College (1927–1929) to obtain premedical course work but returned to the University of Pennsylvania for his final baccalaureate work (1932). Four years later, Greene received his medical diploma from Howard University. He served his internship at Cleveland City Hospital (1937–1939) and surgical residencies at both Douglass Hospital in Philadelphia (1937–1939) and Freedmen's Hospital in Washington, D.C. (1939–1942). From 1942 to 1947, Greene was on the surgical faculty of Howard University Medical School as assistant professor. When the need to establish a department of neurosurgery was evident, Greene was sent to the Montreal Neurological Institute of McGill University, where, working under Wilder Penfield (1891–1976), he completed a two-year residency in neurosurgery (1947–1949). Returning to Howard University, Greene was named chief of the division of neurosurgery (1949–1957) and later chairman of the department of surgery (1955–1957). As the first professor of neurosurgery at Howard, Greene greatly improved the status of neurosurgery at Freedmen's Hospital and helped consolidate undergraduate teaching and residency training in surgery at Howard University Medical School. He was a diplomate of the National Board of Medical Examiners (1938) and the American Board of Surgery (1943), and the first African-American diplomate of the American Board of Neurosurgery (1953). He died of a myocardial infarction.

Cobb Pilcher (1904–1949) was born in Nashville, Tennessee, and graduated from that city's Vanderbilt University in 1924 and its School of Medicine in 1927. He began his postgraduate training at the Peter Bent Brigham under the leadership of Harvey Cushing and remained in Boston until November 1928. At that time, Pilcher returned to Nashville as an assistant resident in medicine at his alma mater (1928–1929). Beginning in July 1929, Pilcher was appointed an assistant resident in surgery and completed his surgical residency in 1932, after which Barney Brooks, chairman of the department of surgery at Vanderbilt, offered Pilcher a full-time faculty position as instructor in surgery. By this time it was increasingly evident that Pilcher had decided on a career in neurosurgery and that he was being groomed to develop a program in neurosurgery at Vanderbilt. Arrangements were made for him to go to the University of Chicago for three months as a special trainee in neuropathology to work under the direction of Percival Bailey, professor of neuropathology (1932). Returning to Vanderbilt, Pilcher began to publish extensively on the subject of neurosurgery, and although his academic career lasted only sixteen years, he managed to gain an international reputation. He served on the editorial boards of the *Archives of Surgery* and the *Quarterly Review of Surgery*. The textbook that he coauthored with Frederic Bancroft (1880–1963), *Surgical Treatment of the Nervous System* (1946), was a leading text among students, trainees, and neurosurgeons. Pilcher was certified by the American Board of Neurological Surgery in 1940, and seven years later was elected president of the Harvey Cushing Society. In 1946 he was appointed president of the Society of University Surgeons. Pilcher unexpectedly died the day after returning from an extended trip throughout Scandinavia and England. Autopsy did not reveal the actual cause of his death, which remains a mystery to this day.

James Winston Watts (1904–1990) was born in Lynchburg, Virginia, and graduated from the Virginia Military Institute and the University of Virginia School of Medicine. He also trained at Massachusetts General Hospital and studied at Yale University and the University of Pennsylvania. Watts served as chief of neurosurgery at George Washington University from 1935 to 1969 and was the chairman of the department of neurology and neurological surgery from 1954 to 1969. Watts was a pioneer in the use of psychosurgery, and he completed the first frontal lobotomy for agitated depression in the United States in 1936 while working with Walter

Freeman (1895–1972), a neurologist on staff at the George Washington University Hospital. By 1950 Watts had performed more than 1,000 lobotomies to treat severe mental and neurological disorders in the absence of alternative approaches. With the development of psychoactive drugs in the mid-1950s to treat ailments that lobotomies were supposed to address, the procedure was phased out as a standard treatment. Watts authored two books with Freeman, the now classic *Psychosurgery: Intelligence, Emotion, and Social Behavior Following Prefrontal Lobotomy for Mental Disorders* (1942) and *Psychosurgery in the Treatment of Mental Disorders and Intractable Pain* (1950).

Arthur Earl Walker (1908–1995) was born in Winnipeg, Manitoba, and graduated from the University of Alberta, where he also received his medical education. After a year of internship in Toronto, he joined the residency training program in neurology and neurosurgery at the University of Chicago. Under the guidance of Percival Bailey, Roy Grinker, and Stephen Polyak, Walker became a leader in the evolving generation of young neurosurgeons who applied the experimental findings of the neurological sciences to clinical neurosurgery. During World War II he served as chief of neurology at Cushing General Hospital in Framingham, Massachusetts, where he became interested in posttraumatic epilepsy. In 1947 Walker was appointed professor of neurological surgery at The Johns Hopkins Hospital, and in his twenty-five-year tenure at that institution, he helped establish a formal division of neurosurgery with its own residency training program. Following his retirement from The Johns Hopkins, Walker moved to Albuquerque as a professor of neurosurgery at the University of New Mexico School of Medicine. Walker authored more than four hundred research papers and wrote eight textbooks, including *Penicillin in Neurology* (1946), *Posttraumatic Epilepsy* (1949), *Transtentorial Herniation* (1962), *Head Injured Men Fifteen Years Later* (1969), *Trigeminal Neuralgia* (1970), *A Manual of Echoencephalography* (1971), and *Cerebral Death* (1977). In 1938, his monograph *The Primate Thalamus* helped explain the function of that area of the brain. Thirteen years later, in collaboration with colleagues and students, he edited *A History of Neurological Surgery*. Walker was one of the few individuals who was president of the American Association of Neurological Surgery, the American Association of Neurology, and the American Electroencephalographic Society, almost at the same time. In addition, he served as president of the American Academy of Neurosurgery and the Society of Neurological Surgeons.

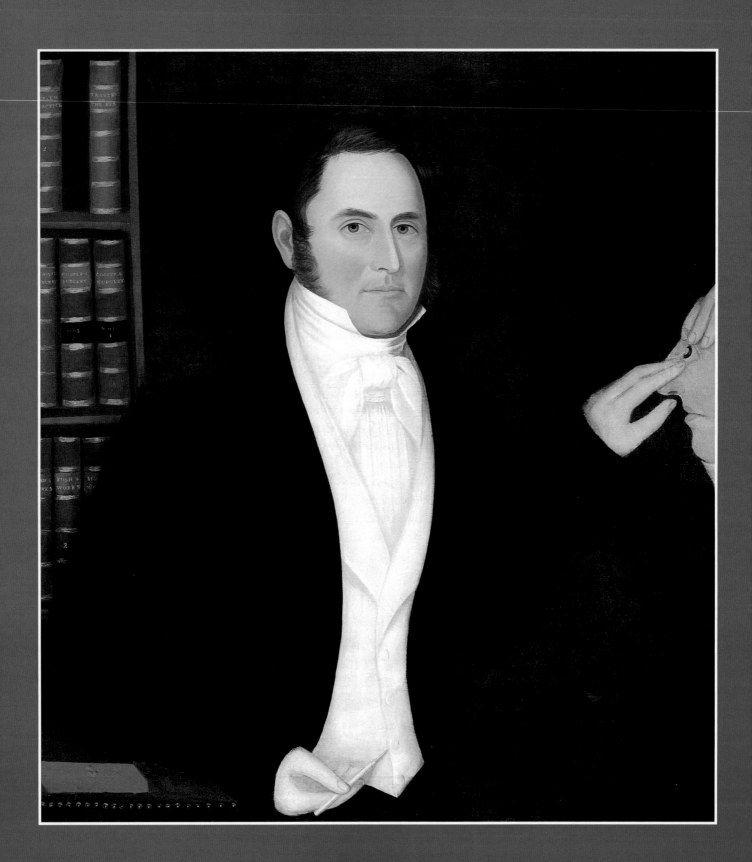

CHAPTER 18

OPHTHALMOLOGIC SURGERY

phthalmology enjoys the longest and most distinguished history of all surgical specialties in the United States, and its evolution can be divided into three broad periods: the first, prior to the mid-1860s, when the American Medical Association first recognized ophthalmology as an area requiring special expertise; the second, from the conclusion of the Civil War to the end of World War I, when national ophthalmologic societies and the concept of ophthalmology as a profession arose; and the third, the 1920s to the present time, with the advancement of modern scientific ophthalmology. Prior to the mid-nineteenth century, there were, strictly speaking, no true American ophthalmologists. Scattered throughout the country, however, were physicians who devoted an unusually large part of their practice to diseases of the eye and could be termed ophthalmologists. Yet, the very fact that in 1805 the Medical and Chirurgical Faculty of Maryland adopted a resolution calling for the granting of "special licenses to dentists and oculists to practice in their respective branches, subjecting them to an examination only on the branches they possess" suggests that in the early nineteenth century "oculists" represented an already recognized branch of medicine.

It is not certain whether these pioneer oculists became such by their own choice or through pressures of the public. However, in 1823, George Frick (1793–1870) authored the country's first textbook on ophthalmology, *A Treatise On the Diseases of the Eye*. It was soon followed by John Gibson's *Condensation of Matter Upon the Anatomy, Surgical Operations and Treatment of Diseases of the Eye* (1832), and Squire Littell's (1803–1866) *A Manual of the Diseases of the Eye* (1837). Numerous pamphlets were also published, primarily on strabismus, by such renowned physicians as John Dix (1813–1884), Alfred Post (1806–1886), James Bolton (1812–1869), and Frank Hamilton (1813–1886). Frick is believed to have been the first American to have generally restricted his practice to diseases of the eye. He received his medical degree from the University of Pennsylvania in 1815 and spent several years in Vienna studying under George Beer (1763–1821). Frick later returned to Baltimore, where he became ophthalmic surgeon at Baltimore General Dispensary, where one of the four patient wards was reserved for his eye cases. By 1840 he had abandoned the practice of ophthalmology, and he spent the remainder of his life in Europe, dying in Dresden. Although Frick's monograph contained little that was original, being largely based on Beer's German textbook *Lehre von den Augenkrankheiten* (1817), a second edition was published in 1826, in London, by an English surgeon, Richard Welbank. Welbank added numerous footnotes and rededicated the work to William Lawrence (1783–1867) but, in recognition of Frick's writing abilities or the summation of Beer's thoughts, left the text essentially unchanged.

1. *(facing page)* "Peter Guernsey, the Eye Doctor." This oil on canvas was painted by Ammi Phillips (circa late 1828). Guernsey (1804–1873) practiced in Dutchess County, New York, where he was well known for his ophthalmologic skills. This portrait is unique among the paintings of early-nineteenth century American physicians in its powerful and graphic expression of Guernsey's occupation, and it is believed to be the earliest portrayal of an American surgeon in the process of examining a patient. Among the volumes occupying Guernsey's bookshelves are the works of Benjamin Rush (1745–1813), Samuel Cooper's (1780–1848) *Practice of Surgery*, Pierre Desault's (1738–1795) *Treatise on Fractures, Luxations, and Other Affections of the Bones*, John Eberle's (1787–1838) *Treatise of the Practice of Medicine* and, most significantly, Benjamin Traver's (1783–1858) *Synopsis of the Diseases of the Eye and Their Treatment* (1825). Phillips was well aware that the placement of fine books in the background appealed to his mostly rural clientele. *(From the Collection of Richard D. Della Penna, M.D., and Mearl A. Naponic, M.D., San Diego, California)*

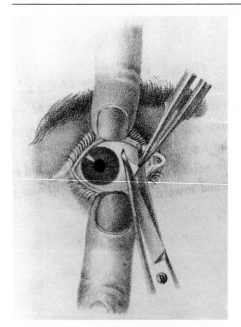

2. In Alfred Post's (1806–1886) *Observations on the Cure of Strabismus* (1841), Nathaniel Currier, of later Currier and Ives fame, served as lithographer for all seven plates, including this "initial stages of an operation to cure strabismus." *(Author's Collection)*

The role of the surgeon in the treatment of eye disease during the first half of the nineteenth century was limited almost exclusively to the cure of cataract, the formation of "artificial pupil," and the evacuation of fluids and foreign matter from the chamber of the eye. Extraction of cataract was an infrequent procedure, performed by only a few skilled men; comminution and depression were the more accepted operations. Occasionally an eye was extirpated for malignancy, but enucleation for other reasons was rarely performed. Despite the lack of a solid cadre of specialists in ophthalmology, by the 1850s a creditable number of special institutions for the treatment of diseases of the eye had been established. Elisha North (1771–1843) opened a private eye infirmary, the country's first, in New London, Connecticut, in 1817 but closed its doors in 1829. The New York Eye Infirmary came into existence in 1820 through the efforts of Edward Delafield (1794–1875) and John Kearny Rodgers (1793–1851). The following year George McClellan (1796–1847) of Philadelphia established the Institution for the Diseases of the Eye and Ear. It was short-lived, lasting no more than three years, and was soon rivaled by the Pennsylvania Infirmary for Diseases of the Eye and Ear (1822). The Infirmary was jointly organized by both prominent citizens and such medical and surgical luminaries as Isaac Hays (1796–1879) and George Wood (1797–1879). It is believed to have remained in existence until the founding in 1830 of the Wills Eye Hospital in 1830. The Wills Hospital physically opened four years later with a staff composed of George Fox (1806–1882), Isaac Hays, Squire Littell, and Isaac Parrish (1811–1852). The Massachusetts Charitable Eye and Ear Infirmary, founded in 1824, is considered to be the country's fifth ophthalmologic institution and had its beginnings through the enterprising work of John Jeffries (1796–1876) and Edward Reynolds (1793–1881).

In the history of ophthalmology in America, several landmark events set the decade of the 1860s apart. In 1863 members of the American Medical Association decided to recognize ophthalmology as an area of special expertise and included it in their Section on Surgery and Anatomy. A decade and a half later, a formal Section on Ophthalmology, Otology, and Laryngology was organized. By 1888 ophthalmology was set apart from the other surgical disciplines and received its own section. In 1864 the American Ophthalmological Society was conceived and organized through the collaborative efforts of Henry D. Noyes (1832–1900) of New York City and Hasket Derby (1835–1914) of Boston. This was a momentous decision, for no specialty medical society existed in the United States before the Civil War, and only one, the Deutsche Ophthalmologische Gesellschaft (1857), preceded it in Europe. Beginning in 1865, papers read at the scientific sessions of the American Ophthalmological Society were informally published in its *Transactions*, but this process was formalized in 1874 when that year's *Transactions* was assigned the title of volume 1. In 1869 the country's first long-lived ophthalmologic periodical not associated with an official body, Jakob Herman Knapp's (1832–1911) *Archives of Ophthalmology and Otology*, was published. However, true honors for publishing the first surgical specialty journal in the United States go to Julius Homberger, who founded *The American Journal of Ophthalmology* in 1862. Unfortunately, the venture folded by its second volume, becoming victim to Homberger's growing mental instability. By 1868 Homberger had been expelled from the American Medical Association for making extravagant claims in published advertisements regarding his supposed ophthalmic skills. The following year he moved to New Orleans and published *Batpaxomyomaxia: A Fight on "Ethics,"* a response to his critics and one of the most bizarre tracts ever written by an American surgeon. Homberger soon became totally insane and died a pauper's death in a Louisiana lunatic asylum.

Specialization in ophthalmology was progressing slowly, but definite advances had occurred. Although few of the physicians on the staffs of the eye infirmaries were true specialists, John Dix of Boston appears to have been the very first to specialize in ophthalmology and otology while working within one of the established ophthalmologic institutions. He paid for an advertisement to this effect in the *Boston Medical and Surgical Journal* about 1840. Elkanah Williams (1822–1888) is given credit for being one of the earliest to limit his practice after settling in Cincinnati in 1855. He was assuredly the first American citizen to hold the title of professor of ophthalmology, receiving such an appointment from the Miami (Ohio) Medical College in 1860. But it was Henry W. Williams (1821–1895) who taught the first organized clinical course in ophthalmology, at Harvard, in 1850. The Williamses were not related, and Henry went on to become the foremost American ophthalmologist of his day and, in 1871, the first professor of ophthalmology at Harvard Medical School.

The last decades of the nineteenth century were marked by a broadening array of clinical ophthalmologic achievements. In 1860 S. Weir Mitchell (1829–1914) experimentally produced cataracts for the first time in a laboratory animal. Six years later Cornelius Rea Agnew (1830–1888), one of the founders of the New York Eye and Ear Hospital, described a new operation for divergent strabismus. That same year, at the third annual meeting of the American Ophthalmological Society, Henry Williams introduced his method for suture of the flap after cataract extraction; he was the first in America to suggest suturing the corneal wound following such an operation. The 1860s ended with Henry Noyes (1832–1900) of New York City investigating the relationship between retinitis and glycosuria. During the early 1870s Edward Loring (1837–1888), an office associate of Cornelius Agnew, gained wide recognition for his continuing work on improving the ophthalmoscope. In 1879 William Thomson (1833–1907), professor of ophthalmology at Jefferson Medical College, described the relationship between astigmatism and chronic headaches. By the early 1880s Jakob Herman Knapp was utilizing cocaine as a local anesthetic in ophthalmologic surgery, specifically for retrobulbar anesthesia. In 1886 John Elmer Weeks (1853–1949) announced, in the *Archives of Ophthalmology*, his discovery of the bacillus that caused acute conjunctival catarrh, or "pink eye." Two years later, George Gould (1848–1922) began to put forth his concept that minute errors of refraction could cause nervous irritation. Speaking before the American Ophthalmological Society in 1893, Knapp demonstrated his "roller-forceps," a small forceps with rollers for blades used to express trachomatous granulations on the palpebral conjunctiva. The century ended with the country's first extensive report (1898) on the use of x-rays in ophthalmologic surgery, authored by William Sweet (1860–1926), a Philadelphia ophthalmologist.

As the specialty of ophthalmology evolved, many textbooks were published. The earliest and most thorough of the mid-nineteenth-century ophthalmologic texts was Henry Williams' 317-page *A Practical Guide to the Study of the Diseases of the Eye; Their Medical and Surgical Treatment* (1862). The next was brought out by Jakob Knapp, who had emigrated in 1868 from Heidelberg, Germany, to New York City, where he established the Ophthalmic and Aural Institute. Within one year's time, he had translated from the German his renowned *Treatise on Intraocular Tumors*. During the early 1870s, nonallopathic physicians began to author ophthalmologic monographs. They included Henry Angell's (1829–1911) *Treatise on Diseases of the Eye; For the Use of General Practitioners* (1870) and Andrew Howe's (1825–1890) *Manual of Eye Surgery* (1874). Angell's *Treatise* was considered, for many years, the standard ophthalmologic text in schools of homeopathy, while Howe was professor of surgery at the Eclectic Medical Institute in Cincinnati. In the middle of the decade, Daniel Bennet St. John Roosa (1838–1908), professor of ophthalmology and otology at the University of the City of New York, and Edward T. Ely (1850–1885), his assistant, authored the well-received *Ophthalmic and Optic Memoranda* (1876), which would go through three more editions. Benjamin Joy Jeffries (1833–1915) wrote *Color-Blindness: Its Dangers and Its Detection* (1879), the first major contribution on the subject by an American surgeon. By the 1880s, a veritable flood of texts was being produced, so much so that more ophthalmologic books were published during the final two decades of the century than in any other medical or surgical specialty. The century concluded with the massive *An American Text-Book of Diseases of the Eye, Ear, Nose and Throat* (1899) by George De Schweinitz (1858–1938), professor of ophthalmology at

Jefferson Medical College, and Burton Randall (1858–1932), clinical professor of diseases of the ear at the University of Pennsylvania.

Despite the presence of the American Ophthalmological Society, its influence was limited by the exclusivity of its total membership, as it was never intended to embrace the broad expanse of practicing ophthalmologists. Instead, the establishment of the American Academy of Ophthalmology and Otolaryngology, whose specific purpose was to bring all ophthalmologists and otolaryngologists into one organization, achieved this goal. It was originally founded in 1896, under the name of the Western Ophthalmologic and Otolaryngologic Society, with Adolf Alt (1851–1920) as its first president, and its name was changed in 1903. The combination of specialties was based on business reasons, not on similarities or overlapping fields: the majority of American ophthalmologists, well into the twentieth century, included otolaryngology in their day-to-day clinical activities. As the meetings of the two combined specialties eventually became too cumbersome, the American Academy of Ophthalmology came into existence in 1978.

At about the turn of the century, questions of adequate training and examinations for ophthalmic specialists were being raised by growing numbers of leaders in American ophthalmology. By the time of World War I, American surgeons had essentially stopped going to Europe for their ophthalmologic education and training. Accordingly, it was deemed necessary to create a quasi-legal authority to judge the qualifications of all practicing American ophthalmologists. Private discussions turned public, and a committee was appointed by the American Ophthalmological Society in 1913 to report on education in the evolving specialty. Chaired by Edward Jackson (1856–1942) of Philadelphia, it found that the United States had fifty-eight specialty hospitals in ophthalmology. Jackson proposed to the Society that any candidate who wished to take a "national" examination to become qualified to practice ophthalmology should have a minimum of one year's preparation in ophthalmologic pathology, refraction, and various other subjects. The following year, another committee was appointed by leaders of the Section on Ophthalmology of the American Medical Association to study the question of forming a national board of ophthalmic examiners. These various initiatives culminated in the formation of a joint committee of the American Academy of Ophthalmology and Otolaryngology, the American Ophthalmological Society, and the Section on Ophthalmology of the American Medical Association, to consider the question of ophthalmic education and certification. Their report in 1915 led to the establishment of the American Board for Ophthalmic Examination in May 1916, the first specialty board to be established in the United States. Following the Academy's annual meeting in Memphis in December 1916, members of the executive committee of the new board examined eleven candidates at the University of Tennessee Medical School. The first certificate, designed by Casey Wood (1856–1920), was awarded to R. S. Lambert. The following year the board was formally incorporated, and its name was officially changed to the American Board of Ophthalmology in 1933.

It was never the purpose of the board to define the requirements for membership in hospital staffs, to gain special recognition or privileges for its diplomates, to state who might or might not practice ophthalmology, or to define the scope of ophthalmic practice. The American Board of Ophthalmology, like all specialty boards, provides candidates with the ability to assess their education and training in relation to their peers. Currently, applicants for board certification in ophthalmology must have completed a postgraduate clinical year in which they have had primary responsibility for patient care in fields such as emergency medicine, family practice, internal medicine, neurology, pediatrics, and surgery. In addition to this single postgraduate year, applicants must have satisfactorily completed an entire formal graduated residency training program in ophthalmology at least thirty-six months long.

In January 1995, of the approximately 621,000 total physicians in active practice, 17,145 (2.8 percent) designated themselves as ophthalmologic surgeons. Within this

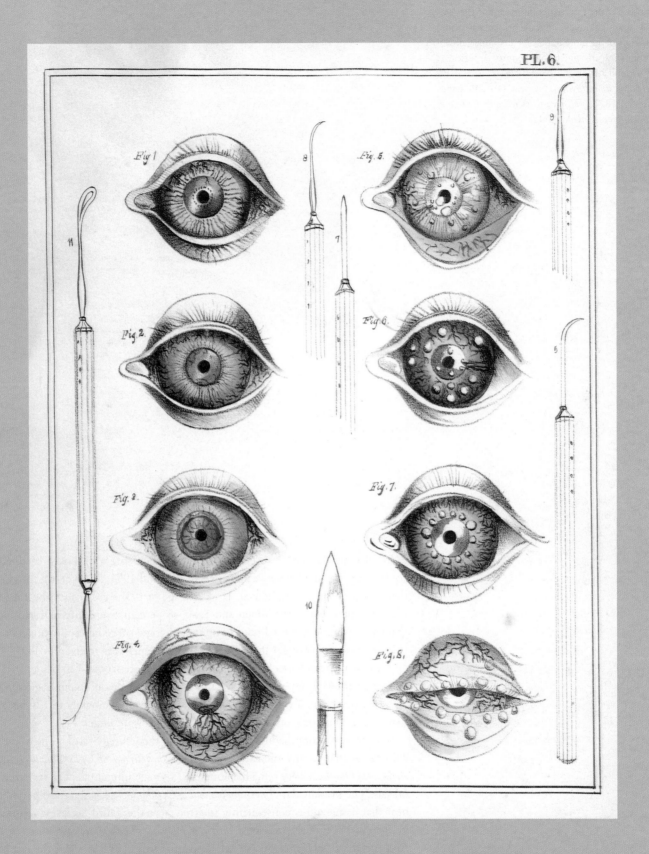

3. Because of its poor arrangement and lack of conciseness, John Mason Gibson's *Condensation of Matter Upon the Anatomy, Surgical Operations and Treatment of Diseases of the Eye* (1832) had little effect on the overall direction of American ophthalmology. Still, it remains the country's first fully illustrated ophthamological textbook, and its hand-colored plates give it a striking appearance. (*Author's Collection*)

4. William Horner's description of a small muscle at the internal commissure of the eye-lids (pars lacrimalis musculi orbicularis ocule) was one of the more important anatomical obser-vations in early nineteenth-century America. It was published in the *Philadelphia Journal of the Medical and Physical Sciences* (vol. 8, pages 70–80, 1824). *(Historical Collections, College of Physicians of Philadelphia)*

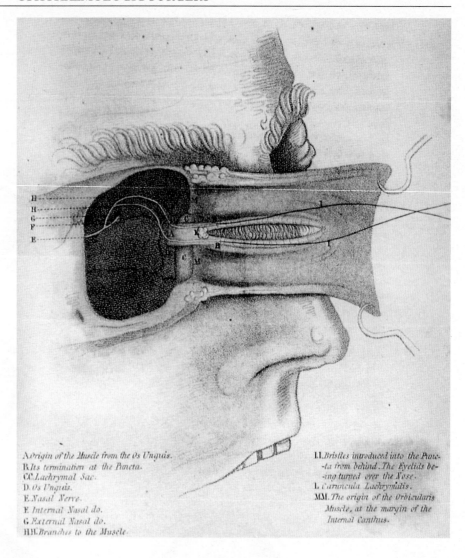

A.*Origin of the Muscle from the Os Unguis.*
B.*Its termination at the Puncta.*
CC.*Lachrymal Sac.*
D.*Os Unguis.*
E.*Nasal Nerve.*
F. *Internal Nasal do.*
G.*External Nasal do.*
HH.*Branches to the Muscle.*

I.I.*Bristles introduced into the Punc--ta from behind. The Eyelids be--ing turned over the Nose.*
L. *Caruncula Lachrymalis.*
MM. *The origin of the Orbicularis Muscle, at the margin of the Internal Canthus.*

cadre of ophthalmologic surgeons, 13,200 (77 percent) were board certified. (By contrast, during the fifteen years between 1980 and 1994, 7,394 certificates in oph-thalmologic surgery were issued, or an average of 493 per year.) Of the 1995 total, 2,025 (12 percent) were women and 1,445 (8 percent) were international medical graduates. Among the total pool of ophthalmologic surgeons, approximately 3,085 (18 percent) were younger than 35; 5,250 (31 percent) were from 35 to 44; 4,430 (26 percent) were from 45 to 54 ; 2,985 (17 percent) were from 55 to 64; and 1,395 (8 percent) were 65 years old and older. Of the 2,025 female ophthalmologic surgeons, 1,590 (79 percent) were under 44, in contrast to the approximately 15,120 male oph-thalmologic surgeons, of whom 6,740 (45 percent) were under 44.

The history of ophthalmologic journalism in the United States is one of the most colorful of that in any specialty. *The American Journal of Ophthalmology* and the *Archives of Ophthalmology* remain among the two most influential peer-reviewed peri-odicals. The present-day *American Journal of Ophthalmology* is the third periodical to bear that name and is consequently referred to as the Third Series. It represents a merger, in 1918, of the previous *American Journal of Ophthalmology* (edited by Adolf Alt), *Annals of Ophthalmology* (six sets of editors from 1891 to 1917, the last having been Meyer Wiener and Clarence Loeb), *Ophthalmic Record* (founded in 1891 by Giles C. Savage [1854–1930] and last edited by Casey Wood), *Ophthalmic Year Book* (organized by Edward Jackson in 1904 and last edited by Jackson, T. B. Schneiderman, and William Zentmayer), *Ophthalmic Literature* (also begun by Jackson and edited by both him and William H. Crisp (1875–1951)), *Ophthalmology* (founded and first published by Harry V. Würdemann in 1904), and *Anales de Oftalmologica* (founded by M. Uribe Troncoso in 1898 and published in Mexico).

Subsequent to the revamping, Edward Jackson emerged as the first editor-in-chief of the new *American Journal of Ophthalmology*. Jackson relinquished his post in 1920 to William Crisp, who remained until 1931. At that time, Lawrence T. Post, professor and head of the eye department at Washington University and Barnes Hospital in St. Louis, assumed editorial control. Derrick T. Vail succeeded Post and went on to serve for twenty-five years, the longest tenure of any editor-in-chief. In 1965 Vail resigned and was followed by Frank W. Newell (1965–1991), Michael Kass (1991–1993), and Bradley R. Straatsma (1994–??).

The *Archives of Ophthalmology* continued to be privately published by the family of Herman J. Knapp for almost a decade and a half after his death in 1911. The American Medical Association assumed administrative control of the periodical in 1928, but editorial decisions remained under the firm guidance of Arnold Knapp (1869–1956), son of the founder, through 1949. With volume 41, Francis H. Adler assumed the editorship, and he was followed by David C. Cogan in 1960. Henry F. Allen, of Boston, took over in 1968 and remained editor through 1975. Since then, the ophthalmologists in charge and their years of service have included Frederick C. Blodi (1976–1983), Morton F. Goldberg (1984–1994), and Daniel M. Albert (1994–??).

As in other surgical specialties, numerous clinical advances have been made in twentieth-century American ophthalmology. Vard H. Hulen (1865–1939) devised a vacuum method of cataract extraction in 1911, and four years later Arnold Knapp reported one hundred successive extractions of "cataract in the capsule after subluxation with the capsule forceps." Alan Woods (1889–1963), of Baltimore, used an intradermal pigment test in sympathetic ophthalmitis (1925). At about the same time (1927), Frederick Verhoeff (1874–1968), in a presentation before the American Ophthalmological Society, described his "buttonhole iridectomy." Five years later, Ramon Castroviejo (1904–1987), while working at the Edward Harkness Eye Institute in New York City, devised a method of keratoplasty. Theodore Terry (1899–1946), of Boston first described retrolental fibroplasia in 1942.

When opthalmological surgeons were queried by members of the research subcommittee of the *Study on Surgical Services for the United States* (1976) regarding important ophthalmologic surgical contributions from 1945 to 1970, photocoagulation and

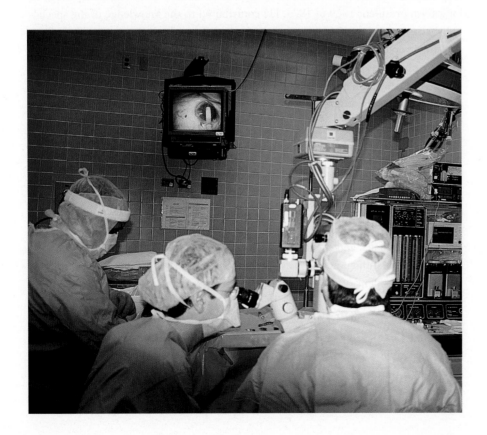

5. Modern cataract surgery requires the aid of a microscope, while minute instrumentation allows micromanipulation inside the eye itself. Through a quarter-inch incision, the ophthalmologic surgeon removes the cloudy lens and replaces it with an artificial device. In most cases no stitches are used, and the patient can return to normal activities in a matter of days. Visualizing the operation on a television screen *(upper left corner)* permits students and residents to better understand the delicate maneuverings. On the monitor can be seen the phacoemulsification device that breaks up and simultaneously removes the faulty lens. *(Courtesy of Stanley B. Burns, M.D., and The Burns Collection and Archive, and with the permission of Stephen Obstbaum, M.D.)*

surgery for retinal detachment and disease were considered to be of first-order importance. Fluorescein fundus angiography, intraocular microsurgery, binocular indirect ophthalmoscopy, and cryoextraction of cataract were deemed of second-order importance, and corneal transplantation and contact lenses were of third-order importance.

The writing of the history of ophthalmology has been well served by numerous American ophthalmologists. Alvin Hubbell (1846–1911) authored *The Development of Ophthalmology in America, 1800 to 1870* (1908), and Wendell Hughes wrote a carefully documented history, *Reconstructive Surgery of the Eyelids* (1943). Recent publications include George Arrington's *A History of Ophthalmology* (1959), Wilbur Rucker's *A History of the Ophthalmoscope* (1971), and George Gorin's impressively detailed *History of Ophthalmology* (1982). The following biographical vignettes provide a brief review of the lives of several individuals who have contributed to the historical development of American ophthalmologic surgery.

BIOGRAPHIES OF OPHTHALMOLOGIC SURGEONS

Henry Willard Williams (1821–1895), born in Boston, attended Boston Latin School and matriculated at Harvard Medical School (1844–1846). He interrupted his medical schooling to study in Europe (1847–1849), where he became interested in ophthalmology while working with Julius Sichel (1802–1868) in Paris, Friedrich Jaeger (1784–1871) and Anton Rosas (1791–1855) in Vienna, and William Lawrence (1783–1867), John Dalrymple (1804–1852), and James Dixon (1814–1896) in London. Returning to the United States, Williams received his Harvard medical degree in 1849. From 1850 to 1855 he was instructor in the theory and practice of medicine in the proprietary Boylston Medical School, and concurrently taught a private class for Harvard medical students interested in eye disease. After a few years of practice, Williams limited himself to ophthalmic work and in 1864 was appointed ophthalmologic surgeon to Boston City Hospital, where he remained for almost three decades. In 1866 Williams was named lecturer in ophthalmology at his alma mater, and five years later, he was promoted to professor of ophthalmology, the first such appointment at Harvard. Williams was a pioneering ophthalmologist, who helped establish the American Ophthalmological Society in 1864 and served as its long-term president 1869 to 1873. He contributed to the knowledge of the specialty by writing on operations for cataract, the use of anesthetic in eye surgery, and the value of atropine instead of mercury as a treatment for iritis. He was among the first in the United States to recognize the clinical value of the ophthalmoscope (invented in 1851 by Hermann von Helmholtz (1821–1894)). Williams was a prolific author, whose popular textbooks include *A Practical Guide to the Study of the Diseases of the Eye: Their Medical and Surgical Treatment* (1862), *Recent Advances in Ophthalmic Science* (1866), *Our Eyes and How to Take Care of Them* (1871), and *The Diagnosis and Treatment of the Diseases of the Eye* (1882). His son, Charles Herbert Williams (1850–1918), became a well-recognized ophthalmologist in his own right.

Elkanah Williams (1822–1888) was born in Lawrence County, Indiana, and received his undergraduate education at Indiana Asbury University (now DePauw), graduating in 1847. He initially studied medicine as an apprentice to Isaac Denson in Bedford, Indiana, and eventually matriculated at the University of Louisville. He came under the influence of Tobias Richardson (1827–1892), a well-known surgeon and future president of the American Medical Association (1878), and received his medical diploma in 1850. The following year, Williams attended an additional course of lectures at the University of Louisville given by Samuel D. Gross. Determined to make diseases of the eye his specialty, Williams practiced in Bedford for two years in order to better his finances and then moved to Europe. With the recent invention of the ophthalmoscope, he was among the first Americans to use the new instrument while studying in Berlin, Paris, and Vienna. Returning to the United States in 1855, Williams settled in Cincinnati, opened a practice devoted

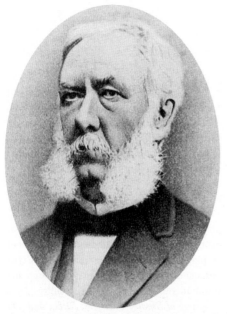

6. Henry Willard Williams. *(Historical Collections, College of Physicians of Philadelphia)*

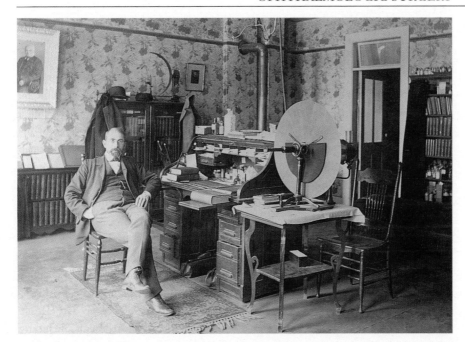

7. A proud ophthalmologist sits among his prized specialized instruments, including visual field devices and perimeters (circa 1905). *(Courtesy of Stanley B. Burns, M.D., and The Burns Collection and Archive)*

solely to ophthalmic conditions, and founded a charitable clinic for eye care at the Miami Medical College. During the Civil War he was an assistant surgeon at the U.S. Marine Hospital in Cincinnati. With the conclusion of hostilities, Williams was appointed professor of ophthalmology at Miami Medical College, the first chair of this specialty in the United States. Among the earliest American physicians to specialize in diseases of the eye, Williams furthered the trend toward ophthalmologic specialization through his effective teaching and operating. Although not a prolific writer, he did serve as editor of the *Lancet and Observer* in Cincinnati (1867–1873). Williams was president of the Ohio Medical Society in 1875 and the International Ophthalmological Congress in New York City in 1876.

Cornelius Rea Agnew (1830–1888) was born in New York City, received his bachelor of arts from Columbia University in 1849, and graduated from that city's College of Physicians and Surgeons in 1852. While attending medical school he also studied with J. Kearney Rogers (1793–1851), who for many years was surgeon to the New York Hospital and the New York Eye and Ear Infirmary. Agnew took postgraduate training as a house surgeon (1852–1854) at the New York Hospital and then moved to the area south of Lake Superior, where he practiced for a year in Houghton, Michigan. In early 1855 he was appointed surgeon to New York Eye and Ear Infirmary and immediately returned to his native city. Aware that he needed further training for his new duties, Agnew traveled to Europe and studied in Dublin, London, and Paris. Returning to America, he was appointed surgeon-general of New York State and medical director of the New York Volunteer Hospital. During the Civil War Agnew was a prominent and vocal member of the U.S. Sanitary Commission. Focusing ever greater amounts of time on diseases of the eye and ear, Agnew established an ophthalmic clinic in the College of Physicians and Surgeons in 1866. Two years later he founded the Brooklyn Eye and Ear Hospital and, in 1869, the Manhattan Eye and Ear Hospital. In the latter year, Agnew was elected to the clinical professorship of diseases of the eye and ear in his alma mater, a position he held until his death. His most important clinical contribution was describing a method of operating for divergent squint in 1866. He remains associated with the Agnew-Verhoeff incision for release of pus in the lacriminal sac in acute phlegmonous dacryocystitis. Among his many honors were the presidencies of the Medical Society of the State of New York (1874) and the American Ophthalmological Society (1874–1878).

Jakob Hermann Knapp (1832–1911) was born in Dauborn, Germany, and received his medical degree from the University of Giessen in 1854. After studying with many of the founders of modern ophthalmology in England, France, and

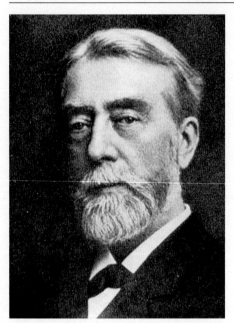

8. Jakob Hermann Knapp. *(Historical Collections, College of Physicians of Philadelphia)*

Germany, Knapp was admitted to the medical faculty at Heidelberg in 1859. Three years later he founded the University Eye and Ear Hospital in Heidelberg, and in 1865 he was named professor of ophthalmology. Despite achieving this position at a relatively early age, Knapp emigrated to America, took up residence in New York City in 1868, and opened the Ophthalmic and Aural Institute. At the same time he established the *Archives of Ophthalmology and Otology*. In 1869 Knapp was elected a member of the American Ophthalmological Society, and within ten years of his arrival in the United States he was appointed the first chairman of the American Medical Association's Section on Ophthalmology. From 1882 to 1888 he served as professor of ophthalmology at the University of the City of New York and then assumed the same position at the College of Physicians and Surgeons (1888–1902). Knapp became particularly influential because he trained many early specialists in ophthalmology in his New York clinic, some of whom went on to become leaders in the specialty. His most important book was *A Treatise on Intraocular Tumors, From Original Observations and Anatomical Investigations* (1869). Although most of his clinical activities centered on ophthalmology, Knapp also devoted time to ear diseases and authored *A Clinical Analysis of the Inflammatory Affections of the Inner Ear* (1871). A remarkably prolific writer, he invented several ophthalmic instruments, including lid forceps, roller forceps used for treating trachoma, a needle-knife for cataract operations, a headrest for the Helmholtz ophthalmoscope, and an individually designed operating chair.

Henry Dewey Noyes (1832–1900), born in New York City, graduated from New York University in 1851 and the College of Physicians and Surgeons in 1855. After serving three years on the resident staff of the New York Hospital, and studying for a year in Europe, Noyes began a private practice in New York City. Specializing in diseases of the eye and ear, he became an assistant ophthalmic surgeon at the New York Eye and Ear Infirmary (1859–1864). In five years he advanced to ophthalmic surgeon, a position he continued to fill until 1900, serving as executive surgeon between 1875 and 1898. From 1868 to 1892 Noyes was professor of ophthalmology and otology at Bellevue Hospital Medical College, and of ophthalmology alone from 1892 to 1900. He was one of the founders of the American Ophthalmological Society and served as its president from 1878 to 1884. Noyes was among the earliest in this country to employ cocaine as a local anesthetic in eye operations, but he is best remembered as the researcher who described the relationship between retinitis and glycosuria. His most prominent written works are *A Treatise on Diseases of the Eye* (1881) and *A Textbook on Diseases of the Eye* (1890).

Daniel Bennett St. John Roosa (1838–1908) was born in Bethel, New York, and attended Yale University but never graduated because of poor health. Instead, he moved home, began to study medicine, and received his degree from the University of the City of New York in 1860. After an internship at New York Hospital, he served for a short time as an assistant surgeon in the Civil War. Roosa spent a year of study in Europe and, returning to New York City, entered private practice devoted to diseases of the eye and ear (1865). A well-respected teacher for almost forty-five years, Roosa served as professor of ophthalmology and otology at his alma mater for eighteen years, and from 1883 to 1908 he taught the same subjects at the New York Post-Graduate Hospital. He was one of the founders of both the Manhattan Eye and Ear Hospital and the Brooklyn Eye and Ear Hospital. Among his many honors were serving as president of the American Otological Society (1874–1876) and being a founding member of the American Neurological Association. Eventually, Roosa limited his practice to ophthalmic diseases, and he served as second chairman of the Section on Ophthalmology of the American Medical Association (1881). He was a prolific author, whose textbooks included *A Vest-Pocket Medical Lexicon* (1865), *A Practical Treatise on the Diseases of the Ear, Including the Anatomy of the Organ* (1873), *Ophthalmic and Optic Memoranda* (1876), *The Determination of the Necessity for Wearing Glasses* (1887), *A Clinical Manual of Diseases of the Eye, Including A Sketch of its Anatomy* (1894), *Defective Eyesight: The Principles of* *its Relief by Glasses* (1899), *Handbook of the Anatomy and Diseases of the Eye and Ear* (1904), and *A Textbook of the Diseases of the Ear, Nose and Pharynx* (1905).

Abner Wellborn Calhoun (1845–1910) was born in Newnan, Georgia, and received most of his early education from private tutors. He initially studied medicine with his father but soon moved North and matriculated at Jefferson Medical College, where he graduated in 1869. Calhoun went into practice with his father, but he desired further training and spent two years in Europe, studying mainly with the Austrian otologist Adam Politzer (1835–1920) while completing additional work in Berlin and London. Returning to the United States, Calhoun settled in Atlanta and became an associate of Willis Westmoreland (1828–1890). Within one year's time (1874), Calhoun was invited to become a member of the faculty of the Atlanta Medical College, where he held the chair of diseases of the eye, ear, and throat. Fifteen years later he was voted president of the new Atlanta College of Physicians and Surgeons, a position he held until his death. Calhoun was one of the few oph-

9. Drawn on stone by J. Queen with P. S. Duval serving as lithographer, this plate from Joseph Pancoast's *Treatise on Operative Surgery* (1844) demonstrates the removal of a cataract. In this particular illustration the operations of depression, or couching, and division and solution are shown. (*Author's Collection*)

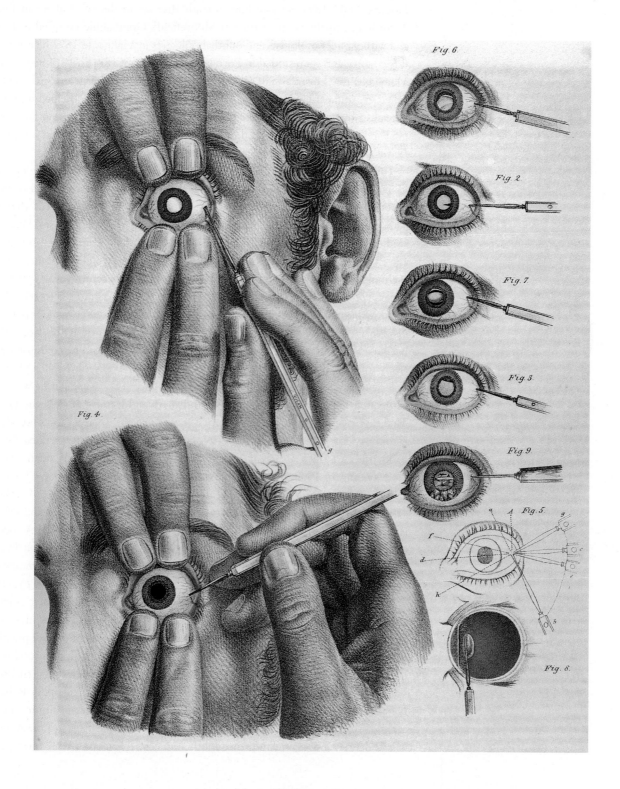

thalmologists practicing in the deep South and, despite not being well published, managed to secure a far-flung clinical reputation. Among his many honors were serving as chairman of the American Medical Association's Section on Ophthalmology (1904) and as president of the Medical Society of Georgia for several terms. At the time of his death, he held the A. W. Calhoun Chair of Ophthalmology, Otology, and Laryngology at the Atlanta College of Physicians and Surgeons and was oculist and aurist to Grady, St. Joseph's, and Wesleyan Memorial Hospitals. His son and grandson, F. Phinizy Calhoun, Sr., and F. Phinizy Calhoun, Jr., both followed in his footsteps, becoming professor and chairman of the Department of Ophthalmology, Emory University School of Medicine, of which the Atlanta College of Physicians and Surgeons was a forerunner.

James Alfred Spalding (1846–1938) was born in Portsmouth, New Hampshire, and graduated from Dartmouth College in 1866 and Harvard Medical School in 1870. Spalding was partially deaf, and while he was at Harvard, Oliver Wendell Holmes (1809–1894) advised him to study diseases of the eye and ear in Europe. Accordingly, Spalding spent time at Moorefield's Ophthalmic Hospital in London and with pioneer otologists and ophthalmologists in Vienna. In 1872 he returned to this country and soon settled in Portland, Maine. From 1881 to 1914 he was on the Maine General Hospital staff as ophthalmologist and aural surgeon. Spalding established eye and ear clinics in Augusta, Bangor, and Portland and helped train young specialists throughout the state. He was a strong advocate for a state eye and ear hospital and an institute for the deaf. He was a prolific writer, whose works included the *Life of Dr. Lyman Spalding* (1917) and *Maine Physicians of 1820* (1929).

John Elmer Weeks (1853–1949), born in Painesville, Ohio, graduated from the University of Michigan School of Medicine in 1881. After a brief trial of private practice, he moved to New York City and began an internship at that city's Almshouse and Workhouse Hospital. Interested in ophthalmic diseases, Weeks also studied under J. Hermann Knapp (1882) at the Ophthalmic and Aural Institute. In 1884 Weeks traveled to Europe, where he resided in Berlin and took courses in ophthalmologic surgery, pathology, and bacteriology. On his return to New York City, Weeks commenced the first course given in bacteriology. From 1885 to 1887, Weeks spent additional time working with Knapp, and during those years he reported the discovery of the bacillus that causes "pink eye," now known as the Koch-Weeks bacillus. Weeks started a private practice in 1887 but did not devote himself exclusively to ophthalmology until a decade later. In 1888 Weeks joined the ophthalmologic staff of the Vanderbilt Clinic in New York City. Two years later he was named surgeon at the New York Eye and Ear Infirmary and lecturer at Bellevue Hospital Medical College, working under Henry Noyes. At the Infirmary, Weeks founded the laboratory for pathology and bacteriology that was subsequently named for him. From 1892 to 1899, Weeks was professor of ophthalmology at Woman's Medical College, and in 1900 he assumed a similar position at Bellevue (later New York University), remaining until he became professor emeritus in 1921. Weeks was actively involved in the politics of organized American ophthalmology and served as chairman of the Section on Ophthalmology of the American Medical Association (1902), president of the American Ophthalmological Society (1921), and chairman of the American Board of Ophthalmology (1923). His textbooks included *Diseases of the Eye, Ear, Throat, and Nose* (1892) and the lengthy *Treatise on Diseases of the Eye* (1910).

Edward Jackson (1856–1942), born in West Goshen, Pennsylvania, graduated from Union College in Schenectady, New York, in 1874 and the University of Pennsylvania School of Medicine in 1878. For six years he was in general practice in West Chester, Pennsylvania, but following a postdiphtheric paralysis involving ocular accommodation, Edward began his lifelong study of ophthalmology. In 1884 he joined the staffs of both the Wills Eye Hospital and the Philadelphia Polyclinic Hospital, advancing to professor of ophthalmology at the latter institution in 1888 and surgeon at Wills two years later. In 1894 Jackson was chairman of the American Medical Association's Section on Ophthalmology. That same year, owing to his wife's illness from tuberculosis, the family moved temporarily to Denver, where they settled permanently in 1898. From 1905 to 1921, Jackson was professor of ophthalmology at the University of Colorado. Few surgeons have ever been so involved with the organization of American ophthalmology as Jackson. In 1903 he was president of the American Academy of Ophthalmology and Otolaryngology, and nine years later he became president of the American Ophthalmological Society. He was the first to organize a postgraduate course in ophthalmology (1912) and, unquestionably, was the principal founder and guiding force behind the establishment of the American Board of Ophthalmic Examinations, serving as its first chairman (1914–1919). For many years he served as a director of the National Society for the Prevention of Blindness. Jackson's principal clinical achievements included descriptions of skiascopy (retinoscopy) (1895) and the practical application of the principles of cross-cylinders to the measurement of astigmatic errors (1893–1907). An influential writer and editor, he founded *Colorado Medicine* (1903), *Ophthalmic Year Book* (1904–1917), *and Ophthalmic Literature* (1911–1917) and was first editor-in-chief of the *American Journal of Ophthalmology* (1918–1928). Among Jackson's textbooks are *Essentials of Refraction and the Diseases of the Eye, and Essentials of Diseases of the Nose and Throat* (1890), *Skiascopy and its Practical Application to the Study of Refraction* (1895), and *A Manual of the Diagnosis and Treatment of the Diseases of the Eye* (1900).

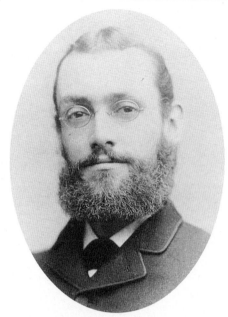

10. Edward Jackson. *(Historical Collections, College of Physicians of Philadelphia)*

Casey Albert Wood (1856–1942) was born in Wellington, Ontario, Canada, and educated at the Ottawa Collegiate Institute (1874) and the University of Bishop's College in Montreal, from which he received his medical diploma in 1877. For a few years following graduation, Wood practiced medicine in Montreal while serving as professor of pathology and chemistry at his medical alma mater and as attending physician at Western Hospital. In 1886 he took further training at the New York Eye and Ear Infirmary and Post-Graduate School, and for two years (1888–1889) he studied in Berlin, Paris, Vienna, and the Royal London Ophthalmic Hospital (Moorfields). Returning to the United States in 1890, Wood set up practice and worked on the staffs of several Chicago hospitals, including Cook County, Alexian Brothers, and Passavant Memorial. From 1890 to 1899 he was professor of clinical ophthalmology at the Chicago Post-Graduate Medical School, and from 1899 to 1906 was in a similar position at the University of Illinois. In 1906 Wood moved his clinical practice to Northwestern University as professor of clinical ophthalmology. He remained until 1908, when he reentered private practice, but from 1913 to 1917 he was once again professor of clinical ophthalmology at the University of Illinois. During World War I he served in the U.S. Army Medical Corps in hospitals in Ohio and Washington, D.C., where he trained workers in dealing with blind soldiers. An indefatigable worker, Wood edited the *Annals of Ophthalmology* (1896–1898) and the *Ophthalmic Record* (1897–1918) and, in 1918, was appointed to the editorial board of the *Annals of Medical History*. Among his honors were serving as chairman of the Ophthalmology Section of the American Medical Association (1898) and as president of the American Academy of Ophthalmology and Otolaryngology. An influential and popular teacher and a prominent practitioner, Wood authored numerous articles in ophthalmologic journals and wrote several well-received textbooks: *Lessons in the Diagnosis and Treatment of Eye Diseases* (1891), *The Eye, Ear, Nose and Throat Yearbook* (1902), *The Common Diseases of the Eye; How to Detect Them and How to Treat Them* (1904), *A System of Ophthalmic Therapeutics* (1909), the two-volume *A System of Ophthalmic Operations* (1911), and the eighteen-volume *American Encyclopedia and Dictionary of Ophthalmology* (1913–1921). The last twenty years of his life were devoted to ornithology and book collecting and led to his authoring *The Fundus Oculi of Birds, Especially as Viewed by the Ophthalmoscope* (1917) and *An Introduction to the Literature of Vertebrate Zoology* (1931).

Carl Koller (1857–1944) was born in Bohemia and received his medical degree from the University of Vienna in 1882. He completed an internship at Vienna's Allgemeines Krankenhaus (1883–1884), and after serving in the Medical Corps of the Austrian Army, he studied with the Leyden-based Hermann Snellen

(1834–1908). Koller was appointed as assistant at the Utrecht Eye Hospital in Holland (1885–1887) and in 1887–1888 lived in London. While an intern at the Allgemeines Krankenhaus 1884 he demonstrated the value of cocaine as a local anesthetic in ophthalmic surgery, thus inaugurating the era of local anesthesia for operations in all branches of surgery. For various personal and political reasons, Koller emigrated to the United States in 1888, where he excelled as a surgeon and ophthalmologist in private practice. Most of his professional life was spent on staff at the Mount Sinai Hospital in New York City and as consulting ophthalmic surgeon to Montefiore Hospital and the Hebrew Orphan Asylum. Although little involved in the world of organized ophthalmologic surgery, Koller was awarded the first Howe Medal in 1922 from the American Ophthalmological Society.

George Edmund De Schweinitz (1858–1938), born in Philadelphia, graduated from Moravian College in 1876 and the University of Pennsylvania School of Medicine in 1881. He took an internship at Children's and University of Pennsylvania Hospitals (1881–1883), and soon began to practice medicine in Philadelphia. His future medical career was determined when he was appointed assistant to William F. Norris (1839–1901), professor of ophthalmology at the University of Pennsylvania, in 1885. De Schweinitz served as a quizmaster in therapeutics at the Medical Institute of Philadelphia (1882–1887) but began to specialize exclusively in ophthalmology after 1887. He was appointed to the ophthalmology faculty at Philadelphia General Hospital in 1887 and was soon named clinical professor of ophthalmology at Jefferson Medical College. By 1896 he was full professor, a position he retained until 1902. In the latter year, De Schweinitz succeeded Norris at the University of Pennsylvania, and he continued in this post for twenty-two years. De Schweinitz had an impressive curriculum vitae, including terms as chairman of the American Medical Association's Section on Ophthalmology (1896) and as president of the College of Physicians of Philadelphia (1910–1913), the American Ophthalmological Society (1916), the American Medical Association (1922), and the International Congress of Ophthalmology held in Washington, D.C. (1922). During World War I he served in the U.S. Army Medical Reserve Corps, in charge of ophthalmology for the Surgeon General's Office, and was founder and director of the army's school of ophthalmology. A leading American authority on ophthalmology, De Schweinitz advanced knowledge of toxic amblyopias, the pathogenesis of iridocyclitis, the mechanism of papilledema, the effect of intraocular injections of antiseptic substances, and pathology of the eye. He wrote prolifically and included among his textbooks *Diseases of the Eye* (1892), which went through ten editions and was among the most respected ophthalmologic textbooks of its era, *The Toxic Amblyopias: Their Classification, History, Symptoms, Pathology, and Treatment* (1896), *An American Text-Book of Diseases of the Eye, Ear, Nose and Throat* (1899), and *Pulsating Exophthalmos* (1908). De Schweinitz had few hobbies and interests outside of ophthalmology and was never married.

Alexander Duane (1858–1926) was born in Malone, New York, graduated from Union College in Schenectady, New York (1878), and received his medical education at the College of Physicians and Surgeons in New York City (1881). After completing a short internship, he practiced general medicine until 1887. At that time, Duane became associated with George T. Stevens (1832–1921), an ophthalmologist based in New York City. In 1888 Duane moved to Norfolk, Virginia, but stayed only two years and returned to New York City to take postgraduate instruction at J. Hermann Knapp's Ophthalmic and Aural Institute. In 1894 Duane became an assistant in Knapp's office, and this began a professional association that lasted many years. Duane's only formal teaching appointment was a brief one at Cornell Medical School, although he always remained active in postgraduate teaching. A member of the American Board of Ophthalmic Examination, Duane served for two years (1915–1917) but was never certified. He was chairman of the American Medical Association's Section on Ophthalmology (1917) and president of the American

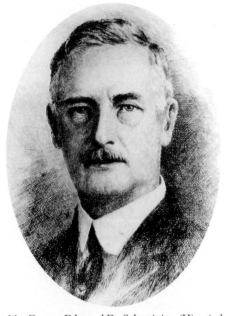

11. George Edmund De Schweinitz. *(Historical Collections, College of Physicians of Philadelphia)*

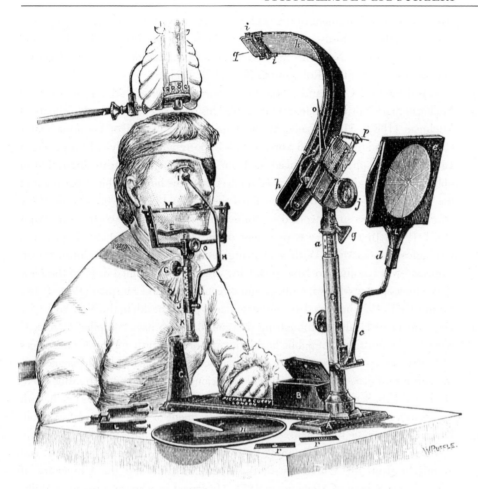

12. In William Norris's (1839–1901) and Charles Oliver's (1853–1911) *Textbook of Ophthalmology* (1893), the proper positioning of a patient to determine field of vision, utilizing a McHardy perimeter, is demonstrated. (*Author's Collection*)

Ophthalmological Society (1923). Duane was a reasonably prolific writer, whose most important monograph was *A New Classification of the Motor Anomalies of the Eye Based Upon Physiological Principles, Together with Their Symptoms, Diagnosis, and Treatment* (1897). He also authored the *Student's Dictionary of Medicine and the Allied Sciences* (1893). During World War I he served as a signal officer on the U.S.S. *Granite State*, where he trained details of men in signaling and quartermaster work. His interest in this subject was connected with his earlier writing of *Rules for Signalling on Land and Sea* (1899), which was used for many years as a textbook in the naval militia.

Harold Gifford (1858–1929), born in Milwaukee, Wisconsin, graduated from Cornell University in 1879 and the University of Michigan School of Medicine in 1882. The major portion of his postgraduate study was in Europe, where he studied in Erlangen and Heidelberg, Germany; Vienna, Austria; and Zurich, Switzerland. Returning to the United States, Gifford settled in Omaha, where he joined the faculty at Omaha Medical College. From 1890–1898 he was lecturer in bacteriology and during the same years was professor of clinical ophthalmology and otology. Gifford was also dean of the faculty (1895–1898) and later professor of ophthalmology and otology (1898–1902). Beginning in 1902, he became associated with the University of Nebraska College of Medicine as associate dean and professor of ophthalmology and otology (1902–1911). In 1911 Gifford was promoted to professor of ophthalmology and otology, and from 1919 to 1925 he was chairman of the department of ophthalmology. Although Gifford did not become a member of the American Ophthalmological Society until 1946, he was a well-respected ophthalmologist and did early research on sympathetic ophthalmia and drainage of the anterior chamber. He was the first to note that organisms in the normal conjunctival sac may become pathogenic when carried into the eye by trauma or operation. Gifford was the first to give a description in English of acute conjunctivitis caused by pneumococcus

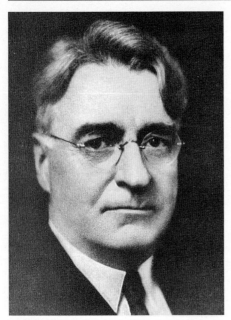

13. Royal Samuel Copeland. *(Historical Collections, College of Physicians of Philadelphia)*

(1896) and the involvement of the ocular conjunctiva with *Sporothrix*. Although not a prolific author, Gifford served as editor of the *Ophthalmic Record* (1897–1915) and was president of the Nebraska State Medical Society. His son was the well-known ophthalmologist Sanford Robinson Gifford (1892–1945).

Royal Samuel Copeland (1868–1938), born near Dexter, Michigan, attended Michigan State Normal College and received his medical education at University of Michigan (1889). He interned at the homeopathic branch of his alma mater (1889–1890) and then pursued a brief course of postgraduate study in Europe. From 1890 to 1895, Copeland practiced medicine in Bay City, Michigan. Interested in ophthalmology and otology, he joined the faculty of the homeopathic department of the University of Michigan and remained there from 1895 to 1908. During those years, Copeland became involved in politics and was elected mayor of Ann Arbor (1901–1903). In 1904 he was president of the American Ophthalmological and Otological Association. With a growing reputation as an able administrator, Copeland was recruited to New York City, where he was named dean of the New York Homeopathic Medical College and director of Flower Hospital (1908–1918). From 1918 to 1922 he served as commissioner of public health in the New York City Department of Health. Although he was considered to have compiled a "mixed" record as commissioner of public health (he fought vigorously for lower milk prices and increased medical treatment for drug addicts, but subjected his department to the corrupt influence of Tammany Hall politicians), he gained enough influence to be elected U.S. Senator from New York. He served from 1922 until his death, with his greatest senatorial achievment being the enactment of the Copeland-Lea Food, Drug, and Cosmetic Bill (1938).

Edward Coleman Ellett (1869–1947) was born in Memphis, Tennessee, and graduated from the University of the South in 1888 and the University of Pennsylvania School of Medicine in 1891. He served as a house surgeon at Wills' Eye Hospital (1891–1893) and then returned to his native city, where he began the private practice of ophthalmology. From 1906 to 1911, he was professor of ophthalmology at the Memphis College of Physicians and Surgeons. Ellett transferred his position to the University of Tennessee College of Medicine, where he remained chairman of the department of ophthalmology until 1922. During World War I he served as a lieutenant colonel in the U.S. Army Medical Corps and commanded a base hospital in France. From 1926 until his death, he was chief of staff at the Memphis Eye, Ear, Nose and Throat Hospital. Ellett was internationally respected as an ophthalmologist, and introduced into the United States such innovations in cataract surgery as the corneoscleral stitch and intracapsular extraction of the cataract. He was closely involved with the formation of the American Board of Ophthalmology (1916), conducting the board's first examinations in Memphis for specialty certification and serving as chairman five times. Among his many honors were the chairmanship of the American Medical Association's Section on Ophthalmology (1914) and the presidencies of the American Academy of Ophthalmology and Otolaryngology (1926) and the American Ophthalmological Association (1932). Although not known as a prolific writer, Ellett managed to exercise great influence on the development of ophthalmology, especially in the South.

Alan Churchill Woods (1889–1963), a native of Baltimore, was the son of Hiram Woods (1857–1931), president of the American Ophthalmological Society in 1920. Alan Woods earned both his bachelor's (1910) and medical (1914) degrees from The Johns Hopkins University, and then pursued an internship at Peter Bent Brigham Hospital. In late 1915 Woods was appointed a fellow in research medicine at the University of Pennsylvania, and shortly thereafter he became an assistant to George de Schweinitz. During World War I Woods was a captain in the U.S. Army Medical Corps, serving in France, and was later transferred to the British Expeditionary Force. Returning to Baltimore in 1919, he joined his father in practice and was appointed instructor in ophthalmology at The Johns Hopkins Hospital. When the

Wilmer Institute was established in 1925, Woods was named associate professor and assistant director under William Wilmer (1863–1936). Nine years later Wilmer retired, and Woods succeeded him as director of the Institute and ophthalmologist-in-chief of The Johns Hopkins Hospital. In 1946 Woods became full professor and retained this rank until his retirement in 1955. Influential both nationally and internationally, he was president of the American Academy of Ophthalmology and Otolaryngology (1947) and the American Ophthalmological Society (1956). During World War II Woods was a civilian consultant to the Surgeon General and served as chairman of the Committee on Ophthalmology of the National Research Council. A prolific contributor to the periodical literature, Woods also authored three textbooks: *Allergy and Immunity in Ophthalmology* (1933), *Endogenous Uveitis* (1956), and *Endogenous Inflammations of the Uveal Tract* (1961).

Sanford Robinson Gifford (1892–1945), son of Harold Gifford, was born in Omaha, Nebraska, and received his education at Cornell University (1913) and the University of Nebraska College of Medicine (1918). During World War I he was in charge of the army's bacteriology laboratory in Base Hospital No. 49 in Allery, France. Following his discharge, and having completed an internship at the Nebraska Lutheran Hospital, Gifford joined his father in practice late in 1919. Seeking further training in ophthalmology, in 1923, Gifford studied in eye clinics and laboratories in Tübingen, Germany; Vienna, Austria; and the Royal Ophthalmic Hospital (Moorfields). Returning to Omaha, he rejoined his father in ophthalmology practice but in 1929 was appointed professor of ophthalmology and chairman of the department of ophthalmology at Northwestern University in Chicago. He also joined the ophthalmologic staffs at Passavant Memorial, Wesley, and Cook County Hospitals. Gifford, a well-known investigator, demonstrated how ocular diseases could be produced by certain bacteria and fungi, and reported the probable etiologic agent of agricultural conjunctivitis, which was then unknown. A respected writer, he was an associate editor of the *Archives of Ophthalmology* during the late 1920s and 1930s and the author of two important monographs, *A Handbook of Ocular Therapeutics* (1932) and *A Textbook of Ophthalmology* (1938). Gifford served as first vice president of the American Academy of Ophthalmology and Otolaryngology in 1943.

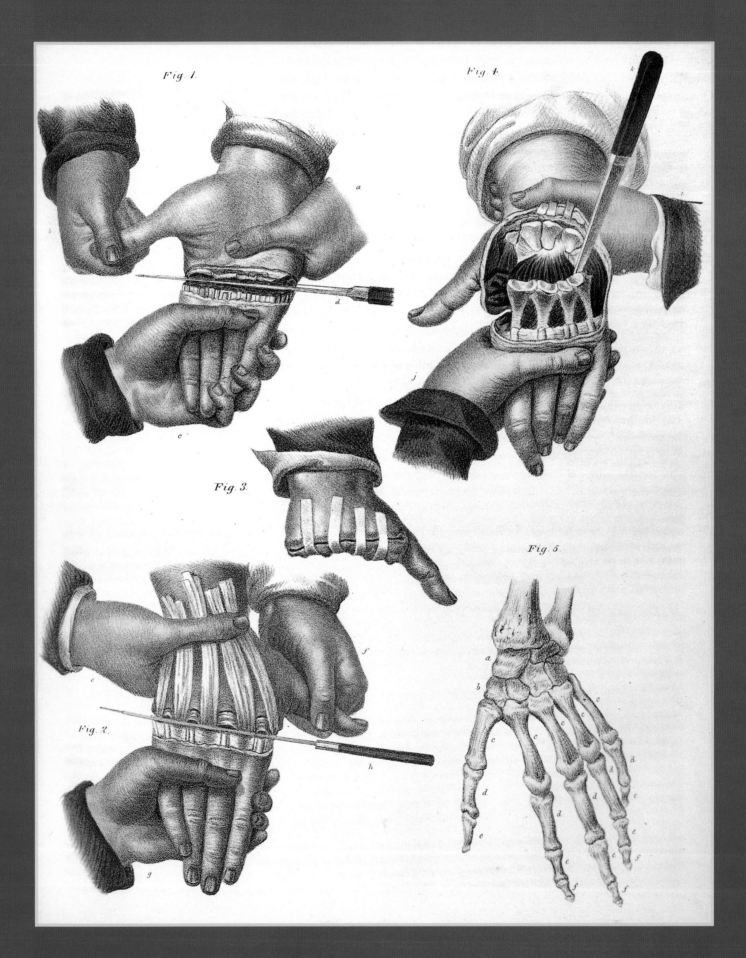

CHAPTER 19

ORTHOPEDIC SURGERY

O f all the surgical specialties in the United States, modern orthopedic surgery has extended its clinical territory most broadly against the backdrop of what previously constituted a general surgeon's clinical activities. When first perceived as a true specialty at the last turn of the century, orthopedics was primarily concerned with congenital bone deformities, particularly the special care of musculoskeletal deformities in children. This is evidenced by the semantic fact that the term *orthopaedy* is derived from two Greek words: *orthos*, straight, and *paidion*, child. Kyphosis, scoliosis, hip joint disease, and bony anomalies, long the cause of overwhelming human suffering, noticeably affected the young, usually as a result of extrapulmonary tuberculosis, osteomyelitis, and other untreatable infections.

Such surgery on bones, joints, and muscles was a direct outgrowth of the widespread use of amputation and the treatment of dislocations and fractures, particularly prominent in nineteenth-century America. Writing in 1876, Samuel D. Gross noted, "Few subjects have been more closely or more thoroughly studied in this country than amputations," "In excision of the bones and joints no country has a better record than ours," "In the treatment of fractures of the long bones, we are, it may fairly be assumed, decidedly in advance of every other nation," and "The reduction of dislocations has been greatly simplified...chiefly through the genius and influence of American surgeons."

Since the time of Gross, orthopedic surgery has absorbed, from the whole of surgery, the management of dislocations and fractures. In addition, orthopedic surgeons have begun to dominate the practice of surgery of the hand, including infection of the extremities and tendon injuries. Such growth is highlighted by the undeniable evolutionary fact that orthopedic surgery has become a surgical specialty unto itself. As various fields of surgery evolved, many surgical specialists continued to work in close collaboration with nonsurgical specialists interested in similar groups of diseases. Pertinent examples include general surgeons and gastroenterologists, pediatric surgeons and pediatricians, cardiac surgeons and cardiologists, neurologic surgeons and neurologists, and urologic surgeons and nephrologists.

In contradistinction are those fields of surgery (i.e., gynecology, ophthalmology, and otorhinolaryngology) that have essentially assumed total therapeutic control of their patients, there being no parallel nonsurgical specialty. However, of all the surgical fields forced to develop free-standing clinical responsibilities, thereby covering a large swath of nonoperative as well as operative care, none exceeded orthopedic surgery in scope and ultimate monetary benefits. Other than the medical specialties of rheumatology and physical rehabilitation and the slowly emerging adjunctive field of sports medicine, the treatment of musculoskeletal disorders has no nonsurgical counterpart in the United States.

1. *(facing page)* "Amputations of the metacarpus" as found in Joseph Pancoast's *A Treatise on Operative Surgery* (1844). *(Author's Collection)*

Unlike other surgical specialties, orthopedic surgery pushed toward formal recognition as a specialty quite early in American surgical history. By the mid-nineteenth century, specialized orthopedic institutions had been established in Boston and New York City. American orthopedic surgery, as a specialized discipline, was less bound to general surgery by years of traditions than were other specialties, and it was quite free to develop independently. Competition, rather than dominance, contributed to its ultimately successful evolution.

Although American orthopedics is said to have begun as a specialized branch of medicine when John Ball Brown (1784–1862) of Boston first opened the Orthopedique Infirmary in 1838, "natural" bonesetters had been present in the colonies for almost two hundred years. In an era when qualified physicians were few, "bonesetters" were individuals who, through innate talent and astute observation of men and animals, had learned the elementary anatomy of muscles and bones and were willing to venture an attempt at repairing common orthopedic emergencies. A bonesetter differed from a cultist or sectarian practitioner in that the craft was entirely empirical. "Natural" bonesetters made no effort to elaborate a theory in order to support or justify their practice. Manipulation was applied directly to the limb or joint, and no other systemic effects were expected.

The bonesetting skill descended in families, passing from father to son and an occasional daughter, much in the manner of other skilled trades. Bonesetters considered their craft to be a natural gift, and they evolved a rich history throughout most of Europe, where they were called *rabouteurs* in France, *Knocheneinrichter* in Germany, *concia-ossi* in Italy, and *algebrista* in Spain. They were also active in the British Isles and their North American colonies, where a considerable element of awe and mysticism surrounded the peculiar talents of these men and women. The most colorful American counterpart of the "natural" bonesetters was the Sweet family of Rhode Island.

The first Sweet in the colonies believed to practice bonesetting was Benoni Sweet (1663–1751), who lived in what is now North Kingston, Rhode Island. Although little is known about the extent of his practice and that of his descendants, they were said to be carrying on a family tradition that had been originally practiced in Wales. By the early part of the nineteenth century, the Sweets' reputation extended up and down the East Coast, so that patients and their families would travel at any time of the year to Rhode Island to have their orthopedic injuries attended to. It has even been stated that Aaron Burr (1756–1836) sent for a member of the Sweet clan to care for his daughter, Theodosia, in New York City. Their familial skill at bonesetting, without any formal medical or surgical training, was remarkable. For over two centuries, members of the Sweet clan treated open and closed fractures, dislocations, and ankylosed joints as well as sprains, bruises, and lacerations. The Sweets remained blacksmiths, farmers, fishermen, laborers, and mechanics, eventually settling throughout New England. Waterman Sweet became particularly successful and, in 1833, went against the family's oral tradition and authored the seventy-five-page *Essay On the Science of Bone-Setting*. Eleven years later he published a sequel, *Views of Anatomy; and Practice of Natural Bonesetting; by a Mechanical Process, Different From all Book Knowledge*. These little appreciated and now rare works, in which various manipulations and the use of emollients, poultices, and other local applications are discussed, represent some of the earliest orthopedic texts published in this country.

The necessity for the Sweets' services began to decrease as more reliable orthopedic innovations from European centers appeared in the United States. In addition, American surgeons were providing technical advances in their own right. Nathan Smith wrote a classic account of osteomyelitis and showed how to trephine for bone necrosis in 1827. Jacob Randolph (1796–1848), son-in-law of Philip Syng Physick, described his father-in-law's method of treating morbus coxarius (hip joint disease) in the *American Journal of the Medical Sciences* in 1830. John Ball Brown popularized tenotomies for clubfeet in 1839. Six years later, Gurdon Buck (1807–1877) per-

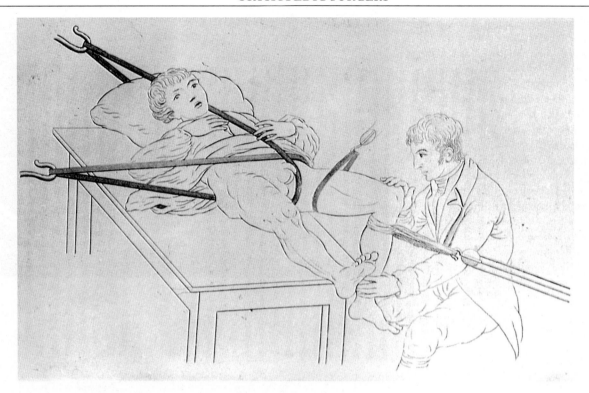

formed one of the more spectacular orthopedic feats by an American surgeon in the first half of the nineteenth century: he treated a kneejoint ankylosed at a right angle and restored it to a nearly straight position by excising a wedge-shaped portion of bone, consisting of the patella, the condyles, and the articular surface of the tibia. Lewis Sayre (1820–1900) resected a hip for ankylosis in 1855.

With regard to fractures and dislocations, the first scientific paper on an orthopedic topic to appear in an American periodical was Physick's case of fracture of the humerus, in which he introduced the use of a seton in the treatment of nonunited fractures (1804). In 1821 John Rhea Barton (1794–1871) detailed "bending" fractures in children. Six years later, John Kearney Rodgers (1793–1851) successfuly wired a previously nonunited fracture of the humerus. Barton described a fracture of the lower articular extremity of the radius in 1838. Working in Buffalo, William Reid (1799–1866) demonstrated the futility of attempting to reduce a dorsal dislocation of the hip by forcible longitudinal traction with pulleys (1852). Instead, the reduction was completed without manipulation At about the same time, Daniel Brainard (1812–1866) developed a special bone drill, or "perforator," which could be introduced subcutaneously to perforate bone ends, thereby simulating a recent fracture and thus stimulating callus formation in nonunited fractures (1854).

Amputations and bony excisions and resections were a class of surgical operations that engaged the technical ingenuity of nineteenth-century American surgeons. Valentine Mott (1785–1865) resected the entire half of a mandible for osteosarcoma in 1822. Two years later, David Rogers (1799–1877) reported on his 1810 excision of most of an upper jaw. Nathan Smith (1762–1829) was the first American to amputate the knee joint (1825). In what has been liberally termed the first successful arthroplasty, Barton perfomed a femoral osteotomy between the greater and lesser trochanters to secure motion in an ankylosed hip (1827). That same year, Mott described the first reported amputation at the hip joint in the country's periodical literature and also provided an account of a successful removal of a left clavicle. In 1852 Henry Bigelow (1818–1890) completed the first excision of the hip joint in America.

Although orthopedics was not yet an organized surgical specialty, several prominent textbooks concerning musculoskeletal diseases had been published by the 1870s. As early as 1830, Samuel D. Gross had written *The Anatomy, Physiology, and*

2. Philip Syng Physick's method of mechanical countertraction to reduce a dislocated femur. This is the earliest report in the American medical literature to describe its use (*Philadelphia Medical Museum*, vol. 1, pages 428–430, 1805) and involves a soft flannel placed between the straps and skin to avoid excoriation. (*Historical Collections, College of Physicians of Philadelphia*)

3. As in all surgical eras, apparati of various importance abounded. The major claim to fame of George Jarvis (1795–1875) was the development of his "surgical adjuster" for fractures and dislocations. It is rare that such complicated medical machinery remains extant after 150 years, but a disassembled Jarvis device *(top)* and a fully employed one as found in Frank Hamilton's *Practical Treatise on Fractures and Dislocations* (1860) *(bottom)* are noted. Jarvis was a superb surgical salesman, although Hamilton noted that he wished the device "would never again be impressed into the service of broken legs" but has often "been used with success in dislocations of the hip as well as in dislocation of the shoulder." *(top: Collection of Alex Peck, Antique Scientifica) (bottom: Author's Collection)*

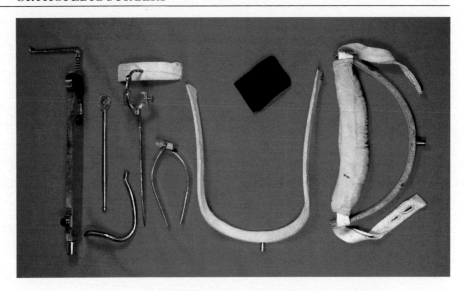

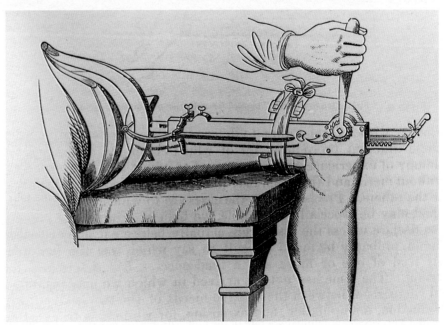

Diseases of the Bones and Joints, the country's first treatise on orthopedics. Three decades later, Frank Hamilton (1813–1889) authored his influential *A Practical Treatise on Fractures and Dislocations*, the first textbook by an American to deal with fractures in depth. During the Civil War, Louis Bauer (1814–1898), founder of the Orthopaedic Institution of Brooklyn (1854), the first orthopedic hospital in the New York City area, gave a series of lectures on orthopedic subjects at the Brooklyn Surgical and Medical Institute. In 1862 these lectures were published in the *Philadelphia Medical and Surgical Reporter*, and two years later they were put in book form: *Lectures on Orthopedic Surgery*. Considered the first true American textbook on orthopedic surgery, the work was also influential on an international level, as it was translated into German, Italian, and Swedish. After the Civil War, George Otis (1830–1881) reported on military orthopedic trauma care with two monographs on amputation at the hip joint (1867) and excision of the head of the femur for gunshot injury (1869).

Two of the country's most prestigious orthopedic hospitals were founded during the 1860s in New York City. Whereas Brown's and Bauer's facilities were privately managed, two institutions were maintained by self-perpetuating boards of trustees: the New York Orthopaedic Dispensary, established by Charles Fayette Taylor (1827–1899), and the Hospital for the Ruptured and Crippled, founded by James Knight (1810–1887). (The latter is presently known as the Hospital for Special Surgery; hernia was included in its original moniker because the orthopedic brace maker also made trusses.) These two institutions became important in the evolution of American orthopedics because, along with the Massachusetts General Hospital, the Hospital of the University of Pennsylvania, and the Jefferson Medical School, they became principal training grounds for the succeeding generation of orthopedic surgeons.

During the 1870s, increasing numbers of textbooks oriented toward orthopedics began to flood the literary marketplace from not only allopathic practitioners but also sectarian surgeons. Andrew Howe (1825–1892), professor of anatomy at the Eclectic Medical Institute of Cincinnati, authored his *Practical and Systematic Treatise on Fractures and Dislocations* (1870), and Edward Franklin (1822–1885), professor of surgery at the Homeopathic Medical College of Missouri, published *The Homoeopathic Treatment of Spinal Curvatures According to the New Principle* (1878). Lewis Sayre (1820–1900), renowned professor of orthopedic surgery, fractures and dislocations, and clinical surgery at Bellevue Hospital Medical College in New York City, compiled the almost five-hundred-page *Lectures on Orthopedic Surgery and Diseases of the Joints* (1876) and followed it a year later with his *Spinal Disease and Spinal Curvature, Their Treatment by Suspension and the Use of the Plaster of Paris Bandage*. The former work was republished almost immediately in England and appeared on the continent in French, German, and Spanish translations. It superseded Bauer's textbook and remained the most important American orthopedic treatise for several decades.

An abrupt transition of orthopedic surgery into an organized surgical specialty occurred in 1887, when, at the instigation of Virgil Gibney (1847–1927) and Newton Shaffer (1846–1928) of New York City, the American Orthopaedic Association was founded. Intended to advance "orthopaedic science and art," the first meeting of the new society took place at the New York Academy of Medicine. Over the next decade and a half, the Association's proceedings were published in a yearly volume known as *The Transactions*, the only American journal dedicated to orthopedic surgery in the nineteenth century. The papers and discussions in *The Transactions* accurately reflect the emerging scientific struggle between older orthopedic concepts, which emphasized the importance of treatment with braces, manipulation, and exercise, and the newer thought, which insisted on including surgical treatment of orthopedic diseases and deformities while stressing the necessity for more accurate knowledge of the pathogenesis of disease processes. Not until the mid-1920s would these two schools of thought be effectively coordinated, at least in major teaching centers. The insistence on including surgical operations as an integral part of the evolving specialty brought surgeons interested in orthopedic diseases into direct professional conflict with general surgeons. Orthopedic surgeons would have to prove that their operative results were superior to those obtained by the nonspecialist, and the ensuing political struggle over turf lasted well into the present century.

Part of this maturation process was reflected in the emboldened scientific writing of this growing cadre of orthopedic surgeons. Edward Bradford (1848–1926) and Robert Lovett (1859–1924) set the tone when they authored the almost eight-hundred-page *A Treatise on Orthopedic Surgery* (1890). The *Treatise* became the most notable contribution of both men, and further editions were published over the next three decades. It was considered the standard orthopedic textbook of its day in most medical schools and had no competition until Royal Whitman (1857–1946) authored his *Treatise on Orthopaedic Surgery* (1901). In 1892 B. F. Parrish described the first successful tendon transplantation. Six years later, Clayton Parkhill introduced external fixation for the treatment of fractures. Robert Osgood (1873–1956) was the first to draw attention to the condition of the tibial tuberosity now referred to as Osgood-Schlatter disease (1903). Arthur Legg (1874–1939) described juvenile osteochondritis deformans in 1910, and one year later, Joel Goldthwait (1866–1961) suggested that lumbago and sciatica might be due to intervertebral disc injury. It was during this pre-World War I period that Russell Hibbs (1869–1932) first utilized spinal fusion to treat scoliosis, while Fred Albee (1876–1945) employed living bone

4. Clayton Parkhill introduced the first bone clamp for external fixation of fractures. Reporting his results to the American Surgical Association (*Annals of Surgery*, vol. 27, pages 553–570, 1898), he used this clinical photograph to show the clamp's appearance at the time of first dressing, six weeks after it had been applied. (*Historical Collections, College of Physicians of Philadelphia*)

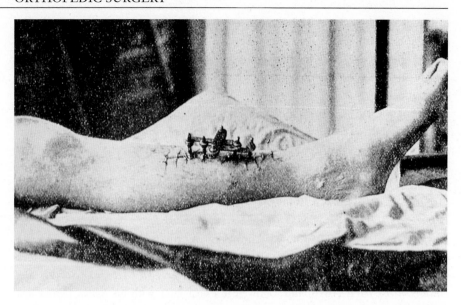

grafts as internal splints, thus introducing bone graft surgery as a planned, carefully designed surgical procedure. Allen Kanavel (1874–1938) produced the first comprehensive treatise on hand surgery, *Infections of the Hand: A Guide to the Surgical Treatment of Acute and Chronic Suppurative Processes in the Fingers, Hand, and Forearm* in 1912. That same year, William Darrach (1876–1948), writing in the *Annals of Surgery*, described his procedure for treatment of anterior dislocation of the head of the ulna. By 1916, Leo Mayer (1884–1972) had completed research on his method of tendon transfer, using tendon sheaths to preserve gliding surfaces.

The first two decades of the twentieth century proved important not only because of technical advances, including recognition of the full value of x-rays to an orthopedist's practice, but also because of an increasing sense of community responsibility for treating the physically handicapped, as is witnessed by the founding of numerous hospital-schools for crippled children. These facilities usually had an orthopedic surgeon as chief of staff, exemplified by DeForest Willard (1846–1910), renowned for his book *The Surgery of Childhood Including Orthopaedic Surgery* (1910) and for his administering the Widener Memorial Industrial Training School for Crippled Children in Philadelphia (1906). Helped by a greater social awareness, expressed in physical rehabilitation programs and social services attached to hospitals and also the beginnings of workmen's compensation laws, the professionalization of the orthopedic surgeon was slowly evolving. H. Winnett Orr (1877–1956), of Nebraska, was a forceful advocate of governmental care for the physically handicapped in a state where a publicly supported orthopedic hospital was in existence by 1910. Despite appearances, government care of the crippled was long overshadowed by the rapid growth of orthopedic facilities based on private charity, such as the first Shriners' Hospital in Louisiana (1922).

Throughout this period of transition leading up to World War I, there was a tremendous growth in orthopedic clubs and societies in Boston (1896), Chicago (1901), and New York (1902). Most importantly, a Section on Orthopedic Surgery was established within the American Medical Association (1912). Orthopedic teaching in medical schools also expanded so much that by 1910, more than one-third of schools included orthopedic surgery as a separate subject or at least combined it with general surgery. One other event from this era proved influential in the growth of American orthopedic surgery: the discontinuance of *The Transactions of the American Orthopaedic Association* and the appearance of the *American Journal of Orthopaedic Surgery*. This step, more than any other, permitted members of the American Orthopedic Association to expand their readership from a self-centered, provincial group to one of more national and international significance.

Membership in the American Orthopaedic Association had been purposely kept exclusive. Nonmembers who were interested in orthopedic subjects had little opportunity to have their papers and case reports published in the scientific literature. By changing the format of the American Orthopaedic Association's journal to include contributions from nonmembers and the printing of abstracts of all orthopedic papers irrespective of their national origin, orthopedic surgery in the United States assumed a new stature. When that wider scope of publication was combined with extraordinary clinical strides, the growth of American orthopedics became phenomenal.

Between the World Wars, the number of young surgeons seeking special training in orthopedic surgery steadily increased, as did both clinical achievements and discoveries in basic science. Royal Whitman reported the first sustained attempt to relieve osteoarthrosis of the hip by surgical means other than fusion (1924). Ernest Codman (1869–1940) and Anatole Kolodny (1892–1957) used statistical and research material gathered from the Registry of Bone Sarcoma of the American College of Surgeons as a means of understanding the pathophysiology of this tumor and updating its nomenclature (1925). During the 1920s, H. Winnett Orr developed a treatment for open fractures involving thorough debridement, reduction of the fracture, and maintenance of the reduction by the technique of pins transfixing the fragments and incorporated into the plaster. Orr's method was described in his monograph *Osteomyelitis and Compound Fractures and Other Infected Wounds: Treatment by the Method of Drainage and Rest*. In 1931 William Baer inaugurated the method of treating osteomyelitis with maggots (larvae of the blow fly), and Marius Smith-Petersen (1886–1953) treated intracapsular fractures of the neck of the femur with a three-flanged nail to prevent rotation of the femoral head. That same year, Michael Burman provided the first description of the arthroscopic appearance of joints other than the knee, and he followed this with another paper on the knee joint (1934). In 1933 Dallas Phemister (1882–1951) utilized epiphysiodesis to inhibit bone growth of a longer leg in the treatment of bony deformities. Codman authored his idiosyncratic and iconoclastically written *The Shoulder* (1934), with its classic study of the rotator cuff. During the mid-1930s, William Mixter (1880–1958) and Joseph Seaton (1901–1963) demonstrated the causal role of intervertebral disc herniation in sciatica. Three important clinical observations were first published in 1939: Marius Smith-Petersen's vitallium cup arthroplasty; Joseph Kite's (1891–1976) method of treating congenital clubfoot by a series of plaster casts and wedgings, without the use of anesthetics, forcible manipulations, or operative procedures; and Arthur Steindler's use of tendon transplantation in the upper extremity. That same year, Willis Campbell (1880–1941) authored *Operative Orthopedics*, one of the most influential American orthopedic textbooks of this century.

With the membership of the American Orthopaedic Association limited to one hundred and fifty individuals, the need for a larger organization to include all qualified orthopedic surgeons became obvious. In order to provide a broad-based organization, several of the more active members of the American Orthopaedic

5. Advertisement from the pages of *The Railway Surgeon* (1918) for an artificial arm. *(Historical Collections, College of Physicians of Philadelphia)*

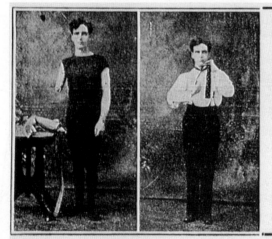

Association met in Chicago in 1933 and founded the American Academy of Orthopaedic Surgeons. The Academy was meant to include every surgeon who could demonstrate a fundamental knowledge of the specialty and whose practice was conducted in an ethical and professional manner, and its first important assignment was to assist in the development of the American Board of Orthopaedic Surgery as the specialty's certifying organization (1934). As a joint venture of the American Medical Association, the American Orthopaedic Association, and the American Academy of Orthopaedic Surgeons, the board defines minimum education requirements in the specialty and aids in stimulating graduate medical education and continuing medical education. Presently, candidates for certification by the American Board of Orthopaedic Surgery are required to have served five years in postdoctoral residency, four of which must be in a program whose curriculum is determined by the director of an accredited orthopedic surgical residency. In 1989, the board also began to award certificates of added qualification in hand surgery.

No discussion of influences on the evolution of American orthopedic surgery during the 1930s can be complete without a mention of poliomyelitis. Because of the crippling paralysis that occured in a certain percentage of patients afflicted with the disease, orthopedic surgeons became increasingly responsible for their overall care. Owing to the direct influence of Franklin D. Roosevelt (1882–1945), himself a victim of the virus when he was barely 40, March of Dimes campaigns were started in the early 1930s, and the National Foundation for Infantile Paralysis was organized in 1938. Through their successful annual fund-raising drives, research grants to orthopedic surgeons became an integral part of the professionalization process and brought about important advances in the surgical treatment of the deformities and crippling paralysis of poliomyelitis.

During World War II, many young surgeons received their initial indoctrination in the care of musculoskeletal injuries. Interest in orthopedic surgery was piqued, the number of orthopedic residencies expanded rapidly, and there was an evident maturation of the specialty. Clinical advances continued in the postwar period, exemplified by Walter Blount's use of epiphyseal stapling to control bone growth (1949), Leslie Rush's medullary fixation of fractures by a longitudinal pin (1949), Earl Brannon's prosthetic device for replacement of destroyed finger-joints (1959), Paul Harrington's rod system for scoliosis and spine fracture surgery (1962), A. B. Swanson's flexible silicone rubber finger-joint prosthesis (1966), and Frank Gunston's total knee replacement, in which the metal and plastic components are held in place with acrylic cement (1971). When orthopedic surgeons were queried by members of the research subcommittee of the *Study on Surgical Services for the United States* (1976) regarding important orthopedic surgical contributions from 1945 to 1970, total hip replacement was considered to be of first-order importance, the Harrington rod instrumentation for scoliosis and compression plating of acute and nonunited shaft fractures were deemed of second-order importance, and pelvic

6. Samuel Milliken (1865–1949) was surgeon in chief of the New York Infirmary for Crippled Children when he authored a classic paper on tendon grafting (*Medical Record*, vol. 48, pages 581–582, 1895). These figures were used to illustrate his epochal attempt to make a "healthy muscle...do the work of one which was completely paralyzed without in any way interfering with its own function." In this particular operation, the tendons of the exterior proprius policis and tibialis anticus were united by continuous suture after their sheaths had been split. (*Historical Collections, College of Physicians of Philadelphia*)

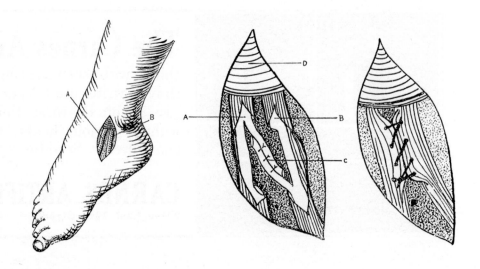

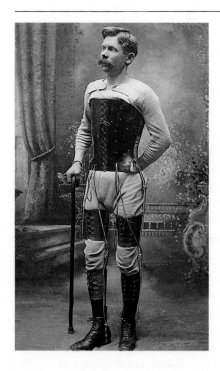

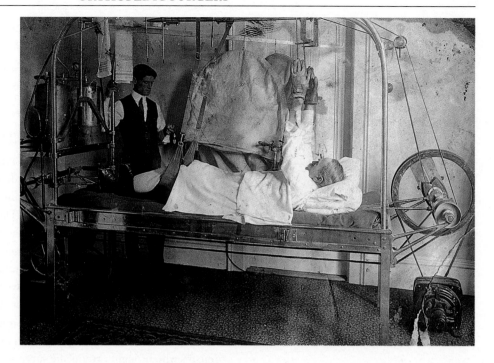

osteotomy for congenital dislocation of the hip and synovectomy for rheumatoid arthritis were termed third-order contributions.

In 1995, of the approximately 621,000 total physicians in active practice in the United States, 21,535 (3.5 percent) designated themselves as orthopedic surgeons. Within this cadre of orthopedic surgeons, 15,325 (71 percent) were board certified. (By contrast, during the fifteen years between 1980 and 1994, 8,226 certificates in orthopedic surgery were issued, or an average of 548 per year.) Of the 1995 total, 600 (2.8 percent) were women and 1,875 (9 percent) were international medical graduates. Among the total pool of orthopedic surgeons, approximately 4,335 (20 percent) were younger than 35; 6,600 (31 percent) were 35 to 44; 5,555 (26 percent) were 45 to 54; 3,625 (17 percent) were 55 to 64; and 1,420 (7 percent) were 65 years old and older. Of the 600 female orthopedic surgeons, 525 (88 percent) were under 44, in contrast to the approximately 20,935 male orthopedic surgeons, of whom 10,410 (50 percent) were under 44.

Presently, the two most influential peer-reviewed orthopedic periodicals are the *Journal of Bone and Joint Surgery*, which represents a continuation of the old *American Journal of Orthopaedic Surgery* and *Clinical Orthopaedics and Related Research*. The more recent editors of the *Journal of Bone and Joint Surgery* and their years of service include William Rogers (1942–1958), Thornton Brown (1959–1978), Paul H, Curtiss, Jr. (1979–1984), and Henry R. Cowell (1985–??). *Clinical Orthopaedics* was founded in 1953, and its editors have been Anthony F. DePalma (1953–1966), Marshall Urist (1966–1993), and Carl Brighton (1993–??).

The written history of orthopedic surgery has been well served by numerous American orthopedists. Robert Osgood authored *The Evolution of Orthopaedic Surgery* in 1925. Edgar Bick (1902–1978) provided a concise and thematic history of orthopedic surgery from the earliest times in his *Source Book of Orthopaedics* (1948) and followed it with *Classics of Orthopaedics* (1976). H. Winnett Orr wrote *On the Contributions of Hugh Owen Thomas of Liverpool, Sir Robert Jones of Liverpool and London, John Ridlon, M.D. of New York and Chicago, to Modern Orthopedic Surgery* in 1949. Alfred Shands (1899–1981) authored *The Early Orthopaedic Surgeons of America* (1970). Joseph Boyes completed *On the Shoulders of Giants, Notable Names in Hand Surgery* in 1976. Recently, Leonard Peltier (born 1920) wrote *Fractures: A History and Iconography of Their Treatment* (1990) and *Orthopedics: A History and Iconography* (1993). A historical report more than one hundred pages long, entitled "Orthopaedic

7. Despite relative advances, orthopedic surgery before the 1890s was generally of a strap-and-buckle nature *(left)*. Since surgical intervention carried the grave risk of infection in bone, or osteomyelitis, orthopedists were forced to evolve elaborate mechanical contraptions to allow their patients to ambulate and use their limbs. The cyanotype print *(right)* shows the complexity needed to make certain devices functional. *(Courtesy of Stanley B. Burns, M.D., and The Burns Collection and Archive)*

Surgery in the United States of America," was authored by Leo Mayer (1844–1972) and appeared in the *Journal of Bone and Joint Surgery* (1950). Historical hagiography aside, the following biographical vignettes provide a brief review of the lives of some individuals who have contributed to the professionalization process of American orthopedic surgery.

BIOGRAPHIES OF ORTHOPEDIC SURGEONS

Henry Gassett Davis (1807–1896) was born in Trenton, Maine, and attended Yale University (1836) and its School of Medicine (1839). While receiving his medical education he also obtained clinical training at Bellevue Hospital in New York City. For fifteen years following graduation, Davis was in general medical and surgical practice in Milbury and Worcester, Massachusetts. During this time he became interested in the treatment of the diseases and deformities of bones and joints. In 1855 Davis moved to New York City, where he confined his clinical activities almost exclusively to those conditions. Within five years his practice had grown so large that he opened a private institution at Madison Avenue and 37th Street, called Dr. Davis's Institute. Davis was a pioneering orthopedic surgeon, founder of the "traction school" of conservative orthopedic surgery, and one of a small group of American surgeons who brought orthopedic surgery from obscurity to recognition as a special branch of the surgical sciences. In his so-called American method of treating joint diseases, fractures, and deformities, continuous "elastic extension" was provided by weights and pulleys, and constituted the bulk of the therapy. His principles of care were elucidated in *Conservative Surgery, As Exhibited in Remedying Some of the Mechanical Causes That Operate Injuriously both in Health and Disease* (1867), considered one of the most notable books in early American orthopedic surgery. Davis's views on many orthopedic conditions and his methods of treatment were far ahead of his time. His professional activities, combined with his writings, made a profound impression on several younger surgeons, most notably Lewis Sayre, Charles Fayette Taylor, and Edward Bradford. Davis retired from his New York City practice in 1869 and resettled in Everett, Massachusetts. He continued his interests in orthopedic diseases and, to within a few years of his death at age 89, attended meetings of the American Orthopaedic Association.

William Ludwig Detmold (1808–1894) was born in Hanover, Germany, and obtained his medical degree from the University of Göttingen in 1830. He served as a surgeon in the Royal Hanoverian Guards while also receiving orthopedic training under Louis Stromeyer (1804–1876) of Hanover. Detmold emigrated to New York City in 1837 and one year later authored a report on several successful operations for "clubfoot by the division of the tendo Achillis," which was published in the *American Journal of the Medical Sciences.* In 1841 he established a public clinic as part of the College of Physicians and Surgeons for the treatment of crippled children. That same year, Detmold received an appointment as a surgeon to Bellevue Hospital. A charter member of the New York Academy of Medicine, he was its vice president from 1853 to 1855. Detmold wrote little but spent a great deal of time administering his clinic. With the outbreak of the Civil War, he assisted in the organization of the U.S. Army Medical Corps, and in 1862 he was named professor of military surgery and hygiene in the College of Physicians and Surgeons. It is stated that from sunrise to noon on the day following the first Battle of Bull Run (July 1861), Detmold amputated seventy-five limbs. Considered a friend of the soldier amputee, he invented a combination knife and fork for one-armed men. The outer edge of the gently rounded utensil was sharp and, with a simple rocking motion, could cut food, which could then be picked up with the three teeth at the end. This implement was supplied by the federal government under the name of the Detmold knife. Following the war and with military surgery losing its prominence, Detmold was made an emeritus professor, a title he held until his death. When New York City's Presbyterian Hospital was organized in 1875, he was named a consulting physician, and he served as president of its medical board from 1880 to 1884. Five years after the American Orthopaedic Association was founded (1887), Detmold was made an honorary member.

James Knight (1810–1887) was born in Taneytown, Maryland, and received his medical education at the Washington Medical College in Baltimore (1832). After pursuing postgraduate training, he moved to New York City (1835) and, within a few years, founded the New York Surgeon's Bandage Institute. From his activities in the design and application of bandages and trusses came his interest in braces and orthopedics, or what he described as "surgico-mechanics." It is also believed that Knight's attraction to orthopedics emanated from a suggestion by Valentine Mott that he devote himself to this field. Accordingly, from 1842 to 1844, Knight assisted Mott in the orthopedic treatment of patients who attended the latter's public clinics of the medical department of the University of the City of New York. As early as 1842, Knight had taken legal steps to establish a hospital for crippled individuals, but not until public awareness was aroused and a fund-raising campaign undertaken (1859–1863) were the articles of incorporation of the New York Society for the Relief of the Ruptured and Crippled filed. Knight assumed leadership in the society and in founding the Hospital for the Ruptured and Crippled, initially using his own house as a hospital. In May 1870, a new building at 42nd Street and Lexington Avenue was occupied, with Knight remaining in charge until his death. Although the institution was not the first orthopedic facility in the United States, it is the first orthopedic hospital to be in continuous operation from its opening to the present day (it is now known as the Hospital for Special Surgery). Knight was one of the last "strap and buckle" pioneers in orthopedics and was so ultraconservative in the utilization of surgical procedures that he refused to have an operating theater placed in the new hospital. His most prominent publication was *Orthopaedia or a Practical Treatise on the Aberrations of the Human Form* (1874). The text mainly dealt with braces, frames, and casts; the only surgical operations mentioned were tenotomies. His other monographs were *The Improvement of the Health of Children and Adults by Natural Means, Including a History of Food and a Consideration of its Substantial Qualities* (1868), and *Static Electricity as a Therapeutic Agent* (1882). At a time when a new generation of orthopedic surgeons were attempting to free themselves from the stigma of being regarded as "mere bandagists" and to justify their professional existence as a separate field from general surgery, Knight remained a surgically conservative autocrat. However, through his advocacy of the expectant plan, or long-term rest for joint lesions, he did manage to establish, for the first time in the country, the ongoing treatment, education, and vocational training of crippled children and adolescents within one institution.

Louis Bauer (1814–1898) was born in Stettin, Prussia, and after university studies in Breslau, Göttingen, and Griefswald received his medical degree from the

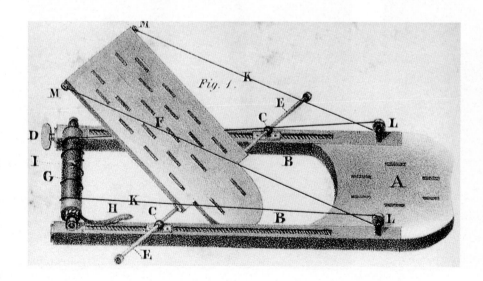

8. William Detmold introduced a clubfoot-extending apparatus modified from a German appliance (*New York Journal of Medicine and Surgery*, vol. 2, pages 1–64, 1840). In his surgical procedure, a narrow-bladed knife was inserted through the skin, and by pressing the scalpel against the constricted tendon fibers the tendon was divided. Forty-eight hours after tenotomy, the foot was placed in an extending apparatus, which stretched the tight structures and helped mold the bones and soft tissues. The footboard had several holes for leather straps to pass through, by which the foot was held to the wood. (*Historical Collections, College of Physicians of Philadelphia*)

University of Berlin in 1838. Bauer became a government district physician in East Prussia and was a pupil of Louis Stromeyer for a few months. A combative personality, Bauer became interested in government and politics and was elected a member of the Prussian House of Representatives. When this parliamentary body was dissolved by government decree, Bauer was falsely accused of high treason and placed in prison. Following his release, the prospect of another arrest caused him to seek political asylum in London, where he established a general medical practice among the growing colony of German expatriates. While living in England, Bauer passed his examination for the Royal College of Surgeons and is said to have served a short while as house surgeon at an orthopedic institution in Manchester. In 1853 he emigrated to the United States and settled in Brooklyn, where he administered to a large colony of former German citizens. Within one year, Bauer organized the German General Dispensary, which was later transformed into the Long Island College Hospital and Medical School (1858). In 1854, Bauer also established the Orthopaedic Institution of Brooklyn, the first orthopedic facility in the New York City area. Seven years later, Bauer was named professor of anatomy and clinical surgery at the Long Island College Hospital, and because of his growing reputation, he was asked to give a series of lectures on orthopedic surgery at the Brooklyn Surgical and Medical Institute. The talks were published in the *Philadelphia Medical and Surgical Reporter* and later reprinted as a textbook, *Lectures on Orthopedic Surgery* (1864). Considered the first "true" orthopedic textbook in the United States, it was published in a second edition in 1868 and was translated into German, Italian, and Swedish. Bauer's other text was *Lectures on Causes, Pathology, and Treatment of Joint Diseases* (1868), consisting of a series of talks delivered at McGill University Medical College. Bauer remained in practice in Brooklyn until 1869, when his strong political views and blunt opinions of other physicians' activities caused him such personal turmoil that he moved to St. Louis, where he became associated with the Humboldt Medical College. When this institution was closed, Bauer undertook to obtain a charter for the College of Physicians and Surgeons (1879), which remained in existence until 1910 and where he served as professor of orthopedic surgery until

9. "Before" and "after" photographs showing the results of treatment for lateral curvature of the spine. These silver prints are extremely important in the history of American surgery, as they along with others in Buckminster Brown's twenty-three-page *Cases of Orthopedic Surgery* (1868) were the first actual photographs used to illustrate an American surgical text. *(Historical Collections, College of Physicians of Philadelphia)*

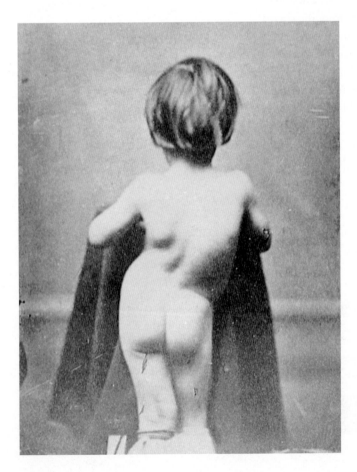
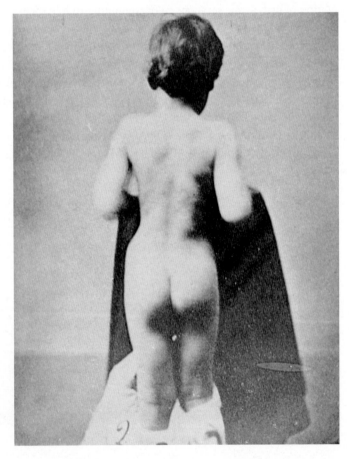

his death. Because of his stormy relationships with so many influential orthopedic surgeons, Bauer was not asked to become a founding member of the American Orthopaedic Association and was never elected an honorary member.

Buckminster Brown (1819–1891), born in Boston, was the son of John Ball Brown (1784–1862) and grandson of John Warren (1753–1815). Buckminster Brown graduated from Harvard Medical School in 1844 and spent 1845–1846 in Europe studying orthopedics under William John Little (1810–1894) in London, Jules Guérin and Sauveur-Henri-Victor Bouvier (1799–1877) in Paris, and Louis Stromeyer in Germany. Returning to Boston, Brown established himself in general practice but limited his clinical activities to orthopedic problems within a few years, being associated with his father at the Boston Orthopedic Institution. Brown also established an orthopedic department in the House of the Good Samaritan, devoted entirely to the treatment of deformities in children. He remained surgeon to this hospital for nineteen years and is regarded as the father of children's orthopedics in America. Brown was especially sensitive to the needs of handicapped children; as a child he had had Pott's disease, which resulted in a spinal deformity and caused him to lead a shut-in existence as a youngster. Although not a voluminous writer, Brown authored several important publications, including *Cases of Orthopaedic Surgery With Photographic Illustrations of the Cases Presented* (1868). This twenty-three-page pamphlet represents the first American orthopedic text to be illustrated with actual photographs, in this case silver prints. He was a charter member of the American Orthopaedic Association and a councilor of the Massachusetts Medical Society. In 1883 Buckminster Brown provided $40,000 to establish the second chair of orthopedic surgery in America, the John Ball and Buckminster Brown Professorship in Orthopaedic Surgery at Harvard University.

Lewis Albert Sayre (1820–1900) was born in Bottle Hill (now Madison), New Jersey, and received his collegiate education at Transylvania University in Lexington, Kentucky (1839). He soon moved to New York City to begin a medical apprenticeship with David Green. There he entered the College of Physicians and Surgeons, from which he received his medical degree in 1842. Following his graduation, Sayre was appointed prosector to Willard Parker (1800–1884), who was then professor of surgery at the College of Physicians and Surgeons. Sayre continued in this capacity for ten years until his appointment as visiting surgeon to Bellevue Hospital. In 1861 Sayre became the chief organizer of the Bellevue Hospital Medical College and, having acquired a reputation for his treatment of bone and joint conditions, was appointed to the orthopedic professorship. This was the first chair of orthopedic surgery in America, and Sayre held the position until 1898 when, following the amalgamation of Bellevue Hospital Medical College with New York University, he became emeritus professor. He was succeeded by his son Reginald Hall Sayre (1859–1929), a well-known orthopedic surgeon in his own right and future president of the American Orthopaedic Association (1903). Lewis Sayre also served as surgeon general of the New York Militia (1845–1861) and held the political position of resident physician (public health officer) of New York City under four different mayors. He improved sanitary conditions in tenements, advocated compulsory vaccination, and established quarantine regulations for the port of New York to prevent the spread of cholera and other communicable diseases. He was a consultant surgeon to many institutions in New York City, including the Charity Hospital on Welfare Island (1859), St. Elizabeth's Hospital, the Northwestern Dispensary, and the Home for Incurables. Known for his skills in treating orthopedic conditions, Sayre completed the second successful resection of the hip joint for tuberculosis in the country (1852) and was the first to utilize plaster of Paris as a support for the spinal column in scoliosis and Pott's disease (1876). He was a respected author, whose textbooks included *A Practical Manual of the Treatment of Club Foot* (1869), *Lectures on Orthopedic Surgery* (1876), and *Spinal Disease and Spinal Curvature, and Their Treatment by Suspension and the Use of the Plaster of Paris Bandage* (1877). A charter member of the New York Pathological Society (1844), the New York Academy of

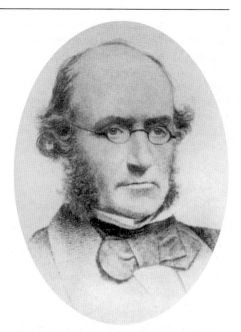

10. Buckminster Brown. *(Historical Collections, College of Physicians of Philadelphia)*

11. Out of concern for maintaining sterility and body fluid precautions, modern orthopedic surgeons often wear full-body "space suits" with air supply. In this hip joint replacement surgery, the surgeon prepares the shaft of the femur to accept the prosthesis. *(Courtesy of Stanley B. Burns, M.D., and The Burns Collection and Archive and the permission of Chitranjans Ranawat, M.D.)*

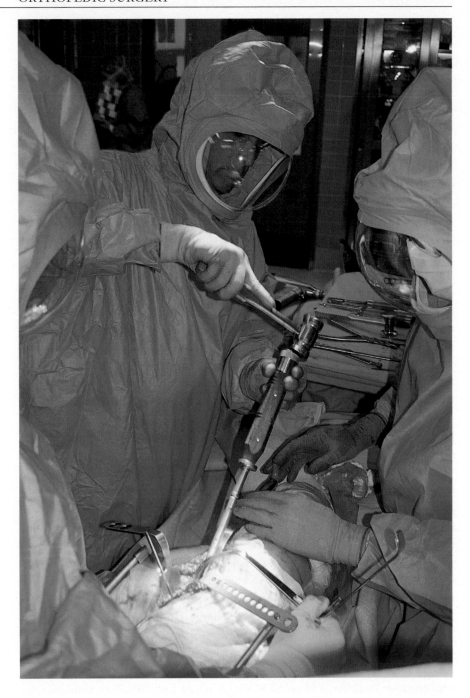

Medicine (1847), the American Medical Association (1847), and the American Surgical Association (1880), he served as president of the American Medical Association in 1880. He urged the membership of the latter organization to publish its own journal, which resulted in the establishment of the *Journal of the American Medical Association* (1882). Although Sayre was elected an honorary member of the American Orthopaedic Association in 1889, he initially opposed the organization of the association, believing that members of the newly proposed society should instead join and become active members of the American Surgical Association.

Charles Fayette Taylor (1827–1899) was born in Williston, Vermont, and attended New York Medical College for one year (1855) but received his medical degree from the University of Vermont in 1856. The following summer, having become impressed with the Swedish system of exercises originated by Peter Henry Ling (1776–1839) of Stockholm, he traveled to London, where he studied therapeutic exercises, or kinesitherapy, with one of Ling's students, Mathias Roth. Ling had developed the ancient Greek art of calisthenics to a science, based on sound anatomic and physiologic principles. He was among those who thought in terms of motions rather than muscles, and believed that the education of the locomotor system was the best way to prevent idiopathic deformities such as scoliosis, round shoulders, hollow back, and weak feet. Returning to the United States in 1857, Taylor introduced the so-called Swedish movements system of therapeutic exercises (in present-day America, the Swedish massage remains a remnant of the system) and went on to invent many machines that increased the effectiveness of the movement cure. From 1857 to 1882, he practiced in New York City. There he was instrumental in establishing the New York Orthopedic Dispensary, from which developed the New York Orthopedic Dispensary and Hospital. Among Taylor's written works were *Theory and Practice of the Movement-Cure; Or, the Treatment of Lateral Curvature of the Spine, Paralysis, Indigestion, Diseases Incident to Women, Derangements of the Nervous System and Other Chronic Affections by the Swedish System of Localized Movements* (1861), *Infantile Paralysis and its Attendant Deformities* (1864), *On the Mechanical Treatment of Disease of the Hip-Joint* (1873), and *Sensation and Pain* (1871). Taylor became well known for his various braces and other orthopedic devices and was honored with medals for his original exhibits at the Paris Exposition (1867), the Vienna Exposition (1873), and the Centennial Exposition in Philadelphia (1876). Taylor sincerely believed that surgery was seldom indicated in the treatment of orthopedic conditions, and his views were so respected that he was made a charter member of the American Orthopaedic Association.

Newton Melman Shaffer (1846–1928) was born in Kinderhook, New York, and commenced the study of medicine in 1863 as a student assistant in the Hospital for the Ruptured and Crippled, working under James Knight. Subsequently, Shaffer obtained his medical degree from the New York University Medical College in 1867. He completed a one-year internship at his alma mater and soon began the practice of general medicine. In 1871 he accepted a position as assistant surgeon in the New York Orthopaedic Dispensary under Charles Fayette Taylor and, following Taylor's resignation (1876) due to failing health, Shaffer succeeded him as surgeon in chief. Four years previously, the administrators of St. Luke's Hospital in New York City had recognized the growing importance of orthopedics and established the first separate orthopedic service in a major general American hospital, under the leadership of Shaffer. In 1882 Shaffer was appointed clinical professor of orthopedic surgery at New York University Medical Center, a position he held until 1886. Shaffer remained without an academic title until 1900. In that year he became the first professor of orthopedic surgery at Cornell University College of Medicine, where he was an emeritus professor from 1913 until his death. He had remained as surgeon in chief at the New York Orthopaedic Dispensary and Hospital until 1898, when he resigned to be succeeded by Russell Hibbs (1869–1932). Among his writings are *Pott's Disease, its Pathology and Mechanical Treatment, with Remarks on Rotary Lateral Curvature* (1879), *The Hysterical Element in Orthopaedic Surgery* (1880), *Brief Essays on Orthopaedic Surgery, Including A Consideration of its Relation to General Surgery* (1898), and *Selected Essays on Orthopaedic Surgery* (1923). Active in the politics of American orthopedic surgery, Shaffer was a charter member and an early president of the New York Orthopaedic Society, which later became the orthopedic section of the New York Academy of Medicine. He was one of the principal organizers and a charter member of the American Orthopaedic Assocation, as well as its second president (1887). Shaffer was chairman of the committee that secured the recognition of orthopedic surgery as a specialty at the Tenth International Medical Congress, held in Berlin in 1890. In addition, he was one of the founders and first chairman of the Orthopedic Section of the American Medical Association and a founding member of the American College of Surgeons. Shaffer was a forceful and combative personality, who regarded himself more as a "mechanician" and tried to relegate operations to general surgeons.

DeForest Willard (1846–1910), born in Newington, Connecticut, attended Yale College (1863) and began his medical education at Jefferson Medical College. As a young child, Willard had been ill with poliomyelitis and was left with a partially paralyzed leg and a clubfoot deformity. In the summer of 1864, D. Hayes Agnew,

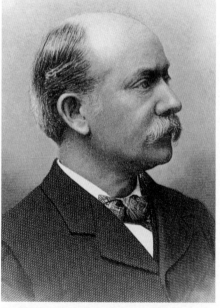

12. Newton Melman Shaffer. *(Historical Collections, College of Physicians of Philadelphia)*

535

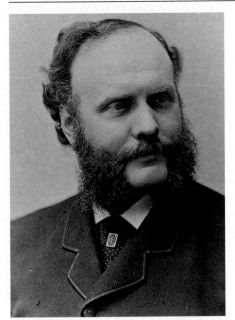

13. DeForest Willard. *(Historical Collections, College of Physicians of Philadelphia)*

professor of surgery at the University of Pennsylvania, performed a tenotomy on Willard's Achilles tendon that resulted in a partial correction of the deformity and made it easier for the young man to walk. Impressed with Agnew's surgical persona, Willard transferred to the University of Pennsylvania School of Medicine, where he eventually received his medical diploma in 1867. In March of that year, he entered Philadelphia General Hospital as a resident physician, where he served for fifteen months. Having completed his training, Willard opened an office for practice in Philadelphia. From this time until his death, he was continuously connected with the anatomical and surgical departments of his alma mater and also served as surgeon to the Presbyterian Hospital. In 1887 Willard was appointed lecturer on orthopedic surgery at the University of Pennsylvania; in 1889, clinical professor; and four years later, full professor. It was he who initially organized the orthopedic department at the university and was instrumental in raising funds for building the Agnew wing of the University Hospital. Of commanding physical girth, Willard served as both president of the American Orthopaedic Association (1890) and the American Surgical Association (1902), and he was chairman of the American Medical Association's Section of Surgery (1902). Among his numerous activities were planning the buildings and serving as surgeon in chief for the Widener Memorial Industrial Training School for Crippled Children in Philadelphia. Of indefatigable energy, Willard was a voluminous writer and contributed numerous chapters on orthopedic surgery to the best-known surgical textbooks of his day. His most important monograph was *The Surgery of Childhood, Including Orthopaedic Surgery* (1910). Willard had one child, DeForest Porter Willard, who became a renowned orthopedic surgeon in his own right, head of the orthopedic department of the Graduate School of Medicine of the University of Pennsylvania, and president of the American Orthopedic Association (1935).

Virgil Pendleton Gibney (1847–1927) was born in Jessamine County, Kentucky, and attended the University of Kentucky in Lexington (1869). The first year of his medical education was taken at the University of Louisville and the second year at Bellevue Hospital Medical Center in New York City, where he received his medical degree in 1871. Following his graduation, Gibney obtained a position as an assistant physician and surgeon under James Knight at the newly constructed Hospital for the Ruptured and Crippled. Seven years later he was appointed house surgeon and in 1883, assistant surgeon. For thirteen years, Gibney physically lived in the hospital and enjoyed a close working relationship with Knight. However, he did not always clinically agree with Knight, who was dogmatic and dictatorial in his methods, especially with regard to the treatment of tuberculous hip disease. Gibney believed that the hip, in the early stage of the disease, should be placed at rest by means of traction (the "American method" espoused by Henry Davis) and that more advanced cases needed operative intervention. Such thinking was anathema to Knight, who taught that the patient should be fitted with a comfortable brace and put through a prescribed daily regimen, including special exercises and dietary manipulation, known as the expectant treatment. In 1884, without Knight's knowledge, Gibney authored the 412-page *The Hip and Its Diseases*, which expressed views contrary to those of his chief. Knight immediately asked for his resignation. Gibney went into private orthopedic practice, but not before first traveling to Europe to study in several orthopedic clinics. From 1884 to 1887, Gibney, in conjunction with William T. Bull and John B. Walker, managed a small private hospital in the neighborhood of their office on Park Avenue and 33rd Street. In 1887 Knight died, and Gibney was asked to return to the Hospital for the Ruptured and Crippled as surgeon in chief. He accepted the offer and went on to change the institution from a facility for crippled children to a hospital fully equipped and staffed for modern orthopedics, separating the hernia department from the orthopedic section. It was Gibney, in that same year of 1887, who helped organized the initial meeting of the American Orthopaedic Association and served as its first president. Twenty-five years later

(1912), Gibney was again elected to the presidency, thus becoming the only member in the history of the association to be so honored twice. He is eponymically remembered for Gibney's fixation bandage: a herring-bone strapping of the foot and leg for sprain of the ankle. When a chair of orthopedic surgery was established at the Columbia University College of Physicians and Surgeons in 1894, Gibney was appointed to be first professor, a position he held until 1917. In 1924, for reasons of health, Gibney resigned as surgeon in chief of the Hospital for the Ruptured and Crippled. He was succeeded by Royal Whitman (1857–1946). In 1969 Alfred R. Shands, Jr. (1899–1981), edited an extensive biography, *Gibney of the Ruptured and Crippled.*

Edward Hickling Bradford (1848–1926) was born in Boston and received his bachelor's (1869), master's (1872), and medical (1873) degrees from Harvard University. He completed a year of postgraduate training at the Massachusetts General Hospital and then spent 1874–1876 in Europe, where he worked in clinics in Berlin, Liverpool, London, Paris, Strasbourg, and Vienna. On returning to Boston in 1876, Bradford opened a general medical practice, but seeing the possibilities of orthopedic surgery, he moved to New York City and studied for a few months at the New York Orthopaedic Dispensary and Hospital under Charles Fayette Taylor. Back in Boston, he received an appointment at the House of the Good Samaritan, working under Buckminster Brown, whom he succeeded four years later as surgeon in chief. Bradford was also appointed to the surgical staff of the Boston City Hospital and the Boston Dispensary, first as surgeon in the outpatient department and later (1885) as visiting surgeon. In 1878 he was named surgeon to the Boston Children's Hospital and, over time, became more closely allied with this institution, becoming its chief surgeon. Two years later, Bradford was appointed to the surgical department of his alma mater with the title of clinical instructor in orthopedic surgery. In 1889 he was promoted to assistant professor and, in 1903, became the first John Ball and Buckminster Brown Professor of Orthopaedic Surgery. He held this title until 1912, when he retired because of age. Bradford was also dean of Harvard Medical School from 1912 to 1918. In 1894, greatly impressed with his earlier visit to the Pio Instituto Rachitici, a special school and hospital for rachitic children in Milan, Italy, Bradford helped found the Boston Industrial School for Crippled and Deformed Children, the first such institution in the United States. He also began the Massachusetts State Hospital School for Crippled Children at Canton (1907) and was chairman of the board of trustees until his death. His most influential written work was *A Treatise on Orthopedic Surgery* (1890), coauthored with Robert Lovett (1859–1924). Considered the standard orthopedic textbook of its day, the textbook went through five editions. A prolific contributor to the surgical literature, Bradford started the "Progress in Orthopaedic Surgery" section in the *Boston Medical and Surgical Journal* (1878) and continued as the editor until 1903. He was one of the founders of the American Orthopaedic Association and its third president (1888), and he was a fellow of the American Surgical Association. His name has long been linked with the Bradford frame for the treatment of spinal disease, an oblong rectangular frame made of pipe, over which are stretched transversely two strips of canvas, permitting the trunk and lower extremities to move as a unit. In his late 50s, Bradford was injured in a bicycling accident and lost the vision in one eye. A decade and a half later, his other eye became affected, resulting in total blindness. At the age of 75, Bradford successfully studied Braille. His oldest son, Robert Fiske Bradford, became governor of Massachusetts.

John Ridlon (1852–1936) was born in Clarendon, Vermont, and received his medical education at the College of Physicians and Surgeons in New York City (1878). He obtained a house officer position at St. Luke's Hospital for two years and, in 1880, received his first orthopedic appointment as assistant to Newton Shaffer at St. Luke's Hospital, later going to the New York Orthopaedic Hospital and

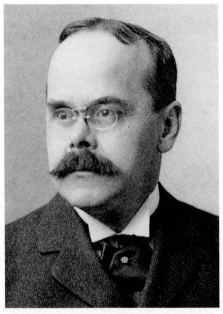

14. Edward Hickling Bradford. *(Historical Collections, College of Physicians of Philadelphia)*

15. Edward Bradford and Elliott Brackett of Boston followed a combined system of frame treatment and plaster of Paris correction for lateral curvature of the spine (*Boston Medical and Surgical Journal* vol. 128, pages 463–468, 1893). They experimented extensively with this apparatus, which was designed to place direct and indirect pressure on the vertebral column during periods of recumbency. (*Historical Collections, College of Physicians of Philadelphia*)

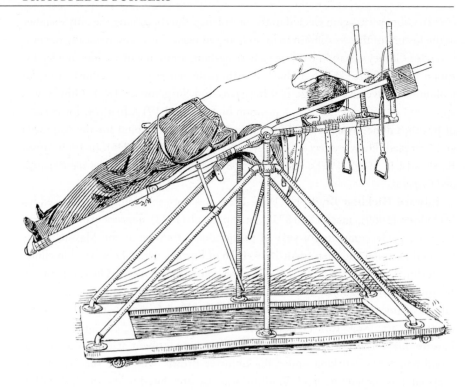

Dispensary. In 1887 Ridlon traveled to Liverpool, England, to work with Hugh Owen Thomas (1834–1891). There he also became friendly with Thomas's nephew and eventual successor, Robert Jones (1858–1933). Returning to New York City, Ridlon made the first Thomas hip splint used in this country. Shaffer immediately ordered the splint removed and, during the ensuing argument, prevented Ridlon's reappointment to St. Luke's surgical staff. Ridlon moved to Chicago (1888), where he became instructor in orthopedic surgery at Northwestern University. One year later he was promoted to full professor, and served for sixteen years. The early years in Chicago proved a disappointment in his attempt to establish a practice, and Ridlon was forced to ask Jones for financial help. The intricacies of the Ridlon–Jones relationship have been described by H. Winnett Orr in his lengthy historical work, *On the Contributions of Hugh Owen Thomas of Liverpool, Sir Robert Jones of Liverpool and London, John Ridlon, M.D., of New York and Chicago, to Modern Orthopedic Surgery* (1949). As a result of their acquaintance and mutual esteem, Ridlon and Jones cooperated between 1892 and 1893 on several jointly authored articles. These reports were reprinted and served as the basis for two textbooks: *Chronic Joint Disease* (1894) and *Lectures on Orthopedic Surgery* (1899). As secretary of the infant American Orthopaedic Association for sixteen years, Ridlon became a powerful force in orthopedic surgery, playing one man against another and openly manipulating its internal affairs. Because of his bitter past experience in New York City, Ridlon was looked upon as a loyal member of what was termed the Western bloc in the American Orthopaedic Association, and went to great lengths to further the careers of such men as Arthur Gillette (1864–1921) of St. Paul, Minnesota and Aaron Steele (1835–1917) of St. Louis.

Royal Whitman (1857–1946), born in Portland, Maine, received his medical education at Harvard University (1882). He served an internship at Boston City Hospital (1883) and also obtained additional training at Cook's School of Anatomy in London (late 1880s), at which time he became a member of the Royal College of Surgeons (1889). During the mid- to late 1880s, Whitman practiced medicine in Boston, but following his return from England, he joined the surgical staff at the Hospital for the Ruptured and Crippled in New York City (1889). He remained at this institution until 1929, eventually serving as successor to Virgil Gibney. Whitman was also adjunct professor of orthopedic surgery at the Columbia University College of Physicians and Surgeons and professor at the New York

Polyclinic Medical School. An early specialist in operative surgery of deformities and diseases of the joints, he developed several techniques for treatment of disorders of the foot and hip that quickly became standard; devised a special metal plate, known as the Whitman plate, for the treatment of flat foot (1889); developed an astragalectomy operation for stabilizing a paralytic foot, especially with calcaneus deformity (1901); originated the "abduction treatment" for fracture of the neck of the femur (1904); and pioneered in the reconstruction operation for nonunited fracture of the hip (1916). Whitman exerted great influence through his clinical teaching skills and the publication of his textbook, *A Treatise on Orthopaedic Surgery* (1901), which by the 1930s had gone through nine editions. In 1895 Whitman was president of the American Orthopaedic Association.

Robert Williamson Lovett (1859–1924) was born in Beverly, Massachusetts, and received his undergraduate (1881) and medical education (1885) at Harvard University. He served as a general house surgeon at Boston City Hospital, but he was mostly interested in orthopedic surgery and spent a few months at the New York Orthopaedic Hospital. When Lovett began practice in Boston (1886), he was appointed surgeon to outpatients at both the Carney and City Hospitals as well as assistant outpatient surgeon at the Children's Hospital. In 1901 he resigned from the Carney and City Hospitals in order to devote all his time to orthopedics. The following year, Lovett was named an assistant in orthopedic surgery at his alma mater, where he advanced through the academic ranks, becoming instructor in orthopedics (1906–1909), assistant professor (1909–1914), and full professor (1914–1915). He finally was named Edward Bradford's successor at the Children's Hospital and the John Ball Brown and Buckminster Brown Professor of Orthopaedic Surgery in 1915, a position he held until his death from cardiac failure. Lovett was also surgeon in chief to the Massachusetts Hospital School for Crippled and Deformed Children in Canton and to the Peabody Home for Crippled Children in Newton. He was a frequent contributor to the surgical literature. Among his textbooks are *A Treatise on Orthopedic Surgery* (1890), coauthored with Bradford; *The Etiology, Pathology, and Treatment of Diseases of the Hip Joint* (1891); *Lateral Curvature of the Spine and Round Shoulders* (1907); and the monumental *Orthopaedic Surgery* (1923), coauthored with Robert Jones. Lovett was a founding member of the American Orthopaedic Association and served as its president in 1898.

Arthur Jay Gillette (1864–1921), born in Prairieville, Minnesota, was educated at Hamline University (1885) and received his medical degree from St. Paul Medical College (1886). He pursued further studies at the New York Polyclinic and graduated from the program there in 1887. Most of Gillette's training was obtained at the New York Orthopaedic Dispensary and Hospital and St. Joseph's Hospital in St. Paul, where he was its first formal intern. Gillette's entire professional career after 1890 was spent in St. Paul, where he limited his practice to orthopedics. In 1897 he was named clinical professor of orthopedics at the University of Minnesota, and the following year, he was promoted to full professor. From 1913 to 1915, he headed the division. Gillette was among the first in the United States to operate for fracture of the neck of the femur (1898). He started the orthopedic department at Ancker Hospital (currently St. Paul-Ramsey Hospital) and worked to establish a state-supported hospital for indigent physically handicapped children, the first such state-supported facility in the country, built in 1910. In 1925, the Hospital for Crippled and Deformed Children was given Gillette's name.

William Stevenson Baer (1872–1931), born in Baltimore, received his bachelor's degree from The Johns Hopkins University in 1894 and his medical degree from the same institution four years later. He was an intern in surgery (1898–1899) and assistant resident in surgery the following year. Having worked with Harvey Cushing at The Hopkins, Baer was recommended by him to William Halsted to take up orthopedics as a specialty. Following Halsted's suggestion, Baer spent the summer of 1900 working in Boston on the orthopedic services at the Massachusetts General and Children's hospitals. Many of the young patients wore plaster body casts as part of their orthopedic therapy. Baer had a body cast placed on himself and wore it all summer long in an attempt to gain the children's confidence by showing them that he, too, was enduring the same discomfort. In September Baer returned to Baltimore with the title of assistant in orthopedic surgery and promptly organized an orthopedic clinic in the basement of The Johns Hopkins Hospital. Baer received little further institutional support from Halsted and was not invited by him to scrub in for orthopedic operations. Accordingly, for many summers thereafter, to further his understanding of orthopedic diseases and their treatments, Baer visited orthopedic clinics throughout Europe, including those of Adolph Lorenz (1854–1946) in Silesia, Vittorio Putti (1860–1940) in Italy, Jacques Calvé (1875–1954) in France, and Robert Jones in Liverpool. In 1905 Baer was advanced to associate in orthopedic surgery, and five years later, to associate professor. His titles notwithstanding, there was a scarcity of orthopedic patients, and the situation led Baer to seek a more active operating service at the Union Protestant Infirmary, working with its surgeon in chief, John Finney. In 1912 the board of managers of the Infirmary decided to open a Children's Hospital School for the treatment of orthopedic problems, with Baer as its head. Utilizing the combined facilities of The Johns Hopkins Hospital and the new Children's Hospital, Baer was eventually able to establish an outstanding orthopedic training program. Not until 1914 was Baer formally listed as "surgeon-in-charge, orthopaedic dispensary" at The Hopkins, and it would be another six years before he was appointed a full visiting surgeon. During World War I Baer was one of three orthopedic consultants to the American Expeditionary Forces on the Western front. Among his most important contributions to the surgical literature was his use of maggots in treating osteomyelitis (1931). His name is eponymically linked with a method of injecting sterilized oil into an ankylosed joint, after the adhesions have been broken up, to prevent their re-formation. Baer was president of the American Orthopaedic Association in 1924.

16. "Minerva Jacket-Neck Cast" by Joseph Hirsch (circa World War II). *(U.S. Naval Historical Center)*

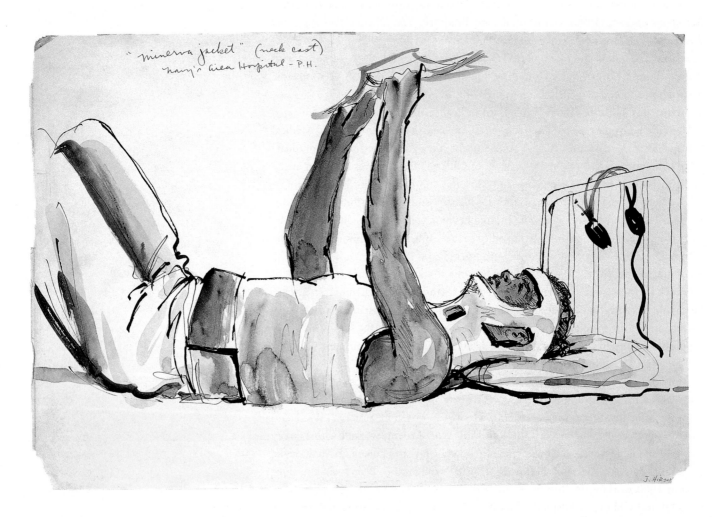

Fred Albee (1876–1945) was born in Alna, Maine, and attended Bowdoin College (1899) and Harvard Medical College (1903). He completed an internship at the Massachusetts General Hospital and entered private practice in Waterbury, Connecticut. Wishing to pursue training in orthopedics, Albee left practice to work as a radiologist and assistant to Virgil Gibney at the Hospital for the Ruptured and Crippled in New York City. Over the next few years, Albee also began working at the New York Post-Graduate Medical School and was named instructor in orthopedic surgery at Columbia University's College of Physicians and Surgeons. He conducted animal research at the Loomis Laboratories and, during operations at the clinics of the New York Post-Graduate Hospital, Bellevue Hospital, Roosevelt Hospital, and the Sea Breeze Hospital, pioneered bone graft surgery as a well-planned operative procedure (1911). In so doing, he became the world's first orthopedic surgeon to employ living bone grafts as internal splints. Albee utilized cutting machines and saws to make inlaid, perfectly fitting grafts, and discussed his findings in the influential monograph *Bone-Graft Surgery* (1915). During and after World War I, he became widely respected for his services to various governments regarding rehabilitative therapies, and he ultimately received decorations from ten foreign countries. He contributed widely to the scientific literature. His other textbooks include *Orthopaedic Surgery for Practitioners* (1908), *Orthopaedic and Reconstruction Surgery* (1919), *Injuries and Diseases of the Hip* (1937), *Bone-Graft Surgery in Diseases, Injury and Deformity* (1940), and *Surgery of the Spinal Column* (1945). Albee's name is eponymically linked with an operation for producing ankylosis of the hip in which the upper surface of the head of the femur is sliced off and the corresponding point of the edge of the acetabulum is squared, so that the two freshened bony surfaces may rest in contact. Among his many teaching appointments were assistant professor of clinical orthopedic surgery at Cornell University Medical School and professor of orthopedic surgery at Columbia University. Albee was president of the American Orthopaedic Association in 1929. Described as an aggressive and egocentric surgeon, Albee authored an autobiography, *A Surgeon's Fight to Rebuild Men* (1943), and his wife, Louella B. Albee, wrote an autobiography of their life together, *Doctor and I* (1951).

Hiram Winnett Orr (1877–1956), born in West Newton, Pennsylvania, attended the University of Nebraska (1885) while also beginning the study of medicine by apprenticing with his uncle, Hudson J. Winnett, in Lincoln, Nebraska. From 1895 to 1899, Orr matriculated at the University of Michigan School of Medicine, where he received his medical degree. He interned at Bellevue Hospital in New York City (1899) and soon returned to Lincoln, joining his uncle in practice. During the summer of 1904, he spent some months in Chicago, working under John Ridlon, professor of orthopedic surgery at Northwestern University. Orr's entire professional life after after 1899 was centered on Lincoln, where he eventually held a multitude of positions. In 1905 he helped formulate legislation for the establishment of the Nebraska Orthopedic Hospital, and he went on to become assistant surgeon and superintendent (1906–1917) and, finally, chief surgeon (1919–1948). From 1923 to 1956, he was also chief consultant and chief orthopedic surgeon to Lincoln General Hospital, Bryan Memorial Hospital, and Veterans Administration Hospital in Lincoln. During his early years he was editor of the *Western Medical Review* (1899–1906), lecturer on the history of medicine at the University of Nebraska College of Medicine (1910–1916), and chief medical inspector of the Lincoln Public Schools (1908). During World War I, Orr was invited to join the Goldthwait Unit of Orthopedic Surgery in England and also served at the Surgical Hospital Center, Savenay, France. He was discharged in 1919 with the rank of lieutenant colonel. During his wartime experience he devised the Orr method for treating osteomyelitis, compound fractures, and other infected wounds. He advocated drainage and rest in wound healing, and developed replacement techniques and control of fragments in fractures by skeletal pin fixation in plaster of Paris and other

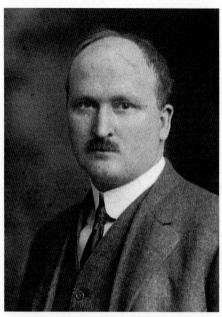

17. Fred Albee. *(Historical Collections, College of Physicians of Philadelphia)*

immobilizing devices. From this work came two textbooks: *Osteomyelitis, Compound Fractures and Other Infected Wounds* (1929) and *Wounds and Fractures: A Clinical Guide to Civil and Military Practice* (1941). Respected for his contributions to the scientific literature, Orr was editor of the *American Journal of Orthopaedic Surgery* (1919–1921). His preoccupation with the history of medicine led to his becoming an ardent book collector and resulted in his writing *On the Contributions of Hugh Owen Thomas of Liverpool, Sir Robert Jones of Liverpool and London, and John Ridlon, M.D., of New York and Chicago to Modern Orthopedic Surgery* (1949). Orr's book collection was donated to the American College of Surgeons, and a fully annotated *Catalogue of the H. Winnett Orr Historical Collection and Other Rare Books in the Library of the American College of Surgeons* was published in 1960. Active in the world of medical politics, Orr was president of the Nebraska State Medical Society (1919) and the American Orthopaedic Association (1936). In addition, he served as chairman of the American Medical Association's Orthopedic Section (1921).

Arthur Steindler (1878–1959) was born in Graslitz, Bohemia, and educated at the University of Prague (1898) and the University of Vienna School of Medicine (1902). He studied for five years (1902–1907) with Edward Albert (1841–1900), Adolf Lorenz, and Carl Friedlander in Vienna, and then emigrated to the United States and became an associate of John Ridlon at St. Luke's Hospital in Chicago (1907–1910) while also working as an orthopedic surgeon at that city's Home for Crippled Children. In 1910 Steindler resettled in Iowa, where he was appointed professor of orthopedic surgery at the Drake Medical School in Des Moines and orthopedic surgeon to the Iowa Methodist and Iowa Lutheran Hospitals. From 1915 to 1948, he was professor and head of orthopedic surgery at the State University of Iowa College of Medicine in Iowa City. Following his retirement from the university, he became chief of orthopedic surgery at Mercy Hospital in Iowa City (1949–1959). Having become a naturalized citizen in 1914, Steindler was a contract surgeon and lieutenant colonel in the U.S. Army Medical Reserve Corps during World War I. A world-renowned orthopedic surgeon and respected teacher, Steindler trained more than two hundred and fifty individuals from all over the world. His knowledge of Latin and modern European languages helped make European orthopedic developments more accessible to American surgeons. He pioneered the treatment of scoliosis by the compensatory method and also developed surgical therapies for various spinal deformities and pes cavus (clubfoot). Kinesiology and the biophysics of locomotion occupied his attention from the mid-1920s on, and he became a leader in reconstructive surgery of the extremities and the use of occupational therapy. A prolific author whose interests spanned all of orthopedics, his nine textbooks include *Reconstructive Surgery of the Upper Extremity* (1923), *Operative Orthopedics* (1925), *Diseases and Deformities of the Spine and Thorax* (1929), *The Mechanics of Normal and Pathological Locomotion of Man* (1935), *Orthopaedic Operations* (1943), and *Kinesiology of the Human Body* (1955). In 1932, Steindler was president of the American Orthopaedic Association.

Willis Cohoon Campbell (1880–1941) was born in Jackson, Mississippi, and had a peripatetic undergraduate life at Millsaps College, Hampden-Sydney College, Roanoke College, and the University of Virginia, receiving his medical degree from the last-named institution in 1904. He initially spent time training as a pediatrician and an anesthetist, but lack of success in starting a practice led him to study orthopedics in Boston, New York, and Europe. Resettling in Memphis, Tennessee (1910), Campbell organized and served as the first chairman of the department of orthopedic surgery at the University of Tennessee (1911–1941). He opened the Willis Campbell Clinic at the university medical center in 1920 and developed this institution into an internationally respected facility, renowned for the excellence of its diagnostic and therapeutic work in orthopedic surgery, as well as for its outstanding postdoctoral training program. In addition, he organized the Crippled Children's

(1919) and Crippled Adults (1923) Hospitals in Memphis and served as their chief of staff until his death. Campbell gained international recognition for many contributions to orthopedic surgery, perhaps the most notable being improved methods of repairing damaged ligaments of the knee, the use of sulfanilamide to prevent infections, the surgical reconstruction of ankylosed joints, and bone grafting to promote healing of nonunited fractures. He was a major leader in organized orthopedic surgery and served as president of the Clinical Orthopaedic Society (1928), the American Orthopaedic Association (1931), the American Academy of Orthopaedic Surgeons (1933), and the American Board of Orthopaedic Surgery (1937–1940). Campbell's three textbooks are regarded as classics: *Orthopedics of Childhood* (1927), *Orthopedic Surgery* (1930), and *Operative Orthopaedics* (1939).

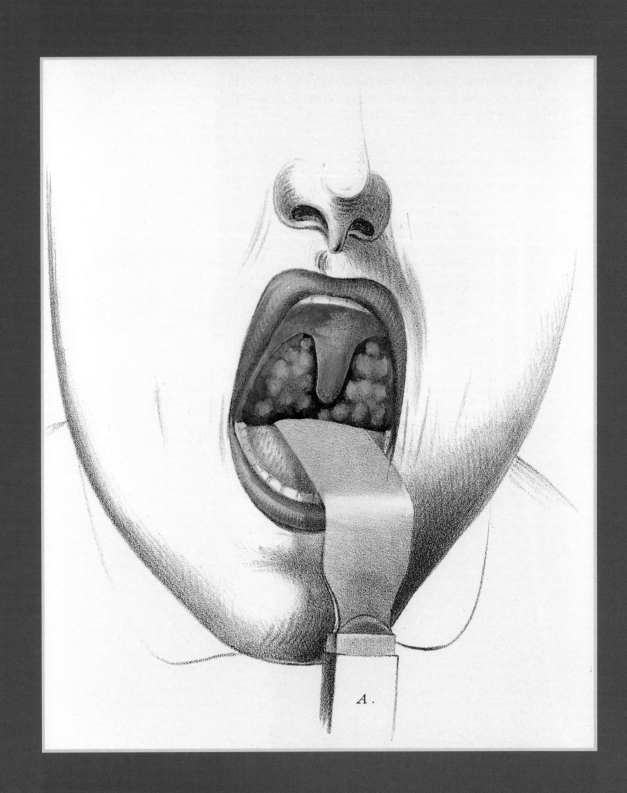

A.

CHAPTER 20

OTORHINOLARYNGOLOGIC SURGERY

lthough otorhinolaryngology did not exist as an organized surgical specialty in the United States until the twentieth century, growing numbers of nineteenth-century physician-surgeons showed an interest in the disparate fields of laryngology, otology, and rhinology. Throughout most of the 1800s, otorhinolaryngology and ophthalmology evolved together, with the old-fashioned eye-ear-nose-throat specialist obtaining much of his clinical information from leaders in Boston, Philadelphia, and New York, who had themselves sought experience in the clinics of London and Paris. This was exclusively an American innovation, but the normality of this relationship was noted in the establishment of such institutions as the New York Eye and Ear Infirmary (1820), the Pennsylvania Infirmary for Diseases of the Eye and Ear (1822), the Massachusetts Charitable Eye and Ear Infirmary (1824), the Baltimore Eye and Ear Institute (1840), the Chicago Eye and Ear Infirmary (1858), and the New Orleans Touro Eye and Ear Infirmary (1876). This assocation of otorhinolaryngology with ophthalmology was enhanced when the executive committee of the American Medical Association authorized, in 1878, establishment of a joint Section on Ophthalmology and Otolaryngology. However, clinical and political imbroglios were already beginning to cause this alignment to weaken, and a decade later, an American Medical Association's Section on Otology, Rhinology and Laryngology received independent status. Aside from the political differences, the simple financial fact was that many otorhinolaryngologists continued to include ophthalmology in their everyday practice, as was noted in the publication of clinically inclusive texts such as George DeSchweinitz's (1858–1938) and Burton Randall's (1858–1932) mammoth *An American Text-Book of Diseases of the Eye, Ear, Nose and Throat* (1899). In certain instances, the ties remained long lasting, as was demonstrated by the American Academy of Ophthalmology and Otolaryngology, founded in 1896, which continued to hold joint meetings of the two specialties well into the 1970s.

Within otorhinolaryngology, laryngology and otology evolved separately throughout most of the 1800's. A gradual melding of the disciplines did not occur until the founding of such organizations as the Section on Otology, Rhinology and Laryngology of the American Medical Association in 1888 and the American Laryngological, Rhinological and Otological Society in 1895. By most accounts, the history of laryngology in the United States and elsewhere formally began with the discovery of the laryngoscope in Europe in the late 1850s. The instrument was introduced into America during the early 1860s, primarily through the efforts of Ernest Krackowizer (1821–1875), an Austrian physician who had emigrated to New York City. He was probably the first physician in this country to visualize the vocal

1. *(facing page)* Horace Green drew this color plate from life and included it in his *Treatise on Diseases of the Air Passages* (1846), the country's first monograph on otorhinolaryngologic surgery. The figure demonstrates tonsillar pathology and an enlarged uvula, which interfered with the patient's breathing. *(Author's Collection)*

cords. While the value of the new methodology was immediately recognized, it was some time before the use of the laryngoscope became widespread. Meanwhile, under the leadership of such individuals as Horace Green (1802–1866), Louis Elsberg (1836–1885), and Jacob DaSilva Solis-Cohen (1838–1927), the study of throat diseases continued.

The primary concern of early otologists was mastoid disease. In most instances, mastoid infections were allowed to develop into "brain fever" unless sufficient local signs were present to suggest that an uncomplicated retroauricular incision and drainage could be accomplished and would suffice as therapy. The first simple mastoidectomy in the United States was completed by Laurence Turnbull (1821–1900) in the early 1860s. Not until the 1870s was trephining of the mastoid process routinely practiced. Even then, infection of the mastoid cell structure often worsened because of forcible irrigations through the trephine opening in an effort to clean out detritus via an existing hole in the tympanic membrane or down the eustachian tube into the throat. As a result, ear infections were often permitted to simply "break out" with the assistance of a hot poultice.

Long before the laryngoscope was introduced or the technical intricacies of mastoidectomy were understood, eminent American physician-surgeons were working in these clinical areas. During the 1820s, Philip Syng Physick improved on his performance of tonsillectomy, previously completed by means of strangulation with a soft wire carried around the tonsillar tissue by a double cannula. By 1828 he had devised an instrument that is the progenitor of all tonsil guillotines, while also describing a forceps "employed to facilitate the extirpation of the tonsil." Samuel Akerly (1785–1845) was active in establishing institutions for deaf-mutes and the blind and, in 1824, authored a pamphlet, *Observations and Correspondence on the Nature and Cure of Deafness, and Other Diseases of the Ears*. Other important contributions to the periodical literature were made by George Lehman (1806–1859) on otitis (1829), George Bushe (1797–1836) on tonsillectomy (1832), Joshua Cohen (1801–1870) on deafness (1841), and Edward Clarke (1820–1877) on aural surgery (1852). A spectacular surgical *tour-de-force* was described by Valentine Mott (1785–1865) when he became the first American surgeon to remove a fibrous growth from the nostril by division of the nasal and maxillary bones (1843). Five years later, Gurdon Buck (1807–1877) reported on "oedematous laryngitis successfully treated by scarifications of the glottis and epiglottis" at a meeting of the American Medical Association. In 1851, Buck performed the country's first known operation for a cancer of the larynx by an external incision. The patient had an epithelial cancer involving the ventricles and vocal cords, the base of the epiglottis, and the aryteno-epiglottic folds, and Buck completed a laryngotracheotomy with partial extirpation of the tumor. The patient eventually had a tracheotomy tube inserted because of extension of the disease, but died of suffocation while attempting to change the cannula (1852).

In 1840 Horace Green startled the medical profession by claiming to be able to pass a sponge-tipped probang, a curved instrument of whalebone ten inches long, into the larynx and thus directly apply medication to the laryngeal mucosa. For the next two decades, he was involved in acrimonious debate over the validity of his research. His textbooks, *A Treatise on Diseases of the Air Passages: Comprising An Inquiry into the History, Pathology, Causes, and Treatment of Those Affections of the Throat Called Bronchitis, Chronic Laryngitis, and Clergyman's Sore Throat* (1846), *Observations on the Pathology of Croup: With Remarks On Its Treatment by Topical Medications* (1849), and *On The Surgical Treatment of Polypi of the Larynx, and Oedema of the Glottis* (1852), were scrutinized in detail. By 1854 the controversy had become so bitter that Green was forced to defend his findings at a public meeting at the New York Academy of Medicine. His talk excited so much heated discussion that the presiding officer was compelled to quell the clamor by appointing a committee to investigate the truth of Green's claims. The committee came to no definitive conclusions, and this seems to have ended the bitter campaign waged against Green. In due time, with acceptance

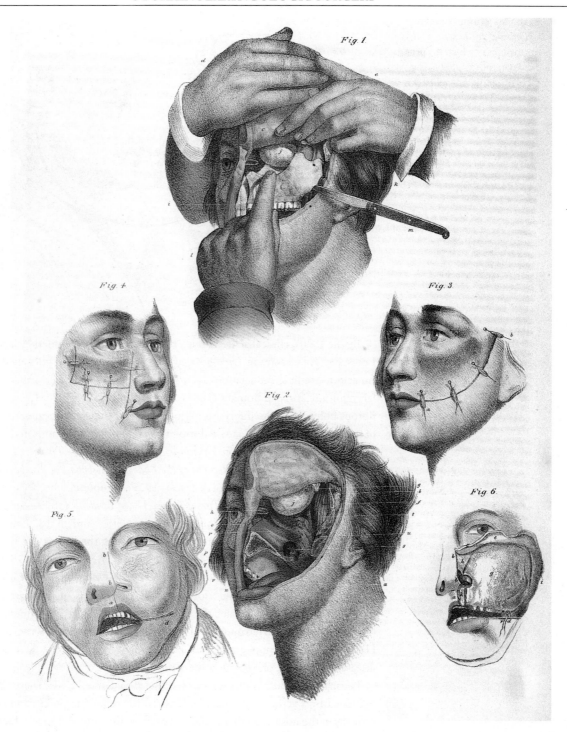

of his research, he became the first physician in this country to confine his practice to diseases of the throat.

James Bryan (1810–1881), professor of surgery at Geneva Medical College in upstate New York, authored the country's first textbook on the ear, (1851). It was eventually followed by Edward Clarke's *Observations on the Nature and Treatment of Polypus of the Ear* (1867). The American Ophthalmological and Otological Society was formed in 1864, mainly among "specialists" in Boston, New York, and Philadelphia. Four years later, those interested in the ear withdrew to form the American Otological Society. These two American societies, limited in membership, antedated all similar groups in Europe and represent the earliest surgical specialty societies in the world. Within a few years, numerous textbooks on otology were being published, including: Laurence Turnbull's *A Clinical Manual of the Diseases of the Ear* (1872), Daniel Bennett St. John Roosa's *A Practical Treatise on the Diseases of the Ear, Including the Anatomy of the Organ* (1873), and Charles Burnett's (1842–1902), *The Ear; Its Anatomy, Physiology, and Diseases* (1877).

2. There are few more terrifying plates in Joseph Pancoast's remarkable *A Treatise on Operative Surgery* (1844) than this view of a resection of the upper jaw. Following in a long tradition of surgical illustrations, the idealized patient is depicted as placid and wide awake while undergoing an operation that must have been completely unbearable in this preanesthetic era. (*Author's Collection*)

547

3. This wood engraving from Laurence Turnbull's *Clinical Manual of the Diseases of the Ear* (1872) shows the manner in which the permeability of the eustachian tube could be diagnosed by a eustachian catheter. (*Author's Collection*)

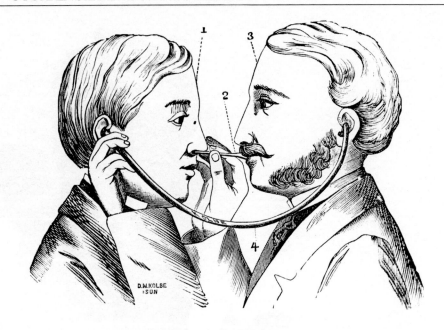

By the 1870s, clinical achievements were being regularly touted by laryngologists. Louis Elsberg's essay on *Laryngoscopal Surgery* (1866) won a gold medal from the American Medical Association. Henry Sands (1830–1888) performed a successful laryngotomy for papillomata (1865), and Jacob DaSilva Solis-Cohen removed a fibrous polyp from the inferior anterior surface of the right vocal cord with the aid of the laryngoscope (1867). Also during this era, Solis-Cohen authored the country's first systematic textbook on laryngology, *Diseases of the Throat: A Guide to the Diagnosis and Treatment of Affections of the Pharynx, Aesophagus, Trachea, Larynx, and Nares* (1872). Francke Bosworth (1843–1925) completed the decade by writing *Handbook Upon Diseases of the Throat for the Use of Students* (1879). American physicians were the first to form laryngologic societies and in 1873 the New York Laryngological Society was founded, mainly through the efforts of Clinton Wagner (1837–1914). Six years later, Elsberg and George Lefferts (1846–1920) were the guiding force behind the American Laryngological Association, the earliest national organization to be established for the study of diseases of the larynx, nose, and throat. In 1873 Wagner opened the first facility exclusively for treatment of nose and throat diseases, the Metropolitan Throat Hospital. That same year, the faculty at Harvard Medical School established a department for instruction in nose and throat disease, the earliest on record in the United States.

During the 1880s, William Jarvis (1855–1895) devised a wire snare that could be tightened by a screw in the handle. Utilized for removing polyps and other sessile growths in the nose and other accessible cavities, this simple device, which was nothing more than a cold wire ecraseur, brought about a new era in intra-nasal surgery. By placement in the hands of both the specialist and general practitioner a safe and easy method for the removal of neoplasms and deformities, modern rhinology was established. Jarvis went on to pioneer the use of cocaine in intra-asal surgery (1884) and an electric light for illuminating the upper air passages (1885), thus making use of the Jarvis snare more practical. In 1882 Ephraim Ingals (1848–1918) described his operation of partial excision of the nasal septum for correction of a deviation. Seven years later, Joseph Bryan (1856–1935) delivered a paper before the Section on Laryngology and Otology of the American Medical Association that contained a classic description of sinusitis. His research into the accessory sinuses stimulated further clinical work in rhinology and culminated with Bosworth's writing the two-volume *A Treatise on Diseases of the Nose and Throat* (1889–1892). It is interesting to note that in the decade since the appearance of his *A Manual of Diseases of the Throat and Nose* (1881), Bosworth changed his emphasis from the throat to the nose by reversing their order in the title. Despite the increasing interest in rhinological surgery, a formal specialty society for rhinology was never organized. Instead, rhinologists tended to also be laryngologists, and rhinologic scientific presentations were usually made at laryngology meetings.

Despite the growing enthusiasm for otorhinolaryngology, formalized clinical instruction in the field(s) was virtually nonexistent in American medical schools until the mid-1880s. Outpatient facilities were primitive and consisted of a few Argand gas burners or some borrowed head mirrors. Clinical lectures made little impression on students busy with general medicine, obstetrics, and surgery. Still, by the early 1890s, practicing physicians were creating a considerable demand for brief preparatory courses (six weeks to four months) in otorhinolaryngology. In many instances, these proprietary courses gave only the most superficial acquaintance with the specialty. Particularly lacking was instruction in head and neck pathology. Similar short-term courses were instituted by English-speaking European surgeons, notably in Berlin and Vienna. American physicians were returning to their home towns with the lucrative imprimatur of "specialist." Only time would demonstrate how many physicians came home from these courses to find, in emergency situations, how poor their basic training in otorhinolaryngology truly was, most notably in difficult operative techniques.

Like other specialty areas, scientific journals were important to the evolution of the field. In 1875 the *Transactions of the American Otological Society* were first published. Other otological journals were also started during the last quarter of the nineteenth century, including the *American Journal of Otology* (1879–1882), edited by Clarence Blake (1843–1919); Jakob H. Knapp's (1832–1911) *Archives of Ophthalmology and Otology* (1869-1900), which was divided into its component sections, the *Archives of Ophthalmology* and *Archives of Otology* in 1879; and James Parker's (1854–1896) *Annals of Ophthalmology and Otology*, which began in 1892 and was separated into the *Annals of Ophthalmology* and *Annals of Otology, Rhinology and Laryngology* in the year of Parker's death. The latter journal continues to remain prominent, and its editors and their years of service include Hannau W. Loeb (1900–1927), Lew W. Dean (1927–1944), Arthur W Proetz (1936–1966), Ben H. Senturia (1967–1981), and Brian F. McCabe, (1982–??).

During the same time period, the *Transactions of the American Laryngological Association* were first being published (1881). Louis Elsberg issued the *Archives of Laryngology* for just four volumes before ceasing publication in 1883. *The Laryngoscope* was founded in 1896 by Max Goldstein (1870–1941). The only periodical devoted to homeopathic otorhinolaryngology was the *Homoeopathic Eye and Ear Journal*, first published in 1895. It was the official organ of the Ophthalmological, Otological and Laryngological Society, an association strictly exclusive to homeopathic physicians practicing otorhinolaryngology. Of more modern journals, the *Archives of Otolaryngology* was established in 1925 by the trustees of the American Medical Association, with George E. Shambaugh, Sr., as the first editor-in- chief. It is one of the most influential of current peer-reviewed journals in otorhinolaryngology, and its name was changed to the *Archives of Otolaryngology–Head and Neck Surgery* in the 1990s to better reflect the clinical areas that now constitute the specialty. Recent editors-in-chief and their years of service are George E. Shambaugh, Jr. (1958–1969), Bobby R. Alford (1970–1979), Byron J. Bailey (1980–1991), and Michael E. Johns (1992–??).

During the last two decades of the nineteenth century, several important clinical events helped bring about further maturation of the specialty. In the mid-1880s, Thomas French (1849–1929), a lecturer on laryngoscopy and diseases of the throat at Long Island College Hospital Medical School, succeeded for the first time in photographing the living larynx. Utilizing "sunlight as the illuminating power," he was able to demonstrate laryngeal pathology that most physicians had never before seen. Joseph O'Dwyer (1841–1898), of New York City, pioneered laryngeal intubation. At a time when tracheotomy was the only method, though ineffective, of treating asphyxiation in diphtheria, O'Dwyer tubes became widespread. Subsequently, the Fell-O'Dwyer method of artificial respiration, in which air was forced into the lungs by bellows through an endotracheal tube, became the most practical method of

4. "Inoperable," A pen-and-ink drawing (circa 1858) by Lucius M. Sargent (1826–1864). Sargent was a house surgeon to the Massachusetts General Hospital when he was appointed "artist to the hospital," which entitles him to be considered the country's first medical illustrator. This scene is unique because it vividly demonstrates the difficulty that American surgeons had in coping with certain disease entities. No known surgeon's skill could help this individual, who appears to have a morbid mandibular growth. Sargent was a brother of Fitzwilliam Sargent (1820–1889), author of *On Bandaging and Other Operations of Minor Surgery* (1848), who in turn was father of the renowned painter John Singer Sargent (1856–1925). Lucius Sargent served as a surgeon in the Civil War, was shot off his horse in an engagement on Meherrin River, Virginia, and died a few days later. (*Courtesy of the Francis A. Countway Library of Medicine*)

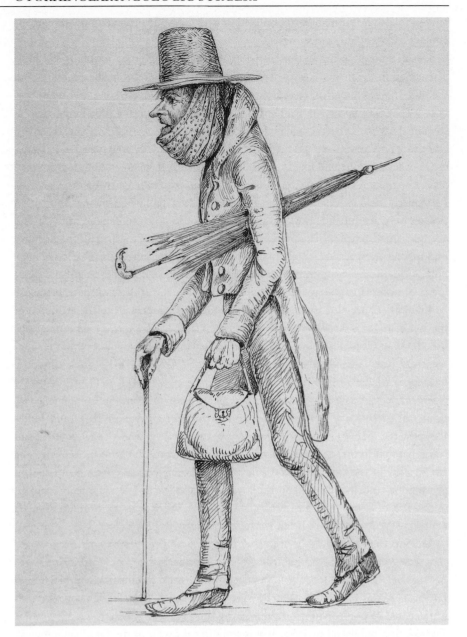

mechanical ventilation in the management of pneumonia. In 1891 Francke Bosworth authored a classic paper on various forms of disease of the ethmoid cells. Two years later, George Caldwell (1834–1918), an instructor in laryngology at the New York Polyclinic Hospital, described an operation of radical exenteration of the contents of the maxillary antrum through an opening made in the supradental (canine) fossa above the second molar tooth. So extensive was the growing interest in otorhinolaryngology that between 1885 and 1900, over thirty-five textbooks were published. Two of the more important were Charles Burnett's two-volume *System of Diseases of the Ear, Nose, and Throat* (1893), the first multiauthored American text on otorhinolaryngology, and Levi Cooper Lane's (1830–1902) almost 1,200-page *The Surgery of the Head and Neck* (1896), the country's first full-length work on head and neck surgery and the first surgical text published in California.

In most respects, otorhinolaryngology at the turn of the century was primarily concerned with the operative intervention, drainage, and control of sepsis in these areas. This was exemplified by Edward Dench's (1864–1936) popularization of the radical mastoidectomy for chronic suppuration within the temporal bone and by the fact that tonsillectomy and adenoidectomy were fast becoming the most common surgical operations performed in America. Most importantly, the careers of several influential full-time otorhinolaryngologists had begun, especially Chevalier Jackson (1865–1958) in Philadelphia and Harris Mosher (1867–1956) in Boston. These clinician-scientists bridged the evolution of otorhinolaryngology from an informal field of specialization within the whole of medicine to a dynamic and fully organized surgical specialty. However, deficiencies in education and clinical performance were still manifest, being particularly noticeable during World War I at the Fort Oglethorpe training center for military otorhinolaryngologists and ophthalmologists. While attempts were made to utilize poorly qualified personnel, serious difficulties arose in Army camps in this country and in base hospitals abroad.

It was evident to leaders in national otorhinolaryngologic societies that improved education and training for the practice of the specialty was imperative. For this reason, an examining body, the American Board of Otolaryngology, was established in 1924. Coming three years after the American Board of Ophthalmology was founded, the American Board of Otolaryngology was the second certifying board formed in the United States. Among those chiefly responsible for the formation was George E. Shambaugh, Sr., who requested that the American Laryngological Society, the American Otological Society, the Triological Society (now known as the American Laryngological, Rhinological and Otological Society), the Academy of Ophthalmology and Otolaryngology (since separated into the American Academy of Otolaryngology—Head and Neck Surgery), and the Section on Laryngology and Otology of the American Medical Association appoint two members each. Members of the Laryngological, Otological, and Triological Societies became the first diplomates of the new board, and the first formal examinations were held in Philadelphia in 1925. Since that time, several other organizations have become sponsors, including the American Broncho-Esophagological Association (1947), the American Society for Head and Neck Surgery (1947), the American Academy of Facial Plastic and Reconstructive Surgery (1971), the American Society of Ophthalmologic and Otolaryngic Allergy (1974), the American Society of Pediatric Otolaryngology (1989), the American Neurotology Society (1991), and the American Rhinologic Society (1994).

A decided improvement in education and training was evident by World War II, when diplomates of the American Board of Otolaryngology secured better recognition and clinical appointments than those without certification status. This era saw several outstanding clinical advances. Robert Lynch devised an operation for the conservative treatment of sinusitis (1924); Arthur Proetz (1888–1966) described the displacement method of treatment of nasal sinusitis (1926); Walter Dandy (1886–1946) formalized his operation for relief of Ménière's syndrome (1928); Maurice Sourdille (1885–1961) published, in the *Bulletin of the New York Academy of Medicine*, a description of the first successful attempt to restore hearing in otosclerosis by fenestration (1937); Julius Lempert (1890–1972) utilized a one-stage fenestration operation to restore hearing in cases of otosclerosis (1938); Samuel Kopetzky (1876–1950) further improved the technique of surgical operations on the labyrinthine capsule (1941); George E. Shambaugh, Jr. (1903–1969) completed research into the surgical treatment of deafness (1942); and Chevalier Jackson and his son Chevalier L. Jackson (1900–1961) authored *Diseases of the Air and Food Passages of Foreign Body Origin* (1937), one of the most comprehensive treatises on the subject ever published.

Currently, the American Board of Otolaryngology defines a certified specialist in this field as one who provides comprehensive medical and surgical care of patients with diseases and disorders that affect the ears, the respiratory and upper alimentary systems, and related structures, and the head and neck in general. Examinees are required to have undergone five years of postgraduate specialty training, which must include one or more years of general surgery and three or more years of otolaryngology–head and neck surgery in approved residency programs. According to guidelines established by the board, the otolaryngologist-head and neck surgeon is responsible for knowing, among various subject areas, the communication sciences, including audiology and speech language pathology; the chemical senses and treatment of allergies; head and neck oncology; and facial plastic and reconstructive surgery.

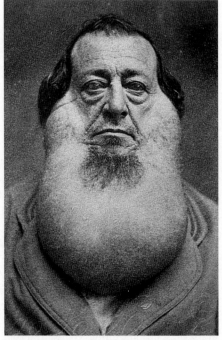

5. An advanced case of cystic hygroma or lymphangioma (circa 1870s). When a growth attained such enormous size it caused difficulty with swallowing and even breathing. This photographic image may have been what Lucius Sargent had in mind when he drew "Inoperable." *(Courtesy of Stanley B. Burns, M.D., and The Burns Collection and Archives)*

In January 1995, of the approximately 621,000 total physicians in active practice in the United States, 8,785 (1.4 percent) designated themselves as otorhinolaryngologic surgeons. Within this cadre of otorhinolaryngologic surgeons, 6,340 (72 percent) were board certified. (By contrast, during the fifteen years between 1980 and 1994, 3,768 certificates in otorhinolaryngologic surgery were issued, or an average of 251 per year.) Of the 1995 total, 595 (7 percent) were women, and 1,095 (12%) were international medical graduates. Among the total pool of otorhinolaryngologic surgeons, approximately 1,760 (20 percent) were younger than 35; 2,540 (29 percent) were 35 to 44; 2,265 (26 percent) were 45 to 54; 1,640 (19 percent) were 55 to 64; and 585 (7 percent) were 65 years old and older. Of the 595 female otorhinolaryngologic surgeons, 510 (86 percent) were under 44, in contrast to the approximately 8,190 male otorhinolaryngologic surgeons, of whom 3,785 (46 percent) were under 44.

When otorhinolaryngologists were queried by members of the research subcommittee of the *Study on Surgical Services for the United States* (1976) regarding important otorhinolaryngologic surgical contributions from 1945 to 1970, surgery for conductive deafness was considered of first-order importance, translabyrinthine removal of acoustic neuroma was deemed of second-order importance, and further development of conservation surgery for laryngeal cancer, nasal septoplasty, and myringotomy and ventillation tube for serous otitis media were termed third-order contributions.

The writing of the history of otorhinolaryngology has not been well served by American authors; only Jonathan Wright (1860–1928) has completed a full-length monograph, *A History of Laryngology and Rhinology* (1914). The following biographies provide a brief understanding of the lives of several American otorhinolaryngologists. However, it should be noted that American otorhinolaryngology, like every other surgical specialty, offers such a plethora of famous names that a certain invidiousness is inevitable in selection. No attempt at a truly general and representative portrayal of the specialty can be provided in the space available.

BIOGRAPHIES OF OTORHINOLARYNGOLOGIC SURGEONS

Laurence Turnbull (1821–1900) was born in Shotts, Lanarkshire, Scotland, and brought to the United States in 1833. He initially studied at the Philadelphia College of Pharmacy (1842), and spent a year working as an apothecary. However, wishing to practice medicine, Turnbull apprenticed with John K. Mitchell (1793–1858) in Philadelphia and matriculated at the Jefferson Medical College in 1845. He served for a year as a resident physician at the Blockley Hospital and by 1857 had gained enough clinical experience to be appointed to the department of diseases of the eye and ear at the Western Clinical Infirmary (later renamed the Howard Hospital). In 1859, Turnbull toured European eye and ear clinics–a tradition he would continue throughout his career. During the Civil War he served at Emory Hospital and Fortress Monroe. Following the conclusion of hostilities, Turnbull rejoined the surgical staff at Howard Hospital and, in 1878, was elected aural surgeon of the Jefferson Hospital. In 1880 he was chairman of the American Medical Association's Section of Ophthalmology, Laryngology and Otology. Although Turnbull's chief work was in ophthalmology and otology, he is remembered as the first American surgeon to author a full-length textbook on anesthesia and its applications, *The Advantages and Accidents of Artificial Anaesthesia* (1878). This was followed by *The New Local Anaesthetic; Hydrochlorate of Cocaine (Muriate of Cocaine), and Etherization by the Rectum* (1885). In 1862 Turnbull reported the country's first performance of a mastoidectomy. Three years later he authored a short pamphlet, *Defective and Impaired Vision, With the Clinical Use of the Ophthalmoscope in Their Diagnosis and Treatment*. Respected as an aural surgeon, Turnbull wrote the almost five-hundred-page *A Clinical Manual of the Diseases of the Ear* (1872) and *Imperfect Hearing and the Hygiene of the Ear* (1881).

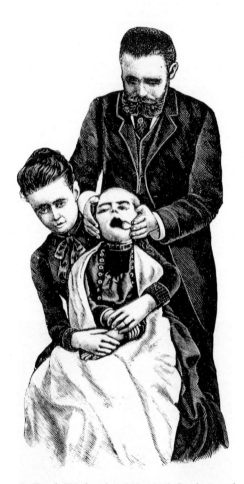

6. Frank Waxham's (1852–1911) *Intubation of the Larynx* (1888) was unusual in that the publisher, Charles Truax, was actually a surgical instrument maker. Waxham was professor of otology, rhinology and laryngology at the College of Physicians and Surgeons in Chicago, where he was an early advocate of intubation in the treatment of diphtheria and croup in children. In the process of perfecting his intubation technique, Waxham began to use tubes made according to his instructions by Truax's manufacturing company. From their designer–manufacturer relationship emerged this monograph on intubation. Without its forty-five engravings, including this one showing the "proper position of patient," physicians could not easily grasp all the details necessary for the procedure to be successful. *(Author's Collection)*

Morris Joseph Asch (1833–1902) was born in Philadelphia and received bachelor's (1852) and master's (1855) degrees from the University of Pennsylvania. The latter year, he also graduated from Jefferson Medical College, and was soon appointed clinical assistant to Samuel D. Gross. In 1861 Asch passed the examination for assistant surgeon of the United States Army, and he was stationed at the surgeon general's office from 1861 to 1862. He subsequently rose in rank to become a medical inspector of the Army of the Potomac and medical director of the 24th Army Corps. He did not formally resign his military commission until 1873, when he entered the practice of medicine in New York City. Largely devoting himself to the study and treatment of diseases of the nose and throat, Asch was appointed surgeon to the throat departments of the New York Eye and Ear Infirmary and the Manhattan Eye and Ear Hospital. He was a founding member of the American Laryngological Association and, for a time, held the position of professor of laryngology at the New York Polyclinic Hospital. His name is eponymically linked with Asch's operation for deviated nasal septum, which utilized "crucial incisions through the convex portion and then overlapped the flaps so as to straighten the septum" (1890).

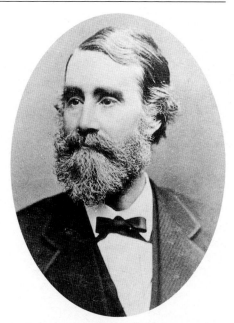

7. Laurence Turnbull. (*Historical Collections, College of Physicians of Philadelphia*)

Louis Elsberg (1836–1885) was born in Iserlohn, Prussia, and brought to the United States at the age of 13. He received his medical degree from Jefferson Medical College in 1857 and completed a short "residency" at the Mt. Sinai Hospital in New York City. Elsberg then traveled to Europe and studied laryngology for a year with Johann Czermak (1828–1873) in Vienna. In 1866, Elsberg's essay *Laryngoscopal Surgery Illustrated in the Treatment of Morbid Growths Within the Larynx* was awarded a prestigious gold medal from the American Medical Association. Seventeen years later, he reported two successful cases of internal esophagotomy, the first to be completed in the country. Most of Elsberg's professional life was spent in New York City, where he served as professor of laryngology at the University Medical College for seventeen years. One of the preeminent early figures in American laryngology, he was the first in the United States to demonstrate in public the laryngoscope for diagnosis and treatment. The short-lived *American Archives of Laryngology* was issued under his editorial guidance (1880–1884). Elsberg was one of the founders of the American Laryngological Association and served as its first president (1879).

Jacob DaSilva Solis-Cohen (1838–1927), born in New York City, graduated from the University of Pennsylvania School of Medicine in 1860. He interned at the Philadelphia Hospital in 1861 and then served in the Medical Corps of the U.S. Navy (1861–1864) and Army (1864–1865). After 1866, Solis-Cohen practiced medicine in Philadelphia, where he was appointed to the electro-therapeutics faculty (1867–1869) and was a lecturer on laryngoscopy and diseases of the throat (1870–1883) at Jefferson Medical College. From 1883 until his retirement from active practice, he was on the faculty of diseases of the throat and chest at the Philadelphia Polyclinic and College for Graduates in Medicine. Solis-Cohen also taught physiology and hygiene of the voice at the National School of Elocution and Oratory in Philadelphia. Through his numerous publications and teaching, Solis-Cohen helped establish laryngology as a surgical specialty in the United States, and he trained many of the leading laryngologists of his time. He was one the first American physicians to study the use of the laryngoscope, and in 1867 he performed one of the earliest excisions of a fibrous polyp from the inferior anterior surface of the right vocal cord with the aid of that instrument. Whether the polyp was cancerous or not remains uncertain, but he is generally given credit for completing the first successful operation for laryngeal cancer. Among his textbooks are *Inhalation: Its Therapeutics and Practice* (1867), *Diseases of the Throat: A Guide to the Diagnosis and Treatment of Affections of the Pharynx, Aesophagus, Trachea, Larynx, and Nares* (1872), *Croup, In Its Relation to Tracheotomy* (1874), and *The Throat and The Voice* (1879). A founder of the American Laryngological Association and its president from 1880 to 1882, he also helped edit the *Archives of Laryngology* for several years.

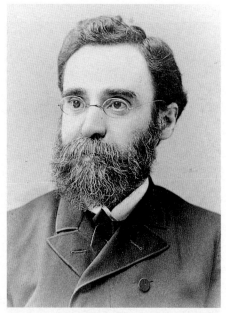

8. Jacob DaSilva Solis-Cohen. (*Historical Collections, College of Physicians of Philadelphia*)

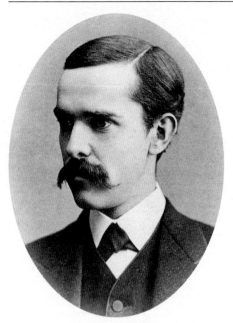

9. Charles Henry Burnett. (*Historical Collections, College of Physicians of Philadelphia*)

Albert Henry Buck (1842–1922), son of Gurdon Buck and born in New York City, received his undergraduate education at Yale University (1864) and a medical diploma from New York City's College of Physicians and Surgeons (1867). After serving a twelve-month internship at the New York Hospital, Buck spent almost three years abroad studying the physiology of the ear in various German and Austrian clinics. Returning to his native city, he was appointed aural surgeon to the New York Eye and Ear Infirmary. He remained associated with this institution for the rest of his professional life. From 1888 to 1904, Buck was also clinical professor of diseases of the ear at the College of Physicians and Surgeons. He proved an important individual in the history of American otorhinolaryngologic surgery because of his writings and his service as president of the American Otological Society in 1879. Buck was one of the most prolific writers among nineteenth-century surgeons, contributing three otologic texts, *Diagnosis and Treatment of Ear Diseases* (1880), *A Manual of Diseases of the Ear* (1889), and *First Principles of Otology* (1899); and various other works, including *A Treatise on Hygiene and Public Health* (1879) and *A Vest-Pocket Medical Dictionary* (1896). He also edited the nine-volume *A Reference Hand-Book of the Medical Sciences, Embracing the Entire Range of Scientific and Practical Medicine and Allied Science By Various Writers* (1886–1893) and jointly edited, with Joseph Bryant (1845–1916), the eight-volume *American Practice of Surgery* (1906–1911). A distinguished scholar and linguist, Buck was interested in the history of medicine and wrote *The Growth of Medicine From the Earliest Times to About 1800* (1917) and *The Dawn of Modern Medicine* (1920).

Charles Henry Burnett (1842–1902) was born in Philadelphia, graduated from Yale University in 1864, and received his medical degree from the University of Pennsylvania in 1867. He was appointed resident physician in the Episcopal Hospital of Philadelphia and, upon completing his one-year term, spent ten months in various hospitals in Europe (1868–1869). Burnett returned to his native city and practiced general medicine for a brief time. Interested in otology, he abandoned his practice and traveled again to Europe, where he worked in the laboratories of Hermann Helmholtz (1821–1894) and Rudolf Virchow (1821–1902) and in the hospital clinic of the Austrian otologist Adam Politzer (1835–1920). Resettling once again in Philadelphia, Burnett established a practice devoted solely to diseases of the ear. In 1882 he was elected professor of diseases of the ear at the Philadelphia Polyclinic Hospital and Medical College. At various other times, Burnett was clinical professor of otology in the Woman's Medical College, aural surgeon to the Presbyterian Hospital, and consulting aurist to the Pennsylvania Institution for Deaf and Dumb and the Philadelphia Hospital for Epileptics. Among his textbooks are *The Ear; Its Anatomy, Physiology, and Diseases* (1877), *Hearing And How to Keep It* (1879), *Diseases and Injuries of the Ear: Their Prevention and Cure* (1889), the two-volume *System of Diseases of the Ear, Nose, and Throat* (1893), and *A Textbook on Diseases of the Ear, Nose and Throat* (1901). For many years, he edited the department of progress of otology in the *American Journal of the Medical Sciences*. Burnett was president of the American Otological Society in 1884.

Emil Gruening (1842–1914) was born in Hohensalza, Prussia (now Inowraclaw, Poland), and emigrated to the United States in 1862. Two years later, he began to study medicine at the College of Physicians and Surgeons in New York City, but his education was temporarily interrupted by the Civil War and his service in the 7th New Jersey Volunteer Infantry. Gruening eventually received his medical diploma in 1867. For the next three years, he pursued postgraduate studies in Berlin, London, and Paris, working especially with Albrecht von Graefe (1828–1870). Returning to New York City in 1870, he was appointed to the surgical staff of the Ophthalmic and Aural Institute, where he was personal assistant to J. Hermann Knapp. From 1878 to 1912, Gruening was ophthalmic surgeon to the New York Eye and Ear Infirmary. He was also on staff at the Mt. Sinai Hospital (1879–1904) and the German (Lenox Hill) Hospital (1880–1904). In addition, he was on the ophthalmology faculty of the New York Polyclinic (1882–1895). Gruening, a pioneer in both ophthalmology and

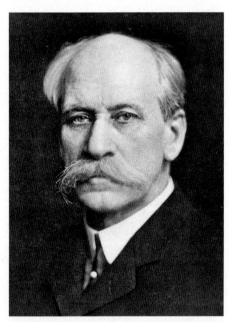

10. Francke Huntington Bosworth. (*Historical Collections, College of Physicians of Philadelphia*)

otorhinolaryngology, helped develop the modern mastoid operation and was among the first to describe and operate successfully upon brain abscesses of otitic origin (1898). He also called attention to the danger of blindness from the consumption of wood alcohol. In 1886 Gruening was president of the New York Ophthalmological Society; in 1903, of the American Otological Society; and in 1910, of the American Ophthalmological Society.

Francke Huntington Bosworth (1843–1925) was born in Marietta, Ohio, and attended Marietta College (1858–1860) but graduated from Yale University in 1862 and the Bellevue Hospital Medical College in 1868. He interned at Bellevue Hospital in 1868 and subsequently began to undertake further training in laryngology. In 1871 he was appointed lecturer on diseases of the throat at his alma mater. Ten years later he became full professor, a position he continued to hold even after Bellevue became united with New York University Medical College (1898) and until he retired from clinical practice. Bosworth was a pioneering laryngologist, who is also credited with having developed the science of rhinology as a well-defined field of surgical specialization. Among his contributions to the scientific literature were a description of a nasal saw to remove septal spurs and other obstructions (1887) and a classic paper on the physiology and pathology of the sinuses (1891). His textbooks include *Handbook Upon Diseases of the Throat for the Use of Students* (1879), *A Manual of Diseases of the Throat and Nose* (1881), the two-

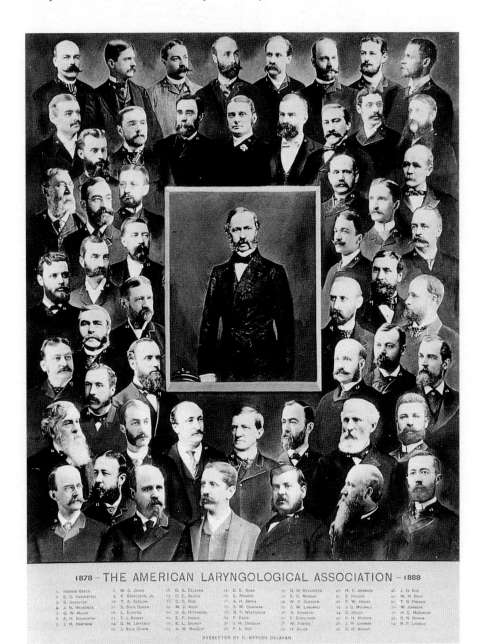

1878 – THE AMERICAN LARYNGOLOGICAL ASSOCIATION – 1888

PRESENTED BY D. BRYSON DELAVAN

11. For the ten-year celebration of its founding, members of the American Laryngological Association were ceremoniously arranged around Horace Green, the "father of American laryngology." (*Historical Collections, College of Physicians of Philadelphia*)

12. Thomas French (1849–1929) was a lecturer on laryngoscopy and diseases of the throat at Long Island College Hospital Medical School in Brooklyn when he perfected a method of photography to depict structures located inside the human body. Subsequently, French was the first to obtain satisfactory photographs of the larynx (*New York Medical Journal* vol. 40, pages 653–656, 1884) and exhibited his work at meetings of the American Laryngological Association. (*Historical Collections, College of Physicians of Philadelphia*)

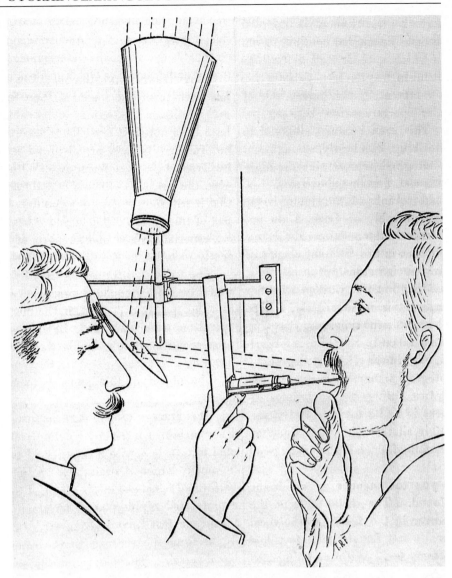

volume *A Treatise on Diseases of the Nose and Throat* (1889–1892), *Taking Cold* (1891), *A Text-Book of Diseases of the Nose and Throat* (1896), and *The Doctor in Old New York* (1898). He was a founder of the New York Laryngological Society (1873) and the American Laryngological Society (1882).

George Morewood Lefferts (1846–1920) was born in Brooklyn, New York, and graduated from the College of Physicians and Surgeons of Columbia University in 1870. He completed an internship at Bellevue and St. Luke's Hospitals and then traveled abroad to pursue further postgraduate training in London, Paris, and Vienna, where he worked with Karl Störk, a founder of laryngology in Europe. From 1871 to 1873, Lefferts was chief of Störk's clinic at the University of Vienna. Returning to the United States, Lefferts began practice in New York City, specializing in diseases of the nose and throat, and was appointed laryngologist to the Demilt Dispensary. In 1874 he established a throat clinic at the New York Eye and Ear Infirmary. He also taught at his alma mater (1873–1904), where he was eventually named professor of laryngoscopy and diseases of the throat. Lefferts was a prolific contributor to medical journals. His most important textbook is *A Pharmacopoeia for the Treatment of the Larynx, Pharynx and Nasal Passages* (1882). In addition, he authored *Diagnosis and Treatment of Chronic Nasal Catarrh, Three Clinical Lectures* (1884). Lefferts was a founder of the New York Laryngological Society (1873) and of the *Archives of Laryngology* (1880). He was also a cofounder and president (1882) of the American Laryngological Association.

Erastus Eugene Holt (1849–1931) was born in Peru, Maine, and graduated from both the Maine Medical School (1874) and New York City's College of Physicians and Surgeons (1875). He interned at Maine General Hospital, where he was its first house doctor, and then entered practice in Portland in 1876. Deciding to specialize in opthalmology and otology, Holt studied these fields in Europe during 1881. Returning to Portland, he founded the Maine Eye and Ear Infirmary in 1886, and remained on its staff until his death. During World War I, Holt was a medical advisor to the governor of Maine and headed a board that examined draftees for military service. A member and frequent officer of numerous local, state, and national professional associations, Holt was a founder of the New England Ophthalmological Society (1886) and the first eye and ear specialist chosen to be president of the Maine Medical Association (1916). He was an incredibly prolific contributor to the surgical literature but never authored a textbook or monograph.

Charles Huntoon Knight (1849–1913), born in Easthampton, Massachusetts, graduated from Williams College in 1871 and the College of Physicians and Surgeons in New York City in 1874. After a few months spent in special study with Thomas Markoe (1819–1901), Knight served a year and a half as intern at the Roosevelt Hospital. In mid-1876, he traveled abroad to further his postgraduate training. Shortly after his return to America, Knight began private surgical practice and soon became associated with Freeman J. Bumstead (1826–1879). By the mid-1880s, Knight's clinical interests were becoming oriented toward diseases of the upper air passages. He served as lecturer on diseases of the nose and throat in the New York Polyclinic Hospital and Medical School from 1888 to 1890 and, during most of the 1890s, was chairman and professor of laryngology in the New York Post-Graduate Medical School. In 1899 he was named professor of diseases of the throat and nose in the Cornell University Medical School, a position he held until 1910. He authored *A Year-Book of Surgery for 1883* (1884), but his most important text was *Diseases of the Nose and Throat* (1903). Knight was secretary (1889–1896) and president (1897) of the American Laryngological Association.

Carl Seiler (1849–1905) was born in Philadelphia, educated at the Universities of Berlin and Pennsylvania, and studied medicine in Heidelberg, Vienna, and Philadelphia, where he received his medical degree in 1871 from the University of Pennsylvania. His interest in laryngology was influenced by his mother, Emma Seiler, who was a noted authority on the voice and the author of *The Voice in Singing* (1868) and *The Voice in Speaking* (1875). Following medical school graduation, Seiler became an office student of Jacob DaSilva Solis-Cohen, and later his first assistant. Seiler was lecturer on laryngoscopy from 1877 to 1895 and chief of the throat dispensary at the Hospital of the University of Pennsylvania for nearly two decades. He was also laryngologist to the German Throat Infirmary and physician in chief to the Union Dispensary. In 1879, Seiler was elected a member of the American Laryngological Association, later serving as its vice president, and was also secretary of the American Medical Association's Section on Otology, Rhinology and Laryngology. Among his written texts are *Handbook of Diagnosis and Treatment of Diseases of the Throat and Nasal Cavities* (1879) and *Compendium of Microscopical Technology* (1881). His name is eponymically linked with a small rod of cartilage attached to the vocal process of the arytenoid cartilage.

William Chapman Jarvis (1855–1895) was born in Fortress Monroe, Virginia, and received his medical education at the University of Maryland (1875). From 1875 to 1877, he pursued postgraduate studies in biology at The Johns Hopkins University while also working in advanced chemistry with Ira Remsen (1846–1927). In 1877 Jarvis moved to New York City, where he began medical practice but soon shifted his clinical focus to laryngology and rhinology. He worked as an assistant on Francke Bosworth's nose and throat service at Bellevue Hospital's outpatient department. In 1881 Jarvis was named lecturer on laryngology at the University of the City of New York (later New York University), and subsequently he became clinical professor of diseases of the throat. Although he rarely participated in organized otorhinolaryngology, Jarvis was one of the specialty's major pioneers. His name is linked eponymically with the Jarvis snare, a wire snare tightened by a screw handle, used for removing polyps and other sessile growths in the nose and other accessible cav-

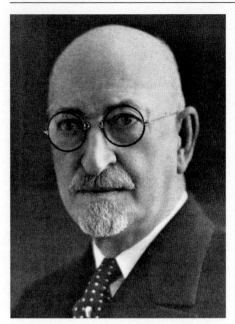

13. Cornelius Godfrey Coakley. (*Historical Collections, College of Physicians of Philadelphia*)

ities. This simple device allowed practitioners to easily extricate neoplasms and deformities. Previously, such growths could not be extirpated except by the use of difficult surgical procedures associated with significant morbidity and mortality. Although Jarvis initially used his snare solely to remove hypertrophic growths, he soon began to utilize it for other problems such as deviated septum. The results were quite impressive and led to the employment of his invention by surgeons throughout the world. Jarvis also pioneered the use of cocaine in intranasal and laryngeal surgery (1884) and suggested the use of an applicator tipped with chromic acid for the treatment of glottic and subglottic growths (1884). In 1885, at a meeting of the New York State Medical Society, Jarvis presented a plan for illumination of the upper air passages by the application of electric light bulbs (Thomas Edison's newly invented mignon lamp) at the focus of the head mirror and the shank of a laryngoscope handle. This was one of the earliest feasible methods of illuminating body cavities. Among his other novel inventions was an electric drill for the correction of deviated septum (1887).

Wendell Christopher Phillips (18571934), born in Hammond, New York, graduated from the Potsdam Normal School in 1879 and the University Medical College of New York University in 1882. Although Phillips had little formal postgraduate training, he soon began the practice of medicine in New York City, where he remained for over half a century. Devoting the majority of his time to diseases of the ear, nose, and throat, he was appointed aural surgeon to the Manhattan Eye and Ear Hospital, where he was a department head for many years. For two decades, he served as professor of otology at the New York Post-Graduate Medical School and Hospital, during which he authored his well-known textbook, *Diseases of the Ear, Nose and Throat* (1910). In 1914 Phillips became an officer of the New York League for the Hard of Hearing, and through his connection with this organization he became the founder, five years later, of the American Federation of Organizations for the Hard of Hearing. The latter organization was instrumental in having school hearing test programs approved by leading medical societies and widely adopted in American public school systems. Phillips took an active and conspicuous part in organized medicine and was elected president of the American Medical Association in 1926. In addition, he was chairman of the American Medical Association's Section of Laryngology, Otology and Rhinology (1923) and was a charter member and president (1907) of the American Laryngological, Rhinological and Otological Society.

Cornelius Godfrey Coakley (1862–1934), born in New York City, attended the College of the City of New York (1884) and received his medical degree from New York University Medical School (1887). After interning at Bellevue Hospital in 1888, he began to practice medicine in his native city and was named director of the histology department at the Loomis Laboratory in 1889. The following year, Coakley was appointed to the anatomy faculty at his alma mater and from 1890 to 1896 was also on the histology faculty. His professional interest changed in the late 1890s, and he joined the laryngology faculty at the University and Bellevue Hospital Medical College (1898–1914), where he eventually became clinical professor of laryngology. From 1914 until his death, Coakley was on the laryngology and otology faculty of the College of Physicians and Surgeons and attending otorhinolaryngologist to Presbyterian Hospital. Best known for his operation of excision of the larynx in cases of cancer, Coakley was president of the American Laryngological Association (1918) and the New York Laryngological Society (1933). He authored *A Manual of Diseases of the Nose and Throat* (1899), which went through four editions and was widely used as a textbook in American medical colleges.

David Braden Kyle (1863–1916) was born at Cadiz, Ohio, and educated at Muskingum College and Jefferson Medical College (1891). A remarkable student, in the autumn of 1891, he was appointed to the chair of pathology in his alma mater, remaining in this capacity until 1896. In the latter year, Kyle was elected professor of laryngology at Jefferson, a position he held until his death. From 1891 to 1893,

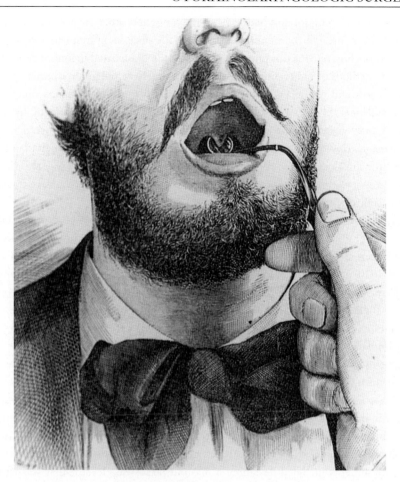

14. Horace Ivins (1856–1899) was a homeopath who lectured on laryngology and otology at Hahnemann Medical College in Philadelphia. This wood engraving is taken from his *Diseases of the Nose and Throat* (1893) and demonstrates the "rhinoscopic mirror in position." (*Author's Collection*)

he was also chief laryngologist, rhinologist, and otologist to St. Mary's Hospital, and later accepted a similar position at St. Agnes Hospital. In 1900 he was president of the American Laryngological, Rhinological and Otological Society and, in 1911, held the same office in the American Laryngological Association. Kyle's chief contribution to the literature of medicine was *A Textbook of Diseases of the Nose and Throat* (1899), of which four subsequent editions were published.

Charles Victor Roman (1864–1934) was born in Williamsport, Pennsylvania, and educated at Hamilton Collegiate Institute, Ontario, Canada (1886) and Meharry Medical College (1899). While at Meharry, he also served an an office assistant to Robert F. Boyd (1858–1912), the first African-American physician with a formal medical degree to practice full-time in Nashville. Following graduation, Roman established a general medical practice in Dallas, Texas, although he became increasingly oriented toward ophthalmologic and otorhinolaryngologic diseases. In 1899 he pursued further training in these fields at the Post-Graduate Medical School and Hospital of Chicago; five years later he studied at the Royal Ophthalmic Hospital and Central London Ear, Nose and Throat Hospital in England. Following his return to the United States, Roman was appointed chairman of ophthalmology and otolaryngology and director of health services at Fisk University and founded the department of ophthalmology and otolaryngology at his alma mater. From 1931 to 1934, he also served as professor of medical history and ethics. Roman was an early leader in African-American medical affairs, both as a founder and editor of the *Journal of the National Medical Association* (1908–1918) and through his efforts as a surgical specialist and observer of medical education at Meharry. In 1934 he authored *Meharry Medical College: A History*.

Chevalier Jackson (1865–1958), born in Pittsburgh, was educated at Western University (1883) and Jefferson Medical College (1886). He studied laryngology in England and, in 1887, began practice in Philadelphia, where he would remain until his death. Although most of Jackson's career was outside the academic arena, he was an influential force in the evolution of modern laryngeal surgery. He developed a

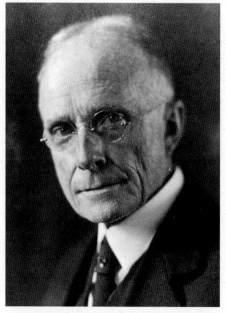

15. Chevalier Jackson. (*Historical Collections, College of Physicians of Philadelphia*)

559

method of removing foreign bodies from the lungs and other air passages by insertion of tubes through the mouth. Jackson initially devised an esophagus scope and later a bronchoscope for this purpose and, in so doing, obviated the more dangerous surgical methods of intervention used at that time. He would go on to train numerous students and physicians in these techniques in his private bronchoscopic clinic in Philadelphia. In 1907 Jackson authored the first textbook on endoscopy, *Tracheo-Bronchoscopy, Esophagoscopy and Gastroscopy*. Ten years later, he reported in the *American Journal of the Medical Sciences* the first removal of an endothelioma of the right bronchus by peroral bronchoscopy. He later completed *Diseases of the Air and Food Passages of Foreign Body Origin* (1937), one of the most comprehensive treatises on the subject ever published.

Francis Randolph Packard (1870–1950) was born in Philadelphia and received his undergraduate (1889) and medical education (1892) at the University of Pennsylvania. He completed a year of postgraduate work with William Osler (1849–1920) at The Johns Hopkins Hospital and then pursued residency training at the Pennsylvania Hospital (1893–1895). In 1895 Packard opened up a medical practice in Philadelphia, but by 1898 his clinical activities were confined to otorhinolaryngologic diseases. Most of his professional career was spent on the otorhinolaryngology faculty of the Philadelphia Polyclinic and College for Graduates in Medicine (later affiliated with the University of Pennsylvania). During the Spanish-American War (1898), Packard was a first lieutenant and assistant surgeon, Second Regiment, Pennsylvania Volunteer Infantry. In 1917–1918 he was an officer in the Medical Corps, U.S. Army, attached to Base Hospital No. 10, Treport, Seine Inférieure, France. The following year, Packard was named chief consultant in otorhinolaryngology, District of Paris. A noted otorhinolaryngologist, whose accomplishments included designing a mastoid periosteal elevator that was widely used for many years, Packard was conspicuously involved in organized medicine and served as president of the American Laryngological Assocation (1930) and the American Otological Society (1936). In 1909 he wrote *A Text-Book of Diseases of the Nose, Throat and Ear*. He is best remembered as a founder of American medical historiography, his most important historical work being the two-volume *The History of Medicine in the United States* (1901). His approach was largely biographical and often failed to distinguish between the important and the trivial. Although he provided little in the way of detailed historical analyses or themes, his books contained a wealth of information, and through his many activities, including the founding and editing of the *Annals of Medical History* (1917–1942), Packard succeeded in arousing an interest in medical history where little had previously existed. Among his other books are *History of the School of Salernum* (1920), *Life and Times of Ambroise Paré* (1921), *Guy Patin and the Medical Profession in Paris in the XVIIth Century* (1925), and *Some Account of the Pennsylvania Hospital* (1938).

Spencer Cornelius Dickerson (1871–1948) was born in Austin, Texas, and educated at the University of Chicago (1897) and Rush Medical College (1901). He interned at Freedmen's Hospital in Washington, D.C. and then established a private medical practice in New Bedford, Massachusetts. In 1907 he moved to Chicago and became affiliated with the Provident Hospital, where he was private surgical assistant to George C. Hall (1864–1930). Dickerson also joined the pathology department, where he remained until 1912. Deciding that his interests lay more with otorhinolaryngology, Dickerson became an assistant in the ophthalmology/otorhinolaryngology department at Rush Medical College (1914–1920). In 1920 he became a member of Provident's ophthalmology and otorhinolaryngology staff, and he was eventually named chairman of the department (1930–1937). Dickerson would go on to train a generation of African-American ophthalmology/otorhinolaryngology specialists at Provident Hospital.

Lee Wallace Dean (1873–1944) was born in Muscatine, Iowa, and received his undergraduate (1894) and medical (1896) education at the State University of Iowa. From 1896 to 1897, he pursued postgraduate work in London and Vienna.

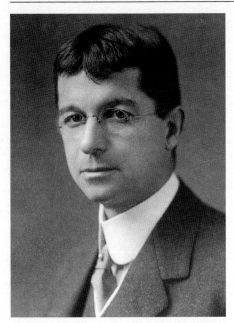

16. Francis Randolph Packard. (*Historical Collections, College of Physicians of Philadelphia*)

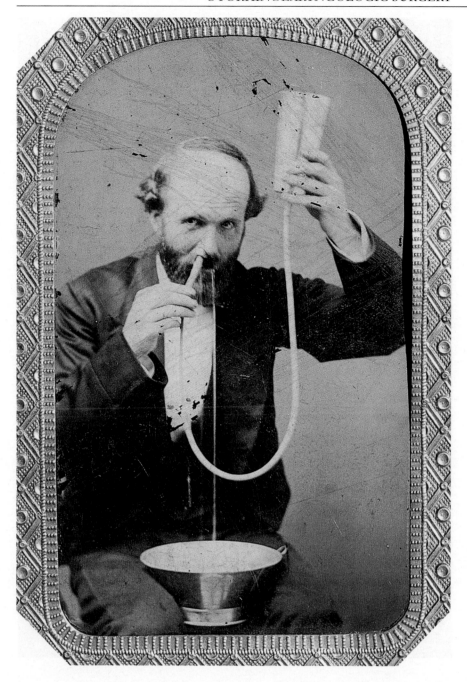

17. In the era after the Civil War, it was not uncommon for physicians to pose for promotional pictures with their new diagnostic and therapeutic tools. The nasal douche was advertised as part of an advisable routine of cleansing and medicating the nasal passages. It was believed that a daily lavage could decrease the incidence of sinusitis and mastoiditis, while for those so afflicted, it could help clear the necrotic debris typically left by the twin ravages of syphilis and tuberculosis. (*Courtesy of Stanley B. Burns, M.D., and The Burns Collection and Archive*)

Returning to his alma mater, Dean joined the anatomy and physiology faculties (1898–1900) and then switched to the otorhinolaryngology and oral surgery faculty, where he remained until 1927. From 1912 to 1927, he was also dean of the medical school. During World War I, Dean was in the U.S. Army Medical Officers' Reserves Corps, and commanding officer of general hospital No. 54 in Iowa City. In 1929 Dean relocated to St. Louis, where he was on the otorhinolaryngology faculty at Washington University and staff otorhinolaryngologist to Barnes, St. Louis Children's, Jewish, and McMillan Eye, Ear, Nose, and Throat Hospitals. He did important research in allergy and sinus disease in children, and he built strong otorhinolaryngology departments at both the State University of Iowa and Washington University. Dean was president of the American Otological Society (1922), the American Laryngological Association (1924), the American Academy of Ophthalmology and Otolaryngology, and the American Laryngological, Rhinological and Otological Society. He also served as editor in chief of the *Annals of Otology, Rhinology and Laryngology* (1927–1944).

James Wilkinson Jervey (1874–1945), born in Charleston, South Carolina, was educated for two years at the University of South Carolina and received his medical diploma from the Medical College of South Carolina in 1897. He began practice in

18. Infection of the ear passages and surrounding sinuses was an important medical problem in the preantibiotic era. Acute and chronic infections could lead to deafness and even spread to the brain, resulting in death. Otolaryngologists were often consulted to treat mastoiditis, as is seen in this photograph (circa 1918). (*Courtesy of Stanley B. Burns, M.D., and The Burns Collection and Archive*)

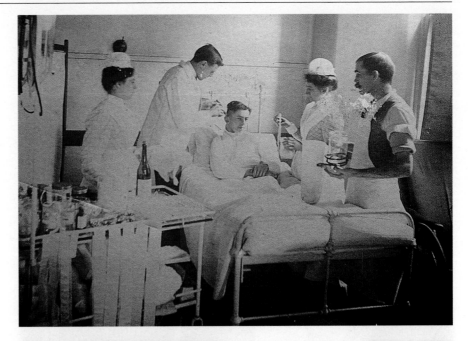

19. Electrocochleography, the first physiologic objective assessment of hearing, being performed at The Johns Hopkins Hospital in 1959. This surgical technique allows otorhinolaryngologists to accurately locate the site of the lesion of hearing loss, and it makes possible the objective assessment of hearing in individuals who cannot be tested by standard behavioral methods. (*Courtesy of Stanley B. Burns, M.D., and The Burns Collection and Archive, and by permission of Robert Ruben, M.D.*)

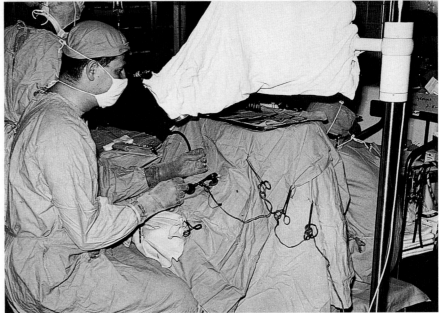

1898, in Greenville, South Carolina, where he established the Jervey Eye, Ear and Throat Hospital. He also organized the Greenville General Hospital and was named chief surgeon to the Piedmont and North Railway Company and oculist to the Southern Railway. A fellow of the American College of Surgeons, Jervey was a diplomate of both the American Board of Ophthalmic Examinations and the American Board of Otolaryngology. An avid speaker and writer, he edited the *Journal of the South Carolina Medical Association* (1908–1912). Jervey served as president of the American Laryngological, Rhinological and Otological Society.

Stanton Abeles Friedberg (1875–1920) was born in Chicago and attended the University of Michigan (1893) and Rush Medical College (1897). He began his work in otorhinolaryngology in 1900, assisting E. Fletcher Ingals (1848–1918). Three years later, Friedberg was appointed to the staff of Cook County Hospital, but in July 1903 he left to study otology and laryngology in Vienna. He returned in 1904, resumed working with Ingals, and was soon appointed attending otorhinolaryngologist to Cook County Hospital (1906–1913). He was also an assistant instructor at his alma mater (1905) and consulting otorhinolaryngologist to the Durand Hospital of the John McCormick Institute for Infectious Diseases (1907). From 1913 to 1919, Friedberg was chief of the eye, ear, and nose department at Cook County Hospital. During World War I, he served eight months in the Base Hospital, Camp Doniphan,

Fort Sill, Oklahoma, and was later stationed in France (1918–1919). In a bizarre twist of fate, Friedberg died of the complications of an operation for mastoiditis.

Samuel James Crowe (1883–1955) was born in Washington County, Virginia, and educated at the University of Georgia (1904) and The Johns Hopkins School of Medicine (1908). He completed a surgical internship and residency at The Johns Hopkins Hospital (1908–1912) and was then asked by William Halsted to attempt to organize a department of otorhinolaryngology. Although Crowe had little experience in the field, he accepted the assigment, but not before first spending four months (summer 1913) in Freiburg, Germany, at the otorhinolaryngology department of Gustav Killian (1860–1921). Returning to Baltimore, Crowe established the first modern clinic of otorhinolaryngology in the United States, and he remained at The Hopkins for his entire professional career. He went on to perform groundbreaking research into the pathophysiology of hearing, and introduced the audiometer into clinical otology. Crowe did the first important research on deafness in humans by correlating hearing impairments, anatomical defects, and injuries in the inner ear. Furthermore, he demonstrated that the growth of lymphoid tissue in and around the eustachian tube was a frequent cause of childhood deafness and developed a method of prevention and treatment using radon, a by-product of radium. Additionally, he recognized that aviators and submariners, who were exposed to sudden changes of air pressure, experienced symptoms comparable to those of children with blockage of the eustachian tubes. During World War II, he established a course at The Hopkins to train medical officers in the use of the nasopharyngoscope and radon therapy. Crowe also developed new operative techniques for tonsillectomy that greatly minimized the occurrence of postoperative pulmonary abscesses (1924). In his most influential paper to the scientific literature, coauthored with Harvey Cushing and John Homans, Crowe provided the first experimental evidence of the relationship between the pituitary body and the reproductive system and demonstrated that hypophysectomy caused genital atrophy (1910).

William Harry Barnes (1887–1945), born in Philadelphia, was the first African American to win a four-year scholarship to the University of Pennsylvania School of Medicine, graduating in 1912. He completed an internship at Douglass and Mercy Hospitals in Philadelphia (1913) and was named assistant otorhinolaryngologist at Douglass Hospital, where he remained until his death. Although Barnes initially was in a general medical practice (1913–1922), the latter years of his career were focused on otorhinolaryngologic diseases. Barnes pursued postgraduate course work at his alma mater in otorhinolaryngologic surgery (1921) and, in 1924 and 1926, completed similar training in Paris and Bordeaux, France. He was also on the otorhinolaryngologic staffs of Mercy and Jefferson Medical School Hospitals and was appointed lecturer in bronchoscopy at Howard University Medical School (1931–1945), which he commuted to from his home in Philadelphia. Barnes was the first African-American physician to be certified by an American surgical specialty board (1927, American Board of Otolaryngology). He was quite active in the National Medical Association, serving as its thirty-seventh president (1936) and performing surgery or giving technical demonstrations and papers. He founded and served as executive secretary of the Society for the Promotion of Negro Specialists in Medicine and was president of the Philadelphia Academy of Medicine and Allied Sciences for three years. Barnes invented a hypophyscope for visualizing the pituitary gland, developed a modification of the Myles lingual tonsillectomy, and devised new operative techniques for opening peritonsillar abscesses and for making incisions in myringotomy.

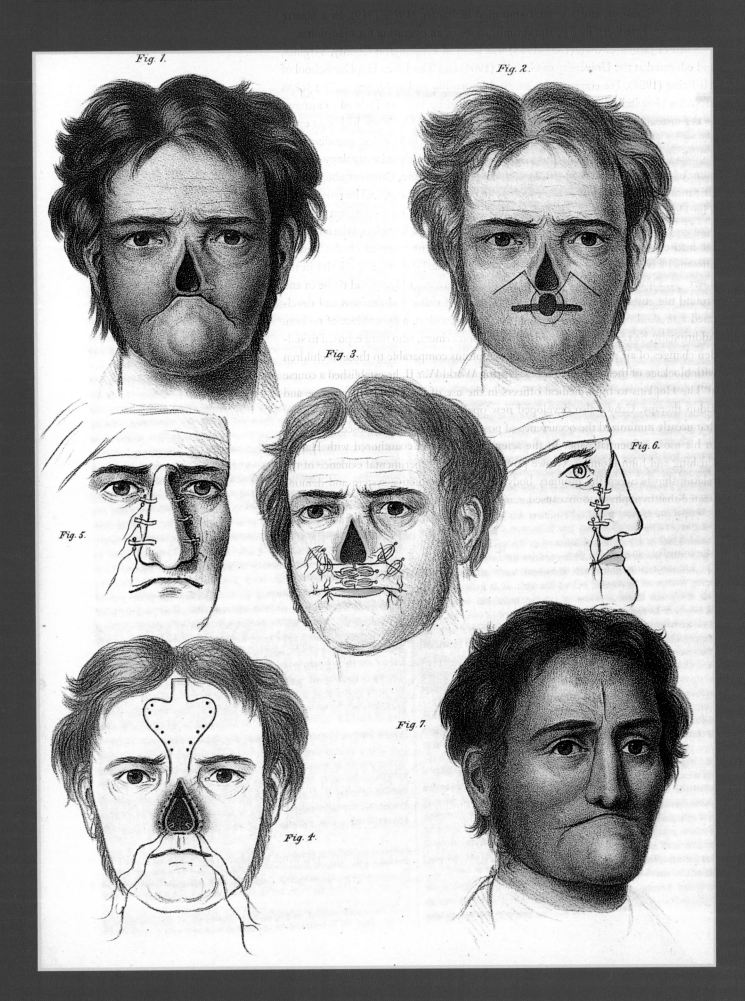

Fig. 1.

Fig. 2.

Fig. 3.

Fig. 5.

Fig. 6.

Fig. 4.

Fig. 7.

CHAPTER 21

PLASTIC SURGERY

n the United States of the 1990s, plastic surgery is both a recognized surgical specialty and a sociocultural phenomenon. Plastic surgeons seemingly garner more media attention than virtually any other medical specialists. Therefore, complete understanding of the evolution and professionalization of plastic surgery requires that the specialty be viewed both from the medical perspective, with regard to its early development and, in its more modern phase, as a measure of society's fascination with the culture of beauty.

Before World War I, plastic surgery as a distinct specialty had a minor impact on the practice of medicine. Some medically astute lay individuals were aware that the surgical correction of congenital and acquired deformities, such as cleft lips and palates, "saddle-noses," and burn sequelae, might be attempted, but the ordinary American remained ignorant of this field of health care. Rhinoplasty ("nose job"), for aesthetic reasons, was virtually unheard of, as were the myriad of other facial procedures (e.g., rhytidoplasty, or surgery for the removal of wrinkles) so common today. Certainly, body sculpting for cosmetic purposes, such as liposuction, abdominoplasty, and breast augmentation or reduction, was unknown. Even the scope of the profession's interest was indeterminate, as witnessed by the confusion concerning the name and, indeed, the anatomic areas of the body to be considered within this supposed surgical discipline. Moreover, who was to be considered a plastic surgeon? Was it, for example, those members of the maxillofacial team assembled at Walter Reed Hospital during World War I, including prosthetic dentists, oral surgeons, ophthalmologists, and otorhinolaryngologists, or instead general surgeons and orthopedic surgeons, who had long considered most plastic and reconstructive operations within their purview?

Unlike other surgical specialties, plastic surgery had not seen any concerted effort to organize a society to meet the specific needs of its practitioners in the nineteenth century. In 1881 the trustees of the American Medical Association authorized a Section on Dentistry, which became known in 1882 as the Section on Dental and Oral Surgery and in 1897 as the Section on Stomatology. This annual meeting was the principal national activity and common gathering place of those interested in the medical and surgical aspects of diseases and malformations of the region of the mouth and jaws, and represented whatever elements of organized plastic surgery could be said to exist in the years up to the 1920s. Still, this is not to suggest that a wide variety of plastic and reconstructive surgical operations were not being performed. It simply meant that such procedures were usually undertaken by physicians who considered themselves all-around surgeons. Yet, some of these surgeons, in the course of their work in general surgery, made important contributions to plastic and reconstructive surgery and began to be conspicuously identified with this growing field.

1. *(facing page)* Facial reconstruction was well advanced by the mid-nineteenth century. Joseph Pancoast demonstrates his "process" of cheiloplasty and rhinoplasty on this 53-year-old patient, who suffered total destruction of the upper lip, the soft parts of the nose, the nasal septum, and the bony turbinates. *(Author's Collection)*

The first article on a plastic surgical topic to be published in an American medical periodical was Isaac Cathrall's (1764–1819) case of "double-hare lip" in 1819. This was soon followed by Nathan Smith's (1762–1829) repair of a cleft palate (staphylorraphy) in 1826, Alexander Steven's (1789–1869) in 1827, and John Collins Warren's (1778–1856) in 1828. These early staphylorraphies were based on the method of Philibert Roux (1780–1854), a Parisian surgeon. However, a decade later, John Peter Mettauer's (1787–1875) paper in the *American Journal of the Medical Sciences* (1837) reported the first repair of a cleft palate utilizing the newer method of Johann Dieffenbach (1792–1847), a German surgeon. That same year, Thomas Dent Mütter (1811–1859) authored the earliest article in our country's scientific literature to deal with operative surgery as treatment for disfigurement from burns. Mütter would go on to develop extensive experience in many areas of reparative surgery, highlighted by his first published description, in the United States (1842), of a pedicle flap.

During the late 1830s, Jonathan Mason Warren (1811–1867) began to report on rhinoplastic operations. In contrast to his later practice, Warren initially utilized the Indian or Brahmin method of rhinoplasty (1837), a technique involving taking a flap from the forehead and twisting it downward to form a new nose. By the 1840s, he was using Gaspare Tagliacozzi's (1545–1599) operation in which the nose is fashioned from the skin of the forearm, which is bound firmly to the face until the flap is solidly united in its new position. Not only was Warren skilled in nasal surgery, but between 1840 and 1860, he was among the more renowned surgeons in the country for closing the complete cleft palate. As a result of Warren's success in devising an "American palatoplastie" (1843) many patients from all parts of the United States were referred to him. At about the same time, Joseph Pancoast (1805–1882) completed his magnificently illustrated *A Treatise on Operative Surgery* (1844), which contained the first extensive section on plastic surgery in an American surgical textbook. Pancoast had a particular interest in taliacotian operations and described a suturing technique involving the union of two edges by a "tongue-and-groove arrangement." In 1847 Frank Hamilton (1813–1886) theorized about using anaplasty, an archaic term for plastic surgery, to heal an ulcer on the calf of a young boy. Hamilton proposed "a plastic operation, with the view of planting upon the center of the ulcer a piece of new and perfectly healthy skin...from the calf of the other leg (having secured the two together)." The patient's family never gave permission for this operation, but seven years later, Hamilton authored his classic paper describing the first use of anaplasty on a laborer for the treatment of old ulcers.

During the Civil War, the most renowned plastic surgical work was completed by Gurdon Buck (1807–1877), particularly his case involving facial reconstructive surgery on Carleton Burgan. Burgan, while serving in the military, developed a rapidly spreading ulcer on his right cheek that resulted in massive tissue loss. Over the course of six months, Buck performed five separate procedures to reconstruct Burgan's face, and Thomas Gunning, a New York City dentist, prepared an artificial "roof" for the mouth and teeth. Buck's interest in reconstructive surgery was further evidenced when he authored the first American work exclusively on the subject: *Contributions to Reparative Surgery; Showing Its Applications to the Treatment of Deformities Produced by Destructive Disease or Injury; Congenital Defects From Arrest or Excess of Development; and Cicatrical Contractions From Burns* (1876). Considered the country's first true textbook on plastic surgery, it is illustrated with some of the earliest engravings to be made from photographs. Buck photographed his plastic surgery patients both before and after surgery so as to demonstrate his results to anyone wishing to consult them.

Also during the late 1860s, David Prince (1816–1889) gave a report to members of the Illinois State Medical Society entitled "Plastics: A New Classification and a Brief Exposition of Plastic Surgery" (1867). Three years later he expanded on this lecture and, in 1871, authored the 240-page text *Plastics and Orthopedics*. Although not well known, Prince's monograph was one of the earliest works in which plastic surgery was treated as a special discipline, apart from the rest of surgery. During the early 1870s, John Hodgen (1826–1882) and D. Hayes Agnew (1818–1892) published reports on their initial research into pinch grafting. Charles Porter (1840–1909), surgeon to the Massachusetts General Hospital, authored a report in the *Boston Medical and Surgical Journal* (1878), which was the first paper on plastic surgery to be illustrated with mechanically reproduced photographs.

As the nineteenth century drew to a close, American surgeons were becoming increasingly innovative in their application of surgical techniques to problems of reconstruction, and they were tentatively beginning the treatment of cosmetic deformities. In 1881 Edward Ely (1850–1885) described the operation of otoplasty. John Roe (1848–1915), of Rochester, New York, authored two influential papers (1887 and 1891) containing the first descriptions of the intranasal approach for corrective rhinoplasty, as well as one of the earliest reports of crude reduction rhinoplasty. In 1892, Robert Weir (1838–1927) wrote a paper on "restoring sunken noses without scarring the face," which marked the beginning of modern step-by-step rhinoplasty. George Howard Monks (1853–1933), a graduate of Harvard Medical School, taught surgical pathology and surgery at Harvard Dental School, where he was professor of oral surgery. In 1898 he authored a report on correcting nasal deformities and disfigurements by surgical operations. Monks described rhinophyma, or "hypertrophic acne," and its surgical treatment and initiated the treatment for bifid nose, "saddleback" nose, and twisted nose. He also emphasized the necessity of comparing before-and-after illustrations with the heads the same size and in the same position, and with the same lighting. That same year, Monks began to popularize the concept of an "island flap" based on a nourishing artery. His many clinical activities in plastic and reconstructive surgery would later become influential in establishing the specialty of plastic surgery. Robert Abbe (1851–1928) described an innovative lip switch flap "for the relief of deformity due to double harelip," which is now known as the Abbe-Estlander operation (1898). He transferred a full-thickness flap from one lip of the oral cavity to fill a defect in the other lip.

Also during the 1880s and 1890s, remarkable progress was being made in skin grafting. John Girdner, in charge of a ward at Bellevue Hospital, described an attempt to treat a burn with skin grafts obtained from a cadaver (1881). E. P. Brewer, of Norwich, Connecticut, discussed the long-term viability of skin removed from a

2. This remarkable plate is from the earliest article (*Boston Medical and Surgical Journal*, vol. 16, pages 69–79, 1837) on rhinoplasty published in the United States. Jonathan Mason Warren utilized both the tagliacotian and the Indian or Brahmin method of nasal reconstruction. (*Historical Collections, College of Physicians of Philadelphia*)

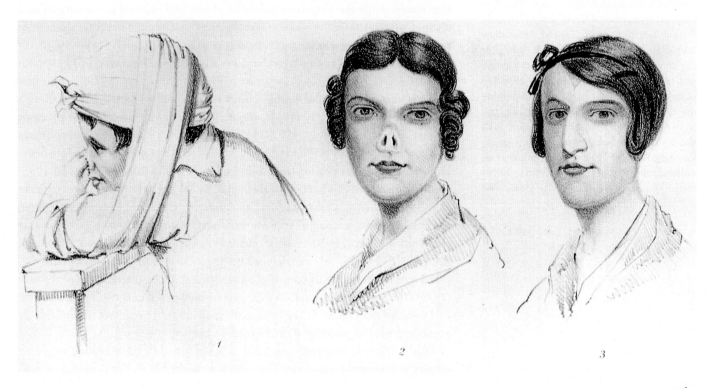

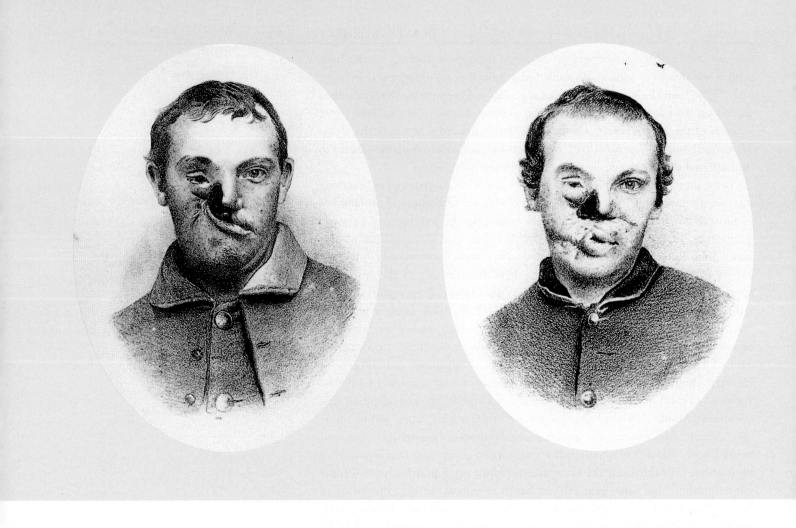

3. Gurdon Buck's skilled reconstruction of Carleton Burgan's deformed face was one of the greatest operative triumphs of nineteenth-century American surgery. While serving in the Civil War, Burgan developed a rapidly spreading ulcer on the right side of his face, resulting in massive tissue loss, presumably from treatment with mercurials for venereal disease. Over the course of six months, Buck completed five separate procedures. The illustrations (*Transactions of the Medical Society of the State of New York*, pages 173–186, 1864) show Burgan prior to the first operation (*left*), after the initial procedure, during which the mouth was reconstructed (*right*), with an improvement of the right angle of the mouth following the second operation (*facing page, left*), and from the front, showing the final result of all the operations (*facing page, right*). Thomas Gunning, a New York dentist, prepared an artificial rubber "roof" for the mouth as well as teeth. (*Historical Collections, College of Physicians of Philadelphia*)

body eighteen hours after death and later used for grafting (1882). In a little-known account from the *Annals of Surgery* (1890), M. E. Van Meter, from Red Bluff, Colorado, described animal-to-man skin grafting that utilized tissue from "two young puppies of the Mexican hairless breed." One year later, George Shrady (1837–1907) suggested, for the first time in the United States, the use of the finger as a medium for transplanting skin flaps from one part of the body to another, particularly in the restoration of a portion of a cheek.

In the years leading up to the World War I, many of the fundamental issues that would shape the long-term future of plastic and reconstructive surgery as a distinct surgical specialty were raised. Interest in cosmetic surgery, apart from reconstructive operations, was increasing. Charles Miller (1880–1950), of Chicago, regarded as both a quack and a plastic surgical visionary, privately published *Cosmetic Surgery: The Correction of Featural Imperfections* (1907), the first book on the subject in the world. This was soon followed by Frederick Kolle's *Plastic and Cosmetic Surgery* (1911), the earliest comprehensive text on cosmetic surgery. John Staige Davis (1872–1946) popularized a new method of splinting skin grafts (1909), and William Luckett (1872–1929) developed the modern operation for the correction of protruding ears (1910). Vilray Blair (1871–1955) reported on closed ramisection of the mandible for micrognathia or prognathism in the *Journal of the American Medical Association* (1909) and, three years later, authored the first detailed treatise on maxillofacial surgery, *Surgery and Diseases of the Mouth and Jaws*. Further work on facial deformities was pursued by John B. Roberts (1852–1924), who introduced the push-back procedure or backward displacement of the velum to ensure adequate speech in congenital clefts of the face (1918). Many of these clinical advances were summarized in Davis' *Plastic Surgery: Its Principles and Practice* (1919), the earliest all-inclusive textbook in the rapidly expanding field of plastic and reconstructive surgery.

World War I is frequently regarded as a watershed in the evolution of plastic surgery as a recognized specialty. Since the war resulted in tens of thousands of hor-

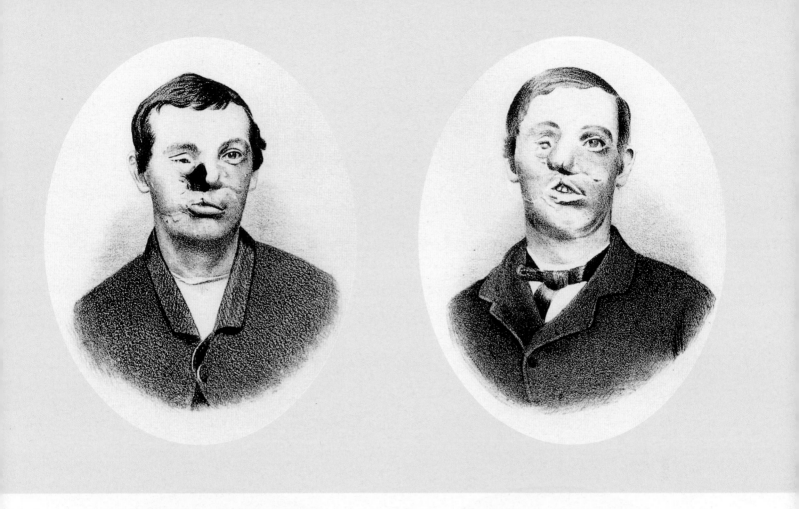

rendous and mutilating injuries, the long-held premise has been that the blossoming of plastic surgery is primarily a medical phenomenon, fueled by war-related advances in reconstructive surgical techniques. There is little doubt that the experiences of World War I, particularly the organization by the U.S. Army of a Section on Head Surgery, with Vilray Blair as chief of plastic surgery, were a turning point in the history of plastic surgery as an organized specialty. However, the war's significance is sometimes overemphasized when it is realized that an impetus toward cosmetic surgery had already been growing for at least two decades and that reconstructive operations were being performed for almost a century before. In the final analysis, the development of modern plastic surgery, unlike that of any other surgical specialty, has to be regarded as more than just a medical phenomenon because cosmetic surgery rapidly became more than just a medical practice. The rest of medicine is concerned with a patient's good health, while plastic surgeons must also be attuned to an individual's outward appearance. As external beauty became an increasingly important part of our culture, the evolution of plastic surgery became affected by both sociologic demands and scientific parameters. Accordingly, the history of plastic century in the post–World War I era must be considered in a societal and cultural as well as a medical context.

With the trench warfare of World War I producing extreme facial injuries, it became evident that some type of interdisciplinary team approach was needed to care for these complex maxillofacial problems. In June 1917, a group of enlisted American surgeons and dentists who had prior clinical experience in managing mutilating head injuries were stationed overseas to work in "specialty teams" under the aegis of the army's Section on Head Surgery. Concurrently, three institutions in this country were specifically designated to handle plastic surgery cases: Jefferson Barracks in Missouri under Blair, Walter Reed Hospital under Robert Ivy, and Fort McHenry under George Schaeffer. Despite the clinical successes during and after the war, the place of plastic surgery as a surgical specialty remained poorly defined, and its separate function on a hospital service was still questioned. In most instances,

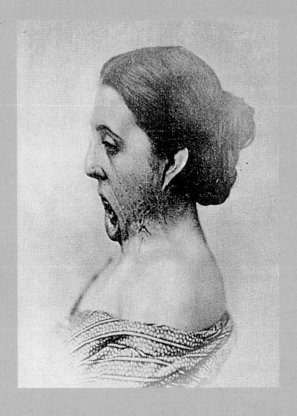
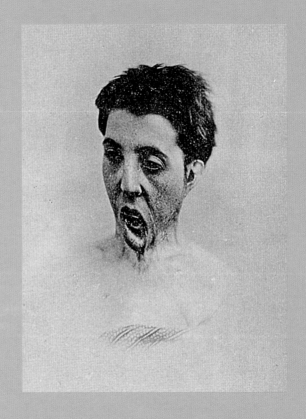
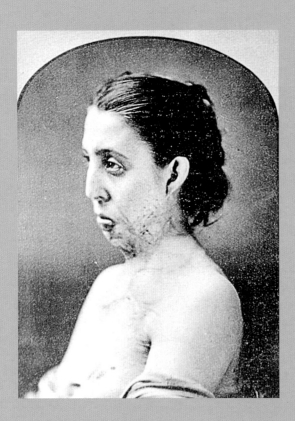
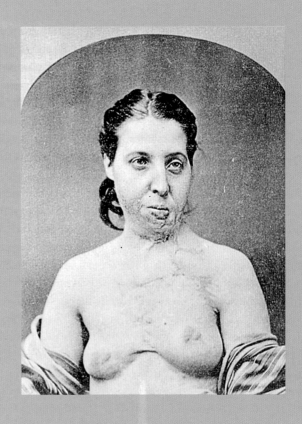

4. Charles Burnham Porter (1840–1909) was a surgeon at the Massachusetts General Hospital when he authored the country's first article on plastic surgery to be published in a periodical (*Boston Medical and Surgical Journal*, vol. 98, pages 423–427, 1878) and illustrated with mechanically reproduced heliotype photographs taken in 1875. Porter's 15-year-old patient underwent five separate procedures to relieve her disfigurement from a burn, as seen in these before-and-after prints. Beginning in 1839, the year of photography's invention, the only way to incorporate photographs into a book or periodical was to physically affix each paper print on a page. By the 1870s, a method had been developed that allowed photographs to be mechanically reproduced by a second printing press. But it was not until the late 1880s that the modern halftone picture made its debut, allowing a photograph to be printed on the same press as the text. (*Historical Collections, College of Physicians of Philadelphia*)

plastic surgical activities continued as a partial activity of the surgical, orthopedic, or some other department. More importantly, only a few surgeons could afford to limit their practice to this still precarious and undefined field on the basis of remunerations.

Despite this uncertainty, some American surgeons returned from World War I eager to organize the new specialty. Blair founded the plastic surgery department at Washington University's Barnes Hospital in St. Louis, the first separate plastic surgical service in the country. On the East Coast, John Staige Davis, following the success of his textbook, was appointed professor of plastic surgery at The Johns Hopkins Hospital, the first person to be so titled. Clearly, a profession was attempting to establish itself, but critical events needed to occur from both an organizational and a qualitative standpoint. As early as 1916, Davis argued that modern surgery had become so vast that no one surgeon could master the entire field, and plastic surgery needed to exist as a separate specialty. At the same time, many so-called plastic surgeons were beginning to graduate from a series of "short courses" given at Walter Reed Hospital under the direction of Robert Ivy. Still, a fundamental question–that of the difference between reconstructive plastic surgery and cosmetic surgery–needed to be settled. How could the cultural value of beauty and the medical value of health be jointly incorporated into a distinct surgical specialty? The issue would not be settled for many decades, and it proved especially divisive during the formative years when plastic surgery was attempting to establish itself as a legitimate branch of American medicine. Such post–World War I debates over legitimacy were limited to the United States; plastic surgery, as an organized and distinct surgical specialty, would not evolve in Europe until after World War II.

By the mid-1920s, rudimentary plastic surgical training programs were scattered throughout the country. However, most training in this field continued with one-on-one preceptorships. At this time a most significant event occurred: the creation of the American Association of Oral Surgeons (1921), the first national organization to include representative plastic surgeons in its constitutiency. The initial membership requirement called for both the M.D. and D.D.S. degrees. The requisite dental degree was dropped in 1923, although fellowship in the American College of Surgeons was added. In 1927 the organization's name was changed to the American Association of Oral and Plastic Surgeons. A decade and a half later, it officially became the American Association of Plastic Surgeons. Like many of the earliest surgical specialty societies, the American Association of Oral and Plastic Surgeons limited its membership. As a result, a more inclusive organization was begun in 1931: the Society of Plastic and Reconstructive Surgery. As its steadily increasing membership rolls included representatives from throughout the country, the name was changed to the American Society of Plastic and Reconstructive Surgery in 1941.

One of the more important steps toward ultimate recognition of the specialty was made when the American Board of Plastic Surgery was formed in June 1937. A year later, it received recognition as a subsidiary of the American Board of Surgery. The final step in the board's evolution was taken in May 1941, when the Advisory Board for Medical Specialties of the American Medical Association afforded the American Board of Plastic Surgery status as a primary specialty board. Presently, among the organizations sponsoring the American Board of Plastic Surgery are the Association of Academic Chairmen of Plastic Surgery, the American Association for Hand Surgery, the American Association of Plastic Surgeons, the American Society for Aesthetic Plastic Surgery, the American Society for Surgery of the Hand, the American Society of Maxillofacial Surgeons, the American Society of Plastic and Reconstructive Surgeons, and the Society of Head and Neck Surgeons. The board states that modern plastic surgery deals with the "repair, reconstruction or replacement of physical defects of form or function involving the skin, musculoskeletal system, cranio-maxillofacial structures, hand, extremities, breast and trunk and external genitalia. It uses aesthetic surgical principles not only to improve undesirable qualities of normal structures but in all reconstructive procedures as well." To be eligible to take the board's examination for certification, applicants must have completed at least three years of general surgical residency training plus two or three years of plastic surgery residency training.

In January 1995, of the approximately 621,000 total physicians in active practice in the United States, 5,205 (less than 1 percent) designated themselves as plastic surgeons. Within this cadre of plastic surgeons, 4,120 (79 percent) were board certified. (By contrast, during the fifteen years between 1980 and 1994, 2,569 certificates in plastic surgery were issued, or an average of 171 per year.) Of the 1995 total, 400 (8 percent) were women and 780 (15 percent) were international medical graduates. Among the total pool of plastic surgeons, approximately 580 (11 percent) were younger than 35; 1,825 (35 percent) were 35 to 44; 1,615 (31 percent) were 45 to 54; 890 (17 percent) were 55 to 64; and 295 (6 percent) were 65 and older. Of the 400 female plastic surgeons, 295 (74 percent) were under 44, in contrast to the approximately 4,805 male plastic surgeons, of whom 2,110 (44 percent) were under 44.

In the years leading up to and through World War II, clinical advances continued unabated. Vilray Blair and James Barrett Brown introduced split-skin grafts for covering large areas of granulating surfaces in 1929. The following year, these surgeons refined the Mirault procedure for repair of cleft lip. In 1939 Earl Padgett perfected a calibrated dermatome to assist in preparing skin grafts. Four years later, Machteld E. Sano reported, in the *American Journal of Surgery*, on the use of fibrin glue for skin grafting. During the war, the Army and Navy established plastic surgery centers, most notably at Valley Forge, Pennsylvania, where reconstructive cases were concentrated and treated by board-certified plastic surgeons. Approximately one-third of the work in plastic surgery was done with free skin grafts, an additional one-third on patients with burns, and the remainder on reconstructive cases. The highlights of wartime advances in plastic surgery included the elimination of tannic acid in the management of burns and the substitution of atraumatic care of the wound, the use of pressure dressings to prevent loss of fluids and blood, early skin grafting, the extensive use of local tissue in repairs, the concept that deep healing can be no better than superficial healing and the development of special surgical procedures for the management of injuries in particular regions, including the palate, jaw, nose, ear, and other parts of the face (the composite free graft from the ear being one notable example).

Greater numbers of plastic surgery textbooks were being published, including *Plastic Surgery of the Breast and Abdominal Wall* (1942) by Max Thorek (1880–1960), *Plastic and Reconstructive Surgery* (1948) by Earl Padgett and Kathryn Stephenson, and *Plastic Surgery* (1950) by Ferris Smith. In order to more easily disseminate the rapidly growing literature on plastic surgery, a monthly journal, *Plastic and Reconstructive Surgery*, was started in 1947 and remains the preeminent peer-reviewed plastic surgical journal. Its editors and their years of stewardship include Warren B. Davis (1946–1947), Robert H. Ivy (1948–1964), Kathryn L. Stephenson (1965–1967), Frank McDowell (1968–1979), and Robert M. Goldwyn (1980–??).

By the 1960s, cosmetic surgery was increasing at a tremendous rate, which reflected the changing mores of beauty in our culture. Whereas once reconstructive surgery constituted the great proportion of plastic surgical operations, cosmetic procedures now command the bulk of the profession's and society's attention. Yet, when plastic surgeons were queried by members of the research subcommittee of the *Study on Surgical Services for the United States* regarding important plastic surgical contributions from 1945 to 1970, no areas were deemed of first-order importance. Silicone and silastic implants were considered of second-order importance, and surgery of cleft lip and palate and surgery of craniofacial anomalies were of third-order importance.

The writing of the history of plastic surgery has been well served by American plastic surgeons. George Dorrance (1877–1948) authored *The Operative Story of Cleft Palate* in 1933 and *The History of Treatment of Fractured Jaws* eight years later. In 1943, Wendell Hughes completed a carefully documented history, *Reconstructive Surgery of the Eyelids*. Maxwell Maltz wrote *Evolution of Plastic Surgery* in 1946. Frank McDowell (1911–1981) edited a chronological five-volume series of plastic surgical indexes (1977–1981) and compiled *The Source Book of Plastic Surgery* (1977). Some of these histories incorporate short biographies into their content, and the following vignettes provide a backward glimpse into the lives of several individuals who have contributed to the evolutionary development of plastic surgery in the United States.

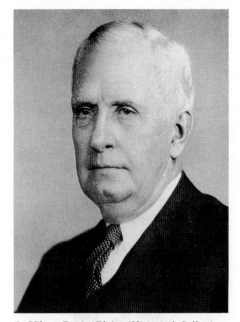

5. Vilray Papin Blair. (*Historical Collections, College of Physicians of Philadelphia*)

BIOGRAPHIES OF PLASTIC SURGEONS

Vilray Papin Blair (1871–1955), born in St. Louis, graduated from Christian Brothers' College in 1890 and St. Louis Medical College in 1893. He pursued an internship at Mullanphy Hospital (1893–1895) and joined the faculty of the Washington University School of Medicine as an instructor in practical anatomy. He advanced through the academic ranks and by 1912 was clinical professor of anatomy. From 1912 to 1927, Blair was an associate and then assistant professor in clinical surgery. In 1927 he was named both professor of clinical surgery and professor of oral surgery. He remained in these positions until 1941, when he became emeritus professor. Six years later, Blair retired from active clinical practice. A pioneer in the development of plastic surgery as a specialty, he played an influential role in the military during World War I, when he was chief of the Section of Oral and Plastic Surgery (1917–1918) and senior consultant in maxillofacial surgery for the American Expeditionary Forces (1918). Following the war, he was named attending specialist in plastic surgery at the Veterans Hospital, Jefferson Barracks, Missouri, and also established the first separate plastic surgery service in the United States at Barnes Hospital. Blair's research and clinical skills led to the improvement of a multitude of surgical techniques for congenital and acquired facial defects. Among his nearly two hundred published papers are such influential reports as a description of a closed ramisection of the mandible for micrognathia or prognathism (1909), the use of split-skin grafts for covering large areas of granulating surfaces (1929), and his modern refinement of Mirault's operation for single harelip (1930). Among his influential textbooks are *Surgery and Diseases of the Mouth and Jaws* (1912), the first comprehensive work on maxillofacial surgery; *Essentials of Oral Surgery* (1923); and *Cancer of the Face and Mouth; Diagnosis, Treatment, Surgical Repair* (1941). Blair was a diplomate of the American Board of Otolaryngology and played a major role in establishing the American Board of Plastic Surgery.

John Staige Davis (1872–1946), born in Norfolk, Virginia, received his undergraduate education at Yale University (1895) and his medical degree from The Johns Hopkins School of Medicine (1899). He served for a year as a house officer at The Johns Hopkins Hospital. In 1900 Davis joined the medical staff at Union Protestant Infirmary, where he pursued further postgraduate training. In 1903 he established a medical practice in Baltimore and six years later joined the surgical faculty at his alma mater. He remained on The Hopkins' surgical staff until his death, although most of his clinical activities were concentrated at the Union Memorial Hospital. Considered the first American surgeon to limit his work exclusively to plastic surgery, Davis was a major contributor to the overall field of plastic and reconstructive surgery, having introduced many of its basic principles and techniques. He perfected the eponymically named Davis graft, in which small sections of full-thickness skin are transplanted to raw areas and allowed to grow together and cover the denuded sections (1909). Davis also developed a technique of utilizing local skin flaps for repairing deformities and blemishes around the face and jaws, and he was quite active in researching the physiology of circulation in skin

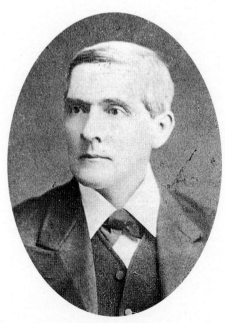

6. John Staige Davis. (*Historical Collections, College of Physicians of Philadelphia*)

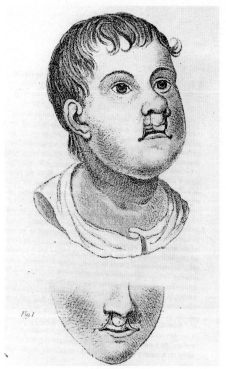

7. Isaac Cathrall's (1764–1819) case of "double hare-lip" in an 11-month-old child was the subject of the first article on a plastic surgical topic to be published in an American medical periodical (*American Medical Recorder* vol. 2, pages 372–373, 1819). (*Historical Collections, College of Physicians of Philadelphia*)

transplantation. He summarized much of his work in *Plastic Surgery: Its Principles and Practice* (1919), a pioneering classic that was widely used for many years. Following the success of his treatise, Davis was named professor of plastic surgery at The Johns Hopkins Hospital, the first such formal academic title in the United States. He helped found and was active in the American College of Surgeons, the American Association of Plastic Surgeons, and the American Board of Plastic Surgery. In 1937 Davis served as vice president of the American Surgical Association, and seven years later he was elected for a two-year term as president of the American Association of Plastic Surgeons.

Frederick Strange Kolle (1872–1929) was born in Hanover, Germany, and received his medical degree from the Long Island College Hospital Medical School (1893), having served as an assistant in the ear department of the Brooklyn Eye and Ear Hospital (1892). He completed an internship at Kings County Hospital (1893–1894) and soon established a private medical practice in Brooklyn (after 1894), while also becoming an assistant physician in the Brooklyn Hospital for Contagious Diseases. Kolle had diverse clinical interests and from 1896 to 1900 was a teacher of electricity in medicine at the Electrical Engineering Institute of Brooklyn. From 1897 to 1902, he was also an associate editor of a monthly periodical, *Electrical Age*, and became radiographer to the Methodist Episcopal Hospital in Brooklyn. For unknown reasons, beginning in 1914, Kolle withdrew entirely from public notice, although it is believed that following World War I, he moved to the Los Angeles area, where he may have done some general practice. Kolle was one of the first x-ray investigators in the United States (1896) and went on to develop numerous radiologic techniques and to invent various devices: the radiometer, the Kolle x-ray switching device, the dentaskiascope, the folding fluoroscope, the x-ray printing process, the Kolle focus tube, and the direct reading x-ray meter. He also became an influential figure in plastic surgery by devising techniques for subcutaneous paraffin injections for cosmetic purposes and by inventing various apparati useful in plastic and reconstructive surgery. Kolle's *Plastic and Cosmetic Surgery* (1911) was the first detailed monograph on cosmetic surgery, although it was predated by a lesser-known work, *Subcutaneous Hydrocarbon Prostheses* (1908). His other texts included *The X-rays, Their Production and Application* (1898), *The Grown Baby Book* (1903), and *The Physician's Who's Who* (1913), a reference work.

George Morris Dorrance (1877–1949) was born in Bristol, Pennsylvania, and graduated from the University of Pennsylvania School of Medicine in 1900. He served an internship and was resident physician at the Hospital of the University of Pennsylvania (1900–1902). Four years later, Dorrance was hired as assistant surgeon to St. Agnes Hospital in Philadelphia and, in 1907, became chief surgeon to that institution. He remained in this position until 1939. Dorrance was also appointed assistant professor of maxillofacial surgery at the School of Dentistry of the University of Pennsylvania in 1917, becoming professor in 1919 and serving until his retirement in 1947. Beginning in 1940, he specialized mainly in cleft palate surgery. During World War I, Dorrance served in the U.S. Army Medical Corps, spending the early part of his service overseas with the Section of Oral and Plastic Surgery in France and England. Later, he was placed in charge of the maxillofacial surgery service at the American Base Hospital No. 11, in Cape May, New Jersey. Dorrance was one of the organizers of the American Board of Plastic Surgery and served as its chairman for two years. In addition, he was president of the American Association of Plastic Surgeons (1936) and the author of two textbooks, *The Operative Story of Cleft Palate* (1933) and the two-volume *The History of Treatment of Fractured Jaws* (1941).

Varaztad Hovhannes Kazanjian (1879–1974) was born in Armenia when it was a province of the Ottoman Empire. Political unrest caused him to emigrate to the United States in 1895. During the next seven years, he worked in a wire mill in

Worcester, Massachusetts, where he mastered the English language and attended Worcester night schools. Becoming an American citizen in 1900, Kazanjian decided to study dentistry and matriculated at Harvard Dental School (1902), graduating in 1905. He soon opened a private dental office in Boston and was also appointed a part-time assistant in prosthetic dentistry at his alma mater. Increasingly interested in maxillofacial surgery, Kazanjian entered medical school at Boston University and completed the second year in 1912, but never returned for the third year. Instead, he accepted the position as head of Harvard's Prosthetic Laboratory. In the early part of World War I, when the First Harvard Unit was organized (1915) to serve with the British forces in France, Kazanjian was appointed dental chief of the unit. Members of the unit were initially stationed at British General Hospital No. 22 in Camiers, near Boulogne, but later were transferred to Hospital No. 20, in the same general area. The British command assigned almost one hundred patient beds to Kazanjian's section, and he remained in charge until 1919. Following his return to civilian life, Kazanjian was appointed professor of military oral surgery at Harvard Dental School, but he soon realized that without a formal medical degree, he could not freely perform in Boston the same surgical procedures he had done in France. Accordingly, he entered the junior year at Harvard Medical School and graduated in 1921, at the age of 42 years. Granted staff privileges at the Massachusetts General Hospital and several other Boston institutions, Kazanjian began a maxillofacial surgical practice, which drew patients from all over the world, including Sigmund Freud (1856–1939), for whom he constructed a facial prosthetic appliance. Named professor of clinical oral surgery at Harvard University in 1922, Kazanjian continued in this capacity until 1941, when he was appointed the first professor of plastic surgery in the history of his alma mater. Kazanjian remained in active private practice until his mid-80s. In 1923 he became a member of the American Association of Plastic Surgeons, and in 1940 he served as its president. Kazanjian authored over 150 professional articles and, in collaboration with his former student John Marquis Converse, wrote the classic plastic surgery textbook, *The Surgical Treatment of Facial Injuries* (1949).

Charles Conrad Miller (1880–1950) was born in New Albany, Indiana, and immediately following high school graduation enlisted as a private in Company C of the Indiana 159th Volunteer Infantry. Expecting to participate in the recently declared Spanish-American War, the unit did little more than six months of stateside bivouacking and was disbanded in November 1898. In 1899 Miller entered the freshman class of the Hospital College of Medicine in Louisville, Kentucky, receiving his diploma in 1902. He moved to Chicago and established a general medical practice that soon became focused on general and cosmetic surgery. In 1907 he even authored an obscure monograph on hernias, *The Cure of Rupture by Paraffin Injections*. Miller soon began improvising surgical procedures to alter facial features, and from 1906 to 1908, he inundated several small county and state medical journals with repetitious articles describing what he termed "featural surgery." During these years he privately published *Cosmetic Surgery: The Correction of Featural Imperfections* (1907), the first book on the subject in the world. Miller was a public relations genius and had little difficulty in finding patients eager to undergo his cosmetic procedures. It was a time of beauty salons and numerous patent nostrums to restore youth, and Miller quietly seized the opportunity to further his practice. All of his various procedures, including blepharoplasties and rhinoplasties, were conducted in an ambulatory setting in his office with the patient under local anesthesia. Between 1908 and 1923, Miller published little, probably because of legal difficulties resulting from his acknowledged ownership of three "quack" drugstores in Chicago, which the *Chicago Daily Tribune* targeted in its campaign against narcotic abuse. In fact, the *Tribune* was the only city newspaper to carry the lurid story, and all charges of selling drugs without a prescription were finally dropped in 1914, when the newspaper's reporter failed to appear in court. Evidently, the unfavorable publicity did not adversely affect

Miller's professional standing in the community, because one year later, he reappeared as editor of *Medicine and Health*, a lay publication. In his new combination home and office, located on the fashionable Near North Side, Miller's "surgical center" prospered and, with the assistance of four nurses, he continued to perform cosmetic procedures. Although he was now too busy to continue writing innumerable journal articles, he did manage to publish two additional cosmetic surgical texts: *Rubber and Gutta Percha Injections; Subcutaneous Injections of Rubber and Gutta Percha for Raising the Depressed Nasal Bridge and Altering External Contours* (1923), and *Cannula Implants and Review of Implantation Technics in Esthetic Surgery* (1926), as well as an expanded version of his cosmetic surgery textbook in 1924. Three years later, Miller's messianic zeal again took hold when he initiated his own journal, *Dr. Charles Conrad Miller's Review of Plastic and Esthetic Surgery*. As he was both editor and sole contributor, the journal's pages were cluttered with advertising coupons relative to Miller's cosmetic surgical practice. The later years of his career are shrouded in obscurity, although it is known that he found time to author several general surgical texts: *Conservative Tonsil Surgery, Safeguarded Thyroidectomy and Thyroid Surgery* (1928), and *The Injection Treatment of Hemorrhoids* (1929). The great economic depression of the 1930s found the character of Miller's surgical practice changing. There was less demand for cosmetic surgery, and Miller himself became disenchanted with "featural problems." In 1930, his childless wife, an invalid for many years, committed suicide. Miller married again, fathered three children, and died of a myocardial infarction in his seventieth year.

Robert Henry Ivy (1881–1974) was born in Southport, England, and came to the United States with the expressed purpose of enrolling in the University of Pennsylvania School of Dentistry. He was awarded a D.D.S. in 1902 and served a dental internship at the Philadelphia General Hospital. Ivy's dental internship experience stimulated his interest in medicine, and he matriculated in the university's school of medicine, graduating in 1907. For the next three years, he served as resident physician at the Episcopal Hospital. In 1910 Ivy entered private practice, and almost immediately he demonstrated an interest in oral and plastic surgery. He became assistant to his uncle, Matthew Cryer, professor of oral surgery at the University of Pennsylvania. During World War I, Ivy was commissioned a captain in the medical corps and was assigned to active duty in the office of the Surgeon General as assistant to Vilray Blair. Ivy helped to formulate plans for the care of maxillofacial injuries and was later ordered to France, where he treated such victims at hospital centers in Clermont-Ferrand and Vichy. Returning to the United States in 1919, Ivy was placed in charge of maxillofacial surgery at the Water Reed Army Hospital. Following his discharge, Ivy joined the surgical staff at the University of Pennsylvania, where his initial appointment was in maxillofacial surgery. In 1943 his title was changed to professor of plastic surgery, and eight years later he retired from active practice and the university. Not content to entirely relax, Ivy accepted an appointment as chief of the newly formed Cleft Palate Division of the Department of Health in Pennsylvania. At the beginning of World War II, Ivy was named a member of the committee on surgery of the National Research Council and chairman of the subcommittee on plastic and maxillofacial surgery. Renowned as a teacher of plastic surgeons, Ivy was one of the organizers of the American Board of Plastic Surgery and was in the founders' group of the American Board of Surgery. He also helped conceive the American Association of Plastic Surgeons, serving as its president in 1928. Ivy's textbooks include *Applied Anatomy and Oral Surgery for Dental Students* (1911), *Applied Immunology* (1915), *Interpretation of Dental and Maxillary Roentgenograms* (1918), *Essentials of Oral Surgery* (1923) coauthored with Blair, and *Fractures of the Jaw* (1931) coauthored with Lawrence Curtis. Ivy was editor in chief of *Plastic and Reconstructive Surgery* from 1946 until 1965. In 1962 he authored an autobiography, *A Link With the Past*.

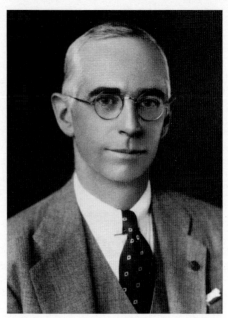

8. Robert Henry Ivy. (*Historical Collections, College of Physicians of Philadelphia*)

Ferris N. Smith (1884–1957), son of a prominent Michigan attorney who later became United States Senator, graduated from the University of Michigan School of Medicine in 1910. He immediately began a "residency" in otorhinolaryngology by joining the surgical service of R. Bishop Canfield, professor of otolaryngology. Because of Smith's early interest in plastic surgical cases, members of the department of general surgery began to refer to him patients with cleft lip and palate, and other facial deformities. After three years of postgraduate training, Smith moved to Grand Rapids, where he established an ear, nose, and throat practice and remained for the rest of his professional life. In 1916, through arrangements made by his father, Smith joined the British Army and began working with Harold Gillies (1882–1960) at Sidcup, England. Both Smith and Gillies made frequent trips to Paris to watch Hippolyte Morestin (1869–1919) perform reconstructive surgical procedures. Having developed numerous French surgical acquaintances, Smith spent many summers after the war conducting a six-week course in plastic surgery in Paris, where he was professor of plastic surgery at the International Clinic. Although not a prolific contributor to the plastic surgical literature, Smith authored two important texts: *Reconstructive Surgery of the Head and Neck in Nelson's Loose-Leaf System* (1928) and *Plastic and Reconstructive Surgery* (1948). Smith was a founding member of the American Board of Plastic Surgery but later dissociated himself from the Board in an argument over whether plastic surgery should be taught by a system of registrars (apprentices) or with residents. Smith trained many individuals as "registrars" at the Blodgett Memorial Hospital in Grand Rapids but never instituted a formal plastic surgical training program. He served as president of the American Association of Plastic Surgeons in 1932.

Joseph Eastman Sheehan (1885–1951) was born in Dublin, Ireland, and brought at a young age to Wallingford, Connecticut. He graduated from Yale Medical School in 1908 and subsequently obtained postgraduate training, first with Theodor Kocher (1841–1917) in Bern, Switzerland, and then in various other cities, including Berlin, Budapest, Heidelberg, London, Paris, and Vienna. He returned to the United States in 1912 and settled in New York City, where he opened a surgical practice. During World War I, Sheehan worked in Sidcup, England, with Harold Gillies. This experience kindled Sheehan's interest in plastic surgery. Maintaining a practice in both New York City and London, Sheehan also was professor of plastic and reconstructive surgery at the New York Polyclinic Medical School and clinical professor of surgery at Columbia University, as well as consultant to various other American and European hospitals. He was certified by the American Board of Otolaryngology and was a founding member of the American Board of Plastic

9. The trench warfare of World War I resulted in devastating gunshot and shrapnel wounds of the exposed head and face. As a result, the field of reconstructive maxillofacial surgery received an enormous impetus through the clinical work of such leading American authorities as Vilray P. Blair and John S. Davis. This series of photographs from the Walter Reed Hospital Maxillofacial Unit illustrates the destructiveness of the injuries and the gratifying results of treatment. (*Courtesy of Stanley B. Burns, M.D., and The Burns Collection and Archive*)

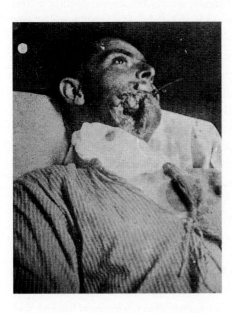
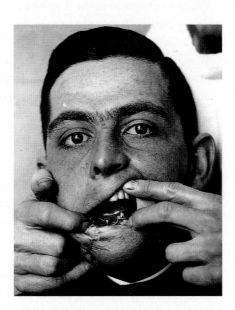
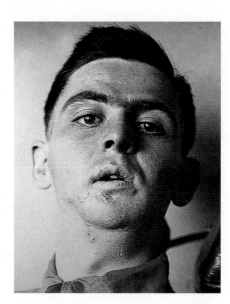

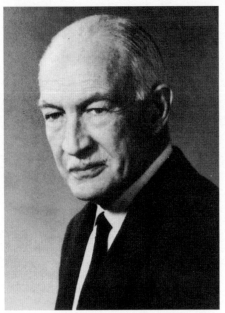

10. Jerome Pierce Webster. (*Historical Collections, College of Physicians of Philadelphia*)

Surgery. Sheehan authored several textbooks, including *Plastic Surgery of the Nose* (1925), *Plastic Surgery of the Orbit* (1927), *A Manual of Reparative Plastic Surgery* (1938), and *General and Plastic Surgery, With Emphasis on War Injuries* (1945). In 1935–1936, he was elected president of the American Association of Plastic Surgeons. A surgical showman and master of public relations, Sheehan was asked by General Francisco Franco of the Spanish National Army to take care of his war wounded during the Spanish Civil War (1936–1939). This resulted in considerable political consternation on the part of his surgical colleagues and eventually caused Sheehan to be labelled a Fascist and declared *persona non grata* in England.

Sumner Leivnetz Koch (1888–1976), born in Cavalier, North Dakota, graduated from Hamline College in 1908 and the Northwestern University School of Medicine in 1914. He interned at the Cook County Hospital (1914–1916) and was invited by Allen Kanavel (1874–1938) to join him in his surgical practice and teaching at the Chicago Wesley Memorial Hospital. During World War I, Koch served in the U.S. Army Medical Corps assigned to the Base Hospital No. 12, the Northwestern Medical School unit, in Camiers Seine Inférieure, France. Following his return to civilian life, Koch continued his association with Kanavel and also organized a hand clinic at Cook Country Hospital. Throughout his professional life, Koch remained in the academic environment of Northwestern University, where he advanced to the rank of professor of surgery. He served from 1923 to 1937 as abstract editor of *Surgery, Gynecology and Obstetrics* and as associate editor from 1937 to 1959. Interested in both hand and burn surgery, Koch served as president of the American Association of Plastic Surgeons (1950) and was a founding member and president of the American Society for Surgery of the Hand.

Jerome Pierce Webster (1888–1974), was born in Ashland, New Hampshire, and graduated from Trinity College in Hartford, Connecticut, in 1910 and The Johns Hopkins School of Medicine in 1914. He began surgical training at The Johns Hopkins Hospital, but his residency was interrupted by World War I, when he served with the U.S. Army Medical Corps in France. Following the end of hostilities, Webster returned to The Hopkins and resumed his postgraduate training. In 1921 he traveled to China as resident surgeon to the recently established Peking Union Medical College. He attained the rank of associate professor of surgery before returning to America in 1926. While in China, Webster began to develop an interest in plastic surgical operations, and in 1928 he spent six months studying with Vilray Blair and James B. Brown in St. Louis. He then furthered his surgical training by relocating to New York City as a fellow in surgery at Columbia University. When the Columbia-Presbyterian Medical Center opened in 1934, Allen O. Whipple, chairman of the department of surgery, asked Webster to organize a division of plastic surgery. Over the next two and a half decades, Webster developed one of the outstanding plastic surgical training programs in the United States. During World War II, he established, in conjunction with his own residency program, one of several army centers in which surgeons and dentists were given an intensive three-month course in the primary care of maxillofacial injuries. After he retired from his professorship in 1954, Webster's principal efforts were directed toward expanding the Webster Library of Plastic Surgery, one of the world's great collections of rare medical books. His interest in plastic surgical history culminated in his writing, with Martha T. Gnudi, *The Life and Times of Gaspare Tagliacozzi, Surgeon of Bologna, 1545–1599* (1950). Webster's professional career was laden with many honors, including the presidency of the American Association of Plastic Surgeons (1941) and the vice presidency of the American Society for Surgery of the Hand (1956). He was one of the founding members of the American Board of Plastic Surgery and served as its chairman from 1947 to 1949.

Earl Calvin Padgett (1893–1946) was born in Greenleaf, Kansas, and educated at the University of Kansas (1916) and the Washington University School of Medicine (1918). From 1919 to 1922, he was a house officer at Barnes Hospital, and then assistant to Vilray Blair in plastic surgery (1923–1924). In 1925 Padgett joined

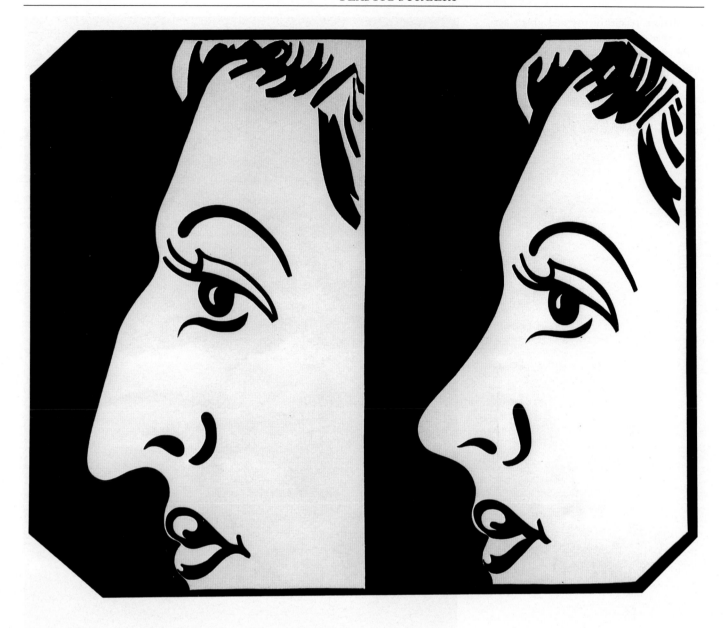

11. "Before and After, 3" (1962) by Andy Warhol (1925–1987). (*Collection of Whitney Museum of American Art, purchased with funds from Charles Simon 71.226, Copyright 1997 Andy Warhol Foundation for the Visual Arts/ARS, New York*)

the surgical faculty at the University of Kansas, and he rose through the academic ranks to become, in 1936, clinical professor of plastic surgery, a position he remained in until his death. His greatest contribution to plastic surgery was his invention of the Padgett-Hood calibrated dermatome. He conceived the idea of bringing and holding the skin to a smooth fixed surface in order to allow a sharp metal blade to be passed at a controlled distance (height), resulting in a large skin graft of uniform thickness (1930). During the 1930s, the device was perfected in collaboration with a University of Kansas professor of engineering, George Hood, and it was used for the first time in 1938. The following year, the invention was fully described in *Surgery, Gynecology and Obstetrics*. There was wide acclaim, and the Padgett-Hood dermatome became a staple with most surgeons. A priority fight erupted when Hood attempted to secure a patent on the device. Many aspects of the story remain shrouded in mystery, although it appears certain that the basic idea was Padgett's. What remains unresolved is who deserves credit for the many engineering changes involved as the dermatome evolved. A prolific author, Padgett wrote three books related to plastic surgery: *Surgical Diseases of the Mouth and Jaws* (1938), *Skin Grafting From a Personal and Experimental Point of View* (1942), and *Plastic and Reconstructive Surgery* (1948), the latter co-authored with Kathryn Stephenson.

Alfred Cyril Callister (1894–1961) was born in Salt Lake City and educated at the University of Utah (1915) and Harvard Medical School (1917). He completed a surgical internship at Boston City Hospital and then a year as resident surgeon

12. Modern reconstructive and plastic surgeons offer a remarkably wide variety of cosmetic improvements. To complete this rhytidectomy, or removal of wrinkles, the surgeon is suturing together what had previously been sagging facial skin. (*Courtesy of Stanley B. Burns, M.D., and The Burns Collection and Archive and the permission of Sherrell J Aston, M.D.*)

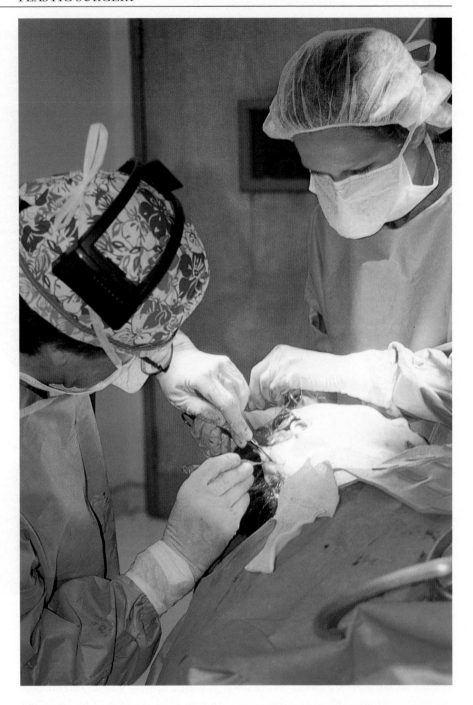

(1918–1919). In 1920 Callister became a physician-surgeon to the County Hospital in Salt Lake City. Four years later, he was named chief of the section of plastic and thoracic surgery at the Latter Day Saints Hospital. He served on the faculty at the University of Utah Medical School (1921–1942), where he was lecturer in hygiene and preventive medicine. During the years of World War II, Callister was dean of the school and also served as procurement and assignment officer for Utah physicians. A 1938 diplomate of the American Board of Plastic Surgery, he was actively involved with virtually all aspects of organized medicine in Utah, including stints as president of the Utah State Medical Association (1941) and as a member of the Utah State Board of Health (1924–1950). His major contribution was taking the leading role in transforming the medical school at the University of Utah from a two-year to a four-year institution (1941–1942). He served as first dean of the reorganized school (1942–1945) and was directly responsible for recruiting the new faculty and integrating the basic sciences with the clinical curriculum. Although he wrote little, Callister's clinical papers dealt mostly with plastic surgical topics, particularly congenital defects of the face.

James Barrett Brown (1899–1971), born in Hannibal, Missouri, received his medical degree from Washington University in 1923. After an internship and a one-year assistant residency at Barnes Hospital in St. Louis, he joined Vilray Blair in the practice of plastic surgery, an association that continued throughout the latter's lifetime. Their joint research activities resulted in the development of the concept of split-thickness skin grafts to cover large granulating surface areas (1929) and a modern refinement of Mirault's procedure for repair of cleft lip (1930). During World War II, Brown served in the U.S. Army, first as senior consultant in plastic and maxillofacial surgery and burns in the European theater of operations. In 1943 he was assigned stateside to the Valley Forge General Hospital, which had been loosely designated as a plastic surgical center. At the conclusion of hostilities (1945), Brown assumed his third military assignment as senior consultant to the Surgeon General of the Army. Eventually, Brown returned to his academic posts at Washington University, where he received a joint appointment as professor of clinical surgery and professor of maxillofacial surgery. On retirement, he was named professor emeritus of plastic surgery. Brown was a prolific author, whose first textbook was *Skin Grafting of Burns* (1943). He went on to author six more works, including *Plastic Surgery of the Nose* (1951), *Neck Dissections* (1954), and *Early Treatment of Facial Injuries* (1964). Active in all aspects of organized surgery, Brown was chairman of the American Board of Plastic Surgery (1946) and president of the American Association of Plastic Surgeons (1954) and the Western Surgical Association (1958). He served on the editorial board of several surgical journals, including *Surgery, Gynecology and Obstetrics; Surgery;* and *Postgraduate Medicine.*

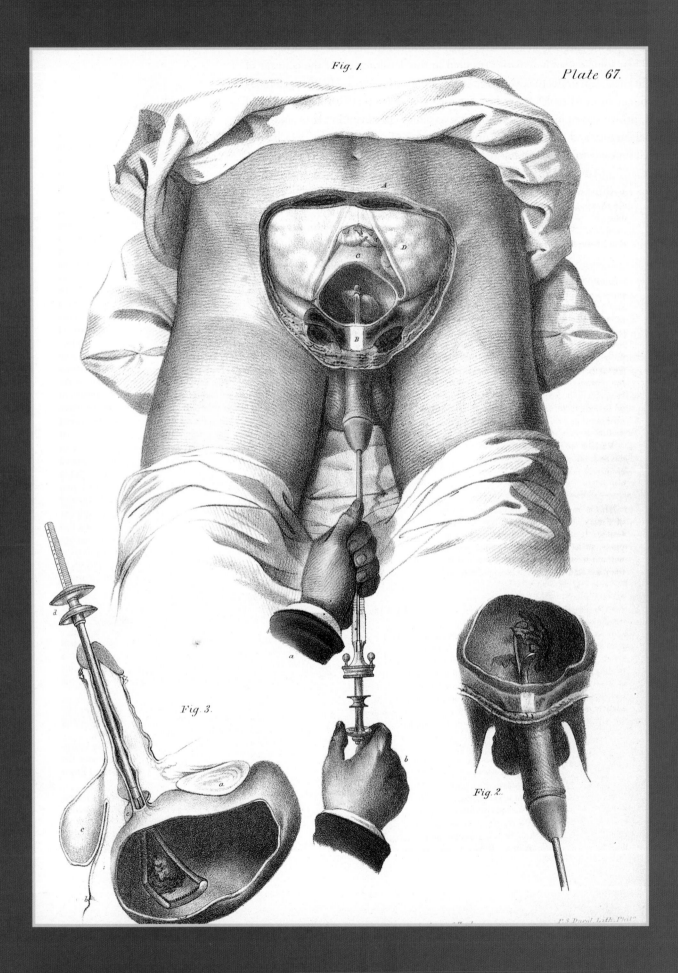

Fig. 1.

Plate 67.

Fig. 3.

Fig. 2.

CHAPTER 22

UROLOGIC SURGERY

Through the beginning of the twentieth century, urology as a specialty was largely dependent on other branches of medicine and surgery. In most instances, the principal source of activity, as well as remuneration, for the so-called urologist was the treatment of venereal diseases and their sequelae. Most commonly, a physician who maintained an interest in urologic diseases functioned generally as a diagnostician of urologic disorders. When a urologic operation was indicated, the patient was customarily referred to another physician with more respectable surgical skills. Accordingly, most of the early contributions to surgery of the urinary organs were made by general surgeons. Attempts at organizing the specialty were limited, other than for the founding of the American Association of Genito-Urinary Surgeons in 1886. No hospitals were strictly devoted to urologic diseases, although beginning in the 1880s, Bellevue Hospital in New York City *ipso facto* contained a urologic ward, owing to the clinical interests of one of its visiting surgeons, Edward Keyes (1843–1924). Not until 1911 would a formal urologic department be opened at Bellevue Hospital, the first such unit in the country.

The development of urology as a primary surgical specialty is traceable, at least in part, to the development of instrumentation that allowed direct visualization of the urinary tract: the cystoscope and urologic endoscopy. However, not until the 1890s was the first modern cystoscope commercially available in the United States. It was modern in the sense that it employed the principle of present-day cystoscopes: an electric source of illumination incorporated into a sophisticated lens system. Before this time, physicians who cared for common inflammations of the anterior and posterior urethra, prostate, and bladder had little more than a crude assortment of bougies, dilators, sounds, and urethratomes available to them. Nineteenth-century American surgeons with an interest in urologic diseases primarily concentrated their activities on two surgical operations: lithotomy (surgical removal of a calculus, especially a vesical calculus) and litholapaxy or lithotrity (crushing of a stone in the bladder and washing out the fragments through a wide-lumen catheter).

The limit of urologic surgical practice in early America is noted in the titles of the first books published on the subject: Robert Muter's 107-page *Practical Observations on the Lateral Operation of Lithotomy* (1824), Alexander Stevens' (1789–1869) *Lectures on Lithotomy* (1838), and Homer Bostwick's (died 1862) compendia, *A Treatise on the Nature and Treatment of Seminal Diseases, Impotency, and Other Kindred Affections* (1847) and *A Complete Practical Work on the Nature and Treatment of Venereal Diseases, and Other Affections of the Genito-Urinary Organs of the Male and Female* (1848). Not until the mid-nineteenth century was the first textbook to provide a systematic approach to genitourinary diseases published: Samuel D. Gross's *A Practical Treatise on the Diseases and Injuries of the Urinary Bladder, the Prostate Gland, and the Urethra* (1851).

1. *(facing page)* Bladder stones were a common surgical problem throughout the nineteenth century. In this plate from Joseph Pancoast's *A Treatise on Operative Surgery* (1844), a lithotripsy (the operation of crushing a stone in the bladder or urethra) by percussion, after the manner of the French surgeon, Leroy d'Etiolles, is demonstrated. *(Author's Collection)*

A quarter of a century later, Gross wrote that "as lithotomists, American surgeons are not surpassed by any in the world," while "lithotrity...has never met with much favour on this continent, a circumstance so much the more surprising when it is remembered how common calculous diseases are in certain sections of the United States." Gross was correct in his assessment, highlighted by Philip Syng Physick's acclaimed lithotomy, in 1831, on Chief Justice John Marshall (1755–1835), Benjamin Dudley's (1785–1870) widely regarded expertise in the operation, and Emil Noeggerath's (1827–1895) introduction of suprapubic cystotomy as a means of removing bladder calculi (1858). However, Gross could not know that in 1878, Henry Bigelow (1818–1890) of Boston would develop a large-caliber evacuation tube to more easily remove bladder debris during lithotrity. Bigelow's improvement of the lithotrite ranks as one of the most memorable contributions to nineteenth-century American surgery. He was adamant that attempts to crush and remove bladder stones should always be completed during a single operation, a procedure he termed litholapaxy. Of prime importance to the success of this method was Bigelow's evacuator, consisting of a powerful rubber bulb and a glass trap beneath for stone fragments. Used with Bigelow's larger catheters, it proved an important advance from prior aspirators and caused lithotrity to become quite popular for a few years.

By the 1850s, operations on the bladder *per se* were being completed with greater frequency. In 1851 Willard Parker (1800–1884) reported on the use of cystotomy as a treatment of irritable bladder. Eight years later, Daniel Ayres (1822–1892), professor of clinical surgery and surgical pathology at the Long Island College Hospital, authored the country's first report of a successful "plastic" operation for exstrophy of the female bladder. Later that year, Gross, writing in the *North American Medico-Chirurgical Review*, noted that Joseph Pancoast (1805–1882) had completed a plastic repair of the bladder in 1858 and that Pancoast's case should be considered the earliest case. During the Civil War, Albert Walter (1811–1876) performed an exploratory laparotomy to repair a bladder rupture caused by a kick to the abdomen (1862). Frank Maury (1840–1879) and Richard Levis (1827–1890) were the most prominent of several surgeons in the 1870s and 1880s who devised ingenious operations for closure of the anterior bladder wall.

At the time of the Civil War, Erastus Wolcott (1804–1880) performed the first recorded nephrectomy, although the patient died two weeks following surgery (1862). Six years later, Henry Bowditch (1808–1892) authored the earliest detailed account of perinephric abscess and its surgical treatment in the American periodical literature (1868). In 1871 John Gilmore (1835–1875) reported the first totally successful nephrectomy. A case of nephrotomy for removal of a calculus was presented in the *New York Medical Journal* in 1873. However, at the Boston City Hospital in 1872, F. E. Bundy and William Ingalls (1813–1903) had removed a large calculus from the right kidney of a female patient via a lumbar incision, the country's first recorded nephrolithotomy. Ingalls did not report this procedure until ten years later, and he never received just recognition for this spectacular feat. By the mid-1880s, operations on the kidney had become so routine that Robert Weir (1838–1927) and Samuel W. Gross (1837–1889) were able to author collective reviews on over one hundred nephrectomies performed in both Europe and the United States.

During the last two decades of the nineteenth century, several seminal events signaled the beginnings of the recognition of urology as a distinct surgical specialty. In 1880 Arthur Cabot (1852–1912) was named clinical instructor of genitourinary surgery at Harvard Medical School. This marked the first time in the country that urologic surgery was officially accorded status in the academic community as a special field apart from the whole of surgery. Six years later, a meeting was held at the New York City residence of Edward Keyes for the purpose of organizing a society devoted to the study of genitourinary and venereal diseases. Twelve "genitourinary surgeons," including Henry Bigelow, John Brinton, Arthur Cabot, Edward Keyes, Fesenden Otis, Roswell Park, and Nicholas Senn, and eight "syphilologists," including Prince Morrow, Frank Sturgis, Robert Taylor, and J. William White, were invit-

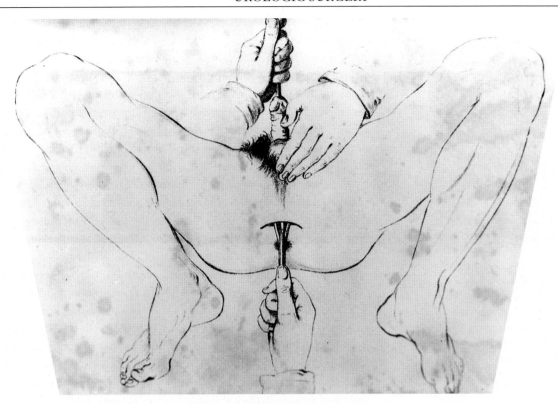

2. Taken from Alexander Stevens' (1789–1869) *Lectures on Lithotomy* (1838), one of the country's earliest monographs on a urologic topic, this plate demonstrates "the mode of introducing the prostatic bisector, directed by the grooved staff from the bottom of the external wound through the prostate gland, into the bladder." (*Author's Collection*)

ed to become founding members of the American Association of Genito-Urinary Surgeons. Realistically, with membership limited to fifty individuals, there was little prospect that this fledgling organization would achieve a position of national prominence and consequent influence any time soon.

From a clinical standpoint, significant advances continued to be made that assured urology's emergence from the shadows of general and gynecologic surgery. In 1884 Fesenden Otis reported the first attempts at utilizing local anesthesia (cocaine placed into the urethra) in urologic surgery. A decade and a half later, Robert Abbe (1851–1928) authored the country's first detailed account, in the *Annals of Surgery*, on the diagnosis of renal calculi by x-ray. At the turn of the century, the introduction of the opaque catheter, a ureteral catheter with a metal stylette, represented the earliest attempt to render the upper urinary tract opaque to roentgen rays. During the 1890s, increasingly complex surgical procedures on the kidneys, ureters, and bladder were devised. Howard Kelly's (1858–1943) important work in genitourinary surgery is often overshadowed by his success as professor of gynecology at The Johns Hopkins Hospital. However, he proved a major figure in the development of urologic surgical techniques. In 1891 he completed a "kolpo-ureterotomy" to permit dilatation of a stricture of the ureter in a female, and removed calcareous material. At the same time, Kelly was perfecting a rudimentary cystoscope to provide direct visual inspection of the female bladder and ureters (1893). One year later, he described an operation for ureterovaginal fistula, in which a uretero–ureteral anastomosis and uretero–ureterostomy were successfully completed. By 1900 Kelly had begun to diagnose bladder calculi by means of scratch marks on a wax-tipped catheter. Also working at The Hopkins, James Brown (1854–1895), who was in charge of the genitourinary dispensary, reported the first ever catherization of the male ureter (1893). That same year, Weller Van Hook (1862–1933), professor of surgery at the Chicago Post-Graduate Medical School, wrote a two-part paper in the *Journal of the American Medical Association* that represented the origin of modern ureteral surgery. Christian Fenger (1840–1902) utilized some of Van Hook's recommendations when he described his operation for stenosis of the ureter at the ureteropelvic junction (1894). All this research enabled George Fowler (1848–1906) and Franklin Martin (1857–1935) to boldly remove a bladder and successfully implant the remaining length of ureters into the rectum (late 1890s).

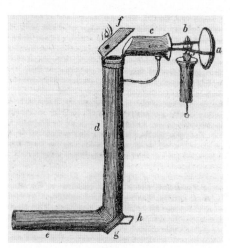

3. John Dix Fisher (1797–1850) devised a rudimentary type of endoscope for viewing the urethra and bladder (*Philadelphia Journal of the Medical and Physical Sciences* vol. 14, pages 409–411, 1827). His instrument for "illuminating dark cavities" used light from a candle, which was then reflected off a series of mirrors onto a looking glass. (*Historical Collections, College of Physicians of Philadelphia*)

It was long appreciated that any progress in the management of diseases of the bladder, kidneys, and ureters depended on an ability to surgically correct obstructions of the bladder neck caused by an enlarged prostate. Because of the prostate's elusive anatomical position, prostatic surgery had proved a technical stumbling block for the surgeon. Not until the mid-1880s did John Gouley (1832–1920) become one of the first American surgeons to obtain extensive experience in performing transurethral prostatic surgery. In 1886 William Belfield (1856–1929), later to become professor of genitourinary surgery at Rush Medical College, performed the first deliberately planned operation for removing obstructing prostatic tissue when he avulsed a pedunculated middle lobe by the suprapubic approach. Three years later, Francis Watson (1853–1942) completed the first median perineal prostatectomy. Eugene Fuller (1858–1930) was the earliest American surgeon to accomplish the removal of both intravesical and intraurethral enlargement of the prostate by the process of suprapubic enucleation (1895).

By the beginnings of the twentieth century, urologic literature had begun to flourish. The first urologic textbook to incorporate surgery in its title was William Van Buren's (1819–1883) and Edward Keyes' *A Practical Treatise on the Surgical Diseases of the Genito-Urinary Organs, Including Syphilis* (1874). Other texts of note included Watson's *The Operative Treatment of the Hypertrophied Prostate* (1888), J. William White's and Edward Martin's *Genito-Urinary Surgery and Venereal Diseases* (1897), and Lemuel Bangs' (1842–1914) and William Hardaway's (1850–1923) massive *An American Textbook of Genito-Urinary Diseases, Syphilis and Diseases of the Skin* (1898). The only periodical dealing strictly with urologic topics in nineteenth-century America was the *Journal of Cutaneous and Genito-Urinary Diseases*. The initial four volumes were simply titled the *Journal of Cutaneous Diseases*; however, at the first annual meeting of the American Association of Genito-Urinary Surgeons (1886), the members elected to have the official report of the transactions of the society published, starting in the fifth volume of the journal, and to incorporate the term "genito-urinary" in its title.

With the turn of the century, urology had already gained sufficient stature as an independent specialty to make evident the need for interchange of ideas among the growing number of urologic surgeons. In 1900 Ramon Guiteras (1859–1917), professor of genitourinary surgery, and his co-workers at the New York Post-Graduate Medical School, formed what was loosely called the New York Genito-Urinary Society. Impelled by a rapidly enlarging attendance, they decided to take on a more formal tone with a wider sphere of activity and transformed themselves into the American Urological Association. Unlike the more exclusive American Association of Genito-Urinary Surgeons, the American Urological Association was founded with the inclusive premise of "receiving into membership all urologists, good and true, of whatever college or hospital connection." In addition, a decided aim was to exclude venereology from the urologic domain. From a political perspective, the most troubling question to face the new organization was whether it should accept the invitation to become an integral part, a genitourinary section as it were, of the American Medical Association. The proposal was debated for seven years and was finally settled at the St. Louis meeting of 1910, when members declined the invitation in a unanimous vote, augural of its wish for continued independence. The trustees of the American Medical Association responded by immediately forming their own Section of Genito-Urinary Diseases. This body held its inaugural meeting in 1912 and had its name changed to the Section on Urology seven years later. Like other American Medical Association surgical sections, it was abolished because of decreasing attendance in the post–World War II era.

Another area of discussion during the early years of the American Urological Association was where the scientific reports presented at its annual meeting should be published. For a time, the papers were submitted to the recently founded *American Journal of Urology*, but beginning with the 1907 convention in Atlantic City, a formal *Transactions of the American Urological Association* was printed in book form under the editorial guidance of Hugh H. Young (1870–1945). Competition with these *Transactions* arose in 1917, when Young began and privately financed the *Journal of Urology*. An important step was taken three years later, when negotiations resulted in the *Journal of Urology* becoming the property of the American Urological Association, to be published by the Williams & Wilkins Company of Baltimore, under the editorship of Young. With the *Journal* declared the official publication of the American Urological Association, every member became an automatic subscriber, as the subscription fee was included in the annual dues. The *Journal of Urology* continues today as the most prestigious of peer-reviewed urologic periodicals, and subsequent editors since the death of Young have included J. A. Campbell Colston (1945–1965), Hugh J. Jewett (1966–1977), William W. Scott (1978–1983), Herbert Brendler (1984–1985), John T. Grayhack (1985–1993), and Jay Y. Gillenwater (1994–??).

Clinical advances continued unabated during the first four decades of the twentieth century and helped bring urology into its modern phase. Francis Hagner (1873–1940) devised the open operation for relief of acute epididymitis (1906). Three years later, Alfred Gray (1873–1932) began to use implantation radium therapy to treat malignant diseases of the bladder. That same year, Leo Buerger (1879–1943) devised a new "direct irrigating observation and double catheterizing cystoscope." In 1910 John Cunningham (1877–1961) developed urethrography, while the modern method of uretero-intestinal anastomosis was being perfected through the experimental work of Robert Coffey (1869–1933). Vesiculography was first demonstrated by Hugh H. Young in 1920. During the 1920s, Joseph McCarthy (1874–1965) invented an oblique pan-endoscope (1923), Earl Osborne (1895–1960) used sodium iodide in uretero-pyelography (1923), and Moses Swick (1900–1985) introduced excretion urography by means of the intravenous and oral administration of sodium ortho-iodohippurate (Hippuran) (1933). Surgery on the kidneys was revolutionized when Alexis Carrel (1873–1944), while working at the Rockefeller Institute in New York City, transplanted a kidney from one animal to another in 1908. Frank Hinman (1880–1961) began his classic work on the surgical treatment of hydronephrosis in 1918. In 1937 Frederic Foley (1891–1966) described a new operation for ureteral stricture at the uretero-pelvic junction. Technical accomplishments in prostatic surgery were advanced by Hugh Young when he described his first radical prostatectomy for carcinoma in 1905. Edwin Beer (1876–1938), writing in the *Journal of the American Medical Association*, discussed his method of utilizing high-frequency current to perform transurethral fulguration of bladder tumors, from which arose the modern operation of transurethral prostatectomy. John Bentley Squier (1873–1948) modified the operation of total suprapubic prostatectomy in 1911, and two years later, Hugh Young described his "punch" prostatectomy operation. In 1920 John Caulk (1881–1938) devised a cautery punch, and during the same period, John Geraghty (1876–1924) improved on Young's perineal prostatectomy. Among the more important textbooks of that era was Alexander Randall's *Surgical Pathology of Prostatic Obstructions* (1931). During World War II, Charles Huggins authored a now classic paper on the treatment of prostatic cancer with stilbestrol (1942), and three years later, he presented his research into adrenalectomy for carcinoma of the prostate.

The final step toward the recognition of urology as a bona fide surgical specialty occurred in 1934 with the organizing of the American Board of Urology. This came about through the concerted efforts of William Braasch (1878–1975), who, at the 1932 meeting of the American Association of Genito-Urinary Surgeons, called attention to the various certifying boards being established in other specialties. He went on to officially request the creation of a board of urology. Two years later, and after considerable political infighting, the American Board of Urology met in Chicago, composed of three representatives each from the American Association of Genito-Urinary Surgeons, the American Urological Association, and the Section of Urology of the American Medical Association. Some six decades later, the current sponsors of the board are the American Urological Association, the American Association of Genito-Urinary Surgeons, the American Association of Clinical Urologists, the Society of University Urologists, the American College of Surgeons, and the Urology Section of the American Academy of Pediatrics. Present-day applicants for certification are required to have a minimum of five years of postgraduate education, of which twelve months must be spent in general surgery and thirty-six months in clinical urology. Of the remaining twelve months, a minimum of six months are to be completed in general surgery, urology, or "other clinical disciplines relevant to urology."

In January 1995, of the approximately 621,000 total physicians in active practice in the United States, 9,725 (1.6 percent) designated themselves as urologic surgeons. Within this cadre of urologic surgeons, 7,435 (76 percent) were board certified. (By contrast, during the fifteen years between 1980 and 1994, 3,822 certificates in urologic surgery were issued, or an average of 255 per year.) Of the 1995 total, 205 (2 percent) were women and 1,805 (19 percent) were international medical graduates. Among the total pool of urologic surgeons, approximately 1,560 (16 precent) were younger than 35; 2,560 (26 percent) were 35 to 44; 2,810 (29 percent) were 45 to 54; 2,000 (21 percent) were 55 to 64; and 795 (8 percent) were 65 and older. Of the 205 female urologic surgeons, 180 (89 percent) were under 44, in contrast to the approximately 9,520 male urologic surgeons, of whom 3,940 (41 percent) were under 44.

The identification of more recent scientific advances to urologic surgery remains a difficult problem. Establishing the important clinical and research advances without the benefit of passage of time can involve undeniable subjectivity. However, when practicing urologists were queried by members of the research subcommittee of the *Study on Surgical Services for the United States* (1976) regarding important urologic surgical contributions from 1945 to 1970, ileal conduit and the effect of hormones on prostate cancer were considered of first-order importance, the treatment of vesicoureteral reflux was deemed of second-order importance, and the diagnosis and treatment of renovascular hypertension and surgery for urinary incontinence were termed third-order contributions.

The history of urology was magnificently detailed in 1933, when an editorial committee of the American Urological Association, composed of Edgar Ballenger, William Frontz, and Homer Hamer, with Bransford Lewis as chairman, produced the now classic two-volume *History of Urology*. This was the first time that an American surgical specialty society undertook such an all-encompassing effort to set forth the history of the profession. Subsequent to that effort, the writing of the history of urology has been minimally served by American urologists. However, Leonard Wershub did author *Urology, From Antiquity to the 20th Century* (1970) and John Herman, *Urology, A View Through the Retrospectroscope* (1973). Surgical history becomes more interesting when the lives of influential personalities are understood. Accordingly, the following brief biographies provide a glimpse into the personal backgrounds of several outstanding American urologic surgeons.

BIOGRAPHIES OF UROLOGIC SURGEONS

Fessenden Nott Otis (1825–1900), born in Ballston Spa, Saratoga County, New York, obtained his undergraduate education at Union College in Schenectady, New York (1849), and his medical diploma from New York Medical School (1852). After serving as an intern at New York City's Charity Hospital, Otis became a surgeon to the Pacific Mail Steamship Company and lived in Panama. He remained in this capacity until 1859, when he returned to New York City and established a general medical-surgical practice. Three years later, Otis was appointed lecturer on genitourinary organs in the College of Physicians and Surgeons. From 1871 to 1890, he was professor of genitourinary diseases at the same institution. During these years, Otis was also president of the medical board of Strangers' Hospital and surgeon to its genitourinary department. In addition, he was consulting surgeon to St. Elizabeth's Hospital, the New York Skin and Cancer Hospital, and the Colored

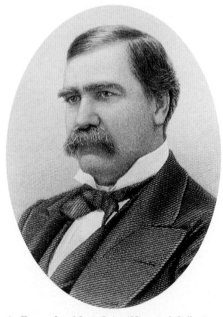

4. Fessenden Nott Otis. (*Historical Collections, College of Physicians of Philadelphia*)

Orphan Asylum. Well known for his contributions to clinical urology, Otis invented the urethrometer (1872) and the dilating urethrotome (1875). His principal writings concerned urologic subjects and included *Stricture of the Male Urethra, Its Radical Cure* (1878), *Clinical Lectures on the Physiological Pathology and Treatment of Syphilis* (1881), *Practical Clinical Lessons on Syphilis and the Genitourinary Diseases* (1883), and *The Male Urethra, Its Diseases and Reflexes* (1888). Otis is best remembered for his paper describing the initial attempts to use local anesthesia in urologic surgery (1884). He was president of the American Association of Genito-Urinary Surgeons in 1891.

Freeman Josiah Bumstead (1826-1879), born in Boston, graduated from Williams College in 1847 and from Harvard Medical School in 1851. He spent a few months in Paris studying venereal diseases and in 1852 settled in New York City, where he opened a general medical practice. He was soon appointed surgeon to the Northern Dispensary (1855) and the New York Eye and Ear Infirmary (1857). Although Bumstead initially devoted the bulk of his clinical activities to diseases of the eye and ear, in 1860 he decided to refocus his practice on venereal diseases. The following year, he was named lecturer on venereal diseases at the College of Physicians and Surgeons, and he was eventually promoted to clinical professor (1867-1871). Among Bumstead's other staff appointments was surgeon to St. Luke's Hospital and the venereal wards of Charity Hospital on Blackwell's Island. His major contribution to the surgical literature is the lengthy *The Pathology and Treatment of Venereal Diseases: Including the Results of Recent Investigations Upon the Subject* (1861). The textbook was so well received that it went through seven editions, the last being in 1904. During the Civil War, Bumstead was an active member of the U.S. Sanitary Commission and authored an important report on venereal diseases in the army and navy.

John Williams Severin Gouley (1832–1920) was born in New Orleans and received his medical education at New York City's College of Physicians and Surgeons (1853). After completing a year as resident physician at Bellevue Hospital, Gouley opened up a general medical practice in Manhattan, where he remained for most of his professional life. He did spend one year in Woodstock, Vermont, as professor of anatomy in the Vermont Medical College (1856). Returning to New York City, Gouley became an office assistant to William Van Buren (1819–1883) but eventually left this position because of a disagreement with Van Buren over which of them had invented the tunnelled catheter. From 1859 to 1861, Gouley was a demonstrator of anatomy in the medical department of the University of New York as well as surgeon to Bellevue Hospital. During the Civil War, he was an assistant surgeon in the U.S. Army Medical Corps, assigned to hospital duty in Washington, D.C. Upon his discharge, Gouley resettled in New York City and joined the surgical staff of St. Vincent's Hospital (1864–1867). Turning his clinical attention to urologic disorders, he was named professor of clinical surgery and genitourinary diseases at the University of New York (1866–1871). For five years he remained without an academic title, but in 1876 he was made professor of diseases of the genitourinary system at the University of New York and consulting surgeon to the Bureau of Medical and Surgical Relief of Outdoor Patients of Bellevue Hospital. One of this country's earliest and most renowned genitourinary specialists, Gouley had a volatile temper, which kept him from becoming a member of the American Association of Genito-Urinary Surgeons. He was an active author, whose clinical textbooks included *Diseases of the Urinary Organs: Including Stricture of the Urethra, Affections of the Prostate, and Stone in the Bladder* (1873), *Diseases of the Urinary Apparatus; Phlegmasic Affections* (1892), and *Surgery of Genito-Urinary Organs* (1907). Among Gouley's other works are *Diseases of Man: Data of Their Nomenclature, Classification & Genesis* (1888) and *Conference on the Moral Philosophy of Medicine* (1906). He remains eponymically linked with a solid, curved catheter used to pass through a urethral stricture.

Lemuel Bolton Bangs (1842–1914) was born in New York City and graduated from the College of Physicians and Surgeons in 1872. While he was in his twenties,

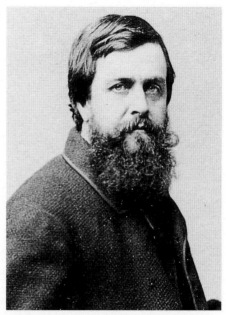

5. Freeman Josiah Bumstead. (*Historical Collections, College of Physicians of Philadelphia*)

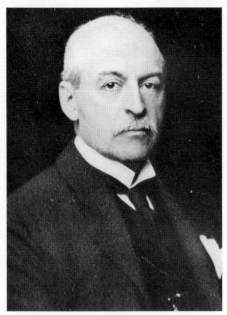

6. Lemuel Bolton Bangs. (*Historical Collections, College of Physicians of Philadelphia*)

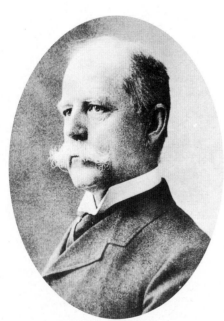

7. Edward Lawrence Keyes. (*Historical Collections, College of Physicians of Philadelphia*)

family financial reversals caused him to interrupt his medical studies and take up business for a few years. After serving an internship at Bellevue Hospital, Bangs took postgraduate courses in Berlin and Vienna. On returning to his native city, Bangs became an office associate of Fessenden Otis and began his clinical activities relative to urologic diseases. Remaining in New York City, Bangs ultimately served as consulting surgeon to Bellevue, Methodist Episcopal, St. Luke's, and St. Vincent's Hospitals. From 1889 to 1894, he was professor of genitourinary diseases at the New York Post-Graduate Medical School and Hospital, and thereafter, emeritus professor; a member of its board of directors, and treasurer of the corporation. For three years (1898 to 1901), Bangs was professor of genitourinary surgery at the Bellevue Hospital Medical School. He contributed frequently to the surgical literature. His only textbook is *An American Textbook of Genito-Urinary Diseases, Syphilis and Diseases of the Skin* (1898), jointly edited with William Hardaway (1859–1923). Bangs served as president of the American Association of Genito-Urinary Surgeons in 1895.

Edward Lawrence Keyes (1843–1924), born in Charleston, South Carolina, graduated from Yale University (1863), and studied medicine at the University of the City of New York (1866). He then spent eighteen months in Europe, mainly at the University of Paris, learning about dermatology, syphilology, and male genitourinary diseases. Returning to New York City, Keyes was appointed professor of dermatology in the Woman's Medical College and lecturer in dematology at Bellevue Hospital, where he taught the first course in dermatology in the United States (1870). During the early 1870s, Keyes became an associate in practice with William Van Buren (1819–1883), who was professor of genitourinary diseases, subsidiary to his professorship of the principles of surgery at Bellevue. In 1875, Keyes was named professor of dermatology, syphilology, and genitourinary surgery at Bellevue, and his ward, though never officially titled a genitourinary one, naturally came to be devoted to this specialty (1877) and was therefore the first specialized facility in America for genitourinary patients. Over the next decade and a half, Keyes's influence as a teacher and clinician became widespread, and he went on to train a whole generation of genitourinary surgeons. After 1885 he was also surgeon to the New York Skin and Cancer Hospital and St. Elizabeth's Hospital. A pioneer in American dermatology and urology, Keyes founded and served as first president of the American Association of Genito-Urinary Surgeons (1887). He introduced the technique of administering continued small doses of mercury in treating syphilis (1877), a method that became standard for over twenty years. In collaboration with Van Buren, Keyes authored *A Practical Treatise on the Surgical Diseases of the Genito-Urinary Organs, Including Syphilis* (1874), the first American book on a urologic topic to incorporate "surgical" in its title. Among Keyes's other works are *The Tonic Treatment of Syphilis* (1877), *The Venereal Diseases, Including Strictures of the Male Urethra* (1880), *The Surgical Diseases of the Genito-Urinary Organs* (1888), *Some Fallacies Concerning Syphilis* (1890), *Venereal Diseases, Their Complications and Sequelae* (1900), and *Diseases of the Genito-Urinary Organs* (1910). His son, Edward Loughborough Keyes, Jr. (1873–1949), (although the two did not share the same middle name, they were referred to as Sr. and Jr.) was professor of urology at Cornell University Medical School and president of both the American Association of Genito-Urinary Surgeons (1912) and the American Urological Association (1915).

Frederick Russell Sturgis (1844–1919), born in Manila, Philippine Islands, graduated from Harvard College in 1864 and Harvard Medical School in 1867. While receiving his medical education, he served one year as a house physician at the Boston City Hospital and in 1866 was house surgeon to the Massachusetts General Hospital. In the fall of 1867, Sturgis relocated to New York City, soon entered into a partnership with Freeman Bumstead, and began to limit his clinical interests to genitourinary and venereal diseases. From 1869 to 1876, Sturgis was also an assistant surgeon at the Manhattan Eye and Ear Hospital. Appointed clinical lecturer on venereal diseases at New York University (1874–1880), he was eventually promoted to professor of diseases of the genitourinary organs and venereal diseases (1881).

However, within a few months, he resigned his professorship at New York University to become professor of venereal and genitourinary diseases in the New York Post-Graduate Medical School and Hospital. From 1882 to 1888, Sturgis was secretary of the faculty, and he later served on the board of directors (1887–1890). Among his other professional positions were surgeon in the department of venereal and skin diseases of the New York Dispensary (1876–1880) and visiting surgeon to the venereal and genitourinary division of the Charity Hospital on Blackwell's Island. Among his written works are *The Student's Manual of Venereal Diseases* (1880) and *Sexual Debility in Man* (1900).

William Niles Wishard (1851–1941) was born in Greenwood, Indiana, attended Wabash College (1870–1872) and graduated from Indiana Medical College (1874). He also received a medical degree from Miami (Ohio) Medical College in 1876. In 1874, Wishard joined his father in a general medical practice in Southport, Indiana, but two years later the younger Wishard moved to Indianapolis, where he remained for the rest of his professional life. For three years (1876–1879), Wishard pursued general practice. In 1879 he was appointed superintendent of the Indianapolis City Hospital, where he was able to perform a considerable number of various surgical operations. In 1883 he was elected to the chair of general medicine at the Medical College of Indiana. With a growing interest in genitourinary diseases and surgery, Wishard took postgraduate training in urology at the New York Post-Graduate Medical School and Hospital (1887) and was a private pupil of both Frederick Sturgis and Eugene Fuller. Returning to Indianapolis, Wishard rejoined the faculty at the Medical College of Indiana, where he was named professor and head of the department of genitourinary surgery. He remained in this position until 1936. During 1888 and 1889, Wishard took time off from his faculty position to attend further postgraduate classes in urology at the Polyclinic in Chicago and in New York City. In 1890 he traveled to Berlin for the International Medical Congress, visited hospitals in Vienna, and saw Max Nitze's (1848–1906) electrically lighted cystoscope for the first time. Wishard also attended clinics in London at St. Peter's Hospital for Stone, St. Bartholomew's Hospital, and St. Thomas' Hospital. As superintendent of the Indianapolis City Hospital, Wishard established the first training school for nurses in the state and, through his fund raising abilities, secured the construction of a new hospital. He developed a rubber catheter bearing his name, as well as other specialized catheters and numerous instruments for urologic surgery. Wishard was one of the country's first surgeons to perform perineal prostatectomy and the earliest to apply cautery under visual observation for reduction of an enlarged prostate (1890). By 1889 he had completed a nephrectomy. The author of numerous articles in the urologic literature, Wishard never wrote a full-length textbook. In 1897 he was the major sponsor behind the Medical Practice Act of Indiana. Among Wishard's many honors were serving as president of the Indianapolis Surgical Society (1890), the Mississippi Valley Medical Association (1895), the Indiana State Medical Association (1898) and the American Urological Association (1905).

Francis Sedgwick Watson (1853–1942), born in Milton, Massachusetts, and graduated from Harvard College in 1875 and Harvard Medical School in 1879. He completed a surgical internship at the Massachusetts General Hospital and then studied in Europe for two years. During the early 1880s, Watson was named surgeon to outpatients at Boston City Hospital and instructor in minor surgery and surgery of the urinary organs at Harvard Medical School. He remained associated with these two institutions for the remainder of his professional life, rising in rank to surgeon in chief at Boston City Hospital and lecturer in genitourinary surgery at Harvard. In 1889 he was also made surgeon to the department of diseases of the genitourinary system at the Boston Dispensary. He resigned from his Boston City Hospital position in 1910. Watson performed the first median perineal prostatectomy in the United States (1889) and subsequently published authoritative articles on the operative treatment of the hypertrophied prostate (1905) as well as extensive reviews on the subject of bladder tumors (1907). Among his many honors were serving as

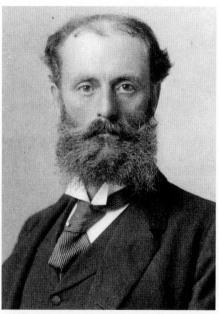

8. Francis Sedgwick Watson. (*Historical Collections, College of Physicians of Philadelphia*)

president of the International Surgical Association's meeting in Moscow (1897), the American Association of Genito-Urinary Surgeons (1897), and the American Urological Association. His two urologic texts are *The Operative Treatment of the Hypertrophied Prostate* (1888) and the two-volume *Diseases and Surgery of the Genito-Urinary System* (1908). In addition, he authored *A Day With the Specialists; Or, Cured At Last; A Tragic Farcelet* (1910) and a privately printed autobiography, *A Bundle of Memories* (1911). In a bit of surgical gossip, Watson, the originator and forceful advocate of perineal prostatectomy, had his own prostate removed by John H. Cunningham (1877–1961) via the suprapubic route.

William Thomas Belfield (1856–1929) was born in St. Louis, and graduated from Rush Medical College in 1878. After serving an internship at Cook County Hospital, he traveled to Europe and spent over two years in postgraduate work in Berlin, London, Paris, and Vienna. Returning to Chicago, Belfield was appointed pathologist at Cook County Hospital (1883–1885) and then staff surgeon (1885–1890), while also serving as surgeon to the genitourinary department at the city's Central Dispensary. In 1886 he performed the first deliberately planned operation for removing obstructing prostatic tissue when he avulsed a pedunculated middle lobe by the suprapubic approach. The following year, he introduced cystoscopy to Chicago surgeons. For many years, Belfield was connected with his alma mater, as professor of bacteriology (1898), associate professor of surgery (1899–1908), professor of genitourinary surgery (1909–1923), and professor emeritus from 1924 until his death. In 1902 he was president of the American Association of Genito-Urinary Surgeons. Belfield is eponymically remembered for vasostomy. He authored one urologic textbook, *Diseases of the Urinary and Male Sexual Organs* (1884). Reported to have been among the first in America to demonstrate the tubercle bacillus and the gonococcus, his other clinical monograph is *On the Relations of Microorganisms to Disease* (1883). Belfield was one of the contributing editors to *The Practical Home Physician: A Popular Guide for the Management of Household Disease* (1884).

Samuel Alexander (1858–1910), born in New York City, graduated from Princeton University in 1879 and Bellevue Hospital Medical College in 1882. Following his internship, he went abroad and studied genitourinary disease in Leipzig, London, and Vienna. Returning to his native city, Alexander began practicing as an associate of Edward L. Keyes. He was also appointed assistant demonstrator of anatomy (1884–1885), clinical lecturer on genitourinary surgery (1886–1889), and professor of genitourinary surgery, dermatology, and syphilography (1889), all at his alma mater. In 1898 Alexander was appointed professor of clinical surgery in the department of genitourinary diseases at Cornell University Medical College. Although considered an expert in the treatment of prostatic hypertrophy, he was not a particularly prolific authority. Alexander was president of the American Association of Genito-Urinary Surgeons in 1902. He died of gangrenous appendicitis.

George Frank Lydston (1858–1923) was born in Tuolumne, California, and received his education at the University of California (1877) and Bellevue Hospital Medical College (1879). He completed an internship at the New York Charity Hospital, remaining there as resident surgeon (1879–1881) while also acting as surgeon to New York State Immigration Hospital on Ward's Island (1881). Lydston relocated to Chicago in 1882 and was appointed lecturer on genitourinary diseases in the College of Physicians and Surgeons (now the University of Illinois School of Medicine). A few years later, he was promoted to professor and served in that capacity until 1890. He was also professor of the principles and practice of surgery and surgical pathology at Northwestern College of Dental Surgery (1886) and surgeon to Cook County Hospital (1893). He was a prolific author, whose clinical textbooks include: *Varicocele and its Treatment* (1892), *Gonorrhoea and Urethritis* (1892), *Stricture of the Urethra* (1893), and *The Surgical Diseases of the Genito-Urinary Tract, Venereal and Sexual Diseases* (1899). In 1914 he began experimental work on testicular transplantation and, three years later, authored *Impotence and Sterility: With Aberrations of the Sexual Function and Sex-Gland Implantation*. Lydston was also professor of sociology and criminology at the Kent College of Law in Chicago and wrote the widely acclaimed *The Diseases of Society (The Vice and Crime Problem)* (1904). Among his literary works are *Addresses and Essays* (1891), *Over the Hookah, the Tales of a Talkative Doctor* (1896), and *Panama and the Sierras; A Doctor's Wander Days* (1900).

Ramon Benjamin Guiteras (1859–1917) was born in Bristol, Rhode Island, attended Harvard College (1878–1879), spent a year and a half traveling in Africa and Europe (1879–1880), and then matriculated at Harvard Medical School (1883). He pursued postgraduate medical studies in Vienna and returned to the United States (1885), settling in New York City, where he was appointed surgeon at the Charity Hospital on Blackwell's Island (now Roosevelt Island). Guiteras served for eighteen months, beginning practice in 1887. Three months later, he was incapacitated by diphtheria, and recuperated for a time in Cuba. In 1888 Guiteras resumed practice, and within five years he was named professor of anatomy and operative surgery at the New York Post-Graduate Hospital and Medical School. He was also consulting surgeon to the Columbus and French hospitals. In the mid-1890s, Guiteras assumed the position of professor of genitourinary surgery at the Post-Graduate Medical School. He is best remembered for being the major organizer of the New York Genito-Urinary Society (1900), the immediate precursor to the American Urological Association (1902). In 1912, Guiteras authored the two-volume *Urology, The Diseases of the Urinary Tract in Men and Women.*

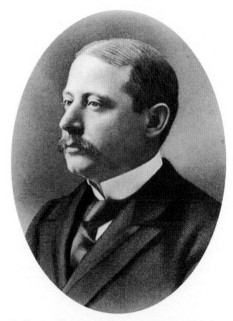

9. Ramon Benjamin Guiteras. (*Historical Collections, College of Physicians of Philadelphia*)

Bransford Lewis (1862–1942) was born in St. Charles, Missouri, and educated at the Missouri Medical College (1884). He served as an intern in the St. Louis City Hospital (1885) and then entered general practice while joining the staffs of the St. Louis City Sanitarium (1886) and the Female Hospital (1887). From 1887-1889, Lewis was an assistant superintendent of the St. Louis City Hospital. In 1889 he was named lecturer on genitourinary surgery at his alma mater. Within one year he had decided to limit his clinical activities to urologic work. Lewis pursued postgraduate urologic training in 1891, in London, Paris and Vienna. During the 1890s, he successively edited the *St. Louis Medical Review* and the *Medical Fortnightly*. At the turn of the century, he resigned his post at Missouri Medical College to accept the position of professor of genitourinary surgery at the Marion-Sims Beaumont Medical College (now St. Louis University School of Medicine), where he remained until his retirement. A prolific contributor to the urologic literature, Lewis wrote only one textbook: *Cystoscopy and Urethroscopy* (1915). He served as chairman of the editorial committee that prepared, under the auspices of the American Urological Association, the two-volume *History of Urology* (1933). In 1907 Lewis was president of the American Urological Association, and two years later he was awarded a gold medal for cystoscopic achievement by the directors of the Louisiana Purchase Exposition.

Hugh Hampton Young (1870–1945), born in San Antonio, Texas, attended the University of Virginia and, in four years' time, received the B.A., M.A., and M.D. degrees (18901–894). He returned to his native city to practice medicine but, realizing his own limitations, decided to pursue further postgraduate education at The Johns Hopkins Hospital. During his first year in Baltimore, Young worked as a graduate student in the surgical dispensary (1894–1895) and, from 1895 to 1898, served as an intern and resident, spending much time on Ward E, where all urologic cases were cared for. In October 1897, William Halsted suggested that Young take charge of the department of genitourinary surgery, and so began the urologic career of the individual considered the founder of modern urology in the United States. Young remained at The Hopkins for the remainder of his professional career, much of it as director of the Brady Urological Institute (1915–1942). During World War I, he was director of urology for the U.S. Army Expeditionary Force and organized urologic clinics for the servicemen, which brought about a marked lowering of venereal disease. Young invented numerous operating instruments and other surgical apparatus. He developed an improved cystoscope and the "punch" prostatectomy operation, the latter being used for "small prostatic bars and contracture of the prostatic orifice." He also devised several innovative surgical procedures for treating genitourinary diseases,

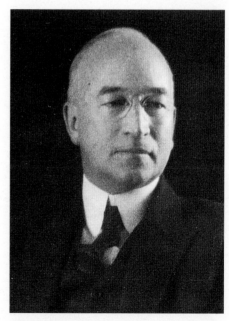

10. Hugh Hampton Young. (*Historical Collections, College of Physicians of Philadelphia*)

including an early perineal prostatectomy (1902), which soon replaced the more dangerous suprapubic approach, and performed the first radical prostatectomy for carcinoma in 1905. Young made pioneer investigations of hermaphroditism and authored the classic text *Genital Abnormalities, Hermaphroditism and Related Adrenal Diseases* (1937). In addition, he developed the drug mercurochrome, which he utilized as an intravenous antiseptic. Quite knowledgeable about infectious diseases, Young was an early advocate of the use of sulfanilamide and other chemotherapeutic drugs in the treatment of venereal disease. His urologic residency program at The Johns Hopkins Hospital became internationally renowned, and Young trained many of the leading urologists of this century. A prolific writer, Young founded (1917) and edited the *Journal of Urology* until his death. Among his clinical texts are *Hypertrophy and Cancer of the Prostate Gland* (1906), *Studies in Urological Surgery* (1906), *Urological Roentgenology* (1928), and *Young's Practice of Urology* (1926). He was president of the American Association of Genito-Urinary Surgeons and the American Urological Association in 1909 and of the International Association of Urology in 1927. *Hugh Young, A Surgeon's Autobiography* was published in 1940.

Hugh Cabot (1872–1945) was born in Beverly Farms, Massachusetts, and educated at Harvard College (1894) and Harvard Medical School (1898). He served a year's internship in the Massachusetts General Hospital and then entered private practice with his much older cousin, Arthur Tracy Cabot (1852–1912), who held the academic title of instructor of genitourinary surgery at Harvard Medical School. The older Cabot had been trained in genitourinary surgery by Henry J. Bigelow (1818–1890), and he, in turn, instructed Hugh Cabot. At first, the younger Cabot engaged in a miscellaneous surgical practice, but he soon confined his clinical activities to his cousin's specialty, which he always called genitourinary surgery instead of urology. By 1909, Cabot was practicing a full range of genitourinary surgery while serving on the surgical staffs of the New England Baptist (1900–1919) and Massachusetts General (1902–1919) Hospitals. In 1910 he was appointed an assistant professor of surgery at his alma mater. Five years later, he served as president of the American Association of Genito-Urinary Surgeons. During World War I, Cabot enlisted with the Harvard unit, Royal Army Medical Corps, British Expeditionary Force, and commanded General Hospital No. 22. Returning to Boston, he found that his practice had withered away and other opportunities seemed lacking. Fortunately, Cabot was appointed professor of surgery and chairman of the department at the University of Michigan School of Medicine (1919). During a four-year tenure in this post, he completely reorganized the surgical department and was so successful in his endeavors that when Victor Vaughan (1851–1929) retired in 1921, Cabot was made dean of the medical school. In 1930 Cabot resigned from his position because of unending dissension that had developed between him and most of the senior medical school faculty. He was promptly invited to join the surgical staff of the Mayo Clinic as head of a surgical section, but with his responsibilities limited to urologic surgery. From 1930 until his retirement in 1939, Cabot served on the Mayo Clinic staff and was professor of surgery at the Mayo Graduate School of Medicine, then part of the University of Minnesota. Following his retirement, Cabot moved back to the Boston area and maintained a small surgical practice. Cabot was a controversial figure in the constant political bickering that marked American medicine of the 1930s. He supported prepayments, group practice, and hospital staff status for all physicians, and he was an advocate of medical insurance plans and even of some degree of socialized medical programs. In 1935 he wrote *The Doctor's Bill*, which exposed the existing methods of financing American health care. He followed this with another critical monograph, *The Patient's Dilemma* (1940). Cabot served as a leading government witness in the 1938–1943 antitrust case against the American Medical Association. He headed White Cross, a Boston health insurance group designed to provide a prepayment plan to finance medical service. His clinical textbooks include *Modern Urology* (1918) and *Surgical Nursing* (1924).

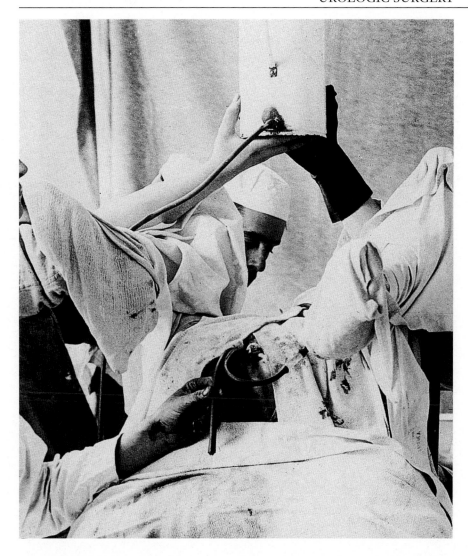

11. Hugh H. Young was one of the pioneers of American urology. In 1902 he performed the first perineal prostatectomy, which soon replaced the more dangerous suprapubic approach. He is shown at the completion of such a case, passing water into the bladder and checking to make sure that the fluid coming out of a second tube located in the bladder is clear. In this way, Young knew there was no ongoing hemorrhage and that the prostatectomy wound was well sealed. (*Courtesy of Stanley B. Burns, M.D., and The Burns Collection and Archive*)

John Bentley Squier (1873–1948) was born in New York City, and received both his undergraduate (1892) and medical (1894) education at Columbia University. He served an internship at St. Luke's Hospital and for the next twelve years was attending surgeon for the City Department of Charities. Focusing his clinical interests on urologic diseases, Squier was appointed professor of genitourinary surgery at the New York Post-Graduate Medical School in 1909, remaining in this capacity until 1924. In 1917 he also became professor of urology at his alma mater and retained this position until his retirement. A prolific contributor to the surgical literature, including an influential report in the *Boston Medical and Surgical Journal* in which he presented a modification of the operation of total suprapubic prostatectomy (1911), he wrote the well-known textbook *Manual of Cystoscopy* (1911). During World War I, Squier served as a major in the Medical Reserve Corps and was also a member of the General Medical Board of the Council of National Defense. He was instrumental in conceiving the plan for the Columbia War Hospital, an emergency facility of over 1,000 beds that was turned over to the federal government in 1917 and became U.S. Army General Hospital No. 1. He enjoyed many honors, including the presidencies of the the American Urological Association (1913), the American Association of Genito-Urinary Surgeons (1920), and the American College of Surgeons (1932).

Gideon Timberlake (1876–1951) was born in Charlottesville, Virginia, and received his medical degree from the University of Virginia in 1902. He served an internship at the Lying-In, Bellevue, and Marine Hospitals in New York City (1903). Timberlake practiced medicine in Charleston, West Virginia, from 1904 to 1907 but decided to study urology under Hugh Young at The Johns Hopkins Hospital. He spent a year working with Young and then opened a urologic practice in Baltimore, where he lived until 1926. For one year, Timberlake was a demonstrator in bacteri-

12. Injuries of the perineum were not uncommon during the Civil War. This photograph from Reed Bontecou's surgical album demonstrates a urologic injury secondary to a gunshot wound. A rudimentary drain has been placed into the bladder to aid the healing process. (*Courtesy of Stanley B. Burns, M.D., and The Burns Collection and Archive*)

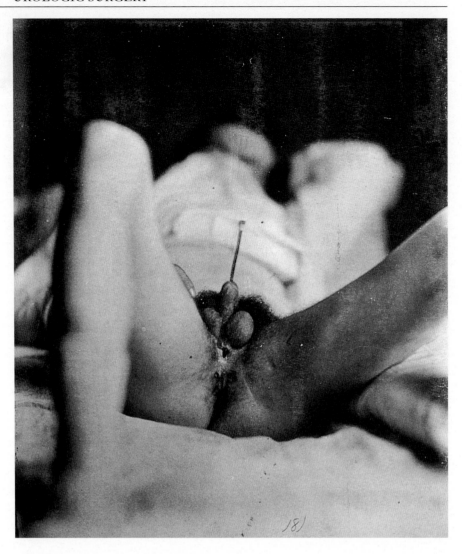

ology at The Hopkins (1909), but in 1910 he joined the urology faculty at the University of Maryland School of Medicine. At the same time, he continued to practice at St. Agnes and Franklin Square Hospitals. During World War I, Timberlake organized and directed the U.S. Army School of Urology at Fort Oglethorpe, Georgia. For a few years after the war, he was on the urologic staff at Walter Reed Hospital in Washington, D.C. From 1926 to 1928, Timberlake practiced urology in Greenville, South Carolina. In 1928 he moved permanently to St. Petersburg, Florida. Timberlake developed numerous urologic techniques and instruments, including an obturator for the resectoscope sheath, a cannula for removing blood clots from the urinary bladder, and electrocoagulation in transurethral prostatic resections. He was a founding member of the American Board of Urology.

William Frederick Braasch (1878–1975) was born in Iowa and received his bachelor's (1900) and medical (1903) degrees from the University of Minnesota. After postgraduate training in pathology (1904–1905), he pursued further training in internal medicine in Vienna. In 1907 Braasch returned to the United States and began his lengthy career at the Mayo Clinic, where he was assigned the task of developing the practice of urology, concentrating on endoscopy. Seven years later, he became the first chairman of the newly formed Section of Urology, a position he maintained for twenty-five years. In 1915 Braasch was named professor of urology in the Mayo Graduate School of Medicine, and he occupied that post until his retirement in 1946. Braasch was a long-standing member of the editorial board of the *Journal of Urology*, contributed over two hundred papers to the surgical literature, and counted among his textbooks *Pyelography (Pyelo-Ureterography)*, *A Study of the Normal and Pathologic Anatomy of the Renal Pelvis and Ureter* (1915), *Urography* (1920), and *Clinical Urography; an Atlas and Textbook of Roentgenologic Diagnosis* (1951). In

1910 he invented the direct vision cystoscope, and a few years later, the prototype of the visual punch for prostatic resection, which ultimately resulted in the Thompson cold punch resectoscope. Braasch was quite active in all aspects of organized medicine and served on the Board of Trustees of the American Medical Association (1940–1948). He was president of the American Urological Association (1921), the American Association of Genito-Urinary Surgeons (1926), and the Clinical Society of Genito-Urinary Surgeons (1933). He is best remembered as the individual who first suggested the idea of establishing the American Board of Urology. In 1969, Braasch authored *Early Days in the Mayo Clinic*.

Herman Louis Kretschmer (1879–1951) was born in Chicago and received an undergraduate degree in pharmacy (1900) and a medical diploma (1904) from Northwestern University. Much of his postgraduate training in genitourinary diseases was pursued at the Pathological Institute in Vienna, Austria, and throughout his career Kretschmer was insistent that the urologist be, in effect, his own pathologist at the operating room table. Establishing a private practice in his native city, Kretschmer was associated with numerous hospitals but remained most closely identified with Northwestern University and Presbyterian Hospital, where his urology service attracted many visiting surgeons. A strong supporter of organized medicine, Kretschmer was chairman of the American Medical Association's Section on Urology (1925) and became the first urologist to be elected president of the Association (1944). Among his many other honors was serving as president of the American Urological Association (1925), the Clinical Society of Genito-Urinary Surgeons (1931), and the American Association of Genito-Urinary Surgeons (1932). Kretschmer was a prime force behind the founding of the American Board of Urology, becoming its first president in 1934 and remaining in this capacity for another decade.

Nathaniel Graham Alcock (1881–1953) born in Platteville, Wisconsin, began his medical education by apprenticing (1902–1903) with L. E. Schmidt, a general practitioner, in Yankton, South Dakota. Alcock later received his bachelor's (1907), master's (1908), and medical (1912) degrees from Northwestern University. After pursuing postgraduate training in genitourinary diseases, Alcock joined the medical faculty at the University of Iowa (1915). In 1922, he was named professor and head of the department of urology. He retired from his academic appointment in 1949, at which time he continued as chief urologist at Mercy Hospital in Iowa City. Alcock contributed significantly to the development of urology as a surgical specialty, especially as a teacher and administrator. In 1932, he was chairman of the Section on Urology of the American Medical Association, and was also president of the Iowa Medical Society (1949). Alcock was among the first of modern urologists to fully comprehend the possibilities of transurethral surgery (1930s), and his operative technique revolutionized the treatment of prostatic disease, reducing a 10 to 25 percent mortality rate to less than 1 percent.

Charles Herbert Garvin (1890–1968) was born in Jacksonville, Florida, and received both his undergraduate (1911) and medical (1915) education at Howard University. He completed a one-year internship at Freedmen's Hospital in Washington, D.C., and began the practice of medicine and surgery as a visiting assistant surgeon at the same institution (1916–1917). During World War I, Garvin joined the U.S. Army Medical Corps and served eleven months in France. At that time, he was the first African-American to receive a commission in the army and the first to study at the Army Medical School in Washington. In 1919 Garvin settled in Cleveland, where he remained in private practice until his death. From 1920 to 1956, he was a staff urologist at the Lakeside Hospital in Cleveland and was also on the urology faculty at Western Reserve University Medical School. Although not well known as a scientific writer, Garvin did author seventeen clinical papers on urology. A crusader for civil rights, Garvin was the first African American to receive an appointment to a Cleveland hospital, which he did by impressing George Crile and his associates with his surgical knowledge. In 1927, when Garvin and his family moved into a new house in a "white" section of Cleveland, it was twice bombed. The

Garvins were not easily frightened, and they went on to remain in that house for forty years. Well known for his involvement in African-American business and community affairs, Garvin was one of the earliest life members of the National Association for the Advancement of Colored People. He was a contributing editor (1943–1949) and member of the editorial board (1959–1968) of the *Journal of the National Medical Association* and compiled the enviable record of having written at least one item for every issue of the *Journal* from 1950 until his death. For over three decades (1931–1964), Garvin served as alumni trustee and then as a regular member of Howard University's board of trustees.

Frederick Eugene Basil Foley (1891–1966) was born in St. Cloud, Minnesota, and educated at Yale University (1913) and the Johns Hopkins School of Medicine (1918). He interned at the Peter Bent Brigham Hospital, where he worked with Harvey Cushing in surgical research. From 1922 to 1960, Foley practiced urology in St. Paul, where he was also professor of urology at the University of Minnesota. In 1929 Foley established the urologic department at the Ancker Hospital in St. Paul. In that same year, he developed the Foley Y plasty for ureteropelvic junction stricture. He invented the inflatable Foley bladder catheter, and his name is therefore one of the most ubiquitous in modern medicine. Later in his career, he devised the Foley urologic operating table (1961).

REFERENCES

BIBLIOGRAPHIES

American College of Surgeons. *A catalogue of the H. Winnett Orr historical collection*. Chicago: American College of Surgeons, 1960.

Austin RB. *Early American medical imprints: a guide to works printed in the United States, 1668–1820*. Washington, DC: US Department of Health, Education, and Welfare, 1961.

Billings JS & Fletcher R. *Index medicus, a monthly classified record of the current medical literature, 1st series*. 21 vols. New York: F Leypoldt, 1879–1899.

Cordasco F. *American medical imprints*, 1820–1910. Totowa, NJ: Rowan & Littlefield, 1985.

Cordasco F. *Homoeopathy in the United States, a bibliography of homoeopathic medical imprints, 1825–1925*. Fairview, NJ: Junius-Vaughn, 1991.

Fulton J & Stanton ME. *The centennial of surgical anesthesia: an annotated catalogue of books and pamphlets bearing on the early history of surgical anesthesia*. New York: Henry Schuman, 1946.

Guerra F. *American medical bibliography*, 1639–1783. New York: Lathrop C Harper, 1962.

Index catalogue of the library of the Surgeon-General's Office, 1st series. 16 vols., 1880–1895; *2nd series*. 21 vols., 1896–1916; *3rd series*. 5 vols., 1918–1925, Washington, DC: US Government Printing Office.

Miller G. *Bibliography of the history of medicine of the United States and Canada, 1939–1960*. Baltimore: The Johns Hopkins Press, 1964.

Morton LT. *Morton's medical bibliography: an annotated checklist illustrating the history of medicine (Garrison and Morton)*. 5th edition, edited by Jeremy M. Norman. Hampshire, Great Britain: Gower, 1991.

BIOGRAPHICAL COMPILATIONS

American Homeopathic Biographical Association. *Biographical cyclopedia of homeopathic physicians and surgeons*. Chicago: American Homeopathic Biographical Association, 1893.

American Medical Association. *Directory of American physicians*. Chicago: American Medical Association, 1906–1996.

Anonymous. *Biographies of physicians and surgeons*. Chicago: JH Beers, 1904.

Appleton's cyclopedia of American biography. 16 vols., New York: D Appleton, 1887–1889.

Atkinson WB. *The physicians and surgeons of the United States*. Philadelphia: Charles Robson, 1878.

Atkinson WB. *A biographical dictionary of contemporary American physicians and surgeons*. Philadelphia: DG Brinton, 1880.

Butler SW. *The medical register and directory of the United States*. Philadelphia: Office of the Medical and Surgical Reporter, 1874. (2nd edition, 1877)

Cleave, E. *Biographical cyclopaedia of homoeopathic physicians and surgeons*. Philadelphia: Galaxy, 1873.

Dictionary of American biography. 21 vols., plus supplements. New York: Scribner, 1943–present.

Flint JB. *Medical and surgical directory of the United States*. New York: JB Flint, 1897.

Francis SW. *Biographical sketches of distinguished living New York surgeons*. New York, John Bradburn, 1866.

Francis SW. *Biographical sketches of distinguished living New York physicians*. New York: GP Putnam & Sons, 1867.

Gross SD. *Lives of eminent American physicians and surgeons of the nineteenth century*. Philadelphia: Lindsay & Blakiston, 1861.

Holloway LM. *Medical obituaries, American physicians' biographical notices in selected medical journals before 1907*. New York: Garland, 1981.

Kaufman M, Galishoff S & Savitt TL. *Dictionary of American medical biography*. Westport, CT: Greenwood Press, 1984.

Kelly HA. *A cyclopedia of American medical biography comprising the lives of eminent deceased physicians and surgeons from 1610 to 1910*. Philadelphia: WB Saunders, 1912.

Kelly HA. *Some American medical botanists commemorated in our botanical nomenclature*. Troy, NY: Southworth, 1914.

Kelly HA & Burrage WL. *American medical biographies*. Baltimore: Norman & Remington, 1920.

Kelly HA & Burrage WL. *Dictionary of American medical biography; lives of eminent physicians of the United States and Canada, from the earliest times*. New York: D Appleton, 1928.

Leonardo R. *Lives of master surgeons*. New York: Froben Press, 1948. (plus Supplement I, 1949)

Master surgeons of America. In: *Surgery, Gynecology, & Obstetrics*, 1922–1939. (Includes more than 150 biographies of American surgeons)

National cyclopedia of American biography. 21 vols., New York: JT White, 1893–1927.

Polk, RL. *Medical and surgical register of the United States*. Detroit: RL Polk, 1886. (Later editions appeared in 1890, 1893, 1896, 1898, 1900, 1902, 1904, and 1906)

Stone RF. *Biography of eminent Americn physicians and surgeons*. Indianapolis: Carlton & Hollenbeck, 1894. (2nd edition, 1898)

Thacher J. *American medical biography: or memoirs of eminent physicians who have flourished in America*. Boston: Richardson & Lord; Cottons & Barnard, 1828.

Watson IA. *Physicians and surgeons of America, a collection of biographical sketches of the regular medical profession*. Concord, MA: Republican Press Association, 1896.

Williams S. *American medical biography: or, memoirs of eminent physicians, embracing principally those who have died since the publication of Dr. Thacher's work on the same subject*. Greenfield, MA: L Merriam, 1845.

BIOGRAPHIES AND AUTOBIOGRAPHIES

Adams HD. *The knife that saves, memoirs of a Lahey Clinic surgeon*. Boston: Countway Library, 1991.

Agnew DH (written by J Howe Adams). *History of the life of D. Hayes Agnew*. Philadelphia: FA Davis, 1892.

Albee FH. *A surgeon's fight to rebuild men, an autobiography*. New York: EP Dutton, 1943.

Allen DP (written by CP Hudson). *The life and times of Dudley Peter Allen*. Cleveland: Cleveland Medical Library Association, 1992.

Atkinson DT: *Texas surgeon, an autobiography*. New York: Ives Washburn, 1958.

Barringer ED. *Bowery to Bellevue, the story of New York's first woman ambulance surgeon*. New York: WW Norton, 1950.

Beaumont W (written by J Meyer). *Life and letters of Dr. William Beaumont*. St Louis: CV Mosby, 1912.

Beaumont W (written by G Rosen). *The reception of William Beaumont's discovery in Europe*. New York: Schuman's, 1942.

Beaumont W (written by G Miller). *Wm. Beaumont's formative years, two early notebooks 1811–1812*. New York: Henry Schuman, 1946.

Beaumont W (written by RB Nelson). *Beaumont: America's first physiologist*. Geneva, IL: Grant House, 1990.

Beaumont W (written by R Horsman). *Frontier doctor: William Beaumont, America's first great medical scientist*. Columbia: University of Missouri Press, 1996.

Bernays A (written by T Bernays). *Augustus Charles Bernays*. St Louis: CV Mosby, 1912.

Bernheim BM. *"Passed as censored."* Philadelphia: JB Lippincott, 1918.

Bernheim BM: *A surgeon's domain*. New York: WW Norton, 1947.

Bigelow HJ. I. *The mechanism of dislocations and fracture of the hip. II. Litholapaxy; or, rapid lithotrity with evacuation*. Boston: Little, Brown, 1900.

Bigelow HJ. *Surgical anesthesia, addresses and other papers*. Boston: Little, Brown, 1900.

Bigelow HJ. *Orthopedic surgery and other medical papers*. Boston: Little, Brown, 1900.

Bigelow HJ. *A memoir of Henry Jacob Bigelow*. Boston: Little, Brown, 1900.

Blalock A (edited by M Ravitch). *The papers of Alfred Blalock*. Baltimore: Johns Hopkins University Press, 1966.

Blalock A (written by WP Longmire). *Alfred Blalock, his life and times*. Private printing, 1991.

Brainard D (written by J Kinney). *Saga of a surgeon*. Springfield: Southern Illinois University, 1987.

Brinton JN. *Personal memoirs of John H. Brinton, major and surgeon USV, 1861–1865*. New York: Neale, 1914.

Brooks B (written by L Rosenfeld). *Barney Brooks, M.D. (1882–1952)*. Nashville: Vanderbilt University Medical Center, 1986.

Brunn H: *Medico-surgical tributes to Harold Brunn*. Berkeley: University of California, 1942.

Bryant H (written by WS Bryant). *Henry Bryant, MD, 1820–1867*. New York: Craftsman, 1952.

Cahan WG. *No stranger to tears: a surgeon's story*. New York: Random House, 1991.

Caleel R. *Surgeon, a year in the life of an inner-city doctor*. New York: Rawson, 1986.

Carson B. *Gifted hands*. Grand Rapids, MI: Zondervan, 1990.

Carrel A (written by WS Edwards & PD Edwards). *Alexis Carrel, visionary surgeon*. Springfield: Charles C Thomas, 1974.

Carrel A (written by TI Malinin). *Surgery and life, the extraordinary career of Alexis Carrel*. New York: Harcourt Brace and Jovanovich, 1979.

Cattell R (written by MC Dunmore). *On the cutting edge*. Plymouth, MA: Jones River Press, 1991.

Christopher F. *One surgeon's practice*. Philadelphia: WB Saunders, 1957.

Churchill ED. *Surgeons to soldiers, diary and records of the surgical consultants allied force headquarters, World War II*. Philadelphia: JB Lippincott, 1972.

Churchill ED. *Wanderjahr, the education of a surgeon*. Boston: Countway Library, 1990.

Cochran J (written by MH Saffron). *Surgeon to Washington*. New York: Columbia University, 1977.

Cole W (written by D Connaughton). *Warren Cole, MD, and the ascent of scientific surgery*. Chicago: Cole Foundation, 1991.

Coller F (written by JO Robinson). *Frederick Amasa Coller, his philosophy, surgical practice, and teachings*. Ann Arbor, MI: National Institute for Burn Medicine, 1987.

Cooley D (written by T Thompson). *Hearts, of surgeons and transplants*. New York: McCall, 1971.

Cooley D (written by H Minetree). *Cooley, the career of a great heart surgeon*. New York: Harper's Magazine, 1973.

Cooper IS. *The vital probe, my life as a brain surgeon*. New York: WW Norton, 1981.

Crile GW (written by G Crile). *George Crile, an autobiography*. Philadelphia: JB Lippincott, 1947.

Crile GW (written by P English). *Shock, physiological surgery, and George Washington Crile*. Westport, CT: Greenwood Press, 1980.

Crile GW, Jr. *The way it was, sex, surgery, treasure, and travel, 1907–1987*. Kent, OH: Kent State University, 1992.

Crosthwait WL (written by E Fischer). *The last stitch*. Philadelphia: JB Lippincott, 1956.

Cullen T (written by J Robinson). *Tom Cullen of Baltimore*. London: Oxford, 1949.

Cushing H (written by J Fulton). *Harvey Cushing, a biography.* Springfield, IL: Charles C Thomas, 1946.

Cushing H (written by E Thomason). *Harvey Cushing, surgeon, author, artist.* New York: Henry Schuman, 1950.

Cushing H (written by P Black). *The surgical art of Harvey Cushing.* Park Ridge, IL: American Association of Neurological Surgeons, 1992.

Cushing H. *Harvey Cushing; seventieth birthday party.* Springfield, IL: Charles C Thomas, 1939.

Cushing H. *The life of Sir William Osler.* Oxford: Clarendon, 1925.

Cushing H. *From a surgeon's journal, 1915–1918.* Boston: Little, Brown & Co., 1936.

Cutler EC (written by R Zollinger). *Elliot Carr Cutler and the cloning of surgeons.* Mount Kisco, NY: Futura, 1989.

DaCosta JC. *Selections from the papers and speeches of John Chalmers DaCosta.* Philadelphia: WB Saunders, 1931.

DaCosta JC. *Poems of John Chalmers DaCosta.* Philadelphia: Dorrance, 1942.

DaCosta JC. *The trials and triumphs of the surgeon and other literary gems.* Philadelphia: Dorrance, 1944.

Dandy W (written by W Fox). *Dandy of Johns Hopkins.* Baltimore: William & Wilkins, 1984.

Davis L. *From one surgeon's notebook.* Springfield, IL: Charles C Thomas, 1967.

Dennis F. *Selected surgical papers (1876–1914).* New York: private printing, 1934.

Dodd, JM. *Autobiography of a surgeon.* New York: Walter Neale, 1928.

Drew, CR (written by CE Wynes). *Charles Richard Drew, the man and the myth.* Urbana: University of Illinois, 1988.

Drew CR (written by DY Croman). *Charles Richard Drew, sprinter in life.* Nashville: Winston-Derek, 1992.

Drew CR (written by S Love). *One blood, the death and resurrection of Charles R. Drew.* Chapel Hill: University of North Carolina Press, 1996

Eloesser L (written by H Shumacker). *Leo Eloesser, MD, eulogy for a free spirit.* New York: Philosophical Library, 1982.

Emmet TA. *Incidents of my life.* New York: GP Putnam's Sons, 1911

Fenger C. *The collected works of Christian Fenger.* Philadelphia: WB Saunders, 1912.

Fenger C (written by E Hirsch). *Christian Fenger.* Chicago: private printing, 1972.

Finney JMT. *A surgeon's life.* New York: GP Putnam's Sons, 1940.

Flexner A. *I remember.* New York: Simon & Schuster, 1940.

Fox R. *Working without a net, memoirs of a small-town surgeon.* West Frankfort, IL: Againcourt-Galen, 1994.

Frazier CH (edited by IS Ravdin, AW Adson, & FC Grant). *Contributions in surgery in honor of CH Frazier.* Philadelphia: JB Lippincott, 1935.

Gerster AG. *Recollections of a New York surgeon.* New York: Paul B Hoeber, 1917.

Gibbon J (written by A Romaine-Davis). *John Gibbon and his heart-lung machine.* Philadelphia: University of Pennsylvania, 1991.

Gibney V (written by A Shands). *Gibney of the Ruptured & Crippled.* New York: Appleton-Century-Crofts, 1969.

Gibson W. *Rambles in Europe in 1839.* Philadelphia: Lea & Blanchard, 1841.

Gross SD. *Autobiography of Samuel D. Gross.* Philadelphia: George Barrie, 1887.

Gunn M. *Memorial sketches of Doctor Moses Gunn, by his wife.* Chicago: WT Keener, 1889.

Hall RJ (written by George Higgins). *Hall of Cottage.* Santa Barbara, CA: Chiron, 1989.

Halsted WS (written by WG MacCallum). *William Stewart Halsted, surgeon.* Baltimore: Johns Hopkins Press, 1930.

Halsted WS (edited by WC Burket). *Surgical papers by William Stewart Halsted.* Baltimore: Johns Hopkins Press, 1934.

Halsted WS (written by G Heuer). *Dr. Halsted.* Baltimore: Johns Hopkins Press, 1952.

Halsted WS (written by S Crowe). *Halsted of Johns Hopkins, the man and his men.* Springfield, IL: Charles C Thomas, 1957.

Hardy JD. *The world of surgery, 1945–1985.* Philadelphia: University of Pennsylvania, 1986.

Herman L. *A surgeon thinks it over.* Philadelphia: University of Pennsylvania, 1962.

Hertzler AE. *The horse and buggy doctor.* New York: Harper & Brothers, 1938.

Hertzler AE. *Ventures in science of a country surgeon.* Halstead, KS: private printing, 1944.

Hibbs RA (written by G Goodwin). *Russell A. Hibbs, pioneer in orthopedic surgery, 1869–1932.* New York: Columbia University, 1935.

Howe AJ. *Miscellaneous papers.* Cincinnati: Robert Clarke, 1894.

Judson A (written by E Judson). *The life of Adoniram Judson, by his son, Edward Judson.* New York: DF Randolph, 1883.

Keen WW. *Addresses and other papers.* Philadelphia: WB Saunders, 1905

Keen WW. *Selected papers and addresses.* Philadelphia: George W Jacobs, 1923

Keen WW (edited by WWK James). *The memoirs of William Williams Keen, M.D.* Doylestown, PA: private printing, 1990.

Kehm R. *The birth of a surgeon.* New York: Vantage, 1982.

John Harvey Kellogg (written by R Schwarz). *John Harvey Kellogg, M.D.* Nashville: Southern Publishing Association, 1970.

Kelly H (written by A Davis). *Dr. Kelly of Hopkins, surgeon, scientist, Christian.* Baltimore: Johns Hopkins Press, 1959.

Kessler HH. *The knife is not enough.* New York: WW Norton, 1968.

Koop CE. *Koop: the memoirs of America's family doctor.* New York: Random House, 1991.

Lahey FH. *Frank Howard Lahey, birthday volume.* Springfield, IL: Charles C Thomas, 1940.

Laroe EK. *Woman surgeon.* New York: Dial, 1957.

Leonardo RA. *American surgeon abroad.* New York: Froben, 1942.

Leonardo RA. *A surgeon looks at life.* New York: Froben, 1945.

Long C (edited by FL Taylor). *Crawford W. Long and the discovery of ether anesthesia.* New York: Paul B Hoeber, 1928.

Long C (written by F Boland). *The first anesthetic, the story of Crawford Long.* Athens: University of Georgia, 1950.

Lydston GF. *Addresses and essays*. Louisville, KY: Renz & Henry, 1892.

Magnuson PB. *Ring the night bell, an autobiography*. London: Heinemann, 1960.

Maltz M. *Doctor Pygmalion, an autobiography*. New York: Thomas Crowell, 1953.

Martin FH. *The joy of living, an autobiography*. Garden City, NY: Doubleday & Doran, 1933.

Martin FH. *Fifty years of medicine and surgery*. Chicago: Surgical Publishing, 1934.

Matas R (written by I Cohn). *Rudolph Matas, a biography*. Garden City, NY: Doubleday, 1960.

Matas R. *Matas birthday volume*. New York: Paul B Hoeber, 1931.

Mayo W & Mayo C. *A collection of papers published previous to 1909*. Philadelphia: WB Saunders, 1912.

Mayo W & Mayo C (written by H Clapesattle). *The Doctors Mayo*. Minneapolis: University of Minnesota, 1941.

Mayo W & Mayo C (written by F Willius). *Aphorisms of Dr. Charles Mayo and Dr. William Mayo*. Rochester, MN: private printing, 1951.

Mayo W & Mayo C (written by G Nagel). *The Mayo legacy*. Springfield, IL: Charles C Thomas, 1966.

Mayo CW. *Mayo, the story of my family and my career*. Garden City, NY: Doubleday, 1968.

McDowell E (written by M Ridenbaugh). *The biography of Ephraim McDowell*. New York: CL Webster, 1890.

McDowell E (written by MT Valentine). *Biography of Ephraim McDowell, the father of ovariotomy*. New York: McDowell, 1897.

McDowell E (written by A Schachner). *Ephraim McDowell, father of ovariotomy and founder of abdominal surgery*. Philadelphia: JB Lippincott, 1921.

McGuire HH (written by J Schildt). *Hunter Holmes McGuire, doctor in gray*. Chewsville, MD: private printing, 1986.

McGuire HH (written by MF Shaw). *Stonewall Jackson's Surgeon, Hunter Holmes McGuire, a biography*. Lynchburg, VA: private printing, 1993.

McGuire S. *Stuart McGuire, an autobiography*. Richmond, VA: William Byrd, 1956.

Monteiro A (written by S Dannett & R Burkart). *Confederate surgeon*. New York: Dodd & Mead, 1969.

Moore FD. *A miracle and a privilege*. Washington: Joseph Henry, 1995.

Morgan E. *The making of a woman surgeon*. New York: GP Putnam, 1980.

Morris RT. *Fifty years a surgeon*. New York: EP Dutton, 1936.

Morton RS. *A woman surgeon*. New York: Grosset & Dunlap, 1937.

Morton RS. *A doctor's holiday in Iran*. New York: Funk & Wagnalls, 1940.

Mott V. *Travels to Europe and the East*. New York: Harper & Brothers, 1842.

Mumford JG. *Surgical memoirs and other essays*. New York: Moffat & Yard, 1908.

Murphy JB (written by L Davis). *J. B. Murphy, stormy petrel of surgery*. New York: GP Putnam's Sons, 1938.

Murphy JB (written by R Schmitz & T Oh). *The remarkable surgical practice of John Benjamin Murphy*. Urbana: University of Illinois, 1993.

Nix JT. *A surgeon reflects*. Shreveport: Louisiana State, 1940.

Nixon PI. *Pat Nixon of Texas*. College Station: Texas A & M, 1979.

Nolen WA. *The making of a surgeon*. New York: Random House, 1970.

Nolen WA. *A surgeon's world*. New York: Random House, 1972.

Ochsner A (written by J Wild & I Harkey). *Alton Ochsner, surgeon of the South*. Baton Rouge: Louisiana State, 1990.

Park R. *Selected papers*. Buffalo: private printing, 1914.

Parson U (written by S Goldowsky). *Yankee surgeon, the life and times of Usher Parsons*. Boston: Countway Library, 1988.

Peacock A. *Globe trotting with a surgeon*. Seattle: Lowman & Hanford, 1936.

Physick PS (written by J Randolph). *A memoir on the life and character of Philip Syng Physick*. Philadelphia: TK & PG Collins, 1839.

Pilcher LS. *A surgical pilgrim's progress*. Philadelphia: JB Lippincott, 1925.

Rosen L. *Memoirs of a surgical houseofficer, Vanderbilt Hospital, 1936–1942*. Nashville, TN: Vanderbilt University, 1991.

Sachs E. *Fifty years of neurosurgery, a personal story*. New York: Vantage, 1958.

Seagrave GS. *Burma surgeon*. New York: WW Norton, 1943.

Seagrave GS. *Burma surgeon returns*. New York: WW Norton, 1946.

Senn N. *Four months among the surgeons of Europe*. Chicago: American Medical Association, 1887.

Senn N. *War correspondence (HispanoAmerican war)*. Chicago: American Medical Association, 1899.

Senn N. *Medico-surgical aspects of the Spanish American War*. Chicago: American Medical Association, 1900.

Sharpe W. *Brain surgeon, an autobiography*. New York: Viking, 1952.

Sims JM. *The story of my life*. New York: D Appleton, 1884.

Sims JM (written by S Harris). *Woman's surgeon*. New York: Macmillan, 1950.

Sims JM (written by D McGregor). *Sexual surgery and the origins of gynecology, J Marion Sims, his hospital, and his patients*. New York: Garland, 1989.

Slaughter FG. *The new science of surgery*. New York: Julian Messner, 1946.

Smith EV. *The making of a surgeon, a midwestern chronicle*. Fond du Lac, WI: private printing, 1942.

Smith N. *Medical and surgical memoirs*. Baltimore: William A Francis, 1831.

Smith N (written by E Smith). *The life and letters of Nathan Smith*. New Haven: Yale University, 1914.

Starzl T. *The puzzle people, memoirs of a transplant surgeon*. Pittsburgh: University of Pittsburgh, 1992.

Stimson L (written by EL Keyes). *Civil War memories*. New York: Knickerbocker, 1918.

Stone HB. *As a man thinketh, a surgeon thinks out loud*. Baltimore: private printing, 1956.

Swinburne J. *A typical American, or incidents in the life of Dr. John Swinburne, surgeon*. Albany, NY: Citizen Office, 1888.

Thomas VT. *Pioneering research in surgical shock and cardiovascular surgery*. Philadelphia: University of Pennsylvania, 1985.

Thorek M. *A surgeon's world*. Philadelphia: JB Lippincott, 1943.

Toland HH (written by L Gottlieb). *Gold mining surgeon.* Manhattan, KS: Sunflower Press, 1985.

Vaughan GT. *Papers on surgery.* Washington: WF Roberts, 1932.

Wangensteen OH (written by L Peltier & JB Aust). *L'étoile du nord, an account of Owen Harding Wangensteen (1898–1981).* Chicago: American College of Surgeons, 1994.

Warbasse, JP. *North star, a contribution to autobiography.* Falmouth, MA: Kendall, 1958.

Warren E. *A doctor's experience in three continents.* Baltimore: Cushings & Bailey, 1885.

Warren J (written by R Truax). *The doctors Warren of Boston.* Boston: Houghton Mifflin, 1968.

Warren J (written by J Cary). *Joseph Warren, physician, politician, patriot.* Urbana: University of Illinois, 1961.

Warren J (written by R Frothingham). *Life and times of Joseph Warren.* Boston: Little & Brown, 1865.

Warren J (written by E Warren). *The life of John Warren.* Boston: Noyes & Holmes, 1874.

Warren JC (written by E Warren). *The life of John Collins Warren.* Boston: Ticknor & Fields, 1860.

Warren JM (written by H Arnold). *Memoir of Jonathan Mason Warren.* Boston: private printing, 1886.

Warren JM (written by R Jones). *The Parisian education of an American surgeon.* Philadelphia: American Philosophical Society, 1978.

Warren JC (written by ED Churchill). *To work in the vineyard of surgery.* Cambridge: Harvard University, 1958.

Weeder RS. *Surgeon, the view from behind the mask.* Chicago: Contemporary Books, 1988.

Welch CE. *A twentieth-century surgeon.* Boston: Massachusetts General Hospital, 1992.

Welch WH (written by S Flexner & J Flexner). *William Henry Welch and the heroic age of American medicine.* New York: Viking, 1941.

Wheeler JB. *Memoirs of a small-town surgeon.* Garden City, NY: Garden City Publishing, 1935.

White CS. *Surgical interlude, recollections and reflections.* Washington: private printing, 1963.

White JW (written by A Repplier). *J William White.* Boston: Houghton Mifflin, 1919.

Williams DH (written by H Buckler). *Doctor Dan, pioneer in American surgery.* Boston: Little Brown, 1954.

Wyeth JA. *With sabre and scalpel.* New York: Harper & Brothers, 1914.

Young H. *Hugh Young.* New York: Harcourt & Brace, 1940.

HISTORY OF SURGERY
(BOOKS AND BOOK CHAPTERS)

Albert DM & Scheie HG. *A history of ophthalmology at the University of Pennsylvania.* Springfield, IL: Charles C Thomas, 1965.

American Association of Genito-Urinary surgeons. *A brief history of the organization and transactions of the American Association of Genito-Urinary surgeons; October 16th, 1886 to October 16, 1911.* New York: private printing, 1911.

American Otological Society. *History of the American Otological Society.* New York: American Otological Society, 1968.

Ballenger EG. *History of urology, prepared under the auspices of the American Urological Association.* Baltimore: Williams & Wilkins, 1933.

Barkley AH. *Kentucky's pioneer lithotomists.* Cincinnati: CJ Krehbiel, 1913.

Berman JK. *The Western Surgical Association, 1891–1900; impressions and selected transactions.* Indianapolis, IN: Hackett, 1976.

Billings JS. The history and literature of surgery. In: *The system of surgery* (edited by F Dennis), vol. 1, pp. 17–144, Philadelphia: Lea Brothers, 1895.

Brewer LA. *The early history and era of development of the Pacific Coast Surgical Association, the first twenty-five meetings, 1926–1954.* Private printing, 1982.

Brewer LA. *The history of the Pacific Coast Surgical Association (1955–1979).* Private printing, 1988.

Blanchard CE. *The romance of proctology.* Youngstown, OH: Medical Success Press, 1938.

Bosk CL. *Forgive and remember: managing medical failure.* Chicago: University of Chicago, 1979.

Brieger GH. From conservative to radical surgery in late nineteenth-century America. In: *Medical theory, surgical practice* (edited by C Lawrence). London: Routledge, 1992.

Brooks SM. *McBurney's point: the story of appendicitis.* New York: AS Barnes, 1969.

Bryan SA. *Pioneering specialists: a history of the American Academy of Ophthalmology and Otolaryngology.* San Francisco: American Academy of Ophthalmology, 1982.

Bryce DP. *The American Laryngological Association, 1878–1978.* Washington: American Laryngological Association, 1978.

Bunker JP, Barnes B & Mosteller F (editors). *Cost, risks and benefits of surgery.* New York: Oxford University Press, 1977.

Clagett OT. *General surgery at the Mayo Clinic, 1900–1970.* Private printing, 1980.

Coates JB. *Medical Department, United States Army; surgery in World War II: volume II, general surgery* (edited by Michael DeBakey). Washington: Office of the Surgeon General, 1955.

Coates JB. *Medical Department, United States Army; surgery in World War II; volume II, activities of surgical consultants* (edited by B Noland Carter). Washington: Office of the Surgeon General, 1964.

Conway H & Stark RB. *Plastic surgery at the New York Hospital one hundred years ago, with biographical notes on Gurdon Buck.* New York: PB Hoeber, 1953.

Curry GJ. *Profiles in trauma.* Springfield, IL: Charles C Thomas, 1969.

Dally A. *Women under the knife, a history of surgery.* London: Hutchinson Radius, 1991.

Davenport H. *University of Michigan surgeons, 1850–1970: who they were and what they did.* Ann Arbor: Historical Center for the Health Sciences, 1993.

Davis L (editor). *Fifty years of surgical progress, 1905–1955.* Chicago: Franklin H Martin Memorial Foundation, 1955.

Davis L. *Fellowship of surgeons, a history of the American College of Surgeons.* Springfield, IL: Charles C. Thomas, 1960.

Dixon EH. *Scenes in the practice of a New York surgeon.* New York: DeWitt & Davenport, 1855.

Dixon EH. *Back-bone, photographed from "the scalpel."* New York: Robert M DeWitt, 1866.

Earle AS. *Surgery in America from the colonial era to the twentieth century: selected writings.* Philadelphia: WB Saunders, 1965.

Earle AS. *Surgery in American from the colonial era to the twentieth century.* New York: Praeger, 1983.

Edmonson JM. *American surgical instruments: the history of their manufacture and a directory of instrument makers to 1900.* San Francisco: Norman Publishing, 1997.

Edmonson JM. Development of the American surgical instrument industry. In: Introduction to a reprinting of Charles Truax's *The Mechanics of Surgery* (1899), pp. vi–xliii. San Francisco: Norman Publishing, 1988.

Flexner JT. *Doctors on horseback: pioneers of American medicine.* New York: Viking, 1937.

Franklin EC. Surgery in the United States. In: *The science and art of surgery, embracing minor and operative surgery; compiled from standard allopathic authorities, and adapted to homoeopathic therapeutics, with a general history of surgery from the earliest periods to the present time,* vol. 1, pp. 25–41, St Louis: Missouri Democrat Book and Job Print, 1867–1873.

Garrison, FH. American surgery. In: *An introduction to the history of medicine with medical chronology, suggestions for study, and bibliographic data,* pp. 498–512, 598–601, and 730–734. Philadelphia: WB Saunders, 1929.

Greenblatt SH (editor). *A history of neurosurgery, in its scientific and professional contexts.* Park Ridge, IL: The American Association of Neurological Surgeons, 1997.

Gross SD. *Report on Kentucky surgery.* Louisville: Webb & Levering, 1853.

Haggard WD. *Surgery, queen of the arts.* Philadelphia: WB Saunders, 1935.

Hart D. *The first forty years at Duke in surgery.* Durham, NC: Duke University, 1971.

Heck CV. *Fifty years of progress: in recognition of the 50th anniversary of the American Academy of Orthopaedic Surgeons.* Chicago: American Academy of Orthopaedic Surgeons, 1983.

Henderson VJ & Organ CH. *Noteworthy publications by African-American surgeons.* Oakland [CA]: private printing, 1995.

Hinman F. *American pediatric urology.* San Francisco: Norman Publishing, 1991.

Hochberg LA. *Thoracic surgery before the 20th century.* New York: Vantage, 1960.

Hodges RM. *A narrative of events connected with the introduction of sulphuric ether into surgical use.* Boston: Little & Brown, 1891.

Hubbell AA. *The development of ophthalmology in America, 1800 to 1870.* Chicago: WT Keener, 1908.

International College of Surgeons. *International College of Surgeons: past, present, and future; six decades of international surgical collaboration.* private printing: International College of Surgeons, 1995.

Johnson ST. *The history of cardiac surgery, 1896–1955.* Baltimore: The Johns Hopkins Press, 1970.

Kagarise MJ & Thomas CG (editors). *Legends and legacies: a look inside: four decades of surgery at the University of North Carolina at Chapel Hill, 1952–1993.* Chapel Hill: Department of Surgery, University of North Carolina School of Medicine, 1997.

Keen WW. *The surgical operations on President Cleveland in 1893.* Philadelphia: George W Jacobs, 1917. (2nd edition, 1928)

Leonardo RA. American surgery. In: *History of surgery,* pp. 297–331. New York: Froben, 1948.

LeVay D. The United States. In: *The history of orthopaedics,* pp. 375–454. Lancs [England]: Parthenon, 1990.

Longmire WP. *Starting from scratch: the early history of the UCLA Department of Surgery.* Pasadena, CA: Castle Press, 1984.

Marr JP. *Pioneer surgeons of the Woman's Hospital: the lives of Sims, Emmet, Peaslee, and Thomas.* Philadelphia: FA Davis, 1957.

Martin JD. *The history of surgery at Emory University School of Medicine.* Atlanta: private printing, 1979.

McDonell K. *The journals of William A. Lindsay, an ordinary nineteenth-century physician's surgical cases.* Indianapolis: Indiana Historical Society, 1989.

Meade R. *A history of thoracic surgery.* Springfield, IL: Charles C Thomas, 1961.

Meade R. *An introduction to the history of general surgery.* Philadelphia: WB Saunders, 1968.

Mengert WF. *History of the American College of Obstetricians and Gynecologists, 1950–1970.* private printing, 1971.

Moore FD. American surgery, progress over two centuries. In: *Advances in American medicine: essays at the bicentennial* (edited by JZ Bowers & EF Purcell), vol 2, pp. 614–684, New York: Josiah Macy, 1976.

Morton CB. *History of the department of surgery, school of medicine, University of Virginia, 1824–1971.* Charlottesville: University of Virginia, 1971.

Mumford JG. American surgery. In: *Surgical memoirs and other essays,* pp. 72–93, New York: Moffat & Yard, 1908.

Mumford JG. Narrative of surgery: a historical sketch. In: *Surgery, its principles and practice* [edited by WW Keen], vol 1, pp. 17–78, Philadelphia: WB Saunders, 1909.

Naef AP. *The story of thoracic surgery.* Toronto: Hogrefe & Huber, 1990.

Newell FW. *The American Ophthalmological Society, 1864–1989: a continuation of Wheeler's first hundred years.* Rochester, MN: The Society, 1989.

Organ C & Kosiba M. *History of the Southwestern Surgical Congress, 1948–1985.* private printing, n.p.n.d.

Organ C & Kosiba M. *A century of black surgeons: the USA experience.* Norman, OK: Transcript Press, 1987.

Orr HW. *Fifty years of the American Orthopaedic Association, golden anniversary meeting.* Omaha, NE: private printing, 1937.

Orr HW. *On the contributions of Hugh Owen Thomas of Liverpool, Sir Robert Jones of Liverpool and London, John Ridlon, MD of New York and Chicago to modern orthopedic surgery.* Springfield, IL: Charles C Thomas, 1949.

Paletta FX & McDowell F. *History of the American Society of Plastic and Reconstructive Surgery.* Baltimore: Waverly, 1963.

Pernick MS. *A calculus of suffering; pain, professionalism, and anesthesia in nineteenth-century America.* New York: Columbia University, 1985.

Pool EH & McGowan FJ. *Surgery at the New York Hospital one hundred years ago.* New York: Paul B Hoeber, 1929.

Ravitch MM. *A century of surgery: the history of the American Surgical Association*. Philadelphia: JB Lippincott, 1981.

Reifler D. *The American Society of Ophthalmic Plastic and Reconstructive Surgery, the first twenty-five years: 1969–1994*. Winter Park, FL: private printing, 1994.

Reilly PR. *The surgical solution, a history of involuntary sterilization in the United States*. Baltimore: Johns Hopkins University Press, 1991.

Rogers SL. *Primitive surgery, skills before science*, Springfield, IL: Charles C Thomas, 1985.

Rodman JS. *History of the American Board of Surgery, 1937–1952*. Philadelphia: JB Lippincott, 1956.

Rutkow IM (editor). *Surgical health care delivery: The Surgical Clinics of North America*. Philadelphia: WB Saunders, (August) 1982.

Rutkow IM (editor). *History of surgery in the United States: The Surgical Clinics of North America, 75th anniversary issue*. Philadelphia: WB Saunders, (December) 1987.

Rutkow IM. *The history of surgery in the United States, 1775–1900: Volume 1, textbooks, monographs, & treatises*. San Francisco: Norman Publishing, 1988.

Rutkow IM. *The history of surgery in the United States, 1775–1900: Volume 2, periodicals and pamphlets*. San Francisco: Norman Publishing, 1992.

Rutkow IM. *Socioeconomics of surgery*. St. Louis: CV Mosby, 1989.

Rutkow IM. *Surgery: an illustrated history*. St Louis: CV Mosby, 1993.

Scott WW. *The Clinical Society of Genito-Urinary Surgeons: a chronicle, 1921–1990*. Baltimore: Williams & Wilkins, 1991.

Shaffer RN. *The history of the American Board of Ophthalmology, 1916–1991*. Rochester, MN: private printing, 1991.

Shands AR. *The early orthopaedic surgeons of America*. St Louis: CV Mosby, 1970.

Shumacker H. *History of the Society of Clinical Surgery*. Indianapolis: Benham, 1977.

Shumacker H. *The Society for Vascular Surgery: a history, 1945–1983*. Manchester, VT: The Society for Vascular Surgery, 1984.

Shumacker HB. *The evolution of cardiac surgery*. Bloomington: Indiana University, 1992.

Smith HH. Historical record of American surgery. In: *A system of operative surgery, based upon the practice of surgeons in the United States*, pp. xvii–cxi, Philadelphia: Lippincott & Grambo, 1852.

Smith HH. History of surgery in the United States and a bibliographical index of American work on subjects connected with the practice of surgery, from the year 1783 to the commencement of the year 1862, and an alphabetical list of American surgeons from the year 1783 to 1860 inclusive: with the titles of their books and papers. In: *The principles and practice of surgery, embracing minor and operative surgery*, vol. 1, pp. 39–61; vol. 2, pp. 727–760, Philadelphia: JB Lippincott, 1863.

Smith S. The evolution of American surgery. In: *American practice of surgery* (edited by JD Bryant & A Buck), vol. 1, pp. 3–67, New York: William Wood, 1906–1911.

Sparkman RS & Shire GT. *Minutes of the American Surgical Association, 1880–1968*. Dallas: Taylor Publishing, 1971.

Sparkman RS. *The Southern Surgical Association, the first 100 years, 1887–1987*. Philadelphia: JB Lippincott, 1989.

Speert H. *Obstetrics and gynecology in America: a history*. Chicago: American College of Obstetricians and Gynecologists, 1980.

Stephenson GW. *American College of Surgeons at 75*. Chicago: American College of Surgeons, 1990.

Stevens A. *American pioneers in abdominal surgery*. Melrose, MA: American Society of Abdominal Surgeons, 1968.

Stockel HH. *The lightning stick: arrows, wounds, and Indian legends*. Reno, NV: University of Nevada Press, 1995.

Surgery, Gynecology and Obstetrics. *Fifty years of surgical progress, 1905–1955*. Chicago: Franklin H Martin Foundation, 1955.

Taylor ES. *History of the American Gynecological Society 1876–1981, and American Association of Obstetricians and Gynecologists, 1881–1981*. St Louis: CV Mosby, 1985.

Thoms H. *Chapters in American obstetrics*. Springfield, IL: Charles C Thomas, 1933.

Wheeler MC. *The American Ophthalmological Society: the first hundred years*. Toronto: University of Toronto, 1964.

Whipple AO. *The evolution of surgery in the United States*. Springfield, IL: Charles C Thomas, 1963.

Wolfe RJ. *Robert C. Hinckley and the recreation of the first operation under ether*. Boston: Boston Medical Library, 1993.

Wigglesworth WC. Surgery in Massachusetts, 1620–1800. In: *Medicine in Colonial Massachusetts, 1620–1820*. Boston: Colonial Society of Massachusetts, 1980.

HISTORY OF SURGERY
(PERIODICAL LITERATURE)

Allen AW. The influence of the American Medical Association on surgery. *American Journal of Surgery* 51:262–266, 1941.

Atwater EC. Of grand dames, surgeons, and hospitals: Batavia, New York, 1900–1940. *Journal of the History of Medicine and Allied Sciences* 45:414–451, 1990.

Aufricht G. The development of plastic surgery in the United States. *Plastic and Reconstructive Surgery* 1:3–25, 1946.

Bacon DR. Surgical heroes: an anesthesiologist's perspective. *Bulletin of the American College of Surgeons* 80:29–36, 1995.

Beacham WD. History of the section on obstetrics and gynecology of the American Medical Association. *Journal of the American Medical Association* 169:1471–1483, 1959.

Beahrs OH. The medical history of President Ronald Reagan. *Surgery, Obstetrics and Gynecology* 178:86–96, 1994.

Berens C. Fifty years of ophthalmology in the United States. *American Journal of Surgery* 51:188–213, 1941.

Berk JB. Early American "do it yourself" surgery. *Contemporary Surgery* 12:41–46, 1978.

Bick EM. American orthopedic surgery. *New York State Journal of Medicine* 76:1192–1197 and 1346–1354, 1976.

Blaisdell FW. Medical advances during the Civil War. *Archives of Surgery* 123:1045–1050, 1988.

Bosniak SL. Ophthalmic plastic and reconstructive surgery in the United States, 1893–1970. *Advances in Ophthalmic and Plastic Reconstructive Surgery* 5:241–281, 1986.

Breinin GM. History of the section on ophthalmology of the American Medical Association. *Archives of Ophthalmology* 84:820–826, 1970.

Brieger GH. American surgery and the germ theory of disease. *Bulletin of the History of Medicine* 40:135–145, 1966.

Brieger GH. A portrait of surgery: surgery in America, 1875–1889. *Surgical Clinics of North America* 67:1181–1216, 1987.

Bryan JH. The history of laryngology and rhinology and the influence of America in the development of this specialty. *Annals of Medical History* 5:151–170, 1932.

Bunker JP. Surgical manpower: a comparison of operations and surgeons in the United States and in England and Wales. *New England Journal of Medicine* 282:135–141, 1970.

Churchill ED. The surgical management of the wounded in the Mediterranean theater at the time of the fall of Rome. *Transactions of the American Surgical Association* 62:268–283, 1944.

Couch NP. On World War II, battlefield surgery, and three wandering consultants. *Bulletin of the American College of Surgeons* 81:21–27, 1996.

Cutler EC. Military surgery—United States Army—European theater of operations, 1944–1945. *Surgery, Gynecology and Obstetrics* 82:261–274, 1946.

Curran JA. Surgical internships over the past fifty years. *American Journal of Surgery* 51:35–39, 1941.

Dannreuther WT. The American Board of Obstetrics and Gynecology, its origin, progress, and accomplishments. *American Journal of Obstetrics and Gynecology* 68:15–19, 1954,

Dennis F. The achievements of American surgery. *Medical Record* 42:637–648, 1892.

Eaton LK. Military surgery at the battle of Tippecanoe. *Bulletin of the History of Medicine* 25:460–463, 1951.

Erichsen J. Impressions of American surgery. *Lancet* 2:717–720, 1874.

Everett HS. The history of the American Gynecological Society and the scientific contributions of its fellows. *American Journal of Obstetrics and Gynecology* 126:908–919, 1976.

Fenton RA. A brief history of otolaryngology in the United States from 1847 to 1947. *Archives of Otolaryngology* 46:153–162, 1947.

Ficarra BJ. The evolution of blood transfusion. *Annals of Medical History* 4:302–323, 1942.

Figg L & Farrell-Beck J. Amputation in the Civil War: physical and social dimensions. *Journal of the History of Medicine and Allied Sciences* 48:454–475, 1993.

Fishbein M. Surgery and the American Medical Association. *American Journal of Surgery* 51:258–261, 1941.

Fogelman MJ. 1880–1890: a creative decade in world surgery. *American Journal of Surgery* 115:812–824, 1968.

Friedberg S. Laryngology and otology in colonial times. *Annals of Medical History* 1:86–101, 1917.

Friedenwald H. The American Ophthalmological Society, a retrospect of seventy-five years. *Archives of Ophthalmology* 23:1–21, 1940.

Gariepy TP. The introduction and acceptance of Listerian antisepsis in the United States. *Journal of the History of Medicine and Allied Sciences* 49:167–206, 1994.

Gilman CM. Military surgery in the American Revolution. *Journal of the Medical Society of New Jersey* 57:491–496, 1959.

Goldsmith HS. Unanswered mysteries in the death of Franklin D. Roosevelt. *Surgery, Gynecology and Obstetrics* 149:899–908, 1979.

Graham AB. An appraisement of the American Proctological Society. *Transactions of the American Proctological Society* 41:170–181, 1940.

Greisman HC. Wound management and medical organization in the Civil War. *Surgical Clinics of North America* 64:625–638, 1984.

Gross SD. A century of American surgery. *American Journal of the Medical Sciences* 71:431–484, 1876.

Haiken B. Plastic surgery and American beauty at 1921. *Bulletin of the History of Medicine* 68:429–453, 1994.

Hall C. The rise of professional surgery in the United States: 1800-1865. *Bulletin of the History of Medicine* 26:231–262, 1952.

Hamilton D. The nineteenth-century surgical revolution–antisepsis or better nutrition? *Bulletin of the History of Medicine* 56:30–40, 1982.

Harris TJ. The early history of otolaryngology in America with special reference to the American Laryngological, Rhinological and Otological Society. *Annals of Otology, Rhinology, and Laryngology* 45:655–665, 1936.

Harvey SD. Effect of the introduction of anesthesia upon surgery. *Journal of the American Dental Association* 32:1351–1357, 1945.

Heaton LD. President Eisenhower's operation for regional enteritis: a footnote to history. *Annals of Surgery* 159:661–664, 1964.

Hirschman LJ. First fifty years of proctology. *American Journal of Surgery* 79:5–12, 1950.

Hughes CW. A review of the late General Eisenhower's operations: epilog to a footnote to history. *Annals of Surgery* 173:793–799, 1971.

Hume EE. The golden jubilee of the Association of Military Surgeons of the United States, a history of its first half-century, 1891–1941. *Military Surgeon* 89:242–538, 1941.

Jain KM, Swan KG, Casey KF. Nobel prize winners in surgery. *American Surgeon* 47:195–200, 1981, and 48:191–196, 287–292, 495–500, & 555–557, 1982

Joy RJT. The natural bonesetters with special reference to the Sweet family of Rhode Island, a study of an early phase of orthopedics. *Bulletin of the History of Medicine* 28:416–441, 1954.

Keen WW. Recent progress in surgery. *Harper's New Monthly Magazine* 79:703–713, 1889.

Kiehn CL. The progression of reconstructive plastic surgery to full maturity as a specialty in World War II. *Plastic and Reconstructive Surgery* 95:1299–1319, 1995.

Kuhns WJ. Blood transfusion in the Civil War. *Transfusion* 5:92–94, 1965.

Lewis CE. Variations in the incidence of surgery. *New England Journal of Medicine* 281:880–885, 1969.

Lobingier AS. The influence of the British masters on American surgery. *American Journal of Surgery* 826–836, 1929.

Longo LD. The rise and fall of Battey's operation: a fashion in surgery. *Bulletin of the History of Medicine* 53:244–267, 1979.

Mann WA. History of the American Journal of Ophthalmology. *American Journal of Ophthalmology* 61:971–984, 1966.

Mason ML. Significance of the American College of Surgeons to progress of surgery in America. *American Journal of Surgery* 51:267–286, 1941.

Matas R. Surgical operations fifty years ago. *American Journal of Surgery* 82:111–121, 1951.

Mayer L. Orthopaedic surgery in the United States of America. *Journal of Bone and Joint Surgery* 32:461–569, 1950.

McDaniel WB. John Jones' introductory lecture to his course in surgery (1769), King's College, printed from the authors' manuscript. *Transactions of the College of Physicians of Philadelphia* (4th series) 8:180–190, 1940.

McDowell JN. Report on the improvements in the art and science of surgery in the last fifty years. *Transactions of the American Medical Association* 13:427–466, 1860.

McGreevy PS. Surgeons at the Little Big Horn. *Surgery, Gynecology and Obstetrics* 140:774–780, 1975.

Miller BJ. The development of heart lung machines. *Surgery, Gynecology and Obstetrics.* 154:403–414, 1982.

Moodie RL. Studies in palaeopathology, XXIV, prehistoric surgery in New Mexico. *American Journal of Surgery* 8:905–908, 1930.

Moore FD. A Nobel award to Joseph E. Murray, MD: some historical perspectives. *Archives of Surgery* 127:627–632, 1992.

Morantz-Sanchez R. Making it in a man's world: the late-nineteenth-century surgical career of Mary Amanda Dixon Jones. *Bulletin of the History of Medicine* 69:542–568, 1995.

Olch PD. Evarts A. Graham, The American College of Surgeons, and the American Board of Surgery. *Journal of the History of Medicine and Allied Sciences* 27:247–261, 1972.

Olch PD. Evarts A. Graham in World War I: the Empyema commission and service in the American Expeditionary Forces. *Journal of the History of Medicine and Allied Sciences* 44:430–446, 1989.

Organ CH. The interlocking of American surgery; an analysis of surgical leadership in the United States, 1945 through 1985. *American Journal of Surgery* 150:638–649, 1985.

Parish LC. Surgeons' Hall–the story of the first medical-school building in the United States. *New England Journal of Medicine* 273:1021–1024, 1965.

Perry T. Surgery in a rural area: 1638–1868. *American Journal of Surgery* 129:347–355, 1975.

Pilcher JE. The annals and achievements of American surgery. *Journal of the American Medical Association* 14:629–636, 1890.

Pollack HM, Cundy KR, Shea FJ. The Babcock surgical clinic. *American Journal of Roentgenology* 166:991–992, 1996.

Pratt LW. A century of progress in otorhinolaryngology. *Bulletin of the American College of Surgeons* 81:27–36, 1996.

Radbill SX. The barber surgeons among the early Dutch and Swedes along the Delaware. *Bulletin of the History of Medicine* 4:718–744, 1936.

Randall P. History of the American Association of Plastic Surgeons, 1921–1996. *Plastic and Reconstructive Surgery* 97:1254–1298, 1996.

Ravitch M. Surgery in 1776. *Annals of Surgery* 186:291–300, 1977.

Reverby S. Stealing the golden eggs: Ernest Amory Codman and the science and management of medicine. *Bulletin of the History of Medicine* 55:156–171, 1981.

Rucker MP. Giles Heale, the Mayflower surgeon. *Bulletin of the History of Medicine* 20:216–231, 1946.

Rutkow IM. William Stewart Halsted and the Germanic influence on education and training programs in surgery. *Surgery, Gynecology and Obstetrics* 147:602–606, 1978.

Rutkow IM. William Halsted and Theodor Kocher: "an exquisite friendship." *Annals of Surgery* 188:630–637, 1978.

Rutkow IM. Valentine Mott (1785–1865), the father of American vascular surgery: a historical perspective. *Surgery* 85:441–450, 1979.

Rutkow IM. The letters of William Halsted and Alexis Carrel. *Surgery, Gynecology and Obstetrics* 151:676–688, 1980.

Rutkow IM. The letters of William Halsted and Erwin Payr. *Surgery, Gynecology and Obstetrics* 161:75–87, 1985.

Rutkow IM. 1) Reference works related to United States surgical history; 2) A chronologic bibliography of American textbooks, monographs, and treatises relating to the surgical sciences, 1775–1899. *Surgical Clinics of North America* 67:1127–1152, 1987.

Rutkow IM. American surgical biographies. *Surgical Clinics of North America* 67:1153–1180, 1987.

Rutkow IM. A history of the Surgical Clinics of North America. *Surgical Clinics of North America* 67:1217–1239, 1987.

Rutkow IM. An experiment in surgical education, the first international exchange of residents: the letters of Halsted, Küttner, Heuer, and Landois. *Archives of Surgery* 123:115–121, 1988.

Rutkow IM. John Syng Dorsey (1783–1818). *Surgery* 103:45–55, 1988.

Rutkow IM. The value of surgical history. *Archives of Surgery* 126:953–956, 1991.

Rutkow IM. How American surgeons introduced radiology into United States medicine. *American Journal of Surgery* 165:252–257, 1993.

Rutkow IM. Railway surgery: traumatology and managed health care in 19th century America. *Archives of Surgery* 128:458–463, 1993,

Rutkow IM. Edwin Hartley Pratt and orificial surgery: unorthodox surgical practice in 19th century United States. *Surgery* 114:558–563, 1993.

Rutkow IM. William Tod Helmuth and Andrew Jackson Howe: surgical sectarianism in 19th century America. *Archives of Surgery* 129:662–668, 1994.

Rutkow IM. William Halsted, his family, and "queer business methods." *Archives of Surgery* 131:123–127, 1996.

Schlicke CP. American surgery's noblest experiment. *Archives of Surgery* 106:379–385, 1973.

Shambaugh GE. Organization of otolaryngology in the United States. *Journal of Laryngology* 81:1273–1277, 1967.

Shapiro HL. Primitive surgery: first evidence of trephining in the Southwest. *Natural History* 27:266–269, 1927.

Sharpe WD. The Confederate States Medical and Surgical Journal: 1864–1865. *Bulletin of the New York Academy of Medicine* 52:373–418, 1976.

Shrady G. American achievements in surgery. *The Forum* 17:167–178, 1894.

Shryock RH. Fame in surgery. *Journal of the International College of Surgeons* 41:511–518, 1967.

Smith DC. A historical overview of the recognition of appendicitis. *New York State Journal of Medicine* 86:572–583 & 639–647, 1986.

Smith DC. Modern surgery and the development of group practice in the midwest. *Caduceus* 2:1–34, 1986.

Smith DC. Appendicitis, appendectomy, and the surgeon. *Bulletin of the History of Medicine* 70:414–441, 1996.

Souchon E. Original contributions of American surgeons to medical sciences. *Transactions of the American Surgical Association* 35:65–171, 1917.

Sparkman RS. The woman in the case, Jane Todd Crawford, 1763–1842. *Annals of Surgery* 189:529–545, 1979.

Stark RB. Surgical care of the Confederate States army. *Bulletin of the New York Academy of Medicine* 34:387–407, 1958.

Stark RB. Immunization saves Washington's army. *Surgery, Gynecology and Obstetrics* 144:425–431, 1977.

Stephenson GW. The College's role in hospital standardization. *Bulletin of the American College of Surgeons* 66:17–29, 1981.

Stevenson L. The surgery of stammering, a forgotten enthusiasm of the nineteenth century. *Bulletin of the History of Medicine* 42:527–554, 1968.

Stookey B. Early neurosurgery in New York: its origin in neurology and general surgery. *Bulletin of the History of Medicine* 26:330–359, 1952.

Tempkin O. The role of surgery in the rise of modern medical thought. *Bulletin of the History of Medicine* 25:248–259, 1951.

Thompson JE. Sagittectomy–first recorded surgical procedure in the American Southwest, 1535: the journey and ministrations of Alvar Nuñez Cabeza de Vaca. *New England Journal of Medicine* 289:1403–1407, 1973.

Tilney NL. Cushing, Cutler and the mitral valve. *Surgery, Gynecology amd Obstetrics* 152:91–96, 1981.

Tilney NL. The marrow of the tragedy. *Surgery, Gynecology and Obstetrics* 157:380-388, 1983.

Tinker MB. America's contributions to surgery. *Johns Hopkins Hospital Bulletin* 13:209–213, 1902.

Trunkey DD. Doctor George Goodfellow, the first civilian trauma surgeon. *Surgery, Gynecology and Obstetrics.* 141:97–104, 1975.

Tyrone C. Certain aspects of gynecological practice in the late 19th century. *American Journal of Surgery* 84:95–106, 1952.

Verhoeff FH. American ophthalmology during the past century. *Archives of Ophthalmology* 39:451–464, 1948.

Viets HR. The earliest printed references in newspapers and journals to the first public demonstration of ether anesthesia in 1846. *Journal of the History of Medicine and Allied Sciences* 4:149–169, 1949.

Wagner FB. The founding fathers and centennial history of the Philadelphia Academy of Surgery. *Annals of Surgery* 192:1–8, 1980.

Wangensteen OH. Surgery and surgical travel groups. *Surgery, Gynecology and Obstetrics.* 147:246–254, 1978.

Warren JM. Recent progress in surgery. *Medical Communications of the Massachusetts Medical Society* 10:267–340, 1864.

Wennberg JE & Gittelsohn AM. Small area variations in health care delivery. *Science* 182:1102–1105, 1973.

Wilson C. American contributions to neurosurgery. *New Orleans Medical and Surgical Journal* 96:140–147, 1943.

Wright JR. The 1917 New York biopsy controversy: a question of surgical incision and the promotion of metastases. *Bulletin of the History of Medicine* 62:546–562, 1988.

Wooden AC. The wounds and weapons of the Revolutionary War from 1775 to 1783. *Delaware Medical Journal* 44:59–65, 1972.

Wynn G. The case book of Dr. Amos A. Evans, surgeon on the frigate "Constitution" in the War of 1812. *Annals of Medical History* 2:70–78, 1940.

HISTORY OF MEDICINE
(BOOKS AND BOOK CHAPTERS)

Abrahams LT. *Extinct medical schools of nineteenth century Philadelphia.* Philadelphia: University of Pennsylvania Press, 1966.

Abrahams LT. *The extinct medical schools of Baltimore.* Baltimore: Maryland Historical Society, 1969.

Adams GW. *Doctors in blue.* New York: Henry Schuman, 1962.

Adams S. *Medical bibliography in an age of discontinuity.* Chicago: Medical Library Association, 1981.

Bauer EL. *Doctors made in America.* Philadelphia: JB Lippincott, 1963.

Bauer LH. *Seventy-five years of medical progress, 1878–1953.* Philadelphia: Lea & Febiger, 1954.

Bell WJ. *The art of Philadelphia medicine.* Catalogue of an exhibition held at the Philadelphia Museum of Art, September 15–December 7, 1965.

Bell WJ. *The colonial physician and other essays.* New York: Science History Publications, 1975.

Blanton WB. *Medicine in Virginia in the seventeenth century.* Richmond, VA: William Byrd Press, 1930.

Blanton WB. *Medicine in Virginia in the eighteenth century.* Richmond, VA: Garrett & Massie, 1931.

Blanton WB. *Medicine in Virginia in the nineteenth century.* Richmond, VA: Garrett & Massie, 1933.

Bloom SW. *The doctor and his patient: a sociological interpretation.* New York: Free Press, 1976.

Bonner TN. *Medicine in Chicago, 1850–1950.* Madison, WI: American History Research Center, 1957.

Bonner TN. *The Kansas doctor: a century of pioneering.* Lawrence: University of Kansas Press, 1959.

Bonner TN. *American doctors and German universities; a chapter in international intellectual relations, 1870–1914.* Lincoln: University of Nebraska, 1963.

Bordley J & Harvey AM. *Two centuries of American medicine, 1776–1976.* Philadelphia: WB Saunders, 1976.

Brieger GH. *Medical America in the nineteenth century.* Baltimore: The Johns Hopkins Press, 1972.

Brooks S. *Civil war medicine*. Springfield, IL: Charles C Thomas, 1966.

Buck AH. *The growth of medicine from the earliest times to about 1800*. New Haven: Yale University, 1917.

Buck AH. *The dawn of modern medicine*. New Haven: Yale University, 1920.

Burrow JG. *Organized medicine in the progressive era: the move toward monopoly*. Baltimore: The Johns Hopkins University Press, 1977.

Calhoun DH. *Professional lives in America: structure and aspiration, 1750–1850*. Cambridge: Harvard University Press, 1965.

Cassedy JH. *Medicine and American growth, 1800–1860*. Madison: University of Wisconsin Press, 1986.

Clarke EH. *A century of American medicine, 1776–1876*. Philadelphia: Henry C Lea, 1876.

Cobb M. *The first Negro medical society, a history of the medico-chirurgical society of the District of Columbia, 1884–1939*. Washington: Associated Publishers, 1939.

Cordasco F. *Medical publishing in 19th century America*. Fairview, NJ: Junius Vaughn, 1990.

Corlett WT. *The medicine man of the American Indians and his cultural background*. Springfield, IL: Charles C Thomas, 1935.

Corner GW. *Two centuries of medicine: a history of the school of medicine, University of Pennsylvania*. Philadelphia: JB Lippincott, 1965.

Cowen DL & Helfand WH. *Pharmacy, an illustrated history*. New York: Harry Abrams, 1990.

Cunningham HH. *Doctors in gray, the Confederate medical service*. Baton Rouge: Louisiana State University, 1958.

Daniels GS. *American science in the age of Jackson*. New York: Columbia University Press, 1968.

Davis NS. *History of medical education and institutions in the United States*. Chicago: SC Griggs, 1851.

Davis NS. *History of the American Medical Association from its organization up to January, 1855*. Philadelphia: Lippincott & Grambo, 1855.

Derbyshire RC. *Medical licensure and discipline in the United States*. Baltimore: The Johns Hopkins Press, 1969.

DeVille KA. *Medical malpractice in nineteenth-century America: origins and legacy*. New York: New York University Press, 1990.

Donahue MP. *Nursing, the finest art, an illustrated history*. St Louis: CV Mosby, 1985.

Duffy J. *The healers: a history of American medicine*. Urbana: University of Illinois, 1976.

Eisenberg RL. *Radiology, an illustrated history*. St Louis: Mosby-Year Book, 1992.

Ficarra B. *Essays on historical medicine*. New York: Froben, 1948.

Fishbein M. *A history of the American Medical Association, 1847 to 1947*. Philadelphia: WB Saunders, 1947.

Freidson E. *Profession of medicine*. New York: Dodd & Mead, 1970.

Garceau O. *The political life of the American Medical Association*. Cambridge: Harvard University Press, 1941.

Gerdts WH. *The art of healing: medicine and science in American art*. Birmingham, AL: Birmingham Museum of Art, 1981.

Gevitz N. *Other healers; unorthodox medicine in America*. Baltimore: The Johns Hopkins Press, 1988.

Gilbert JB. *A bibliography of articles on the history of American medicine compiled from "writings on American history," 1902–1937*. New York: New York Academy of Medicine, 1951.

Gillett MC. *The army medical department, 1775–1818 and 1818–1865*. Washington: Center of Military History, 1981 & 1987.

Goler RI. *The healing arts in early America*. New York City: Fraunces Tavern Museum, 1985.

Gordon MB. *Aesculapius comes to the colonies*. Ventnor, NJ: Ventnor Publishers, 1949.

Grinnell GB. *The Cheyenne Indians, their history and ways of life*. New Haven: Yale University Press, 1924.

Haller JS. *American medicine in transition, 1840–1910*. Urbana: University of Illinois, 1981.

Hirshfield DS. *The lost reform: the campaign for compulsory health insurance in the United States from 1932 to 1943*. Cambridge: Harvard University Press, 1970.

Howell JD. *Technology and American medical practice, 1880–1930: an anthology of sources*. New York: Garland, 1988.

Howell JD. *Technology in the hospital; transforming patient care in the early twentieth century*. Baltimore: The Johns Hopkins University Press, 1995.

Hurd-Mead KC. *Medical women of America: a short history of the pioneer medical women of America*. New York: Froben, 1933.

Karolevitz R. *Doctors of the old west, a pictorial history of medicine on the frontier*. New York: Bonanza Books, 1967.

Kaufman M. *Homeopathy in America: the rise and fall of a medical heresy*. Baltimore: The Johns Hopkins Press, 1971.

Kaufman M. *American medical education: the formative years, 1765–1910*. Westport, CT: Greenwood Press, 1976.

Kett JF. *The formation of the American medical profession, the role of institutions, 1780–1860*. New Haven: Yale University, 1968.

King LS. *Medical thinking: a historical preface*. Princeton: Princeton University Press, 1982.

King LS. *American medicine comes of age, 1840–1920*. Chicago: American Medical Association, 1984.

King LS. *Transformations in American medicine*. Baltimore: The Johns Hopkins Press, 1991.

King WH. *History of homoeopathy and its institutions in America*. New York: Lewis Publishing, 1905.

Landis HRM. *The history of the development of medical sciences in America*. Philadelphia: Lea Brothers, 1901.

Larson MS. *The rise of professionalism: a sociological analysis*. Berkeley: University of California Press, 1977.

Leavitt JW & Numbers RL. *Sickness and health in America: readings in the history of medicine and public health*. Madison: University of Wisconsin, 1985.

Ludmerer KM. *Learning to heal: the development of American medical education*. New York: Basic Books, 1985.

Lyons A & Petrucelli RJ. *Medicine, an illustrated history*. New York: Harry Abrams, 1978.

Marks G & Beatty WK. *The story of medicine in America*. New York: Charles Scribner's Sons, 1973.

Marti-Ibanez F. *History of American medicine*. New York: MD Publications, 1958.

Morais HM. *The history of the Negro in medicine*. New York: Publishers Co., 1967.

Mumford JG. *A narrative of medicine in America*. Philadelphia: JB Lippincott, 1903.

Norris GW. *The early history of medicine in Philadelphia*. Philadelphia: private printing, 1886.

Norwood WF. *Medical education in the United States before the Civil War*. Philadelphia: University of Pennsylvania Press, 1944.

Numbers RL. *Almost persuaded: American physicians and compulsory health insurance, 1912–1920*. Baltimore: The Johns Hopkins University Press, 1978.

Numbers RL [editor]. *The education of American physicians, historical essays*. Berkeley: University of California, 1980.

Nuland SB. *Doctors, the biography of medicine*. New York: Alfred A Knopf, 1988.

Packard FR. *History of medicine in the United States*. New York: Paul B Hoeber, 1931.

Park R. *An epitome of the history of medicine*. Philadelphia: FA Davis, 1898.

Rauch JH. *Medical education, medical colleges, and the regulation of the practice of medicine in the United States and Canada, 1765–1891*. Springfield, IL: HW Rokker, 1891.

Rayack E. *Professional power and American medicine: the economics of the American Medical Association:* Cleveland: World, 1967.

Reverby S & Rosner D. *Health care in America: essays in social history*. Philadelphia: Temple University, 1979.

Risse GB, Numbers RL & Leavitt JW. *Medicine without doctors: home health care in American history*. New York: Science History Publications, 1977.

Rosen G. *Fee and fee bills: some economic aspects of medical practice in nineteenth century America*. Baltimore: The Johns Hopkins Press, 1946.

Rosen G. *The specialization of medicine*. New York: Froben Press, 1944.

Rosen G. *The structure of American medical practice, 1875–1941*. Philadelphia: University of Pennsylvania, 1983.

Rosenberg CE. *The care of strangers, the rise of America's hospital system*. New York: Basic Books, 1987.

Rothstein W. *American physicians in the nineteenth century*. Baltimore: The Johns Hopkins University Press, 1972.

Rothstein W. *American medical schools and the practice of medicine: a history*. New York: Oxford University, 1987.

Rousselot J (editor). *Medicine in art: a cultural history*. New York: McGraw Hill, 1967.

Shafer HB. *The American medical profession, 1783 to 1850*. New York: Columbia University, 1936.

Shryock R. *American medical research past and present*. New York: Commonwealth Fund, 1947.

Shryock R. *Medicine and society in America, 1660–1860*. New York: New York University, 1960.

Shryock R. *Medicine in America; historical essays*. Baltimore: The Johns Hopkins Press, 1966.

Shryock R. *Medical licensing in America, 1650–1965*. Baltimore: The Johns Hopkins Press, 1967.

Sigerist H. *American medicine*. New York: Norton, 1934.

Smith NS. *History of medical education and institutions in the United States, from the first settlement of the British colonies to the year 1850*. Chicago: SC Griggs, 1851.

Smith NS. *History of the American Medical Association from its organization to January, 1855*. Philadelphia: Lippincott & Grambo, 1855.

Starr P. *The social transformation of American medicine*. Basic Books, 1982.

Stevens R. *American medicine and the public interest*. New Haven: Yale University, 1971.

Stone E: *Medicine among the American Indians*. New York: Paul B Hoeber, 1932.

Thompson R. *Glimpses of medical Europe*. Philadelphia: JB Lippincott, 1908.

Toner JM. *Contributions to the annals of medical progress and medical education in the United States before and during the War of Independence*. Washington: Government Printing Office, 1874.

Viets H. *A brief history of medicine in Massachusetts*. Boston: Houghton Mifflin, 1930.

Vogel MJ & Rosenberg CE. *The therapeutic revolution, essays in the social history of American medicine*. Philadelphia: University of Pennyslvania, 1970.

Vogel VJ. *American Indian medicine*. Norman: University of Oklahoma Press, 1970.

Walsh MR. *Doctors wanted: no women need apply: sexual barriers in the medical profession, 1835–1875*. New Haven: Yale University, 1977.

Warner JH. *The therapeutic perspective: medical practice, knowledge, and identity in America, 1820–1885*. Cambridge: Harvard University, 1986.

Whorton JC. *Crusaders for freedom: the history of American health reformers*. Princeton: Princeton University Press, 1982.

Wickes S. *History of medicine in New Jersey, and of its medical men*. Newark, NJ: Martin R Dennis, 1897.

HISTORY OF MEDICINE
(PERIODICAL LITERATURE)

Axelsen DE. Women as victims of medical experimentation: J Marion Sims' surgery on slave women, 1845–1850. *Sage* 2:10–13, 1985.

Bell, WJ. Medical students and their examiners in eighteenth century America. *Transactions and Studies of the College of Physicians of Philadelphia* 4:14–24, 1953.

Bell WJ. Medical practice in colonial America. *Bulletin of the History of Medicine* 31:442–453, 1957.

Bell WJ. Lives in medicine: the biographical dictionaries of Thacher, Williams, and Gross. *Bulletin of the History of Medicine* 42:101–120, 1968.

Bevan AD. The over-crowding of the medical profession. *Journal of the Association of American Medical Colleges* 11:377–384, 1936.

Bick EM. French influences on early American medicine and surgery. *Journal of the Mount Sinai Hospital* 24:499–509, 1957.

Billings JS. The medical journals of the United States. *Boston Medical and Surgical Journal* 100:1–14, 1879.

Billing JS. American inventions and discoveries in medicine, surgery and practical sanitation. *Smithsonian Institute, Annual Report*, Board of Regents, Washington, 1893

Blake JB. Early American medical literature. *Journal of the American Medical Association* 236:41–46, 1976.

Bonner TN. German doctors in America - 1887–1914, their views and impressions of American life and medicine. *Journal of the History of Medicine and Allied Sciences* 14:1–17, 1959.

Bousfield MO. An account of physicians of color in the United States. *Bulletin of the History of Medicine* 17:61–84, 1945.

Brieger GH. Therapeutic conflicts and the American medical profession in the 1860s. *Bulletin of the History of Medicine* 41:215–222, 1967.

Brooks H. The medicine of the American Indian. *Bulletin of the New York Academy of Medicine* 5:264–275, 1929.

Burns CR. Malpractice suits in American medicine before the Civil War. *Bulletin of the History of Medicine* 43:41–56, 1969.

Cassedy JH. The flourishing and character of early American medical journalism, 1797-1860. *Journal of the History of Medicine and Allied Sciences* 38:135–150, 1983.

Cassedy JH. Numbering the North's medical events: humanitarianism and science in Civil War Statistics. *Bulletin of the History of Medicine* 66:210–233, 1992.

Coates JB. The history of the U.S. Army Medical Department in World War II. *Bulletin of the Medical Library Association* 47:264–273, 1959.

Daniels GH. The process of professionalization in American science: the emergent period, 1820–1860. *Isis* 58:151–166, 1967.

Ebert M. The rise and development of the American medical periodical, 1797–1850. *Bulletin of the Medical Library Association* 40:243–276, 1952.

Edwards LF. Resurrection riots during the heroic age of anatomy in America. *Bulletin of the History of Medicine* 25:178–184, 1951.

Estes JW. "A disagreeable and dangerous employment": medical letters from the siege of Boston. *Journal of the History of Medicine and Allied Sciences* 31:271–291, 1976.

Farmer HE. An account of the earliest colored gentlemen in medical science in the United States. *Bulletin of the History of Medicine* 8:599–618, 1940.

Fye WB. The origin of the full-time faculty system, implications for clinical research. *Journal of the American Medical Association* 265:1555–1562, 1991.

Heaton LD. Progress in army medicine: medical progress in World War II. *Maryland Medical Journal* 9:432–438, 1960.

Jones RM. American doctors and the Parisian medical world, 1830–1840. *Bulletin of the History of Medicine* 47:40–65 & 177–204, 1973.

Kaufman M. The admission of women to nineteenth-century American medical societies. *Bulletin of the History of Medicine* 50:251–260, 1976.

Kevles DJ. Into hostile political camps: the reorganization of international science in World War I. *Isis* 62:47–60, 1971.

Keys TE. The development of the medical motion picture. *Surgery, Gynecology and Obstetrics* 91:625–636, 1950.

Kraus M. American and European medicine in the 18th century. *Bulletin of the History of Medicine* 8:679–695, 1940.

Leake C. Medical caricature in the United States. *Bulletin of the Society of Medical History of Chicago* 4:1–29, 1928.

Lesky E. American medicine as viewed by Viennese physicians, 1893–1912. *Bulletin of the History of Medicine* 56:368–376, 1982.

Long PH. Medical progress and medical education during the war. *Journal of the American Medical Association* 130:983–990, 1946.

Madison DL. Preserving individualism in the organizational society: "cooperation" and American medical practice, 1900–1920. *Bulletin of the History of Medicine* 70:442–483, 1996.

Major R. Aboriginal American medicine north of Mexico. *Annals of Medical History* 10:544–551, 1938.

McDaniel WB. The beginnings of American medical historiography. *Bulletin of the History of Medicine* 26:45–53, 1952.

McDaniel WB. A view of nineteenth century medical historiography in the United States of America. *Bulletin of the History of Medicine* 33:415–435, 1959.

Peitzman SJ. "Thoroughly practical:" America's polyclinic medical schools. *Bulletin of the History of Medicine* 54:166–187, 1980.

Richmond PA. American attitudes toward the germ theory of disease (1860–1880). *Journal of the History of Medicine and Allied Sciences* 9:428–454, 1954.

Rosen G. The efficiency criterion in medical care, 1900–1920: an early approach to the evaluation of health service. *Bulletin of the History of Medicine* 50:28–44, 1976.

Rosenberg CE. The American medical profession: mid-nineteenth century. *Mid-America* 44:163–171, 1962.

Twiss JR. Medical practice in colonial America. *Bulletin of the New York Academy of Medicine* 36:538–551, 1960.

Warner JD. The campaign for medical microscopy in antebellum America. *Bulletin of the History of Medicine* 69:367–386, 1995.

Warner JH. The nature-trusting heresy: American physicians and the concept of the healing power of nature. *Perspectives in American History* 11:291–324, 1977.

Warren R. Reflections on nineteenth century German medicine. *American Journal of Surgery* 135:461–468, 1978.

REFERENCE WORKS

Grun B. *The timetables of history, a horizontal linkage of people and events.* New York: Simon & Schuster, 1991.

Urdang L. *The timetables of American history.* New York: Simon & Schuster, 1981.

INDEX

Italic numbers indicate illustrations.
Boldface numbers indicate biographies.

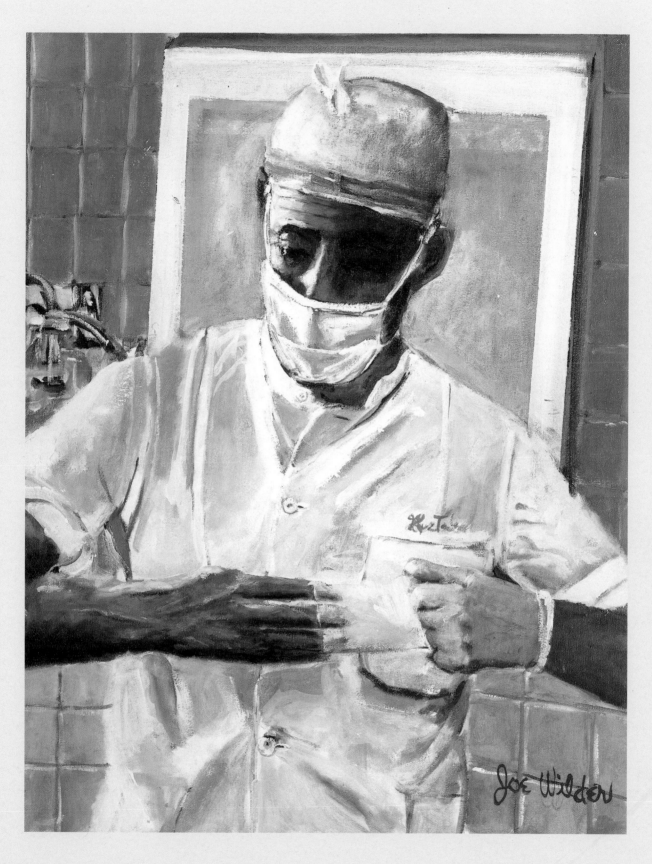

"Removing Gloves." Joseph Wilder portrays a surgeon at the conclusion of a difficult case and at the end of a long day. Painted in 1987 as part of his "Surgeon At Work" series, this clearly shows the weariness of an exhausted physician in his daily surgical struggle to vanquish the foe of disease. The forces of life and death are in constant struggle, and Wilder's canvas is Everyman's surgical stage. Wilder is the doyen of surgeon-painters, and his creative genius declares that medicine must continue as the most scientific of the humanities and remain the most humane of the sciences. *(Collection of the artist)*